Did you look for:

- —Focus of infection
- —OTC medication
- —Tinea pedis
- —Occupational causes

- —Mucosal clues
- —Pets
- —Foreign travel
- —Tumor

Did you:

- —Mentally transpose lesion to another site?
- —KOH?
- —Culture?
- —Do blood studies?
- —Biopsy?

- —Really listen to the patient?
- —Patch test?
- —Challenge with drug or foods?
- —Do stool culture?
- —Use the index in this book?
- —Give up? . . . Don't . . .

ADVANCED DERMATOLOGIC DIAGNOSIS

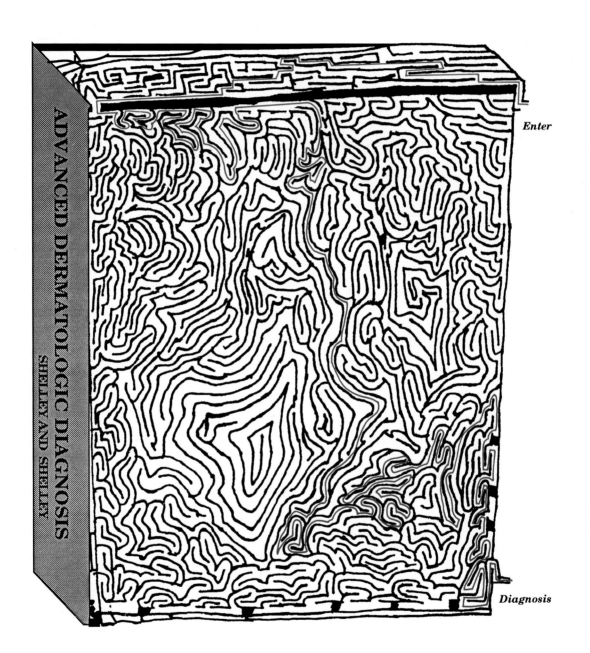

Enter

Diagnosis

ADVANCED DERMATOLOGIC DIAGNOSIS

SHELLEY AND SHELLEY

Tommy Shelley

ADVANCED DERMATOLOGIC DIAGNOSIS

WALTER B. SHELLEY, M.D.
Professor of Dermatology

E. DORINDA SHELLEY, M.D.
Professor and Chief of Dermatology

Division of Dermatology, Department of Medicine,
Medical College of Ohio, Toledo, Ohio

W. B. SAUNDERS COMPANY
Harcourt Brace Jovanovich, Inc.
Philadelphia • London • Toronto • Montreal • Sydney • Tokyo

W. B. SAUNDERS COMPANY
Harcourt Brace Jovanovich, Inc.

The Curtis Center
Independence Square West
Philadelphia, Pennsylvania 19106

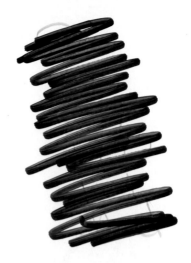

Library of Congress Cataloging-in-Publication Data

Shelley, Walter B. (Walter Brown),
    Advanced dermatologic diagnosis / Walter B. Shelley, E. Dorinda Shelley.—1st ed.
      p. cm.
    Includes bibliographical references and index.
    ISBN 0-7216-3433-8
    1. Skin—Diseases—Diagnosis. I. Shelley, Walter B. II. Shelley, E. Dorinda.
II. Title.
    [DNLM: 1. Skin Diseases—diagnosis. WR 140 S545a]
RL 105.S54 1992
616.5′075—dc20
DNLM/DLC   91-40449

ADVANCED DERMATOLOGIC DIAGNOSIS   ISBN   0-7216-3433-8

Printed in the United States of America.

Last digit is the print number: 9   8   7   6   5   4   3   2   1

To Tommy, Katharine, and Willy

Better than all measures
of delightful sound

Better than all treasures
that in books are found

Acknowledgements

Thought doesn't grow on trees. It grows in the library. We are happy to have enjoyed the richness of diagnostic thought provided by both the Raymon H. Mulford Library of the Medical College of Ohio and the Alfred Taubman Medical Library of the University of Michigan.

Georgiann Monhollen translated our faceless pen tracks into the computer image of a polished typescript.

Lorene Mehling, as our administrative right arm, provided support for every aspect of this undertaking.

John Dyson, Medical Editor *extraordinaire*, gave us the continuing encouragement, advice, and prodding so needed over these past five years.

Lorraine and David Kilmer took our thousands of pages of typescript and magically transformed them into this book for your thoughts to grow on.

The University Museum, University of Pennsylvania, Philadelphia, PA, photographed their sculpture from Kongo, Zaire (p. viii).

To each of these and to you, fond reader, we are grateful.

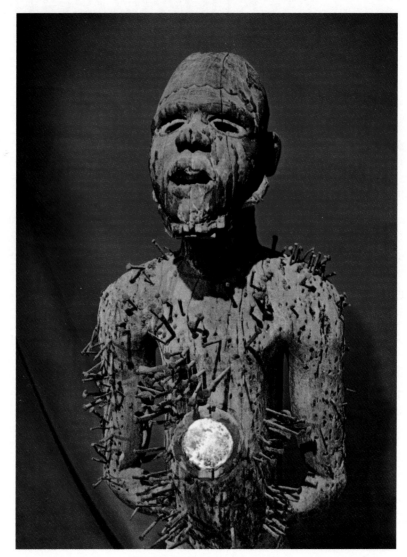

"Do I really need another test?"

Preface

Diagnosis ranges from the delight of the synaptic spark of instant recognition to the distress of seeing, but not quite knowing, what one sees. This is a book to reduce distress. It centers on elusive diagnoses. It summons diagnoses you know but have overlooked. It presents disorders you once knew but have somehow or somewhat forgotten. Finally, it alerts you to rarities you never knew were in the literature. Used properly, this book should be a cure for the anxiety of agnosia and anomia.

This is a workbook for your office desk. It has a clinician-friendly retrieval system, based on a "looks like" principle. The major "lead-in" identifiable lesions, symptoms, or signs are alphabetized. Under these you will find the "reminds me of" crowd to be considered. We have tried to keep the "yawn index" of differential diagnosis as low as possible by presenting interesting cases and keeping tables and lists to a minimum. Photographs are interspersed and themes of typographic variation played. Aphorisms should appear just when you, the reader, begin to nod.

This is a clinician's book. It attempts to bring life and sense into the field of sophisticated differential diagnosis. It presents an "expanded clinical mind," challenging you to be a better diagnostician. It should help you see what's in the skin and what's beneath. Always, it strives to reproduce the excitement generated by the master clinician John H. Stokes, who could summon and justify a dozen reasonable alternative diagnoses for what appeared to the rest of us as a mundane rash. Surely, a computer can out-perform this, but for us its printout is about as interesting and rewarding as last year's list of missing persons.

This is an atlas for stargazing. Dermatology has a far richer legacy of classifiable disease than any other branch of medicine. At the time of Willan nearly two centuries ago the dermatologic heavens boasted only a score of disease constellations. Today, the trained eye discerns several thousand diagnostic constellations. Learn to recognize them. You will become starry-eyed with wonderment and your patients will call you a star.

WALTER B. SHELLEY
E. DORINDA SHELLEY

Contents

xii   Contents

Principia Diagnostica

The Arts of Dermatologic Diagnosis

THE FINE ART OF USING THIS BOOK
THE SCHOLARLY ART OF KNOWING
THE INCOMPARABLE ART OF LOOKING
THE NIMBLE ART OF QUESTIONING
THE QUIET ART OF THINKING

The skin is a diagnostician's delight. Everything to be named is in full view. One has but to look, and recognize. There is none of the groping and searching the internist must endure even to identify the organ afflicted, let alone to make the diagnosis.

So where is the artistry of dermatologic diagnosis if one has but to look and recognize? The artistry comes in recognizing the unrecognizable. It comes in making sense out of a senseless nondescript jumble of nonspecific skin changes. And it comes in the search for the underlying cause, once the disorder has been named. Such artistry derives from special arts:

THE FINE ART OF USING THIS BOOK

Making the correct diagnosis is one of the intellectual joys of medical practice. And here is a book to enhance your enjoyment of daily practice. We have written it to illuminate the diagnostic passageways one must take when the diagnosis cannot be made at the doorway.

This book is a thinking man's guide to the classification of skin disease. Indeed, to think is to classify. Man cannot think of the objects in the world about him without making distinctions, whether they be at the level of the caveman's little rock versus big rock or the physicist's lepton versus baryon.

Your first thoughts on seeing a new patient will center on classification, i.e., diagnosis. This diagnostic process may be one of instantaneous recognition. In this case you have no need for a book, only your eidetic match. But we have written to help when there is no "Augenblick" diagnosis. To do this we have based the book on the principle that all the changes you observe in the skin, whether in part or in toto, remind you of one or more diagnoses. It is around these "lead" diagnoses that the book is crafted as a thesaurus. Each lead can take you alphabetically to a cluster of "look alikes." Here, you will find by means of annotated references, examples, and photographs the singular features and the decisive laboratory tests needed for the differentiation of morphologically similar diseases.

This is not a book for the novice in nosology. If the patient's constellation of history, symptoms, and skin changes suggests nothing to you, this book will be as worthless as Roget's dictionary of synonyms is for one who cannot spell. Moreover, this is not a book of histopathology but rather one of the gross patterns of clinicopathology.

This book does not promise diagnoses "without tears." Searching for the right diagnosis can be an arduous, treacherous, and lengthy undertaking. Unlike birds, bees, and butterflies, skin diseases do not breed true. Yet we try to sight and identify several thousand "species." All these may and do vary in configuration, location, and color. They may hide in black skin. They may have multifaceted lives, changing their form with treatment and waxing and waning as they are modulated immunologically. They may come in a forme fruste, as well as in atypical confounding sports. And

1

they may be but reaction patterns—wherein the cause itself is the only real diagnosis. Small wonder that the taxonomy of birds, bees, and butterflies is the greater science and the nosology of diseases the greater art.

This is a personal approach to diagnosis, written by two clinicians for but one clinician, namely, you. We have searched the world's literature to bring you instructive examples of sparkling dermatologic diagnostic insight. We have sought to avoid dull, lifeless, computer-generated lists that would lie asleep on your bookshelf. Instead of putting you to sleep, we hope to awaken you to the diversity of dermatologic diagnosis.

THE SCHOLARLY ART OF KNOWING

Of the arts of diagnosis, knowing is surely the greatest. But how is one to know? One must be taught. Search out a master diagnostician for your guide. Have him show as many diseases as possible. Have him point out the obvious as well as the subtle distinguishing features. Have him name the changes, the patterns, and the diseases. Memorize them. Challenge your mind to recall them visually whenever you see their names in print.

Expand your portfolio of identifiable images by traveling to the library. The journals, books, and especially the modern color atlases provide an invaluable extension of your diagnostic horizon. Search out Kodachrome libraries of authentic dermatoses and view them repeatedly until you can instantly recognize each one. The great hematologist Hal Downey annually assessed his diagnostic skill by reading blood smears of 600 authentic cases. Only when he had a perfect score on all 600 did he feel competent to read new slides from referring physicians.

Above all, go to staff rounds, clinical patient presentations, and dermatologic offices and clinics for continuing exposure to the obscure, the exotic, and the variant. Make your own visual diagnosis before peeking at the history, laboratory findings, or the presenter's diagnosis.

Learn the habits and habitats of disease. Look for distribution patterns telling you whether the disease is of internal or external origin. Watch for certain localization sites that almost spell the diagnosis, e.g., the chin with its dental sinus, the scalp with its kerion. Recognize the perverse inverse distribution of pityriasis rosea. Firm up your grasp of diseases that may thrive and limit themselves to the intertriginous sites, such as psoriasis.

The art of knowing is the art of the visual memory. You can never see too many patients, too many atlases, or too many Kodachromes. Your brain has a limitless capacity to store images if you will but stretch it. Using it is not abusing it. And frequent recall of these images keeps them sharp and bright.

To see and to remember is to know.

THE INCOMPARABLE ART OF LOOKING

This would seem to be the simplest of the arts, and yet its simplicity beguiles one into neglect. To reach the level of art, looking must be a skillful active undertaking. You must be clearly wide awake and ready for the challenges of inspection. You must think as you look. What is there? What is not there? We recall a medical class of 125 students, each of whom was asked to examine a patient's abdomen. Only 3 of the 125 saw that the patient had no umbilicus, the other 122 being blinded by their suppression of the inconsistent. They saw, but did not perceive, the scar where the umbilicus had been resected.

One must be curious and look at things not brought to your attention by the patient. Look at the moles. Are they dysplastic? Look for sun damage. Is there precancerous change? Look for dry skin. Is it of recent onset? Look for hyperhidrosis in the handshake and in the clothing. Ask questions of yourself as you look. There is no art in looking at the skin passively.

The art of looking calls for attention to the overlooked areas. And this cannot be done casually. It must be done with bubbling curiosity. Does the scalp harbor nits, psoriasis, or hair dye? We recall the frantic call of a neurosurgeon in the operating room. About to do a craniotomy, he saw a scalp covered with surgical "stop signs." All had escaped detection by his medical student, intern, and resident in their comprehensive history and physicals. By shaving the patient's head, his nurse dramatically revealed florid psoriasis that would have been evident on simple inspection of an area of parted hair.

Your curiosity should lead you to pull back the ears for evidence of seborrheic dermatitis and early basal cell carcinoma. Have the patient close his eyes while you open yours to lesions on the upper eyelids hidden from the patient's binocular view. We recall noting a basal cell carcinoma on the right upper eyelid of a patient with hand dermatitis. Not only was the patient unaware of it, but so was the resident who had taken her lengthy history. Although we sent the resident back in three times "to find" the skin cancer, he never did find it.

The mouth is a cave that can be filled with diagnostic treasures the patient never knew were there! Does the patient have caries, leukoplakia, or candidiasis? Is there an iatrogenic hairy tongue? Are there Koplik spots? Is there sialorrhea or xerostomia? Do you see lichen planus on the buccal mucosa? Are the faucial tonsils enlarged, erythematous, or studded with pustules? And how about the lingual tonsils? Is the pharynx inflamed? Such an examination calls for excellent lighting, a tongue blade for exposure, and methodical stepwise assessment of the half-dozen sites of diagnostic signs in the mouth. Don't forget that the tongue blade is not transparent. It can cover lesions as well as uncover them.

Patients dislike disrobing, but if you are in a diagnostic corner you must examine all 2 m^2 of the cutaneous landscape. Look under the breasts, in the axillae, down in the gluteal cleft, as well as at the perineum and under the scrotum. These areas may offer clues to the presence of psoriasis, seborrheic dermatitis, erythrasma, or syphilis.

The nails are the only place where the patient's dermatologic history is preserved for more than 30 days. The fingernails reveal the past 5 months and the toenails the past 18 months. Look for the dystrophy of former injuries. Assess the patient's cutaneous age by the striations. Let the Beau's lines alert you to the patient's past health. "Usure des ongles" speaks even more vividly than the patient as to months of incessant pruritus.

We have been stressing the art of seeing what the patient doesn't see. Nowhere does the patient "see" less than on his feet. We have had scores of patients deny the presence of the very tinea pedis that accounted for their generalized pruritus, urticaria, hand dermatitis, or generalized eczematous trichophytid. Look and scrape.

The modes of looking at the patient's lesions are many. Shift from one to another and use as many of these as necessary to make the diagnosis:

The First Look

The first look is best made without benefit of history, without prejudice of former diagnoses, and without bias of laboratory data. A diagnosis can be made in $\frac{1}{25}$ second if it is a simple matter of recognition, so that the art of knowing sometimes replaces the art of looking. Looking at the patient's problems should be done only under excellent light. Dark cocktail lounges or curbstones on cloudy days are no place to examine nevi. The retinal input and your diagnostic output are directly proportional to the available lumina. No cardiologist listens to the heart where steam pipes are pounding, and no dermatologist should "listen" to the skin in twilight. Likewise, the cardiologist does not listen through an overcoat, so be sure that makeup is removed, as well as nylon hose.

The Second Look

Take a second long look after you have queried the patient, examined the laboratory data, and grasped some possible diagnoses. The retina can process data from 50,000 points in one field. Use it now to look at details of the lesions.

The Global Look

Avoid peephole dermatology. Insist on seeing as much as possible of the patient's skin. Stand back, perceive the patterning of distribution, look for satellite lesions. Look at the big picture. We will always remember our experience in residency when we were presented a case of unexplained hand dermatitis. The patient, a 12-year-old boy, averred his skin elsewhere was absolutely normal. Our professor simply said, "Drop your pants," and there to our amazement and embarrassment was a penis covered with scabietic burrows.

The Magnified Look

The unaided eye is excellent for the global look, but for close inspection use a magnifier. We prefer an Optivisor loupe with a power of 2.7×. Interestingly, for a few months we tried a Zeiss operating scope with a range of powers up to magnification of 180× and found that none of these powers gave us the information we derived from the simple loupe. With the higher powers, we could not see the trees for the leaves. Possibly, if one spent years learning to recognize surface lesions under high power, the operating scope would be a valuable diagnostic tool.

The Tactile Look

See with your fingers. Palpate with your fingers. Only in this way can you sense early scleroderma, the faint ring of granuloma annulare, or the rough skin of the atopic. Palpate for lymph nodes, and palpate for the enlarged nerves of leprosy. Your fingers will tell you if a lesion is bound down. They will also speak to elastosis and tell you the extent of a lipoma. Let your fingers do the looking for what your eyes can't see. Touch remains a unique way of looking.

The Wood's Light Look

Visible light does not make all things visible. The presence of fluorescent compounds, elaborated by certain pathogenic bacteria and fungi, is revealed only by using the ultraviolet light in Wood's light. With a wavelength peaking at about 360 nm, it converts the invisible to the visible. It is invaluable for looking at erythrasma with its coral-red emission and tinea capitis with its greenish hues. Furthermore, porphyrins in teeth are dramatically displayed under Wood's light. Wood's light also allows one to see areas of subtle hypopigmentation by accentuating the contrast between melanized and hypomelanized skin. A suspicion of the ash-leaf macules of tuberous sclerosis calls for its use, as does a fading tinea versicolor.

Wood's light enables evaluation of patient compliance in taking tetracycline, since the drug is excreted in the sebum and can thus be visualized at the follicular pores. Likewise, it permits detection of fluorescent contact sensitizers on the skin. It can be used to monitor the use of creams and lotions containing fluorescent drugs or compounds.

Its use as distractor for the children in your practice is also real. Looking at their clothing and skin in the darkened room can bring the hush of magic. No less effective is the painting of their warts with a fluorescent acridine orange tincture. Successful use of Wood's light depends on three essentials: a totally dark room, a totally dark-adapted retina, and a light operating at full power. One must wait several minutes in the dark for the eye to adapt and for the lamp to reach full power. In this respect, you see more with a larger, stronger lamp than with a small weak unit.

The Positional Look

Changing the position of the patient and of the light can bring new insights. We have found atrophic areas of skin on the abdomen, evident only when the patient was supine. We became aware of the pedal papules of herniated fat only when the patient was standing. We have observed glomus tumors evident only with the arm dependent. Sometimes cross-lighting or even subdued lighting is essential for seeing the lesions. This is true for spotting lichen spinulosus, the early regrowth of hair, or faint vitiligo. Changing the patient's position can change your diagnostic position.

The Diascopic Look

Viewing the lesion under oil or through a glass slide pressed against the skin is valuable. The two techniques may be combined to give a better, though limited, view past the epidermis. The Wickham's striae of lichen planus and the distorted nail fold capillaries of collagen diseases are two types of lesions best viewed under oil. The glass slide pressed against the skin exposes more of the dermal changes: telangiectasia, granulomas, and the rarely seen apple jelly nodule of lupus vulgaris. Diascopy is a special form of looking at the skin by looking into it.

The Manipulative Look

There are a few minor manipulative maneuvers one can do to improve the art of looking.

Remove scales and crusts to see if erosions or ulcers lie beneath.

Scrape a scaling lesion for the capillary bleeding of the Auspitz sign.

Subsect an eschar to see if there is pus below.

Use a hair blower on the patient's head to really see the scalp.

Shave off the top layer of nail plate to see how deep the pigment is.

Inject Xylocaine or saline into a suspect basal cell carcinoma to enhance its gross morphology.

Apply vinegar for 2 minutes to genital skin to visualize warts.

The Kodachrome Look

For a higher level of diagnostic insight, use Kodachromes. Just as the pathologist magnifies his view of the skin with the microscope, we "magnify" our view with the projector. Projected on a bigger-than-life screen, your patient's lesions often display new diagnostic possibilities. Such stretching of the patient's skin on the screen can stretch your mind. For convenience, we keep a Caramate 4000 viewer in our office.

The Deeper Look

Do a biopsy!

The Informed Look

In the real world of busy practice it is impossible to look everywhere in every way. Thus the informed look is the one most practiced. It is the art of looking where the diagnostic gold is. It is a marvelous skill that comes from experience. Some do it intuitively and become the master diagnosticians. But for most of us it is the conscious effort to look away from the patient's presenting lesion or complaint for other visual clues. Here are some examples:

Look for nits in the scalp of the patient with generalized pruritus.
Look for the buccal mucosal lesions of lichen planus in the patient with strange excoriated lesions.
Look for the hirsutism of porphyria in the patient with scrapes and bruises on the hands.
Look for herpetic lesions in the patient with erythema multiforme.
Look for tinea pedis in the patient with dyshidrosis.

The Longitudinal Look

Look at the patient's lesions next week, and next month, and 3 months later. It will surely lengthen or shorten your differential. In summary, never approach a patient with a look of indifference. Don't be a "lumper." Be a problem solver. Look for the diagnosis using all the ways of looking you can. Such a mission takes time and energy, but above all it takes an intense, sustained interest in finding the answer. None of your diagnostic challenges deserves a look that is less comprehensive.

THE NIMBLE ART OF QUESTIONING

Why Take a History?

You don't take a history to identify a flower, a flea, or a friend. So why take a history when confronted with a skin disease? You do it because medical diagnosis extends well beyond the sterile taxonomy of biologic classification. It is an exercise in problem solving. Not only does the diagnosis have to be as precise and limiting as possible, but it must be explicative. It must explain, and it must look to the cause. For this all-embracing discipline of diagnosis, the history is essential.

What Does the History Do?

It confirms or weakens your initial impression.
A baby with bullous lesions suggests a diagnosis of urticaria pigmentosa, and a history of such lesions present since birth supports the diagnosis.

It deletes untenable diagnostic hypotheses.
Blisters on the dorsal aspect of a patient's hands suggest porphyria cutanea tarda, but the history of a burn yesterday excludes this diagnosis.

It suggests new diagnoses.
The patient's history of diabetes mellitus may elicit a sudden awareness of bullous dermatosis of diabetes.

It awakens you to derivative or secondary diagnoses.
A history of an atopic child with flaring after contact with a wool rug suggests an irritant dermatitis.

It finds causes.
The history of flares of a hand eruption after the patient has eaten ham sandwiches may explain a dyshidrosis of years' duration.

It provides diagnostic guidance in management.
A history of bullae following "sulfa" administration cautions you on your prescriptive approach.

How Is the History Taken?

Carefully! Take time. Take notes.

Take a complete history. Learn the details of the course, therapy, personal health, medications, surgery, allergies, family history, occupation, hobbies, menses, habits. One of the most common errors is to assume that the patient doesn't do things you don't do.

Avoid spot history taking. It leaves holes in your head, as well as in your history. The wild, inspired question may make the diagnosis on occasion; however, like a "hole in one," it does not win many diagnostic golf games.

Be interested. Be curious. Even a mental yawn is strictly forbidden. Lean forward and learn:
What does the patient feel is the cause?
What makes it better?
What makes it worse?

Find out the patient's symptoms. This provides real diagnostic help. If it doesn't itch, it can hardly be contact dermatitis.

Analyze the response to treatment. If it didn't respond to dapsone, dermatitis herpetiformis is unlikely. Likewise, no response to ketoconazole eliminates the diagnosis of candidiasis.

Amplify your history if the diagnosis is a reaction pattern. Don't be satisfied with insurance form diagnoses such as contact dermatitis, drug eruption, or urticaria. The history can be your best friend in finding the cause, i.e., the ultimate diagnostic triumph. Remember, lots of people can identify a poppy in a pasture, but it takes a diagnostician to find out how it got there.

Connect the history to your working diagnosis. The stomatitis patient must tell you about toothpaste, dentures, lozenges, mouthwashes, chewing gum, breath fresheners, cinnamon cookies, dental visits, cigarettes, cigars, snuff, and all kinds of other stuff. Pay special attention to "medicines" that are not prescription. Patients often don't tell you about pain pills, headache pills, antihistamines, nonsteroidal anti-inflammatory drugs (NSAIDs), laxatives, minerals, sinusitis sprays, eye drops, tranquilizers, sleeping pills, and artificial sweeteners. We recall a girl with pseudotumor cerebri and hair loss who failed to tell a score of physicians and medical students that she was taking massive doses of vitamin A. She thought of it as a food.

Let your history taking be a teaching device. Alert the patient to what you are thinking. One of our patients had no clues for us concerning a hand eruption, but we kept asking her about foods. On the next visit she had the answer. It was caused by Cherry 7-Up, which she proved by challenge. Indeed, she then realized that her hand eruption had begun the summer that Cherry 7-Up was introduced. Challenges with plain 7-Up, Cherry Coca-Cola, and Coca-Cola were all negative. In this case, didactic history taking led to the ultimate etiologic diagnosis and cure but required an incubation period.

Learn about the patient's environment and habits. Does he have parakeets, rabbits, turkeys? Does he have an aquarium? Exactly what chemicals are in his work place? How does he clean his skin? Exactly how much alcohol does he drink? Does he bathe three times a day? How about recreational drugs, vitamins, contraceptives? In the world of the difficult diagnosis, you simply can't know too much. We know of one puzzling eruption due to the perfume in the tampons used by the patient.

Question the relatives, the nurses, and friends. We recall puzzling cellulitis in a baby. The nurses observed that whenever the mother entered the hospital room the baby screamed. This led to the discovery that the mother was injecting turpentine into the child's buttocks.

Question the patient alone. Many embarrassing, yet diagnostically significant, answers never come out in the presence of a parent, spouse, friend, or medical student. Ask me no questions in public and I will tell you no lies.

Keep enlarging your history data base with every visit. Never stop questioning. Rephrase and repeat queries about aerosols, perfumes, and incense. That perplexing pruritus may be due to mites from the birds' nest that is outside the patient's bedroom window air conditioner. A history is never complete until you have the diagnosis and the patient has the cure.

THE QUIET ART OF THINKING

One look and the clinician said, "Erythrokeratoderma variabilis." How did he ever think of that? The answer is—he knew. No amount of brilliant reasoning, inductive logic, or analysis of the history and laboratory data can match the diagnostic prowess of those who possess instant recognition. It is said that the master chess players recognize as many as 50,000 chess patterns, whereas the average player possesses a repertoire of only 1000. Without doubt, the master dermatologist has a repertoire of thousands of patterns of skin disease, one of which may instantly match with the patient's unknown problem and produce the diagnosis. But what do you do if there is no instant recognition?

The answer is to think, think, think. It is akin to the answer given the man who asked how to get to Carnegie Hall: "Practice, practice, practice." Just as one cannot practice without a violin, one cannot think without facts. Thinking demands that you have facts that you have stored, facts that you have generated from looking at the lesions and listening to the patient, facts from securing laboratory data, and facts from directing your reading. Given this mix, the synapses begin to flash and you delve deeper into your memory bank. You see new possibilities, and you generate new ideas on how to proceed diagnostically.

Such thinking can be facilitated, enhanced, and enriched by certain conscious maneuvers:

Keep your initial list of diagnostic possibilities small.
  Three or four diagnoses are about all the brain can effectively process.

Avoid overloading your mental circuits.
  Too many details blow the fuses. Ignore the anomalous and focus on a few major findings in the skin, in the history, and in the laboratory data.

Challenge your brain with questions.
  Is there a pattern that suggests atypical pityriasis rosea?
  Has the problem recurred in the same site, as a nonpigmenting drug eruption would?
  Is it limited to an area known to favor fungal infection?

Transpose the lesion to another site. This generates new thoughts. Would the erythema of the scrotum suggest steroid-induced rosacea if it occurred on the face?

Transpose your problem to another age group . . . to another sex . . . to another occupation.

Imagine that the history is wrong.
  Could the patient be forgetful? Deceitful?
  Could the lesion be factitial?
  Has it been there for months, not days?

Generate new ideas. Think of the various causes of skin disease:
  contactants?   infection?   douches?   spermicidal jellies?
  drugs?   diabetes?   tampons?

Think of new tests. Don't be inhibited from doing a palmar biopsy, an HIV antibody test, endocrine assays.

Don't lock into one diagnosis.
  Challenge yourself to think of others. Could it be leprosy? Could it be vasculitis?
  The "hypothesis hop" is preferable to the same old waltz.

Allow time for delayed recognition.
  After all, you can't name every one of your friends on instant sight. Sometimes the diagnosis will come in a flash only when you sit down to write the referring doctor.

Keep reading and dipping into your atlases, texts, and journals.
  Serendipity can work wonders.

Next visit, approach the patient as a consultant.
  Look at the problem through fresh eyes, critical for things you didn't see or ask about before.

Be confident.
  Don't bury your brain in a shroud of despair. Stay alive with a "working" diagnosis, if nothing else.

Keep generating new facts.
  Watch for new lesions, new associations, new laboratory tests. One may eventually prove to be the key to the lock.

Remember, there is more than meets the eye in dermatologic diagnosis.
  There is thinking. It is hard work, but it is marvelous therapy for any diagnostician distraught because the pathologist doesn't know what the matter is, either. So think when the patient is with you, think when the patient is not with you, and let your brain think about it when you are not even thinking about it.

Thinking is a gentle, quiet art of diagnosis that can be practiced anytime, anywhere.

Reflections

PHILOSOPHICAL OBSERVATIONS ON DIAGNOSIS
THE PRINCIPLES OF DIAGNOSIS
OBSERVATIONS OF CLASSIFICATION
DIAGNOSTIC AIDS
THE CERTAINTY OF UNCERTAINTY IN DIAGNOSIS
SOURCES OF ERROR
DIAGNOSTIC PLOYS

PHILOSOPHICAL OBSERVATIONS ON DIAGNOSIS

Cutler P: Problem Solving in Clinical Medicine: From Data to Diagnosis, 2nd ed., Baltimore, Williams & Wilkins, 1985, 603 pp.

There is no more important field in medicine than diagnosis. Without it, we are charlatans or witch doctors treating in the dark with potions and prayers.

Kassirer JP, Gorry GA: Clinical problem solving: A behavioral analysis. Ann Intern Med 1978; 89:245–255.

Statements that individuals make about their problem-solving behavior are often incomplete, misleading, or even incorrect. In any event, the strategies of experts vary considerably.

Barrows HS, Feltovich PJ: The clinical reasoning process. Med Educ 1987; 21:86–91.

No two doctors will follow the same path of inquiry with the same problem, since one's strategy is oriented to the initial data and guided by hypotheses and an investigational approach that represents a personal accumulation of experience and understanding.

The mind is capable of processing data almost instantaneously and of undertaking problem solving at an unconscious level. Do not think that the mental processes underlying pattern recognition of a dermatologic lesion must be very simple. They simply are not.

Hamm RM: Clinical interaction and clinical analysis: Expertise and the cognitive continuum. *In* Dowie JA, Elstein AS (eds): Professional Judgment: A Reader in Clinical Decision Making. Cambridge, Cambridge University Press, 1988; pp 78–105.

It takes 20 minutes on teaching rounds to arrive at a tentative diagnosis, but only 15 seconds of talking with a new patient for an experienced clinician to arrive at the same point. This illustrates the two ends of our cognitive continuum of diagnostic thinking, the one being analytical, the other intuitive.

Schön DA: The reflective practitioner: How professionals think in action. New York, Basic Books, Inc., 1983, 374 pp.

The hallmark of the **best clinicians** is their ability to "reflect in action." Particularly valuable are the reflections that suggest an "experiment." Thus, when the practitioner reflects in action he becomes a researcher in the practice context. He can construct a new theory of his unique case. It is here that the art of practice in uncertainty and uniqueness makes linkage with the scientist's art of research.

The most important part of **clinical expertise** comes in the form of "knowledge in action." In contrast to "knowledge for action," which can be acquired from books or colleagues, this sort of knowledge is revealed only in action—

in the doing of the task, whether it be tightrope walking or clinical diagnosis. There is no reason to expect the performer to be able to articulate it or even for outside observers to be able to capture and make it into knowledge for action by others.

The clinician's knowing is tacit, implicit in his pattern of action and in his feel for clinical problems. Each clinician recognizes disease in ways beyond his description. Each clinician makes judgments for which he cannot state criteria. Each clinician displays skills for which he cannot state the rules and procedures. Neither we nor the clinician can tell how once we know a person's face we can recognize it out of a thousand, indeed, out of a million faces.

The physician seeing innumerable variations of a small number of diseases develops a **repertoire** of **expectations, images,** and **techniques.** He learns what to look for and how to respond to what he finds. He becomes less and less subject to surprise. His knowing in practice becomes increasingly tacit, spontaneous, and automatic. But this can have negative effects. As his practice becomes more repetitive and routine, he may miss important opportunities to think about what he is doing. He may be drawn into patterns of error that he cannot correct. And if he learns to be selectively inattentive to phenomena that are outside his knowledge-in-action, he may suffer from boredom, indeed "burnout." The **antidote is reflection.** It will make new sense of situations of uncertainty or uniqueness that he may now allow himself to experience.

It is essential that clinicians avoid being locked into a view of themselves as technical experts who can find nothing in the world of practice to occasion reflection. They must cast off their skillful, selective inattention to the unusual. They must move beyond junk categories and situational control. They must lose their fear of uncertainty and welcome it as a call for reflection and new action. It can bring excitement back to a tired practice.

Steckel RJ: Research in medical diagnosis: Neglected national problem. AJR 1984; 143:919–921.

Cost-containment in medical care demands accurate diagnoses made without undue delay.

Eraker SA, Politser P: How decisions are reached: Physician and patient. *In* Dowie JA, Elstein AS (eds): Professional Judgement: A Reader in Clinical Decision Making. Cambridge, Cambridge University Press, 1988, pp 379–394.

Both patients and physicians find decisions involving trade-offs between health care and money to be extremely distasteful.

Albert DA, Munson R, Resnik MD: Reasoning in Medicine. An Introduction to Clinical Inference. Baltimore, Johns Hopkins University Press, 1988, 263 pp.

Two professors of philosophy and an internist have written this book. It is a splendid volume for stimulating self-scrutiny of how we think and how we should think. You will come away with new understanding of inductive logic, the workhorse of medical reasoning.

In essence, the **clinician** remains the **best diagnostic instrument,** whether he functions as a detective, a gambler, or an artist in making the diagnosis.

Hoffbrand BI: **Diagnostic process.** Lancet 1987; 1:278–279.

Whether or not a diagnosis is reached, the diagnostic process of talking to and touching the patient, with perhaps a test or two, should be used for its therapeutic content.

THE PRINCIPLES OF DIAGNOSIS

Haxthausen H: How are dermatological diagnoses made? Trans St. Johns Hosp Dermatol Soc 1950; 30:3–13.

Diagnosis is the art of exaggerating the important details of location, arrangement, color, and form while ignoring all the rest.

Beautyman W: Newman's *Grammar of Assent* and the diagnostic process. Perspect Biol Med 1982; 25:472–478.

Recognition works by **instant analogy** once the disease has been scanned by the experienced observer. It does not proceed as a conscious logical reasoning process. Indeed, it finds verbal reasoning far too cumbersome for its purposes.

Kundel HL, La Follette PS: Visual search patterns and experience with radiological images. Radiology 1972; 103:523–528.

The eyes rove over a scene in jumps (coarse saccades), hovering for about 0.2 second at one location while a burst of neural impulses is passed from the retina to the higher centers. The **perception** of the visual world then results from a **complex interplay** of received **sensations** and **information** stored in **memory**. The eyes are directed to various regions, but large areas of most visual scenes are not sampled by the sensitive fovea. As a result, much of our information is obtained from the less acute periphery of the retina or supplied by memory. Improvement in the search comes from having complete familiarity with the abnormal features of the object of search, as well as knowing the normal background that envelops it. It is like spotting a friend in a crowd.

Riegelman RK: Dethroning the detective theory of diagnosis. Postgrad Med 1981; 70 (Nov):239–244.

Contrast the detective solving a murder mystery and the doctor making a diagnosis:

The detective must solve the crime, whereas the doctor often finds it unnecessary and impractical to ascertain a specific diagnosis. Admitting that a problem is of unknown cause is often better medicine than subjecting the patient to the risks of diagnosis.

Time may be against the detective, but for the doctor, observation is a way of using **time as a diagnostic test** (e.g., allowing the vesicles of chickenpox to appear).

The detective should leave no stone unturned, but for the doctor **diagnostic testing** should be **sharply focused**, not of the genre "if you can think of it, order it."

The detective will find but one criminal, but the doctor finds that most patients with multiple problems have multiple diseases. The principle of **diagnostic parsimony** appeals to the physician's intellect, but limits his diagnoses.

The detective must find a solution that is certain, whereas in medicine nothing is certain but biopsy and autopsy, and that certainly is not always true.

The detective identifies the criminal and knows he is responsible for the crime. Meanwhile, the doctor makes a diagnosis such as gallstones, but this does not necessarily explain the patient's symptoms. A diagnosis can be significant and yet irrelevant to the patient's problems.

The fictional detective avoids the obvious criminal in search of a better story. The doctor must avoid the pursuit of the zebra and be satisfied to find the common dray horse at the hitching post. He should not do a work-up for carcinoid syndrome in a 50-year-old woman with hot flashes.

Finally, the detective never stumbles onto a solution, whereas the physician who keeps an open mind and a thoughtful approach may well stumble upon a diagnosis not considered before.

Ramsay DL, Benimoff A: The ability of primary care physicians to recognize the common dermatoses. Arch Dermatol 1981; 117:620–622.

A single high-quality color transparency of each of the 20 most frequently encountered or serious skin diseases was shown to a group of 285 primary care physicians and to a group of 30 academic dermatologists. They were asked to record their best diagnosis without benefit of history or laboratory studies. The primary-care physician score was 54% and the dermatologist score 96%.

You can name only what you recognize.

Elstein AS, Shulman LS, Sprafka SA: Medical Problem Solving: An Analysis of Clinical Reasoning. Cambridge, Mass., Harvard University Press, 1978, 330 pp.

The results of 5 years of research at Michigan State University:

Examination of the patient provides cues that are clustered or "chunked" to allow memory retrieval of matching disease patterns (diagnostic possibilities or hypotheses).

These **working hypotheses**, always small in number, narrow the problem-solving space that must be searched for a solution. Continuing examination allows validation, rejection, or addition of other diagnostic hypotheses. The generation of hypotheses is invaluable in focusing one's memory on the case at hand. Likewise, the formation of hypotheses directs an economical search for information and serves as an organizational device for the storage and recall of information in the physician's memory.

Most diagnoses are made by routine means, not by brilliant insight or creativity. Avoid making snap diagnoses.

The most common error in diagnostic thinking is to assign new information to existing hypotheses rather than to create new hypotheses or remember the information separately. This results from the physician's very human need to perceive problems as having limited degrees of complexity. Physicians do not show a consistently uniform profile of competence in diagnosis. Competence remains a variable reflecting knowledge, prior clinical exposure, and interest in any given specific problem situation.

Van Damme B: **Diagnostic process**. Lancet 1987; 1:279.

Making a diagnosis is more than making a label: Several modes and levels can always be discerned. There are different levels of precision. Thus, "cancer" is not an acceptable diagnosis. It must be refined for type of tumor, degree of differentiation, level of invasion, presence of metastasis, and so on. In other instances the diagnosis may be etiologic (e.g., gonococcal infection), pathogenetic (e.g., hyperthyroidism), or it may describe a single symptom (e.g., anemia) or delineate a group of symptoms (e.g., oculocerebrorenal syndrome of Lowe).

Schwartz S, Griffin T: Medical Thinking. The Psychology of Medical Judgment and Decision Making. New York, Springer-Verlag, 1986, 277 pp.

Experts are not ones with better memories, greater perceptual skills, or deeper thoughts. **Experts** are the ones who have their **knowledge efficiently organized**.

"Although much of the information used in clinical decision making is objective, the physician's values (a belief that pain relief is more important than potential addiction to pain-killing drugs, for example) and subjectivity are as much a part of the clinical process as the objective finding of laboratory tests."

Tyrer JH, Eadie MJ: The Astute Physician. How to Think in Clinical Medicine. Amsterdam, Elsevier Scientific Publishing Co., 1976, 200 pp.

Evidence, knowledge, and reasoning are the three legs of the stool on which clinical diagnosis rests. "Ear, eye, and hand are the Holy Trinity of clinical observation and are frequently used in combination."

"In history taking, the physician should clearly distinguish between evidence of facts, and evidence offering opinions about facts, as is the case in a court of law."

"In general, the greater the number of relevant facts that can be established about a patient's illness, the more one can reduce the number of single diagnoses that can explain these facts."

"What the patient says should not necessarily be accepted at face value." Histories often become unreliable in disability cases, in which symptoms may be either exaggerated or concealed.

"**History taking involves more than listening** to the statements of the patient because the physician does not take a history with his eyes shut. He notices how old the patient appears, how he walks into the room, whether he is thin or fat, and sometimes much more. . . ."

"The meaning of what a person sees depends on his past experience and education as well as on his interest and attention. . . . Observation is selective. **One perceives what one is interested in.**"

"When an abnormality is present, one finds it much more readily if one knows *what* to search for and *where* to search. In general, it is much easier to find the answer to a problem if one asks oneself the right questions."

"Abnormality may comprise the presence of phenomena normally absent, as well as the absence of phenomena normally present."

Utilization of the physician's sense of touch via **palpation** reveals unique important information, such as:

    provocation of pain, tenderness, or hyperalgesia
    temperature
    size, consistency, and depth of a mass
    palpable vibrations and rubs
    blood vessel pulsations
    mobility of joints
    blanching of erythema
    edema (pitting on pressure)
    fluctuation of a swelling that contains fluid
    tendon reflexes (with a percussion hammer)
    dimensions of a swelling or anatomic structure (using a tape measure)
    skin texture (smooth, rough, scaly)
    abnormal moistness or dryness

Elstein AS, Bordage G: Psychology of clinical reasoning. *In* Dowie JA, Elstein AS (eds): Professional Judgement: A Reader in Clinical Decision Making. Cambridge, Cambridge University Press, 1988; pp 109–129.

Given the limited information processing capabilities of the brain, one is required to:

    represent the problem simplistically

select the data carefully
process the data serially
think rationally

Newman JH: An Essay in Aid of a Grammar of Assent, 1870; Reprinted Garden City, N. Y., Doubleday & Co., 1955, pp 261–262.

More than 100 years ago Cardinal Newman wrote: "There are physicians who excel in the *diagnosis* of complaints; though it does not follow from this, that they could defend their decision in a particular case against a brother physician who disputed it. They are guided by natural acuteness and varied experience; they have their own idiosyncratic modes of observing, generalizing and concluding; when questioned, they can but rest on their own authority, or appeal to the future event."

Dodwell PC: Human pattern and object perception. *In* Held R, Leibowitz HW, Teuber H-L (eds): Handbook of Sensory Physiology, Vol. 8. New York, Springer-Verlag, 1978; 8:523–548.

Interest and **attention** affect the way we perceive things and the way we report them.

Higgins RM: The process of diagnosis. Lancet 1987; 1:1146–1147.

The process of diagnosis has more to do with the **physician's patience**, **obsessiveness**, and **willingness to take risks** than with intellectual thought processes.

Grant J, Marsden P: The structure of memorized knowledge in students and clinicians: An explanation for diagnostic expertise. Med Educ 1987; 21:92–98.

Memory is a highly personalized tool that the experienced clinician constantly redesigns and improves. Both its form and function reflect its daily use in diagnostic work. This is the secret of the master's performance superiority over the beginner who has but a "general issue" memory tool.

Waldenström JG: Necessary diagnostic pigeonholes—defense of taxonomy in medicine as well as in botany. Acta Med Scand 1978; 203:145–147.

Young doctors must learn and remember as many clinical pictures as possible, with a number of characteristic features from each. It is not the details but the total picture or **Gestalt** that they must learn. A patient with aphasia is described who, despite the loss of ability to recognize or name any letters in the alphabet, could read easily when he saw the letters grouped to form words.

Cotterill JA: Dermatological games. Br J Dermatol 1981; 105:311–320.

It is possible to be ill without having a disease, and likewise it is possible to have a disease without being ill. Diagnosis is never the ultimate goal line in the game of patient study, but rather the starting line for good management. You will live as a physician not by diagnosis alone, but by making and acting upon a complete assessment of the **emotional**, **social**, and **occupational effects of the disease** on the patient.

Clendening L, Hashinger EH: Methods of Diagnosis. St. Louis, CV Mosby Co., 1947, 868 pp.

"The most frequent and by all odds the **most serious mistake** in the physical examination is to **find a sign that is not present**. . . . When he has found a sign, he is committed to something. . . . It commits the diagnostician (and the patient) to serious consequences, [such as] unnecessary options. It takes courage and experience to say, "The heart [or skin] is normal." We make these mistakes because of lack of self assurance and fear of being shown up by rival consultants. The patient may also lead us astray by having so many symptoms that we feel we must find something to account for them."

Turning over an essential part of the examination to someone else is working with false data.

OBSERVATIONS ON CLASSIFICATION

Feinstein AR: Clinical Judgment. Baltimore, Williams & Wilkins, 1967, p 85.

"**Dermatology** has continued to maintain its own **taxonomy**—a colorful cornucopia of concatenating cutaneous classification. Dermatologists, luckier than most other clinicians, can constantly see and touch the disease they diagnose in the skin, and so the dermatologist still makes diagnoses based on what he, rather than the pathologist, observes. The diagnostic vocabulary of dermatology is doubtlessly over-cluttered and sometimes seems strange to other clinicians, but the taxonomy is effective."

Asher R: Making sense. Lancet 1959; 2:359–365.

We overemphasize certain **syndromes** by giving names to them and overlook others probably just as important because we have not christened them. (This from the pen of the scholar who named Munchausen's syndrome and thereby ended its anonymous travels.)

McCormick JS: Diagnosis: The need for demystification. Lancet 1986; 1434–1435.

Diagnosis of physical disease is based on recognition, similar to the botanist's recognition of a plant. It is not an adventure in science, but in **taxonomy**. As such it calls not for imagination and scientific hypothesis, but for facts and precise identification.

Jacquez JA, (ed): The Diagnostic Process. Ann Arbor, Mich., Malloy Lithographing, Inc., 1964, 391 pp.

A **diagnosis** is a **probability statement** within a taxonomic scheme largely derived from a stochastic, sequential process of eliminating and ordering of possibilities. It depends on pattern recognition to a large degree. It still is unclear as to the minimum number of points needed to identify a pattern. How does one label the information we call diagnosis? Should it be descriptive, etiologic, physiopathologic, or chemical?

In medicine, the reality of the individual patient and the abstraction of a disease or diagnosis form two poles of an axis, along which the physician's mind shuttles during the process of making a diagnosis. The **bias of classification** leads to overlooking or not reporting certain cases that cannot be diagnosed because they seem to lie between two diseases or between health and well-defined disease.

Miller MC III, Westphal MC Jr, Reigart JR II: **Mathematical models** in **medical diagnosis**. New York, Praeger Publishers, 1981, 187 pp.

A heuristic adventure for the mathematically oriented physician interested, for example, in **cluster analysis**, a process leading to formal, planned, purposeful, and scientific classification. The word *clustering* has many synonyms: numerical taxonomy, taximetrics, taxonorics, morphometrics, botyrology, nosology, nosography, systematics, biosystematics, and pattern recognition.

Green G, Defoe EC Jr: What is a **clinical algorithm**? Clin Pediatr 1978; 17:457–463.

An algorithm is a rule of procedure for solving a clinical problem. It is a flow chart of step-by-step instructions telling what information to seek and in what order. It can be used to guide general physicians, paramedical personnel, or the public in making a diagnosis. Ten clinical algorithms would cover 75% of all the problems seen in a primary pediatric practice.

Oliver JH Jr: Crisis in **biosystematics** of **arthropods**. Science 1988; 240:967.

The study and prevention of arthropod-associated disease demands expertise in the identification and classification of not only the disease but also the carrier organisms. This latter field of biosystematics is not adequately funded, so that few have been trained or supported to make the subtle distinctions between *Ixodes dammini* (the primary tick vector of Lyme disease) and *I. scapularis*. Similarly, few have the capabilities of DNA probes or chromosome banding needed to identify the six species of the *Anopheles gambiae* complex of mosquitoes responsible for one million deaths each year due to malaria. Support for this special area of diagnosis must come from the public, not the patient.

Waldenström JG: Necessary diagnostic pigeonholes—defense of taxonomy in medicine as well as in botany. Acta Med Scand 1978; 203:145–147.

A patient who had severe pains in his foot had consulted many doctors but none had exactly diagnosed the condition. Finally there was one who really understood and told the patient that he had a typical "pied douloureux"; the fact that somebody obviously understood made the patient feel ever so much better.

Wong A J-W: Recognition of general patterns using neural networks. Biol Cybern 1988; 58:361–372.

Aircraft identification is now within the range of the pattern-recognition capabilities of a computer employing a mathematical model of a network of neurons, with synaptic strengths as the memory matrix. (Can recognition of skin disease be far behind?)

Sun M: Botany bids for the "big science" league. Science 1987; 237:967–968.

There are 17,000 species of plants in North America that are now to be catalogued in an 11-volume encyclopedia. In its taxonomic dossier, each plant will have a list of its various names and a description of its looks and locations. (Surely, the *Flora Cutaneorum Mundi* deserve a similar compilation!)

DIAGNOSTIC AIDS

Ackerman AB, Cockerell CJ: Cutaneous Lesions: Correlations from microscopic to gross morphologic features. Cutis 37: 137–138, 1986.

Here are the 20 words you need to describe fundamental skin lesions (apart from color and consistency):

macules	scale—crusts
patches	eschars
papules	atrophies
plaques	keratoses
nodules	erosions
tumors	ulcers
vesicles	fissures
bullae	burrows
pustules	cords
crusts	telangiectases

Note: The following useful terms describe special types of fundamental lesions. We often leapfrog over the fundamental lesion (to the consternation of the neophyte) and use these terms:

abscesses	infarcts
cysts	lichenification
desquamation	milia
ecchymoses	pigmentation
excoriations	sclerosis
exudates	scars
gangrene	sphacelus (eschar)
hematomas	vegetations
hemorrhages	wheal

Hutchinson R: An address on the principles of diagnosis. Br Med J 1928; 1:335–337.

"Diagnosis is based on an accurate interpretation of symptoms and signs . . . symptoms are elicited by taking the history and by the cross-examination of the patient upon it. This is the patient's contribution to the making of the diagnosis. . . . There is usually one symptom that troubles the patient more than any other . . . the "**presenting symptom**" . . . and special attention should always be given to it. . . . The detection of signs depends upon observation and training in clinical methods of investigation. . . . Having elicited the symptoms and signs which are present, knowledge is necessary in interpreting them, for without knowledge one is 'mind-blind'. . . . After observation and knowledge comes judgement as a factor in the making of a diagnosis. . . . We can increase our powers of observation by training and practice . . . and our knowledge by study and experience . . . but **judgement** seems to be an inborn faculty. . . . **Clinical instinct** is, in truth, simply a power of rapid instinctive judgement . . . much the same as 'common sense' and closely allied to a sense of humour, which is the same thing as a sense of proportion. Those who lack it are apt, in making a diagnosis, to fail to see the wood for the trees. . . . The effect of an error in judgement is wholly bad, as it shakes the self confidence that is really necessary to the exercise of prompt and accurate decision. . . . For some time after a "howler" one is afraid to come to a decision in any difficult case. . . . Fortunately, however, the diagnostician has a happy knack of forgetting his own mistakes whilst remembering those of other people."

"Having made your diagnosis, should you communicate it to the patient? Certainly not always, nor in all circumstances. . . . Sometimes, in fact, one would a little rather not know the exact name of his complaint, as if he does he is pretty sure to look it up in a medical dictionary. . . . If the prognosis is good, there is no reason why the patient should not know the name of the disease; if bad, a little judicious vagueness is wiser . . . It is not every patient who is fit to be told the whole truth about his disease."

Dr. Hutchinson also discusses some common diagnostic pitfalls:

Just when you think you are most scientific with the latest laboratory studies, you are most likely to make a mistake.

Be aware that "common things" occur most commonly. Don't diagnose rarities.

Don't make a diagnosis at once, to be regretted at last.

Be careful in making any diagnosis of a disease you want to see or to study.

Don't mistake a label for a diagnosis: a label like gastritis or neuritis is not a diagnosis.

Try to account for all the clinical features by assuming the presence of only one pathologic process whenever possible. Don't diagnose two diseases simultaneously in the same patient.

Walk the diagnostic tightrope between overconfidence and excessive caution.

Look at the problem with a **fresh, open mind**, unbiased by the opinions of others.

When significant new signs or laboratory data appear, **be prepared to change your diagnosis**.

You will not always be right in your diagnosis, for disease does not always play the game.

Eddy DM, Clanton CH: The art of diagnosis: Solving the clinicopathological exercise. N Engl J Med 1982; 306:1263–1268.

To explain a patient's myriad of elementary findings of clinical, historical, and laboratory origin is such a monumental cognitive task that the diagnostician falls back on a simpler and more heuristic approach. He selects one or possibly two findings, focuses on this pivot, and temporarily ignores all the other findings.

Simel DL: Playing the odds. Lancet 1985; 1:329–330.

Successful gamblers would make **good diagnosticians**. They always "**play the odds**" rather than the "rule out" or "need to know" game. Abstruse formulas are provided for medical gambling.

Kundel HL, Wright DJ: The influence of prior knowledge on **visual search strategies** during the viewing of chest radiographs. Radiology 1969; 93:315–320.

Given 20 seconds to read a chest radiograph, experienced observers use a strategy for search that reflects what is seen and what might be seen.

Fulop M: Teaching **differential diagnosis** to beginning clinical students. Am J Med 1985; 79:745–749.

Difficult diagnostic problems make you think:

congenital	neurologic
genetic	psychiatric
infectious	iatrogenic
immunologic	traumatic
endocrinologic	neoplastic

Gale J: Some cognitive components of the diagnostic thinking process. Br J Educ Psychol 1982; 52:64–76.

The diagnostic thinking process is not a unique form of thinking, but is rather characteristic of adult cognition. Review the following components of your approach to **improve diagnostic skills**. It is this **self-awareness** and self-monitoring in daily practice that can facilitate remediation, correction of errors, and inefficiency of thinking.

1. Prediagnostic interpretation of data
2. Diagnostic interpretation of data

3. Judgment of the need for further inquiry
4. Search for specific features of disease
5. Reinterpretation of clinical information with or without new data
6. Active confirmation of interpretation
7. Active elimination of an interpretation
8. Postponement of confirmation or elimination
9. Interview of a patient as directed by the patient, by the diagnosis, or by the general area
10. Failure to make a specific or general inquiry.

Coulehan JL, Block MR: The medical interview: A primer for students of the art. Philadelphia, FA Davis Co., 1987, 221 pp.

An exquisite account of the art of using the patient as a consultant.

Some patients magnify symptoms to ensure a complete work-up that will not miss cancer. Others minimize symptoms in the hope of being reassured. Diagnostic tests may be therapeutically valuable and reassuring, particularly when they are normal. **Touching the patient**, even briefly, helps to establish better understanding and more empathic communication in the relationship between patient and physician. Doctors who do this are perceived as spending more time with patients and explaining things much better.

Empathy consists of **listening to** and **understanding** the total communication of the patient as expressed through **words, feelings**, and **gestures**. It is not an emotional state of feeling sympathetic or feeling sorry for someone. Because understanding is the core concept of objectivity, the empathic scientific physician is the one most likely to obtain an accurate history. When a physician uses the term *poor historian* to describe a patient, he may be saying, "The history is unclear because *I'm* a poor historian."

Lookingbill DP: Yield from a complete skin examination. Findings in 1157 new dermatology patients. J Am Acad Dermatol 1988; 18:31–37.

Among other things, complete skin examinations revealed:

hidden rashes of help in making diagnosis	1.8%
hidden rashes unrelated but significant	3.3%
malignant tumors	2.0%
dysplastic nevi	2.3%

It was concluded that the overall yield of significant incidental findings in 15% of patients would appear to justify a **total skin examination** for all new patients. Only 4% of 1157 new patients declined a total skin examination. Modesty and infirmity appeared to be the major reasons for refusal. One elderly woman refused by saying, "Young man, I didn't get to be 91 by taking off my clothes for just anybody."

In this study, 55 patients had incidental skin tumors suspicious for malignancy, with 22 (2%) malignant tumors confirmed by biopsy. This included 20 basal cell carcinomas, half of which were on covered areas (trunk, legs). Dysplastic nevi were suspected in 25 (2 to 3%) of the patients, but were confirmed by biopsy in only 4 of 11 patients. Neurofibromatosis was newly diagnosed in 2 patients, and AIDS was discovered in 1 patient because of a biopsy showing Kaposi's sarcoma. The most common "**hidden**" **rash** severe enough to warrant therapy was **tinea pedis**, followed by tinea versicolor and tinea cruris. Did you check your patient's feet today?

Nutt JJ: Early signs of orthopedic conditions. Ann Intern Med 1940; 14:1050–1064.

The expression of the face and eyes, especially the eyes, is replete with signs for physicians if they will but recognize them. The face reflects pain, ache, and apprehension, and the good diagnostician is adept at interpreting the **facial expressions** of the patient.

"The all-seeing eye, the sensitive finger, the trained ear, and the knowing nose are still most helpful instruments in making diagnoses."

Hobus PPM, Schmidt HG, Boshuizen HPA, Patel VL: Contextual factors in the activation of the first diagnostic hypotheses: Expert-novice differences. Med Educ 1987; 21:471–476.

In arriving at an initial diagnosis, experienced physicians, unlike the beginners, make extensive use of "**context**" information: sex, age, risk factors of work, behaviors, heredity, appearance, prior diseases, medications.

Einterz EM: **Cultural barriers** and the diagnostic process. Lancet 1987; 1:1434.

Medical history-taking in nonwestern illiterate societies provides the challenge of linguistic and cultural barriers. The Tivs in central Nigeria complain of witches attacking them in the night and show scratch marks on their arms as proof. Others describe dysuria as "biting of the penis." Their concept of time reflects the absence of watches and calendars. Thus, a week may be but 4 days, and conversely a child of 2 years may be said by his mother to be 10.

Fitzgerald FT, Tierney LM: The bedside Sherlock Holmes. West J Med 1982; 137:169–175.

The accuracy and adventure of differential diagnosis is enhanced by looking for diagnostic leads and **clues** in the patient's **clothing, jewelry,** and **possessions**.

Here is a sampling:

    suitcase sign—expects to be hospitalized
    tie patterns—may indicate hobbies worthy of query
    fit of clothing—weight changes
    too warmly dressed—hypothyroidism
    rings too tight—edema, acromegaly
    purseful of "sourballs"—xerostomia of Sjögren's syndrome
    reading material—educational level

See this article for a remarkable lesson on how much an internist can deduce by examining not the patient but what is around him. Elementary, my dear Watson. His pockets filled with licorice explain his myopathy!

Bradburn NM, Rips LJ, Shevell SK: Answering autobiographical questions: The impact of memory and inference on surveys. Science 1987; 236:157–161.

Memory recall is **improved** by

1. Giving the patient sufficient time between questions
2. Providing cues such as possible answers
3. Asking first about most recent events
4. **Repeating key questions** at **each visit**

But remember, some information can never be recalled.

Michelson HE, Bovenmyer DA: A case for diagnosis. Arch Dermatol 1966; 93:250.

There is an old axiom in Vienna dermatology that if you cannot make a diagnosis you must make a good description, and the better the description the more apt one is to arrive at a diagnosis.

In other words, the best way to approach an obscure diagnostic problem is to **write down a good description** of what can be seen in the skin. (The eye sees more when it has to report to the hand.)

Cutler P: Problem Solving in Clinical Medicine: From Data to Diagnosis, 2nd ed. Baltimore, Williams & Wilkins, 1985, pp 161–163.

Algorithms (printed flow charts) should not be regarded as a problem-solving panacea. They are little more than prefabricated dendrograms that serve as recipes for a mindless cook. They are rigid, difficult to write, can inhibit independent thinking, and are often so intricate as to require a compass and guide.

Neuhauser D: Careful thinking. AJR 1982; 139:849–854.

We are passing out of the era of medical thinking when good clinical judgment was a charismatic "gift of the gods." Today's formal medical thinking involves national computer programs that cross reference symptoms and diseases using probabilities. Artificial intelligence diagnostic programs are likewise evolving.

No longer is a test a test. It is viewed now from the standpoint of relevancy, accuracy, sensitivity, specificity, and cost. No longer is the bias of the senior physician revered. The new god is **decision analysis** with its explicit rules of logic and quantitation. No longer are possible diagnoses simply listed. Each is now assigned a rank order based on probability data. No longer do we hear the baroque music of a Richard Cabot case report. The modern beat comes with the hum of the computer disc. If you want to play for the new generation of students, take lessons on the computer.

Waldrop MM: Toward a unified theory of cognition. Science 1988; 241:27–29.

All cognition involves some sort of problem solving. The traditional techniques we use are:

trial and error (leap and then look)

hill climbing (do whatever seems best at the time)

means-ends analysis (If I am over here and my goal is over there, I should try to reduce the difference.)

All of these have been incorporated into computers for years. Thus there are general problem-solving computers and there are highly specialized computers (e.g., Mycin) for the diagnosis of infectious disease. But none of these could rise above the knowledge programmed into them.

Today there is a new computer program, Soar, which can learn from experience. When it reaches an impasse in problem solving, that is, when it does not know what to do next, it automatically sets up a subgoal to resolve the impasse. When it succeeds, it goes back to the original channel of problem solving, but bringing with it a new "chunk" of knowledge that it encodes. As a result, it will never suffer that particular impasse again. In a specific example, Soar took 1731 steps to solve an original problem, but astonishingly only 7 steps to solve that same problem on a second run. This proved it had become a self-taught expert. For medical diagnosis, use the program called Neomycin-Soar.

Schwartz WB, Patil RS, Szolovits P: Artificial intelligence in medicine. Where do we stand? N Engl J Med 1987; 316:685–688.

Artificial intelligence programs still cannot act as a reliable consultant on medical problems, but they can generate a long list of diagnostic possibilities. Such a list fails in narrowing the diagnostic focus, although it does succeed in bringing otherwise overlooked diseases to the clinician's attention.

Haynes RB, McKibbon KA, Fitzgerald D, et al: How to keep up with the medical literature. IV: Using the literature to solve clinical problems. Ann Intern Med 1986; 105:636–640.

Scanning many **journals** for articles of great clinical pertinence is like skimming the cream off the medical literature. It provides breadth rather than the depth needed for a special problem case.

The following guide should help you in solving a specific diagnostic problem in your day-to-day clinical practice. These are the routes to in-depth knowledge:

1. Consult your textbooks, yearbooks, monographs, and atlases. You bought them, use them.
2. Look in your file of "tear-outs," Xerox copies, reprints of recent articles. You don't have a file? Start one today. Good articles are best retrieved when torn out and filed by you.
3. **Consult an expert.** If there is none locally, call long distance, send Kodachrome prints, and history abstract.
4. Browse through that file of unread journals on your desk or go to the library for a serendipitous stroll through the stacks. It's a form of medical lottery.
5. Look in *Index Medicus* under the subject heading skin disease for the exotic or under an appropriate diagnostic heading such as urticaria. You can scan all the titles for the past 5 years in 30 minutes of your lunch hour.
6. Order a specific Medline Search to bring up all the references available up to the past few weeks. Alternative diagnostic search systems are available, but this is generally the broadest based, reflecting the holdings of the National Library of Medicine in Bethesda.

You now should know more about your patient's problem than anyone else in the world.

Cullen K: Personal view. Br Med J 1982; 284:502.

Gifted doctors like reading the journal reports of case conferences as an automatic check on their clinical sharpness. As our learning demands some effort, the choice of what should be stored merits a special kind of shrewdness if we are to **avoid cluttering** up our **memory** with junk.

Levene GM, Goolamali SK: Diagnostic Picture Tests in Dermatology. London, Wolfe Medical Publications, 1986, 126 pp.

There are 186 color plates for diagnosis and quizzing.

THE CERTAINTY OF UNCERTAINTY IN DIAGNOSIS

Katz J: Why doctors don't disclose **uncertainty**. *In* Dowie JA, Elstein AS (eds): Professional Judgement: A Reader in Clinical Decision Making. Cambridge, Cambridge University Press, 1988, pp 544–565.

Physicians generally hold to the view that when their ship sails on the high seas of medical uncertainty, patients prefer to believe the captain has charts, compass, and sextant, even though he may actually have none of these.

Macartney FJ: Diagnostic logic. Br Med J 1987; 295:1325–1331.

In the field of medical diagnosis, we are not in the business of establishing the foundations of scientific knowledge. Hence, in the real world of patient care, we do not have to be certain the diagnosis is correct. All we need to know is that if we manage the patient on the assumption that our diagnosis is correct, the patient will do better than if any other diagnosis is assumed.

Barondess JA: The impossible in medicine. Perspect Biol Med 1986; 29:521–529.

The impossible dream in medicine is certainty. Always there is diagnostic uncertainty, which often is heightened by:

the presence of more than one disease
the intrusion of distractor symptoms and signs
a poor history due to language barriers, an obtunded patient, and the like
the indeterminant effects of prior therapy
the nonexistence of confirmatory diagnostic tests
the fact that **undescribed diseases still exist**
the limitations of diagnostic tests

The **skillful clinician** is the one who can **disregard** the **trivial** nonspecific **complaints** of the patient as well as the **irrelevant laboratory findings**. He is the one who can develop a patterned cluster of clinical data that leads in a reductionist fashion to a diagnosis. His skill comes only after years of clinical practice.

Gale J, Marsden P: Medical Diagnosis, from Student to Clinician. Oxford, Oxford University Press, 1983, 218 pp.

The problems of diagnosis are not neat and tidy problems. Each one is different. Each one requires judgment. There are no externally set criteria against which "accuracy" of diagnosis can be measured.

Brown GW: Bayes' formula. Conditional probability and clinical medicine. Am J Dis Child 1981; 135:1125–1129.

Bayes' formula, used to bring mathematical precision into the field of telling the **probability** of **diagnostic relationships**, stems from the ruminations of a Presbyterian minister, Reverend Thomas Bayes, more than 200 years ago in southern England. Whether he was calculating the chances of salvation or not we do not know, but today his probability formula is more cited than used in diagnosis.

Balla JI: The **Diagnostic Process**: A Model for Clinical Teachers. Cambridge, Cambridge University Press, 1985, 150 pp.

"Many clinicians will abhor the idea that uncertainty may creep into medical decision making. . . . However, when we speak of decision making as we do here, we will have made the basic assumption that our information sources may be incomplete or incorrect and we are indeed facing uncertainty."

The flight from the uncertainty of the diagnostic process leads the scientific analyst to look at rational models that cover most situations in which decisions have to be made through the diagnostic process. These problems may be examined through the lens of:

Symbolic logic:
Present the information in a symbolic manner, using letters of the alphabet for rigorous logical thinking. Alternatives include Venn diagrams for mathematical congruency and set theory for finer discrimination.

Bayes's theorem:
> An analysis of known probability as a measure of subjective belief in the likelihood of a diagnosis.

Gambles:
> Guidance by consideration of what is the probability of winning or losing, as well as what is the magnitude of the gain or loss.

Weighting of Cues:
> A subjective assessment of the significance of the history, physical, and laboratory findings, allowing strong cues to favor or negate a diagnosis.

Decision trees:
> These visualize courses of diagnostic action as long branches of a tree with the insertion of probabilities to provide a basis for a logical temporal sequence.

All of these are viewed by most clinicians as cumbersome mathematics of medicine. Ideally, all of the above are used intuitively by the experienced clinician in his flight from diagnostic uncertainty.

Eddy DM: Variations in Physician Practice: The Role of Uncertainty. *In* Dowie J, Elstein A (eds): Professional Judgement: A Reader in Clinical Decision Making. Cambridge, Cambridge University Press, 1988; pp 45–59.

Uncertainty, biases, errors, and differences of opinions, motives, and values weaken every link in the chain that connects a patient's actual condition to the selection of a diagnostic test.

Observer variation makes for much diagnostic uncertainty: 22 physicians were asked to note cyanosis in 20 patients, in whom the absolute diagnosis was made by oximetry. Only 53% of the physicians diagnosed cyanosis in subjects with extremely low oxygen content, and 26% saw cyanosis in subjects with normal oxygen levels. Physicians vary in their ability to observe the signs, symptoms, and findings of even well-defined diseases.

One of the easiest ways to fit a **large problem** in our minds is to **lop off huge parts** of it. But there is uncertainty as to which parts to lop off.

Moskowitz AJ, Kuipers BJ, Kassirer JP: Dealing with uncertainty, risks, and tradeoffs in clinical decisions: A cognitive science approach. Ann Intern Med 1988; 108:435–449.

Physicians do not conceive and solve clinical problems by "growing a decision tree in their heads." They actually develop a sequence of decisions based on available, yet incomplete, information.

Bosk CL: Occupational rituals in patient management. N Engl J Med 1980; 303:71–76.

Strategies used by physicians **to manage** the inevitable **uncertainties** facing them:

Hedged assertions in the form of approximations ("It is approximately . . .") and shields ("As far as I can tell right now . . .")

Probability reasoning with numerical estimates of diagnostic likelihoods

Facing the patient not as an uncertainty but as a research opportunity to learn something new

Request for consultation provides an immediate payoff, but the response poses the risk of aggravating the uncertainty

Socratic teaching in which interchange at rounds leads to more tests

Deciding not to decide provides a "wait-and-see" tranquilizer for the uncertain.

Gallows humor in which laughter is the only response to an absurd situation

Hyperrealism involves a mix of detachment, resignation, helplessness, and anger.

SOURCES OF ERROR

Asher R: **Malingering.** Trans Med Soc London 1959; 75:34–44.

"The pride of a doctor who has caught a malingerer is akin to that of a fisherman who has landed an enormous fish." Malingering is the imitation, production, or encouragement of illness for a deliberate end, with the patient quite conscious of what he is doing and quite cognizant of why he is doing it. It is the planned fraudulent faking of illness and is very rare. It should be **diagnosed with great caution**, as many examples of apparent malingering have turned out to be cases of organic disease.

The author's personal case of misdiagnosis: One Sunday afternoon the author dressed his 2-year-old daughter and took her for a walk. She kept falling to the left. She walked with a ridiculous scissors gait and frequently fell to the ground. She cried and said she had pain. To the father, it was obviously sheer devilment, a malignant aggressive demonstration against the father figure. When the mother returned she undressed the child for her evening bath. There was a sudden cry, "Do you realize you've put both her legs through the same hole in her knickers?"

Dowie JA, Elstein AS (eds): Professional Judgement: A Reader in Clinical Decision Making. Cambridge, Cambridge University Press, 1988, 565 pp.

Clinicians look with suspicion on any attempt to dissect and define their clinical judgment, but here is a golden collection of reprints of 30 classic articles that place the doctor under a microscope.

Focusing on the **diagnostician's failures**, they saw these four flaws:

1. Failure to retrieve the correct hypothesis from memory: Learn to restructure and reformulate for new diagnostic insight as the problem solving proceeds; **avoid entrapment by the initial hypothesis**.
2. Pursuit of exotic diagnoses at the expense of the more probable: Suppress your desire to make "the diagnosis of the year"; concentrate on day-to-day diagnoses.
3. Misinterpretation of data: Value negative findings, ignore the irrelevant, and show parsimony in collecting data.
4. Lack of appreciation of statistical properties of clinical evidence: Recognize that a series provides a firmer footing than that one vivid memorable case; realize that the predictive value of a "diagnostic" test is poor in an area where the disease is rare; avoid making diagnoses based on wishful thinking or on overconfidence.

Jackson R: The importance of being visually literate. Observations on the art and science of making a morphological diagnosis in dermatology. Arch Dermatol 1975; 111:632–636.

Three **common failures**:

1. **Looking** intently at **too few sites**. You can focus closely only on an area the size of a dime at arm's length. Detailed vision demands that image fall on the fovea, thereby eliminating 99.9% of the visual field.

2. **Looking with an improper frame of mind. Boredom, disinterest, fatigue**, lack of confidence, or medication you are taking keeps visual images from reaching the cortical recognition center.
3. **Looking without hypothesizing.** Diagnostic synthetic constructs demand something be added to or subtracted from the often imperfect image the patient presents. Recognition demands the cortical cybernetics of positive and negative feedback into the visual process.

"Once clinical information is received, it is probably impossible to suppress. The age-old dermatological practice of looking first and talking afterwards is probably based on the same phenomenon. Your accuracy of diagnosis may be higher if you approach your visual examination without preconceived ideas."

Dimsdale JE: Delays and slips in medical diagnosis. Perspect Biol Med 1984; 27:213–220.

You have **impaired diagnostic abilities**:

1. When the patient comes from a group (racial, professional, or otherwise) with which you are uncomfortable
2. When the patient's behavior makes **you feel uncomfortable or angry**
3. When the patient is too close to you (colleague, family member)
4. When the patient's illness itself makes you uncomfortable

Tuddenham WJ: Visual search, image organization and reader error in roentgen diagnosis. Studies of the psychophysiology of roentgen **image perception**. Radiology 1962; 78:694–704.

Three experienced radiologists studying a collection of chest films "overlooked" 20 to 30% of findings that they as a group later judged to have been reportable. (Let the dermatologic diagnostician beware.)

Arkes HR, Saville PD, Wortmann RL, Harkness AR: Hindsight bias among physicians weighing the likelihood of diagnoses. *In* Dowie JA, Elstein AS (eds): Professional Judgement: A Reader in Clinical Decision Making. Cambridge, Cambridge University Press, 1988, pp 374–378.

Diagnostic accuracy may be compromised by knowledge of previous diagnoses or studies. This is the "**hindsight**" **bias** that leads a physician to agree with what another doctor had thought or done rather than analyzing available data independently.

Reducing doctors' errors. Br Med J 1977; 1:1178–1179.

The constant rapid flow of large quantities of often irrelevant information impairs one's diagnostic performance.

Phillips WC, Scott JA, Blasczcynski G: Statistics for diagnostic procedures. II: The significance of "no significance": What a negative statistical test really means. AJR 1983; 141:203–206.

Often "**no significant difference**" means *not* that the groups are identical, but rather that they are *too small*. Don't forget that the medical literature is skewed toward positive findings, since neither authors nor journals wish to publish negative results.

Campbell EJM: The diagnosing mind. Lancet 1987; 1:849–851.

In most teaching hospitals, layers of staff review, **gamesmanship**, and the struggle for status promote mindless diagnostic work-ups.

Diagnosis: Logic and psycho-logic. Lancet 1987; 1:840–841.

Humans are often illogical and inefficient in using information, frequently make wrong deductions, ignore evidence, overemphasize irrelevancies, and are inconsistent, both with others and with themselves. Beware!

Kaplan MM: Weekly clinicopathological exercises. Case 27-1988. N Engl J Med 1988; 319:37–44.

At one of these conferences years ago, Franz J. Ingelfinger was analyzing the findings on a patient with malabsorption. He reasoned flawlessly and arrived at the logical and best diagnosis. But it was wrong. His concluding remark to the pathologist was, "You may have had the correct diagnosis, but I have the better one."

Kassirer JP: Diagnostic reasoning. Ann Intern Med 1989; 110:893–900.

The **formulation of hypotheses** is an essential initial step in any diagnostic reasoning process. Such hypotheses form a context within which further information-gathering takes place. Your short-term memory capability limits the number of actively considered hypotheses to about **seven**. These, in turn, are continually assessed, dismissed, or verified. The initiation or triggering of such hypotheses is dependent upon a few observations made by you.

The reasoning process used in arriving at a diagnosis involves three distinct strategies. Any one or all may be used in a specific problem-solving situation.

Strategy 1: Probabilistic reasoning. This approach involves an assessment of the probability of the clinical findings or laboratory tests being diagnostic. (Thus, a silvery scale triggers a diagnosis of the common disease psoriasis.) It is a way of dealing with the uncertainty that is present in the world of disease. In its highest form, probabilistic reasoning allows quantitative mathematical expression based on scientific data derived from observations on large population groups. But most commonly it expresses itself in such terms as very common, common, uncommon, rare, extremely rare.

Probabilistic reasoning encounters problems in that test results are neither positive nor negative, but a continuous variable; nor can a disease be simply considered as present or absent. Its varying stages exhibit a spectrum of findings in the history, the physical examination, and in the laboratory data. Finally, in probabilistic thinking, the failure to consider all the possible diagnoses may result in a failure to consider the correct diagnosis.

Probabilistic reasoning does give you the power of statistics to make a creditable diagnosis. It allows you to **weigh the significance of test results**. Thus, whenever the likelihood of a given disease is extremely high, a negative test result does not exclude the presence of the disease unless the test is highly sensitive. Conversely, if the pretest probability of a disease is extremely low, a positive test can be disregarded or viewed as a false-positive unless the test is highly specific.

Strategy 2: Causal reasoning. This centers on reasoning based on a knowledge of the pathophysiology of disease. (Thus the patient's complaint of pruritus triggers a diagnosis of contact dermatitis.) Causal reasoning relies on **cause-and-effect relationships**. It permits diagnostic assessment of congruity of duration and magnitude between response and stimulus (when and to what degree was the patient exposed to poison ivy?). It permits extrapolation to further testing and data gathering for verification, validation, or dismissal of a given diagnosis. It allows for the critical search for discrepancies as well as confirmatory findings. This type of reasoning provides you with diagnostic confidence arising out of its richness of exploratory power.

Strategy 3: Deterministic reasoning. This is the ordinary everyday diagnostic thought process of following the known rules of rubric that if certain conditions are met, then the correct diagnosis must follow. When parallel rules compete, either will win or lose on its strength and relevance. Such reasoning being governed by rules is amenable to expression in a one- or two-page branching algorithm. Most such **algorithms**, i.e., thought flow charts, are designed to direct thinking in a logical rigid path to either the correct diagnosis or at least to the correct interpretation of a single test. They force you to ask and answer questions you might neglect or forget. However, in complex medical problems, algorithms fail, trapped in their own tangle of intertwining branches. Other defects become evident.

1. Algorithms cannot handle uncertainty that is inherent in every history, physical examination, or laboratory test.

2. Algorithms have the flaws of the faulty or limited experience of the author or composer.

3. The entry point may be the same for disparate clinical conditions, yet the pathways appropriate for only one disease. Thus, following a diagnostic pathway for urinary tract infection is worthless and misleading for study of the patient with vaginitis. Still both of these diseases have an entry point of dysuria.

4. Most **algorithms** are **unsuitable** for patients **with multiple complaints** or complex interrelated tests. Algorithms don't permit the shading, the fudging, the intuitive slanting, and the provisional suppositions so dear to a clinician's diagnostic heart.

All in all, the algorithm is usually much too black and white for the colorful world of clinical practice.

Kassirer JP, Kopelman RI: Cognitive errors in diagnosis: Instantiation, classification of consequences. Am J Med 1989; 86:433–441.

Physicians are guilty of the following **cognitive diagnosis errors**:

Failure to even think of the correct diagnosis, given the trigger of observations.

Failure to select the relevant or significant symptom for study in depth.

Failure to consider the common disease as the likely diagnosis.

Failure to appreciate that **a positive test for a very rare disease is likely to be a false-positive one**. (These are the times the hoof beats are heard as those of a zebra.)

Failure in causal reasoning. A 61-year-old woman with hypertension developed **purpura** of the **hands** and **toes** several days after cardiac catheterization. Her physician carried out extensive immunologic studies, performed renal arteriography as a reason for evidence of vasculitis. The nephrologist promptly made the correct diagnosis of catheter-induced **atheroembolism**.

Failure to doubt a clinical axiom, such as missing the diagnosis of a painful bleeding peptic ulcer because "bleeding ulcers don't hurt."

Failure to verify the diagnosis, i.e., failure to recognize that the findings were inconsistent with the disease.

No-fault errors as in the case of a disease presenting in a completely atypical, unrecognizable form.

Yoon Y, Brobst RW, Bergstresser PR, Peterson LL: A connectionist expert system for dermatology diagnosis. Expert Systems 1990; 4:22–31.

DESKNET is a computer tool designed for the instruction of medical students in the diagnosis of papulosquamous skin disease.

Its use enhances the student's information-gathering and utilizing skills in the diagnostic process. DESKNET generates knowledge via a connectionist expert system in which the implicit knowledge of an expert is utilized, but not expressed explicitly. It does not use the conventional rule-based system that allows explanation of the decisions taken. Thus, DESKNET is a three-layered neural network system wherein a back propogation algorithm generates its own knowledge base from patient's cases. The computer is given the clinical signs as an input layer and an expert's diagnosis as the desired output layer. The hidden middle layer generates a pattern of weighted intercommunications constituting an implicit specification of decision criteria. This is done by excitatory or inhibitory connections with the layers above and below.

Tinea corporis, tinea versicolor, and seborrheic dermatitis were diagnosed with a success rate of over 80%. However, psoriasis was recognized only 30% of the time, apparently in view of its high capacity to resemble the other diseases. Obviously, DESKNET won't be opening an office, quite yet.

Burton JL: The logic of dermatologic diagnosis. Clin Exp Dermatol 1981; 6:1–21.

Geoffrey Dowling had uncanny diagnostic skills based on his remarkable visual memory. Yet a diagnostician is not limited to pattern recognition. There are 15,000 different symptoms, signs, and investigations potentially available for processing by the physician's brain. But note, the human mind can attend to only seven items of information simultaneously.

Numerical taxonomy deserves a place in classifying dermatologic disease. It is based on the statistical estimation of the **resemblance between patients**, so that patients who most resemble each other can be clustered into groups that differ from each other. The many disease indicants of a series of patients are recorded, and their resemblance to each other is computed and expressed numerically as a coefficient of similarity that varies from zero to unity. A score of 1 indicates perfect agreement, i.e., the two patients are identical. A score of 0 shows they are completely different. Tedious calculations performed by computer eventually allow groups of patients, most resembling each other, to be defined. Such numerical taxonomy is superior to the intuitive process carried out by experienced clinicians since:

1. It is objective, not biased by the more memorable cases.
2. It forces clinicians to think and define diagnostic criteria exactly.
3. It allows integration of data of different types with quantitative expression of importance.
4. It allows the computer to analyze data and increase greatly diagnostic discrimination.

Finally, in an ideal world, we should know the specificity and sensitivity of every sign, symptom, and test result that we use. But in our real world, we can still make only our best guesses. And some "guessers" are better than others. We call them the better diagnosticians.

Diagnostic Ploys

1. **Transposition** as an aid to diagnosis:

   Mentally transpose the lesion:
     to different areas
     to a different distribution pattern
     to a different age group
     to the opposite sex
     to a different race

2. **Lesional focus** as an aid to diagnosis:
     focus on a primary lesion
     focus on a representative area
     mentally expand its distribution or size
     mentally reduce its distribution or size

3. **History** as an aid to diagnosis:
     since birth, familial trait: genetic
     known exposure to illness: contagious
     cyclic: menses, seasonal
     nocturnal: neutropenia
     occupation, hobbies: specific contactants, hazards
     pets: allergy to parasites, mites, fleas
     travel: endemic disease
     history may be wrong: new diagnosis

4. **Etiology** as an aid to diagnosis:

   Could it be:
     a drug sensitivity
     a contact sensitivity
     an autoimmune disease

   Could it be due to a:
     virus
     bacteria
     spirochete
     fungus
     insect
     animal

   Is it factitial?
     fingernail
     teeth
     chemicals
     physical agent

Your diagnostic horizon will surely widen as you spend time looking, thinking, questioning, testing, and reading.

HOW TO MAKE A DIAGNOSIS

We saw a nail so loose	We called it onycholysis
It was hanging by a cuticle	We called it onycholysis totalis
It was a nail so black	We called it onycholysis totalis noir
It was twisted and thick	We called it onycholysis totalis noir et dystrophica
It was of cause unknown	We called it onycholysis totalis noir et dystrophica idiopathica
The patient asked if it is cancer	We replied gravely, "No it's only onycholysis totalis noir et dystrophica idiopathica benigna."
It had never been seen before	So now we call it onycholysis totalis noir et dystrophica idiopathica benigna of Shelley.

Diagnosis is so easy, once you get the hang of it.

Don't Just Stand There and Look: Do Something

See	Skin test
Smell	Study hair
Scrape	Study sebaceous gland
Swab	Study sweat gland
Stain	Study vessels
Strip	Study blood, urine, feces
Slice	Size up the patient
Slit	Search with instruments
Soak	Search for more information
Sample	Solve it

And you will have to do something if the diagnosis doesn't come from a glance. You will have to work, to gather numerous bits and pieces of information, to sort out the irrelevant, to arrange and rearrange the pieces, to finally perceive the mosaic pattern we call the diagnosis. It is not a passive act. Here are a score of things to do.

SEE

You've listened, and now's the time to look. Stand back and see the big picture. See what you can see. What is the **patterning**, the **distribution**, the areas that are clear? Are the photo areas specifically involved? Does it limit itself to the areas of physiologic dryness, or is it limited to the seborrheic zone? Does it favor the stasis areas? Keep looking and asking. Is it zosteriform, unilateral, quadratic, banded? Is it limited to glabrous skin?

Come in closer. Are there vesicles, pustules? Is it follicular? Do you see filiform spines? What do you see in the **mouth**, the **conjunctiva**, the **glans penis**, the **vagina**? Separate the **toes**. Look for tinea pedis. The patient will disclaim a lifetime of fungal scaling of the soles, which now may be the source of a follicular "id." Look at the **nails**. Have they the polish of "usure des ongles," the pits of alopecia areata, the oil spots of psoriasis, the ragged edge of onychophagia? Look in the **pubic hair** and in the **scalp** for pediculi causing generalized pruritus. Are there islands of uninvolved skin as seen in the erythroderma of pityriasis rubra pilaris?

Look where the patient points, and look where he doesn't. The patient with a hand eruption may fail to show you the scaling crusted lesions of scabies on the penis. Look for carcinomas and for warts the patient has accepted unknowingly. **Behind the ears**, the **closed eyelid**, and the **back** are terra incognita to the patient. Do not neglect these sites. Here the diagnosis is easy. What is hard is remembering to look.

Move the light. Shadow the lesion, spotlight it, and now magnify it.

Epstein E: **Magnifiers** in dermatology: A personal survey. J Am Acad Dermatol 1985; 13:687–698.

> Although the pathologist lives in a world magnified 100 to 1000 times, the clinician does not benefit from a highly magnified view of the patient. Even 10- to 20-power magnification of a lesion, while it provides a dramatic sight, does not aid in diagnosis. Indeed, it may hinder, confuse, and frustrate. Even at $15\times$ the depth of field is so small (2 mm) that only part of the lesion is in focus. And it is a focus that comes and goes even as the patient breathes

or grimaces. Furthermore, the lens must be less than an inch from the skin, so that one has a restricted working distance.

The most useful magnification for detailed clinical inspection is $3\times$ to $4\times$. Lower magnification, although useful in surgery, does not provide much more information than inspection with the unaided eye.

The single lens **hand-held magnifier** is the simplest and least expensive. An example is the Bausch and Lomb Hastings $5\times$ magnifier. To go to a binocular system, use of the **headband-mounted Optivisor** with a magnification of $2.75\times$ is recommended.

For an elite system use the expanded-field **binocular loupe** (Designs for Vision). Here two small magnifying telescopes are attached to spectacle frames or a headband. They give far greater working distance than the single lens loupe. The $3.5\times$ is ideal, not being too heavy or bulky, except in price.

We personally use a headband loupe with dual $2.5\times$ power lenses. It brings us a world just two and a half times life size. It is a special world we have lived in for years. Its creatures are not too big and not too small. For special features an $8\times$ hand lens may be employed. More impressive to the patient but not necessarily more helpful to you is the binocular surgical stereomicroscope with a 200-mm lens system with built-in light source and a Contax automatic 35-mm camera. Excellent visualization of the skin, and particularly of pigmented lesions, is obtained by using the Dermatoscope (Dermatologic Lab and Supply, Council Bluffs, IA 51503). By placing a drop of mineral oil on the skin surface the epidermis becomes translucent. Reflective glare is reduced by covering the oil with glass. An oil/glass interface allows a better view of epidermal and superficial dermal changes. It magnifies 10 power.

> Katz HI, Prawer SE, Mooney JJ, Samson CR: Pre-atrophy: Covert sign of **thinned skin**. J Am Acad Dermatol 1989; 20:731–735.
>
> Viewing the skin with an $8\times$ **hand lens** following application of **mineral oil** and a coverslip permits early recognition of **epidermal atrophy**. In the atrophic sites that develop, for example, after application of superpotent steroids, one can see the normally hidden subpapillary vascular channels.

Next, look at the skin under Wood's light.

> Jillson OF: Wood's light: An incredibly important diagnostic tool. Cutis 1981; 28:620–626.
>
> With a good high-intensity **Wood's light** you have a new dimension for visual diagnosis. You can see:
>
> fungi shining **blue green**, but it won't let you see the nonfluorescing *Trichophyton tonsurans* or *verrucosum*, only the common *Microsporum canis* and the now rare *Microsporum audouinii*.
>
> an otherwise inapparent tinea versicolor in an antecubital space, in the diaper area, and even the form localized to the hair follicles. Look for the **yellow-white** or **copper-orange** hue.
>
> *Pseudomonas aeruginosa* colonization of the ear canal, toe webs, or scrotum. Look for the **blue** of the fluorescein formed by these bacteria.
>
> the *Corynebacterium minutissimum* colonization in erythrasma. Look for a brilliant **coral-red** fluorescence between the toes, in the groin, and in the axillae.
>
> pigment changes essentially invisible in ordinary light. Look for the leaf-shaped **white** macules pathognomonic of tuberous sclerosis and present also in genetic carriers of the trait.

the earliest signs of pigment return in treated vitiligo so valuable in encouraging the patient.

Wood's light is truly an "ultra" diagnostic aid.

Harber LC, Bickers DR: Photosensitivity Diseases. Principles of Diagnosis and Treatment, 2nd ed. Philadelphia, B.C. Decker, Inc., 1989, pp 421–433.

Don't just look at skin but also look at **urine**, **stool**, and **blood** extract under Wood's light if porphyria is suspected. Rapid screening tests for office use (quantitative clinical laboratory determinations required for definitive diagnosis):

1. Urine

    Direct Wood's light inspection: **Reddish-orange** fluorescence indicative of large amounts of porphyrins (uroporphyrin or coproporphyrin)

    More dramatic if acidify (10 drops of glacial acetic acid to 4 ml urine) and extract with 1 ml of amyl alcohol. Upper alcohol layer will show pink fluorescence. Such a positive crude assay is indicative of a porphyric state (porphyria cutanea tarda, erythropoietic porphyria, hepatoerythropoietic porphyria, variegate porphyria, hereditary coproporphyria).

2. Stool

    Direct Wood's light inspection will show fluorescence if large amounts of porphyrin present.

    Can enhance by extraction with mixture of equal parts of amyl alcohol, glacial acetic acid, and ethyl ether (4 ml to pea-sized stool specimen). Mix this extract with 1.5 N hydrochloric acid (2 ml). HCl layer will show **red fluorescence**.

3. Red Blood Cells

    Wood's light examination of whole blood extraction (2.5 ml of mix of ethyl ether 5 parts and glacial acetic acid 1 part, added to 10 ml blood. Mix, decant, add 0.5 ml of 3 N HCl). Lower layer will show intense **red fluorescence** in patient with erythropoietic protoporphyria or hepatic erythropoietic porphyria.

    In erythropoietic porphyria the offending uroporphyrin is not extracted, since it is water soluble. To detect this marker, mix 1 ml of blood with 3 ml of methanol-sulfuric acid (20:1). Such a positive red cell extract will show **red-pink fluorescence**.

Transilluminate the **nose**, **ear**, or **finger** to determine extent of a mass such as a carcinoma. Using a strong **red light** is preferable, since only the red wavelengths penetrate through the corium.

For viewing the capillaries, the nail fold is ideal, since here the capillaries are seen parallel to the skin surface, thus permitting visualization of the capillary loops in their entirety.

Minkin W, Rabhan NB: Office **nailfold capillary microscopy** using ophthalmoscope. J Am Acad Dermatol 1988; 7:190–193.

1. Place a drop of mineral oil on the nail fold of the fourth finger.
2. Hold the ophthalmoscope (set at +40) close, but not in contact with oil.
3. Thus provided with 10 × magnification, one visualizes normal capillaries as thin regularly spaced loops in a row perpendicular to the nail.
4. In **scleroderma** the loops are enlarged and dilated, as well as being disorganized and indeed absent in areas.

5. In **lupus erythematosus** the loops are tortuous and meandering, but not dilated. At times they resemble glomeruli.
6. The method is not suitable for capillary study in black-skinned persons or in nail folds traumatized by manual labor or by cuticular manipulation.

McKiernan FE: Water-soluble gels in narrowfield **nail fold capillary microscopy**. Arthritis Rheum 1986; 29:304.

Use **K-Y jelly** for translucency and the 20-diopter lens of an ophthalmoscope for viewing.

Slaaf DW, Tangelder GJ, Reneman RS, et al: A versatile incident illuminator for intravital microscopy. Int J Microcirc Clin Exp 1987; 6:391–397.

Not only **capillaries**, but also **venules**, can be visualized in the **nail fold** skin by using Ploempak incident illuminator in conjunction with a Leitz microscope. Red cells appeared dark on a light background, permitting calculation of their flow velocity. The illuminator consists of a special mirror (50% reflectance and 50% transmittance) mounted at 45 degrees to the optical axis of the microscope.

Changes in location and **size** of lesions provide valuable clues for diagnosis. Record the exact location and size in your chart. Use either freehand drawings or **anatomic rubber stamps**. A complete set of such stamp dyes, outlining every area of the body, is available from Dermatologic Lab and Supply, Council Bluffs, IA 51503. Using them will focus your thinking on what you record. To mark lesions or patch and skin test sites invisibly use **fluorescent marking pens** (Dermatologic Lab and Supply). This allows you to follow urticarial and other lesion regressions or extensions for the 2 weeks between visits. The patient does not see the marks, but you do under Wood's light.

The **ruler** is as essential as the pen in keeping records. Use it to measure progress and relapse. Measuring the volume of ulcers, such as decubitus ulcers, is an important maneuver, since often the perimeter may give no indication of changes in size. Thus, the **syringe** joins the ruler as an important handmaiden to diagnosis. Finally, the **Tumorimeter** (Dermatologic Lab and Supply) provides accurate measurement of irregular lesions in square centimeters.

Mohs FE, Snow SN, Kivett WF, et al: **Anatomic rubber stamps** of the face and body to document procedures: One picture is worth a thousand words. J Dermatol Surg Oncol 1990; 16:280.

Large rubber stamps provide appropriate regional outline imprints in your chart. This allows accurate rapid documentation of the exact anatomic sites of your patient's lesions. Such records enhance your diagnostic skill in recognizing the distribution, patterning, and course of lesions.

Shelley WB: **Clinical measurement pen**. Arch Dermatol 1983; 119:364–365.

A centimeter–scored adhesive strip on your pen facilitates the measuring and recording of the size of lesions.

Tüzün Y, Yazici H: A method of measuring skin lesions. Arch Dermatol 1981; 117:192.

Mark the circumference of a lesion or skin test induration with an ordinary **ball-point pen**. Place a **piece of paper** immediately **over the marking**, thus transferring the outline. This can then be kept as a record for evaluation of any change in the lesion or skin test. It also lends itself to the precision of quantitation by planimetry.

Here's a technique for recording the dimensions of what you and your camera can't see, but what you can palpate. It also allows the patient to assist you by reproducing the outline of delayed urticarial reactions for later inspection.

Berg W, Traneroth C, Gunnarsson A, Lossing C: A method for measuring pressure sores. Lancet 1990; 335:1445–1446.

To **measure** the **volume** of a **pressure sore**, cover it with a tight, transparent, adhesive film, inserting an air vent needle at highest point. Inject an isotonic saline, measuring amount of saline to fill the cavity.

To complete the sizing of the ulcer, **trace** with pen the **circumference** on the **plastic film** before removing it.

Finally, you will see more if you **photograph** the patient and **project** the Kodachromes **on a large screen**. These magnified and fixed images, studied in the absence of the turbulence of patient distractions and visual interruptions, provide new diagnostic insights.

Katz HI, Hien NT, Prawer SE, et al: A **three-dimensional photography** system for dermatological diagnosis. J Am Acad Dermatol 1983; 8:850–856.

Stereoscopic photography permits a three-dimensional reproduction of your patient's lesions for later diagnostic review and for consultation. Stereoscopic viewing is superior to looking at the usual two-dimensional photographs.

Kopf AW, Rivers JK, Slue W, et al: Photographs are useful for detection of malignant melanomas in patients who have dysplastic nevi. J Am Acad Dermatol 1988; 19:1132–1134.

Total body photographs (numbering 24) permit clear distinction between the relatively stable **dysplastic nevus** and the progressively changing **malignant melanoma**.

Nelson GD, Krause JL (eds): **Clinical Photography** in Plastic Surgery. Edinburgh, Churchill Livingstone, 1988.

Here is a practical guide on how to record what you can't adequately describe. It describes equipment and techniques. See the Macbeth color chart to ensure correct exposure for color matching of skin tones.

SMELL

Detection of disease by smell has proven to be of limited value. The modern examining room is a well-ventilated, air-conditioned area that rapidly removes most diagnostic odors. The patient today consults the physician much earlier in the course of the disease, often before the odor has developed. In other instances the odor is masked by perfumes.

Another reason for the stunted growth of olfactory diagnosis is the physician's reluctance to really smell the patient. Some physicians are virtually anosmic, while others rapidly adapt to an odor initially ignored by them. And, indeed, in many patients the odor may be episodic and not present at the time of consultations.

It is essential to make an accurate assessment as to the presence or absence of odor. Most of the patients who consult us concerning an odor suffer from a delusion rather than a malodor.

Nonetheless, the odor of **rotten fish** is real and is diagnostic for the fish odor syndrome (**trimethylaminuria**). It is an odor that leads to an asocial life, yet may not be present unless the patient is challenged with an oral dose of 4 teaspoons of choline (obtained at health food stores). Like the majority of odors, it is generated by bacteria. In this instance, however, there is a congenital or acquired inability to degrade the malodorous gas, trimethylamine, generated by the gut bacteria and absorbed from the gut.

In contrast to this rarity is the **pungent odor** diagnostic of the unwashed, unperfumed **axilla** or **perineum**. Here the skin bacteria generate the odor (3-methyl-2-hexanoic acid) by acting upon **apocrine sweat**. In rare instances, infection within the gland itself, i.e., hidradenitis suppurativa, may be the source of the axillary or genital odor. **Malodorous feet** are diagnostic of bacterial overgrowth in the presence of hyperhidrosis. "**Bad breath**" suggests a diagnosis of gingivitis or failure to brush or floss food particles away from between the teeth. But, it also can be a sign of the presence of pus.

Foul odors can emanate from the **nose** as a result of an intranasal foreign body, from the **ear** with infection, and from the **vagina** in *Gardnerella* vaginitis with bacterial growth. Any moist, exudative, or vegetative skin lesion, as well as an ulcer, supports a heavy bacterial population with a resultant odor.

Hayden GF: **Olfactory diagnosis** in medicine. Postgrad Med 1980; 67(4):110–118.

Most physicians can recognize more than 100 aromatic substances. Approach the patient with an "open nose" and you may find 100 clues as listed herein.

SCRAPE

Let me count the ways I scrape thee. Scrape for a KOH, for staining, for culture, and scrape for the diagnostic sign of dermographism, for the Darier's sign of mastocytosis or the pseudo-Darier sign of smooth muscle growths. Scrape the blister base for the Tzanck test and swab the vagina for *Trichomonas*. Scrape for the wandering *Sarcoptes* mite and scrape under the fingernails of factitial dermatitis patients for incriminating epidermal shreds. And finally, scrape the pruritic patient for the sheer pleasure it brings him!

Any specimen obtained by your scraping can be permanently mounted by simply adding a drop of cyanoacrylate glue and a coverslip. This is great for making teaching slides.

Jacobs PH: 13 commandments for **potassium hydroxide** direct **preparations**. Cutis 1989; 44:368.

1. Clean area of contaminants such as cotton fibers, pollen, spores.
2. If dry, add drop of water to prevent scales flying into air.
3. Scrape edge of lesion.
4. Do not scrape deeply enough to produce bleeding points.
5. Scrape enough to get a large amount of scales.
6. If vesicle is present, remove roof. Place it and scrapings from its undersurface on glass slide.
7. If **tinea versicolor** is suspected, scrape scaly spots, not just edge.
8. If nail, secure material from throughout nail.
9. Scrape facial lesions, since tinea faciei can mimic many dermatoses.
10. In **black-dot ringworm** of scalp, remove broken hair with curet, needle, hemostat, or scalpel.
11. Scan slide on microscope with low power. Confirm at 450 $\times$.

12. There are only two situations demanding a potassium hydroxide prep-
    aration:
    a. When you know the patient has a fungal infection.
    b. When you know he doesn't.
13. Thou shalt not forget to culture.

Shelley WB, Wood MG: The **white spot target** for microscopic examination of **nails** for
fungi. J Am Acad Dermatol 1982; 6:92–96.

Microscopic examination of dystrophic fingernails and toenails for pathogenic
fungi can be facilitated by (1) sampling an area of whitish discoloration of
the nail plate, (2) employing a Gillette Super Blue Blade to secure a thin
slice of friable material within the white spot (this material is truly a fungal
culture), and (3) immersing the specimen in **xylene** for instant clearing and
reading. Some deep nail-plate or -bed infections require removal of the plate
and adherent bed for histologic examination with PAS staining.

We prefer xylene to KOH, since it clears more rapidly and is less damaging to the
microscope.

Shelley WB, Wood MG: New technique for instant visualization of **fungi** in **hair**. J Am
Acad Dermatol 1980; 2:69–71.

Physical fragmentation of hair by hammering the specimen placed between
metal surfaces (e.g., two halves of razor blade) allows instant visualization of
any fungi present. Xylene is used for clearing.

Monod M, Baudraz-Rosselet F, Ramelet AA, Frenk E: **Direct mycological examination**
in dermatology: A comparison of different methods. Dermatologica 1989; 179:
183–186.

Direct examination of specimens cleared with KOH (or NaOH) 10 to 30%
gently heated for 30 seconds is the most widely used method of searching
for fungi.

More sophisticated and time-consuming techniques include:

1. Conventional microscopy with staining:
   provides color contrast
   alternate stains:

   > Congo red 0.3% in sodiumlaurylsulfate 5%
   > Parker Quink blue-black and 30% KOH, equal parts
   > Chlorazol black E in DMS0 and 5% KOH, 1 to 9
   > Methylene blue 1.5% in ethanol (95%), mix with water, 1 to 9
   > Cotton blue 2% in equal parts water, phenol, lactic acid

2. Phase microscopy: provides better optical contrast
3. **Fluorescent microscopy** provides brilliant fluorescent staining of polysaccharides of hyphae, spores, and yeast. Fluorochromes used:

   > Blancophor P 0.1% in 15% KOH
   > Calcofluor White, requires two steps
   > Uvifex 2 B, requires two steps

   Must use 400 to 440 nm wavelength

Precision, sensitivity, and ease of reading are best achieved with **fluorescent staining**.
It permits even a single spore to be easily found. What is hard is finding a fluorescent
microscope.

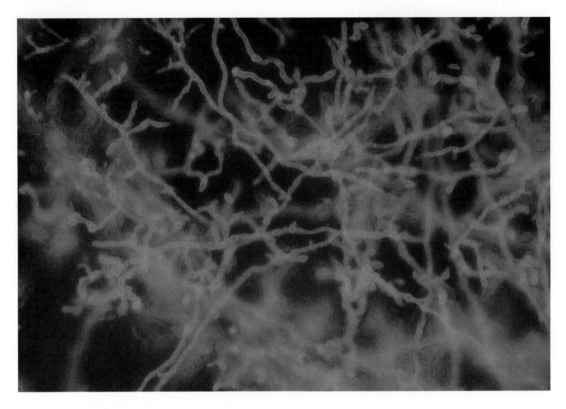

Reque PG, Lorincz AE: Supravital **microscopic fluorescent technique** for the detection of **tinea capitis**. Cutis 1988; 402:111–114.

Add a drop of buffered 0.2 mM **acridine orange** solution (pH 7.2, citrate-phosphate buffer) to skin scrapings or hair clippings on a glass slide. Apply a glass coverslip and seal the edges with melted paraffin. Examine immediately using a fluorescent microscope (436-nm excitation filter, 490-nm barrier filter) for fluorescent hyphae, spores, or conidia. Sometimes exact species may be identified from characteristic macroconidia or microconidia. *Malassezia furfur* may also be identified.

A stock solution of 2.0 mM purified acridine orange in deionized water can be kept refrigerated for many months. A working solution is prepared by adding buffered filtered saline.

Borchers SW: Moistened gauze technic to aid in the diagnosis of **tinea capitis**. J Am Acad Dermatol 1985; 13:672–673.

Tap-water moistened gauze is firmly rubbed over the affected area of scalp. Broken hairs are removed from the gauze with a 22-gauge needle and subjected to both KOH examination and culture for analysis of suspect cases of tinea capitis. This beats plucking!

Head ES, Henry JC, Macdonald EM: The cotton swab technic for the culture of dermatophyte infection: Its efficacy and merit. J Am Acad Dermatol 1984; 11:797–801.

The problem: Secure a specimen for fungal study from eyelid of an unruly child.

The available tools:

scalpel blade no. 15

microscopic slide
hairbrush
toothbrush
piece of stiff rag
agar plate contact
vinyl adhesive tape

The best tool: sterile moist cotton swab

The technique:

Rub swab vigorously over active part of lesion.
Streak swab over culture medium.

The results: Matched fungal cultures, one by swab, one by scrape, on each of 110 subjects showed no difference in culture results.

For a kinder, gentler approach, use the swab. It is patient-friendly.

Basal J: Curets for dermatophyte cultures. J Am Acad Dermatol 1985; 12:728.

Use a no. 6 curet to obtain material.

Elewski BE, Hazen PG: The superficial mycoses and the dermatophytes. J Am Acad Dermatol 1989; 21:655–673.

Detailed directions on how to culture and identify the couple of dozen pathogens out of the 100,000 species of fungi known to inhabit our world. If the patient's **hair fluoresces**, the **fungus** is an **ectothrix** growing on the outside of the hair and is one of these **four species** of *Microsporum*: *M. canis*, *M. andouinii*, *M. distortum*, or *M. ferrugineum*.

Folkers E, Vreeswijk J, Oranje AP, Duivenvoorden JN: Rapid diagnosis in **varicella** and **herpes zoster**: Re-evaluation of direct smear (Tzanck test) and electron microscopy including colloidal gold immuno-electron microscopy in comparison with virus isolation. Br J Dermatol 1989; 121:287–296.

Tzanck smear test (the Netherlands technique):

Take scrapings from the base of vesicles, pustules, or erosions, smear on glass slides, and air dry. Fix in methanol.
Stain 0.5 minute with Hemacolor.
Dip five times in methanol, three times in eosin, and three times in thiazine.
Rinse with water, air dry, and apply a permanent mounting medium and coverglass.
Examine under light microscopy. Look for characteristic herpetic–induced nuclear changes in epidermal cells (enlargement, multinucleation, crowding of nuclei with molding, margination of nuclear chromatin, ground-glass appearance, intranuclear inclusions with halo).

A positive test indicates herpetic infection but cannot distinguish between varicella-zoster and herpes simplex infection.

Pitfalls: In older pustular lesions, keratinocyte may be necrotic with loss of nuclear detail. In very early lesions, changes may not have evolved to diagnostic levels.

Immunoelectron microscopy:

Scrape vigorously with a vaccinostyle and place in a plastic sampling tube containing moistened gauze.

Freeze at $-25°C$ (normal freezer).

Homogenize with sterile sand and then centrifuge.

Adsorb virus particles (in the supernatant) on the carbon side of collodion–carbon-coated nickel grids.

Stain with gold-tagged, polyclonal antibodies against varicella-zoster virus (VZV).

Look for gold particles in the varicella-zoster viral cores and envelopes.

A positive test rules out herpes simplex virus, cytomegalovirus, and Epstein-Barr virus. An answer is obtained within hours, whereas viral culture may require several weeks.

If the test is negative for VZV, herpes simplex virus (HSV) can be identified and typed by using specified HSV monoclonal antibodies and then gold tagged rabbit–anti-mouse antibodies.

Overall results (positive tests):

Tzanck test	91%
Viral isolation	80%
Direct electron microscopy	80%
Colloidal gold immunoelectron microscopy	95%

Feldman SR, Woosley JT: Use of Sedi-Stain for the diagnosis of **elastosis perforans serpiginosa**. J Am Acad Dermatol 1989; 20:1137–1138.

A simple procedure to corroborate the clinical diagnosis of elastosis perforans serpiginosa is the microscopic examination of a **potassium hydroxide (10%)**–treated **scraping** of a representative keratotic papule. The preparation reveals matted hyphae-like fibers. These can be stained not only with the Giemsa but also by the **Sedi stain**. The latter is a simple commercial office stain (Clay Adams, Franklin Lakes, NJ) used routinely in urinalysis staining. This stain colors the extruded elastic fibers initially as blue and, in time, a persistent bright red.

Dutz W, Kohout E: Dermatologic diagnosis using the hemocytometer and the dental broach. Int J Dermatol 1982; 21:410.

Insert and rotate **dental burr** in **crusted** or **ulcerative lesion** to secure sample for stab culture, plating, or direct smear. Far better than a cotton swab. Valuable in diagnosis of leishmaniasis, leprosy, yaws, and anthrax.

Dupre A, Viraben R: Congenital smooth muscle nevus with follicular spotted appearance. J Am Acad Dermatol 1985; 13:837–838.

A 17-year-old girl had a **slightly pigmented** 10-cm **congenital plaque** on the left thigh. It contained numerous confetti-like spotted, **pigmented**, **lenticular papules** with central **follicular orifices**. Upon **rubbing**, the lesions became **transiently elevated** (pseudo-Darier's sign), giving the clue that this could be a nevus of contractile smooth muscle. Biopsy confirmed that the perifollicular papules represented smooth muscle hyperplasia.

SWAB

A swab of an open lesion, a purulent area, pharynx, or vagina, as well as other mucosal surfaces, can provide material for staining or culture of pathogenic bacteria, viruses, fungi, or protozoa.

Aly R, Maibach HI: Clinical **Skin Microbiology**: Pathogenic **Bacteria** and Pathogenic **Viruses**. Springfield, Ill., Charles C Thomas, 1978, p 133.

A "how-to" book on smearing, staining, growing, and knowing pathogens.

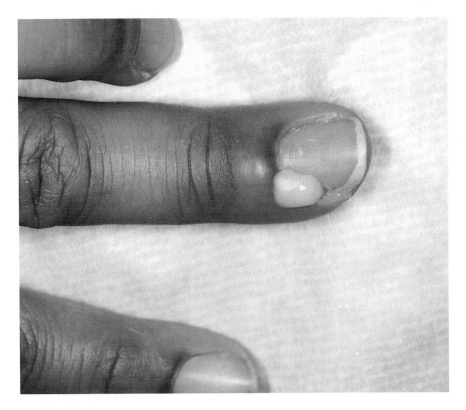

Frey D, Oldfield RJ, Bridger RC: A Colour Atlas of **Pathogenic Fungi**. London, White
Medical Publications, Ltd, 1979, p 168.

An exquisite set of portraits of "criminal" fungi seated on Petri dishes.

Versteeg J: Color Atlas of Virology. Chicago, Year Book Medical Publishers, Inc., 1985,
p 240.

To make a **virus diagnosis**:

1. Take the specimen from the right place, at the right time, and the right
   way.
2. **Secure epithelium** that has been really rubbed. The virus lives within
   the cell; **mucus and secretions are of *no* value.** (Many viruses are to be
   found only in the first few days.)
3. Transport rapidly in medium or keep at 4°C. (Many viruses die in 30
   minutes unless they are in special medium.)
4. Stool culture also may be necessary, for enteroviruses may be the cause.
5. Be patient. The report will not come for days or weeks. (The laboratory
   will inoculate the specimen in cell culture, embryonated eggs, or animals, and just as it was in the patient there is another incubation period.
   Serologic methods require 7 to 10 days for diagnostic rise in IgM.)

Krieger JN, Tam MR, Stevens CE, et al: Diagnosis of **trichomoniasis**: Comparison of
conventional wet-mount examination with cytological studies, cultures, and monoclonal antibody staining of direct specimens. JAMA 1988; 259:1223–1227.

1. Secure vaginal specimens with Ayre wooden spatula or endocervical
   specimen by rotating two cotton-tipped applicators within canal.
2. Gently agitate in saline, remove, and touch to center of slide.

3. Scan at $100\times$ and then $400\times$ for motile protozoa (trichomonads). The number of *Trichomonas vaginalis* organisms in three high-power fields is recorded for positive specimens.
4. Viewing must be done at once, since organisms lose diagnostic motility on cooling.

This **wet mount technique** was not diagnostic in 40% of 88 infected women.

A second method involves a smear of the specimen on a glass slide, immediate fixation with 95% ethyl alcohol, and staining with the **Papanicolaou stain**. Here the trichomonas organism is pale staining, pear to round, and 8 to 20μ in size. Again this technique failed to identify 44% of the infected group.

Culture on both Feinberg-Whittington medium and Diamond's TYI-S-33 allowed isolation of the trichomonas from all 88 infected women. Yet it is impractical in the clinical setting, requiring days for growth. The preferred diagnostic maneuver was **direct immunofluorescence** using monoclonal antibodies. Here the alcohol-fixed slide could be stained and read within an hour or at one's leisure during the following month if the specimen slide was kept at $-20°C$. Only 14% of the culture-proven infections were missed by this antibody stain.

STAIN

To learn the rate at which the dead stratum corneum is being shed, stain the skin with a 5% preparation of the fluorescent dye dansyl chloride in white soft paraffin. This is done by keeping the salve in place for 24 hours. The **stratum corneum turnover time** is the time required for complete extinction of the fluorescence in the skin surface. Examination with a fluorescent lamp is done daily for as long as required, in some instances for 21 days. Less sophisticated but still useful information may be obtained by using a fluorescent marker pen to stain deep into the stratum corneum and the Wood's light to observe its disappearance.

> Finlay AY, Marshall RJ, Marks R: A fluorescence photographic photometric technique to assess stratum corneum turnover rate and barrier function in vivo. Br J Dermatol 1982; 107:35–42.
>
> An objective method in which densitometric measurement of the dansyl chloride shedding is done by photography.

Likewise, staining or bleaching the hair permits estimation of the rate of growth as one measures the rate at which unstained hair appears. Again, a fluorescent dye may be applied from a **fluorescent marker pen** available in artists' supply shops.

STRIP

It is possible to strip off layers of the stratum corneum with simple Scotch tape. Better for this are the precoated adhesive microscope slides (Durotak slides, Dermatologic Lab and Supply, Council Bluffs, IA 51503). Thus, specimens can be secured, stained, and viewed for the presence of fungi, bacteria, ectoparasites, or foreign bodies, such as plant spines. We prefer the **cyanoacrylate stripping technique**. We add a small drop of Krazy Glue or analogue to a glass slide. This is pressed firmly into the skin to be stripped and kept in place for 1 minute and 10 seconds. Then, careful removal of the slide from the skin provides a dry sheet of superficial stratum corneum firmly adherent to the slide. Visualization of the undersurface, the hair follicles, and any **Demodex** present is facilitated by adding a drop of xylene and a coverslip.

Goldschmidt H, Kligman AM: Exfoliative cytology of human horny layer; methods of cell removal and microscopic techniques. Arch Dermatol 1967; 96:572–576.

An adhesive cement (3M EC791) on a glass slide, when briefly pressed on dry skin and using a rocking motion, will remove 10,000 to 100,000 cells of the stratum corneum. There is excellent orientation, unlike what is seen in a scraping.

The slides are best viewed after staining. Fixation is not required, since these corneocytes have been "fixed" in their normal process of undergoing cell death. The cells are "stain resistant," so staining times must be extended by a factor of 5 to 10. These stains are valuable: Giemsa or Gram for bacteria, PAS for fungi, Papanicolaou for nuclei, and Masson's silver for melanin.

An alternate and convenient way of securing sheets of corneocytes is the application of **double stick tape**. This can be applied to not easily accessible sites, and then applied to the slide for viewing. (Today, the Durotak Adhesive [Dermatologic Lab and Supply, Council Bluffs, IA 51503] is the most popular pressure-sensitive tape used for this purpose.)

Goldschmidt H, Thew MA: **Exfoliative cytology** of **psoriasis** and other common dermatoses: Quantitative analysis of parakeratotic horny cells in 266 patients. Arch Dermatol 1972; 106:476–483.

By means of adhesive slides, sheets of the outer corneocytes of a variety of dermatoses were removed and stained (Giemsa). Psoriasis was distinctive in showing many nucleated cells (parakeratosis) as well as many cells with residual nuclear halos only. Leukocytes were also found within the corneocytes.

Aylesworth R, Baldridge D: **Feather pillow dermatitis** caused by an unusual **mite**, *Dermatophagoides scheremetewskyi*. J Am Acad Dermatol 1985; 13:680–681.

Three weeks of tiny red, pruritic papules of the scalp and forearms in this 21-year-old man were traced to small creatures he himself trapped under clear plastic tape, while they were crawling over his skin.

Under the microscope, the creatures were identified as psoroptid mites, specifically *Dermatophagoides scheremetewskyi* Bogdanoff 1864. A thorough search of the patient's home revealed their lair to be three feather pillows. When these **pillows** were **shaken over** a piece of **dark paper**, a shower of white mites descended upon the paper.

Removal of the pillows (which were years old and had been stored in a relative's basement) produced prompt abatement of the patient's pruritus. However, it returned in full measure a few days later. Spraying the bed and apartment with Raid gave no help, but Diazinon solution (0.5%) applied to the cracks and corners plus 3% malathion to all sites of human contact resulted in the elimination of the mites and a cure.

This mite has been spotted before on feather pillows, kapok, monkey food, a bed, and a sparrow's nest, as well as on rats, mice, and bats.

Keirans JE, Litwak TR: **Pictorial key** to the adults of **hard ticks**, family Ixodidae (Ixodida; Ixodoidea), east of the Mississippi River. J Med Entomol 1989; 26:435–448.

Have the patient bring the tick or extracted biting part on adhesive tape for comparison with this pictorial guide.

Jacobs DS, Kasten BL Jr, Demott WR, Wolfson WL: Laboratory Test Handbook, 2nd ed, with key word index. Baltimore, Williams & Wilkins, 1990, pp 724–725.

To make the diagnosis of **pinworm** infestation (*Enterobius vermicularis*), make a Scotch tape stripping of perianal area several hours after retiring or early in morning before bowel movement. The clear Scotch tape is placed sticky side out over the end of a glass slide and pressed firmly against mucocutaneous surface after spreading anal folds. Pinworm eggs, female worms, or parts of them may be seen on microscopic examination.

SLICE

The **Gillette Super Blue Blade** provides full-thickness biopsies of the stratum corneum, invaluable in your search for fungi, acari, and foreign bodies. We dislike the crude designation of *shave biopsy* and refer to the procedure as **subsection**.

Shelley WB, Wood MG: The **stratum corneum biopsy** for instant visualization of **fungi**. J Am Acad Dermatol 1980; 2:56–58.

1. Carefully select a biopsy site at the very edge of the suspected tinea lesion. The edge should show fine, thin scaling and should not be erosive or covered with heavy scale or crust. Alternatively, an ideal site is one in which superficial vesiculation is evident.
2. While the skin is held taut, a horizontal specimen of the selected stratum corneum is obtained by a gentle sawing motion of half of a Gillette Super Blue Blade.
3. The stratum corneum is transferred from the blade to a glass slide and covered with a drop of **xylene** and a coverslip.
4. View under low or medial power with lowered substage condenser. Hyphae present are seen immediately because of the instant clearing effect of xylene.

Permanent mounts can be made by using cyanoacrylate (Krazy Glue) in place of xylene. The urge to build a better "fungus trap" is always present. The "blade-and-xylene" examination is fast and fun.

Martin WE, Wheeler CE Jr: Diagnosis of human **scabies** by **epidermal shave biopsy**. J Am Acad Dermatol 1979; 1:335–337.

Locate a papule, burrow, or blister that has not been excoriated. (Examine in station order: interdigital areas, wrists, elbows, anterior axillary folds, beneath breasts, pelvis, penis, scrotum, buttocks, thighs, popliteal spaces, and ankles.)

Raise a likely site between your (gloved) forefinger and thumb and "saw" the top off the lesion using a no. 15 scalpel blade held parallel to the skin. (If the patient is an infant or hyperkinetic child, try finding a "surrogate" lesion for analysis on an older family member.)

Place the specimen in immersion oil on a slide, place a coverslip, and scan under low power for scybala, eggs, and mites.

The Gillette Super Blue Blade also provides an excellent surface of cut tissue for **touch preparations** in the evaluation of tumors, inflammation, or microorganisms.

Barr RJ: **Cutaneous cytology**. J Am Acad Dermatol 1984; 10:163–180.

A superb guide on how to look at the cells that constitute the skin lesion that puzzles you. In your own office you can learn to rapidly discern certain viral, fungal, and malignant changes. It is monolayer cell "touch-and-go" pathology in contrast to full-dress biopsy pathology. Herein, you find another niche for the morphologist. With this technique he can get his "sections" without sectioning. Precise details are provided for **Papanicolaou** and polysciences multiple **stains** as well as a 1-minute **Giemsa**.

Held JL, Berkowitz RK, Grossman ME: Use of **touch preparation** for rapid diagnosis of **disseminated candidiasis**. J Am Acad Dermatol 1988; 19:1063–1066.

On the fourth day of induction chemotherapy for myelogenous **leukemia**, this 46-year-old woman developed fever and neutropenia. Intensive antibiotic therapy was followed 48 hours later by an **erythematous maculopapular eruption**, presumed to be a drug allergy to allopurinol. This was stopped, but 6 days later a new crop of erythematous papules appeared. Most of these had a central white spot.

The diagnosis was quickly obtained when a touch preparation was made from **4-mm punch biopsy**. This was done by lightly but firmly **touching the dermal surface** of the specimen **to a glass slide**. A Gram stain revealed mycelia and budding yeast forms. A diagnosis of systemic candidiasis was made and the Hickman catheter removed at once and amphotericin therapy begun. A month later the patient's candidiasis had been cured, her leukemia was in remission, and she was discharged.

Although the blood culture, urine culture, and biopsy culture each grew *Candida tropicalis*, the skin biopsy specimen, even on periodic acid–Schiff staining of step sections, failed to reveal any organisms.

Any hospitalized patient who is febrile, neutropenic, and deteriorating despite intravenous antibiotics may have systemic candidiasis. The touch preparation provides the clinician an extremely rapid means of making a provisional diagnosis of candidiasis. Either a Gram stain or KOH preparation may be used. In doing the test, one must be alert to the fact that *Pityrosporum* may be present and show up as budding yeast forms. However, distinction is made by noting that there are no hyphae or multiple budding seen with the pityrosporum organism. The touch of only the undersurface of the specimen eliminates confusion with nonpathogenic yeast or fungi on the stratum corneum.

A "touch" in time can save diagnostic time.

Sven KC, Yermakov V, Raudales O: The use of **imprint technic** for rapid diagnosis in post-mortem examinations: A diagnostically rewarding procedure. Am J Clin Pathol 1976; 65:291–300.

Press glass slide firmly on cut surface of selected tissue for a few seconds, or if non-neoplastic, smear scalpel scraping on slide. Fix at once in 95% ethyl alcohol for 10 seconds. Stain with H and E as for frozen section. Ready to read in 3 minutes.

Finally, superficial biopsies are all that is needed for certain diagnostic tests such as identification of the virus in orf.

SLIT

A slit and squeeze can express all sorts of material for diagnosis, extending through milia, microcysts, molluscum contagiosum to leprosy. It is especially useful in assessing those tiny troublesome little things (TTLT syndrome) on milady's face. Use a no. 11 scalpel tip.

Shelley WB, Burmeister V: Office diagnosis of **molluscum contagiosum** by light microscopic demonstration of **virions**. Cutis 1985; 36:465–466.

Slit open the molluscum and extract the pearly core, and squash it between two glass slides. Add a drop of Sedi-Stain (Clay Adams, Parsippany, NJ 07054) and a coverslip. Scan under "high dry" magnification for myriads of tiny dark particles that are stained molluscum virions. They may also be seen within the molluscum bodies, which are distinctive oval-shaped infected keratinocytes with flattened displaced nuclei.

If the slide is rinsed or flushed after the Sedi-Stain is applied, all of the virions and your diagnostic skill go down the drain.

Composition of Sedi-Stain:

crystal violet	0.10%
safranin 0	0.25%
ammonium oxalate	0.03%
ethyl alcohol (SD-3A)	10. 0%
water and stabilizers	89.62%

Sehgal VN, Joginder MB: **Slit-skin smear** in **leprosy**. Int J Dermatol 1990; 29:9–16.

For direct visualization and quantitation of *Mycobacterium leprae*, a variety of techniques are available.

1. Incise skin squeezed between thumb and finger. Scrape a slit 2 mm deep and 5 mm long for transfer to slide. This is the preferred method.
2. Snip a small piece of skin and crush on slide.
3. Press slide against lesions, making 10 successive smears on same area of slide.
4. Scrape nasal mucosa or smear from ulcer.
5. Blow nose content into sheet of cellophane, and smear mucus with cotton swab.

Fixation: Air dry—fix in heat for 5 minutes (40° to 50°C), or hold over flame.

Stain: Ziehl-Neelsen stain or fluorescent stain (phenol-auramine)

Read: Beaded red rods lying singly or in clumps against a blue background

Negative smears do not preclude leprosy.

SOAK

Soaking the skin in tap water will often reveal the presence of a hidden wart. And soaking the skin in 5% acetic acid (vinegar) solution brings genital warts into full display. Soaking the hands provides information on the autonomic function. Finally, soaking off crusts and debris may reveal the presence of an unsuspected ulcer.

Rosenberg SK, Greenberg MD, Reid R: Sexually transmitted papillomaviral infection in men. Obstet Gynecol Clin North Am 1987; 14:495–512.

Soak the genital area for 5 minutes with **vinegar-saturated gauze**.

Inspect under 10 to 16× magnification for areas of acetowhitening.

The white points are warts and if not detected prior to soaking are considered subclinical.

Of 199 male partners of women with proven warts, 99 had warts evident on direct visualization, but 47 more had **subclinical warts** perceived only after the vinegar soak. It is noteworthy that many of the 99 were completely unaware of any lesions.

Biopsy specimens of 20 subclinical lesions (5 penile and 15 scrotal) were sent for Southern blot hybridization with probes for human papillomaviral types 6, 11, 16, 78, and 31. Eight of the samples showed HPV DNA. The others did not.

Rapaport M: **Vinegar elucidation** of **warts**. J Am Acad Dermatol 1990; 22:147.

Milia, furrows, and small cysts also show focal whitening upon application of vinegar, pointing up the need for clinical experience in using the vinegar test for subclinical warts.

Elliott RB: **Wrinkling** of the skin in **cystic fibrosis**. Lancet 1974; 2:108.

The skin of children with cystic fibrosis wrinkles within a couple of minutes upon **immersion in tap water**. This wrinkling occurs far more rapidly than in normal children and a "3-minute bowl of water" test might be a cheap diagnostic screening test.

Braham J, Sadeh M, Sarova-Pinhos I: **Skin wrinkling** on **immersion of hand**. A test of sympathetic function. Arch Neurol 1979; 36:113–114.

The wrinkling of the skin experienced on immersion of the hands in warm water depends on an **intact sympathetic pathway**. No wrinkling was observed in 12 patients 2 days after a sympathectomy, and 2 patients with unilateral sympathetic paralysis associated with Horner's syndrome showed no palmar wrinkling on the affected side.

Soaking the hand is thus a convenient, reliable bedside test for assessing the integrity of the sympathetic nerve supply to the hand.

SAMPLE

Take a sample. Take a **biopsy**.

When you are puzzled, this is the single most important thing you can do. But remember, the pathologist does best with something distinctive. Look for something distinctive for biopsy. We spend more time picking a site for biopsy than we do in doing the biopsy. Remember also, if the skin change is not homogeneous, the larger excisional biopsy wins. It provides more information, fewer negative reports. Avoid the trephine and subsection biopsy in these instances.

A superficial biopsy may miss the deeper plasma cell infiltrate of syphilis, the malignant cells of melanoma, or underlying panniculitis. Eosinophilic fasciitis as well as necrotizing fasciitis can be missed even with a full-thickness skin biopsy. Again, only with **deep biopsy** will you identify the insidious calcifying aponeurotic fibroma. Go for the gold. Go deep.

Avoid unnecessary trauma to the skin specimen you are taking. Use sharp disposable trephines. Do not use hemostats or stretch the skin by pulling it out. Cut cleanly. Fix at once, since autolysis begins when you cut the blood supply. Tightly close the specimen bottle to prevent leakage. If specimen is to be mailed, ensure against freezing by proper packaging.

Let the pathologist know the history, how the lesions looked, and what other skin changes were present, and label the site precisely. Act as if he were at your side. He needs to integrate your gross pathologic view with his microscopic pathologic findings. Help him and he will help you.

Ask for a **special stain** when you are looking for something special, like mucin, amyloid, or spirochetes. **Immunofluorescence** studies help in diagnosing dermatitis herpetiformis and lupus states. **Monoclonal antibody stains** come to the forefront in identifying cellular infiltrates and immunocompetence. They also allow precision in identifying the forms of epidermolysis bullosa.

In a widespread heterogeneous eruption, multiple biopsies are better than multiple consultations.

No superficial biopsies on melanoma suspects.

Remember all biopsies leave scars. If you can, pick an inconspicuous site.

> Robinson JK: Fundamentals of **Skin Biopsy**. Chicago, Year Book Medical Publishers, Inc., 1986, 124 pp.
>
> Here are the details on how, why, when, and where to take a proper biopsy.

> Telfer NR, Dalziel KL, Colver GB, Dawber RPR: **Nail biopsy**: Indications, techniques, results. Br J Dermatol 1989; 121 (suppl 34):65.
>
> For evaluation of nail dystrophies
>
> > A narrow (<3 mm) longitudinal biopsy extending from the distal inter-phalangeal joint to fingertip and dissected off underlying bone
> > Sample from lateral aspect to facilitate suturing.
> > Carefully realign lunula.
> > Stain with PAS as well as H & E.
>
> For evaluation of discrete lesions
>
> > Use trephine through nail plate or nail bed alone after removal of plate.
> > Reflect proximal nail fold before biopsy of nail matrix, or pterygium may result.
> > No suture is needed if 3-mm specimen taken.
> > Pigmented lesion biopsies must include matrix, since melanocytes are found only in this site.
>
> Anticipated diagnoses: lichen planus, nevus, glomus tumor, lymphoma, squamous cell carcinoma, and malignant melanoma
>
> Contraindication to nail biopsy: diabetes, peripheral vascular disease, immunocompromised patient

> Logan ME, Zaim MT: **Histologic stains** in dermatopathology. J Am Acad Dermatol 1990; 22:820–830.
>
> Your pathologist can do more than stain with hematoxylin for DNA and with eosin for the cytoplasm and connective tissue. He can stain for:
>
> collagen
> > van Gieson's stain
> > Masson trichrome
>
> elastin (not stained by H & E)
> > acid orcein
> > Verhoeff
> > Gomori aldehyde fuchsin
>
> reticulum (type III collagen)
> > Gomori silver nitrate
>
> carbohydrate
> > alcian blue
> > colloidal iron
> > toluidine blue
> > periodic acid–Schiff (PAS)

When you want him to look for something special, ask for something special in the way of stains.

protein (amyloid)
   Congo red
   crystal violet
   thioflavine T
lipid
   Sudan black B
   oil red O
melanin and mineral
   Fontana-Masson (for melanin)
   dopa reaction (for tyrosinase)
   Perls' Prussian blue (for iron)
   Von Kossa (for calcium)
   alizarin red S (for calcium)
mast cells
   Giemsa
   Leder reaction
microorganisms
   Gram (acetone decolonizes permeable walled bacteria, viz. gram-negative)
   Ziehl-Neelsen (mycobacteria)
   Fite (lepra bacillus)
   Warthin-Starry (spirochetes, Donovan bodies, cat scratch bacteria)
   Gomori's methenamine (fungi)
   silver nitrate

On occasion, you will need **transmission electron microscopy**, and for **detection of metallic elements** the **scanning electron x-ray probe techniques** are invaluable.

Newton GA, Sanchez RL, Swedo J, Smith EB: Lafora's disease: The role of skin biopsy. Arch Dermatol 1987; 123:1667–1669.

There are a number of **invisible dermatoses** not evident to the physician or patient, but readily seen by the pathologist. A biopsy of seemingly normal skin may quickly reveal abnormal **metabolic deposits** similar to those in muscle, brain, and liver.

A 16-year-old girl had attacks of generalized convulsions for 8 months, along with progressive incoordination and weakness and deterioration of her school performance. Extensive hospital studies were normal, but the onset of myoclonic seizures at this age suggested **Lafora's disease**, a progressive neurometabolic disorder transmitted by autosomal recessive inheritance. Skin biopsy confirmed the diagnosis, showing characteristic PAS-positive inclusions in eccrine sweat duct cells. These Lafora bodies can also be seen in apocrine glands and cutaneous nerves and are demonstrable in PAS-stained frozen sections (for rapid diagnosis).

Other invisible dermatoses with **pathognomonic inclusion bodies** include: lipofuscinoses, neuronal ceroid; glycogenosis II (Pompe's disease); leukodystrophies.

Jaworsky C, Murphy GF: **Special techniques** in dermatology. Arch Dermatol 1989; 125:963–974.

Although the hematoxylin-eosin–stained section is the mainstay of dermatopathology, look at the specialized approaches your **pathologist** can use to help you.

Morphologic analytic techniques

1. 1-µm section analysis
2. Transmission electron microscopy
3. x-Ray probe microanalysis at an ultrastructural level
4. Digital image analysis for quantification

Functional analytic techniques

1. Immunofluorescence, direct biopsy; indirect serum
2. Immunohistochemical markers for nuclear, cytoplasmic, and surface
3. Molecular biologic techniques; DNA hybridization; restriction enzyme analysis; karyotyping

And soon we will have the fabulous **polymerase chain reaction** (PCR) for detecting the invisible traces of the pathogen's DNA.

Wang N, Minassian H: The formaldehyde-fixed and paraffin embedded tissues for diagnostic transmission **electron microscopy**: A retrospective and prospective study. Human Pathol 1987; 18:715–727.

That fine structure can be studied retrospectively for infective agents, foreign particles, or organelles associated with neoplasms is demonstrated.

Bergfeld WF, McMahon JT: Identification of foreign metallic substances inducing hyperpigmentation of skin: Light microscopy, electron microscopy, and x-ray energy spectroscopic examination. Adv Dermatol 1987; 2:171–183.

x-Ray energy spectroscopy examination allows specific identification of silver, gold, and mercury, as well as other foreign metals in biopsy specimens of skin.

Sipe JC, O'Brien JS: Ultrastructure of skin biopsy specimens in lysosomal storage diseases: Common sources of error in diagnosis. Clin Genet 1979; 15:118–125.

There are 35 known **lysosomal storage diseases**, evidence of which can be obtained in many instances by a skin biopsy, thus obviating need for biopsy of the brain or viscera. When possible, specific enzyme assays should also be performed prior to making a final diagnosis.

Avoid these pitfalls:

1. **Biopsy technique**
   Do not clamp, squeeze, mince, compress, or use a hemostat on the tissue. A punch biopsy is adequate.
   Lift the specimen out by piercing it with the 26-gauge needle on the syringe used to administer the local anesthetic.
   Do not delay for a second getting the specimen into fixative.

2. **Fixation**—processing problems
   Avoid a large specimen and thus inadequate penetration of the fixative.
   Preferred fixative: chilled 5% glutaraldehyde–4% paraformaldehyde in 0.2 M sodium cacodylate buffer, pH 7.2, for 4 to 6 hours.
   Avoid errors in dehydration.
   Avoid inadequate embedding.

3. Interpretative errors
   Be aware of normal structures:
      Osmium tetroxide–reactive lipid structures that look like membranous "myelin figures"
      Mast cell inclusions that are laminated and resemble the fingerprint or curvilinear bodies of Batten's disease
      Melanosomes within melanocytes, simulating glycogen storage disease

        Unmyelinated axons, synaptic terminals, and Schwann cell processes that may contain dense core vesicles suggesting C-type viral particles or cytoplasmic inclusions

        Endothelial cells with pinocytotic vesicles resembling lysosomes

        Leukocytes with organelles resembling the inclusions of neuronal ceroid-lipofuscinoses

        Myoepithelial cells of eccrine glands with pinocytotic vesicles resembling lysosomes

        Sebaceous glands with large cytoplasmic lipid droplets resembling lysosomes

        Fibroblasts with assorted vacuoles and vesicles

        Epidermal keratinizing cells with multivesicular bodies

4. Do not use cultured fibroblasts for electron microscopic identification of lysosomal storage material. Interpretation is difficult and unreliable.

Fleming KA, Venning V, Evans M: **DNA typing** of **genital warts** and diagnosis of **sexual abuse** of children. Lancet 1987; 2:454.

DNA typing of the anal warts in this 5-year-old boy proved identical to that of warts on his right hand, thus eliminating genital warts as evidence of child abuse.

Gedde-Dahl T Jr, Wuepper KJ (eds): Prenatal diagnosis of heritable skin diseases. Curr Probl Dermatol 1987; 16:1–216.

An overview of the subject as of 1985:

Newer advances in biopsy possibilities include DNA typing of warts to identify the precancerous forms as well as the source of transmission in possible cases of child abuse. Another area of diagnostic help is the prenatal diagnosis of heritable skin disease. It is now possible at certain centers to make a prenatal diagnosis of the various types of:

    epidermolysis bullosa
    ichthyosis
    oculocutaneous albinism
    hypohidrotic ectodermal dysplasia
    xeroderma pigmentosum
    Cockayne's syndrome
    Bloom's syndrome
    Menkes' syndrome
    dyskeratosis congenita
    sickle cell anemia
    hemophilia
    neurofibromatosis
    cystic fibrosis
    alpha-antitrypsin deficiency

The advances are so rapid as to necessitate continuing consultation with one of the thousand genetic counselors now serving the United States.

SKIN TEST

The classic skin test is the epicutaneous **patch test** in which potential sensitizers are placed in occlusive contact with the patient's skin for 48 or more hours. In case contact photosensitivity is suspected, the patch test sites are then irradiated with ultraviolet light (UVA) and read again in another 48 hours. Equally important is phototesting of the skin for intrinsic photosensitivity states. Here, hot quartz mercury vapor lamps, fluorescent tubes, or the high-intensity metal halide lamp (330 to 460 nm) is used to determine the degree of sensitivity (minimal erythema dose) or to replicate the disease (e.g., solar urticaria, persistent light reaction).

Intradermal tests are used, but less often. These include the **scratch** and **prick tests** so popular with allergists. Intradermal injections of progesterone, estrone, acetylcholine, mecholyl, and norepinephrine are also used in assessing selected autoimmune states. Likewise the **tuberculin test**, lepromin test, and Kveim test, as well as trichophyton, *Candida*, streptokinase/streptodornase, and histoplasmin tests are done. Innumerable mold and bacterial antigens are also available. Even a saline skin test serves as a diagnostic test for Behçet's disease.

Fransway AF: Epicutaneous patch testing: Current trends and controversial topics. Mayo Clinic Proc 1989; 64:415–423.

Details on exactly what to do, what to test, and how to read.

Reasons for false-positive readings:
use of irritant substance
pressure and edging irritation
tests done on irritable skin
mistaking pustular and urticarial reactions for positive test

Reasons for false-negative readings:
too low a concentration or inappropriate vehicle
too brief a contact (patch fell off)
failure to reproduce original conditions, such as sweating, sunlight exposure
failure to read later at 72 to 96 hours
failure to do photopatch test
concurrent steroid or ultraviolet light therapy

Adverse reactions:
induction of sensitization
flare of primary dermatitis
persistent positive test
induction of Koebner response
hyperpigmentation or hypopigmentation
infection, necrosis, scarring
anaphylaxis

de Groot AC: **Patch Testing**: Test Concentrations and Vehicles for **2800 Allergens**. New York, Elsevier, 1986, 295 pp.

An all-inclusive vade mecum for assessing contact sensitivity to that unusual compound.

Harber LC, Bickers DR: Photosensitivity Diseases: Principles of Diagnosis and Treatment, 2nd ed. Philadelphia, B.C. Decker, Inc., 1989, pp 395–405.

Phototesting

Light source:

Appropriate fluorescent tubes or hot quartz mercury vapor lamp. Must provide wavelength (action spectrum) responsible for photodermatosis. This is usually UVA, except for **persistent light reactor**, which **requires UVB**.

Westinghouse FS fluorescent **sunlamp** emits continuous spectrum between 275 and 380 nm with a peak at 315.

Black light tubes provide UVA range (320 to 400 nm).

Hot quartz lamps provide discontinuous spectrum of both UVA and UVB.

Metal halide lamps provide UVA and visible light (330 to 460 nm). Technique: stepwise irradiation dosage.

Purpose:

Determine **minimal erythema dose** and replicate photodermatosis in test area.

Photopatch testing

Light source:

Bank of black light (UVA lamps) fluorescent tubes or hot quartz mercury lamp with **window glass** interposed to **remove UVB**.

Technique:

Duplicate contact allergen patches applied under occlusive cover.
Remove one set at 48 hours and read.
Irradiate these sites **with half** the **minimal erythema dose** (or 1 to 5 J/cm^2).
Cover area again.
Remove covers of both sets at 96 hours, read and compare.
Photopatch test is positive if irradiated site is positive and nonirradiated site is negative.

Hazards

Same as standard patch tests
False-positives and false-negatives reflect inappropriate amount or type of irradiation.

Dahl MV: Clinical Immunodermatology, 2nd ed. Chicago, Year Book Medical Publishers, Inc., 1988, p 114.

Intradermal skin test panel for T-cell defect in immunity:

Tuberculin, 0.1 ml 5 IU. If negative, repeat with 250 TU.
Candidin, 0.1 ml 1:100 (Hollister Stier) (for infants 1:10)
Trichophytin, 0.1 ml 1:100 (Hollister Stier) (for infants 1:10)
Tetanus toxoid 0.1 ml 1:100

Failure to respond to all four of these suggests a lack of normal immune competence.

Gilhar A, Winterstein G, Turani H, et al: Skin hyperactivity response (pathergy) in **Behçet's disease**. J Am Acad Dermatol 1989; 21:547–552.

One tenth of 1 ml of sterile **saline solution** was injected **intradermally** in the forearm of 11 patients with Behçet's disease. The next day 10 showed a diagnostically significant pustule in the center of an erythematous zone at the injection site.

A saline injection thus provides a simple test for the skin hyperreactivity (pathergy) so characteristic of Behçet's disease.

Extracutaneous skin testing can be done by **oral or parenteral challenges** with suspected **drugs** and **foods**. The hazard here is much greater, and usually the cautious clinician awaits inadvertent exposures to accomplish such "testing." This is especially true in all instances of bullous drug eruptions. However, the ready availability of steroid therapy makes oral challenges with minute doses more feasible and plausible, especially in the case of drugs essential to the patient's well-being.

And don't forget simple skin **testing for sensation** with needle and cotton wisp. To miss a diagnosis of leprosy for want of a demonstration of anesthesia is deplorable. And check sensitivity to **heat** and **cold**. Lastly, test for **capillary fragility**.

> Jacobs DS, Kasten BL Jr, DeMott WR, Wolfson WL: Laboratory Test Handbook, 2nd ed, with key word index. Baltimore, Williams & Wilkins, 1990, pp 377–378.

Test for **capillary fragility** with negative-pressure suction cup or Rumpel-Leede tourniquet test. A **suction cup** is applied to skin for 1 minute. Least negative pressure required to produce petechiae is measure of capillary resistance. Alternatively, **blood pressure cuff** is applied at pressure halfway between diastolic and systolic for 5 minutes. Number of **petechiae** indicates capillary resistance. The test may be positive immediately before or after menstruation.

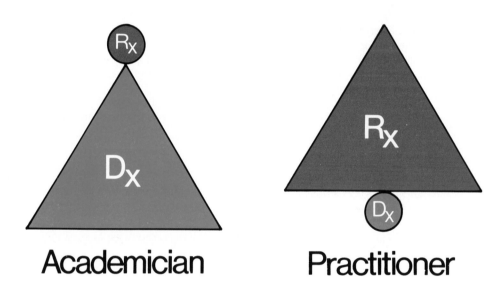

STUDY HAIR

The patient with a hair problem wants you to do more than stand there and look. And there is lots to do.

> Caserio RJ: Diagnostic techniques for hair disorders. Part III: Clinical hair manipulations and clinical findings. Cutis 1987; 40:442–448.

Hair pluck

Do not shampoo for week before to accurately assess telogen phase.
Clamp 50 to 60 hairs immediately adjacent to scalp with rubber-tipped hemostat and forcibly extract.
Cut hairs at upper side of hemostat.
Place hair bulb ends on double-sided tape or between slides.
Count number of anagen hairs and number of telogen hairs.
Normal: 85% anagen, 15% telogen.
Diagnostic
    Telogen effluvium: more than 20% telogen
    Trichotillomania: no telogen hairs present

Hair pull

Grasp cluster of hairs between left thumb and ring fingers.

Using index and third finger, hold hairs taut for separation and count of 60 hairs.

Grasp these hairs at scalp between right thumb and index finger, and exert sliding traction.

If more than four hairs come out, it favors diagnosis of telogen effluvium, alopecia areata, or hereditary thinning.

Hair counts

Patient **collects all hairs** on pillow, in sink, comb, brush, and shoulders, as well as in shampoo (nylon net over drain).

Place hairs in plastic bag, label the day and the shampoo used, then count at leisure.

Do this for 14 consecutive days.

Bring bags to office for physician to check bulb type, shaft abnormalities, and morphology of distal tip.

Normal loss: 50 to 100 hairs a day and 200 to 250 hairs on days of shampoo. If shampoo is done daily, normal loss is 100 hairs a day.

Part width

Make coronal parts with patient's comb.

Compare width with that in occipital area.

Widened parts speak to significant hair loss.

Hair growth window

Shave 2- by 2-cm area of scalp.

Cover with Op-site or Duoderm for 7 days.

Physician removes dressing and measures hair length.

Normal: Hair should be 2.5 mm long.

Useful in patients who claim hair has stopped growing.

Hair feathering

Grasp distal 2 to 3 cm end of hairs.

Give brisk pull.

Appearance of **short broken hairs** is indicative of **hair shaft defect**.

Viewing hair

Direct look for short (4- to 10-mm), darkly pigmented hair frayed at distal tip with narrowed nonpigmented stalk

When plucked, entire exclamation-point hair visible, wherein telogen bulb is dot of exclamation point

Diagnostic for **alopecia areata**

Contrast

Part hair.

Place index card with white or black felt contrast surface.

Short miniature hairs can be readily seen.
Good for evaluating hair growth stimulants.

Scalp biopsy

Avoid cosmetic areas as well as skin over temporal and occipital arteries.
Clip hair in 1-cm square area.
Inject lidocaine (1% with epinephrine, 1.5 ml) intradermally.
Aspirate before and during to avoid intravascular injection.
Wait 20 minutes for vasoconstrictor effect.
Paper-tape-down uncut hairs in vicinity.
Obtain full-thickness **6-mm punch** specimen.
Angle punch parallel to hair shaft emergence angle.
Close with 4-0 proline suture.
Halve specimen for routine and immunofluorescence studies.

Shelley WB: Hair examination using **double stick tape**. J Am Acad Dermatol 1983;
8:430–431.

Mounting hairs on glass slides to which double-stick transparent tape has
been previously applied permits swift systematic examination of the immobilized hair shaft. In addition to study of cuticular structure, the hairs can
be observed for changes in diameter associated with disease, malnutrition,
and cytotoxic agents.

Entire hairs can be permanently stored in this manner by simply adding a
large coverslip. (An alternative is the use of Durotak slides, Dermatologic
Lab & Supply, Council Bluffs, IA 51503.) These ready-to-use precoated
slides have peel-off paper backing over the pressure-sensitive adhesive.

Baden HP, Kubilus J, Baden L: A **stain** for plucked **anagen hairs**. J Am Acad Dermatol
1979; 1:121–122.

The internal root sheath of plucked anagen hairs stains a distinctive red when
immersed in a drop of DACA (1% dimethylamino-cinnamaldehyde in 0.5 N
HCl). The color results from a reaction with the citrulline in the sheath. By
contrast, the hair bulb of plucked **club hairs** stains only a faint orange.

Culbertson JC, Breslau NA, Moore MK, Engel E: **Sex chromatin determination** from
hair. JAMA 1969; 207:560–561.

Pluck terminal hair. **Stain** with freshly filtered **aceto-orcein** (30 sec, 65°C).
Slice off bulb, and slide root sheath off. Compress sheath under coverslip to
get monolayer of cells. Look for solid dark chromatin body in nuclei (oil
immersion 1250×) (65% of hair sheath cells will show sex chromatin body
in women, but only 2% in males).

STUDY SEBACEOUS GLAND

The easiest way to assess sebum secretion is to place a glass slide on the skin, remove
it, and observe the amount of visible oil. Equally direct is the application of cigarette
paper to the skin. The oil absorbed becomes apparent as spots on the paper. Gravimetric methods are possible, but difficult because of the small quantities involved.
Other methods involve an absorbent tape and instrumentation.

Nordstrum KM, Schmus HG, McGinley KJ, Leyden JJ: **Measurement** of **sebum output**
using a lipid absorbent tape. J Invest Dermatol 1986; 87:260–263.

Cleanse skin

Apply Seb-U-Tape (CuDerm Corp., Dallas, Texas) (microporous polymeric film with adhesive backing).

Leave in place 1 hour.

Number and size of black spots reflect sebum secretion.

Can record photographically and also quantitate by image analysis.

Saint Léger D, Berrebi C, Duboi C, Agache P: The lipometre: An easy tool for rapid quantitation of skin surface lipids (SSL) in man. Arch Dermatol Res 1979; 265:79–89.

The **lipometre** is an electronic device based on principle that ground glass becomes translucent once coated with lipids. Using a sapphire plate placed against the skin for 15 seconds, it gives a direct reading of the collected lipid as $\mu g/cm^2$.

STUDY SWEAT GLAND

The diagnosis of **anhidrosis**, whether generalized, localized, random, or "areata," is difficult in the temperate climates. Its significance extends from classifying ectodermal defects to assessing autonomic denervation due to surgery or disease, such as the neuropathy of diabetes mellitus. To make the diagnosis calls for stimulating the gland and visualizing sweat. The usual stimulant is heat or exercise. In the office this is difficult. So often the diagnosis is missed unless the patient is carefully queried. In children with **ectodermal defects** a bout of fever may lead to all sorts of studies for infectious disease when the true cause is anhidrotic heat intolerance.

A simple stimulus is the **intradermal** injection of 0.05 ml of 1% **acetylcholine** or **pilocarpine**. Visualization is aided by prior painting of the skin with **iodine** solution (3% iodine in ethanol) followed by application of **starch or paper** held in contact momentarily. The purple dots indicate sweating, which carries the iodine into the starch, producing the color change.

The use of iodinated starch as described below is a superior method, since skin is not stained.

For **quantitation of sweating**, tared weighings of Webril gauze pads kept in place for 30 minutes provide a gravimetric method. Also available is an instrument (Evaporimeter, Servo Med, Inc., 78 Lee St., Warrenton, VA 22186) that provides a digital readout of water evaporation from the skin. Its dual probe allows simultaneous recording of control areas.

The diagnosis of **cystic fibrosis** is facilitated by sweat analysis for an increase in electrolytes and osmolality, reflecting a diminished sweat gland function.

Sato KT, Richardson A, Timm DE, Sato K: One-step **iodine starch method** for direct visualization of **sweating**. Am J Med Sci 1988; 295:528–531.

Add 1 gm of iodine crystals to 500 gm of soluble starch (S-516, Fisher Scientific).

Allow to stand for few days at room temperature (starch becomes light yellow brown).

Store in tightly capped bottle (stable for years).

Spray iodinated starch on area to be studied.

Sweat droplets are visualized as discrete, dark-purple dots.

Wipe powder away and repeat for consecutive readings.

Juhlin L, Shelley WB: **A stain** for **sweat pores**. Nature 1967; 213:408.

Apply a 5% solution of *o*-**phthalaldehyde** in xylene to skin. Within 3 minutes each sweat gland orifice is stained black, permitting counts. The stain remains for about a week and does not wash off, but can be removed by Scotch tape stripping.

Berg D, Weingold DH, Abson KG, Olsen EA: **Sweating** in **ectodermal dysplasia syndromes**: A review. Arch Dermatol 1990; 126:1075–1079.

Here you will find a superb review of all the **tests of sweating** with full literature citations. Accurate evaluation of sweating permits not only effective diagnosis and classification of ectodermal dysplasia syndromes, but also aids in genetic counseling by potential detection of carrier states.

Ryder REJ, Marshall R, Johnson K, et al: **Acetylcholine sweatspot test** for autonomic denervation. Lancet 1988; 1:1303–1305.

Inject 0.1 ml of 1% acetylcholine intradermally. Coat skin with 2% iodine in absolute alcohol. Apply thin layer of starch in arachis oil (100 gm/100 ml). Absence of dark spots occurs in **diabetic neuropathy**. Optimal time for photography is 6 minutes.

Hatzis J, Varelzidis A, Tosca A: Sweat gland function in **dermatophytosis**. Arch Dermatol Res 1982; 273:1–7.

Fungal infection is among the many scaling eruptions in which **sweat excretion** is **reduced** because of poral blockage.

Carter EP, Barrett AD, Heeley AF, Kuzemko JA: Improved **sweat test method** for the diagnosis of **cystic fibrosis**. Arch Dis Child 1984; 59:919–922.

Sweat osmolality was increased in 39 patients with cystic fibrosis: 220 to 416 mmol/kg compared to 62 to 196 mmol/kg in 34 controls.

Sweat sodium concentrations were elevated in these cystic fibrosis patients: 60 to 150 mmol/liter compared to 9 to 72 mmol/liter in the controls.

These parameters are most easily measured using the Macroduct unit for sweat inducer (**pilocarpine iontophoresis**) and a Macroduct sweat collector. Analysis can be done using a vapor pressure osmometer, a sweat conductivity analyzer (Sweat-Chek), or a sodium or chloride microanalyzer (Wescor Inc, 459 South Main Street, Logan, Utah 84321).

STUDY VESSELS

In no area is there a wider range of instruments for visualization and measurement than in the cutaneous vasculature. You can study it from the simple direct view of nail fold capillaries to the sophisticated photo plethysmography.

Ryan TJ: Dermal vasculature. *In* Skerrow D and Skerrow CJ (eds): Methods in Skin Research. New York, John Wiley & Sons, 1985, pp 527–558.

To see **blood vessel patterning**, press on skin with blunt probe or curet ring. This disperses the veil of tissue fluid that partially obscures the upper dermal blood vessels.

Ryan TJ: **Measurement of blood flow** and other properties of the vessels of the skin.

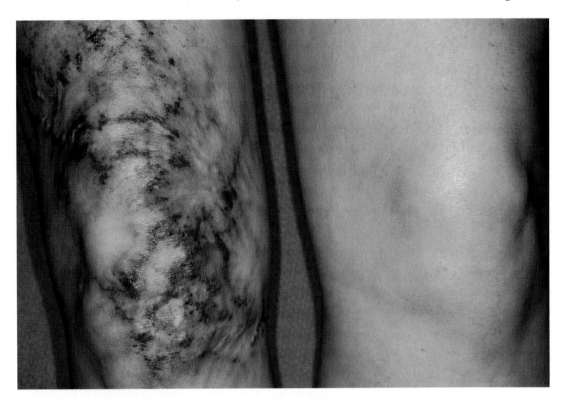

In Jarrett A (ed): The Physiology and Pathophysiology of the Skin. New York, Academic Press, 1973, vol 2, pp 653–679.

Assess circulation time:

Subpapillary plexus filling time: Pressure on the surface of the skin causes pallor and empties subpapillary venous plexus. Sudden release is followed by filling of the plexus and a normal return of color in 1 to 2 seconds.

Elevation of limb well above heart level results in blanching. Upon dropping the limb to well below heart level, the vessels in the skin fill and the skin appears flushed within 10 to 15 seconds.

Occlude circulation by inflation of **sphygmomanometer cuff** for 5 to 15 minutes. On release, skin flushes within 5 seconds, and this fades after 15 seconds.

Prick histamine 1:1000 into skin. Wheal develops within 3 minutes, whereas wheal will not develop on ischemic skin or may take over 5 minutes to develop.

Ryan TJ: Cutaneous circulation. *In* Goldsmith LA (ed): Biochemistry and Physiology of the Skin. New York, Oxford University Press, 1983, pp 817–877.

A **light stroke to the skin** in some disorders results in development of whiteness some 10 to 15 seconds later. Such **white dermographism** may be due to a release of local vasoconstrictor agents in the upper dermis, or a response of contractile elements in the capillary pericytes following stretch, or swelling of endothelial cells, thereby obstructing inflow. It is typically seen in **atopic eczema**.

Fronek A: Noninvasive diagnostics in **vascular disease**. New York, McGraw-Hill Book Co., 1989, 608 pp.

A classic on how to assess every aspect of your patient's vascular status. Especially valuable is the section on **testing** in **Raynaud's disease**.

Young AE: Investigation of **vascular malformations**. *In* Mulliken JB, Young AE (eds): Vascular Birthmarks: Hemangiomas and Malformations. Philadelphia, W. B. Saunders Company, 1988, pp 128–140.

Do nothing when there are no clinical indications for interventional treatment, because even a single blood test can be a frightening experience for a child.

The following studies are valuable to assess the need for treatment:

1. Clinical assessment: The **Nicoladoni-Branham test**.

    Occlude arterial inflow by pneumatic cuff while measuring pulse rate for a full minute before and after inflation.

    If rate fall is in excess of 10/minute, the test is positive and indicates a large **arteriovenous fistula** in the limb.

2. **Plethysmography**

    Quantify blood flow in limb by strain gauge, impedance, gravimetric or water bath displacement methods. This detects increased blood flow through fistulas.

    Measure pulse volume. It will be higher above and below an arteriovenous fistula.

    Cannulate leg vein, connect to transducer, and measure **venous pressure** to see if sufficiently high to indicate vein atresia or obstruction that is surgically amenable.

    Immerse lower leg in water bath while patient exercises by knee bends. Normally, foot volume drops. Repeat exercise after applying tourniquet below knee to prevent reflux of blood down **superficial veins**. If deep veins are inadequate there will be low expelled volume. Second, if there is reflux in **deep veins**, there will be rapid refilling.

3. **Doppler assessments**

    Detect **velocity** and **direction of flow** using pencil-sized ultrasound transducers operating at 5 to 10 MHz.

4. Radiographic assessments

    Arteriography will demonstrate early venous filling and arterial enlargement, both hallmarks of arteriovenous fistulas.

    Isotopes can locate sites of **thrombosis**. Also, after injection of labeled macroaggregated albumin particles larger than 10 μ into the artery, the amount measured in the lung indicates the amount that bypassed the capillaries and went through an arteriovenous fistula.

    The location of **bleeding** from **gastrointestinal vascular anomalies**, if suspected in the presence of anemia, can be located by **scintigraphy** (^{99m}Tc sulfur colloid).

    Radioactive colloidal compounds injected intradermally permit assessment of function of the **lymphatics**—distinguishing **lymphedema** from venous edema.

5. **Thermography**

    Of limited value, but impressive elevations of temperature in areas over **arteriovenous fistulas**. Use thermoprobe, thermocamera (infrared-sensitive film) or heat-sensitive plastic sheets (liquid crystals).

6. Blood-gas analysis

    Not helpful, since raised PO_2 in femoral vein may be result of varicose veins as well as fistulas.

7. Biopsy

Only if worried about possible presence of sarcoma or angiokeratomas.

8. Coagulation studies

Platelet count is **down** or a consumptive coagulopathy is seen in venous abnormalities. Fibrinogen is taken up in abnormal vessels and when patient is in a hemorrhagic state. Look for increased prothrombin and partial thromboplastin times.

The advantage of referring to the very model of a modern vascular laboratory is evident.

Ryan TJ, Cherry GW: The assessment of **vascular abnormalities** of the **leg**. Recent Adv Dermatol 1986; 7:87–101.

The leg is poorly supplied with microvessels and hence is especially dependent on an adequate venous and arterial blood supply.

If the patient is **over 40 years** of age, a lifetime of the erect or feet-down posture produces **venous disease** with ulceration. If the patient is **over 70**, begin to look for **arterial disease** and its **ulcers**.

With *venous ulcers*, always look for contributory factors or diabetes mellitus, cellulitis, trauma, infection, rheumatoid arthritis, or immune complex disease.

Arterial ulcers, i.e., **ischemic** ulcers, are small and shallow. Usually they are seen over the metatarsal heads on the lateral and medial sides of the feet. Aiding in the diagnosis is the **loss of hairs** from the **dorsum** of the **feet** and **toes**. The patients often complain of aches and cramps (**intermittent claudication**) following moderate exercise. Pain at night in bed relieved by lowering the legs is another sign of arterial disease.

In contrast to assessing the subtleties of venous flow defects, primary assessment of the arterial function centers on a forceful palpable arterial pulse.

Palpate for reduced **pulses** or absence of pulses in the dorsalis pedis, posterior tibial, popliteal, and femoral arteries. **Elevate the feet** for 2 minutes, **then** suddenly place them in a **dependent position**. Failure to see color return in 15 seconds indicates moderate arterial ischemia, whereas periods greater than 30 seconds are indicative of severe ischemia.

The diagnosis of **acute deep-vein thrombosis** is most readily made by **phlebography**. However, physical examination for venous valvular incompetence is made by manually compressing with one hand the saphenous veins while gently feeling with the other hand any consequent distal dilatation due to retrograde flow through incompetent valves. Tapping the veins in the thigh similarly transmits a pulse to the hand palpating the veins at the level of the calf.

Assess the retrograde filling by elevating the leg and digitally compressing the proximal end of the long saphenous vein; have the patient stand, and 20 seconds after veins above fill, release digital pressure. Sudden retrograde filling indicates long **saphenous vein incompetence**. By compressing the popliteal space similarly, competence of the short saphenous vein can be assessed. Alternatively, the use of an **ultrasound Doppler unit** will allow you to localize not only **venous valvular incompetence** but also **incompetent perforator veins**.

STUDY BLOOD, URINE, FECES

See the chapter on The Inner Game of Laboratory Diagnosis.

SIZE UP THE PATIENT

It was the rule of the master diagnostician Henry Michelson to **first determine if the patient was sick** or not. For this, a careful history is invaluable, but you can do more. Measure the blood pressure, weight, and temperature. Look for pharyngitis, tonsillitis, dental caries. Check for lymphadenopathy. Order a health profile, including a urinalysis. Look for other leads into special diagnostic tests. What does the skin suggest? Should he have a general physical examination? Does he have a paraneoplastic syndrome? Does he need a chest x-ray, gastrointestinal series, guaiac test, or stool culture? Should he have a test for HIV infection?

Villaverde MM, MacMillan CW: **Fever:** From Symptom to Treatment. New York, Van Nostrand Reinhold Company, 1978, 597 pp.

Febrile diseases with **dermatologic symptoms** may begin in three ways:

1. **Influenza-like onset:** fever, chills, aches, asthenia, general malaise, pharyngolaryngeal discomfort, conjunctivitis, and nasal discharge

measles	rickettsialpox
rubella	dengue fever
epidemic typhus	coccidioidomycosis
murine typhus	tularemia
Rocky Mountain spotted fever	

2. **Febrile onset:** fever, chills, and malaise begin simultaneously with the rash

varicella	rat-bite fever
herpes simplex	relapsing fever
herpes zoster	psittacosis
scarlet fever	toxoplasmosis
typhoid fever	leptospirosis
variola	

3. Localized skin symptoms: lesions that become more conspicuous

Q fever	filariasis
yellow fever	lymphogranuloma venereum
cellulitis	phlebitis
erysipelas	abscess
sunburn	glanders (farcy)
trichinosis	

The **syndrome fever** is an aggregate of pyrexia, tachycardia, hyperpnea, concentrated urine, and other vasomotor, gastrointestinal, or nervous symptoms. Anorexia, weakness, chilliness, or malaise may be prodromal to the elevation of body temperature.

Axillary or inguinal temperature is about 0.5°C (1°F) less than oral temperature, and rectal about 0.5°C more.

Fever patterns are a valuable aid in diagnosis:

1. Sustained: constantly elevated above normal
2. **Remittent:** fluctuates from higher to lower levels, but is constantly above normal.
3. Intermittent: the daily lower level is below the normal 37°C.
4. **Relapsing:** one or more days of normal temperature alternating between days of fever
5. **Hyperthermia:** the higher peaks reach 40°C (105°F)
6. Septic (hectic): marked oscillations of temperature with chills and sweating

7. Febricula: elevation of temperature only slightly evident and symptoms barely noticeable.

Staphylococcal infections usually cause remittent fever, whereas **streptococcal infections** cause sustained fever. **Severe chills** are seen mainly in the following:

malaria	typhoid fever	recurrent fever
variola	tonsillitis	scarlet fever
erysipelas	pneumonia	influenza
measles	epidemic typhus	

Phlebitis, cholecystitis, urinary tract infection, visceral abscesses, hemolytic crises, and incompatible blood transfusions may also be heralded by chills.

Most **febrile illnesses with rashes** in **children** start with **erythematous macules** at predictable locations: the face, neck, trunk, wrists, or ankles. The macules then become **papular** or coalesce to produce a uniform erythematous rash.

measles	typhoid fever	scarlet fever
epidemic typhus	psittacosis	relapsing fever
German measles	leptospirosis	toxoplasmosis
murine typhus	erysipelas	cellulitis
Rocky Mountain spotted fever	rickettsialpox	sunburn
dengue		

Other febrile rashes, especially in children, are **vesicular**:

varicella	herpes simplex
herpes zoster	variola
severe erysipelas	severe sunburn

Ulcers develop from papules or inflamed lymph nodes in:

rickettsialpox (black eschar)	lymphogranuloma venereum
rat-bite fever	glanders
abscess	(farcy)
tularemia	

Profuse sweating accompanies chills in:

malaria	typhoid
measles	dengue
pneumonia	trichinosis
miliaria rubra	

Characteristic skin reactions of febrile diseases:

erythema nodosum: coccidioidomycosis
erythema multiforme: coccidioidomycosis
local ulceration: rat-bite fever
jaundice:

leptospirosis	hepatitis
Q fever	cholangitis
yellow fever	pancreatitis

inflamed veins: phlebitis
tremor ± suppuration: abscesses

Febrile diseases by geographic distribution:

United States
eastern:
Rocky Mountain spotted fever
toxoplasmosis
midwest:
histoplasmosis

northwest:
  Rocky Mountain spotted fever
western:
  plague
  relapsing fever
southwest:
  coccidioidomycosis
south:
  leprosy
  malaria
  blastomycosis
Hawaii
  leprosy
Alaska
  trichinosis

Tropical diseases
  malaria
  variola
  yellow fever
  schistosomiasis
  dengue
  filariasis
  leprosy

Central America
  yellow fever
  trypanosomiasis

kala-azar
schistosomiasis
South America
  plague
  kala-azar
  trypanosomiasis
  yellow fever
  schistosomiasis
Africa
  plague
  yellow fever
  kala-azar
  relapsing fever
  trypanosomiasis
  schistosomiasis
Europe and former USSR
  relapsing fever
  plague
  all others
Asia
  yellow fever
  cholera
  plague
  dengue
  relapsing fever
  kala-azar
  melioidosis

Laboratory tests for **fever**:

erythrocyte sedimentation rate (active infection, liver disease)
complete blood count
blood cultures (bacterial and viral)
cultures of sputum, feces, throat, wounds, discharge, spinal fluid, urine,
  pus
serology: antibodies, complement, fixation, hemagglutination
ECG
skin biopsy
radioisotope scans
x-rays

Serologic studies are **diagnostic** in:

influenza
parainfluenza
varicella
measles
poliomyelitis
smallpox
herpes simplex
infectious mononucleosis
dengue
herpangina
acute respiratory disease (ARD)
endemic typhus
trench fever
rickettsialpox
streptococcal infections
cholera
tularemia

melioidosis
leptospirosis
trichinosis
herpes zoster
rabies
aseptic meningitis
acute febrile respiratory illness
  (AFRI)
yellow fever
murine typhus
Rocky Mountain spotted fever
salmonellosis
brucellosis
plague
toxoplasmosis
syphilis
schistosomiasis

Centor RM, Meier FA, Dalton HP: **Throat cultures** and **rapid tests** for diagnosis of **group A streptococcal pharyngitis**. Ann Intern Med 1986; 105:892–899.

Two techniques may be used:

1. Culture swab specimen obtained from posterior pharynx using blood agar plate. Time required—24 to 48 hours.
2. Extract group A carbohydrate from swab of pharynx using acid or enzyme. Use antibody in commercial kit to identify this streptococcal carbohydrate by means of agglutination or EIA (enzyme-linked immunosorbent assay). Time required, 7 to 70 minutes.

Note: **Chlamydia** cause 20% of adult pharyngitis and *Mycoplasma* cause 10%. Other causes are rare.

Rojeski MT, Gharib H: Nodular thyroid disease; evaluation and management. N Engl J Med 1985; 313:428–436.

The best initial diagnostic step for **evaluation** of a **nodular thyroid** is fine-needle aspiration biopsy performed by an experienced physician and interpreted by an experienced cytopathologist. Laboratory tests, ultrasound, and radionuclide imaging (thyroid scans) cannot distinguish between benign and malignant nodules.

Physical characteristics and duration of a thyroid nodule are poor predictors of malignancy. The neck should be carefully examined for lymph nodes. A history of exposure to ionizing radiation is an important risk factor for cancer. Thyroid disease is usually not associated with thyroid cancer, although lymphoma is increased with Hashimoto's thyroiditis.

Ravin A: Tachycardia and **sensitivity to heat** as indications for basal metabolism rate determination. Ann Intern Med 1941; 15:478–486.

Thyrotoxicosis is probably **not present** if the patient has a pulse rate below 96, expresses indifference to heat and cold, prefers heat, or complains of **cold hands** and **feet**.

Canti G: A Colour Atlas of Sputum Cytology: The Early Diagnosis of Lung Cancer. Chicago, Year Book Medical Publishers, Inc., 1988, 181 pp.

An excellent display in color of what can be seen in a **scraping** of **oral mucosa**. Preparation should be fixed while still wet in 95% alcohol and stained by the Papanicolaou method. Plates show multinucleate giant cells of herpes simplex, budding yeasts, and fungal hyphae, as well as contaminant vegetable cells and the spidery forms of stellate hairs from the leaves of plane trees (sycamores and maples).

Markell EK, Voge M: **Medical Parasitology**, 6th ed. Philadelphia, W.B. Saunders Company, 1986, 383 pp.

Look for *Giardia lamblia,* worms, and *Entamoeba histolytica* in stools.

Moss AA, Hanelin LG: **Occult malignant tumors** in **dermatologic disease**. The futility of radiologic search. Radiology 1977; 123:69–71.

Radiologic search for tumors should be guided by specific clinical findings suggesting a carcinoma in a particular organ. The appearance of **dermato-myositis**, polymyositis, **bullous pemphigoid**, or dermatitis herpetiformis does not call for all-out, indiscriminate radiologic surveys for an occult malignant tumor.

Council on Scientific Affairs: Positron emission tomography: A new approach to brain chemistry. JAMA 1988; 260:2704–2710.

We have had the CAT scan, and now we have the newest PET: positron emission tomography. It gives unique aid in demonstrating malignant tumors, epilepsy, strokes, and dementia.

Salimi Z, Vas W, Tang-Barton P, et al: Assessment of **tissue viability** in **frostbite** by ^{99m}Tc pertechnetate scintigraphy. Am J Roentg Ray Soc 1984; 142:415–419.

Injection of pertechnetate in antecubital vein allows viewing and recording of tissue viability on oscilloscope.

SEARCH WITH INSTRUMENTS

Instruments can vary from a simple glass slide for measuring **skin extensibility** to complex scanning electron microscopy. In the first instance, the slide is attached to the skin by cyanoacrylate adhesive and the extensibility of the skin recorded on a protractor when torsion is applied. In the latter case, hairs can be examined diagnostically at magnifications up to $20,000\times$.

Below is a sampling of instruments and what you can do with them. It is like looking through a gardener's tool catalogue. You may not buy anything, but it's fun to look.

Leveque J-L (ed): **Cutaneous Investigation** in Health and Disease: Noninvasive Methods and Instrumentation. New York, Marcel Dekker, Inc., 1989, 439 pp.

When the patient asks "Isn't there another test you could do?", this is the book for you. It tells you exactly how to assess:

1. Skin surface topography

    visualization (regression test of Kligman)
    macrophotography (violet-blue lighting)
    replicas (silicone rubber, Beagley-Gibson grading)
    sticky slide specimen (adhesive-tape strip)
    instrumentation (scan densitometry, profilometry, stylus, multidirectional, computerized image)

2. Desquamation and keratinocyte cohesiveness

    dansyl chloride stratum corneum renewal time
    desquamation: corneocyte loss

3. Frictional properties

    gravity load
    deceleration of rotating probe
    deflection of a spring

4. Skin surface pH

    colorimetric
    buffer capacity
    potentiometric

5. Hydration status

    impedance (resistance to alternating current)
    conductance
    capacitance

6. Transepidermal water loss

      chamber technique
        open
          electrohygrometer
          thermal conductivity cell
          infrared water vapor analyzer
          dew point hygrometer
          electrolytic water vapor analyzer
          dielectric permittivity
        closed
          gravimetric
      electromagnetic probe
      infants
        urine osmolarity
        body weight

7.   Skin surface lipids

      solvent extraction
      gravimetric (cigarette paper)
      ground-glass technique
      betonite clay technique
      Seb-U-tape
      qualitative
        thin-layer chromatography
        gas chromatography

8.   Skin thickness

      micrometer skin fold
      xeroradiography, useful only on forearm
      ultrasound pulse
        A scan
        B scan
      nuclear magnetic resonance imaging

9.   Mechanical properties

      tensile
      torsional
      elevation
      indentation
      suction
      vibration

10.   Melanin

      reflectance spectroscopy (red light to avoid hemoglobin absorption band)

11.   Erythema

      monochromatic photography

12.   Skin temperature

      thermocouples
      resistance thermometers
      liquid crystal films
      infrared thermography

13.   Thermal conductivity

      hematron transducer

14.   Microcirculation

      O_2 electrode
      laser Doppler flowmetry

capillary microscope
fluorescence videomicroscopy, videodensitometry
capillary pressure
fluorescence microlymphography
indirect lymphography
photoplethysmography

What more could a patient ask for?

Marks R: Device and rule. Clin Exp Dermatol 1985; 10:303–327.

The description and interpretation of skin lesions increasingly call for instrumentation to provide quantitative data. The clinician's sensory organs provide invaluable data and are the cornerstone for gross diagnosis. Yet the clinician suffers **verbal inadequacy.** He cannot communicate the enormous bits of information provided by his eye scan of the patient's skin disease. His eye surely outruns his tongue. Likewise, his sensory input quickly overloads his memory system. The clinician also suffers from inability to perceive the subclinical, the invisible, the inapparent.

Instruments available today to **enhance diagnostic grasp** are:

skin color reflectance spectrophotometers
scanning densitometers for skin contour
photographic image analyzers
xeroradiography
ultrasound skin-thickness measurement
dermographometers
Doppler flowmeter (laser, ultrasound)
desquamators for cell loss
evaporimeters for water loss
lipometers for sebum secretion

The clinician is as an astronomer who can sight the stars and constellations, but the clinicians must have the radiotelescope, the infrared telescope, and the x-ray telescope to diagnose the universe.

Skerrow D, Skerrow CJ (eds): **Methods** in **Skin Research.** New York, John Wiley & Sons, 1985, 673 pp.

How to **measure** and **analyze:**

surface lipids
hair
epidermal cells
skin microbiology
skin permeability
photosensitivity

Marks RM, Barton SP, Edwards C (eds): The **physical nature** of the **skin.** Boston, MTP Press Limited, 1988, 219 pp.

How to measure:

skin contour	skin thickness
subjective	biopsy
replicative	skin fold
optical	x-ray
photographic	magnetic resonance
	ultrasound
	skin hydration

skin blood flow
   light microscopy
   infrared thermography
   microwave thermography
   thermal conductance
   plethysmography (photoreflectance)
   isotope clearance
   fluorescence
   laser Doppler
   pulsed ultrasound Doppler

Gibbons RD, Fiedler-Weiss VC: Computer-aided quantification of **scalp hair**. Dermatol Clin 1986; 4:627–640.

How to count hairs, other than one by one.

Engel J-M, Flesch U, Stüttgen G (eds): Thermological Methods. Weinheim, Germany, VCH, 1985, 326 pp.

This monograph details all of the methods of **measuring skin temperature**. **Liquid crystal systems** are the most popular for dermatologic use.

Note:

   Areas of incipient or subclinical **urticaria** can be detected by finding loci of elevated temperature.

   Sites of former **contact dermatitis** or positive patch tests have a persistent elevation in skin temperature.

   Skin temperature is lower in areas of third-degree burns, and areas of **necrosis** can be identified by noting cool border.

   Sclerodermatous skin is hotter because of reduction in thermal buffer of fat.

   Malignant but not benign **tumors** show increased surface temperature. Benign tumors such as lipomas show cooler skin because of heat buffer.

   Skin temperature is lower over joints.

   Smoking a **cigarette** lowers the temperature of hands by 3°C.

   Skin temperatures can be displayed now in form of isotherms showing resolutions of differences as small as 0.1°C.

Stüttgen G, Flesch V: Dermatological **thermography**. Weinheim, Germany, VCH, 1985, 177 pp.

A fascinating color atlas of infrared portraits of skin lesions. It provides all the diagnostic information a dermatologist can secure from modern thermographic sensors.

Simons DG: Fibrositis/fibromyalgia: A form of **myofascial trigger points**? Am J Med 1986; 81 (suppl 3A):93–98.

A pressure threshold meter (model PTH-AFZ, Pain Diagnostics and Thermography, Great Neck, New York) permits you to measure the pressure required to elicit **pain** in tender areas, e.g., **Dercum's disease.**

Huch R, Huch A, Lübbers DW: Transcutaneous PO_2. New York, Thieme-Stratton, Inc., 1981, 170 pp.

A detailed guide on how to measure oxygen exchange and pressure through the skin.

Serup J: Non-invasive quantitation of psoriasis plaques—measurement of **skin thickness** with 15 mHz pulsed **ultrasound**. Clin Exp Dermatol 1984; 9:502–508.

The thickness of **psoriatic plaques** was measured using an ultrasound probe.

Solomons AM: Estimation of "**epidermal**" **thickness** using an impedance method. Bioeng Skin 1987; 3:281–285.

Conductance measurements at 1 kHz made between an ECG electrode on the skin and an inserted acupuncture needle allowed measurement of the thickness of keratinized epidermis.

Kalis B, DeRigal J, Léonard F, et al: In vivo study of **scleroderma** by non-invasive techniques. Br J Dermatol 1990; 122:785–791.

Ultrasound A-scan echography, displayed on an oscilloscope, permits measurement of **skin thickness**. The value is derived from an ultrasound pulse being reflected from the dermis-fat interface, using the speed of ultrasound at 1605 m/sec.

A **twistometer**, using a low torque (30×10^{-4}Nm) applied by a disc fixed to the skin by double-sided adhesive tape, allowed the angle of rotation to be displayed automatically.

These two tools provided the most exact and useful data for showing an increase in thickness and a decrease in extensibility in progressive scleroderma.

Measurement of blood flow using a laser-Doppler velocimeter and the transcutaneous PO_2 using a Roche Kontron apparatus were not as useful.

Physical measurement of the skin can provide prognostic as well as diagnostic aid.

Crowe DM, Willard MS, Murahata RI: Quantitation of erythema by reflectance spectroscopy. J Soc Cosmet Chem 1987; 38:451–455.

Erythema can be **quantitated** by employing a fiberoptic bundle attached to a scanning spectrophotometer. Such **reflectance spectroscopy** adds precision in assessing skin irritants.

Webster JG (ed): Encyclopedia of Medical Devices and Instrumentation. New York, John Wiley & Sons, Inc., 1988, vol 1–4, 4000 pp.

The state of the science of **instrumentation** in **studying skin** and all that's within.

Dermascan A (Network Marketing, P.O. Box 5246, Evanston, IL 60204) is an instrument that measures **skin thickness** noninvasively by **ultrasound**.

The Imex Pocket-Dop II (IMEX Medical Systems, Inc., 6355 Joyce Drive, Golden, CO 80403) is a **hand-held Doppler unit** for diagnosing **occlusive vascular conditions**, taking difficult blood pressures, and detecting weak pulses. Intriguing to the pediatric patient.

A laserflow blood perfusion monitor (TSI, Inc., 500 Caroigan Road, St. Paul, MN 55164) allows measurement of the microcirculation **blood flow** in millimeters/minute/100 gm of tissue.

Addison LA, Fischer PM: The **office laboratory**, 2nd ed. Norwalk, Conn, Appleton and Lange, 1990, 464 pp.

Complete guide to setting up a diagnostic laboratory within your own office. But recall, you will be under federal scrutiny.

SEARCH FOR MORE INFORMATION

If you want an interesting practice, bring interesting ideas into your practice. And where do they come from? Reading, listening, and thinking.

The most fertile source of ideas is the monumental **Index Medicus** (National Library of Medicine, 8600 Rockville Pike, Bethesda, Maryland 20894). Published every month and cumulatively indexed every spring, this multivolumed encyclopedic survey is a genie that can stretch your diagnostic horizon. You can open it either to subject or to the name of a speaker you have heard.

For those who prefer keyboard tapping over page turning, **MEDLINE** provides computer access to this same diagnostic genie. It covers the medical literature since 1966 and provides it on a constantly updated series of compact discs, with not only video viewing but also printouts. With experience and the use of carefully selected key words, MEDLINE crossmatches concepts and pulls more articles than you will find on direct use of *Index Medicus*. Furthermore, abstracts of articles can be provided and printed out.

A variety of entries into MEDLINE are available. One of the most popular is **Paper Chase** (350 Longwood Ave., Boston, MA 02115, 1-800-722-2075). To access this you need a personal computer or terminal, a telephone line, and a modem. It can bring consultants from all over the world into your office, each on the bidding of your keyboard. And you have a quarter of a million subject headings from which to choose your panel of consultants.

Another reference source, but more difficult to use in print form, is the SCI (**Science Citation Index**, Institute for Scientific Information, Inc., 3501 Market Street, Philadelphia, PA 19104). Here the author is the primary entry point and reference given for each paper that cites his primary publication. This permits tracking of the development of knowledge along specific paths. Alternatively, one may use the **SCI Permuterm Subject Index**, with subject words leading to the authors. Thus, one can enter under the author W.B. Shelley or under the subject psoriasis. The *Science Citation Index* is published bimonthly and is cumulatively indexed every year and every 5 years. For easy use, it also comes on compact disc, bringing you the authors and subjects of more than 3100 science journals.

Some of the best diagnostic thoughts come serendipitously while browsing in a library. But denied this form of grazing, access to or a subscription to **Current Contents: Clinical Medicine** (ISI, 3501 Market Street, Philadelphia, PA 19104) is wondrously stimulating. Every week it brings you a photocopy of the table of contents of the world's most important dermatologic journals, as well as hundreds of the other medical journals. More than that, there is an abstract of what your patients are reading in the public press, as well as a continual listing of the new medical books and their contents. As we write this we see in the August 20, 1990, issue that *Dermatologica* 1990; 181:5–7, has an article on **idiopathic recalcitrant facial flushing syndrome** by Tur, Ryatt, and Maibach. We have just such a patient. Now, a call to the library or a card to ISI in Philadelphia will bring us a reprint. You can thus bring excitement and vigor into your practice by reading *Current Contents: Clinical Medicine* every Thursday morning. It is the Journal of Journals.

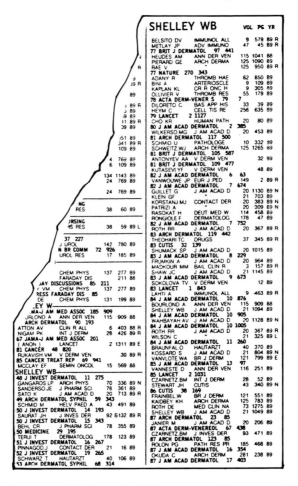

Finally, read and compare the hazards of doing something versus doing nothing.

Flegel K, Obseasohn R: Adverse effects of diagnostic tests: A study of the quality of reporting. Arch Intern Med 1982; 142:883–887.

There is little literature monitoring of the **hazards** of **diagnostic test procedures**, but here are the adverse effects associated with **liver biopsy** as reported in 32 articles:

pain
hypertension
periumbilical discoloration
bacteremia
pneumothorax
needle fracture with liver remnant
arteriovenous fistula
hematoma
hemobilia
hemoperitoneum
hemorrhage requiring transfusion
bile peritonitis
bile pleuritis
septicemia
hepatic artery aneurysm

Does your methotrexate patient really need that liver biopsy?

SOLVE IT

Don't just stand there. Do something. And here's how you do it:

Pariser DM, Caserio RJ, Eaglstein WH: **Techniques** for **Diagnosing Skin** and **Hair Disease**, 2nd ed. New York, Thieme Medical Publishers, Inc., 1986, 208 pp.

Follow these clear directions and illustrations on what to do and exactly how to do it, plus precisely what it means.

Jacobs PH, Anhalt TS: Handbook of **skin clues** of **systemic disease**. 2nd ed. Philadelphia, Lea & Febiger, 1987, 123 pp.

Use this check list of what to do and what to order. Outlined for each symptom and sign.

Shelley WB: On **solving clinical problems**. Cutis 1984; 34:426–428.

Listen to the patient.
Know the literature.
Use the laboratory.

Be imaginative.
Hospitalize.
Seek serendipity.

Don't give up!

The Inner Game of Laboratory Diagnosis

General Principles
The Routine Health Profile
Dermatologically Relevant Laboratory Tests
Dermatologic Health Profile
General Reference Works

GENERAL PRINCIPLES

Order diagnostic tests only when the results

can enhance your awareness of the nature and extent of your patient's disease
can affect your therapy
can allay the patient's real fears
can protect you from the threat of a malpractice suit
can provide necessary confirmation

Be aware of the **limitations** of **diagnostic tests**:

false-positives in healthy patients or in patients with other diseases
false-negatives in patients who have the disease in its early or late stages or in an atypical form
laboratory error, mislabeling, misreading, mishandling, misrecording, or misreporting

Remember that new tests are initially viewed to be more sensitive and more specific than they may prove to be upon study of a larger random population of healthy and sick people.

Diagnostic tests are most useful when you consider that the probability of a disease being present is intermediate, i.e., neither high nor low. If the probability in your estimate is high, you will disregard the negative result, believing that the test is not sufficiently sensitive. If, on the other hand, you feel the disease is highly unlikely, you will disregard the positive result, believing that the test is not sufficiently specific. Thus, a high degree of clinical certainty always overrides the uncertainty of the laboratory data.

The greater the number of different diagnostic tests done, the greater the chance of getting false-positive or irrelevant leads. Your patient's test value may fall outside the cover of the bell curve and not sound an alarm of disease. The possibilities for laboratory error increase in the automated multiple-screen procedures. When in doubt, repeat the test on a single value request. Don't forget that drugs interact not only with each other but also with laboratory tests. Medication can lead to false laboratory values. The elevated thyroid test results in patients taking oral contraceptives are an oft-cited example.

Take into account the effect of food. The fasting state is mandatory for tests such as serum iron and serum triglycerides, but not cholesterol. Other examples of the effect of foods include the need to restrict bananas when testing the urine for 5-hydroxyindoleacetic acid excretion. If in doubt, check with your laboratory.

Keep your laboratory testing sharply focused. Let your clinical suspicions be the determinant in requesting a test. Too many tests are mindlessly ordered, resulting in "**laboratory lottery**" with that one chance in a million of winning a diagnosis. Use common sense to blend medical sense with economic sense. Take time to ask, "If I were this patient, would I want this test enough to pay for it out of my own pocket?" Take clinical pride in making out that laboratory slip.

Mellinkoff SM: The physician of tomorrow. JAMA 1977; 237:1952–1962.

Is there a seasoned physician who has not seen some patients subjected to the wrong tests, at the wrong times, for the wrong reasons, at great expense, and with disastrous results because the original history was taken clumsily or carelessly?

Williams SV, Eisenberg JM: Help with diagnostic decisions. Ann Intern Med 1982; 97:444–445.

Normal limits are set to **include 95%** of **normal people**. The other 5% are outliers with false-positive tests that lead to worry and anxiety in patients and, at times, to further tests that can be inconvenient, expensive, and risky. Furthermore, to ignore what you "feel" is a false-positive, or to act incorrectly on the basis of it, is to incur legal risk.

Sensitivity indicates how often the test is **positive in disease** (PID), i.e., the proportion of patients with the disease in question for whom the test result is abnormal. **Specificity** indicates how often the test is **normal in health** (NIH), i.e., the proportion of individuals without the disease who show a normal test.

Predictive value answers the question: If the test is positive, what is the probability that the patient has the disease? This is derived from considering not only the sensitivity and specificity, but also the incidence of the disease in your patient population. The higher the probability of the disease, the higher the positive predictive value.

Cebull RD, Beck JR: Biochemical profiles: applications in ambulatory screening and preadmission testing of adults. Ann Intern Med 1987; 106:403–413.

Criteria for usefulness of diagnostic screening tests:

Will the test detect disease that would otherwise remain undetected?

What are the test's risks, sensitivity, specificity, cost, and patient acceptance?

Will earlier detection have a favorable impact on the patient's psychological well-being?

Is therapy more effective in an early stage of the disease?

What are the nonmedical consequences of diagnostic labeling? What is the impact on the individual?

Note that the probability that a *healthy* person will have normal results on all tests in a biochemical profile is 95% for a profile of only one test, 74% for 6 tests, and 36% for 20 tests. Should you do 100 tests, the probability drops to 0.6%. (Enough tests can prove that anyone is sick.)

Cebul RD: The **likelihood ratio** and diagnostic tests. Ann Intern Med 1986; 104:888–889.

$$\text{Likelihood ratio} = \frac{\text{proportion of diseased patients with result}}{\text{proportion of nondiseased patients with result}}$$

This ratio is a valuable quantitative expression of the discriminating ability of a diagnostic test no matter whether the test is being reported as negative, indeterminate, positive, or in milligrams per deciliter. As an example, if 36 of 45 patients with pulmonary embolism have a positive test and 15 of 44 controls show the same positive test, the likelihood ratio is 2.35, i.e., the test is more than twice as likely to occur in the patient with the embolism as in the normal.

Phillips WC, Scott JA, Blasczcynski G: **Statistics for diagnostic procedures**. How sensitive is "sensitivity"; how specific is "specificity"? AJR 1983; 140:1265–1270.

Clinical questions and their answers:

Given a positive test, what are the chances your patient has the disease? Given a negative test, what are the chances your patient does not have the disease?

The answers require the positive and also the negative predictive values for the test. Such values are calculated by means of **Bayes' theorem** using the three parameters:

1. Sensitivity (S):

    probability of a positive test in a patient with that disease

2. Specificity (s):

    probability of a negative test in a patient without the disease

3. Prevalence of disease (P):

    proportion of patients in test population who actually have the disease

$$\text{Thus, positive predictive value} = \frac{PS}{Ps = (1 - P)(1 - s)}$$

Note: (1) The more prevalent the disease, the higher the predictive value of the test; (2) although the Bayesian theory is mathematically sound, the results in clinical medicine are not uniformly good, largely because precise data on the three variables in the equation are not available.

Narins RG, Cohen JJ: Bicarbonate therapy in severe acidosis. Ann Intern Med 1988; 108:311.

Today's decisions must be based on interpretations of currently available studies, imperfect as they may be.

Schreiber MH: Wilson's law of diminishing returns. AJR 1982; 138:786–787.

Know when the diagnostic party is over and stop ordering studies to confirm the obvious. Wilson's law puts it best: "The more times you run over a dead cat, the flatter it gets."

Rang M: The **Ulysses syndrome**. Can Med Assoc J 1972; 106:122–123.

The normal range in laboratory investigations excludes the upper and lower 2.5%. As a result, 5% of the normal population will be labeled abnormal. These false-positives are obtained for clinical as well as histopathologic observations. If the physician is not suspicious and critical of the odd-ball report or value, the patient may be launched on a **needless voyage of testing** and further study. He now has the Ulysses syndrome with its attendant mental, physical, and financial strains. This sequence of studies and more studies eventually results in a return to awareness that the patient is normal. It has been named the Ulysses syndrome, since it is reminiscent of Ulysses' 20 years of unnecessary adventures in an attempt to return to his point of departure.

The cause of the syndrome is excessive use of testing: 66% of persons having 20 tests done will have at least one abnormal result, often the first sign of the Ulysses syndrome.

Contributing factors are (1) mass screening; (2) indifferences to costs, shouldered by the invisible third party; (3) residents carrying out investigative overkill to avoid staff criticism; (4) laboratory request forms offering such a feast of tests that the doctor orders more than he can digest.

And, we would add, the diagnostician must avoid not only the Ulysses syndrome, but also the **Charybdis syndrome** of not going out to sea at all.

THE ROUTINE HEALTH PROFILE

She said her doctor told her she had an undisclosed disease.

Patients with puzzling, perplexing, pellicle problems love to have tests done. Even when they have a condition well known to you, they have a deep intuitive fear that something is wrong inside. They need the reassurance of "negative blood and urine." Furthermore, screening tests are never amiss. They may reveal some serious problem entirely unrelated to the skin and as yet completely asymptomatic. Modern instrumentation makes it possible to secure the 30 to 40 values in a complete blood count, urinalysis, and blood chemistry profile almost for the same cost as a single, isolated value such as cholesterol. It is currently a patient's best diagnostic bargain.

Here are a few of the dermatologic diagnoses that may spring into your mind when you scan the data on your patient's health profile or chemscreen.

Eosinophils	Parasites, hypereosinophilic syndrome, eosinophilic fasciitis, tryptophan syndrome, drug reaction
Erythrocytes	Polycythemia vera
Neutrophils	Infection, Sweet's syndrome, cyclic neutropenia
Platelets	Purpura, immune reaction
Calcium	Sarcoidosis, granulomas
Cholesterol	Xanthomas
Glucose	Diabetes mellitus, glucagonoma, necrobiosis lipoidica
Hepatic enzymes	Urticaria, Gianotti-Crosti syndrome, drug intolerance
Rapid plasma reagin	Syphilis, lupus
T_4	Hypo- or hyperthyroidism
Sedimentation rate	Infection, Hodgkin's disease, arteritis
Uric acid	Tophi, psoriasis

Shapiro MF, Greenfield S: The **complete blood count** and leucocyte differential count. An approach to their rational application. Ann Intern Med 1987; 106:65–74.

The complete blood count should be reserved for sick people. It is not useful as a routine screen for the general population or in individuals in whom no abnormality is suspected. Even the patient who asks for it needs to be taught to think probabilistically.

Use it when there is a suspicion of a primary hematologic disorder. Use it to detect and to monitor the adverse effect of the drug you are prescribing, e.g., dapsone.

Cebul RD, Beck JR: Biochemical profiles: Applications in ambulatory screening and preadmission testing of adults. Ann Intern Med 1987; 106:403–413.

Illustrative Associations:

Albumin, decreased	Liver disease, nephrotic syndrome, malnutrition
Blood urea nitrogen, increased	Renal disease
Calcium, increased	Sarcoidosis, bone disease (Paget's), hyperparathyroidism
Cholesterol, increased	Familial hypothyroidism, hepatitis
decreased	Liver disease, malabsorption, hyperthyroidism
Alkaline phosphatase, increased	Liver disease, bone disease
Lactic dehydrogenase, increased	Hemolysis, thromboembolism, inflammation, malignant disease
Glucose, increased	Diabetes mellitus, steroids, hyperthyroidism, glucagonoma
Potassium, increased	Renal failure, acidosis
decreased	Steroids
Protein, increased	Liver disease, lymphoma, collagen-vascular disease
Sodium, increased	Thromboembolism, steroids, diabetes insipidus
decreased	Volume depletion, antidiuretic hormone excess

Rosen MA: **C-reactive protein:** A marker of **infection, inflammation,** tissue damage, and malignancy. Diag Clin Test 1990; 28(May):18–22.

The **acute-phase response** occurs in a wide variety of systemic infections, inflammations, immune responses, trauma, and malignant disease. The dominant feature is a burst of **hepatic activity**, signaled by a several-hundredfold increase in one of its products, viz., C-reactive protein. Only 2% of these elevations are due to skin disorders, whereas **malignant neoplasms** account for more than 30%.

Sox HC, Liang MH: The **erythrocyte sedimentation rate** guidelines for rational use. Ann Intern Med 1986; 104:512–523.

This most venerable of tests makes a very small contribution in screening for disease or in detecting infection, cancer, or connective tissue disease. Should it be **elevated**, a history and physical examination usually disclose the cause. Significantly in the patient suspected of having **temporal arteritis** (tender reddened nodules along temporal artery, jaw claudication, transient monocular blindness), an elevated sedimentation rate is virtually a sine qua non for diagnosis.

Lambert RE, Fainstat M: Elevated **erythrocyte sedimentation rate**: Common clinical correlations. *In* Louis AA (ed): Handbook of Difficult Diagnosis. New York, Churchill Livingstone, 1990, pp 424–433.

When the sedimentation rate is **low**, think drugs, hemoglobinopathies, menses.

When the sedimentation rate is a surprise, think of the possibility of error, e.g., blood too warm, rate high; blood too cool, rate low. When the sedimentation rate is elevated, remember that this reflects the presence of scores of disease states all neatly listed in this review.

Beganovic S: The **erythrocyte sedimentation rate**. Ann Intern Med 1987; 107:425.

In **elderly patients**, elevated sedimentation rates may be attributed to occult infection, especially urinary tract, Hodgkin's disease, renal carcinoma, tuberculosis.

Fletcher RH: **Carcinoembryonic antigen**. Ann Intern Med 1966; 104:66–73.

Carcinoembryonic antigen (CEA) is one of a class of oncofetal antigens normally present in fetal life that reappears in high concentration in patients with certain **malignant tumors**, especially epithelial. Because the sensitivity and specificity of the CEA family of glycoproteins are low, the presence of this antigen cannot be used as a solitary screening test for colorectal carcinoma. A variety of unrelated conditions led to **elevated CEA** levels in the plasma. These include **smoking**, liver disease, inflammatory bowel disease, and renal failure.

However, higher CEA levels in the presence of known cancer indicate a more extensive tumor and a poorer prognosis. Furthermore, a rise in the plasma CEA level in a patient after treatment does signal a **recurrence of the tumor**. Hence, it has value in prognosis and in postsurgical monitoring.

Noppen M, Schandevijl W, Musch W, Vincken W: **Sarcoidosis** and **hypercalcemia**. Ann Intern Med 1986; 105:143–144.

In a 47-year-old woman with asthma, surgical removal of a superior mediastinal mass containing sarcoid granulomas caused the serum calcium to decrease from 11.2 to 8.4 mg/dl (normal 8.5 to 10.2). Hypercalcemia may have been due to increased circulating 1,25-dihydroxyvitamin D, resulting from aberrant 1-alpha-hydroxylase activity in sarcoid tissue.

Hoffman VN, Korzeniowski OM: **Leprosy**, hypercalcemia, and elevated serum calcitriol levels. Ann Intern Med 1986; 105:890–891.

Hypercalcemia in granulomatous diseases probably results from ectopic production of calcitriol by granulomas.

McPherson ML, Prince SR, Atamer ER, et al: **Theophylline-induced hypercalcemia**. Ann Intern Med 1986; 105:52–54.

Hypercalcemia was found in 11 of 60 patients hospitalized with theophylline toxicity. As theophylline levels fell, serum calcium levels returned to normal. In normal volunteers, propranolol reversed the increase in serum calcium induced by therapeutic levels of theophylline, suggesting that an adrenergic mechanism is involved.

Coggeshall J, Merrill W, Hande K, Prez RD: Implications of hypercalcemia with respect to diagnosis and treatment of lung cancer. Am J Med 1986; 80:325–328.

Don't forget **lung cancer** as a cause of **hypercalcemia**. The tumor is usually large and incurable. Symptoms of hypercalcemia include anorexia, nausea, vomiting, lethargy, confusion, and stupor.

Kaufman RE: Trichiniasis: Clinical considerations. Ann Intern Med 1940; 14:1431–1460.

With significant **eosinophilia**, look for the following:

trichinosis	asthma	psoriasis
Taenia echinococcus	urticaria	pollinosis
angioneurotic edema	serum sickness	scarlet fever
eosinophilic leukemia	rheumatic fever	eczema
periarteritis nodosa	polycythemia vera	infectious
pemphigus	drug sensitivity	mononucleosis
Hodgkin's disease	foreign protein injections	intestinal helminths
secondary syphilis	familial eosinophilia	

Scheitlin WA, Frick PG: **Hypophosphataemia:** A pathognomonic sign in **gram-negative septicaemia.** Lancet 1964; 2:102.

Serum phosphate levels ranged from 0.7 to 3.4 mg/100 ml in six patients with renal disease and septicemia due to *Proteus vulgaris* (2), *Escherichia coli* (3), and *Salmonella typhimurium* (1). The cause of the acute hypophosphatemia is unknown. It has been seen elsewhere only in voluntary **sustained hyperventilation**.

Kolesnick RN, Gershengorn MC: **Thyrotropin-releasing hormone** and the pituitary: New insights into the mechanisms of stimulated secretion and clinical usage. Am J Med 1985; 79:729–739.

If **hyperthyroidism** is suspected, but results of other tests are equivocal, check the TRH (thyrotropin releasing hormone) stimulation test. This hypothalamic hormone **regulates TSH** (thyrotropin) but not prolactin. **Results** are **altered** by anorexia nervosa, depression, iodine contrast administration, and **drug therapy** (steroids, oral contraceptives, lithium, dopamine agonists, and antagonists).

Multiple **causes of hyperthyroidism** are listed, including iodides and malignant disease with thyroid stimulators (choriocarcinoma, hydatidiform mole, embryonal carcinoma of testes, and pituitary tumor).

Hart G: **Syphilis tests** in diagnostic and therapeutic decision making. Ann Intern Med 1986; 104:368–376.

Although a **darkfield examination** of a suspect primary lesion of syphilis (indurated, painless, solitary) or of a scarified or moist secondary lesion is ideal for the diagnosis, most physicians do not have facilities or expertise. Nonetheless, a **capillary tube containing exudate** is suitable for sending to a laboratory, and the use of fluorescein-labeled anti-*Treponema pallidum* globulin permits sharp distinction from the saprophytic nonpathogenic spirochetes.

The **titered VDRL** is now the **serologic test of choice** for diagnosing syphilis. A titer of less than 1:8 at 1 week raises doubt as to the presence of syphilis. When the test remains negative or of low titer at 1 and 3 months, syphilis is highly unlikely. A rising titer confirms the diagnosis of secondary syphilis.

Routine **cerebrospinal fluid assessment** for syphilis is not warranted. It is reserved for patients with syphilis and neurologic abnormalities, for infants who appear to have congenital syphilis, or for patients showing relapse after treatment.

DERMATOLOGICALLY RELEVANT LABORATORY TESTS

There are innumerable laboratory tests that can be done to aid in making a diagnosis. Here is a list of some of the more critical ones arranged according to the suspected diagnosis. The references following give you more in-depth help.

DISEASE	TESTS
Acquired immunodeficiency syndrome (AIDS)	HIV serology
	Lymphocyte subset enumeration
	HIV culture
Acrodermatitis enteropathica	Zinc
Acrodynia	Mercury (blood, urine, hair, nails)
Acromegaly	Growth hormone
Actinomycosis	Aerobic, anaerobic, and fungal culture of abscess
Addison's disease	Adrenocorticotrophic hormone

Disease	Tests
	ACTH response test
	Cortisol, plasma
Alcoholism	Blood alcohol
Alopecia	Heavy metal screen: blood, urine
	Iron, TIBC
	Amino acid screen: urine, plasma
	Biotinidase, serum
Amebiasis	Ova and parasites, stool
Angioedema	C4 complement
	C1 esterase inhibitor
Antibiotic-associated colitis	*Clostridium difficile*
	toxin assay
Antiphospholipid antibody syndrome	Anticardiolipin antibody
Argininosuccinic aciduria	Ammonia, blood
	Argininosuccinic acid: plasma, urine
Arthritis, rheumatoid	Rheumatoid factor
Ascariasis	Ova and parasites, stool
Ataxia-telangiectasia	Chromosome analysis
	IgA, IgG, IgM
Atopic dermatitis	IgE antibodies
	Radioallergosorbent (RAST) tests
Autoimmune disease	ANA
	Immune complexes
	Cryoglobulin
Bacteremia	Blood culture
Bacteriuria	Urine culture
	Leukocyte esterase, urine
Blastomycosis	*Blastomyces* antibody
Bromoderma	Bromide
Bullous eruption	Viral culture
	Virus detection by fluorescent antibody
	Pemphigus, pemphigoid antibodies
Candidiasis	Blood culture
	Candida antibody
Carbon monoxide poisoning	Carboxyhemoglobin
Carcinoid	Serotonin
Carotinemia	Carotene
Cellulitis	Culture
Coccidioidomycosis	Serology
Cold sensitivity	Anti-DNA
	ANA
	Cold agglutinins
	Cryofibrinogen
	Cryoglobulin
Congenital disorders	Chromosome analysis
Connective tissue disease	Autoantibodies
	Mitochondrial antibodies
Creeping eruption	Eosinophilia
Cryptococcosis	Cryptococcus antigen and antibody titers
	Sputum, CSF culture
Cushing's syndrome	Cortisol, urine, plasma
	Urinary ketosteroids
Cyanosis	Methemoglobin
Cytomegalovirus	Culture
	Monoclonal antibody
Dapsone intolerance	G6PD
Down's syndrome	Chromosome analysis (blood)
Endocrine status	Luteinizing hormone
	Follicle-stimulating hormone
	Estradiol, testosterone, T_3, T_4, TSH
	Prolactin, progesterone

continued

Disease	Tests
Eosinophilic fasciitis	Eosinophilia
	Hypergammaglobulinemia
	Sedimentation rate
Erythema infectiosum	Serology
	(Specialty Laboratories, Inc.,
	Santa Monica, CA 90404,
	1-800-421-7110)
Fabry's disease	α-Galactosidase, serum
	Fibroblasts (skin Bx)
Filariasis	Filaria in blood
Fish-odor syndrome	Trimethylamine, urine
Flushing	Bradykinin
	Histamine
	Prostaglandins
	Serotonin
	Serotonin metabolite (5 HIAA)
	Substance P
Folate deficiency	Folic acid: serum, RBC
Galactorrhea	Prolactin
Gianotti-Crosti syndrome	Hepatitis B, parainfluenza, EBV panel,
	Coxsackie
Giardiasis	Ova and parasites, stool
Glucagonoma	Glucagon, plasma
Health status	Chemistry profile
	Sedimentation rate
	C-reactive protein
Hepatitis	Hepatitis A antibody IgM
	Hepatitis B surface antigen
	ANA
Herpes virus infection	Virus culture
	Direct immunofluorescent stain
	Antibodies
Herpes zoster	Virus culture
	Antibodies
Hirsutism	Dehydroepiandrosterone sulfate, serum
	Testosterone
	Prolactin
	Cyclosporine
	Estradiol
Histoplasmosis	Sputum: washings, culture
	Complement fixation, serology
Hurler's disease	α-L-Iduronidase (leukocytes)
Hyperthyroidism	Thyroxine (T_4)
Hypothyroidism	Thyroid antimicrosomal antibody
	Thyroid-stimulating hormone (TSH)
Immune status	Immunoglobulins IgE, IgG, IgA, IgM
	T and B cell labeling
Inborn errors of metabolism	Amino acid screen: plasma, urine
Infectious mononucleosis	Monospot test
	Epstein-Barr virus antibodies
Jaundice, hemolytic	Coombs': direct, indirect
Lead poisoning	Lead
Leg ulcer	Cryoglobulin
	Cryofibrinogen
	Cold agglutinins
	Coagulation screen
	Immune complexes
	Phospholipid antibody
	Zinc
Leishmaniasis	Serologic test
Lymphogranuloma venereum	*Chlamydia* antibodies

DISEASE	TESTS
Mastocytosis	Histamine, blood
	Bone marrow
Measles	Viral culture
	Serum antibodies
Menkes' syndrome	Copper, serum
Mercury poisoning	Mercury: blood, urine
Metal poisoning	Aluminum
	Arsenic
	Cadmium
	Chromium
	Copper
	Gold
	Lead
	Lithium
	Manganese
	Mercury
	Thallium
	Zinc (serum or urine screen)
Microfilariasis	Microfilariae, blood
Neurosyphilis	FTA-ABS, serum
	VDRL, spinal fluid
Nongonococcal urethritis	*Chlamydia* culture
Panniculitis	Amylase, serum
	Lipase
	α_1-Antichymotrypsin
	α_1-Antitrypsin
Pemphigus	Serology
Pharyngitis	Culture for group A beta-hemolytic streptococci, *Corynebacterium diphtheriae*
	Stain for *Chlamydia trachomatis*
Pheochromocytoma	Catecholamines
Porphyria	Porphyrins, urine
	Porphobilinogen, urine
	Protoporphyrin, RBC
	δ-Aminolevulinic acid, urine
Pregnancy	Human chorionic gonadotropin, serum
Prostate cancer	Prostate-specific antigen (PSA), serum
Psoriasis	Streptococcal antibodies (Mayo Clinic)
	Methotrexate, serum
Purpura	Platelet count
	Factor VIII
	Bleeding time
Raynaud's disease	Cold agglutinin titer
Rocky Mountain spotted fever	Antibodies
Rubella	Serology
Rubeola	Serology
Sarcoidosis	Angiotensin converting enzyme (ACE)
	Calcium
Scarlet fever	Group A streptococci latex screen, serum
	Throat culture for group A β-hemolytic streptococci
Scleroderma	Scl-70 antibody
Scurvy	Ascorbic acid: serum, plasma
Sjögren's syndrome	SS-A (Ro), SS-B (La) antibodies
Sporotrichosis	Skin culture
Streptococcal infection	Group A streptococci latex screen
Stress states	Catecholamines: norepinephrine, epinephrine, dopamine
Syphilis	Darkfield
	RPR, VDRL
	FTA-ABS, serum

continued

Disease	Tests
Systemic lupus erythematosus	ANA
	Anti-DNA
	Antibodies to extractable nuclear antigens
Thrombosis, infarct	Coagulation factor survey
	Protein C
	Protein S
Thrush	Throat culture
Vaginitis, vaginosis	Herpes simplex
	Neisseria gonorrhoeae culture
	Trichomonas preparation
	Bacterial culture
Varicella	Viral culture
	Varicella-zoster antibodies
Vasculitis	Immune complexes
	Cryoglobulins
	ASO titer
Viral infection	Culture, serology:
	Cytomegalovirus
	Enterovirus
	Epstein-Barr virus
	Herpes simplex virus
	Influenza virus
	Mumps virus
	Parainfluenza virus
	Respiratory syncytial virus
Virilization	Testosterone
Xanthoma	Cholesterol
	Triglycerides
	Lipid panel

Bacterial Infections

> Wentworth BB (ed): **Diagnostic procedures** for **bacterial infections**. Washington, DC, American Public Health Association, 1987, 868 pp.
>
> This book takes you well beyond smear and culture. It is a complete, detailed guide on the laboratory diagnosis of bacterial infections.

> Aronson MD, Bor DH: **Blood cultures**. Ann Intern Med 1987; 106:246–253.
>
> The blood culture is the only test used to define bacteremia. To be successful, it calls for large-volume samples (10 to 30 ml) taken on at least three different occasions, under rigorously sterile conditions. The large volume of blood required comes from the fact that 1 ml contains less than 30 colony-forming units. The need for multiple cultures reflects the intermittent nature of bacteremia, analogous to the spiking of fevers. The sterile conditions relate to avoidance of contaminant nonpathogenic organisms on the skin and elsewhere. Nonetheless, 2 to 3% false-positives occur. But in immunocompromised patients the normally harmless nonpathogen becomes pathogenic. When **transient bacteremia** plays a role in eliciting skin disease, as in **vasculitis, psoriasis,** or **purpura**, it is important to know:
>
> 1. Bacteremia occurs in up to 85% of patients having a **dental procedure**. Usually it occurs in the first 1 to 5 minutes and clears by 15 minutes.
> 2. Bacteremia occurs in the course of localized infections or when infected tissue is manipulated or surgically drained. (The **infected gallbladder** thus could be responsible for bacteremic pulses. We recall a patient with **recalcitrant hand eczema** not cured until she had a cholecystectomy.)
> 3. Bacteremia even occurs with innocuous-appearing events, such as **tooth brushing** and **bowel movement**. (Recall that the **stool is 25% bacteria**. We had a patient with adult **acneiform folliculitis** cured by the simple

remedy of a tablespoon of mineral oil per day. Averting a rough passage through the bowels may have averted pathogenic bacteremia.

Komaroff AL: Urinalysis and urine culture in women with **dysuria**. Ann Intern Med 1986; 104:212–218.

Urinalysis will reveal the hallmark of urinary tract infection, viz., the presence of telltale **leukocytes**. Such pyuria is clinically significant if there are 2 to 5 leukocytes per high power field.

Flushing

Grahame-Smith DG: What is the cause of the **carcinoid flush**? Gut 1987; 28:1413–1416.

Measure levels during flushing attack:

bradykinin	Plasma
(Interscience Institute, Inglewood, CA 90301, 800-421-7133)	
histamine	Blood, urine
(Smith Kline, BioScience Labs, St. Louis, MO 63146, 800-665-7525)	
prostaglandins	Plasma
(thromboxane B_2)	
(prostacyclin [6-keto-$PGF_{1\alpha}$]	
(Mayo Medical Labs, Rochester, MN 55905, 800-533-1710)	
serotonin	Serum
(5-hydroxytryptamine)	
serotonin metabolite	Urine
(5-hydroxyindoleacetic acid) 5-HIAA	
(Nichols Institute Reference Laboratories, San Juan Capistrano, CA 92675, 800-553-5445)	
substance P	Plasma
(Smith Kline Labs, St. Louis, MO 63146, 800-669-7525)	

Fungal Infection

Frey D, Oldfield RJ, Bridger RC: A Colour Atlas of **Pathogenic Fungi**. London, Wolfe Medical Publications, Ltd., 1979, 168 pp.

If you can grow it, you can identify it with this book and a microscope at your side. Magnificent full-color gross and microscopic portraits of all the pathogenic fungi you could ever see world wide.

Immune Disease

Peter JB: The Use and Interpretation of Tests in Clinical Immunology, 6th ed. Omaha, Interstate Press, 1989, 89 pp.

A valuable paperback that provides clinical insight into all the tests that can be done on a patient with immune disease. It is fully referenced, and the writing is sharply focused. The author is the president of Specialty Laboratories, Inc. (2211 Michigan Avenue, Santa Monica, CA, 1-800-421-7110).

Beutner EH (ed): Handbook of Clinical Relevance of Tests. Buffalo, Immco Diagnostics, 1989, 24 pp.

Another paperback of value in knowing what to order and what it means for vesiculobullous disease and connective tissue diseases.

In **vesiculobullous disease**, serum shows:

intercellular antibodies in more than 90% of patients with pemphigus (all forms)

IgG class **basement membrane zone (BMZ) antibodies**:
in about 70% of patients with bullous pemphigoid
in 10% with cicatricial pemphigoid
in 25% with epidermolysis bullosa acquisita
in none with hereditary epidermolysis bullosa
HG: special IgG class BMZ antibody: in 50% with herpes gestationis
IgA class BMZ antibodies: in 10% with linear IgA bullous dermatoses
IgA class EmA (endomysial antibodies): in 70% with dermatitis herpetiformis

Details are given on the significance of the antibodies to (1) nuclei (ANA), (2) native DNA, DNP, histone, (3) extractable nuclear antigens (ENA): SM, RNP, SS-A (Ro), SS-B (La), Scl-70, Jo-1, PCNA, Ku, (4) phospholipids (lupus anticoagulant).

Use ANA titers (>160) and patterns (peripheral) as screen for **systemic lupus erythematosus (SLE)**.
Native DNA as well as SM antibodies are diagnostic of **SLE** when found.
Histone antibodies suggest **drug-induced lupus**.
RNP antibodies indicate **mixed connective tissue disease**.
SS-A (Ro) and SS-B (La) antibodies suggest **Sjögren's syndrome**.
Scl-70 antibodies are marker for **scleroderma**, occurring in nearly half of the cases.
Jo-1 antibodies are marker for **polymyositis**.
Antibodies to Ku (Ki) and PCNA are of little clinical value.
Antibodies to phospholipids (lupus anticoagulant) occur in patients with **phlebitis, thrombosis, livedo, ulcers, ischemia, necrosis**.

For a copy, write Immco Diagnostics, 963 Kenmore Avenue, Buffalo, NY 14223.

Kaye BR, Fainstat M: **Antinuclear antibodies**. *In* Louis AA (ed): Handbook of Difficult Diagnosis. New York, Churchill Livingstone, 1990, pp 434–448.

Although a positive antinuclear antibody test is a diagnostic criterion for systemic lupus erythematosus (SLE), it is **not specific** for the disease. A positive test is seen in many other infectious, hematologic, hepatic, pulmo-nary, rheumatologic, and neoplastic diseases, as well as being induced by many drugs.

Note: Some "ANAs" are not antibodies to nuclear antigens, but are really antibodies to cytoplasmic, ribosomal, or nucleolar proteins.

A **homogeneous** patterning suggests a drug etiology as well as SLE.

A **speckled** pattern is the most common and shows the widest range of causes.

The **peripheral** pattern is seen with a wide variety of conditions exhibiting double-stranded DNA reactivity.

The **nucleolar** pattern more often suggests scleroderma or Raynaud's disease.

The positive ANA test tells you something is broke, but it sure doesn't tell you what to fix.

Henriques HF III, Phillips TM: **Immune complex assays:** A clinical and laboratory review. Am Clin Products Review, Oct. 1987, pp 28–31.

Antibody (made up of any or all five immunoglobulins, IgA, IgD, IgE, IgG, IgM) binds to an antigen, resulting in an immune complex. This promotes invader recognition and activation of the cellular immune system. The size of the immune complex macromolecule determines whether the complex will be **soluble or circulating**. Its size, as well as anatomic hemodynamic factors and the presence of IgG receptors, determines its deposition and its pathogenicity. These complexes have a pathogenic role in systemic lupus erythematosus, thrombocytopenia, and serum sickness, as well as rheumatoid arthritis.

There are nonspecific assays for quantification of these immune complexes, but none for specific quantitation. The commonly available antigen-nonspecific assay is the C1q binding (**ELISA**) assay. The **Raji cell assays** remain very expensive, involving cell cultured lines of lymphoma cells with many cell surface receptors for C3.

Complement is a series of **enzymes** (C1–C9) that bind to the immune complex. These complement factors allow the antibody to either destroy the antigen (unknown) or attach to the macrophage for presentation to the cellular immune system. Thus, complement provides the bridge between cellular and serum immune systems. The initiating complement C1q recognizes the tail position (Fc) of the antibody and initiates a cascade of sequential complement component activation.

Council on Scientific Affairs: In vitro **testing for allergy**. Report II of the Allergy Panel. JAMA 1987; 258;1639–1643.

Circulating immune complexes are not of diagnostic value at this time.

Complement (total hemolytic CH_{50}, C3, C4) is used to evaluate and follow up patients with **lupus erythematosus** and with **necrotizing vasculitis**. It is also useful to detect individuals with a genetic lack of this defense system or of its inhibitor.

IgE correlates in a general way with sensitivity to allergens. Watch for its elevation in IgE myeloma, hyperimmunoglobulinemia, **staphylococcal abscess syndrome**, parasitic disease, and allergic bronchopulmonary aspergillosis.

T- and B-lymphocyte cell assays permit (1) evaluation of past immune capabilities, (2) characterization of **leukemias** and **lymphomas**, (3) evaluation of immune deficiencies.

No testing procedure can replace an adequate clinical history and careful physical examination.

Yates VM, Kerr REI, Frier K, et al: Early diagnosis of **infantile** seborrhoeic dermatitis and atopic dermatitis: Total and specific IgE levels. Br J Dermatol 1983; 108:639–645.

It is possible to **distinguish atopic and seborrheic dermatitis** in infants before the classic clinical features have evolved. This is done by performing the radioallergosorbent (**RAST**) tests for **egg white** and **milk antibodies**.

All nine atopic infants studied had a positive RAST to egg white and seven of the nine to milk: Not one of 27 patients with infantile seborrheic dermatitis showed positive tests. Measuring the **IgE level** also permits distinguishing these two diseases, but to a lesser degree of accuracy. The IgE level was above normal in 8 of 9 infants with atopic dermatitis, whereas only 2 of 27 infants with seborrheic dermatitis showed elevated IgE levels.

Dahl MV: Clinical Immunodermatology, 2nd ed. Chicago, Year Book Medical Publishers, Inc., 1988, 422 pp.

Details on laboratory evaluation of immune function with such pearls as (1) **quantitative immunoglobulin levels** are better than immunoelectrophoresis in uncovering immunoglobulin deficiency; (2) **total hemolytic complement** (**CH_{50}**) is the best test for screening classic pathway complement deficiency or dysfunction; (3) the number of **small lymphocytes** in a blood smear is a gross reflection of the number of **circulating T cells**.

Tests to evaluate patient's **immune status**:

> **Humoral (B-cell–dependent)**
> quantitative IgG, IgM, IgA, IgE
> peripheral blood B-cell count
> Total hemolytic complement (CH_{50})
> X-ray of pharynx and chest

> **Cell mediated (T-cell–dependent)**
> peripheral blood T-cell count
> intradermal skin test
> dinitrochlorobenzene (DNCB) sensitization
> Helper T4/suppressor T8 T-cell ratio

> **Effector cell function**
> Rebuck skin window technique
> irritant patch test
> neutrophil count
> nitroblue tetrazolium test

Bos JD: Skin immune system (SIS). Boca Raton, Fla, CRC Press, Inc., 1990, 501 pp.

The master background reference for understanding immune disease of the skin.

Be alert to **primary immunodeficiency skin diseases** revealed by laboratory study:

> low T- and B-cell counts
> agammaglobulinemia
> hypogammaglobulinemia
> IgA deficiency
> hyperimmunoglobulin E syndrome
> growth hormone deficiency
> kappa-chain deficiency
> phagocyte function defect
> > neutrophil-6-phosphate
> > dehydrogenase deficiency
> > myeloperoxidase deficiency
> > leukocyte adherence deficiency
> transcobalamin II deficiency
> complement deficiencies
> > $C1_q$, $C1_r$, C2, C3, C4, C5, C6, C7, C8 α, β, γ or C9 deficiency
> > C1-inhibitor deficiency
> > factor I, factor H
> > properdin
> chromosomal abnormalities
> metal transport defects (low zinc)
> orotic aciduria
> biotin–dependent carboxylase deficiency
> purine-nucleoside phosphorylase deficiency
> adenosine deaminase deficiency

Lyme Disease

Duffy J, Mertz LE, Wobig GH, Katzmann JA: Diagnosing Lyme disease: The contribution of serologic testing. Mayo Clin Proc 1988; 63:1116–1121.

The paucity of *Borrelia burgdorferi* spirochetes in the skin lesions of Lyme disease makes both culture and histologic visualization by stain a rare event. Accordingly, the only laboratory assistance of real usefulness is the detection of circulating antibodies to *B. burgdorferi*.

A single specimen is sufficient for the currently popular **ELISA test**. In the early stages, only half of the cases will prove positive. Subsequent tests are not satisfactory, since the immediate treatment-instituted as well as the disease-induced immunosuppression abrogates the diagnostic antibody response. The test is not infallible because of the background value of antispirochetal and cross-reacting antibodies.

A **positive serologic test** for Lyme disease is **not essential to the diagnosis**.

Nutrition

Roe DA (ed): **Nutrition** and the Skin. New York, A.R. Liss, Inc., 1986, 199 pp.

Twenty **vitamin** and **mineral assays** for detection of deficiency syndromes in skin:

ascorbic acid	niacin
biotin	protein
cobalamin (vitamin B_{12})	pyridoxine
calcium	riboflavin
copper	thiamine (B_1)
essential fatty acids (RBC triene/tetraene ratio)	vitamin A
folic acid	vitamin D
iodine	vitamin E
iron	vitamin K
magnesium	zinc

Humphries LL, Adams LJ, Eckfeldt JH, et al: Hyperamylasemia in patients with **eating disorders**. Ann Intern Med 1987; 106:50–52.

Increased serum amylase is common (35%) among patients with bulimia and anorexia nervosa, but usually does not signal pancreatitis. If serum lipase and pancreatic isoamylase activities are normal, the amylase is of salivary gland origin and further work-up for pancreatitis is unnecessary.

Neldner KH: Zinc nutriture and the skin. *In* Roe DA (ed): Nutrition and the Skin. New York, A.R. Liss, Inc., 1986, pp 131–149.

Disorders and conditions producing **zinc-deficiency dermatoses**:

dietary–high fiber, **alcohol**, parenteral feeding
gastrointestinal–**gastrectomy**, bowel resection, blind loop syndromes, malabsorption
traumatic–surgery, burns
malignant disease–all types
infection–parasitic
renal disorder–dialysis, nephrotic syndrome, renal tubular disease
iatrogenic–antimetabolite drugs, chelation therapy
genetic–acrodermatitis enteropathica, **diabetes mellitus**
miscellaneous–hemolytic anemia, collagen vascular disease, **pregnancy**

It pays to think zinc when looking at a strange dermatitis. Order a **plasma level** determination, but be sure that rubber stoppers are not used and that the specimen doesn't hemolyze. Red cells and rubber stoppers are zinc rich!

Parasitic Diseases

Marshall EK, Voge M: Medical Parasitology, 6th ed. Philadelphia, W.B. Saunders Company, 1986, 383 pp.

To make the diagnosis:

Examine the stool:

> Wet film, sedimentation or flotation techniques for concentration, stained slides, and culture (*Entamoeba histolytica*).
> Do not examine stools after barium enema. Wait 1 week.
> Avoid antibiotics for a whole month before examination.
> Avoid antacids, milk of magnesia, kaolin, or bismuth medication.
> Do not use mineral or castor oil for purgation.
> If Fleet's enema is used, discard first-movement specimen.

Examine the blood:

> **Fresh blood** preparation must be thin so red cells don't obscure visualization. Look for whiplike motions of microfilariae or undulating trypanosomes.
> **Stained thin blood films** permit visualization of trypanosomes, microfilariae, and intracellular malarial parasites.
> Thick blood films are also useful.
> Parasitic infections account for only 4% of cases of **eosinophilia** (more than 5% eosinophils). Half of all cases are due to **atopic disease** or **lymphoma**.

Examine **tissue smears**:

> Look for *Leishmania* or *Toxoplasma*.
> Animal inoculation rarely used.

Examine **serologic tests**:

amebiasis	schistosomiasis
toxoplasmosis	cysticercosis
leishmaniasis	hydatid disease
Chagas' disease	trichinosis

Porphyria

Harber LC, Bickers DR: Photosensitivity Diseases. Principles of Diagnosis and Treatment, 2nd ed. Philadelphia, B.C. Decker, 1989, pp 421–433.

Data from the porphyrin laboratory:

DIAGNOSIS	PORPHYRIN	SPECIMEN
porphyria cutanea tarda	uroporphyrin I & III	urine
hepatoerythropoietic porphyria	protoporphyrin IX	RBC
	isocoproporphyrin	feces
erythropoietic porphyria	uroporphyrin I	urine
erythropoietic protoporphyria	protoporphyrin IX	RBC
variegate porphyria	porphobilinogen	urine
acute intermittent porphyria	porphobilinogen	urine
hereditary coproporphyria	coproporphyrin	feces

Details are provided for testing procedures and normal ranges.

Syphilis

Luger AFH: **Serologic diagnosis of syphilis:** Current methods. *In* Young H, McMillan A (eds): Immunological Diagnosis of Sexually Transmitted Diseases. New York, Marcel Dekker, Inc., 1988, pp 249–274.

A definitive 25-page review.

1. Tests using **lipoidal antigens**:

   > In 1941, Mary Pangborn isolated cardiolipin from ox hearts. It is a diphospholipid that is inert, but upon the addition of lecithin and choles-

terol becomes serologically active, reacting with the "**reagins**" or **Wassermann antibodies** in the sera of patients with syphilis. These reagins are autoantibodies against components in mitochondrial membrane.

The one lipoidal antigen test that has supplanted all the rest of the "Wassermann tests" is the **VDRL** (Venereal Disease Research Laboratory) test, developed at the CDC in Atlanta in 1946.

The antigen is 0.03% cardiolipin, 0.21% lecithin, and 0.9% cholesterol in saline solution. The addition of heated serum containing the antibodies of syphilis induces microscopically visible flocculation. Serially doubling the serum dilution provides a quantitative essay, whereas the highest dilution that can be classified as reactive is reported as the titer. The result is available in 40 minutes. For the Rapid Plasma Reagin test (**RPR**), charcoal is added to the antigen and the test read on a plastic card in 5 minutes.

The test usually becomes positive 4 to 5 weeks after infection. One in a hundred of the patients with secondary syphilis show a negative test when undiluted serum is used, but on further dilutions the test becomes positive (**prozone phenomenon**).

Following adequate treatment of a patient **in the first few months** of the disease, the **VDRL becomes nonreactive in 6 to 12 months**. If treatment is given later, the reactivity may be present up to 5 years later. Indeed, one in five may still have reactive tests 30 to 35 years later. Proper treatment ordinarily ensures a fourfold drop in titer at 3 months, whereas a fourfold increase in titer indicates treatment failure or reinfection.

In the untreated individual, the test will spontaneously reverse in 25 to 40% of instances over a period of years.

Nonspecific reactivity, i.e., the **biologic false-positive** (BFP), occurs in less than 1% of all sera examined, but in 5 to 8% of all reactive samples. It is **caused mainly by IgM autoantibodies (rheumatoid factor)** and is thus seen in autoimmune disease. Nearly half of patients with **systemic lupus erythematosus** have a positive VDRL. It is also found in patients with increased turnover of nucleic acids, as in **infectious mononucleosis**, viral pneumonia, malignant disease, **leprosy**, psittacosis, and **malaria**.

2. Tests using *Treponema pallidum* **antigen:**

For the greatest sensitivity and specificity, the pathogen itself (or fragments) is used as the antigen. The test remains positive, since it is so sensitive in detecting the specific diagnostic IgG antibody. The treponemal antigen allows two basic test procedures:

A. Fluorescent treponemal antibody absorption (**FTA-ABS**) test

In this test, *Treponema pallidum*, harvested from rabbit orchitis and acetone fixed on slides, is the antigen. The serum to be tested is first diluted in a sorbent of Reiter treponemes to remove the antibodies against nonpathogenic treponemes. The serum is then placed on the slide and incubated to allow the antibodies to attach to the pathogenic treponemes. These antibodies are visualized by adding a fluorescein isothiocyanate-labeled antiglobulin, which attaches to them and can be seen by means of a fluorescent microscope. The intensity of fluorescence is graded from 1 to 4 plus. Quantitation is undertaken using a serial trebling dilution of sera starting at 1:5, and usually the test is scored only as reactive or nonreactive at a 1:5 dilution.

This test becomes reactive at least 1 to 2 weeks before all other tests. Because of this and its high specificity and sensitivity it is the most reliable test available in doubtful cases.

B. *Treponema pallidum* hemagglutination assay (**TPHA**) and the micro-hemagglutination with *T. pallidum* antigen test (**MHA-TP**)

In this test, sheep erythrocytes treated with formalin and coated with an ultrasonicate of orchitis–derived *T. pallidum* serve as the antigen. The serum is first incubated in a diluent containing the nonpathogenic (Reiter) treponemes and rabbit testicular tissue and also extracts of sheep and beef erythrocytes. It is then incubated for 18 hours with the *T. pallidum*–coated red cells, which agglutinate in the presence of the specific antibody to *T. pallidum*. Sera are recovered at 1:80 dilution, with quantitation made by serial doubling dilutions from 1:80 to 1:5120. This test is the most sensitive and most specific method for detecting antibodies to *T. pallidum*. The margin of error is between 0.008% false-nonreactive and 0.07% false-reactive findings. It generally remains positive for life.

A variant of the TPHA test is the microhemagglutination test with *T. pallidum* antigen (MHA-TP), which is much less expensive as it requires smaller amounts of reagents.

C. Solid phase hemadsorption (**SPHA**) test

The same reagents required for the MHA-TP test are used in the solid phase hemadsorption test (SPHA) to detect antitreponemal IgM antibodies (IgM-SPHA). The wells of polystyrene microtiter plates are coated with μ chain–specific serum (anti-IgM). The patient's serum is added and incubated for 30 minutes. After rinsing, the MHA-TP test is performed. The serum IgM binds to the walls of the wells, and antitreponemal IgM reacts with the TPHA antigen. The test is reactive if agglutination occurs at a dilution greater than or equal to 1:8.

3. **Detection of IgM antibodies:**

Specific tests for IgM antibodies include:
a. 19S-IgM-FTA-ABS
b. IgM-SPHA
c. IgM-ELISA (enzyme-linked immunosorbent assay)

Reactivity indicates either **new or active infection** and the need for treatment. These IgM antibodies are the first demonstrable sign of a humoral response to *T. pallidum* and are detectable at the **end of the second week of infection**. IgM titers decline rapidly after adequate treatment, and **persistence indicates treatment failure**. Antitreponemal IgM in the CSF indicates neurosyphilis, provided that the blood/CSF barrier function is normal.

4. Diagnosis of **neurosyphilis**:

A **lumbar puncture** or cisternal puncture is essential in patients with reactive serum tests but no history of infection with *T. pallidum*, particularly if these findings persist unchanged after treatment. The findings of abnormal CSF cytology and elevated protein (Dattner-Thomas formula, cell count $>5 \times 10^6$/liter, and total protein above 0.45 gm/liter) indicate inflammation without a specific cause. However, restoration of these findings to normal is the first indication of the effectiveness of treatment. Traditional diagnostic criteria for neurosyphilis are inadequate because of atypical presentations and the finding that CSF VDRL tests are nonreactive in 30 to 47% of patients with active neurosyphilis.

The **diagnosis of neurosyphilis** can be **established** by:
a. Treponemal hemagglutination (TPHA) index above 100
b. *T. pallidum* agglutination (TPA) index above 2
c. CSF IgM-SPHA test reactivity

    d. CSF IgM-ELISA test reactivity

The **diagnosis of neurosyphilis** is **excluded** by:

    a. CSF TPHA or CSF MHA-TP tests nonreactive

    b. CSF FTA-ABS test nonreactive

5. Diagnosis of **congenital syphilis**:

The detection of **IgM antibodies** for **T. pallidum** is essential for the diagnosis of congenital syphilis and indicates the need for treatment. IgM reactivity of serum in the newborn is proof of prenatal infection.

Thromboses, Intravascular Clotting

DeMott WR: Coagulation. *In* Jacobs DS, Kasten BL, DeMott WE, Wolfson WL: Laboratory Test Handbook, 2nd ed, with key word index. Baltimore, Williams & Wilkins, 1990, pp 369–437.

A complete survey of what can be done in a modern coagulation laboratory. These often-expensive tests are best ordered under the direction of a hematologist.

With a patient who has **thrombotic disease** it is simplest to order the **hypercoagulable state coagulation screen**. This commonly includes antithrombin III, protein C, protein S, factors VII and XII, and a platelet aggregation determination. For assessment of **disseminated intravascular coagulation**, an **intravascular coagulation screen** is ordered. This includes a platelet count, fibrinogen, thrombin time, partial thromboplastin time, dilute clot lysis, fibrin breakdown products, and a blood smear to detect microangiopathic changes in the red blood cells.

Strickler H, Lammle B, Furlan M, Sulzer I: Heparin-dependent *in vitro* aggregation of normal platelets by plasma of a patient with **heparin-induced skin necrosis**: Specific diagnostic test for rare side effect. Am J Med 1988; 85:721–724.

Heparin can induce **thrombocytopenia, deep-vein thrombosis**, and **skin necrosis** at the **site** of its **subcutaneous injection**. The syndrome, HATT, can be detected by adding the patient's heparinized plasma to platelet-rich plasma preparations from normal individuals. The patient's plasma will induce a diagnostic rapid consistent aggregation of the normal platelet suspensions. The etiologic factor is a circulating immunoglobulin in the patient's blood.

Suchman AL, Griner PF: Diagnostic uses of the activated partial thromboplastin time and prothrombin time. Ann Intern Med 1986; 104:810–816.

Of all the tests known to assess the **ability of blood to clot**, the two best are the activated **partial thromboplastin time** and the **prothrombin time**. If the results of both tests are normal, no further study of the coagulation system is necessary.

Note that the prothrombin time measures the activity of factor VII, the coagulant made by the liver and whose synthesis is inhibited by warfarin (**Coumadin**). Patients taking warfarin usually have monthly determinations of **prothrombin time** to monitor the required therapeutic dose. Alternatively, when **heparin** is used as a direct anticoagulant, therapy is monitored by the activated **partial thromboplastin time**.

Rick ME: **Protein C** and **protein S**. Vitamin K-dependent inhibitors of blood coagulation. JAMA 1990; 263:701–703.

Young patients with **venous thrombosis**, those with recurrent thrombosis without other obvious causes, and all those with family histories of thrombotic disease should be screened for deficiencies of protein C and protein S.

Coumadin skin necrosis and **ulcers** develop because of capillary thrombosis as a result of Coumadin's impairing the synthesis of protein C. Liver disease is another cause of deficiency in both protein C and protein S.

Viral Disease

Versteeg J: Color Atlas of Virology. Chicago, Year Book Medical Publishers, Inc., 1985, 240 pp.

A wonderful color tour through the land of **laboratory virology**.

Lee PC, Hallsworth P: Rapid viral diagnosis in perspective. Br Med J 1990; 300:1413–1418.

Herpes simplex virus

Culture in permissive cell lines permits visual evidence of the presence of the virus in 99% of cases by the fourth day.

Enzyme immunoassay kits permit same-day diagnosis with 95% sensitivity and 100% specificity.

Varicella-zoster virus

Culture is unsatisfactory.

Monoclonal antibody kit permits rapid detection with a 92% sensitivity.

Electron microscopy provides presumptive diagnosis since only in zoster is the virus found in such large numbers.

It does not distinguish the HZV from other herpes viruses.

Cytomegalovirus

Centrifugation-enhanced culture is the method of choice.

Monoclonal antibodies allow detection the same day using leukocytes.

Epstein-Barr virus

Best test is Paul-Bunnell assay for **heterophile antibodies**. It involves a rapid slide agglutination procedure using horse or sheep red cells. False-positives occur at rate of 7%.

Enzyme immunoassay kits now use Epstein-Barr viral antigen trapped in nuclear extract for detecting IgM and IgG antibodies.

Human immunodeficiency virus

Kits use viral antigen bound to plastic to bind and assay serum IgM and IgG antibodies.

Agglutination kits will now give usually reliable results in 30 minutes.

Western blot assay is the gold standard, but technically very difficult.

Note that latent period between infection and appearance of antibodies is usually less than 3 months, but may last for years. Antigen assays are the only alternative during this window period. These are based on enzyme immunoassays.

Chlamydia trachomatis

This is a bacterial pathogen traditionally cultured by viral laboratories. Currently, immunoassays (enzyme) or immunofluorescence allow detection of *Chlamydia* antigen.

Papilloma virus

The dream is that the **polymerase chain reaction** will amplify the DNA segment from a single wart virus gene to a level readily detectable by ethidium bromide staining or hybridization.

DERMATOLOGIC HEALTH PROFILE

TEST	ASSOCIATION
☐ ACE	Sarcoidosis
☐ Aminoacids	Metabolic error
☐ Ammonia	Metabolic error
☐ α_1-Antichymotrypsin	Pruritus, cholinergic urticaria
☐ α_1-Antitrypsin	Panniculitis
	Painful nodules
	Angioedema
	Factitial-like "diggers"
☐ Biotinidase	Hair loss
☐ Coagulogram:	Thrombosis
☐ Antithrombin III	Thrombosis
☐ Protein C	
☐ Protein S	
☐ C1 esterase	Hereditary angioedema
☐ Cold agglutinins, cryoglobulin, cryofibrinogen	Cold sensitivity
☐ Complement CH_{50}	C1q, second, third, fourth, fifth components
☐ EBV antibodies	Connective tissue disease
☐ Endocrine screen:	
☐ Testosterone	Hair loss, hirsutism
☐ DHEA	Hair loss, hirsutism
☐ Estrone	Hair loss, hirsutism
☐ Prolactin	Hair loss, hirsutism
☐ FTA-ABS	Syphilis
☐ α-Galactosidase	Fabry's disease
☐ Glucagon	Glucagonoma
☐ Glucose-6-dehydrogenase	Dapsone sensitivity
☐ HIV antibodies	AIDS
☐ Hepatitis screen	Hepatitis, urticaria
☐ Human chorionic gonadotropin	Pregnancy
☐ IgE	Atopy
☐ Lyme test	*Borrelia* infection
☐ Pemphigus antibodies	Pemphigus
☐ Porphyrin screen:	Photosensitivity
☐ Urine	
☐ Stool	
☐ RBC	
☐ Scl-70 antibody	Scleroderma
☐ Streptococcal antibodies	Psoriasis
☐ Substance P	Flushing
☐ Tyrosine	Keratoderma
☐ Vitamin assays	Nutrition and therapy
☐ A	
☐ B_1	
☐ B_2	
☐ B_6	
☐ B_{12}	
☐ C	
☐ D	
☐ E	
☐ Zinc	Acrodermatitis enteropathica

A photocopy of this can be checked as appropriate and given to the laboratory.

SCREENING PANELS AND PROFILES

☐ Amino acid screen	M
☐ Cellular immunity panel	SK
☐ Coagulation screen	SK
☐ Complement evaluation	SK
☐ Fungus group (systemic)	SK
Aspergillus, Blastomyces, Coccidioides, Cryptococcus, Histoplasma	
☐ Hepatitis	M
☐ Hirsutism	N
☐ IgE (RAST) antibody panels	M
☐ Seasonal inhalants—grasses, trees, weeds	
☐ Nonseasonal inhalants—animals, house dust, mites, molds, smoke	
☐ Foods—dairy, fish, fruit, greens, meats, nuts, vegetables, chocolate, coffee	
☐ Other—penicillin, insulin (5 types), insects, parasites—*Ascaris, Echinococcus*	
☐ Inborn errors of metabolism	M
☐ Lipid panel	N
☐ Lipoprotein profile	M
☐ Liver panel	SK
☐ Lupus panel	SK
☐ Lymphadenopathy panel	SK
☐ Maculopapular rash (adenovirus, rubella, rubeola)	SK
☐ TORCH (congenital infection)	SK
☐ Thyroid antibody screen	M

M = Mayo Clinic Laboratories
SK = Smith Kline Bioscience Laboratories
N = Nichols Institute Reference Laboratories

GENERAL REFERENCE WORKS

Butterworth T, Cawley NS: **Laboratory diagnosis**. Clin Dermatol 1986; 4:1–140.

The key laboratory findings for **525 skin diseases** and syndromes are presented in a succinct alphabetized fashion according to disease and in a second section according to test.

Jacobs PH, Anhalt TS: Handbook of Skin Clues of Systemic Disease, 2nd ed. Philadelphia, Lea & Febiger, 1991, 150 pp.

A "what-to-look-for" and "**what-to-order**" book with alphabetized entries according to disease.

Jacobs DS, Kasten BL, DeMott WR, Wolfson WH: **Laboratory Test Handbook with key word index**, 2nd ed. Baltimore, Williams & Wilkins, 1990, 1244 pp.

The one book to have if you're having only one. A marvelously heuristic guide to interpretative analysis of chemical, serologic, and microbiologic data, with a key word index to advise you what to order.

Pearls—The most relevant reference ranges are those provided by your laboratory. **Most tests do not have sharp cut-off points between normal and abnormal.** Many values are altered by posture, exercise, food, age, weight, and medicine.

Infants and **young children** have their own normal ranges.

Pregnancy increases alkaline phosphatase. **Contraceptives** increase T_4.

Have patient in **fasting state** for iron, iron-binding capacity, potassium, lipids, blood sugar, B_{12}-folate levels.

Caffeine elevates catecholamine levels.

A **traumatic venipuncture** produces hemolysis and may invalidate coagulation tests, as well as give spurious high values for serum AST and ALT, LDH, acid phosphatase, bilirubin, and magnesium.

Urethral catheterization, sex, menstruation can be responsible for a few red cells in urine.

Blood taken after **exercise** will show high CPK.

Some values show **circadian rhythms** (e.g., eosinophils low in afternoon), so comparisons require samples taken at same time of day.

Hand clenching with tourniquet increases potassium.

Prolonged contact with clot or a lipemic specimen introduces errors.

Instruments in the laboratory may go wrong, always obeying Murphy's law, third corollary: "If there is a possibility of several things going wrong, the one that will cause the most damage will be the one to go wrong." Remember, there is always the possibility that the patient is healthy, and it's the laboratory that is unhealthy.

Wallach J: Interpretation of Diagnostic Tests: A Synopsis of Laboratory Medicine, 4th ed. Boston, Little, Brown & Co., 1986, 825, pp.

Superb, easy-to-use handbook of specific laboratory examinations, as well as what to look for in disease of organ systems. It also has a special section on **drug interference in laboratory testing**. This paperback can be carried in your white-coat pocket, giving you "skin-manship" on rounds.

Note diagnostic value of **color of sweat**:

brown:	ochronosis
red:	rifampin
blue:	copper, occupational exposure
blue-black:	chromhidrosis

Sox HC Jr: Common Diagnostic Tests. Use and Interpretation. Philadelphia, American College of Physicians, 1987, 380 pp.

Essay type accounts of the meaning behind your everyday general laboratory tests.

Siest G, Galteau M-M: **Drug Effects on Laboratory Test Results**: Analytical Interferences and Pharmacologic Effects. Littleton, Mass, PSG Publishing Co., Inc., 1988, 528 pp.

A book on how to judge the validity of laboratory analyses from a drug-polluted blood stream.

Tietz NW (ed): Textbook of Clinical Chemistry. Philadelphia, W.B. Saunders Company, 1986, 1919 pp.

A mammoth tome that tells you all—biochemistry techniques, values, interpretation, metabolic pathways, and history.

Leavelle DE: **Mayo Medical Laboratories Interpretive Handbook**, 6th ed. Rochester, Minn, Mayo Medical Laboratories, 1990, 277 pp.

Here is an invaluable source of succinct, clearly understandable data on what tests can be done, how they are done, and what they mean. The appendices include a complete list of 34 lysosomal storage disorders, their clinical features, and their specific diagnostic enzyme deficits. Also listed are the seven types of porphyria and the diagnostic tests recommended for each. Using this will improve your diagnostic game!

The Compleat Diagnostician's Bookshelf

Many of my colleagues go to meetings to listen to presentations, but I prefer to read because I can better direct my attention than if I am at the mercy of the speaker.

JOSHUA LEDERBERG

No diagnostic resource is more invigorating than a personal library into which you can dip and dive every day. A daily dip and dive are a must to bring to mind both the old and the new. Scan the atlases to enhance your instant recognition of those rare expressions of disease in skin. Dive deep into the monographs, texts, and journals for help with that puzzling patient. You will find it. Even the titles will call forth serendipitous and fruitful thoughts.

DO I SEE WHAT IS THERE?

Jackson R: Morphological Dermatology: A Study of the Living Gross Pathology of the Skin. Springfield, IL, Charles C Thomas, 1979, 338 pp.

A book to teach you how to see what others can't.

CAN I FIND IT IN AN ATLAS?

Du Vivier A: Atlas of Clinical Dermatology. Philadelphia, W.B. Saunders Co., 1986.

Scanning over a thousand of these clinical photographs is a good "warm-up" for any clinical diagnostic race. Each photo here should be as recognizable as an old friend. If not, make new friends.

Bork K, Bräuninger W: Diagnosis and Treatment of Common Skin Diseases. Philadelphia, W.B. Saunders Co., 1988, 247 pp.

Another superb "warm-up" book with color pictures of 400 more friends.

Bhutani LK: Colour Atlas of Dermatology. 3rd ed. Kent, England, Quest Meridien Ltd., 1986, 209 pp.

A classic collection of life-size color portraits of skin disease as seen in India.

Ferrandiz C: Clinical Atlas of Dermatology. Chicago, Year Book Publishers, Inc., 1987, 128 pp.

If you haven't many dermatologic acquaintances, start here.

Korting GW, Denk R: Differential Diagnosis in Dermatology. Philadelphia, W.B. Saunders Co., 1976, 767 pp.

If your friends look alike, use this atlas of 720 color photos of look-alikes.

Chessel GSJ, Jamieson MJ, Morton RA, et al (eds): Photo Dx, an Aid for the Study of Physical Diagnosis. Vols. 1–4, Chicago, Year Book Medical Publishers, Inc., 1984.

A paperback series with illustrations and quizzes on 776 patients.

Anonymous: 400 self-assessment picture tests in clinical medicine. Chicago, Year Book Medical Publishers, Inc., 1984, 280 pp.

More diagnostic color pictures culled from 40,000 examples found in over 100 specialty atlases.

Levene GM, Goolamali SK: Diagnostic Picture Tests in Dermatology. London, Wolfe Medical Publications, Ltd., 126 pp.

A glance favors the prepared mind; here is a small atlas to enhance your glance by preparing your mind.

Du Vivier A: Atlas of Infections of the Skin. Philadelphia, J.B. Lippincott, 1991, 128 pp.

Practice on these 236 full-color portraits.

Larsen WG, Adams RM, Maibach HI (eds): Color Text of Contact Dermatitis. Philadelphia, W.B. Saunders Co., 1992, 238 pp.

Scan this for 170 examples in vivid color of the hazards of exposure to contactants both epidermally and enterally.

IS YOUR PATIENT BLACK?

Rosen T, Martin S: Atlas of Black Dermatology. Boston, Little Brown and Company, 1981, 179 pp.

Invaluable guide, full of insight and wisdom, with a self-assessment quiz that is humbling for those who only see white patients.

Basset A, Liautaud B, Ndiaye B: Dermatology of Black Skin. New York, Oxford University Press, 1986, 114 pp.

A pocketbook of color plates to help you see the lesion behind the melanin.

Basset A, Maleville J, Basset M, Liautaud B: Infectious and Parasitic Diseases on Black Skin. London, Science Press Ltd., 1988, 116 pp.

A treasure of 230 color photographs from the hot, humid tropics.

McDonald J, Scott DA (eds): Dermatology in Black Patients. Dermatol Clin 1988; 6:343–496.

For the inexperienced, diagnosis of skin lesions in blacks is difficult because of the propensity of the black epidermis and dermis to proliferate. As a result, one sees unexpected follicular hyperkeratosis, lichenification, plaques, and nodules. In children, vesiculobullous reactions abound, and in adults, ulcers.

IS YOUR PATIENT YOUNG?

Zitelli BJ, Davis JW (eds): Atlas of Pediatric Physical Diagnosis. St. Louis, C.V. Mosby Co., 1987.

An absolutely superb giant color display of what you can learn by examining the skin of sick children. Browsing here is guaranteed to raise your "instant recognition index."

Caputo R, Ackerman AB, Sison-Torre EQ, Hirsch E: Pediatric Dermatology and Dermatopathology, A Text and Atlas. Philadelphia, Lea & Febiger, 1988.

Two hundred more color plates for your mental file.

Meneghini CL, Bonifazi E: An Atlas of Pediatric Dermatology. Chicago, Year Book Medical Publishers, 1985, 172 pp.

The more you look, the more you learn.

Weinberg S, Prose NS: Color Atlas of Pediatric Dermatology. 2nd ed. New York, McGraw-Hill, 1990, 264 pp.

The latest.

Hurwitz S: Clinical Pediatric Dermatology. A Textbook of Skin Disorders of Childhood and Adolescence. Philadelphia, W.B. Saunders Co., 1981, 481 pp.

Our favorite.

Schachner LA, Hansen RC (eds): Pediatric Dermatology, Vols. 1 & 2. New York, Churchill Livingstone, 1988, 1641 pp.

52 experts join together to give you the last word on the little ones and their big problems.

IS YOUR PATIENT OLD?

Marks R: Skin Disease in Old Age. Philadelphia, J.B. Lippincott Co., 1987, 276 pp.

A fine color tour of the aging terrain.

Korting GW: Geriatric Dermatology. Philadelphia, W.B. Saunders Co., 1980, 194 pp.

Another atlas in excellent color.

Newcomer VD, Young EM (eds): Geriatric Dermatology. Clinical Diagnosis and Practical Therapy. New York, Igaku-Shoin, 1989, 700 pp.

92 experts provide diagnostic aid in recognizing what's new with who's old.

Monk BE, Graham-Brown RAL, Sarkany I (eds): Skin Disorders in the Elderly. London, Blackwell Scientific Publications, 1988, 340 pp.

Identification insight from Great Britain on aged skin.

COULD MEDICATION BE THE CAUSE?

Bork K: Cutaneous Side Effects of Drugs. Philadelphia, W.B. Saunders Co., 1988, 422 pp.

Invaluable classic with over 400 superb color plates of all that drugs can do to the skin.

Dukes MNG, Beeley L (eds): Side Effects of Drugs Annual 13. A Worldwide Yearly Survey of New Data and Trends. New York, Elsevier, 1989, 532 pp.

Complete annual coverage of all the latest reports of drug reactions in the skin and elsewhere.

COULD YOUR PATIENT HAVE AIDS?

Penneys NS: Skin Manifestations of AIDS. Philadelphia, J.B. Lippincott Co., 1990, 210 pp.

A number one book on the number one diagnostic challenge in your practice. Exquisite color plates ranging from cryptococcosis of the tongue to linear Kaposi's sarcoma.

Weismann K, Petersen CS, Søndergaard J, Wantzin GL: Skin Signs in AIDS. Copenhagen, Munksgaard, 1988, 173 pp.

Another atlas to heighten your awareness of the innumerable skin signs pointing to AIDS.

Farthing CF, Brown SE, Staughton RCD: Color Atlas of AIDS and HIV Disease. 2nd ed. Chicago, Year Book Medical Publishers, Inc., 1988, 115 pp.

Extends your diagnostic vision to other organs as well as skin.

Friedman-Kien AE (ed): Color Atlas of AIDS. Philadelphia, W.B. Saunders Co., 1989, 155 pp.

An instructive pictorial view from the man who first discerned Kaposi's sarcoma as an index sign of an immune deficit in young homosexual men.

HAS YOUR PATIENT BEEN IN THE TROPICS?

Peters W, Gilles HM: A Colour Atlas of Tropical Medicine and Parasitology. 3rd ed. Boca Raton, FL, CRC Press, Inc., 1988, 240 pp.

750 pictures to guide you through the unusual snail-, soil-, and sneeze-mediated diseases of the tropics.

Canizares O (ed): Clinical Tropical Dermatology. London, Blackwell Scientific Publications, 1975, 464 pp.

Well-illustrated, comprehensive text.

Binford CH, Connor DH (eds): Pathology of Tropical and Extraordinary Diseases, 2 Vols. Washington, Armed Forces Institute of Pathology, 1976.

Another excellent resource on the cutaneous and extracutaneous hazards of life in the tropics.

Simons RDG, Marshall J (eds): Essays on Tropical Dermatology. Amsterdam, Excerpta Medica Foundation, 1969, 276 pp.

A wonderful scholarly reference source on the skin diseases of the tropics.

Pettit JHS, Parish LC: Manual of Tropical Dermatology. New York, Springer-Verlag, 1984, 260 pp.

Comprehensive survey with unique index of clinical signs, symptoms, and sites and their associated diseases, e.g., in urticaria, look for filariasis, schistosomiasis, and dracunculosis.

HAS YOUR PATIENT BEEN TO THE OCEAN?

Fisher AA: Atlas of Aquatic Dermatology. New York, Grune & Stratton, 1978, 113 pp.

If your patient caught it in the water, look here.

Halstead BW: Poisonous and Venomous Marine Animals of the World. 2nd ed. Princeton, NJ, Darwin Press, 1988, 1456 pp.

An unparalleled work, lavishly illustrated, providing the minutest detail of what marine life can do to human skin.

DOES ANYONE ELSE IN THE FAMILY HAVE IT?
HAS IT BEEN PRESENT SINCE BIRTH?

Alper J: Genetic Disorders of the Skin. Chicago, Mosby/Year Book, 1991, 378 pp.

The latest.

Buyse ML (ed): Birth Defects Enclopedia. Dover, MA, Center for Birth Defects Information Services Inc., 1990, 1892 pp.

The comprehensive, systematic illustrated reference source for diagnosis, delineation, etiology, biodynamics, occurrence, prevention, and treatment.

McKusick VA: Mendelian Inheritance in Man: Catalogs of Autosomal Dominant, Autosomal Recessive, and X-linked Phenotypes. 8th ed. Baltimore, The Johns Hopkins University Press, 1988, 1626 pp.

The Bible. If it isn't in here, it isn't.

Gorlin RJ, Cohen MM Jr., Levin LS: Syndromes of the Head and Neck. 3rd ed. New York, Oxford University Press, 1990, 1620 pp.

2300 photographs with details of 400 new syndromes. Unsurpassed visual coverage.

Nyhan WL, Sakati NA: Diagnostic Recognition of Genetic Disease. Philadelphia, Lea & Febiger, 1987, 754 pp.

A black and white illustrated overview.

Gomez MR (ed): Neurocutaneous Diseases. A Practical Approach. London, Butterworths, 1987, 387 pp.

A superb, syndrome-laden reference text.

Der Kaloustian VM, Kurban AK: Genetic Diseases of the Skin. New York, Springer-Verlag, 1979, 339 pp.

Browsing here can be very rewarding for rare sightings such as the whistling face.

IS IT WORK RELATED?

Adams RM (ed): Occupational Skin Disease. 2nd ed. Philadelphia, W.B. Saunders Co., 1990, 706 pp.

A masterpiece to help you find exactly what's irritating and what's allergenic in patients' work environments, whether they be baker, butcher, or candlestick maker.

Maibach HI (ed): Occupational and Industrial Dermatology. 2nd ed. Chicago, Year Book Medical Publishers, 1987, 477 pp.

Another excellent source with wide coverage from plastics to forestry products.

Lenga RE (ed): The Sigma-Aldrich Library of Chemical Safety Data. Edition II, Vols. 1 & 2. Milwaukee, WI, Sigma-Aldrich Corporation, 1988, 4097 pp.

Safety data on 11,000 compounds your patient may question.

COULD COSMETICS BE THE CAUSE?

Nater JP, de Groot AC: Unwanted Effects of Cosmetics and Drugs Used in Dermatology. 2nd ed. New York, Elsevier, 1985, 522 pp.

Exquisitely detailed account of the chemistry of what your patient is applying and what can happen that isn't pretty.

IS THE DIET AT FAULT?

McLaren DS: A Colour Atlas of Nutritional Disorders. London, Wolfe Medical Publications, Ltd., 1981, 109 pp.

A picture tour of what happens when people are starved for vitamins, minerals, and protein, or lack the enzymes to use them.

Roe DA (ed): Nutrition and the Skin. New York, Alan R. Liss, Inc., 1986, 199 pp.

Helps you remember the importance of the essential fatty acids and the nonessential food additives.

Brostoff J, Challacombe SJ (eds): Food Allergy and Intolerance. London, Balliére Tindall, 1987, 1032 pp.

Comprehensive, ranging from blackberry purpura to peanut butter urticaria.

Metcalfe DM, Sampson HA, Simon RA: Food Allergy. Cambridge, MA, Blackwell Scientific Publications Inc., 1991, 418 pp.

More food for thought.

DOES SUNLIGHT MAKE IT WORSE?

Harber LC, Bicker DR: Photosensitivity Diseases. Principles of Diagnosis and Treatment. 2nd ed. Philadelphia, BC Decker, Inc., 1989, 442 pp.

Enlightens you on everything you want to know about genetic, metabolic, phototoxic, photoallergic, neoplastic, destructive, photoaggravated, and idiopathic photosensitivity disease.

De Leo VA (ed): Photosensitivity Diseases. Dermatol Clin 1986; 4:167–343.

Light on the subject from 26 authorities.

Frain-Bell W: Cutaneous Photobiology. New York, Oxford University Press, 1985, 244 pp.

The essence of the 15-year clinical diagnostic experience of the director of a photomedicine institute.

CAN IT BE "NERVES"?

Koblenzer CS: Psychocutaneous Disease: A Practical Guide to Clinical Evaluation and Management. Orlando, FL, Grune & Stratton, Inc., 1987, 352 pp.

Details on diagnosing the interplay along the neuroectodermal axis.

WHAT AREA IS INVOLVED?

Scalp

Rook A, Dawber R: Diseases of the Hair and Scalp. 2nd ed. London, Blackwell Scientific Publications, 1991, 625 pp.

Here's where you'll find pearls; for example, hair loss following the lines of the cranial sutures should make you think of the Hallermann-Streiff syndrome.

Baden HP: Diseases of the Hair and Nails. Chicago, Year Book Medical Publishers, Inc., 1987, 236 pp.

Color plates of what to see in the scalp and at your fingertips.

Nails

Scher RK, Daniel CR III (eds): Nails: Therapy, Diagnosis, Surgery. Philadelphia, W.B. Saunders Co., 1990, 320 pp.

A marvelous new survey in color.

Zaias N: The Nail in Health and Disease. 2nd ed. Norwalk, CT, Appleton & Lange, 1990, 255 pp.

A classic reference revised and expanded from Mr. Nail himself.

Baran R, Dawber RPR (eds): Diseases of the Nail and Their Management. London, Blackwell Scientific Publications, 1984, 469 pp.

Everything you could want to know.

Samman PD, Fenton DA: The Nails in Disease. 4th ed. Chicago, Year Book Medical Publishers, Inc., 1986, 215 pp.

A valuable black and white pocket book for ready reference.

Oral Mucosa

Pindborg JJ: Atlas of Diseases of the Oral Mucosa. 4th ed. Philadelphia, W.B. Saunders Co., 1985, 357 pp.

The ultimate source.

Cawson RA, Eveson JW: Oral Pathology and Diagnosis, 1987, 330 pp.

Another excellent source.

Laskaris G: Color Atlas of Oral Diseases. New York, Thieme Medical Publishers, Inc., 1988, 314 pp.

A flip and scan help.

Beaven DW, Brooks SE: A Color Atlas of the Tongue in Clinical Diagnosis. Chicago, Year Book Medical Publishers, Inc., 1988, 256 pp.

A book to stick your head in, before the patient sticks out his tongue.

The Eye

Spalton DJ, Hitchings RA, Hunter PA: Atlas of Clinical Ophthalmology. Philadelphia, J.B. Lippincott Co., 1984.

Everything concerning the eyelid inside and out, in brilliant color.

Griffith DG, Sacasche S: Cutaneous Abnormalities of the Eyelid and Face: An Atlas with Histopathology. New York, McGraw-Hill, 1987, 500 pp.

A tour de force of facial problems.

Ostler HB, Dawson CR, Okumoto M: Color Atlas of Infectious and Inflammatory Diseases of the External Eye. Baltimore, Urban & Schwarzenberg, 1987, 166 pp.

A focus on blepharitis.

The Ear

Bull TR: A Colour Atlas of ENT Diagnosis. Revised 2nd Edition. Chicago, Year Book Medical Publishers, Inc., 1987, 256 pp.

For an in-depth color look into the ear, nose, and throat.

Hawke M, Jahn AF: Diseases of the Ear: Clinical and Pathologic Aspects. Philadelphia, Lea & Febiger, 1987.

The best-ever guided trip down the external auditory canal.

The Face

Mann TP: Colour Atlas of Pediatric Facial Diagnosis. Norwell, MA, Kluwer Academic Publishing, 1989, 195 pp.

A fantastic aid.

The Hand

Berry TJ: The Hand as a Mirror of Systemic Disease. Philadelphia, F.A. Davis, 1963, 216 pp.

Detailed differential lists of hand signs of internal disease.

Loesch DZ: Quantitative dermatoglyphics. Classification, Genetics and Pathology. Oxford, Oxford University Press, 1983, 441 pp.

How to read palms for a genetic diagnosis.

Legs and Feet

Samitz MH: Cutaneous Disorders of the Lower Extremities. 2nd ed. Philadelphia, J.B. Lippincott Co., 1981, 266 pp.

How to get into diagnosis, feet first.

Young JR, Graor RA, Olin JW, Bartholomew JR (eds): Peripheral Vascular Diseases. St. Louis, Mosby/Year Book, 1991, 790 pp.

Over 500 illustrations to give you a leg up on the problem.

Levy SW: Skin Problems of the Amputee. St. Louis, Green, 1983, 304 pp.

What to expect.

The Genitalia

Ridley CM (ed): The Vulva. New York, Churchill Livingstone, 1988, 363 pp.

An important contribution to regional diagnosis.

Hewitt J, Pelisse M, Daniel BJ: Diseases of the Vulva. New York, McGraw-Hill, 1991, 213 pp.

Another look.

Wisdom A: Color Atlas of Sexually Transmitted Diseases. Chicago, Year Book Medical Publishers, Inc., 1989, 296 pp.

A good overview.

Parish LC, Sehgal VN, Buntin DM: Color Atlas of Sexually Transmitted Diseases. New York, Igaku-Shoin Medical Publishers Inc, 1991, 184 pp.

The latest with 184 photos.

Bhutani LK: Colour Atlas of Sexually Transmitted Diseases. New Delhi, Mehta Offset Works, 1986, 160 pp.

Exquisite, unforgettable, large color plates.

Veins and Lymphatics

Browse NL, Burnand KS, Thomas ML: Diseases of the Veins: Pathology, Diagnosis, and Treatment. Baltimore, Edward Arnold, 1988, 704 pp.

A visible component of skin and what can go wrong.

Kinmonth JB: The Lymphatics: Surgery, Lymphography and Disease of the Chyle and Lymphatic Systems. 2nd ed. Baltimore, Edward Arnold, 1982, 440 pp.

The definitive work in the field.

YOU HAVE DIAGNOSIS BUT NEED TO REFINE IT

Acne

Cunliffe WJ: Acne. Chicago, Year Book Medical Publishers, Inc., 1989, 400 pp.

Look here for species identification.

Plewig G, Kligman AM: Acne and Acnelike Disorders. New York, Springer-Verlag, 1992, 600 pp.

A monographic masterpiece.

Atopic Dermatitis

Rajka G: Essential Aspects of Atopic Dermatitis. New York, Springer-Verlag, 1989, 261 pp.

Everything you could want to know from the guru of atopy.

Ruzicka T, Ring J, Przybilla B: Handbook of Atopic Dermatitis. New York, Springer-Verlag, 1991, 496 pp.

New insights.

Schwanitz HJ: Atopic Palmoplantar Eczema. New York, Springer-Verlag, 1988, 144 pp.

Details on one of our commonest problems.

Bacterial Infection

Findlay GH: The Dermatology of Bacterial Infections. Chicago, Year Book Medical Publishers, Inc., 1987, 370 pp.

Substance with style: The thinking man's guide to recognition of the clinical faces of bacterial infection.

Behçet's Syndrome

O'Duffy JD, Kokmen E: Behçet's Disease, Basic and Clinical Aspects. New York, Marcel Dekker, Inc., 1991, 696 pp.

The complete guide.

Birthmarks

Mulliken JB, Young AE: Vascular Birthmarks: Hemangiomas and Malformations. Philadelphia, W.B. Saunders Co., 1988, 483 pp.

Of every three children born, one will have a vascular birthmark. And for every child seen with a birthmark, this book is an invaluable reference.

Ryan TJ, Cherry GW (eds): Vascular Birthmarks: Pathogenesis and Management. New York, Oxford University Press, 1987, 203 pp.

Good section on clinical relevance.

Bean WB: Vascular Spiders and Related Lesions of the Skin. Springfield, IL, Charles C Thomas, 1958, 372 pp.

When a blood vessel puzzles, find the answer here.

Blistering Diseases

Wojnarowska F, Briggaman RA (eds): Management of Blistering Diseases. New York, Raven Press, 1990, 308 pp.

All the blister family is here and they tell you how to manage naming them.

Cancer

Mackie RM: Skin Cancer: An Illustrated Guide to the Aetiology, Clinical Features, Pathology, and Management of Benign and Malignant Cutaneous Tumours. Chicago, Year Book Medical Publishers, Inc., 1989, 346 pp.

A classic in color. A joy to hold and to own.

Berenbein BA: Pseudocarcinoma of the Skin. New York, Plenum Publishing Corp., 1985, 276 pp.

Details on what looks like cancer but isn't, e.g., bromoderma, blastomycosis.

Contact Dermatitis

Fisher AA: Contact Dermatitis. 3rd ed. Philadelphia, Lea & Febiger, 1986, 954 pp.

A magnificent encyclopedic work that can transform you into a Sherlock Holmes.

Cronin E: Contact Dermatitis. London, Churchill Livingstone, 1980, 915 pp.

Another monumental work, England's answer to "the Fisher" and a brilliant one indeed.

Maibach HI, Mennét (eds): Nickel and the Skin: Immunology and Toxicology. Boca Raton, FL, CRC Press, Inc., 1989, 223 pp.

Exhaustive treatise on the most common cause of allergic contact dermatitis.

Foussereau J, Benezra C, Maibach HI: Occupational Contact Dermatitis. Clinical and Chemical Aspects. Philadelphia, W.B. Saunders Co., 1982, 452 pp.

For those specialized work related problems.

Jackson EM, Goldner R (eds): Irritant Contact Dermatitis. New York, Marcel Dekker, Inc., 1989, 240 pp.

More insight into diagnosis of nonallergenic dermatitis.

Benezra C, Ducombs G, Sell Y, Foussereau J: Plant Contact Dermatitis. St. Louis, C.V. Mosby Co., 1985, 353 pp.

Whether the cause be dandelions, meadowgrass, or tulips, this book shows you in full color how to recognize the plant and the dermatitis.

Mitchell J, Rook A: Botanical Dermatology Plants and Plant Products Injurious to the Skin. Vancouver, Greenglass Ltd., 1989, 787 pp.

Encyclopedic reference work unadulterated by pictures.

Frosch PJ, Dooms-Gossens A, Lachapelle J-M, et al: Current Topics in Contact Dermatitis. New York, Springer-Verlag, 1989, 613 pp.

A jewel piece with such gems as the case of presumed mycosis fungoides actually due to a contact dermatitis caused by brown trousers.

Ectodermal Dysplasia

Freire-Maia N, Pinheiro M: Ectodermal Dysplasias: A Clinical and Genetic Study. New York, Alan R. Liss, Inc., 1984, 251 pp.

Every ectodermal dysplasia syndrome you can think of and a lot more. Essential guide for precision in diagnosing and classifying all ectodermal defects.

Endocrine Problems

Besser GM, Cudworth AG (eds): Clinical Endocrinology. An Illustrated Text. Philadelphia, J.B. Lippincott Co., 1987.

The ultimate reference on all your patient's endocrine status. A delight in color and thought.

Epidermolysis Bullosa

Priestley GC, Tidman MJ, Weiss JB, Eady RAJ (eds): Epidermolysis Bullosa: A comprehensive Review of Classification Management and Laboratory Studies. Crowthorne, UK, DEBRA, 1990, 198 pp.

Detailed help from 52 investigators.

Filariasis

Offesen EA: Filariasis. New York, John Wiley & Sons, 1987, 305 pp.

Details on a tropical disease affecting over 130 million people.

Fungal Disease

Rippon JW: Medical Mycology. The Pathogenic Fungi and Pathogenic Actinomycetes. 3rd ed. Philadelphia, W.B. Saunders Co., 1988, 795 pp.

The ultimate reference with pearls such as (1) the cluster of cases of blastomycosis in a group of school children, traced to their nature outing to a beaver dam; (2) a city-wide epidemic of histoplasmosis involving over 100,000 cases; (3) one stray cat in Moscow accounting for tinea capitis in over 100 children.

Roberts SOB, Hay RJ, Mackensie DWR: A Clinician's Guide to Fungal Disease. New York, Marcel Dekker, Inc., 1984, 252 pp.

A reader-friendly guide to diagnosis of both the superficial and the systemic.

Grigoric D: Medical Mycology. Toronto, Ontario, Hans Huber Publishers, 1987, 187 pp.

A splendid large format color tour of fungi as you see them in the clinic and in the lab.

Hirsutism

Greenblatt RB, Mahesh VB, Gambrell RD (eds): The Cause and Management of Hirsutism. Park Ridge, NJ, Parthenon Publishing Group, 1987, 227 pp.

A literate answer to why women have beards.

Ichthyosis

Traupe H: The Ichthyoses: A Guide to Clinical Diagnosis, Genetic Counseling, and Therapy. New York, Springer-Verlag, 1989, 253 pp.

You can't tell one scale from another without this book. A treasury of taxonomy.

Infectious Disease

Emond RTD: Color Atlas of Infectious Diseases. Chicago, Year Book Medical Publishers, Inc., 1974, 384 pp.

A vade mecum of common bacterial, fungal, and viral contagions.

Insect Bites

Alexander JO: Arthropods and Human Skin. New York, Springer-Verlag, 1984, 422 pp.

If you don't know whether it was a 6- or an 8-legged pathogen, run for this book.

Kaposi's Sarcoma

Ziegler JL, Dorfman RF: Kaposi's Sarcoma: Pathophysiology and Clinical Management. New York, Marcel Dekker, Inc., 1988, 266 pp.

More on a tumor whose time has come.

Gottlieb GJ, Ackerman AB (eds): Kaposi's Sarcoma: A Text and Atlas. Philadelphia, Lea & Febiger, 1988, 330 pp.

Kaposi's sarcoma inside and out.

Leprosy

Jopling WH, McDougall AL: Handbook of Leprosy. 4th ed. London, Heinemann Professional Publishing, 1988, 180 pp.

Four times a classic.

Lupus Erythematosus

Wallace DJ, Dubois EL (eds): Dubois' Lupus Erythematosus. 3rd ed. Philadelphia, Lea & Febiger, 1987, 775 pp.

To aid you in recognizing every variant of a most varied disease.

Lymphomas

Burg G, Braun-Falco O: Cutaneous Lymphomas, Pseudolymphomas and Related Disorders. New York, Springer-Verlag, 1983, 542 pp.

Beautifully illustrated color guide through lymphoma land, with views of everything classifiable from parapsoriasis to insect bite pseudolymphoma.

Melanoma

Bolch CM, Milton GW: Cutaneous Melanoma. Philadelphia, J.B. Lippincott Co., 1985, 538 pp.

How to tell the bad black spots.

Mycetoma

Mahgoub E, Murray IG: Mycetoma. London, William Heinemann Medical Books, Ltd., 1973, 132 pp.

Complete, succinct picture of all aspects of fungal tumor of the subcutaneous tissue.

Pathology

Stevens A, Wheater PR, Lower JS: Clinical Dermatopathology. A Text and Colour Atlas. New York, Churchill Livingstone, 1989, 195 pp.

A marvelous juxtaposition of color plates showing what you can see on and in the skin. These clinical windows into the pathology below provide lots of fun.

Pigmented Lesions

Maize JC, Ackerman AB: Pigmented Lesions of the Skin. Clinicopathologic Correlations. Philadelphia, Lea & Febiger, 1987, 328 pp.

Exquisite, comprehensive survey ranging from the benign freckle to the malignant melanoma, and from the lichen planus–like keratosis to the reticulated pigmented anomaly of the flexures (Dowling-Degos).

Pruritus

Gatti S, Serri F: Pruritus in Clinical Medicine. New York, McGraw-Hill, 1984, 112 pp.

An Italian slant on why your patient itches.

Psoriasis

Mier PD, van de Kerkhof PCM (eds): Textbook of Psoriasis. New York, Churchill Livingstone, 1986, 292 pp.

All of the varieties of psoriasis are corralled within 27 pages. Peeking through the fence you will see elephantine psoriasis and psoriasis ostracea, as well as generalized pustular psoriasis induced by progesterone and nummular eczema evolving into plaque psoriasis.

Roenigk HH, Maibach HI (eds): Psoriasis. 2nd ed. New York, Marcel Dekker, Inc., 1991, 992 pp.

Incomparable detail on diagnosis.

Sarcoidosis

Izumi C (ed): Sarcoidosis. Philadelphia, J.B. Lippincott Co., 1986, 175 pp.

Multifaceted monograph.

Scleroderma

Black CM, Myers AR (eds): Systemic Sclerosis (Scleroderma). New York, Gower Medical Publishing Limited, 1985, 459 pp.

Help from an international viewpoint.

Jablonska S: Scleroderma and Pseudoscleroderma. 2nd ed. Warsaw, Polish Medical Publishers, 1975, 640 pp.

The hard-core reference for classifying scleroderma patients.

Sjögren's Syndrome

Talal N, Moutsopoulous HM, Kassan SS (eds): Sjögren's Syndrome: Clinical and Immunological Aspects. New York, Springer-Verlag, 1987, 299 pp.

The best available book on Sjögren's syndrome and how it attracts the attention of rheumatologists, immunologists, ophthalmologists, and dentists, as well as dermatologists!

Vitiligo

Ortonne J-P, Mosher DB, Fitzpatrick TB: Vitiligo and Other Hypomelanoses of Hair and Skin. New York, Plenum Medical Book Company, 1983, 638 pp.

A vast survey with special attention to the diagnosis of hypomelanosis due to chemicals.

Urticaria

Czarnetski BM: Urticaria. New York, Springer-Verlag, 1986, 189 pp.

A model for monograph mavens and a decision maker in diagnostic dilemmas.

Warts

Bunney MH: Viral Warts: Their Biology and Treatment. New York, Oxford University Press, 1982, 99 pp.

Diagnostic wisdom from the doyenne of the wart world.

DOES YOUR PATIENT HAVE MEDICAL PROBLEMS?

Stein JH (ed): Internal Medicine. 3rd ed. Boston, Little, Brown and Co., 1990, 2460 pp.

This magnificent summation of all of medicine will help satisfy your every curiosity about your patient's internal disease.

Samiu AH, Douglas RG Jr., Barondess JA (eds): Textbook of Diagnostic Medicine. Philadelphia, Lea & Febiger, 1987, 900 pp.

Want to explore your patient's noncutaneous complaint? Want to learn how the internist uses the laboratory? This book is the answer.

Dieppe PA, Bacon PA, Bamji AN, Watt I: Atlas of Clinical Rheumatology. Philadelphia, Lea & Febiger, 1986, 387 pp.

A giant color atlas of what the skin does in rheumatoid disease. Invaluable reference.

Calin A: Differential Diagnosis in Rheumatology: An Atlas for the Physician. Philadelphia, J.B. Lippincott Co., 1984, 220 pp.

A case study approach to diagnostic dermatology, using 200 patients in the rheumatology clinic. Great color.

Jelinck JE (ed): The Skin in Diabetes. Philadelphia, Lea & Febiger, 1986, 237 pp.

The varied cutaneous faces of diabetes mellitus.

Levin ME, O'Neal LW (eds): The Diabetic Foot. 4th ed. St. Louis, C.V. Mosby Co., 1988, 362 pp.

Close analysis of the *locus minoris resistentiae* of the diabetic.

CAN YOU BE THE FIRST TO RECOGNIZE YOUR PATIENT HAS INTERNAL DISEASE?

Braverman IM: Skin Signs of Systemic Disease. 2nd ed. Philadelphia, W.B. Saunders Co., 1981, 965 pp.

The master reference.

Callen JP, Jorizzo J, Greek KE, et al: Dermatological Signs of Internal Disease. Philadelphia, W.B. Saunders Co., 1988, 383 pp.

The skin signs of internal disease presented in the context of the major medical specialties: hematology/oncology, metabolic disease, gastroenterology, infectious disease, rheumatology, and general medicine.

Hurwitz S: The Skin and Systemic Disease in Children. Chicago, Year Book Medical Publishers, Inc., 1985, 416 pp.

The skin as a diagnostic window for disease in little tots.

Sharvill DE: Skin Signs of Systemic Disease. Philadelphia, J.B. Lippincott Co., 1988, 85 pp.

Looking through the skin when you look at it.

THE TIME HAS COME TO EXAMINE

Swartz MH: Textbook of Physical Diagnosis. History and Examination. Philadelphia, W.B. Saunders Co., 1989, 646 pp.

A wonderfully innovative text on how to examine the skin (and other organs).

STILL NO ANSWER, USE THESE REFERENCE TEXTS

Champion RH, Burton JL, Ebling FJG (eds): Rook/Wilkinson/Ebling Textbook of Dermatology. 4 volumes, 5th Edition. London, Blackwell Scientific Publications, 1992, 3160 pp.

A day in the clinic without this is a day without the sunshine of knowledge.

Demis DJ (ed): Clinical Dermatology. 4 loose leaf volumes, Annual Update. Philadelphia, J.B. Lippincott Co., 1988, 4748 pp.

Our Encyclopedia Dermatologica. 357 authors, 5000 photos. Wow. How did they ever proofread it?

Fitzpatrick TB, Eisen AZ, Wolff K, et al (eds): Dermatology in General Medicine. Textbook and Atlas. Two volumes, 3rd ed. New York, McGraw-Hill Book Co., 1987, 2641 pp.

Another great diagnostic probe.

Braun-Falco O, Plewig G, Wolff HH, Winkelmann RK: Dermatology. New York, Springer-Verlag, 1989, 1100 pp.

An English translation of a great German classic.

Moschella SL, Hurley HJ (eds): Dermatology. Two volumes, 3rd ed. Philadelphia, W.B. Saunders Co., 1992, 2271 pp.

A four-star reference for diagnostic thoughts from the clinicians.

Habif TP: Clinical Guide to Diagnosis and Therapy. 2nd ed. St. Louis, Mosby-Year Book, 1990, 776 pp.

A diagnostic tour-de-force by a single author. Winner of the American Medical Writers Association Award for Excellence. Better than life; color photos of 822 patients.

Sams WM, Lynch PJ (eds): Principles and Practice of Dermatology. New York, Churchill Livingstone, Inc., 1990, 1013 pp.

The newest; sure to be a winner with 73 contributors, 588 crisp color illustrations.

Arnold HL, Odom RB, James WD: Andrews' Diseases of the Skin: Clinical Dermatology. 8th ed. Philadelphia, W.B. Saunders Co., 1990, 1062 pp.

These three distinguished dermatologists have brought this eighth edition of an "old master" to the epitome of erudition. The color in this book is not in its illustrations, but in its writing and in its wisdom. A clinical book by clinicians and for clinicians.

BOOKS FOR SPECIAL HELP ON DIFFERENTIAL DIAGNOSIS

Lazarus GS, Goldsmith LA: Diagnosis of Skin Disease. Philadelphia, F.A. Davis Co., 1980, 506 pp.

Lesion shape and color-oriented diagnosis.

Ashton R, Leppart B: Differential Diagnosis in Dermatology. Philadelphia, J.B. Lippincott Co., 1989, 300 pp.

An algorithmic approach.

Lebwohl M (ed): Difficult Diagnoses in Dermatology. New York, Churchill Livingstone, 1988, 450 pp.

Problem-oriented differential diagnosis.

Louis AA (ed): Handbook of Difficult Diagnosis. New York, Churchill Livingstone, 1990, 777 pp.

Contains an 80-page nugget of diagnostic analysis of over a dozen significant dermatologic problems. Very helpful checklists.

Wilkinson DS, Mascaro JM, Orfanos CE (eds): Clinical Dermatology. The CMD Case Collection. New York, Schattauer, 1987, 393 pp.

Instructive color-illustrated accounts of very rare cases presented at the World Congress of Dermatology in Berlin.

Grollnick H, Stadler R: Dia-Klinik: New York, Schattauer, 1987, 118 pp.

More world congress, world-class varieties in full color, but text is in German.

YOU ARE REFERRED A CASE OF CARRINGTON-LIEBOW SYNDROME. WHERE TO LOOK IT UP?

Magalini SI, Magalini SL, de Francisci G: Dictionary of Medical Syndromes. 3rd ed. Philadelphia, J.B. Lippincott Co., 1990, 1042 pp.

Over 3000 syndromes and eponyms, not to be found in the typical medical dictionary.

Jablonska S: Illustrated Dictionary of Eponymic Syndromes and Diseases and Their Synonyms. Philadelphia, W.B. Saunders Co., 1969, 335 pp.

Valuable for its photos.

Plunckett ER: Talk Name and Trade Diseases. Stamford, CT, Barrett Book Company, 1978, 352 pp.

From ampoule snapper's thumb to alkali itch, from scrumpox to scribe's palsy. They're all there and defined.

Thornton SP: Ophthalmic Eponyms. An Encyclopedia of Named Signs, Syndromes and Diseases in Ophthalmology. Birmingham, Alabama, Aesculapius Publishing Company, 1967, 324 pp.

A rich mine of information about naming eyebrow, eyelid, and ear anomalies.

Jablonska S: Illustrated Dictionary of Dentistry. Philadelphia, WB Saunders Co., 1982, 919 pp.

If it's a dental syndrome, use page 765 and beyond.

HOW CAN I ORGANIZE MY RECORDS, REPRINTS, AND SLIDES BY DIAGNOSIS?

Lamberg S: Retrieval System for Dermatological Photographs. 3rd ed. Buffalo, Westwood, 1989, 54 pp.

How to bring order out of the chaos of your slide collection and thereby enhance retrieval.

HOW CAN I CODE MY DIAGNOSIS FOR BILLING?

U.S. Department of Health and Human Sciences: The International Classification of Diseases. 9th Revision. Clinical Modification ICD-9-CM. 4th ed, Two Volumes. Washington, U.S. Government Printing Office, 1992, 2096 pp.

The standard reference.

Anon: Abridged Version of ICD-9 & CPT Codes for Dermatologists. Blue Bell, PA, Dermik Laboratories, Inc., 1991, 32 pp.

A pocketful of CPTs.

Brown CS (ed): SNODERM: Systematized Nomenclature of Dermatology. Baltimore, Waverly Press, Inc., 1978, 290 pp.

An alternate coding system.

HOW CAN I KEEP UP?

Read, read, read:

Journal of American Academy of Dermatology
Archives of Dermatology
International Journal of Dermatology
Cutis
The Schoch Letter
Skin and Allergy News

British Journal of Dermatology
Clinical and Experimental Dermatology
Acta Dermato-Venereologica
Dermatologica
Contact Dermatitis
American Journal of Contact Dermatitis
Pediatric Dermatology

Review, review, review:

Advances in Dermatology, Vols 1–6, Year Book Publishers
Clinics in Dermatology, Vols 1–7, J.B. Lippincott Co.
Current Problems in Dermatology, Vols 1–19, Karger
Current Problems in Dermatology, Vols 1–6, Year Book Publishers
Dermatologic Clinics, Vols 1–9, W.B. Saunders Co.
Recent Advances in Dermatology, Vols 1–8, Churchill Livingstone
Seminars in Dermatology, Vols 1–8, W.B. Saunders Co.

Listen, listen, listen:

Dialogues in Dermatology
American Academy of Dermatology
Local, state, national, international meetings

HOW CAN I KEEP UP MY SPIRITS?

Manning PR, DeBakey L: Medicine, Preserving the Passion. New York, Springer-Verlag, 1987, 297 pp.

Inspiring specific techniques for pursuing the fun and excitement of lifelong learning. An antidote for "burn out."

THE COMPLEAT DIAGNOSTICIAN'S QUINTESSENTIAL BOOKSHELF

Rook/Wilkinson/Ebling Textbook of Dermatology
Bork, Cutaneous Side Effects of Drugs
Hurwitz, Clinical Pediatric Dermatology
Penneys, Skin Manifestations of AIDS
McKusick, Mendelian Inheritance in Man
Adams, Occupational Skin Diseases
Rook and Dawber, Diseases of Hair and Scalp
Baran R, Barth J, Dawber R, Nail Disorders
Fisher, Contact Dermatitis
Braverman, Skin Signs of Systemic Disease

Sources and Resources

ALLERGEN EXTRACTS

Intradermal, scratch, prick, multitest diagnostic pollens, house dust, molds, epidermals, ingestants, insects, mites.

Allergy Laboratories of Ohio
623 East 11th Avenue
Columbus, OH 43211
1-800-654-5439

Center Laboratories
35 Channel Drive
Fort Washington, NY 11050
1-800-2-CENTER

Hollister-Stier
P.O. Box 3145
Spokane, WA 99220
1-800-541-3782

CAMERAS

Lester A. Dine, Inc.
100 Milbar Blvd.
Farmingdale, NY 11735
1-516-454-6100

Complete close-up camera equipment.

CATALOGUES

Dermatologic Buying Guide
Dermatologic Lab and Supply
201 Ridge Street, Suite 205
Council Bluffs, IA 51503
1-800-831-6273

This 103-page catalogue answers every need of the dermatologic diagnostician for:

fungal culture media
KOH preparations
stains
Durotak slides
biopsy instruments and sutures
nail nippers
razor blades
Wood's lamps
MED testers
marking tools and pens
tumorimeters
dermatoscopes
loupes
magnifiers
lamps
books: 250 titles to give diagnostic help

Cole-Parmer Instrument Company
7425 North Oak Park Avenue
Chicago, IL 60648
1-800-323-4340

computer software
conductivity meters
Doppler flow meters
heaters
magnifiers
microscopes, cameras
pH testers

temperature measuring devices
tensile testers
timers
ultraviolet lamps
water analysis test kits
weather measurement devices

DIAGNOSTIC LABORATORIES

Mayo Medical Laboratories
200 First Street, Southwest
Rochester, MN 55905
1-800-533-1710

See

1992 Test Catalogue for over 365 pages of tests done by them.

1992 *Tissue and Special Stains Catalogue* for over 130 pages of dermatopathology services. This includes detection of direct and indirect immunofluorescence, immunofluorescent antibodies, as well as monoclonal antibody staining for T-cell subsets, B cells, and histiocytes. They also do immunoperoxidase stain for herpes simplex virus, both types 1 and 2, as well as the Warthin-Starry stain for spirochetes and Donovan bodies in tissue. X-ray microanalysis is also done for detection of heavy metals.

Genetics Catalogue: provides assays for cytogenetics and molecular genetic (DNA probe) studies.

Mayo Medical Laboratories: **Interpretative Handbook** gives interpretative data for each diagnostic test.

Pediatrics Catalogue: Tests specially adapted to pediatric-aged patients.

Communique: Newsletter regularly updating laboratory services available.

If your patient can't go to Mayo's, at least his blood, urine, stool, and skin can.

Nichols Institute Reference Laboratories Test Catalogue 1990
26441 Via de Anza
San Juan Capistrano, CA 92675
1-800-553-5445

147 pages of available tests, including:

alpha-1 antitrypsin
polymerase chain reaction
    PCR techniques
immune deficiency
    panel I, II
immune activation panel
T-cell subset panel
T and B cells subset panel
leukemia panels

lipid panels
toxicology
trace elements in blood and urine
aluminum and selenium in serum/plasma
chromosome studies
prostate specific antigen
parathyroid hormone levels
RAST tests for pollens, foods, plants, and insect allergies

Smith Kline Bio-Science Laboratories Directory of Services
11636 Administration Drive
St. Louis, MO 63146
1-800-669-7525

Nationwide outpatient service, collection centers. Directory of 283 pages provides comprehensive list of laboratory tests done as well as panels for screening.

Roche Biomedical Laboratories Directory of Services 1989
3600-A Woodpark Blvd.
Charlotte, NC 28206
1-800-438-6915

National network of patient services. Directory of 300 pages provides complete list of tests available, including tryptophan plasma level, 150 specific food allergen sensitivity tests, and chromosome analysis.

DORA 87: Hicks JM, Young DS. Directory of rare analyses. Washington, D.C., American Association for Clinical Chemistry, Inc., 1987, 447 pp.

For that rare analysis look here (Directory on sale at the American Association for Clinical Chemistry, Inc., 1725 K Street, N.W., Washington, D.C. 20006). The Directory lists hundreds of smaller, highly specialized laboratories doing unique, valuable analysis; thus:

for trimethylamine in urine (fish odor syndrome), call

Metabolic Laboratory
Arkansas Children's Hospital
804 Wolfe Street
Little Rock, AR 72202
1-501-370-1300

for α, β, or γ melanocyte stimulating hormone, the release inhibiting factor (MIF) and melatonin determinations, as well as somatostatin, call

Interscience Institute
944 West Hyde Park Blvd.
Los Angeles, CA 90302
1-800-421-7133

Specialty Laboratories, Inc.
2211 Michigan Avenue
Santa Monica, CA 90404
1-800-421-7110

Specializing in immunologic assays, including Parvovirus B19 infection (erythema infectiosum), multiple autoantibodies, and antineutrophil cytoplasm antibodies.

DIAGNOSTIC SLIDES OF SKIN DISEASE

American Academy of Dermatology
P.O. Box 192
Evanston, IL 60204

Thirteen hundred and fifty 35-mm color transparencies available from their National Library of Dermatologic Teaching Slides. Available in 27 taxonomic groups of 50 slides each.

"DO SOMETHING" DIAGNOSTIC KITS

Eastman Kodak Company
Clinical Products Division
Rochester, NY 14650
1-800-445-6325 (ext. 450)

SureCell Line
Herpes simplex virus test kit–Office test with answer 12 minutes after taking swab
Chlamydia test kit–Office test with answer 21 minutes after swab or urine sample
Strep A test kit–Rapid office test for presence of Group A Streptococcus
hCG-urine test kit–Detection of pregnancy 2 minutes after urine sampling. This is a visual immunoassay for human chorionic gonadotropin (hCG) produced by placenta.

For details on sensitivity and specificity of these four kits, see Tilley LJ: Test Kits for Rapid Routine Testing, American Clinical Laboratory 1990; 9:20–31.

ELECTRON MICROSCOPY

Mayo Clinic Medical Laboratories
  200 First Street, SW
  Rochester, MN 55905
  1-800-533-1710

EXAMINING LIGHTS

  Light Technology Systems
  16760 Stagg Street, No 211
  Van Nuys, CA 91406

  Medical Illumination, Inc.
  12734 Branford Street, Suite 1
  Arleta, CA 91331

GENETIC RESOURCES

  Genetic Test Catalogue
  Mayo Medical Laboratories
  200 First Street, Southwest
  Rochester, MN 55905
  1-800-533-1710

A treasure chest of tests and studies you can do for your patient with genetic disease.

  International Directory of Genetic Services, 9th Edition, 1990, 75 pp.
  Lynch HT and Hoden RH: March of Dimes Birth Defects Foundation
  White Plains, NY 10605
  1-402-280-2972

List of genetic centers and geneticists available for consultation around the world.

  Murray JC, Toriello HV: Guide to North American Graduate and Postgraduate Training
  Programs in Human Genetics. American Society of Human Genetics, 1990, 66 pp.
  9650 Rockville Pike
  Bethesda, MD 20814
  1-301-571-1825

Another consultation resource near you.

  Membership 90–91 Directory
  American Society of Human Genetics, 1990, 166 pp.
  9650 Rockville Pike
  Bethesda, MD 20814
  1-301-571-1825

Names and addresses.

IMMUNOFLUORESCENT STUDIES

Immco Diagnostics
  963 Kenmore Avenue
  P.O. Box 903
  Buffalo, NY 14223
  1-800-537-TEST
Immunodermatology Program
  Wright State University
  P.O. Box 927
  Dayton, OH 45401
Mayo Medical Laboratories
  200 First Street, SW
  Rochester, MN 55905
  1-800-533-1710

See: Tissues and Special Stains Catalogue, 1990; 130 pp. Provides comprehensive service with innumerable stains available, including immunofluorescence.

INFECTIOUS DISEASE OR DISEASE CLUSTERS

Centers for Disease Control
1600 Clifton Road
302 Freeway Park EO6
Atlanta, GA 30333

IONTOPHORESIS UNITS

General Medical Company
1935 Armacost Avenue
Los Angeles, CA 90025

LectroPatch Iontophoresis Unit for introduction of test substances.

LITERATURE SEARCH

Index Medicus at your medical library.
MEDLINE search by your medical library.
PaperChase
   Center for Clinical Computing
   Beth Israel Hospital
   Boston, MA 02215
   1-617-732-5925

User-friendly, self-instructional online biographic retrieval system for your personal use. Requirements: personal computer, modem, printer. For more details see: Wolffing BK, Computerized Literature Searching in the Ambulatory Setting Using PaperChase, Henry Ford Hospital Medical Journal, 1990; 38:57–61.

DERM/DDX
   American Academy of Dermatology
   Dermatology Services, Inc.
   1567 Maple Avenue
   Evanston, IL 60204-3116
   1-708-869-3954

A computerized diagnostic aid that allows you to enter symptoms to get a list of probable diseases or to enter a diagnosis to get a list of other applicable diseases that could be considered.

PATCH TESTS

Hermal Pharmaceutical Laboratory, Inc.
163 Delaware Avenue
Delmar, NY 12054
1-800-HERMAL-1

Allergen Patch Test Kit–20 selected allergens, Finn chambers, ScanPor Tape
Omniderm Inc
8400 Darnley Rd
Montreal, Quebec, Canada
H4T, M4
1-514-340-1114

TroLAB Patch Test. Allergens: 278 substances.

PATHOLOGY

Consultants

A. Bernard Ackerman, M.D.
New York University
530 First Avenue #7J
New York, NY 10016

Wilma F. Bergfeld, M.D.
Department of Dermatology and Pathology
Cleveland Clinic Foundation
9500 Euclid Ave.
Cleveland, OH 44106

Martin Brownstein, M.D.
2 North Plandome Road
Port Washington, NY 11050

Robert Freeman, M.D.
Department of Dermatology
Southwestern Medical School
5323 Harry Hines Blvd.
Dallas, TX 75235

Loren E. Golitz, M.D.
Dermatology Department 0148
Denver General Hospital
777 Bannock Street
Denver, CO 80204

James H. Graham, M.D.
Department of Pathology
Scripps Clinic and Research Foundation
10666 North Torrey Pines Road
La Jolla, CA 92037

John T. Headington, M.D.
Department of Pathology
University of Michigan
School of Medicine
Med Sci, Box 0602
Ann Arbor, MI 48109

Waine C. Johnson, M.D.
137 South Easton Road
P.O. Box 8
Glenside, PA 19038

Philip LeBoit, M.D.
Department of Dermatology and Pathology
University of California, San Francisco
501 HSW–Pathology
San Francisco, CA 94143

John C. Maize, M.D.
Medical University of South Carolina
Department of Dermatology
171 Ashley Avenue
Charleston, SC 29425

Neil S. McNutt, M.D.
New York Hospital
Dermatopathology (F-340)
525 East 68th Street
New York, NY 10021

Amir H. Mehregan, M.D.
Pinkus Dermatopathology Laboratory
1314 North Macomb
P.O. Box 360
Monroe, MI 48161

Martin C. Mihm, Jr., M.D.
Massachusetts General Hospital
Department of Dermatopathology
Boston, MA 02114

Daniel Richfield, M.D.
Department of Dermatology and Pathology
University of Cincinnati
128 LaFayette Lane
Cincinnati, OH 45220

Alvin R. Solomon, M.D.
Department of Dermatology
Emory University School of Medicine
207 Woodruff Memorial Research Bldg.
Atlanta, GA 30322

Richard K. Winkelmann, M.D.
Mayo Clinic Scottsdale
13400 East Shea Blvd.
Scottsdale, AZ 85259

RADIOMETERS

International Light, Inc.
17 Graf Road
Newburyport, MA 01950

SURGICAL INSTRUMENTS

Mill-Bilt Instrument Company
2145 West Central Avenue
Toledo, OH 43606

Miltex Instrument Company, Inc.
6 Ohio Drive
Lake Success, NY 11042

Robbins Instruments, Inc.
2 North Passaic Avenue
P.O. Box 441
Chatham, NJ 07928

ULTRASOUND EQUIPMENT

Taberna Pro Medicum
P.O. Box 80
Sudbury, MA 01776

Digital ultrasound imaging system.

Abscess

Abscess is a term dermatologists share with all of medicine, meaning a focal collection of pus that results from liquefactive necrosis of tissue anywhere in the body. In the skin it presents as a nodule, with the prototype skin abscess being the common boil. Most abscesses are caused by pyogenic organisms, particularly staphylococci. This battleground of bacteria, debris, and leukocytes is surrounded by a wall of granulation tissue and proliferating myofibroblasts, in contrast to the spreading battle scene of streptococci, which cannot be contained and continuously expands as a cellulitis.

If the abscess wall ruptures, a sinus may result, through which large amounts of pus may discharge. Just as "where there's smoke, there's fire," where there's a sinus, there's an abscess. Alternatively, the abscess roof may erode, leaving an ulcer with a necrotic floor that sloughs. Some abscesses never drain or erode but simply involute, leaving a calcified fibrotic scar.

The soft fluctuant nature of a nodule or mass, its location, and the purulent material obtained on needle aspiration readily permit the diagnosis of "abscess," which can then be subclassified into such categories as furuncle, pilonidal cyst, pyoderma gangrenosum, acne abscess, and hidradenitis suppurativa. The dermatologist can further identify it by naming the location—whether it be breast or perianal, orbital, or otic. The *International Dictionary of Medicine and Biology* devotes six pages to naming abscesses.

The real challenge is in discerning hidden abscesses and finding the causes of obvious ones. With sudden idiopathic facial swelling, think of a dental abscess; and in patients with sepsis, think of an embolic abscess. Look for underlying Crohn's disease, osteomyelitis, fat necrosis, and foreign body reactions. Don't forget the factitial abscess. Patients may not tell you of the milk, feces, soap, or other pyogenic foreign materials they or one of their multiple "personalities" may have injected into their skin.

Even harder to suspect is the abscess of child abuse. We recall unexplained tender red draining abscesses of a baby's bottom. While the infant was hospitalized an astute nurse noted that the baby screamed each time shortly after the arrival of the "loving" mother. The next day when the infant started to scream, the nurse burst into the room and discovered the mother with a syringe, injecting turpentine into her child's buttocks.

The abscess wall should be studied histologically for necrotic tumor, molluscum contagiosum, foreign bodies, and parasites such as amebae, filariae, and worms. The abscess contents must be cultured for aerobic and anaerobic bacteria, candida, dermatophytes, and deep fungi. Only then will you have a proper diagnosis—shorter, it is hoped, than the internist's diagnosis of "uncomplicated superior surface lateral left lobe amebic liver abscess" syndrome (known as USSLLLALA syndrome—the longest acronym in medicine!).

Face

Boudreau S, Hines HC, Hood AF: **Dermal abscesses** with *Staphylococcus aureus*, cytomegalovirus and acid-fact bacilli in a patient with acquired immunodeficiency syndrome (**AIDS**). J Cutan Pathol 1988; 15:53–57.

A 34-year-old homosexual man with AIDS had multiple crusted papules of his face and arms, resembling molluscum contagiosum. Skin biopsies revealed a central dermal abscess with large clusters of gram-positive loci surrounded by neutrophils, granular necrotic material, and granulation tissue. One papule also contained intranuclear cytomegalic inclusions and acid-fast bacilli, presumed to be the *Mycobacterium avium-intracellulare* cultured from his bone marrow. Bacterial cultures of skin lesions grew *Staphylococcus aureus*. He soon died of *Pneumocystis carinii* pneumonia.

In immunosuppressed patients, look for multiple infectious agents in each skin lesion.

Macomber WB, Wang MK-H, Gottlieb E: Cutaneous **lesions of dental origin** simulating skin cancer. GP 1956; 14:81–85.

A 53-year-old woman had a 4-month history of a 1.5-cm depressed adherent ulcer on the left chin, fixed to the mandible. There was surrounding inflammation, induration, and crust formation, and a small amount of thin purulent drainage issued from a sinus opening. A probe passed easily into an alveolar abscess in the mandible in an area of carious teeth of the left lower jaw, seen on x-ray. Tooth extraction and curettage of the abscess cavity were curative, although a scar on the chin from the cutaneous scar had to be revised.

A chronic alveolar abscess usually develops insidiously, often at some distance from the affected tooth. The abscess originates at the apex of an infected tooth or retained root, and slowly penetrates and destroys surrounding bone. Eventually a subperiosteal abscess forms, which most often drains intraorally.

External drainage to the skin may alternatively occur, depending on gravity and the anatomic location of the infected tooth, with a resulting chronic draining cutaneous sinus. The abscess cavity becomes filled with granuloma-like tissue (**dental granuloma**), which may spread to the sinus opening. The wall of the sinus becomes fibrotic, with fixation of the skin to the bone. Early drainage is purulent, but later becomes serosanguineous and finally serous. Crust formation occurs, particularly after alternate drainage is established inside the mouth.

The lesion begins as a small nodule that grows slowly and progressively and finally ulcerates. It becomes crusted and bleeds easily on trauma, with granulomalike tissue. The surrounding skin becomes indurated and adherent to underlying bone. Such a lesion may persist for years, with no hint of a deep-seated etiologic factor. However, tenderness of a tooth to bite or percussion on the suspected side of the mandible suggests an underlying abscess, as do swelling and tenderness of the overlying bone. A cordlike structure extending from the sinus opening to the alveolus may be palpable inside the mouth. Enlarged submaxillary or submental nodes may also be present.

After the crust is cleaned off, the sinus opening may be visible and should be explored with a fine malleable metal probe. This may lead to the diseased tooth. Diagnostic evaluation should also include x-ray of the jaw bones and intraoral x-rays, as well as careful dental examination. A culture and smear for actinomycosis are also advisable. The injection of contrast material into

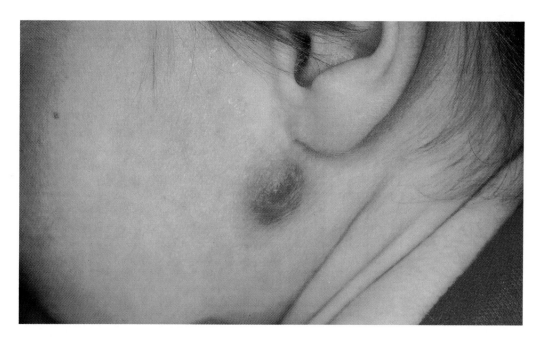

the sinus tract may also help to delineate the extension of the sinus to the jaw.

The differential diagnosis of the dental sinus includes:

thyroglossal sinus   epidermoid cyst
actinomycosis   basal cell epithelioma
branchial fistula   squamous cell epithelioma
salivary fistula

Scott MJ Jr, Scott MJ Sr: Cutaneous **odontogenic sinus**. J Am Acad Dermatol 1980; 2:521–524.

After plucking several hairs from her chin, a 46-year-old woman developed a 5-mm indentation with a 2.5-mm umbilicated red papule at its base, just to the right of the submental region. It had been present for 2 weeks. There was no sinus tract, and nothing could be expressed. The teeth in the mandibular frontal areas were not sensitive to percussion. She denied dental problems, foreign travel, or exposure to the vectors of anthrax, oriental sore, or actinomycosis. Antibiotic therapy on two occasions was without effect. A dental x-ray showed a well-circumscribed radiolucent area at the root of the mandibular right cuspid, suggesting an odontogenic sinus. She resisted the diagnosis because of its therapeutic implications, but after 4 months during which time pus could sometimes be expressed from the lesion, the involved tooth was extracted. The nodule promptly disappeared, leaving only a slight hyperpigmented indentation after 3 months.

The differential diagnosis of a dental sinus centers on:

osteomyelitis of the facial bones (often multiple sinuses)
foreign bodies (A small splinter of windshield glass following a car accident or an embedded hair in a barber may years later produce a sinus tract.)
congenital fistulas (A branchial cleft fistula localizes on the anterior border of the sternocleidomastoid muscle; a thyroglossal fistula is near the midline inferior to the hyoid bone.)
granulomas (Dental disease and sinus tract are absent.)

Winstock D: Four cases of external facial **sinuses of dental origin**. Proc R Soc Med 1959; 52:749–751.

Discharging facial sinuses of dental origin are uncommon. The most common type is a median mental sinus associated with a lower incisal apical abscess; it resembles an infected sebaceous cyst. Sinuses on the cheek have been mistaken for epidermoid cysts, infected acne cysts, actinomycosis, and carcinoma.

A 15-year-old girl had a transient toothache followed by the appearance of a bluish area on her right cheek. Four months later she had a reddish-purple nodule with a central punctum from which pus could be expressed by gentle pressure. The surrounding skin was dimpled and partially adherent to the deep tissues. Inside her mouth, a firm cord was palpable from the upper right premolar sulcus to the sinus. Extraction of the upper right first premolar, which was abscessed, was curative.

A 22-year-old man developed a discharging "cyst" on his left cheek 4 weeks after removal of the upper left second premolar. It was excised three times over the next 2 years but kept recurring. Four years after the tooth extraction he had an acute flare-up, and x-rays disclosed a retained abscessed root. Removal of this root stopped the drainage, and excision of the skin lesion 2 months later revealed a chronic inflammatory sinus.

It is advisable to examine the teeth in all cases of discharging facial lesions that persist despite treatment for a nonspecific dermal abscess.

Cioffi GA, Terezhalmy GT, Parlette HL: Cutaneous draining **sinus tract**: An odontogenic etiology. J Am Acad Dermatol 1986; 14:94–100.

For 5 years a 20-year-old woman had a draining lesion under her chin. Three surgical excisions had yielded microscopic diagnoses of cellulitis and granulation tissue. Treatment with topical and systemic antibacterial agents, as well as topical steroids, had been of little help.

At the time of examination, a submental node was palpable, and the lower right incisor was darkened, mobile, and sensitive to percussion. X-rays disclosed a periapical abscess. Within 21 days of root canal therapy, the submental skin lesion had healed.

A literature review of 137 cases of chronic dental infection with a suppurative sinus tract disclosed that swelling and pain are usually absent, and patients are unaware of any dental problems. The best treatment is root canal therapy, although extraction is also curative. Diagnostic ignorance often leads to surgery, radiation therapy, and treatment with ineffectual systemic antibiotics over a period of years.

McCluer CFA, Jr., Burns RE: **Dental** abscess with **sinus tract** formation. Arch Dermatol 1961; 83:941–944.

Dental abscess may be ruled out only by intraoral films of the entire mandible and maxilla. Extraoral dental films are not adequate.

The nearest tooth to the skin lesion is not necessarily the tooth involved by abscess. Pus may dissect beneath the periosteum for some distance before exiting into the skin.

Fascial planes and muscle groups of the face and neck influence the course of sinus tracts to the skin. Dental abscesses from the upper jaw usually drain about the zygomatic and infraorbital area, while those of the lower jaw usually track to the chin, neck, and submaxillary areas. However, any tooth can drain in almost any location.

A dental abscess most commonly drains through an intraoral fistula, located on the palate, either side of the mandible or maxilla, or in the antrum or nasal cavity. Even an edentulous patient may have an abscess and sinus tract due to an incomplete extraction.

Wolff A, Kitchen G, Bennett R: Sports medicine quiz. Injury to nose. Aust Fam Physician 1987; 16:922.

A 15-year-old footballer was accidentally punched on the nose during a match. The nose did not bleed, but was quite tender, and later in the day the youngster could not breathe freely though the nose. Five days later he felt unwell and anorexic, with pain in his face and throbbing in the nose. Ten days after the injury he was febrile, and his nose was red and hot. The nostrils were completely obstructed by a bulging red septum.

The diagnosis was **nasal septum abscess**, which developed in a hematoma (formed between the two sheets of mucoperiosteum covering the septum). No fracture of the bony septum was seen. Treatment consisted of surgical drainage of the abscess under general anesthesia, and intravenous antibiotics for *Staphylococcus aureus* found in the pus.

Nasal septum abscess may be life-threatening, as the infection readily passes to the orbit or cavernous sinus through thrombosing veins. Necrosis of cartilage and bone may cause depression of the nasal bridge.

Schache DJ, Stebbing A, Rees M: Congenital **pilonidal sinus of the nose**. NZ J Surg 1989; 59:511–512.

A 13-year-old schoolboy had a discharging sinus on the bridge of his nose, noted immediately after birth. During childhood it had intermittently become inflamed and discharged pus and hairs. Excision revealed a hair-filled sinus with granulation tissue at the base.

Unique, however, was the presence of hair follicles in the squamous epithelium of the superficial portion of the sinus, which presumably acted as the source of hairs in the sinus. The sinus tract was nearly 2 inches long.

Rud J: **Cervicofacial actinomycosis**. J Oral Surg 1967; 25:229–235.

A 33-year-old woman developed a painless 10-cm left submandibular abscess, which was hard and infiltrated, and red and swollen in the center with a tendency to perforate. She was afebrile. Five months previously she had had oral surgery with removal of a partially impacted lower left third molar.

Incision of the abscess yielded thick yellow pus with small granules, but no actinomycetes or threads. A culture grew *Actinobacillus actinomycetemcomitans* and *Bacteroides corrodens*. Penicillin was curative, although not until a second abscess 3 cm behind the initial one had perforated.

If a dental infection develops into a hard subcutaneous swelling with perforation through the skin, actinomycosis should be suspected. Most dental infections develop into submucous abscesses, which perforate intraorally.

Cervicofacial actinomycosis presents as abscesses that tend to form fistulas. The anaerobic microbes are saprophytes in the oral cavity but flourish in the anaerobic conditions that occur in extraction sockets, impacted teeth, jaw fractures, periodontal pocket formation, and periapical osteitis.

Das DK, Bhatt NC, Khan VA, Luthra UK: **Cervicofacial actinomycosis:** Diagnosis by fine needle aspiration cytology. Acta Cytol 1989; 33:278–280.

Two patients with sebaceous-cyst–like swelling of the left parotid gland and right maxillary regions underwent fine-needle aspiration cytology, as did a third man with a submandibular swelling.

Smears showed inflammatory cells and gram-positive balls or aggregates of *Actinomyces* in fine granules with radiating filaments. A Gomori silver methenamine stain confirmed the cytodiagnosis.

Scalp

Razzouk A, Collins N, Zirkle T: Chronic extensive **necrotizing abscess** of the **scalp**. Ann Plast Surg 1988; 20:124–127.

A chronic draining purulent ulcer on the scalp calls for bacterial and fungal cultures, as well as plain x-ray films of the skull to assess soft tissue swelling, periosteal reaction, and the possible presence of a foreign body, osteomyelitis, or tumor.

Scalp abscesses are rare because of the rich blood supply of the head. Most of them are acute, following traumatic scalp lacerations, puncture wounds, or needle electrode insertion for fetal monitoring. These usually resolve quickly with antibiotic treatment. In contrast, postsurgical scalp ulcers may become chronic as a result of extensive purulent fibrosis of the scalp. The subaponeurotic layer of the scalp is loose and scanty, allowing rapid spread of infection with empyema. The periosteum becomes very thick (up to 2.5 cm) with dense fibrosis and foci of necrosis and inflammation.

A subgaleal abscess occurs as a soft fluctuant mass with local tenderness and adjacent erythema and induration. Puffiness of the eyelids and lymphadenopathy may also be present. Purulent drainage from a sinus tract or a chronic nonhealing ulcer warrants operative intervention.

Nichter LS, Thomas DM, Atkinson J, et al: **Scalp infections** in black children: Think **kerion**. Plast Reconstruct Surg 1987; 80:717–719.

A 19-month-old black girl with seborrheic dermatitis of the scalp since birth developed swelling and erythema of the scalp with multiple subcutaneous abscesses draining yellow pus over 70 percent of her scalp. Her temperature was 104°F, white blood count 30,800, and erythrocyte sedimentation rate 74; wound and blood cultures for bacteria and fungi were negative. She did not improve with intravenous antibiotics. After two surgical procedures, including incision and drainage, and elevation of supragaleal flaps and placement of drainage catheters, a surgical fungal culture showed *Trichophyton tonsurans*. She was then treated with griseofulvin and systemic steroids and became afebrile after 1 day.

This child had a kerion, with boggy inflammation, yellow folliculopustules, and crusts. The Wood's light examination is negative for fluorescence with *T. tonsurans*, but a KOH examination will reveal an endothrix infection with chains of spores within the hair follicle. Inflammatory lesions are difficult to culture and may require two or three repeat cultures.

Berne B, Venge P, Öhman S: **Perifolliculitis capitis** abscedens et suffodiens (Hoffman). Complete healing associated with oral zinc therapy. Arch Dermatol 1985: 121:1028–1030.

Tender suppurating nodules had been present on the scalp of a 24-year-old man for 1 year. He had an 8- by 12-cm area of alopecia covered with erythematous fluctuant suppurating nodules with intercommunicating sinuses, from which *Staphylococcus aureus* was isolated. The entire scalp had numerous similar smaller lesions. A biopsy specimen showed a dense inflammatory infiltrate. Blood studies, including neutrophil phagocytosis, migration, bactericidal functions, and serum zinc level, were entirely normal. However, neutrophil chemotactic activity was reduced. Perifolliculitis capitis abscedens et suffodiens was diagnosed.

Within 3 weeks of the starting of oral zinc sulfate therapy (400 mg/day) the nodules had disappeared, hair growth occurred, and neutrophil function returned to normal. After 6 months the scalp was healthy with a full complement of hair. Zinc therapy was discontinued, and there was no relapse in the following 5 years.

Note: all this was achieved in the complete absence of antibiotic or steroid therapy.

Goldstein N, Tuazon CU, Lessin L: **Carbuncles** caused by ***Candida albicans***. J Am Acad Dermatol 1986; 14:511–512.

One month prior to hospitalization a 16-year-old white girl with diabetes and neutropenia had small (2 mm) indurated lesions in the scalp. Aspirates grew *Candida albicans*, believed to be contaminants.

The lesions enlarged, coalesced, and became painful, forming five 4- by 5-cm indurated crusted lesions with local alopecia. Repeat aspirates showed *C. albicans*, finally believed to be pathogenic. Flucytosine and surgical debridement were curative. However, 6 months later the patient returned with a *C. albicans* perinephric abscess.

Trust the laboratory personnel to find the pathogens, and then believe them when they do.

Breathes there a dermatologist with soul so dead,
Who never to himself has said,
"What the hell is that?"

Axilla

Richards M, Hurse A: **Corynebacterium pseudotuberculosis** abscesses in a young butcher. Aust NZ J Med 1985; 15:85–86.

For 6 weeks an 18-year-old butcher in Australia had had severe headache, fever, profuse sweats, and swelling in his right axilla and right epitrochlear area. His work involved handling offal, and he frequently had cuts on his hands. Pus removed from large abscesses in the axilla and epitrochlear area showed no organisms, and cultures were negative.

A biopsy of the abscess wall on the arm showed vascular fibrous tissue with granulation tissue. A repeat Gram stain of pus was negative, but a small isolate of *Corynebacterium pseudotuberculosis* was recovered after 4 days. Despite treatment with tetracycline and erythromycin, he developed a 6-cm abscess in the 13th week of illness, which was excised but subsequently drained for 5 months. Eventually, all of the abscesses healed.

Veterinarians recognize *C. pseudotuberculosis* as a cause of lymphadenopathy ("cheesy gland") in sheep and goats, and isolated ulcers and abscesses in cattle and horses. This aerobic pleomorphic gram-positive bacillus grows slowly and resembles a diphtheroid contaminant on culture. Therefore, any "diphtheroids" isolated from an abscess in workers handling offal and hides should be treated with suspicion.

Murray-Leisure KA, Egan N, Weitekamp MR: Skin lesions caused by **Mycobacterium scrofulaceum**. Arch Dermatol 1987; 123:369–370.

A 32-year-old man with systemic lupus erythematosus controlled by steroid therapy developed three deep nodules on the right thigh, buttock, and posterior axilla. He did not feel ill and was afebrile, without lymphadenopathy. Three weeks later the lesions were nodular and fluctuant, and the 3- by 2-cm thigh lesion had ulcerated. Incision and drainage of the axillary abscess yielded copious pus with no organisms on Gram's stain and no aerobic or anaerobic growth on routine media. Oral erythromycin for 2 weeks caused no improvement.

Two weeks later a skin biopsy from the edge of the nonhealing axillary ulcer showed granulomatous inflammation with giant cells and a few acid-fast organisms. Another **subcutaneous nodule** developed on the right thigh 4 weeks later, and needle aspiration yielded pus with numerous acid-fast bacilli, identified as *Mycobacterium scrofulaceum*, a slow-growing mycobacterium. Treatment with isoniazid and rifampin for 9 months cleared the lesions, despite in vitro drug resistance of the organism.

Vellodi C: Subcutaneous **Salmonella** abscess—an unusual manifestation of salmonellosis. J R Soc Med 1990; 83:190.

An 86-year-old man developed a small, hard swelling in the left posterior axillary line, overlying the site of pleural aspiration done 6 months before for pleural effusion. It grew and burst 2 weeks later, discharging thick purulent blood-stained fluid that grew out *Salmonella typhimurium* phage type 12. The source of the infection was not detected. Although the patient was elderly and generally debilitated, he made a remarkable recovery with antibiotics, which cleared the abscess and pleural effusion.

Soft tissue abscesses due to salmonellosis are rare and usually related to infection of the gastrointestinal tract. In this case, however, the abscess localized at a site of previous surgical trauma. Carrier states of *Salmonella* other than *S. typhi* are rare, but in this patient carrier status could not be ruled out, since his stool and urine were not cultured prior to antibiotic therapy.

Aird I: **Pilonidal sinus** of the **axilla**. Br Med J 1952; 1:902–903.

A 34-year-old man had a small sinus in the right axilla, which had intermittently discharged pus for 6 months. No axillary lymph nodes were palpable. Cultures for tuberculosis were negative. Over the next 2 years surgical excision was done three times for multiple draining sinuses and subcutaneous induration, which always recurred until radical excision of the floor of the axilla was performed.

The diagnosis remained uncertain until two small hairs with a surrounding foreign body reaction were found in a sinus tract. Interestingly, he had previously undergone two operations for pilonidal sinuses in the sacrococcygeal area.

A Glossary of Skin

Macule:	A stain that won't come off in rain
Papule:	A bump that may decide to clump
Nodule:	A lump much bigger than a bump
Pimple:	A dimple upside down, that's simple
Vesicle:	A dewdrop caught and held so taut
Bulla:	A blister where the ivy kissed her
Pustule:	An elder blister gone to fester
Wheal:	A hive where once a bedbug hugged her
Comedo:	A tiny baby zit, that's it
Burrow:	A place to hide a mite inside
Scale:	A dancing squame that has no shame
Crust:	A skin that's bust and gone to rust
Erosion:	A place where skin has lost its face
Ulcer:	A pit in which bacteria sit
Fissure:	A crack in skin that's out of whack
Scar:	The mending—that's the ending

E. Dorinda Shelley
Walter B. Shelley

(From JAMA 262: 2917, 1989.)

Breast

Rench MA, Baker CJ: Group B streptococcal **breast abscess** in a mother and **mastitis** in her **infant**. Obstet Gynecol 1989; 73:875–877.

Postpartum endemic mastitis occurs in 1 to 5% of women. Breast abscesses are rare, occurring in about 10% of patients with mastitis, and during lactation are usually caused by *Staphylococcus aureus*.

Mastitis is rare in infants and is caused most frequently by *S. aureus* and *Escherichia coli*.

A fissure in the nipple of the left breast was followed by erythema, warmth, and pain of the entire left breast in a 38-year-old woman with a newborn son who was being breast-fed. Despite antibiotics, she developed chills and fever and a large abscess, which grew out group B streptococcus. The 12-day-old baby also developed swelling, erythema, and warmth of the left breast, with breast exudate that grew the same organism.

Only about 25% of breast abscesses are preceded by a nipple fissure, but pain from the fissure interrupts normal feeding and leads to milk stasis and bacterial growth. The lactating breast responds by localizing the infection, which impairs vascular perfusion and delivery of antibiotics to the abscess site.

Rudoy RC, Nelson JD: **Breast abscess** during the **neonatal** period. A review. Am J Dis Child 1975; 129:1031–1034.

A typical breast abscess in a neonate is unilateral, begins on day 8 to 10 of life, and is caused by *Staphylococcus aureus*. Systemic toxicity is usually absent, and most patients have a temperature less than 37.8°C (100.0°F). Surgical drainage yields about 10 ml of pus.

In this study of 39 infants, *Salmonella* and *Escherichia coli* were found in 4 patients, while 32 infants had *Staphylococcus aureus*; 84% of abscesses started during the first 3 weeks of life. Physiologic breast enlargement, especially in girls, may be an important predisposing factor.

The etiologic agent may be quickly identified by a Gram stain of purulent material expressed from the nipple or obtained by needle aspiration or incision and drainage.

An important complication is reduction in breast size, seen in adulthood.

Habif DV, Perzin KH, Lipton R, Lattes R: **Subareolar abscess** associated with squamous metaplasia of lactiferous ducts. Am J Surg 1970; 119:523–526.

Women with inverted nipples may also have inflamed comedones and infected sebaceous cysts (epidermal inclusion cysts) of the nipples. These lesions represent dilated portions of the nipple ducts that have undergone squamous metaplasia. Rupture of the ducts leads to foreign body abscesses with bacterial invasion.

In normal lactiferous ducts there is an abrupt transition from squamous to columnar epithelium approximately 1 to 2 mm underneath the epidermal surface of the nipple. Keratin may accumulate within the lumen of the proximal ducts, causing dilatation or rupture with subareolar abscess formation.

Crile G, Chatty EM: Squamous metaplasia of lactiferous ducts. Arch Surg 1971; 102:533–534.

A 35-year-old woman had an undrained abscess of the left breast just lateral to the areola and a draining sinus similarly located on the right breast. She had had 20 operations in 13 years for breast abscesses and fistulas. Always the abscesses and draining fistulas recurred, pointing at the periphery of the areola.

Periareolar abscesses are almost always caused by squamous metaplasia with hyperkeratosis of the terminal portions of the lactiferous ducts. The squamous epithelium of the ducts exfoliates, like the lining of an epidermal inclusion cyst. White keratin accumulates in the ducts. When the nipple is squeezed, the toothpaste-like material can be expressed, resembling worms with the unpleasant odor of a wen. The ducts tend to rupture, causing inflammation with foreign body giant cells. The proper treatment is surgical excision of the peripheral ducts.

Autoimmune panniculitis may also cause breast abscesses, responsive to oral prednisone treatment.

Gannon MX, Crowson MC, Fielding JWL: **Periareolar pilonidal abscesses** in a hairdresser. Br Med J 1988; 297:1641–1642.

A 21-year-old woman who had been a women's hairdresser for some years had recently begun to cut men's hair. She then began developing periareolar inflammation on both breasts, followed by numerous breast abscesses over a 3-month-period. Tissue removed at biopsy showed periductal mastitis. The lesions were unresponsive to antibiotics.

The woman gave a history of having to remove short hairs protruding from her nipples at the end of a working day. A clump of short hairs was then found within an abscess, and in a subsequent abscess digital pressure from within the abscess cavity extruded hair through the mammary ducts. By this technique hair was cleared from the ducts and recurrence of abscesses stopped. Biopsy revealed birefringent foreign material, identified as hair, in the wall of the abscess cavity.

This type of pilonidal disease of the areola is rare, but it has also been reported in a canine beautician and sheepshearers' assistants who carry wool close to their breast. Use of protective clothing or plasters is curative.

Hanson PJV, Thomes JM, Collins JV: ***Mycobacterium chelonei*** and **abscess** formation in soft tissues. Tubercle 1987; 68:297–299.

A 46-year-old English woman developed a 10-cm red, hot, tender swelling in the left breast over a 1-week period. The regional lymph nodes were not enlarged. Inflammatory carcinoma was suspected, but tissue obtained by needle biopsy revealed noncaseating granulomas and acid-fast bacilli. *Mycobacterium chelonei* was isolated on Löwenstein-Jensen medium after 6 weeks.

Treatment with isoniazid, rifampicin, and pyrazinamide reduced the size of the abscess but did not prevent two more abscesses from forming in the same breast. Tetracycline caused no further improvement, but administration of erythromycin and trimethoprim for 5 months cleared the lesions.

M. chelonei is a rapidly growing species of mycobacteria found in soil, house dust, and domestic water supplies (resistant to chlorination). Infection occurs where the skin is broken, resulting in a wartlike lesion or soft tissue abscess. Surgical incisions and injection sites have been infection sites.

Wilson ME: **Wegener's granulomatosis** presenting as **breast abscess**. Am J Med 1987; 83:1168.

A 39-year-old mother of five developed fever and a 5-cm erythematous tender mass on her right breast. Surgical drainage yielded 15 ml of thick green non-foul-smelling pus. Cytologic study showed only polymorphonuclear leukocytes, with no organisms or malignant cells. All cultures (bacterial, fungal, mycobacterial) were negative. Antibiotics did not help.

Her history revealed that 2 months earlier she had oral surgery to remove a retained left molar root, followed by left maxillary sinusitis and pain in the right cheek, unresponsive to antibiotics. Tissue taken from the maxillary sinus showed necrotizing granulomatous vasculitis with eosinophilic infiltrates and giant cells. Repeat surgical drainage and biopsy of the rapidly enlarging breast abscess showed identical pathologic findings, consistent with Wegener's granulomatosis. She improved rapidly with prednisone and cyclophosphamide therapy.

In a patient with a "sterile" breast abscess that is unresponsive to antibiotics, obtain a biopsy!

Medicine is a science of uncertainty and an art of probability. One of the chief reasons for this uncertainty is the increasing variability in the manifestations of any one disease.

Sir William Osler

Katz BJ, Kalter DC, Bruce S: **Subcutaneous nodules** in a man diagnosed as having tuberculosis. Arch Dermatol 1988; 124:121–124.

A 27-year-old black man had multiple tender, raised erythematous subcutaneous nodules for 2 months on the arms, legs, neck, and trunk. They began as small "pimples" that gradually enlarged to 2 to 5 cm and became fluctuant and warm, discharging light yellow serosanguineous material. Five months before he had had a nonproductive cough, low-grade fever, night sweats, anorexia, and weight loss. A presumptive diagnosis of pulmonary tuberculosis was based on a chest x-ray that showed a right upper-lobe reticulonodular infiltrate and a PPD test positive at 20 mm, although sputum cultures were negative for acid-fast bacilli. Treatment with rifampin, isoniazid, and pyrazinamide failed, and he lost 22 pounds over a 5-month period.

Aspiration of a fluctuant nodule revealed yellowish granules suggestive of actinomycosis, and culture yielded a facultative aerobe of the *Actinobacillus* species, commonly found in **actinomycosis**. Long-term treatment with penicillin was successful.

Always consider actinomycosis with:

> draining sinuses or recurrent abscesses
> exudates containing gram-positive rods that do not grow on aerobic culture.
> sulfur granules in the exudate or biopsy specimen. It may explain other systemic problems involving the chest, brain, bone, liver, and kidneys. Actinomycosis may be associated with false-positive tuberculin skin tests.

Serologic and cutaneous testing for actinomycosis is variable and not recommended. Anaerobic cultures of pus or sulfur granules on glucose agar or brain-heart infusion medium at 37°C for 2 to 4 days result in 1- to 2-mm white glistening nodular colonies with irregular margins. Multiple synergistic anaerobes may be present, including *Actinobacillus actinomycetemcomitans*. A Gram stain reveals lobulated masses of pleomorphic gram-positive bacilli, some of which are long slender branching filaments with pseudohyphae.

Sulfur granules develop when a polysaccharide protein substance from inflamed tissue cements the organisms (filaments) together. Granular colonies in the center of the nodules may have radiating mycelial filaments, surrounded by liquefactive necrosis, polymorphonuclear leukocytes, and granulation tissue with calcification. The granules vary from white to yellow and are 0.25 to 2 mm in diameter. To recover them from a lesion, place a gauze dressing over an open wound overnight, as the granules will adhere to the dressing. They may also be found by aspirating pus into a tube and gently rolling the tube, leaving granules on the sides. Cultures of sulfur granules give a higher rate of organism recovery than do cultures of pus alone. Sulfur granules are also found in infections due to *Nocardia brasiliensis* and to some *Streptomyces* species, and in botryomycosis and mycetoma.

McCarty MJ, Whitlock WL, Dietrich RA: Cutaneous signs of cardiopulmonary disease. **A red hot sternal mass.** Chest 1989; 96:924–926.

For 5 days a 65-year-old woman had a slowly enlarging red tender mass over the midsternal area. For 2 months she had also had malaise, nonproductive cough, low-grade fevers, and a 9-kg weight loss. The tender mass on her sternum was 9.5 by 9.5 cm. Fine-needle aspiration yielded scant amounts of turbid serosanguineous material, which revealed **actinomycosis** on Gram stain. Cultures confirmed the presence of *Actinomyces israelii*.

Chest x-ray examination and computed tomography of the chest showed a pulmonary parenchymal process and large mass in the anterior mediastinum extending through the anterior chest wall with sternal cortical erosion.

Treatment for 12 months with penicillin cleared all of her lesions.

Helm TN, Mazanec D: **Disseminated aspergillosis** presenting as a **skin abscess**. Cleve Clin J Med 1990; 57:92–94.

A 58-year-old black woman with pulmonary and cutaneous sarcoidosis had taken prednisone (20 mg daily) for 4 years. She then developed pain in the right lower paralumbar region, exacerbated by movement. After $3\frac{1}{2}$ months a 6- by 4-cm firm moveable mass appeared in the same area. Over the next 2 weeks it enlarged to 10 by 10 cm and became markedly erythematous and tender. Drainage of the subcutaneous abscess yielded 50 ml of pus, which grew *Aspergillus fumigatus*. Her back pain was immediately relieved.

She had no complement fixation antibodies to *Aspergillus*, although immuno-diffusion studies showed bands of identity to all types of *Aspergillus* studied. *Aspergillus fumigatus* was also cultured from her lungs and sinuses. Despite treatment with amphotericin B, she soon died. Presumably the skin infection was secondary to systemic aspergillosis.

The presence of unrelenting lower back pain at rest should suggest an infectious or malignant cause, particularly in older patients. In immunosuppressed patients, infection should be a primary consideration.

van Durme DJ, Holder CD, Brownlee HJ: **Gonorrhea** presenting as a **subcutaneous abscess**. J Fam Pract 1989; 29:675–678.

A 70-year-old woman developed sudden pain and swelling around the right scapula, with a 5- by 8-cm deep subcutaneous fluctuant area visible 2 weeks later. There was no increased warmth or overlying skin charge. Computed tomography revealed a 4- by 10-cm fluid collection, and needle aspiration performed under CT guidance revealed pus with gram-negative diplococci. Surgical drainage produced 150 ml of thick pus, which grew out *Neisseria gonorrhoeae* (β-lactamase negative).

She shared a bed with her daughter, who had been treated for gonorrhea 10 months before. Possibly a break in skin integrity allowed the organism to enter. She denied any sexual activity for 20 years. Her health was generally poor because of diabetes, hypothyroidism, alcoholic cirrhosis, and rheumatoid arthritis treated intermittently with prednisone.

Benson PM, Roth RR, Hicks CB, Brisker J: **Nodular subcutaneous abscesses** caused by *Candida tropicalis*. J Am Acad Dermatol 1987; 16:623–624.

For 2 days a 33-year-old white man with acute myelocytic leukemia had had multiple 1- to 2-cm skin-colored slightly tender, firm, freely mobile nodules on the thorax, abdomen, and extremities. He was afebrile, but had vague proximal muscle myalgias.

An incisional biopsy specimen revealed a small abscess cavity with thick purulent material in the subcutaneous fat. A KOH preparation showed numerous hyphal elements, pseudohyphae, and blastoconidia, consistent with *Candida* species. Gram's stain and routine bacterial cultures were negative. Fungal cultures grew *Candida tropicalis*.

History revealed that 10 days prior to onset of the nodules he had had a febrile episode with diffuse myalgias and a papular erythematous exanthem. Fungal cultures of blood, urine, and a skin biopsy had been negative, but this could have represented systemic candidemia. *Candida tropicalis* may be more virulent than *C. albicans*.

Don't forget to use a KOH preparation on pus from an abscess—it could be lifesaving.

Clery AP, Clery AB: **Pilonidal disease** of the **umbilicus**. Br J Surg 1963; 50:666–668.

A 34-year-old male tailor's cutter complained of pain and discharge from the umbilicus. One year previously he had had a small pustule of the umbilicus, which healed in a few days. Ten months later the umbilical suppuration recurred. Examination revealed a well-built man covered with dark hairs on his abdomen and limbs. Two tufts of black hair protruded from the umbilicus, amid purulent discharge, and the surrounding skin was red and inflamed.

Omphalectomy confirmed the clinical diagnosis of pilonidal sinus. A coiled mass of black hairs was found within a cavity lined by granulation tissue.

Most cases of pilonidal sinus of the umbilicus have occurred in unusually hirsute men. A diagnosis of pilonidal sinus should be strongly considered whenever a patient with excessive body hair complains of recurrent navel suppuration.

Patey D, Williams ES: **Pilonidal sinus** of the **umbilicus**. Lancet 1956; 2:281–282.

A 26-year-old Indian student with a dense growth of dark tough hair on the abdomen had exuberant granulations around a discharging sinus in the folds of the umbilicus. A protruding tuft of hairs was extracted from the sinus, but it did not heal. At surgery, about 300 hairs were found in a 2-cm-long pilonidal sinus. All of the hairs had the same orientation, with the root ends directed deeply.

This type of sinus may be an uncommon variety of the common granulomatous sinus of the umbilicus resulting from accumulation of dirt, clothing fragments, and epithelial debris in the umbilical depression.

Crosby DL: **Pilonidal sinus** of the **suprapubic** region. Br J Surg 1962; 49:457–458.

An 18-year-old girl had a 10-month history of a "discharging boil" at the upper border of the mons pubis. It began like a boil, but failed to heal, and drained yellow offensive material intermittently. She had had other boils and frequently rode horseback.

Examination revealed a sinus opening at the upper border of the mons pubis, from which pus could be obtained. A subcutaneous tract was palpable passing down to the vulva, and a metal probe passed easily through the sinus, exiting just anterior to the clitoris. During surgery, a short compact cylinder of hairs was extruded. Histologic examination revealed infected granulation tissue, and a pilonidal sinus was diagnosed. The etiologic role of horseback riding was probably minor.

Jarasius B: **Pilonidal sinus** of the **pubis**. Med J. Aust 1985; 143:322.

A 36-year-old woman had recurrent abscesses of the pubic region for 3 years. There were always a small erythematous macule or sinus and frequently a small amount of serous discharge. A small sinus was found in the midline on the mons pubis, with a slightly tender 2- by 1-cm lump deep to this. A probe disclosed a 2-cm-long sinus tract lined with granulation tissue and containing numerous hairs. Excision of the sinus tract confirmed a pilonidal sinus.

Careful inquiry failed to reveal any activity, such as horseback riding, which might have been causally related. Only four cases of pilonidal sinuses of the pubic area had been reported previously.

Arms

Canales FL, Newmeyer WL III, Kilgore ES Jr.: The treatment of **felons** and paronychias. Hand Clin 1989; 5:515–523.

A felon is an abscess with a given name. Basically, it is a palmar closed-space infection of the distal pulp of the finger that leads to abscess formation. It begins with throbbing pain, tension, and swelling of the entire pulp. Usually, but not always, the patient can recall an injury with a sliver of wood or glass, or a minor cut. Even a blood test fingerstick can be responsible, i.e., the fingerstick felon.

Usually, *Staphylococcus aureus* is the responsible pathogen. Initially there is little but inflammation and cellulitis; however, abscess formation soon occurs, especially in the immunocompromised patient. The tissue pressure mounts, as the pus cannot exit from the closed compartment. Tissue perfusion is compromised, leading to ischemic necrosis of both skin and periosteum and finally bone. Osteitis, osteomyelitis, and suppurative flexor tenosynovitis may ensue.

Immediate antibiotic administration and drainage by longitudinal incision into the terminal palmar pulp (but not crossing the flexion crease) are recommended following the early diagnosis.

The word *felon* comes from the old French term for a villain and, in turn, felony, an act done by a villain. And so to miss the diagnosis of a felon might indeed be a felony.

Borghans JGA, Stanford JL: *Mycobacterium chelonei* in abscesses after injection of diphtheria-pertussis-tetanus-polio vaccine. Am Rev Resp Dis 1973; 107:1–8.

Most cases of **injection abscesses** caused by rapidly growing mycobacteria are due to *Mycobacterium ranae* (fortuitum).

In 47 children in the Netherlands, 50 abscesses developed after they received DPTP vaccine. Each lesion started as a lump at the injection site from 1 to 13 months (mean 3 months) after the injection. The lumps were painless, but after 6 weeks a 1- to 4-cm abscess formed. Only six abscesses drained spontaneously, and the rest required incision and drainage. There was no fever or lymphadenopathy.

Skin biopsies revealed fistulating subcutaneous inflammation with a few epithelioid granulomas. Acid-fast rods were found with Ziehl-Neelsen stain in one of six lesions. After this, a more intensive search for mycobacteria was carried out, with prolongation of routine cultures and use of special culture media at 30° and 37°C. Tiny whitish growth appeared on blood agar plates 4 days after inoculation. Short acid-fast rods were present in these colonies. *M. chelonei* was eventually identified.

Several children in this outbreak were skin tested with the following antigens:

old tuberculin (OT)
PPD F (*ranae*)
PPD A1 (*avium*)
PPD Gause
PPD Glaze (American strain of *M. chelonei*)

All skin tests were negative except for PPD Glaze, which was reactive in several children.

Patients with chronic focal infective lesions on the arms or legs should be carefully questioned about injections. Often a long interval has elapsed between the injection and abscess formation, so that the patient may not relate the two events. Specimens from their lesions should be examined microscopically and culturally for acid-fast organisms.

Brandrup F, Asschenfeldt P: *Molluscum contagiosum*-induced **comedo** and secondary **abscess** formation. Pediatr Dermatol 1989; 6:118–121.

A 9-year-old boy had recurrent fluctuating abscesses of the forearms for 1 month, leading to surgical excisions. A bluish red abscess, resembling an acne cyst, was present on the left forearm, along with two black open comedolike lesions about 1 mm in width. He also had typical small waxy papules of molluscum contagiosum scattered on his trunk and extremities. He was not atopic.

Cultures taken of pus showed either no growth or only a few micrococci. Gram stains revealed many polymorphonuclear leukocytes, epithelial cells, and a few cocci. No search for molluscum bodies was made.

Biopsy of a slightly inflamed comedo revealed typical molluscum bodies in the deep part of the epidermis within the lower portion of a pilosebaceous follicle. The comedolike plugging was thought to be a reaction pattern secondary to the viral infection.

History revealed that the primary lesion was a comedo, which became pustular and cystic a few days after attempts to squeeze out the contents. Presumably the inflammatory reaction represented a foreign body reaction.

Philipsen EK, Larsen S, Jensen KD: **Subcutaneous abscesses** and pulmonary infiltrate due to **Actinomyces** infection. Case report. Acta Chir Scand 1988; 154:675–677.

A 56-year-old man developed three simultaneous abscesses of his left upper and lower arm, right foot, and left calf. They began as 15-cm-long moderately tender swellings without redness, but soon became painful, red, and indurated. He also had a nonproductive cough, and a right upper lobe infiltrate was noted on x-ray.

Drainage of thick malodorous yellow pus from the abscesses showed no growth. However, microscopy of a biopsy specimen from the arm swelling revealed *Actinomyces* grains. Treatment with penicillin for 6 months was curative. His poor oral hygiene was blamed as the source of the infection, via both aspiration and hematogenous spread.

No routine serologic tests are available for *Actinomyces*. The gram-positive filamentous bacterium is difficult to culture, requiring 4 to 6 days of anaerobic incubation at 37°C on blood agar. The bacteria form macroscopic "sulfur granules" composed of intertwined filaments.

Okano M: Primary cutaneous **actinomycosis** of the **extremities**: A report from Japan. Cutis 1989; 44:231–233.

A 30-year-old Japanese man had three discrete oval erythematous fluctuant lesions on the left upper arm and right thigh. Incision of the 6-cm moist lesion on the thigh revealed fluid with many yellowish granules. Biopsy specimens showed granulation tissue with abscesses and sulfur granules containing gram-positive branching bacilli that were not acid-fast. Aerobic and anaerobic cultures were negative. Oral minocycline was curative.

Although apparently no trauma preceded any of the lesions, this patient had cerebral palsy, so that his saliva could have reached the sites of the lesions, causing actinomycosis.

Nocardiosis was ruled out by the bacilli's lack of acid fastness (Ziehl-Neelsen stain) and the negative aerobic culture.

Novick NL, Tapia L, Bottone EJ: **Invasive *Trichophyton rubrum*** infection in an immunocompromised host. Case report and review of the literature. Am J Med 1987; 82:321–325.

A 28-year-old Colombian man with a renal transplant developed nail dystrophies of his fingers and toes and a diffuse pruritic rash on his upper back about 1 year after surgery. Two years later he noted two small pimple-like lesions on his right leg, which slowly grew and became exquisitely painful to touch. He also developed intractable pruritus, scaly soles, and annular erythematous patches with active scaling borders on his groin, inner thighs, and buttocks. In addition, he had six dusky reddish purple, smooth, fluctuant lesions (4 to 10 cm) on his right arm and right leg. They were cool, but very tender, with no surrounding erythema or edema.

Biopsy specimens from the fluctuant lesions revealed neutrophilic abscess cavities in the deep dermis and subcutis surrounded by early granulation tissue. PAS stain revealed scattered hyphae in the stratum corneum and upper follicular infundibulum. Cultures of pus showed no growth on routine bacterial and mycobacterial media but grew *Trichophyton rubrum* on Sabouraud's medium. A KOH preparation of pus, as well as a Gram stain, revealed irregular septate hyphae. *T. rubrum* also grew from his groin, buttocks, and dystrophic fingernails.

Invasive *T. rubrum* infections are rare and nearly always preceded by chronic cutaneous *T. rubrum* lesions. Tissue invasion is attributed to alteration in host resistance. Delayed-type hypersensitivity correlates with resistance to infection, whereas immediate hypersensitivity correlates with persistent chronic infection.

It would seem prudent to give antifungal therapy prior to immunosuppression in any patient with a chronic *T. rubrum* infection.

Kelly SE: Multiple **injection abscesses** in a diabetic caused by ***Mycobacterium chelonei***. Clin Exp Dermatol 1987; 12:48–49.

Four painful indurated subcutaneous lesions on both thighs of an 18-year-old Pakistani diabetic girl resulted from an inadequately sterilized needle and syringe used for insulin injections. The lesions ulcerated, with sinus formation and discharge of pus. Skin biopsy samples showed a dense dermal and subcutaneous fat infiltrate, with lymphocytes, plasma cells, histiocytes, and several poorly formed epithelioid granulomas. A single mycobacterium bacillus was identified with auramine-O staining, and prolonged culture of tissue from the biopsy yielded a scanty growth of *Mycobacterium chelonei*. The lesions healed rapidly with rifampicin therapy. The organism was also sensitive to clofamine and erythromycin.

M. chelonei produces nonpigmented colonies on Lowenstein-Jensen medium after 12 to 14 weeks. Most strains are resistant to standard tuberculous therapy but are often sensitive to erythromycin and cephalosporins. The organism causes mainly soft tissue infections in humans and has previously been reported to cause injection abscesses.

Singh G, Singh M: Erythromycin for **BCG cold abscess**. Lancet 1984; 2:979.

Six weeks after BCG vaccination a 4-month-old girl had a 3- by 2-cm fluctuant lesion at the site. A similar subcutaneous cold abscess was seen in a 3-month-old boy 2 months after BCG administration. Aspiration of both abscesses yielded acid-fast bacilli on Ziehl-Neelsen stain and no other organism on culture. Treatment with erythromycin for 15 days was curative.

If it's indescribable, photograph it.

Bello EF, Posalski I, Pitchon H, Bayer AS: **Fasciitis** and **abscesses** complicating **lipo-suction**. West J Med 1988; 148:703–706.

A 43-year-old woman who had undergone suction lipectomy of the abdomen and thighs developed fever, rigors, and excruciating pain at both thigh lipo-suction sites 2 days later. After 5 more days she was hospitalized with sepsis and moderate ecchymoses of the proximal one third of the left medial and posterolateral thigh, with overlying erythema and edema. The right thigh was tender and ecchymotic with erythema and edema of the right lateral area. Despite antibiotics, she became icteric, and her right thigh remained extremely swollen. Computed tomography on the sixth hospital day showed intense soft tissue inflammation and a fluid collection in the posterior aspect of the right thigh. Extensive fasciitis and multiple loculated abscesses were incised and drained, with cultures showing *Klebsiella pneumoniae* and *Escherichia coli*. She recovered with continuing administration of antibiotics but still had induration without tenderness 3 months later.

Amazingly, infectious complications after liposuction are rare, occurring in approximately 0.6%. Other complications include hypesthesia, seroma, edema, pigmentation, pain, hematoma, and skin sloughing, with an overall complication rate of about 9%.

Fleming MG, Milburn PB, Prose NS: *Pseudomonas* **septicemia** with **nodules** and **bullae**. Pediatr Dermatol 1987; 4:18–20.

A 12-year-old girl who was receiving prednisone (60 mg/day) for systemic lupus erythematosus became febrile (temperature 41°C) and was hospital-ized. Five days later she developed bullae (clear and hemorrhagic) and mul-tiple 1- to 3-cm erythematous indurated nodules on the trunk and extrem-ities. A biopsy specimen from the edge of a bulla revealed an abscess cavity filled with neutrophils, Gram stain negative. Fluid from a bulla, however, revealed gram-negative rods, proven to be *Pseudomonas aeruginosa*.

The source of her septicemia was a cavitating pseudomonal pneumonia. De-spite intravenous antibiotics, she died 11 days after admission.

The hematogenous dissemination of *P. aeruginosa* may lead to nodules, bul-lae, and subcutaneous abscesses. Pathologically, they differ mainly in the level of the dermis or subcutis at which bacterial proliferation and tissue necrosis occur. **Ecthyma gangrenosum**, pathognomonic of *Pseudomonas* sep-ticemia, is a similar lesion, which becomes necrotic and ulcerates. An ery-thematous macule that becomes indurated and then bullous or pustular, it finally sloughs to form a gangrenous ulcer with an erythematous halo.

Bullous lesions in sepsis may also be caused by *Escherichia coli*, *Aeromonas hydrophila*, and *Vibrio* species.

Nugteren-Huying WM: Primary cutaneous **actinomycosis**. Br J Dermatol 1989; 121:801–802.

Abscesses and **draining sinuses** recurring for 2 years in the right leg of this 29-year-old man had failed to respond to antibiotics, and bacterial cultures were uniformly negative.

Despite the failure to culture *Actinomyces*, actinomycosis was diagnosed by demonstrating filamentous organisms in the biopsy material and by culturing *Actinobacillus actinomycetemcomitans*, a fellow traveler with *Actinomyces israelii*, the true gram-positive anaerobic bacterial cause of actinomycosis.

Intravenous penicillin for 6 weeks followed by a year of oral penicillin was curative.

The diagnosis here gave the physician and the patient the strength to persist and conquer.

Hendrick SJ, Jorizzo JL, Newton RC: **Giant *Mycobacterium fortuitum* abscess** associated with systemic lupus erythematosus. Arch Dermatol 1986; 122:695–697.

A 36-year-old woman with systemic lupus erythematosus had dusky red nodules of the calves for 6 months, which ulcerated and gradually healed with scarring. A biopsy specimen showed a nonspecific granulomatous infiltrate, and fungal and mycobacterial cultures were negative. Three weeks later her left buttock became swollen, red, and tender. This time a biopsy specimen showed deep septal panniculitis with vascular involvement consistent with erythema nodosum. Numerous acid-fast bacteria were found on special staining, and within a week the culture of her abscess showed acid-fast bacteria, later identified as *Mycobacterium fortuitum*. Surgical incision and drainage down to muscle with conjoint antibiotic therapy (doxycycline, ethambutol) resulted in healing over the next 15 months.

The presence of acute systemic lupus erythematosus and immunosuppression with prednisone set the stage for these organisms to produce widespread abscesses. This was disseminated disease, not the localized inoculation form seen in patients who have scraped their hand on an aquarium. Be aware of the abscess-producing potential of these acid-fast organisms, and beware that one negative culture does not rule out your diagnosis.

Manji N, Hulyalkar AR, Keroack MA, et al: Cutaneous **pseudo abscesses**: An unusual presentation of severe **pancreatitis**. Am J Gastroenterol 1987; 83:177–179.

A 53-year-old white man with a history of alcohol abuse was acutely ill, with a temperature of 39°C and firm 1- to 4-cm nontender nodules on his thighs, legs, buttocks, and upper arms. A tender fluctuant 6-cm area was present on the dorsal aspect of the right hand, and similar smaller lesions occurred on the dorsal aspect of the left hand and right Achilles tendon.

Incision of the right-hand lesion yielded 70 ml of thick brown fluid with few leukocytes and no organisms on Gram stain or culture. Wet mount showed multiple fat globules. His serum amylase and lipase values were elevated, and computed tomography revealed an enlarged head of the pancreas.

Results of skin biopsy of a nodule showed fat and collagen necrosis consistent with **nodular panniculitis**. Fluid aspirated from a fluctuant area had an amylase value of 3240 IU/liter.

He died on the 38th hospital day of peritonitis, acute pancreatitis, and fat necrosis.

O'Malley BP, Minuk T, Castelli M: **Buttock abscess** complicating **Crohn's disease**. J Can Assoc Radiol 1989; 40:51–52.

A 25-year-old woman with Crohn's disease developed severe low back pain, fever, chills, and a warm fluctuant tender 5-cm mass in the medial right buttock. Her white blood count was 20,600, and she had mild tenderness in the right lower abdomen.

Sonographic examination of the right buttock revealed gas in the buttock mass, as well as in the right pelvis. A barium follow-through study outlined a fistulous tract extending from the terminal ileum to the buttock lesion. At surgery, the terminal ileum was found to be perforated, and there was an abscess in the right pelvis that extended through the greater sciatic foramen into the soft tissues of the right buttock.

Computed tomography was diagnostic in another similar case, showing gas bubbles in an abscess and elucidating the location and extent of the problem.

Watch out for fistulas communicating with the skin in Crohn's disease, particularly from a retroperitoneal abscess. The fistula site may be quite remote from an occult gastrointestinal perforation.

Soe GB, Gersten LM, Wilkins J, et al: **Infection** associated with [**computer**] **joystick** mimicking a spider bite. West J Med 1987; 146:748.

A 17-year-old right-handed boy was hospitalized with fever (temperature 101.7°F) and a grossly edematous indurated violaceous left hand. Incision and drainage of the web space between the second and third fingers yielded gross pus that grew *Staphylococcus aureus*.

History revealed that he spent most of his time playing his favorite kung fu video game, which involved use of a ball-shaped joystick in his left hand. He developed blisters on the left palm, which were then rubbed off, resulting in infection and abscess formation.

Neuromuscular complications of video games include:

"pseudovideoma"
"Pac-Man phalanx"
"firing-finger syndrome"
"Space Invaders wrist"
seizures

Perhaps video game players should wear gloves to protect their palms, similar to golfers and baseball players, who also need a firm grip on their sticks!

Pruzansky ME, Remer S: **Abscesses** of the **hand** associated with **otopharyngeal infections** in children. J Hand Surg 1986; 11A:844–846.

Abscesses of the hand may result from hematogenous spread of infection from an ear, the throat, or the upper respiratory tract. Surgical decompression is often necessary to arrest the closed-space infection.

A 15-month-old Hispanic girl had fever (temperature 104°F), right otitis media, and diffuse swelling of the left hand with tense erythematous, shiny skin over the thenar eminence. Left epitrochlear and axillary nodes were palpable. Blood cultures grew *Hemophilus influenzae*. Despite immobilization, elevation, and intravenous antibiotics, the redness and swelling increased, and surgical drainage of the thenar space was required. Wound cultures were negative. She recovered uneventfully.

An 8-year-old boy had fever (temperature 104°F), pharyngitis, erythema and injection of the right ear, and swelling and erythema of the dorsal area of the left hand and wrist. Fluctuance was palpable over the dorsal area of the hand, and the fingers were swollen. Axillary lymph nodes were enlarged. Throat and blood cultures grew group A beta hemolytic *Streptococcus*. After 5 days of intravenous antibiotics, the hand swelling continued. Surgical drainage was performed on the extensor tenosynovium and subaponeurotic space.

Blinkhorn RJ, Strimbu V, Effron D, Spagnuolo PJ: "Punch" **actinomycosis** causing **osteomyelitis** of the **hand**. Arch Intern Med 1988; 148:2668–2670.

A 51-year-old man confronted a burglar in his home and struck him with his right fist, knocking out two of his adversary's teeth. He suffered a laceration over his right second metacarpophalangeal joint, which was followed by swelling and pain the next day. Self-administered penicillin for a week caused improvement, but 6 weeks later there was increasing pain and swelling, unresponsive to tetracycline. Two months after the encounter there was an area of swelling, warmth, and fluctuance dorsally over the distal right second metacarpal, with a zone of surrounding induration and erythema. An x-ray of the hand showed osteomyelitis of the right second metacarpal. In the operating room, incision of the abscess yielded thick yellow-brown pus with pinhead-sized white gritty granules, and a bone biopsy was obtained. Numerous branching filamentous gram-positive rods were present, and *Actinomyces israelii* was cultured along with three other organisms. Treatment with high-dose penicillin for 1 year was curative.

Actinomycosis should be suspected when a **human bite injury**, especially a punch injury, is followed by a chronically draining sinus.

Currie AR, Gibson T, Goodall AL: **Interdigital sinuses** of **barbers' hands**. Br J Surg 1953; 41:278–286.

Interdigital sinuses in various stages of development were found in 10 of 77 barbers examined from 18 different shops. Short sharp hairs accumulate in finger webs, which are moist and sticky with soaps, hair creams, and sweat. The webs between the second and third and third and fourth fingers on the right hand are most commonly involved. The hairs penetrate the epidermis and induce inflammation, sinus formation, and sometimes abscesses. Multiple **pits** in the **finger webs** may mark the entrances to sinuses.

In the early stage, which is marked by a shallow pit, careful removal of all hairs from the finger web each night will be curative. If infection has occurred, however, surgical excision is necessary to remove the granulomatous reaction at the deep tip of the sinus.

Rand C: Cocktail stick injuries: Delayed diagnosis of a **retained foreign body**. Br Med J 1987; 295: 1658.

A 32-year-old housewife and a 12-year-old girl both stepped on wooden **cocktail sticks** while walking barefoot on a carpet. Each of them pulled out the protruding stick and assumed that the entire stick had been removed. However, they did not remember the length of the stick or whether the piece removed was pointed at both ends. A similar episode occurred with a $1\frac{1}{2}$-year-old girl who fell onto a cocktail stick, which entered the hypothenar eminence of her hand.

All three subsequently had draining sinuses, abscesses, and pain for months. Several antibiotics were helpful but not curative. Cure came only with surgical removal of the retained cocktail sticks, which, although measuring 3 to 7 cm in length, were not visible on radiologic study.

Moral: If a broken stick has been removed from a wound, surgical exploration should be carried out. Antibiotics will mask the signs of a retained foreign body.

Faergemann J, Gisslen H, Dahlberg E, et al: ***Trichophyton rubrum* abscesses** in immunocompromised patients. A case report. Acta Derm Venereol 1989; 69:244–247.

A 72-year-old man with a myelodysplastic syndrome being treated with prednisolone (100 mg/day) developed multiple dark erythematous scaling lesions on his left foot and lower leg. Some lesions had ulcerated, resembling vasculitis. He also had dry scaly soles (KOH-positive) and toenail changes. A skin biopsy specimen revealed granulomatous infiltrates and septated hyphae and arthrospores in the deep dermis. No fungi were seen in the stratum corneum.

Trichophyton rubrum was cultured from both the biopsy and skin scales from the foot.

T. rubrum abscesses should be suspected in all immunocompromised patients with signs of superficial dermatophyte infections.

Diagnostic chance favors the prepared mind.

Krajden S, Burul CJ, Fuksa M: *Campylobacter jejuni* associated with a **perirectal abscess**. Can J Surg 1986; 29:228.

Most (80%) perirectal abscesses arise in the six to ten anal glands that empty into the anal canal at the dentate margin. The infection begins in the plane between the internal (visceral) and external (somatic) sphincters and progresses caudally to form the common low variety of perianal abscess.

The abscesses usually reveal mixed infections of anaerobes (particularly *Bacteroides fragilis*) and gram-negative enteric bacilli.

In this case, however, a 64-year-old woman with an acute perirectal abscess had experienced diarrhea and abdominal pain 2 weeks before. Culture of pus from the abscess revealed *Campylobacter jejuni*, which commonly causes acute enteritis. This organism requires specific media and culture conditions for isolation, so that the laboratory should be notified to look for it in any perianal abscess in a patient with preceding enteritis.

Taylor BA, Hughes LE: Circumferential **perianal pilonidal sinuses**. Dis Colon Rectum 1984; 27:120–122.

Recurrent perianal abscesses, having no connection with the anorectum, may represent pilonidal sinuses.

A 34-year-old man who had had four episodes of perianal abscesses over 18 months was examined under anesthesia. In addition to large first-degree hemorrhoids he had several fleshy skin tags at the anal verge, almost completely encircling the anus. In the intersphincteric groove adjacent to the skin tags, there were several pits containing hair fragments and sebaceous material. The pits were connected by a subcutaneous tract, almost completely encircling the anus. There was no communication with the anorectum. A circumferential strip of skin and subcutaneous fat was removed, along with all tracks and skin tags. Histologic examination revealed tracks lined by granulation tissue and containing hairs, typical of pilonidal sinuses.

Mortensen NJ, Thomson JP: **Perianal abscess** due to *Enterobius vermicularis*. Dis Colon Rectum 1984; 27:677–678.

Perianal abscesses may arise from:

posterior fissure in ano
infection of anal hematoma
anal gland infection with intersphincteric abscess (most common cause)
Crohn's disease
tuberculosis

In an 11-year-old boy with recurrent perianal abscesses, **threadworms** were found within the anal crypts, lower rectum, and an intersphincteric abscess. Ova of *Enterobius vermicularis* were also present in the abscess wall on histologic examination. He had not complained of pruritus ani, a common symptom of threadworm infestation.

Doberneck RC: **Perianal suppuration:** Results of treatment. Am Surg 1987; 53:569–572.

Perianal suppuration includes the spectrum of perianal disease from cryptitis through abscess and fistula formation. It is a common cause of pain and disability and merits serious attention. Most patients present with perianal abscess.

All patients deserve treatment of abscesses under general or spinal anesthesia to enable more thorough evaluation and superior drainage. Office drainage of perianal abscess under local anesthesia may seem to be more cost-effective but often ultimately is followed by recurrences and fistula formation.

This study includes 101 patients with perianal suppuration treated surgically at the University of New Mexico.

Nelson RL, Prasad ML, Abcarian H: **Anal carcinoma** presenting as a **perirectal abscess** or fistula. Arch Surg 1985; 120:632–634.

Acute or chronic perianal suppuration cells for operative exploration with biopsy of all abscesses and fistulas. This is necessary to effectively treat the abscess and rule out inflammatory bowel disease and anorectal carcinoma.

The chronic fistulas and abscesses caused by **hidradenitis suppurativa** in the perianal area pose a high risk of hidden squamous cell carcinoma. Older patients with perianal disease for more than 15 years are particularly at risk.

Perianal abscesses may also be caused by the extension of a rectal cancer into the perianal and ischiorectal tissues or by an adenocarcinoma associated with a chronic anal fistula.

Slater DN: **Perianal abscess:** "Have I excluded leukaemia?" Br Med J 1984; 289:1682.

Two patients with classic perianal abscesses were found after surgery to have acute myeloblastic leukemia.

A complete blood count with differential white cell count should be done in patients with perianal abscess to exclude leukemia. Surgical excision might not be the optimal treatment.

Winslett MC, Allan A, Ambrose NS: **Anorectal sepsis** as a presentation of occult rectal and systemic disease. Dis Colon Rectum 1988; 31:597–600.

All patients with anorectal sepsis should have an adequate examination under anesthesia. This should include biopsies of the wall of the abscess and the rectal mucosa. Cultures of pus should be obtained, and help differentiate between fistulas (with "gut-specific" bacteria) and simple abscesses.

In this study of 233 patients at three teaching hospitals, approximately 60% had simple perianal abscesses and 33% had ischiorectal abscesses. Only a few patients had fistula in ano. Only 11% had associated minor anal disease, including hemorrhoids, fissures, and intractable pruritus ani.

Brewer NS, Spencer RJ, Nichols DR: Primary **anorectal actinomycosis**. JAMA 1974; 228:1397–1400.

Protracted draining **perianal sinuses** unresponsive to surgical therapy should suggest actinomycosis. Nine cases are reported from the Mayo Clinic, including eight men, five of whom were diabetic. All patients except one had multiple draining sinuses. Sulfur granules were observed at surgery in seven cases. One patient had a perianal mass that proved to be an actinomycotic abscess.

Woody induration is a major clue, along with sulfur granules in the purulent drainage and recurrent fistulas without inflammatory bowel disease. Infection with *Actinomycosis israelii* will be missed unless anaerobic cultures are obtained.

Perianal fistulas are most commonly associated with chronic ulcerative colitis, diabetes mellitus, and regional enteritis. Less common underlying conditions include tuberculosis, rectal carcinoma, trauma, malnutrition, hidradenitis suppurativa, hypogammaglobulinemia, and diverticulitis.

Harris GJ, Metcalf AM: Primary **perianal actinomycosis**. Report of a case and review of the literature. Dis Colon Rectum 1988; 31:311–312.

An 81-year-old diabetic woman had had multiple perianal abscesses 40 years earlier, treated surgically. Her disease was then quiescent until new abscesses appeared 18 months prior to admission. She now had a firm irregular mass in the right posterolateral quadrant with extension to the posterior midline. The anal sphincter tone was normal, and there was no adenopathy.

Aspiration of the mass yielded serosanguineous fluid with small yellow crystals. A Gram stain was negative, but aerobic cultures grew mixed enteric flora, and anaerobic isolation showed probable *Actinomyces* species. Treatment with intravenous ampicillin and surgical exploration was successful.

If you don't look at the feet and you don't look in the mouth, you may be putting your foot in your mouth.

Bartholin's Gland

Word B: Office treatment of cyst and **abscess** of **Bartholin's gland duct**. South Med J 1968; 61:514–518.

"The very name of Bartholin is surrounded by a degree of excitement, and for the past three centuries has enlivened the imagination of mankind with thoughts of the delights of earthly lust."

Bartholin's glands are paired vulvovaginal glands that are buried five layers beneath the surface of the vulvar mucosa. Each gland is drained by a duct about 1 inch long and empties into the vestibule on the lateral external midportion of the hymenal ring. When the duct becomes blocked at the vestibular orifice, continuing secretion from the gland expands the duct lumen, resulting in a cyst of the duct and eventual abscess on the posterior region of the vulva. A cyst or abscess is located immediately beneath the skin and vestibular mucosa and does not extend deeply to involve the gland.

The function of Bartholin's glands appears to be the continuous supply of a slippery secretion for lubrication of the vestibular surface. The glands do not function before puberty, possibly accounting for vulvar synechiae seen in little girls. Unilateral excision of Bartholin's gland results in a dry scaly vestibular wall on the affected side, resembling skin rather than mucosa. Vulvectomy causes similar dryness because of the loss of Bartholin's glands.

The differential diagnosis of other lesions in the posterior region of the vulva includes:

carcinoma of Bartholin's gland	hydrocele of the canal of Nuck
enterocele	fibroma (diverticular apparatus)
perineal hernia	pudendal hematoma
ischiorectal abscess	metastatic carcinoma
sebaceous cyst	

Davies JA, Rees E, Hobson D, Karaylannis P: Isolation of *Chlamydia trachomatis* from **Bartholin's ducts**. Br J Vener Dis 1978; 54:409–413.

For more than 240 years, inflammation of Bartholin's ducts has been known to be a manifestation of venereal diseases.

Exudate from Bartholin's duct is obtained by introducing a finger into the vagina and massaging the length of the duct. The exudate may be yellow (mucopurulent), white (mucoid), cloudy mucus, or clear mucus.

In this study of 30 women in a venereal disease clinic in Liverpool, *Neisseria gonorrhoeae* was found in the Bartholin's duct exudate in 24 patients and *Chlamydia trachomatis* was similarly found in 9 patients. Concurrent infection with both organisms occurred in 7 patients.

Matseoane S, Harris T, Moscowitz E: Isolated endometriosis in a **Bartholin gland**. NY State J Med 1987; 87:575–576.

A 29-year-old woman had a 4- × 3-cm firm rubbery mass in the left Bartholin gland. She noted recurrent **swelling** of the gland **during menses**. Twice previously the gland had been incised and drained to reduce swelling. Excision of the mass revealed endometriosis within a Bartholin gland. She had no evidence of abdominal or pelvic endometriosis.

Think of endometriosis in any "cyst" that enlarges during the menses.

Brook I: Aerobic and anaerobic **microbiology of Bartholin's abscess**. Surg Gynecol Obstet 1989; 32–34.

This is a review of bacterial cultures from 28 women over a 10-year period. The Bartholin's gland abscesses were surgically incised and drained at Walter Reed Army Medical Center and the Naval Medical Center, Bethesda.

Look for: *Bacteroides* species (21 cases)   *Neisseria gonorrhoeae* (4 cases)
                 Escherichia coli (6 cases)

Hueston JT: The **aetiology** of **pilonidal sinuses**. Br J Surg 1953; 41:307–311.

A pilonidal sinus is a subcutaneous cavity that contains hair and is lined by granulation tissue. It communicates with the surface by a sinus tract lined by squamous epithelium and is caused by the penetration of loose hairs from the exterior into the subcutaneous tissues. The hair fragments induce inflammation and a foreign body reaction, with eventual deep abscess formation.

Most patients are men, ages 20 to 25 years, with stiff dark wiry hair and greasy skin. Sedentary occupations, such as riding in or driving vehicles with rigid suspensions, which subject the sacrococcygeal region to repeated minor trauma, are often implicated. Hot climates and the accumulation of sweat and epithelial debris in the natal cleft favor the penetration of loose hairs, sharper ends first, into enlarged hair follicles in the midline. There are usually two or more small pits in the midline over the sinus cavity, and secondary lateral openings are common.

The acquired pilonidal sinus must be distinguished from the following developmental conditions:

postanal dimple
congenital dermal sinus
postanal dermoid
sacrococcygeal dermoid

Brearley R: **Pilonidal sinus**. A new theory of origin. Br J Surg 1955; 43:62–68.

Natural movements of the buttocks produce a cigarette-rolling action that twists loose hairs into a bundle and drills them obliquely through the skin. Suction forces produced by separation of the buttocks then draw the hairs inward, producing a sinus.

An 18-year-old girl was seen with an abscess between the left great and second toes. She worked in a factory upholstering chairs and was found to have horsehair between her toes. She knew other girls with the same condition. Presumably, penetration of the horsehairs between the toes led to pilonidal sinuses of the **toe webs**.

Page BH: The entry of hair into a **pilonidal sinus**. Br J Surg 1969; 56:32.

Here is experimental proof that a hair will work its way into a pilonidal sinus from the outside, provided it is aligned root-first in the mouth of the sinus. The rough scales on the hair thus point upward toward the top, and the hair cannot move in the opposite direction.

A young woman with a sacrococcygeal pilonidal sinus had two of her scalp hairs engaged in the mouth of her sinus: the root end of one hair (which was knotted at the other end) and the tip of another hair. She then walked around for 30 minutes, which showed that the knotted hair had become very much shorter. After 3 hours the knot had almost entered the mouth of the sinus, whereas the other hair had become completely disengaged.

Brook I: Microbiology of infected **pilonidal sinuses**. J Clin Pathol 1989; 42:1140–1142.

In 75 patients with pilonidal sinuses, aspirates of pus revealed:

anaerobic bacteria only in 58 (77%)
aerobic bacteria only in 3 (4%)
mixed aerobic and anaerobic in 14 (19%)

Among 147 anaerobes isolated, the predominant organisms were *Bacteroides*   151 sp and anaerobic cocci. Aerobes isolated included *Escherichia coli*, *Proteus* sp group D streptococcus, and *Pseudomonas* sp.

This study highlights the predominance of anaerobic bacteria in infected pilonidal sinuses. The polymicrobial nature of the isolates probably indicates synergy among the different bacterial strains. Treatment should include antibiotics such as clindamycin, cefoxitin, metronidazole, imipenem, or the combination of a β-lactamase inhibitor and a penicillin.

Griffin SM, McEvilly W, Cole TP: **Pilonidal sinus** of the **penis**. Br J Urol 1990; 65:422–424.

A 29-year-old uncircumcised married man developed a 2 by 1.5 cm ulcer of the ventral corona adjacent to the glans penis. It followed a small abscess that had appeared 7 months previously. Although cultures revealed *Candida albicans* and *Staphylococcus aureus*, treatment with antifungal and antibiotic agents did not help. The ulcer was indurated with a rolled border, bled on contact, and was infected. Venereal disease test and chest x-ray results were negative.

The lesion was excised under general anesthesia, revealing a sinus tract containing necrotic debris and hair. The sinus was lined by squamous epithelium and granulation tissue, typical of a pilonidal sinus.

Haworth JC, Zachary RB: **Congenital dermal sinuses** in children. Their relation to pilonidal sinuses. Lancet 1955; 2:10–14.

A congenital dermal sinus may lead from the skin over the skull or spine to some part of the central nervous system or its coverings. Sometimes it ends in a dermoid cyst or teratoma within the skull or spinal canal. A few hairs may protrude from the sinus, and it may be surrounded by a hemangioma. Warning signs may result from infection, leading to **meningitis** or an abscess. Enlargement of a **dermoid cyst** at the end of the sinus tract may also cause pressure effects, resulting in paresthesias and paralysis. **Coccygeal sinuses** are the most common sinuses in children.

An 11-month-old baby boy developed purulent discharge from a small sinus over the sacrum, which was followed at age 1 year by *Proteus* meningitis. He recovered with antibiotics, but the sinus again drained creamy material, and the surrounding skin became red and hard, with a raised granulomatous area just below the sinus. A swab from the sinus grew *Proteus*. Surgery revealed a 7-cm-long sinus tract that led into the dura and finished as a continuation of the filum terminale.

A 4-month-old baby boy was noted to have a 4-cm soft, slightly raised, reddish zone over the lower lumbar spine, with a sinus in the center. The spinous processes were impalpable at this site, but there was a lateral bony ridge. When the baby was 11 months of age the sinus tract was uneventfully excised and led down through a spina bifida into the dura in the upper lumbar spine.

A 13-month-old baby boy was hospitalized with his third attack of meningitis due to *Escherichia coli*. Over the fourth lumbar vertebra there was a small sinus with a tuft of protruding hair, surrounded by a capillary hemangioma. Surgery revealed a sinus that led into the subarachnoid space and ended in an infected dermoid cyst, which compressed the dorsal lumbar cord, causing flaccid paralysis of the legs and incontinence of urine and feces. After surgery, he had residual weakness and anesthesia of the legs and incontinence.

Doubting your diagnosis is a first step to certainty.

Shewring DJ, Rushforth GF: A bizarre **postoperative wound infection**. Br Med J 1990; 300:1557.

Three months after hemiarthroplasty of the left knee, a 73-year-old woman had an inflamed wound. Twenty milliliters of yellow pus was drained from an abscess cavity that did not appear to communicate with the joint. Culture of the pus yielded *Pasteurella multocida*. When the patient was more closely questioned, she revealed that she had had her **dog lick** the wound to promote healing after part of the wound had broken down 3 weeks previously.

Infection with *P. multocida* is a common sequel to dog or cat bites, but here was one from a dog lick. The laboratory can help you take a better history!

Diagnostic Aids

Fine BC, Sheckman PR, Bartlett JC: **Incision** and **drainage** of soft-tissue **abscesses** and bacteremia. Ann Intern Med 1985; 103:645.

Transient bacteremia, as long as 20 minutes after the procedure, often occurs after incision and drainage of cutaneous abscesses. Blood cultures were positive in six of ten patients tested, and four of the patients had more than one organism in the blood.

Patients at risk for endocarditis should be treated accordingly.

Glen DL: Use of **hydrogen peroxide** to identify internal opening of **anal fistula** and perianal abscess. Aust NZ J Surg 1986; 56:433–435.

Hydrogen peroxide produces frothing on contact with tissue and an expanding bubbling efflux. Injection of small amounts (0.5 to 0.2 ml) along fistulous tracts and into perianal abscesses was helpful in finding internal openings on the dentate line.

Presumably this technique would be useful in other types of cutaneous abscesses.

Chaudary RR, Ramanathan K: The use of **computed tomographic scanning** to diagnose sterile **gluteal abscesses**. NY State J Med 1987; 87:233–234.

An 8-year-old boy had a firm, mobile, slightly tender mass with skin fixation on the left buttock. The right buttock was also slightly enlarged without any focal mass.

Radiologic evaluation with soft tissue films showed subcutaneous masses with rim-like calcifications. Computed tomography of the midpelvis demonstrated fat/fluid levels in rounded cystic gluteal masses bilaterally.

Further history disclosed that he had diabetes insipidus and had been receiving vasopressin tannate in **peanut oil injections** until 2 years previously. The diagnosis was sterile gluteal abscesses secondary to the peanut oil.

The scan was extremely helpful in ruling out other causes of gluteal masses, including hematoma, abscesses, parasitic cysts, and necrotic tumors.

Porter JA, Loughry CW, Cook AJ. Use of the **computerized tomographic scan** in the diagnosis and treatment of **abscesses**. Am J Surg 1985; 150:257–262.

Computed tomography has revolutionized the diagnosis and treatment of abscesses. It is the "diagnostic procedure of choice" in the diagnosis of abscesses.

It often enables percutaneous abscess drainage and relief of sepsis without the morbidity of a laparotomy.

Wall SD, Fisher MR, Amparo EG, et al: **Magnetic resonance imaging** in the evaluation of abscesses. AJR 1985; 144:1217–1221.

Magnetic resonance imaging (MRI) demonstrated a more clear delineation of the extent of inflammatory changes than did computed tomography (CT). MRI also showed the abscess as a collection distinct from the surrounding structure, whereas with CT the abscess often blended in with the surrounding tissue (unless it contained air).

A disadvantage of MRI was that it did not show calcification. It also could not differentiate abscesses from other fluid collections and necrotic tumors.

Koelbel G, Schmiedl U, Majer MC, et al: Diagnosis of **fistulae** and **sinus tracts** in patients with Crohn disease: Value of **MR imaging**. AJR 1989; 152:999–1003.

In patients with **Crohn's disease**, magnetic resonance imaging with T1-weighted images clearly showed cutaneous openings of fistulas as defects in the subcutaneous fat. Sinus tracts or fistulas were demonstrated by MRI in 14 of 17 patients. All of these patients were known to have fistulas by other tests: barium, sinographic, MR, CT, and sonography.

T2-weighted images showed fluid collections within the fistulas, localized fluid in extraintestinal tissues, and inflammatory changes within muscles.

Is your patient being overtreated and underdiagnosed?
Is your patient being overdiagnosed and undertreated?

Acanthosis Nigricans

Black velvet is the fabric you use to make a diagnosis of acanthosis nigricans. It is not a difficult diagnosis. The striking symmetry, localization on the neck and axillae, and black velvet texture are distinctive. Its early pigment change may suggest other diagnoses, such as the "dirty neck" of atopic dermatitis. In infants the thickened skin changes that appear later may suggest ichthyosis hystrix.

The true challenge is in finding the cause. Most often acanthosis nigricans is seen in very obese pubertal or prepubertal children, in whom it is a marker for elevated insulin levels. After menarche it may be associated with elevated testosterone levels, irregular menses, and hirsutism. Measure insulin and testosterone levels.

In a patient who is not obese and who has no family trait of the disease, look for endocrinopathies and rare congenital syndromes. It may be as simple as hypothyroidism. Have an endocrinologist and pediatrician review the child. Is there an insulinoma?

Next, look for a drug as a cause. We have seen acanthosis develop with a large intake of nicotinic acid, but other drugs may be responsible, such as steroids and oral contraceptives. The latter regularly elevate insulin levels.

Most importantly, if no other cause is found and the patient is older, comprehensive studies must be undertaken to find an underlying malignant condition. It is usually an adenocarcinoma in the intestinal tract or abdomen. X-rays and CT are invaluable. Acanthosis nigricans can be a paraneoplastic process, and it is your job to find the neoplasm. If it is not found, "black velvet" may be the patient's shroud.

Diagnosis

Rendon MI, Cruz PD, Sontheimer RD, Bergstresser PR: **Acanthosis nigricans:** A cutaneous marker of tissue **resistance to insulin.** J Am Acad Dermatol 1989; 21:461–469.

Hyperpigmented, velvety to verrucous hyperkeratotic plaques occur symmetrically in the axillae, nape, and flexural areas. They can involve the entire skin, including the palms, soles, and mucous membranes.

If the onset is before the age of 10 years, suspect a familial form (autosomal dominant). Also look for congenital anomalies:

> Alström syndrome
> ataxia telangiectasia
> Bloom syndrome
> Crouzon's disease (craniofacial dysostosis)
> Lawrence-Seip syndrome (total lipodystrophy)
> leprechaunism
> Prader-Willi syndrome
> Rabson's syndrome
> Rud's syndrome
> syndrome of acral hypertrophy and muscle cramps

If the onset is severe and sudden, look for underlying malignant disease (gastric, ovarian, uterine).

If the onset is mild but sudden, suspect a drug such as nicotinic acid or diethylstilbestrol.

If the onset is insidious, suspect obesity and high insulin levels, and *order* a plasma insulin level determination.

The finding of elevated insulin levels (even in the presence of normal blood sugar levels) indicates a type A or type B syndrome of insulin resistance. In type A the testosterone level is elevated, and there is virilization. In type B there is also testosterone elevation, but no virilization. Look for autoimmune syndromes and antibodies to insulin receptors.

Resistance to the action of insulin stems from pharmacologic or immuno-mediated defects in insulin receptors on the postreceptor pathway, with resulting compensatory excretion of excessive insulin. Binding of insulin to insulin-like growth factor receptors on keratinocytes leads to the epidermal proliferation of acanthosis nigricans. Excessive insulin may likewise bind to ovarian tissue, with resulting increased production of androgens.

"Hyperinsulinemia" and acanthosis nigricans also occur in obesity because of a decrease (down regulation) of insulin receptors.

Certain tumors secrete insulin-like hormones, with resulting acanthosis nigricans.

In ancanthosis nigricans, look for insulin as the growth hormone behind it all.

Stuart CA, Pate CJ, Peters EJ: Prevalence of **acanthosis nigricans** in an unselected population. Am J Med 1989; 87:269–272.

The posterior area of the neck of every child in the sixth and eighth grades of the public schools in Galveston, Texas, was examined during the state-mandated health survey for scoliosis.

Acanthosis nigricans was found in 7.1% (101) of 1412 children examined, a much higher number than anticipated. It was equally distributed between boys and girls and was most common in children with severe obesity. Biopsy was not necessary to confirm the diagnosis, as the skin changes were typical. Based on experience, the back of the neck was consistently the most severely affected area in acanthosis nigricans.

The greatest prevalence was at age 12, which is consistent with reports that acanthosis nigricans occurs at or before the start of puberty. It was much more common among Hispanics (5.5%) and blacks (13.3%), than whites (only 2 of 440 children). Differing rates of obesity did not seem to account for the prevalence differences between the ethnic groups.

The severity of skin lesions correlated with excessive insulin secretion. **Hyperinsulinemia** leads to obesity, non–insulin-dependent diabetes mellitus, hypertension, ovarian dysfunction, excessive androgen secretion, and atherosclerosis. Acanthosis nigricans thus may be a cutaneous marker of great medical significance.

Curth HO, Aschner BM: Genetic studies on **acanthosis nigricans**. Arch Dermatol 1959; 79:55–66.

Benign acanthosis nigricans may be difficult to differentiate from ichthyosis hystrix in some childhood cases. Acanthosis nigricans has soft ridges, a predilection for the axillae, and exacerbation at puberty. **Ichthyosis hystrix** has dry keratoses and plantar and palmar keratoderma and improves in summer. These two conditions may occur in the same family or together in the same patient.

Pseudoacanthosis nigricans is benign and associated with obesity. It begins when obesity develops and disappears when the patient returns to normal weight. The skin changes are usually slight, with mildly elevated dark ridges on the neck and axillae in darkly pigmented obese persons. Familial cases have been observed. Mechanical factors may play a role.

Flier JS: Metabolic importance of **acanthosis nigricans**. Arch Dermatol 1985; 121:193–194.

Acanthosis nigricans is associated with either a malignant internal tumor or tissue resistance to insulin.

Adult patients with new-onset acanthosis nigricans should have a careful search for an **occult tumor**, which may not become clinically evident until years later. Gastrointestinal tract neoplasms are the most common. Presumably, some tumors produce epidermal growth factor as well as products that activate insulin-like growth factors or related receptors in the skin, leading to the characteristic brown velvety hyperkeratotic plaques in the axillae, posterior neck area, and other flexural areas.

Acanthosis nigricans is common in all clinical conditions in which insulin action at the cellular level is markedly reduced. This includes obesity, types A and B syndrome of insulin resistance, leprechaunism, and a variety of endocrinopathies.

Insulin can bind to and activate receptors for growth-promoting peptides (insulin-like growth factors). In **hyperinsulinemia**, increased insulin binding to receptors promotes metabolism and growth of cells, including epidermal cells that overgrow and produce complex folding (papillomatosis).

Hall JM, Moreland A, Cox GJ, Wade TR: **Oral acanthosis nigricans:** Report of a case and comparison of oral and cutaneous pathology. Am J Dermatopathol 1988; 10:68–73.

Oral acanthosis nigricans appears as numerous skin-colored warty papules of the lips and labial commissures. The filiform papillae of the tongue also become hypertrophied, producing a deeply fissured papillomatous surface. The buccal mucosa and palate show only a diffuse uneven surface or velvety white appearance. Even the gingiva may show nodules, resembling fibromas.

Note that intraoral lesions are not pigmented and are more common in association with malignant disease. They do not occur in the absence of cutaneous acanthosis nigricans. Hyperkeratotic changes in the palms and soles are also frequently associated.

The clinical differential diagnosis for **papillomatous lesions** of the **oral mucosa** includes:

Goltz-Gorlin syndrome (retardation, pigmentation, telangiectasias, anomalies of the eyes and extremities)

Cowden's disease (facial trichilemmomas, abnormalities of thyroid, central nervous system, gastrointestinal tract, and musculoskeletal system)

pyostomatitis vegetans (ulcerative colitis or other gastrointestinal disturbance)

lipoid proteinosis (yellowish plaques and nodules in mouth and skin, onset early in life)

Wegener's granulomatosis (gingival nodules, multisystem granulomatous disease)

multicentric reticulohistiocytosis (nodules on head and neck, polyarthritis)

The **velvety white** appearance on the **buccal mucosa** in some patients with acanthosis nigricans may suggest:

pachyonychia congenita (cutaneous signs, nail dystrophy)

dyskeratosis congenita (cutaneous signs, nail dystrophy)

hereditary benign intraepithelial dyskeratosis (white plaques on cornea, biopsy with intracytoplasmic inclusions)

leukoedema

white sponge nevus

Sedano HU, Gorlin RJ: **Acanthosis nigricans**. Oral Surg 1987; 63:462–467.

Neoplastic associations

Of associated tumors, 75% are abdominal adenocarcinomas, of which 60% arise in the stomach. Other adenocarcinomas seen are in the intestine, uterus, pancreas, breast, lung, and bladder.

Non-neoplastic associations.

insulin-resistant syndromes:
Type A: genetic defects in insulin receptor
Type B: autoantibodies to insulin receptor
Type C: defect at postreceptor level
Obesity
endocrinopathies
Addison's disease
Stein-Leventhal syndrome
Prader-Willi syndrome
Alström's syndrome
hyperthyroidism and hypothyroidism
pinealomas
congenital syndromes
Bloom's syndrome
Crouzon's disease
cutis gyratum (Beare)
autosomal dominant type
clinically suggests ichthyosis hystrix, present at birth or later
drug-induced
diethylstilbestrol
nicotinic acid
topical nicotinic acid
miscellaneous
lupoid hepatitis

juvenile Paget's disease of bone (osteoectasia)
pemphigus vulgaris

Flier JS, Young JB, Landsberg L: **Familial insulin resistance** with acanthosis nigricans, **acral hypertrophy**, and **muscle cramps**. N Engl J Med 1980; 303:970–973.

A sister and brother are described with **axillary acanthosis nigricans**, enlargement of the hands, and severe muscle cramps of the arms, legs, and trunk. The 30-year-old woman also had signs of masculinization with balding and hirsutism, polycystic ovaries, and enlarged kidneys. Both patients had high fasting insulin levels with insulin resistance and had normal levels of growth hormone and somatomedin C.

The acral hypertrophy resembled **acromegaly**, in which growth is believed to be stimulated by somatomedins, a family of growth-promoting peptides whose secretion is controlled by growth hormone. Since the levels of growth hormone and somatomedin C were normal in these patients, insulin was probably the culprit. High levels of insulin can stimulate growth through low-affinity binding to receptors for somatomedin-like peptides.

The presence of acanthosis nigricans, unexplained muscle cramps, or acral enlargement without an excess of growth hormone calls for a search for insulin resistance, regardless of the state of glucose tolerance.

Endocrinopathy

Richards GE, Cavallo A, Meyer WJ III, et al: Obesity, **acanthosis nigricans**, insulin resistance and **hyperandrogenemia**: Pediatric perspective and natural history. J Pediatr 1985; 107:893–897.

A study of 22 children with acanthosis nigricans revealed **hyperinsulinemia**. Fasting insulin levels were 2.5 times those of obese controls, and 10 times those of lean controls (49.8 μU/ml versus 19.6 μU/ml and 5.25 μU/ml, respectively). Affected patients were obese (5.7 SD above the mean for age), and as the obesity increased the acanthosis nigricans worsened. After menarche, the girls suffered hyperandrogenemia, with **menstrual irregularities** and **hirsutism**.

Acanthosis nigricans is a genetic syndrome appearing in obese families, and its presence alerts the clinician to search for other affected family members. It occurs in 50% of morbidly obese children. But obesity is not the only association. Acanthosis nigricans occurs in other fat disorders (partial lipodystrophy, lipoatrophic diabetes) and endocrine diseases (Cushing's syndrome, acromegaly, leprechaunism, and Robson-Mendenhall syndrome with pineal and adrenal hyperplasia and diabetes mellitus). It also should be anticipated in patients with insulin receptor antibodies and a wide range of malignancies in older patients.

Hisler BM, Savoy LB: **Acanthosis nigricans** of the **forehead** and **fingers** associated with **hyperinsulinemia**. Arch Dermatol 1987; 123:1441–1442.

Asymptomatic darkening of the forehead and neck for 7 years led a 64-year-old obese man to seek medical attention. The lesions were hyperpigmented velvety plaques of the forehead, elbows, dorsal interphalangeal joints, axillae, and posterior area of the neck. Acanthosis nigricans was confirmed by biopsy. He also had palmar and plantar hyperkeratosis.

Despite normal blood sugar, he had a greatly elevated fasting serum insulin level of 89 μU/ml, (normal 7 to 25 μU/ml). There were no antibodies to insulin, indicating tissue resistance to insulin. Since insulin binds to and activates receptors for growth-promoting factor (thereby favoring cell growth), the high insulin levels were felt to account for the acanthosis nigricans.

Shuttleworth D, Weavind GP, Graham-Brown RAC: **Acanthosis nigricans** and diabetes mellitus in a patient with Klinefelter's syndrome: A reaction to **methyltestosterone**. Clin Exp Dermatol 1987; 12:288–290.

A 32-year-old male, complaining of loss of libido and infertility, was found to have testicular atrophy, low serum testosterone levels, and the karyotyping of Klinefelter's syndrome.

After 11 years of treatment with methyltestosterone (250 mg every 3 weeks) he was noted to have multiple skin tags of the neck and axillae and thickened velvety pigmented axillary skin confirmed as acanthosis nigricans on biopsy. He was also found to have diabetes mellitus with insulin resistance.

Iatrogenic **hyperandrogenism** probably caused these changes, including insulin resistance and diabetes. Acanthosis nigricans has not been previously reported in Klinefelter's syndrome, which has hypogonadism. However, it is associated with hypergonadism in the polycystic ovary syndrome and goes into remission following reduction in androgen levels.

Methyltestosterone must be added to the list of drugs capable of inducing acanthosis nigricans—stilbestrol, nicotinic acid, and corticosteroids.

Flier JS, Eastman RC, Minaker KL, et al: **Acanthosis nigricans** in **obese women** with **hyperandrogenism**. Characterization of an insulin-resistant state distinct from the Type A and B syndromes. Diabetes 1985; 34:101–107.

Acanthosis nigricans was seen in 5% (15 of 300) of women being studied for hyperandrogenism thought to be due to the **polycystic ovarian syndrome**. All were obese and insulin resistant, as assessed by hyperinsulinemia when fasting and after oral glucose administration. None were diabetic, and all had normal fasting plasma glucose levels with only minimally impaired glucose tolerance on testing. Insulin receptor antibodies were absent.

Acanthosis nigricans is a cutaneous marker for severe tissue resistance to insulin, which may be caused by:

antibodies to insulin receptors (type B syndrome, patients with autoimmune features)
genetic defects in receptor or postreceptor function (type A syndrome, thin women with hyperandrogenism and no immune features).
obesity (obese women with hyperandrogenism).

Evaluation of cases of acanthosis nigricans should include antibodies to insulin receptors and studies of insulin receptors in fresh and cultured cells.

Dunaif A, Graf M, Mandeli J, et al: Characterization of groups of **hyperandrogenic women** with **acanthosis nigricans**, impaired glucose tolerance, and/or hyperinsulinemia. J Clin Endocrinol Metab 1987; 65:499–507.

Evaluation of 62 hyperandrogenic women revealed actanthosis nigricans in 29%, most of them obese.

Hyperandrogenism and hyperinsulinemia are closely related in the **polycystic ovary** (PCO) **syndrome**, independent of obesity. If obesity is present, however, 50% of PCO women have acanthosis nigricans, associated with more profound **hyperinsulinemia**.

PCO was diagnosed in 46 women, 28 of whom were obese. PCO was diagnosed if a woman with hirsutism had chronic oligomenorrhea or amenorrhea in association with hyperandrogenism (elevations of one or more plasma androgen levels). PCO represents a common disorder of insulin action, but only obese PCO women are at risk for impairment of glucose tolerance, independent of the presence of acanthosis nigricans.

Hyperandrogenic women without PCO did not have hyperinsulinemia or abnormal glucose tolerance tests.

Given JR, Kerber IJ, Wiser WL, et al: Remission of **acanthosis nigricans** associated with **polycystic ovarian disease** and a stromal luteoma. J Clin Endocrinol Metab 1974; 38:347–355.

A 17-year-old black nulligravida had **secondary amenorrhea**. Her menses had been regular from age 11 to 15 years, when they abruptly ceased. She then gained weight, developed **hirsutism**, and noted dark thick coarse skin on her face, neck, back, axillae, and antecubital fossae, consistent with acanthosis nigricans.

Endocrine work-up revealed markedly elevated plasma androstenedione and testosterone levels, as well as elevated urinary 17-ketosteroid levels. Laparotomy revealed polycystic ovarian disease and a stromal luteoma (lipoid cell tumor). Despite ovarian wedge resection, the acanthosis nigricans eventually worsened, and plasma androgens increased. Cyclical treatment with a combination-type oral contraceptive (norethindrone 2 mg, mestranol 0.1 mg) for 2 years almost completely cleared the acanthosis nigricans. The massive androgen production by the ovaries was thus successfully suppressed by estrogen.

Benign acanthosis nigricans has been associated with several endocrine and metabolic disorders:

acromegaly   Prader-Willi syndrome
diabetes mellitus   Laurence-Moon-Bardet-Biedl syndrome
Cushing's disease   polycystic ovarian disease

Winkelmann RK, Scheen SR, Jr., Underdahl LO: **Acanthosis nigricans** and **endocrine disease**. JAMA 1960; 174:1145–1152.

Among 57 patients with acanthosis nigricans seen at the Mayo Clinic from 1935 to 1956, 18 had associated malignant disease and 9 had an associated endocrinopathy. Pituitary adenomas, polycystic ovaries, adrenal insufficiency, and diabetes mellitus were the main endocrine problems found. Other cases associated with Cushing's disease, hypothyroidism, and hyperthyroidism are cited.

In **Addison's disease**, seen in two cases, the hyperpigmentation obscured the acanthosis nigricans, which could easily have been missed.

Kahn CR, Flier JS, Bar RS, et al: The **syndromes** of **insulin resistance** and **acanthosis nigricans**. N Engl J Med 1976; 294:739–745.

Two distinct clinical syndromes are described with acanthosis nigricans: severe insulin resistance and decreased insulin binding to its receptors. All patients are females, and the majority are black. The glucose tolerance tends to remit, and ketoacidosis is rare.

Type A: Seen in young **teenagers** with **hirsutism**, polycystic ovaries, clitoral enlargement, coarse features, and accelerated growth. Patients often have **multiple skin tags**. Primary amenorrhea and increased plasma testosterone may be present.

Type B: Occurs in **middle-aged women** with **alopecia**, arthralgias, enlarged salivary glands, proteinuria, leukopenia, increased gamma globulin and erythrocyte sedimentation rate, and **positive ANA** and **anti-DNA antibodies**. An immunologic disease is suggested.

The fasting glucose and glucose tolerance test may be normal, and not all patients have symptoms of hypoglycemia. Only a plasma insulin measurement or a direct insulin tolerance test will detect severe insulin resistance. If the blood sugar level is elevated, oral hypoglycemic agents and high doses of insulin have little effect on blood sugar levels.

Atkinson AB, Kennedy L, Andrews WJ, et al: Diverse endocrine presentations of the syndrome of **acanthosis nigricans** and **insulin resistance**. J R Coll Physicians Lond 1989; 23:165–169.

Endocrine evaluation of eight cases of acanthosis nigricans and insulin resistance included the following serum tests:

LH (luteinizing hormone)
FSH (follicle-stimulating hormone)
growth hormone
TSH (thyroid-stimulating hormone)
prolactin
total thyroxine
cortisol
insulin
insulin antibodies
insulin receptor antibodies
glucose
oral glucose tolerance test
insulin infusion test (euglycamic clamp)

Widespread endocrine abnormalities were found, varying from extreme growth retardation and juvenile hypothyroidism in two children to gonadotropin deficiency in an adult male. The **pubic** and **groin areas** tended to be more severely affected than the axillae with **acanthosis nigricans**.

Acanthosis nigricans should be carefully looked for in endocrine patients and in patients with hirsutism and/or menstrual irregularities. Such patients should be screened for diabetes mellitus and autoimmune disease.

Ober KP: **Acanthosis nigricans** and insulin resistance associated with **hypothyroidism**. Arch Dermatol 1985; 121:229–231.

For 1 year an obese 15-year-old boy had had diffuse hyperpigmentation and acanthosis nigricans around the neck and in the axillary, antecubital, and inguinal areas. His thyroid gland was easily palpable, with a thyroxine (T_4) level 2.1 μg/dl (normal 5 to 11.5), triiodothyronine (T_3) resin uptake 17.8% (normal 28 to 35%), and thyrotropin (TSH) level greater than 56 μU/ml (normal <10). A fasting serum glucose level was 86 mg/dl, but serum insulin level was 118 μU/ml (normal <12).

Treatment of his primary hypothyroidism with thyroxine resulted in weight loss, reversal of hyperinsulinemia, and resolution of the acanthosis nigricans.

Dix JH, Levy WJ, Fuenning C: Remission of **acanthosis nigricans, hypertrichosis,** and **Hashimoto's thyroiditis** with thyroxine replacement. Pediatr Dermatol 1986; 3:323–326.

A 13-year-old mildly obese girl initially developed darkening of her heels, umbilical region, and posterior area of the neck over an 18-month-period. Dark velvety verrucous lesions were also present under the breasts, in the axillae, and on the extensor surfaces of the elbows and ankles. In addition, increased hair growth was prominent over the posterior neck area and dorsal spine. Her thyroid gland was firm and symmetrically enlarged. The relaxation phase of the Achilles reflex was delayed.

Laboratory evaluation revealed hypothyroidism: T_4-RIA 2.0 μg/ml (normal 5.5 to 11.5), T_3U 28% (normal 35 to 45), T_7 0.6 (normal 1.9 to 5.2), TSH-RIA 41 UIU/ml (normal < 7.0). Hashimoto's thyroiditis was confirmed with elevated microsomal (1:1600) and thyroglobulin (1:320) antibodies. Normal studies included a 2-hour glucose tolerance test with insulin levels, serum testosterone, luteinizing hormone, follicle-stimulating hormone, UA, and ANA. Her hemoglobin was 11.4 gm.

After 3 months of levothyroxine (0.15 mg daily) therapy the acanthosis nigricans had nearly disappeared, and the excessive hair growth on her back had resolved. A similar result is seen in hypothyroid dachshund dogs, who develop acanthosis nigricans, which improves with thyroid therapy.

In some cases, hypothyroidism appears to be directly involved in the pathogenesis of acanthosis nigricans.

Rare diagnoses are rarely made, unless you think of them.

Drug Etiology

Fleming MG, Simon SI: **Cutaneous insulin reaction** resembling **acanthosis nigricans**. Arch Dermatol 1986; 122:1054–1056.

Symmetrical 6- by 8-cm round hyperkeratotic hyperpigmented plaques with a pebbly verrucous surface appeared on the anterior area of the thighs of a 57-year-old diabetic. They resulted from years of injecting beef-pork insulin into these sites and nowhere else. Once the insulin was given at other sites on a rotational basis, the lesions began to resolve without local therapy. They resembled acanthosis nigricans clinically and histologically.

This finding focuses our attention on the role of insulin, insulin receptors, and insulin antibodies in the pathogenesis of true acanthosis nigricans.

Randle HW, Winkelmann RK: **Steroid-induced acanthosis nigricans** in dermatomyositis. Arch Dermatol 1979; 115:587–588.

A 22-year-old woman, in whom **dermatomyositis** was originally diagnosed at age 4 years, was treated with oral steroids for 9 years. She had severe **calcinosis cutis**. Prior to discontinuation of the steroids her menses started, and she developed hyperpigmentation and verrucose epithelial hyperplasia of the axillae, groin, and neck. Her appearance was cushingoid, and her stature was short but she was not obese. Three years after the steroids were stopped she began to grow normally, and 7 years after this there was pronounced regression of the acanthosis nigricans.

Five other cases are cited in which acanthosis nigricans developed in patients taking long-term steroids.

Curth HO: **Acanthosis nigricans** following use of **oral contraceptives**. Arch Dermatol 1975; 111:1069.

A 36-year-old woman, mother of two children, had acanthosis nigricans of the axillae, neck, and groin. She had been taking oral contraceptives for 8 years and continued to take them for 2 more years. Repeated work-ups for malignant disease were negative. She then discontinued the oral contraceptive drugs, and 5 years later her acanthosis nigricans was almost completely resolved.

Other cases are reported in which use or exposure to **diethylstilbestrol** was associated with the development of acanthosis nigricans. Therefore the role of estrogens in acanthosis nigricans may be important.

Banuchi SR, Cohen L, Lorincz AL, Morgan J: **Acanthosis nigricans** following **diethylstilbestrol** therapy. Occurrence in patients with childhood muscular dystrophy. Arch Dermatol 1974; 109:545–546.

Two brothers with childhood muscular dystrophy, ages 11 and 13 years, were treated with diethylstilbestrol (5 mg daily) for 18 months. After approximately 7 months of treatment, hyperpigmentation was noted on the neck, chest, axillae, nipples, areolae, navel, linea alba, groin, and dorsal area of the feet of both boys. Material from a skin biopsy in one boy showed acanthosis nigricans.

In all, six boys (age 5 to 17 years) were similarly treated with diethylstilbestrol. All developed **gynecomastia** and **hyperpigmentation** of the areolae, nipples, navel, linea alba, and scrotum, but only the two brothers developed acanthosis nigricans.

Greenspan AH, Shupack JL, Foo S-H, Wise AC: **Acanthosis nigricans**-like hyperpigmentation secondary to **triazinate therapy**. Arch Dermatol 1985; 121:232–235.

A 42-year-old woman developed brownish hyperpigmentation with surrounding erythema in the axillae and groin. It had appeared 5 weeks after intravenous therapy with the investigational cancer chemotherapeutic agent triazinate, a folic acid antagonist, used to treat her medulloblastoma. The pigment resolved spontaneously, but subsequent courses produced velvety hyperpigmentation characteristic of acanthosis nigricans. By the fifth weekly dose of the fourth course of this chemotherapy, the hyperpigmentation had extended to the popliteal fossae, inframammary and breast regions, perioral area, and hands. A biopsy confirmed acanthosis nigricans.

It is likely that the induced **folate deficiency**, and not the tumor, was responsible for the acanthosis nigricans. Folate and vitamin B_{12} deficiency are well documented causes of hyperpigmentation. Niacin, diethylstilbestrol, and corticosteroids are also known to induce acanthosis nigricans.

Other skin changes reported with triazinate include erythroderma, mucositis, stomatitis, erythema of the extremities, desquamation in the groin and penis, and hyperpigmentation over the infused veins.

You have to be wrong often enough to learn how to be right.

Malignancy

Rigel DS, Jacobs MI: **Malignant acanthosis nigricans:** A review. J Dermatol Surg Oncol 1980; 6:923–927.

By the time a neoplasm is discovered in cases of acanthosis nigricans, it is usually highly malignant and has metastasized, with a rapidly fatal outcome.

In this review of 277 cases, 75% of the tumors were intra-abdominal carcinomas, particularly of the stomach. Other tumors included squamous cell carcinomas, lymphomas, and sarcomas.

The axillae were the most common sites of involvement with acanthosis nigricans. Other locations included the dorsal area of the hands, knuckles, fingers in entirety, palms and soles (hyperkeratosis), and mucous membranes. Rarely, the entire skin is involved.

Andreev VC, Boyanov L, Tsankov N: **Generalized acanthosis nigricans**. Dermatologica 1981; 163:19–24.

A 62-year-old man developed increasing pruritus of the back and extensor surfaces of the arms and legs over 3 months. Warty growths then began to appear on the backs of the hands. Extensive investigation for occult malignant disease revealed advanced inoperative **gastric carcinoma** with intra-abdominal metastases. While the itch continued unabated, confluent warty growths appeared in the perioral and perianal areas, and the axillary and groin skin became darkened and thickened with a mamillated hyperkeratotic surface. The palms and soles also developed punctate pearly hyperkeratosis, with fissures and a yellow-gray color. Numerous **seborrheic keratoses** of the chest, back, and extensor surfaces of the extremities joined the parade of new lesions, along with many new filiform and common **warts** in the axillary folds, trunk, and extremities. The oral mucosa did not escape this new growth invasion, as the mucosa became covered with florid, granular, papillomatous growths.

A diagnosis of generalized acanthosis nigricans was made, with full recognition also of the **Leser-Trélat** sign. The patient's wide range of paraneoplastic skin changes was presumably due to a circulating growth hormone produced by tumor cells.

The pruritus never yielded until shortly before death, 6 months later.

Jacobs MI, Rigel DS: **Acanthosis nigricans** and the **sign** of **Leser-Trélat** associated with adenocarcinoma of the gallbladder. Cancer 1981; 48:325–328.

A 56-year-old woman lost 20 lb in 1 month, in association with nausea, vomiting, and abdominal distress. Three months earlier she had noted progressive darkening of the axillae, sides of the neck, and groin, in addition to a sudden eruption of crops of pruritic warty lesions. The keratoses (0.2 to 0.5 cm) varied from skin-colored to brown and were present on the malar area, dorsal surface of the hands, and extensor aspects of the arms.

Biopsy specimens revealed acanthosis nigricans and seborrheic keratosis. The acanthosis nigricans was extensive, also involving her antecubital fossae, abdomen, lower back, genital area, and inner thighs, in addition to her neck and axillae.

Metastatic adenocarcinoma was found in her liver, proven at autopsy 3 months later to be from the **gallbladder**. This type of malignant tumor causes more than 6000 deaths per year in the United States and constitutes nearly 5% of all malignanct tumors.

The sign of Leser-Trélat is considered by some to be part of the spectrum of malignant acanthosis nigricans. The **seborrheic keratosis** lesions appear suddenly, increase rapidly in number and size, and are pruritic.

Curth HO, Hilberg A, Machacek GF: The site and histology of the cancer associated with **malignant acanthosis nigricans**. Cancer 1962; 15:364–382.

Malignant acanthosis nigricans differs from other types of acanthosis nigricans by sometimes involving the mouth and causing palmar/plantar keratoses.

In this histologic review of 42 tumors associated with malignant acanthosis nigricans, almost all tumors were adenocarcinomas.

Benign acanthosis nigricans with cancer is a different syndrome, as the dermatosis is not activated by the tumor.

Muramatsu T, Matsumoto H, Yamashina Y, et al: **Pemphigus foliaceus** associated with **acanthosis nigricans**–like lesions and **hepatocellular carcinoma**. Int J Dermatol 1986; 25:459–460.

A 54-year-old Japanese man developed mildly pruritic erythematous erosions, crusts, and blisters in the axillae. They subsequently spread to his scalp, face, trunk, and extremities. Three months later they evolved into hyperpigmented hyperkeratotic plaques in the axillae and groin. The **Nikolsky sign** was positive, and small flaccid bullae were present in the scaly crusted hyperpigmented verrucous lesions.

A skin biopsy specimen from a verrucous lesion resembled acanthosis nigricans, while a biopsy specimen from an erythematous vesicular lesion revealed superficial acantholysis at or near the granular layer. Pemphigus foliaceus was confirmed through direct and indirect immunofluorescence.

The eruption cleared with oral steroids, but 1 year later the eruption reappeared, and computed tomography revealed an intrahepatic tumor. He died of hepatocellular carcinoma 7 months later. His serum **α-fetoprotein** level was originally normal but had increased to 555.7 ng/ml (normal 0 to 2.5) at the time of diagnosis. His circulating intercellular antibodies were originally 1:20, then normal during treatment, and finally 1:160.

Gautam HP: **Malignant acanthosis nigricans** associated with **squamous cell carcinoma** of the **bronchus**. Ann Thorac Surg 1969; 7:481–485.

For 6 months a 65-year-old man had noticed progressive roughness and **thickening** of his **palms** and **soles**, as well as warty lesions on the backs of his hands. Discrete, firm, pigmented warty excrescences were present on the dorsal aspect of the hands and flexural area of the forearms. He also had intense **itching** of diffuse symmetrical yellowish-brown hyperkeratosis of the fingers, palms, soles, and feet.

He was a heavy smoker, but had no symptoms apart from the dermatosis. Marked **finger clubbing** was present, along with poor air entry into the left lower chest. Chest x-ray revealed a large mass in the left lower lobe, which on palliative pneumonectomy was a poorly differentiated squamous cell carcinoma with node metastases. Following surgery, the itching disappeared and the dermatosis significantly regressed.

Hage E, Hage J: **Malignant acanthosis nigricans**—a para-endocrine syndrome. Acta Derm Venereol 1977; 57:169–172.

A 71-year-old woman had typical acanthosis nigricans of the flexural areas along with numerous wartlike verrucous papules on the dorsal aspect of the hands, arms, trunk, and abdomen. **Condyloma acuminata–like lesions** were present around the mouth and on the eyelids. Later, her palms and nipples became dry and hyperkeratotic. Many lesions resembled **warts** but had no similarity to the seborrheic keratoses seen in the Leser-Trélat sign. Specimens from skin biopsies showed only acanthosis nigricans.

Exploratory laparotomy revealed a diffuse infiltrating **gastric carcinoma** that involved the entire stomach wall and had metastasized. One week after total gastrectomy the skin lesions showed regression, but the patient died a few weeks later.

Menzies DG, Choo-Kang J, Buxton PK, Campbell IW: **Acanthosis nigricans** associated with **alveolar cell carcinoma**. Thorax 1988; 43:414–415.

A 61-year-old retired miner had a 5-month history of **itching** and a 6-week history of progressive dyspnea on exertion. He had smoked 20 cigarettes a day for more than 40 years. Examination revealed hyperpigmented velvety plaques in the axilla, groin, and neck; hyperpigmented nipples; and **hyperkeratosis** of the **palms** and **soles**. There was no lymphadenopathy, but chest x-rays showed bilateral infiltrates, and there were widespread crepitations in his chest. A transbronchial biopsy specimen revealed alveolar cell carcinoma. The patient died 4 months later.

To date, eight cases of adenocarcinoma of the lung and five cases of squamous cell carinoma of the lung have been reported in association with acanthosis nigricans.

Brown J, Winkelmann RK, Randall RV: **Acanthosis nigricans** and **pituitary tumors**. Report of eight cases. JAMA 1966; 198:619–623.

Pituitary tumors commonly cause the following skin changes:

hypertrichosis
hyperpigmentation
fibromas
hypertrophy of skin and mucous membranes
acromegaly or gigantism
acanthosis nigricans

The art of diagnosis is the art of delicate debridement of irrelevant symptoms and signs.

Acne

The hallmark of acne is the comedo, but the marks of acne are the papule, the cyst, and the scar. As perhaps the most common of all skin diseases, acne is regularly diagnosed by the public, but the physician needs to make observations on the cause. This may range from maternal androgens in the infant with comedones, to friction from a back pack in tropical acne, to steroids in the transplant patient's explosive papulopustular acne of the trunk. Although acne vulgaris is a universal announcement of adolescence, it may occur at any time. Thus, the 86-year-old woman receiving androgens for treatment of malignant disease may have the "acne face" of sweet 16.

The pitfalls of differential diagnosis include failure to recognize gram-negative folliculitis, as well as *Pityrosporum* or *Candida* folliculitis. There may also be failure to perceive drug-induced acne, resulting from lithium, Dilantin, or contraceptives. Even the exotic may confuse. One of our patients with acne maintained that a cyst on his left cheek was migratory. On biopsy, it proved to be a dirofilarial infection.

Similarly, the role of hair greases and oily sun screens, as well as foods such as nuts and kelp, must not be ignored. Miliaria rubra of the back and rosacea of the face pose a diagnostic challenge at times. But the greatest challenge in any acne patient remains the awareness and assessment of what the patient puts on the skin, takes as medication, eats, or exposes the skin to in the work place or on vacation.

Varieties

Bedi TR, Bhutani LK: **Familial comedones** (a case report). Indian J Dermatol 1974; 20:6–7.

A 33-year-old Indian housewife had multiple asymptomatic **blackheads** and pitted scars over the face, neck, trunk, buttocks, and extensor aspects of both extremities. They began symmetrically at the age of 5 years on the elbows and knees and at age 18 spread to her face, neck, and upper trunk. New lesions kept appearing, and old lesions healed with pigmentation and pitted scars. The lesions were worse during summers, premenstrually, and post-partum. She also had severe asthma in winter.

Examination revealed multiple comedones and pigmented pitted scars over the entire body except for the palms, soles, and flexors of the extremities. Multiple tiny sebaceous cysts were present on the eyelids, forehead, and cheeks.

Her family history revealed seven other members with multiple comedones, many of whom also had asthma. The mode of inheritance was autosomal dominant.

Ganor S, Sacks TG: A comparison of the flora of the **comedones** of acne vulgaris and comedones in elderly people. Dermatologica 1969; 138:1–9.

The comedones of acne vulgaris and comedo senilis are morphologically identical, although inflammatory papules and pustules do not develop from the latter.

The striking finding in this study was that about 60% of **senile comedones** contained *Pityrosporum* **species** yeasts, including *P. ovale* and *P. orbiculare*. *Corynebacterium* species are found much less frequently in senile comedones than in the comedones of acne.

Agins JRG: **Grouped periorbital comedones**. Br J Dermatol 1964; 76:158–164.

In a study of 2037 hospitalized patients in Malta, 113 (5.6%) were found to have five or more grouped comedones in the periorbital area.

Females with grouped comedones were all found to be suffering from kidney or urinary system disease, hypertension, or diabetes mellitus. Overall, 81.4% of the patients had **urinary tract disease**. Malignant disease accounted for 15% of cases.

Burket JM, Storrs, FJ: **Nodulocystic infantile acne** occurring in a kindred of steato-cystoma. Arch Dermatol 1987; 123:432–433.

At 18 months of age a little girl developed deep red-brown cysts and nodules of the forehead and cheeks. There were also comedones, small papules, and pustules of the chin. She had not had neonatal acne, and there was no history of creams, oils, or grease having been applied to her face. Extensive endo-crinologic studies revealed no evidence of virilization. Her family history revealed that six members of her family had **steatocystoma multiplex**, including her mother, grandmother, and great-grandfather. Her 6-week-old brother also had mild neonatal acne, with comedones and milia since birth. Skin biopsy specimens of the patient revealed only cystic acne, with no evidence of steatocystoma multiplex.

Over a 5-month period the nodulocystic lesions worsened, despite treatment with oral erythromycin and topical antibiotics. She was then treated for 5 months with 13-cis-retinoic acid (0.5 to 1.0 mg/kg/day). This was followed by striking improvement, but not until 6 weeks after discontinuation of the drug. During treatment, her hair growth was retarded, and she became sullen, cranky, and withdrawn, signs that reversed after the drug was stopped.

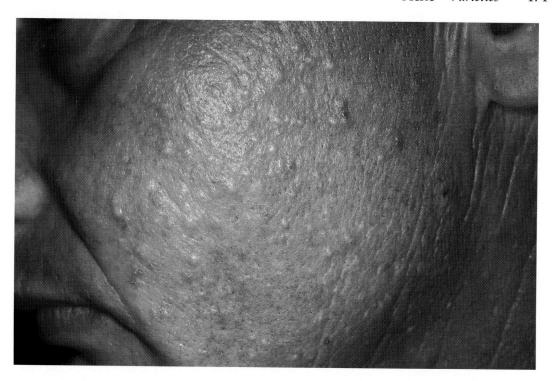

Hughes BR, Cunliffe WJ: An **acne naevus**. Clin Exp Dermatol 1987; 12:357–359.

A large discrete area over the left anterior aspect of the chest was the localizing site of papular and cystic acne lesions in a 17-year-old boy who had had increasingly severe acne for 2 years on the face, back, and left chest. Since birth, he had had an abnormal patch of skin on his left chest. This site, labeled an acne nevus, had a sebum excretion rate 3.5 times that of the normal right anterior aspect of the chest. It also had many more comedones than the contralateral control site.

Chicarilli ZN: **Follicular occlusion triad: Hidradenitis suppurativa, acne conglobata,** and **dissecting cellulitis** of the **scalp**. Ann Plastic Surg 1987; 18:230–237.

A 59-year-old man had had extensive papulocystic lesions and draining sinuses since his late 20s. At one point his scalp was severely involved with localized alopecia over the **nodules** and **sinuses**, but the dissecting cellulitis had become quiescent, leaving residual firm ridges over the vertex. Other sites of involvement included the neck, trunk, axillae, buttocks, and genitourinary and perianal areas. Cultures of sinuses repeatedly grew *Staphylococcus aureus*.

He had not been able to sit down for 10 years because of severe pain in the buttocks and perianal area, and he also had to wear a diaper on account of the numerous draining sinuses. A 7-cm ulcer of the left buttock, from which previous biopsies showed "acute and chronic inflammation and granulation tissue," proved to be a **squamous cell carcinoma** after multiple deep biopsies. In addition, dozens of carcinomas in situ and invasive squamous cell carcinomas involved nearly every sinus tract and communicating fistula examined in the large specimen removed.

Occult malignancy should be suspected in any locally persistent draining sinus. In lesions suspicious for malignancy, repeated incisional biopsies or an excisional biopsy should be done before accepting an incongruous diagnosis of "atypical pseudoepitheliomatous hyperplasia."

Leiferman KM, Groover RV, Dicken CH: **Acne fulminans** and **myositis**. Cutis 1984; 34:249–251.

A 15-year-old boy with a shawl distribution of ulcerative, exudative painful acne lesions, which spared his neck and face, was hospitalized because of back pain, generalized myalgias, arthralgias, and inability to walk. Four months earlier he had developed **severe necrotic acne** of the shoulder girdle, unresponsive to minocycline (150 mg/day). For 5 weeks he had been having intermittent **fevers**, anorexia, and malaise and had lost 9 kg in weight. Laboratory studies revealed persistent leukocytosis up to 18,000/μl, hemoglobin 10.9 gm/100 ml, sedimentation rate of 73 mm/hr, and negative blood cultures.

Acne fulminans with myositis was diagnosed, and steroid therapy brought relief.

This rare distinctive form of acne develops rapidly on the chest and back of adolescent boys. **Polyarthralgias** are common. It is not a form of acne conglobata, which is characterized by cysts rather than necrosis.

Initially this patient's inability to walk was perceived as a conversion reaction in a socially disturbed teen-ager. However, electromyographic studies demonstrated a true myopathy.

McAuley D, Miller RA: **Acne fulminans** associated with **inflammatory bowel disease**. Report of a case. Arch Dermatol 1985; 121:91–93.

A 29-year-old man suddenly developed erythematous papules and nodular indurated crusted necrotic skin lesions on his face, jaw, and neck. His chest and back were spared. The slightest touch produced excruciating pain.

Despite treatment with oral antibiotics, he developed chills and fever (temperature to 39°C) and was soon hospitalized. Blood and skin cultures were negative, and intravenous antibiotics for 3 days did not help. Skin biopsy showed focal areas of edema in the superficial dermis and a mild mononuclear cell infiltrate around the pilosebaceous units. Direct immunofluorescence disclosed IgG, IgM, and IgA deposits in the stratum corneum, with C_3 in dermal vessel walls. Oral prednisone (100 mg/day) was started, and 36 hours later he became afebrile.

In a few days, however, he developed arthralgias in the elbows, knees, and ankles, as well as diffuse abdominal pain, vomiting, and bowel movements containing bright red blood. Crohn's disease was diagnosed after surgical exploration revealed an inflamed terminal ileum. He subsequently did well, with clearing of his skin while taking prednisone (20 mg/day) and sulfasalazine (4 gm/day).

Gonzalez T, Gantes M, Bustabad S, Diaz-Flores L: **Acne fulminans** associated with **arthritis** in monozygotic twins. J. Rheumatol 1985; 389–390.

A 14-year-old boy suddenly developed multiple, confluent, crusted ulcers over his face, lateral aspect of the neck, shoulders, and upper back. He also had weight loss, severe arthritis of the knees and left wrist, joint pains, and fever (temperature to 39°C). His WBC was 16,900 with 78% segmented neutrophils, and ESR was 123 mm/hr.

One month later, his identical twin was hospitalized with nearly identical findings.

These cases illustrate the role of genetic susceptibility in the association of acne fulminans with biopsy-proven synovitis.

Benhamou CL, Chamot AM, Kahn MF: Synovitis-acne-pustulosis-hyperostosis-osteomyelitis **syndrome (SAPHO)**. A new syndrome among the spondyloarthropathies. Clin Exp Rheumatol 1988; 6:109–112.

Acne conglobata, acne fulminans, hidradenitis suppurativa, and **palmoplantar pustulosis** may exhibit similar osteoarticular findings with a pseudoseptic pattern. Aseptic **osteomyelitis** is usually present at some stage, with inflammatory involvement of medullary bone.

Acne rheumatism occurs mainly in teen-agers. The most common symptoms are pain and enlargement of the sternum, proximal clavicle, and first ribs, i.e., anterior chest-wall involvement. Sacroiliitis and sclerotic spondylitis also occur. Hyperostosis and osteosclerosis are commonly seen on x-rays of the chest and spine.

Madsen JL: Scintigraphic detection of **clavicular hyperostosis** in a patient with **fulminant acne**. Clin Nucl Med 1988; 13:345.

A 15-year-old boy developed upper chest pain 6 months after the onset of fulminant acne.

Bone imaging of the upper trunk 2 hours after intravenous injection of Tc-99m methylene diphosphonate (MDP) showed intense activity within both clavicles. Three months later x-ray examination showed hyperostosis in the same area. Biopsies from both clavicles did not reveal malignant disease or microorganisms.

Clavicular hyperostosis and fulminant acne constitute a rare but well-described entity. Bone imaging may offer the diagnostic clue.

Jemec GBE, Rasmussen I: Bone lesions of **acne fulminans**. Case report and review of the literature. J Am Acad Dermatol 1989; 20:353–357.

Acne fulminans affects young men in their teens and occurs after a period of mild acne vulgaris. Large confluent necrotic areas with gelatinous debris suddenly appear, with no comedones or cysts. They are very tender and lead to a characteristic bent-over posture.

The clinical picture is that of septicemia, but most cultures are negative and the effects of antibiotics are uncertain.

Osteomyelitis usually affects the epiphysis of the long bones and only rarely the clavicles.

An immune mechanism is suspected as the cause of **arthralgias** and **hematuria**, but circulating immunocomplexes and immunoglobulin deposition in skin are not consistently found.

Massa MC, Su WPD: **Pyoderma faciale**: A clinical study of twenty-nine patients. J Am Acad Dermatol 1982; 6:84–91.

The following clinical features were revealed in the 29 patients seen at the Mayo Clinic from 1969 to 1980:

> female predominance (all patients!)
> sudden onset after teen-age years with rapid progression of lesions
> facial lesions only
> absence of systemic complaints (except fatigue)
> intense erythematous to purple discoloration, cysts, swelling, spontaneous purulent drainage, lack of comedones
> marked scarring

Laboratory findings: bacterial cultures negative or contain a variety of skin contaminants; no gram-negative organisms; two cases with *Staphylococcus aureus*.

Differential diagnosis:

> gram-negative acne (culture distinguishes).

acne conglobata (males, multiple comedones, prolonged course, trunk and face involved).

acne rosacea (telangiectasia, papules, pustules, no cysts).

Leyden JJ: **Low serum iron levels** and moderate anemia in **severe nodulocystic acne**. Reversal with isotretinoin therapy. Arch Dermatol 1985; 121:214–215.

In 24 males (18 to 21 years old), severe nodulocystic acne of the face and trunk was evaluated for oral isotretinoin therapy. Low serum iron levels were found in 75% and mild anemia in 25%. Ferritin levels were elevated, but transferrin saturation was normal.

The patients were felt to have the anemia of chronic disease resulting from cutaneous inflammation, rather than an iron-deficiency state. Storage iron is held within ferritin, a protein molecule that in serum parallels the concentration of storage iron within the body. Increased serum ferritin helps to rule out iron deficiency and is common in inflammatory states.

Treatment with isotretinoin for 5 months led to normal iron levels and correction of anemia in these patients, perhaps as a result of reversal of chronic severe inflammation.

Pérez-Villa F, Campistol JM, Ferrando J, Botey A: **Renal amyloidosis** secondary to **acne conglobata**. Int J Dermatol 1989; 28:132–133.

A 62-year-old man had suffered from acne conglobata of the back, buttocks, and abdomen since the age of 20 years. One year previously proteinuria was detected, followed 5 months later by **renal failure**.

Kidney and rectal biopsies were positive for amyloid, in contrast to a skin biopsy, which showed only follicular keratinization, inflammation around follicles, and dermal abscesses, but no amyloid.

Despite hemodialysis he developed anuria and died of an intracranial hemorrhage 35 days after being hospitalized.

Since the patient had no evidence of Bence-Jones protein or serum or urine monoclonal immunoglobulins, he appeared to have secondary amyloidosis induced by severe acne conglobata for 40 years. Reactive systemic amyloidosis is often associated with chronic skin infection and suppuration.

Whipp MJ, Harrington CI, Dundas S: Fatal **squamous cell carcinoma** associated with acne conglobata in a father and daughter. Br J Dermatol 1987; 117:389–392.

Acne conglobata mainly affects men and begins insidiously after puberty with comedones, cysts, abscesses, and draining sinus tracts. The back, buttocks, and chest are particularly involved, although other sites include the neck, shoulders, abdomen, face, thighs, and upper arms. **Abscesses** break down to form intercommunicating ulcers and sinus tracts, and healing occurs slowly with pitting and **keloid bridge scars**.

Acne conglobata is linked pathogenetically with hidradenitis suppurativa and dissecting cellulitis of the scalp in the "follicular occlusion triad." Squamous cell carcinoma is a recognized complication of these conditions and is often rapidly fatal. Careful follow-up of acne conglobata patients is therefore indicated.

A 56-year-old woman with widespread abscesses on the buttocks, axillae, and back since age 18 developed a painful rapidly enlarging **ulcer crater** on her right loin. It was 3 cm deep with a shaggy proliferative margin and had multiple satellite nodules in a 25- by 10-cm area. Despite radiation treatment of this well-differentiated squamous cell carcinoma, she died 4 months later. Her father also had had acne conglobata and died similarly of squamous cell carcinoma at the age of 55 years.

Tosti A, Guerra L, Bettoli V, Bonelli U: Solid **facial edema** as a complication of **acne vulgaris** in twins. J Am Acad Dermatol 1987; 17:843–844.

A pair of 14-year-old identical male twins had severe papulopustular acne of the face associated with pronounced centrofacial edema.

The edema started in both boys in the same month, 1 year after the onset of acne. They were both taking minocycline (100 mg/day); there was no improvement when the drug was stopped. The edema was nontender and noninflammatory, being most marked in the **periorbital** areas and **base of the nose**. It was worse in the morning and decreased by the end of the day.

Extensive blood tests were normal except for elevated ASO titers, 1500 and 750 U, respectively (normal 0 to 200). Skin biopsies revealed only acne vulgaris, with no mucin deposition. Direct immunofluorescence was negative. Systemic steroids for 2 weeks did not improve the edema. Topical and oral antibiotics caused moderate resolution of the acne but not the facial edema.

Inherited factors may be involved in this unusual complication of acne vulgaris.

Frank SB: Uncommon aspects of common acne. Cutis 1974; 14:817–822.

A nice review of many types of unusual acne.

"Hippie acne" occurred under the headbands worn by hippies.

The same phenomenon (**acne mechanica**) occurs on the neck of concert violinists, resulting from irritation by the chin rest.

Mills OH, Kligman AM: **Acne mechanica**. Arch Dermatol 1975; 111:481–483.

Mechanical forces may intensify acne. These include pressure, tension, friction, stretching, rubbing, pinching, and pulling.

Rubbing of the skin by clothing, football pads, and belts, as well as rubbing of the back during driving of trucks, all exacerbate acne.

Let an atlas take some of the diagnostic weight off your shoulders.

External Causes

Ancona AA: Occupational acne. *In* Adams RM (ed): Occupational Medicine: Occupational Skin Disease. Philadelphia, Hanley & Belfus, Inc., 1986, pp 229–236.

Oil acne is the most common form of **industrial acne**. It is caused by greases and insoluble cutting oils containing a high percentage of mineral oil. Machine-tool operators in the metal industry are most commonly affected.

Insoluble oils generally contain a high percentage of refined petroleum oil, a small amount of animal or vegetable oil, sulfur, and preservatives. Technical oils apparently replace skin lipids and interfere with keratinization, inducing hyperkeratosis and follicular plugging, followed by pilosebaceous unit inflammation. Microorganisms in oils do not play a significant role.

Lesions are usually inflammatory pustules and papules on exposed sites, such as the forearms and dorsal aspect of hands, in direct contact with coolants. Oil-soaked clothing may also induce lesions, particularly on the abdomen and thighs. The course is chronic, and there may be associated **melanosis**, photosensitivity, and skin cancer.

Coal tar acne results from airborne fumes given off by hot pitch or other tar oils and distillation by-products. The lesions are almost purely comedones, particularly on the malar areas, and tend to clear fairly rapidly after exposure ceases. **Photosensitivity**, smarting and watering of the eyes, and heavy pigmentation may be associated problems.

Taylor JS: The pilosebaceous unit. *In* Maibach HI (ed): Occupational and Industrial Dermatology, 2nd ed. Chicago, Year Book Medical Publishers, Inc., 1987, pp 105–120.

Occupational exposure to cutting oils, coal tar oils, pitch, or creosote may induce **acne**. Likewise, heat, friction, and harsh detergents may be acnegenic. The most specific occupational acnegen remains the halogenated aromatic compound group. This includes the halogenated naphthalenes and biphenyls. Some are present in herbicides.

Fulton JE Jr., Kligman AM: Aggravation of acne vulgaris by topical application of corticosteroids under occlusion. Cutis 1968; 4:1106–1109.

Topical steroids may initially decrease erythema, pain, and cyst size in severe inflammatory acne. Over 2 to 6 months, however, severe flares are likely, signaled by a striking increase in closed comedones followed by inflammatory papules. The process may be subtle, with a gradual increase in comedones over several months.

Experimental acne may be reliably reproduced in acne-prone areas by the application of potent topical steroids to normal skin under Saran Wrap. Steroid-induced comedones rupture early, resulting in small inflammatory papules.

Litt JZ: **McDonald's acne.** Arch Dermatol 1974; 110:956.

Youngsters working in **fast-food restaurants** where they are in constant contact with hot cooking oils and greases develop "McDonald's acne." Marked acne often appears suddenly on the face and chest, especially during the summer months. It also clears dramatically when the person stops working there.

Should this be covered under the workers' compensation law?

Das M, Misra MP: **Acne** and **folliculitis** due to **diesel oil.** Contact Dermatitis 1988; 18:120–121.

A 28-year-old man who had been an automobile mechanic for 15 years had a 5-year history of comedones and pustules on his forearms, dorsal aspect of the hands, and anterior midthighs. He worked with diesel oil and frequently wiped his hands on the front of his trousers. He complained of intermittent itching and burning of both his skin and eyes.

In addition to acne and folliculitis, other signs of **diesel oil toxicity** included hepatomegaly, azoospermia, and psychological disturbances.

Similar lesions have been reported in oil-field workers, oil refiners, and paraffin-pressmen, who also developed **furuncles** and **carbuncles** in addition to folliculitis, pustules, and comedones on the fingers, dorsal aspect of the hands, and forearms.

Frankel EB: **Acne** secondary to **white petrolatum** use. Arch Dermatol 1985; 121:589–590.

A 15-minute nightly **massage** of petrolatum into the right cheek of a 21-year-old woman led to the appearance of comedones and then erythematous papules and pustules. Massage had been prescribed by her neurologist to alleviate Bell's palsy of that area, and she accomplished it with white petrolatum.

The left side of the face remained entirely clear of acne.

Know your patients' habits to know why they have acne.

Plewig G, Fulton JE, Kligman AM: **Pomade acne**. Arch Dermatol 1970; 101:580–584.

Among 735 Negro men examined with regard to daily use of scalp creams and oils, about 70% of long-term users of pomades had acne.

The eruption involved the forehead and temples and consisted of numerous closely set uniform follicular papules with occasional papulopustules. The papules were **closed comedones**.

Pomades are weak acnegens. It generally takes a year or more of daily use to produce the eruption. Lesions rarely go beyond the closed comedo stage.

Srinivas CR, Padhee A, Balanchandran C, et al: **Comedones** induced by **coconut oil** in a borderline tuberculoid lesion. Int J Lepr Other Mycobact Dis 1988; 56:471–472.

A 42-year-old Indian woman developed comedones within a hypopigmented anesthetic patch of tuberculoid leprosy on one knee. A biopsy specimen showed hyperkeratosis and follicular plugging, as well as tuberculoid granulomas. Because the affected site was dry, she was in the habit of massaging coconut oil into it.

Coconut oil thus joins cutting oils and various cosmetics as being comedogenic.

Plewig G, Kligman AM: Induction of acne by topical steroids. Arch Dermatol Forsch 1973; 247:29–52.

Cases of **steroid acne** appear to be identical clinically whether elicited topically, orally, or parenterally.

Its most notable feature is the rapid evolution of numerous dull-red dome-shaped papules that are uniform in size and shape. It is never nodulocystic but may be pustular. Comedones are absent in the early phase, but may appear several weeks later. Lesions heal without scarring. Stinging and burning may be a problem.

Postacne sufferers are much more likely to develop steroid acne than are normal controls.

In young acne-prone adults topical steroids under continuous occlusion will induce many small follicular papules after 7 to 14 days, which reach maximum size by 3 weeks. They begin to regress 1 week after exposure is stopped, and after 3 weeks they are insignificant except for closed comedones.

Mills OH, Kligman AM: **Acne detergicans**. Arch Dermatol 1975; 111:65–68.

The obsessive use of soaps four to six times daily by acne patients may aggravate the disease and spread it to unusual locations.

Hjorth N, Sjølin K-E, Sylvest B, Thomsen K: Acne aestivalis—**Mallorca acne**. Acta Derm Venereol 1972; 52:61–63.

This distinctive form of acne occurs mainly in young women slightly older than the usual group of acne sufferers. It starts in spring or summer and lasts 3 to 6 months despite therapy. There is a history of **sunbathing**, with or without sunscreens. Scandinavian patients tend to get it after a Mediterranean holiday.

The eruption is symmetrical and localized to the face, sides of the neck, upper chest, and shoulders. Primary lesions are 1- to 3-mm large, hard, pink or pale, dome-shaped papules with narrow red halos. Comedones and pustules are rare. The papules may be closely set or sparse. They tend to itch after sun exposure, possibly from sweating or heat. Miliaria rubra was not observed.

The causative role of sunscreens is suspected, but unproven.

Tindall JP: **Chloracne** and chloracnegens. J Am Acad Dermatol 1985; 13:539–558.

Chloracne is an acneiform eruption that heralds systemic poisoning by aromatic chlorinated hydrocarbons of varying structure. Its distinctive distribution favors the area below and to the **outer side of the eye** and **behind the ear**. The nose is remarkably resistant and may be the only uninvolved site on the face. In contrast, the **penis** and **scrotum** are common sites of involvement with acneiform lesions.

In severe cases, the shoulders, chest, back, buttocks, and abdomen become involved. The hands, feet, forearms, and legs are generally exempt, but the axillae can be involved in those who have simply ingested or inhaled the chloracnegen.

The latent period between contact and clinical signs is 2 to 4 weeks and the duration of lesions may vary from 6 months to over 30 years. The initial lesion is the comedo, and the diagnosis of chloracne can be made by seeing as few as a dozen **comedones** in the malar crescent area. Eventually every follicle may contain a comedo, giving the skin a grayish appearance. The lesions progress to become small pale **yellow cysts** and then large cysts. **Cold abscesses** also occur, particularly on the back of the neck, trunk, and buttocks. The degree of inflammation is usually far less than in cystic acne. Scarring occurs, ranging from fine pitting, as in **atrophoderma vermiculatum**, to deep scars.

Porphyria cutanea tarda has been reported concomitantly (herbicide manufacture). Erythema and edema of the face, possibly due to **photosensitivity**, have occurred in Europe, followed by hyperpigmentation of the face. **Generalized hyperpigmentation** also occurs and may involve the nails, conjunctiva, and mucous membranes. **Hypertrichosis** may be seen with the pigmentation, suggesting hepatic porphyria. Fine **follicular hyperkeratosis** on the upper trunk, neck, and flexural areas was reported from Japan. Hyperhidrosis of the palms and soles also may occur. **Granuloma annulare–like** lesions on the dorsal aspect of the hands and palms have been reported from Europe, probably induced by chlorinated hydrocarbons.

Ophthalmic chloracne refers to conjunctivitis and the conversion of meibomian glands into squamous cysts filled with cheesy material. The meibomian glands, with the eyelashes, are analogous to pilosebaceous units.

Sources of contact range from insulation waxes (Halowax) and contaminated dairy foods (PCB, PBBs, polyhalogenated biphenyls) to insecticides, fungicides (dioxins), and herbicides (azobenzenes).

Systemic findings in **poisoning** from **chlorinated hydrocarbons** include:

weight loss	edema of all four limbs
liver damage	increased triglycerides
hepatic porphyria	headache, fatigue, irritability, insomnia
hyperhidrosis of **palms** and **soles**	impotence
nausea, vomiting, diarrhea	peripheral neuropathy
joint pains	persistent bronchitis, dyspnea

Caputo R, Monti M, Ermacora E, et al: Cutaneous manifestations of tetrachlorodibenzo-p-dioxin in children and adolescents. Follow-up 10 years after the Seveso, Italy, accident. J Am Acad Dermatol 1988; 19:812–819.

On July 10, 1976, a cloud of finely dispersed tetrachlorodibenzo-p-dioxin (TCDD) settled down over 200 acres, including thousands of people, animals, and foodstuff in Seveso, Italy. It had come from an accident in a chemical plant processing sodium trichlorophenate.

The immediate effect on exposed skin was erythema and edema, especially of the face and limbs. It occurred only in those directly under the visible cloud, and only in those under age 20 years. The lesions appeared within 2 hours and faded in 2 weeks, leaving mild hyperpigmentation. Vesiculobullous and **necrotic lesions** also appeared on the **fingertips** and occasionally the knees and buttocks of children playing in TCDD-contaminated soil. Vesicular and pink papulonodular lesions were also seen on the upper trunk and arms in a few children. They appeared 2 weeks after the accident and faded in about 10 days.

The late lesions were those of **chloracne**, evident within 2 months, although new cases continued to appear for up to 8 months after the accident. Open comedones and pale yellow cysts particularly affected the cheeks and ears but also the nape of the neck and axillae. The centrofacial area was always spared.

In severe cases involving nonexposed areas, hyperkeratotic papules and comedones were seen on the arms and legs. A few children also developed **granuloma annulare–like** lesions or **erythema elevatum diutinum–like** lesions on the hands and fingers. The chloracne lesions slowly involuted over 2 to 3 years, leaving marked atrophic scarring in many cases.

The toxic cloud of Seveso was an "acne rain" for all the children under it. Chloracne was the most reliable and typical sign of poisoning by TCDD, especially in prepubertal children and adolescents, and was the most sensitive indicator of environmental pollution.

Orris P, Worobec S, Kahn G, et al: **Chloracne** in **firefighters**. Lancet 1986; 1:210–211.

Firefighters are exposed to a variety of burning materials (plastics, tars, woods) that probably include chloracnegens, such as polychlorinated and polybrominated compounds.

Two firefighters with multiple comedones are presented, both of whom had been exposed to burning silicon tetrachloride. A 52-year-old man had multiple open **comedones** in the **periorbital**, preauricular, neck, and right axillary areas, as well as multiple inflamed pustular cysts over the shoulders. A 50-year-old man had multiple open and closed comedones in the periorbital and malar areas.

Chloracne (halogen acne) is a persistent form of acne that is very resistant to treatment. It may be impossible to differentiate from acne vulgaris, both clinically and histologically.

Known causes of chloracne include:

polyhalogenated naphthalenes
biphenyls
dibenzofurans
dibenzodioxins
tetrachloroazoxybenzene
tetrachlorobenzene

Cole GW, Stone O, Gates D, Culver D: **Chloracne** from pentachlorophenol-preserved wood. Contact Dermatitis 1986; 15:164–168.

For 6 months a 32-year-old white man had been developing multiple small yellow-white papules diffusely over his entire body, with occasional inflamed papules. The malar and postauricular areas were covered with numerous 2- to 3-mm **keratin cysts**. His trunk, buttocks, thighs, and lower legs were also involved. Skin biopsy revealed a keratin cyst that communicated with the skin surface, consistent with chloracne.

The culprit proved to be the PCP-pretreated lumber he worked with in constructing piers for small-boat marinas. Within 9 months of starting this work he noted a papular acneiform eruption. When working with the wood he wore only shorts and shoes, often lying atop the lumber for considerable periods to measure it. Thus he routinely disregarded safety precautions for skin protection.

PCP (pentachlorophenol) is a popular bactericide and fungicide used to preserve wood and is impregnated into the wood under high pressure in a vacuum. The amount of preservative per cubic foot may be stamped on the lumber.

Guldager H: **Halothane allergy** as cause of **acne**. Lancet 1987; 1:1211–1212.

A 27-year-old woman developed an acneiform eruption on her face 2 weeks after starting work as a nurse anesthetist. Tetracycline and a steroid cream did not help. Four months later she had similar lesions affecting her whole body after administering a halothane anesthetic.

Skin biopsy revealed spongiose skin and subepidermal edema with infiltration of polymorphonuclear leukocytes, consistent with an allergic skin reaction.

She was transferred to work in an intensive care unit, but every time she came in contact with a patient who had just had halothane anesthesia a widespread acneiform eruption recurred within a few hours.

Halothane hepatitis has been reported to be a delayed hypersensitivity reaction, and the skin reaction may be similar.

Acne occurring in **operating room staff** may represent halothane allergy and should be looked into.

Zatulove A, Konnerth NA: **Comedogenicity testing** of **cosmetics**. Cutis 1987; 39:521.

Acne in women past the age of 25 years is increasing, possibly because of the increased use and incorrect removal of cosmetic creams, lotions, and makeup.

Cosmetic scientists at Estee Lauder and other cosmetic firms test new products and their ingredients for comedogenicity using the ear of the New Zealand white rabbit, an extremely sensitive test model. Over a 3-week period, 15 applications of test product (0.05 ml) are placed on the internal base of the right ear of each rabbit. The left ear acts as the control. Each ear is observed for follicular hyperkeratosis and comedones, and biopsies on day 19 are sectioned transversely and evaluated for acanthosis, keratosis, and keratin plugging.

The high level of sensitivity of the **rabbit ear assay** may unfairly condemn some potential cosmetic ingredients. Therefore, consumer use tests are often run simultaneously for 3 weeks.

Mills OH, Porte M, Kligman AM: Enhancement of comedogenic substances by ultraviolet radiation. Br J Dermatol 1978; 98:145–153.

About one of five acne patients gets worse with sun exposure. This apparently results from ultraviolet radiation having a potentiating effect on comedogenic substances.

Increased comedogenicity with **ultraviolet radiation** was demonstrated in the rabbit's ear using human sebum, sulfur, cocoa butter, squalene, and coal tar to produce comedones. Similarly in humans, coal tar and squalene plus ultraviolet light increased the size of experimentally induced microcomedones.

Although **sunbathing** often produces immediate beneficial effects in acne with more rapid resolution of pustules, the long-term effects may be adverse because of the creation of new comedones.

Adriaans B, du Vivier A: **Acne** in an **irradiated area**. Arch Dermatol 1989; 125:1005.

A 44-year-old woman who had had acne as a teenager had a left simple mastectomy with axillary clearance performed for an intraductal carcinoma of the breast. A local recurrence on the left chest was treated with radiation therapy (45 Gy from a cobalt-60 machine). One month after completing therapy she developed papules, pustules, and comedones localized to the area of radiotherapy.

Presumably, irradiation produced follicular inflammation and hyperkeratosis, with decreased shedding of keratinocytes, increased adherence of these cells, and bacterial proliferation. Localized follicular comedones and pustules resulted.

If you find yourself in deep water, row for the nearest consultant.

Internal Causes

Papa CM: **Acne** and hidden **iodides**. Arch Dermatol 1976; 112:555–556.

In patients with pustular inflammatory acne, look for a high-iodide diet; such foods are produced in fast-food snack establishments. This may be the true cause of "**McDonald's acne**."

Also look for **kelp** ingestion, which occurs with tablets used for weight control and with "natural vitamins." Two cases of teenagers with mild comedonal acne are cited, in whom crops of abscess-like inflammatory pustules and papulonodules developed on the face, neck, shoulders, and back shortly after they started taking kelp tablets. The lesions cleared within several weeks after stopping the seaweed supplement, which is high in iodides.

Heydenreich G: Testosterone and anabolic steroids and **acne fulminans**. Arch Dermatol 1989; 125:571–572.

A 21-year-old body builder, who had previously had slight facial acne, began taking large amounts of **testosterone** and **anabolic steroids** to increase his muscle mass. After 4 weeks, tiny pustules appeared on his face and shoulders, followed in a few more weeks by erythema, infiltration, tenderness, and ulceration with thick crusts. After 2 months, tender oozing ulcers and nodulocystic lesions covered his face, back, shoulders, neck, upper arms, chest, and underarms. He felt ill and lost weight.

Prednisone (25 mg daily) administration was then started. Relief was dramatic, but the prednisone had to be continued for 3 months because of the development of fever, malaise, and a flu-like syndrome whenever it was stopped. The disease activity stopped 6 months after it had started, leaving scars and keloids.

Skin biopsy showed acute, suppurative folliculitis, both deep and superficial types. Repeated bacterial cultures showed *Staphylococcus albus*.

Acne vulgaris and the worsening of acne vulgaris are probably common complications of the misuse of testosterone and anabolic steroids. These drugs increase the sebum excretion rate in men, which in turn increases the population of *Propionibacterium acnes*. Possibly, this bacterium, or an associated antigen, triggers an immunologic reaction leading to acne fulminans.

Cook TJ, Lorincz AL: Absence of **steroid acne** in **children**. A clinical study. Arch Dermatol 1964; 89:442–445.

A study of 133 patients receiving long-term high doses of corticosteroids showed that children under the age of 10 years did not get steroid acne.

Among 65 such patients ages 0 to 9 years, only one girl developed acne and facial oiliness, and this did not occur until 2 weeks after she was also given an androgen. Children 10 to 12 years old are somewhat more likely to develop steroid acne, which occurred in 25% of 32 patients. Only two children had facial oiliness.

In the teenage group, 18 of 19 patients (95%) demonstrated steroid acne. As in the other groups, many complained of marked dryness. Facial oiliness was seen in only six patients (31.6%).

In contrast to steroid acne, **hypertrichosis** is a common finding in children taking steroids. It occurred in 75% of the 0- to 9-year-old group, 65% of the 10- to 12-year-old group, and 37% of the teenage group.

Traupe H, von Mühlendahl KE, Bramswig J, Happle R: **Acne** of the **fulminans** type following **testosterone therapy** in three excessively tall boys. Arch Dermatol 1988; 124:414–417.

The pathogenic role of testosterone in acne is underscored by the appearance of acne fulminans in three teenagers who were being treated with intramuscular injections of testosterone enanthate (250 mg/week or 500 mg every 2 weeks) to close the epiphyses. The severe **ulcerative acne** with fever, malaise, **polyarthralgias**, and weight loss appeared after 7 to 12 months of injections. In two of the patients, treatment with isotretinoin precipitated **pyogenic granuloma-like** lesions as previously observed in acne conglobata. The disease persisted for 3 to 4 months after testosterone was discontinued.

Tucker S, Buell J, Fisher HR: **Luteoma** of **pregnancy**: Case report. Am J Obstet Gynecol 1975; 121:282.

During the seventh month of pregnancy a 33-year-old black woman developed **severe cystic acne** of the forehead and coarse **facial hair** on the chin. Clitoral enlargement and deepening voice had been noted at 3 to 4 months' gestation. At the time of delivery by cesarean section, wedge biopsies were done of very large bilateral cystic ovaries, which revealed luteinized cysts rather than a focal tumor. Following delivery, the acne resolved with scarring over several months.

Luteoma of pregnancy is a benign ovarian tumor that usually presents as an adnexal mass during pregnancy. It may cause **masculinization** of the mother and female fetus through elaboration of androgenic hormones. The tumor regresses following pregnancy, with androgen levels rapidly returning to normal. Tests for abnormal androgen production should be done during pregnancy.

Oliwiecki S, Burton JL: **Severe acne** due to **isoniazid**. Clin Exp Dermatol 1988; 13:283–284.

A 43-year-old man with pulmonary tuberculosis (sputum culture = *Mycobacterium avium-intracellulare*) had a left upper lobectomy 9 months after he started taking standard doses of rifampicin, ethambutol, pyrazinamide, and isoniazid. Five months after surgery, while still taking rifampicin (600 mg/day), isoniazid (300 mg/day), and ethambutol (1000 mg/day), he developed a severe acneiform eruption of comedones and pustules on his back, shoulders, and buttocks, which was unresponsive to treatment with oxytetracycline for 3 months. He had no past history of acne. One month after discontinuation of isoniazid the acne began to improve, and 2 months later it had completely cleared, despite continuing treatment with rifampicin and ethambutol.

The acne had begun 15 months after he started taking isoniazid. This is consistent with other reports of acne developing after prolonged treatment with the drug. Since isoniazid is a structural analogue of niacin (nicotinic acid), it may induce follicular plugging similar to that seen in pellagra. The late onset of severe acne should suggest a search for a causative drug.

Lowe L, Herbert AA: **Cystic** and **comedonal acne**: A side effect of **etretinate therapy**. Int J Dermatol 1989; 28:482.

During the seventh week of treatment with etretinate for psoriasis, a 33-year-old man developed numerous clogged comedones on the chin, jawline, and lateral aspect of the neck, as well as tender inflammatory cysts on the back and posterior aspect of the neck. The lesions had cleared one month after the drug was discontinued.

Acne has been documented to be a side effect of etretinate in approximately 1.5% of patients in clinical trials.

Menter A, Boyd A: **Cystic acne** in psoriatic patients undergoing **etretinate therapy**. J Am Acad Dermatol 1988; 18:751–752.

A 30-year-old man with generalized inflammatory psoriasis had excellent clearing with etretinate (75 mg/day). However, after 6 weeks of treatment he developed severe cystic acne on his back, chest, stomach, axillae, and thighs, with sparing of his face and neck. Etretinate was stopped after 12 weeks of treatment, and the acne then cleared over a 3-month period.

A 44-year-old man with pustular and extensive inflammatory plaque psoriasis was started on etretinate (25 mg bid). After 2 weeks he developed mildly pruritic inflammatory acne cysts on his back, posterior aspect of the arms, and ankles. The eruption cleared with topical erythromycin lotion, although the etretinate was continued.

Bernhard JD: **Acne cosmetica** following successful treatment with oral isotretinoin. Arch Dermatol 1985; 121:26.

A 19-year-old woman with cystic acne of the face, chest, and back had been successfully treated with oral isotretinoin (80 mg/day) for 4 months.

Five months later she had a new facial "rash," consisting of numerous closed comedones and tiny pustules on her forehead. She had been using a new **oily hair conditioner** and was believed to have acne cosmetica.

Patients with acne should be warned that treatment with Accutane does not make them "immune" to factors known to provoke acne cosmetica.

Vexiau P, Gourmel B, Julien R, et al: Severe acne-like lesions caused by **amineptine overdosage**. Lancet 1988; 1:585.

Very **severe acne**, including large cysts, was seen in five patients taking large doses of the **tricyclic antidepressant** amineptine (survector). Lesions were most prominent on the face, back, and chest but also occurred on the arms, legs, and perineum. Treatment with isotretinoin for 6 to 18 months caused no improvement.

After discontinuation of the drug, the lesions had disappeared in only one patient after 3 months. Amineptine metabolites were recovered from matter inside a facial lesion, suggesting that the drug may accumulate in the cutaneous lesions and slowly be released, accounting for continuing lesions after the drug had been stopped for several months.

Some patients have so much wrong with them that any diagnosis will do.

Dubrow TJ, Lesavoy MA: **Acne of the heel:** Acne vulgaris complicating a free vascularized latissimus dorsi musculocutaneous flap. Ann Plast Surg 1989; 23:349–351.

A 27-year-old man with severe acne scarring on his back sustained a large left-heel avulsion in a motorcycle accident. Heel coverage was accomplished with a latissimus dorsi free flap with vascular pedicle, and all wounds healed without difficulty.

One year later in the **graft site** on the heel he developed huge clustered **multipored blackheads**, large **acne cysts**, and draining nodules and sinuses discharging sanguineous and purulent material. The acne on his back had also reactivated, with diffuse pustules and comedones surrounding the donor scar. Despite intravenous antibiotics the large heel pustules continued to form, and 10 months later heel debridement was performed, and a cross-leg flap was attached. Healing was successful, and no acne had formed at the site in a 3-year follow-up.

This may have been an example of **acne mechanica**, due to weight bearing on skin not accustomed to prolonged pressure. Donor-site acne scarring should be considered a contraindication to free mucocutaneous flap transfer in young patients.

Dekio S, Imaoka C, Jidoi J: **Candida folliculitis** associated with **hypothyroidism**. Br J Dermatol 1987; 117:663–664.

Slightly pruritic follicular erythematous papules and pustules covered the face of a 49-year-old housewife for 2 months. The papules, but not the pustules, accompanied comedones. She was also hypothyroid, with puffy, pale, and dry facial skin. A KOH–Parker Quink ink preparation of a pustule and papule showed many hyphae, and culture proved the pathogen to be *Candida albicans*. Bacterial cultures were negative. She had no oral, genital, or other signs of candidiasis. In hypothyroidism the sebaceous glands secrete less sebum than normal, possibly leading to a decreased normal flora of lipophilic organisms and replacement by *Candida albicans*, which produced folliculitis.

Leyden JJ, Marples RR, Mills OH Jr, Kligman AM: **Gram-negative folliculitis**—a complication of antibiotic therapy in acne vulgaris. Br J Dermatol 1973; 88:533–538.

In most acne patients, therapy with an effective antibiotic produces gradual improvement over 4 to 6 weeks. In contrast, in gram-negative folliculitis, the response to antibiotics is very rapid, with either rapid exacerbation (due to overgrowth of resistant organisms) or rapid improvement. Skin biopsy shows an intrafollicular abscess without comedo formation.

There are two distinct varieties of gram-negative folliculitis:

> **superficial pustules** with **red bases** grouped around the nose, associated with lactose–fermenting gram-negative rods
> **deep nodules** and **cysts** on the face, caused by *Proteus* infection

Many cases occur in older acne patients who have been taking antibiotics for prolonged periods. The reservoir of gram-negative organisms appears to be the nasal mucosa, and culturing the anterior nares may be helpful. The use of **hexachlorophene-containing soaps** may also contribute to overgrowth of gram-negative bacteria.

Lambert WC, Bagley MP, Khan Y, Schwartz RA: **Pustular acneiform secondary syphilis.** Cutis 1986; 37:69–70.

For 6 weeks a 28-year-old homosexual Hispanic man had noted an erythema-   185 tous pustular acneiform eruption on his face, chest, back, and extremities. A few lesions involved the scalp, and two were on his left sole. He had been under treatment with female hormones (medroxyprogesterone acetate and Premarin). The acneiform eruption proved to be secondary syphilis (STS titer 1:256, spirochetes in skin biopsy seen with Warthin-Starre stain).

Clues to alert you that an eruption is syphilis and not acne:

short duration
occurrence after usual "acne age"
comedones and scarring absent
wider distribution, including scalp
indolent papules with more crust than pus

Shelley WB, Wood MG: **Acneiform herpes simplex.** Cutis 1981; 27:475–478.

A 31-year-old woman suddenly had two tender **acneiform papules** appear in the left paranasal area. Concurrently she had developed grouped vesicles on the right upper lip. She had had repeated similar episodes. Occasionally the acneiform papulopustular lesions appeared independently of the vesicular lesions.

Vesicular herpes simplex was confirmed by biopsy on the lip. The acneiform lesions proved to be a papular form of herpes simplex, with giant multinucleate cells in a setting of epidermal destruction and marked dermal inflammatory response.

This rare form of herpes usually occurs as a **small group of papules**, always recurring at the **same site** on the chin. The lesions are episodic, often appearing premenstrually or with stress. They clear in 7 to 14 days without scarring.

Today the possibility of acneiform herpes simplex calls for the prophylactic (also diagnostic) use of systemic acyclovir therapy.

Lee S, Kim J-G, Kang JS: **Eruptive vellus hair cysts.** Arch Dermatol 1984; 120:1191–1195.

A 21-year-old man considered the multiple 1- to 4-mm follicular papules on his anterior chest to be acne. They had been present for 1 year. White cheesy material could be expressed from the lesions by gentle squeezing. Skin biopsy showed squamous cell–lined cysts in the upper and mid-dermis, containing laminated and amorphous keratin and vellus hairs.

Vellus hair cysts are **yellowish** or **reddish-brown papules**, either grouped or scattered, with smooth or crusted surfaces. White comedo-like lesions with pinpoint surfaces are also seen. They mimic acne, folliculitis, perforating papular dermatosis, and keratosis pilaris. They occur at any age, but often begin in childhood or young adulthood. Spontaneous regression is common. Although the major site of predilection is the **anterior chest**, they may be seen also on the arms, legs, face, neck, and groin.

The cyst walls may rupture, producing granulomatous inflammation with foreign body giant cells. The histologic differential diagnosis includes:

epidermal cysts
steatocystoma multiplex
milia
dermoid cysts
pilar cysts

Price M, Russell Jones R: **Familial dyskeratotic comedones.** Clin Exp Dermatol 1985; 10:147–153.

A 44-year-old man had suffered with a widespread hyperkeratotic comedolike eruption since age 14. It was most pronounced around the **waist, thighs, buttocks, penis**, and over the **knuckles**. His scrotal skin was thickened, with a tendency to develop fissures. One brother had a similar eruption, but no one had the disorder in the two preceding generations.

Skin biopsy of a hyperkeratotic papule revealed a deformed follicular orifice with a parakeratotic plug and acantholysis with occasional dyskeratotic cells in the follicle wall. A scrotal lesion showed considerable acantholysis with the dilapidated brick-wall appearance of Hailey-Hailey disease, and also dyskeratosis with numerous large prematurely keratinized cells.

The comedones, dominant inheritance, and focal acantholytic dyskeratosis make this eruption unique.

Focal acantholytic dyskeratosis is also seen in:

Darier's disease
benign familial pemphigus
transient acantholytic dermatosis
warty dyskeratoma
persistent acantholytic dermatosis

Read more, and you'll diagnose more.

Acrodermatitis Enteropathica

Think of acrodermatitis enteropathica when there is a pediatric history of conjoint skin and bowel problems. It is an easy diagnosis in an **unhappy baby** with **florid candidiasis**, **perioral** and **perianal dermatitis**, **sparse hair** growth, and chronic **diarrhea**. The child may have a low intake of zinc (cow's milk) or an inherited defect in the intestinal transport of zinc.

Think of zinc deficiency in an adult with **hyperalimentation**, **chronic alcoholism**, **intestinal malabsorption**, or **pregnancy**. The patient may be receiving zinc-poor intravenous feedings or have a very poor diet. Zinc deficiency is especially hard to diagnose in an adult who has only a few perianal erosions, mild paronychia, recurrent folliculitis and impetigo, and questionable hair loss.

We have no specific diagnostic marker, yet acrodermatitis enteropathica is essentially a "zincopenic" dermatitis. Finding a low serum zinc level or observing a rapid therapeutic response to oral zinc strengthens the clinical diagnosis immeasurably. However, there are pitfalls, as zinc levels in blood may be contaminated by a zinc-rich rubber stopper or instrumental error. Also, a noncompliant patient may not take the prescribed zinc, or an infant may "spit up" an oral dose.

Occasionally a patient with signs of zinc deficiency will have normal zinc levels. Supportive evidence for zinc deficiency may then be obtained by electron microscopy of small-bowel biopsies; capillary gas-liquid chromatography determination of plasma essential fatty acids, which are poorly absorbed in acrodermatitis enteropathica; and zinc absorption tests using radioisotopes (^{65}Zn or ^{69m}Zn).

Zinc is an essential component of more than 40 different enzymes, so that zinc deficiency causes multienzyme defects and multisymptomatic disease. The most metabolically active tissues in the body (hair, leukocytes, and gut) soon feel the effects of zinc malabsorption or zinc mal-intake. Hair grows poorly, yeast and bacterial infections thrive in the face of weakened leukocyte defenses, and the gut becomes irritable, with 10 or more liquid stools a day.

Think of "zincopenia" to explain alopecia, ulcers, infections, and a host of strange unexplainable skin changes. Zinc ranks with biotin as a truly essential element in both cutaneous health and disease.

If you think zinc, you'll order zinc.

Van Wouwe JP: Clinical and laboratory diagnosis of **acrodermatitis enteropathica**. Eur J Pediatr 1989; 149:2–8.

A masterful sweep of 179 acrodermatitis enteropathica patients in the literature and the author's clinic revealed:

1. In **infants** up to 2 months, the prominent symptom is **diarrhea**. Throughout infancy, mood changes, anorexia, dermatitis, and neurologic changes were common.
2. In **toddlers** and school children, **recurrent infections**, **alopecia**, nail deformations, and growth retardation were prevalent.
3. In adults, **miscarriages** and birth defects occur.
4. The severity may wax and wane, with the patient sometimes being symptom free. At menarche, complete remission may occur spontaneously.
5. Uncommon features such as ophthalmic (photophobia, poor vision), cerebral, or hepatic involvement may be overlooked, with a fatal outcome. The untreated disease has a 20% mortality. **Zinc depletion** also impairs keratinization, epiphyseal ossification, myelination of neuronal axons, pancreatic exocrine secretion, gonad maturation, and immunity.

6. The laboratory diagnosis is of limited help. Although mean zinc levels (serum, urine, hair) are about 50% of normal, there is a 15% overlap with health controls. Moreover, low zinc levels are found in other diseases. In vivo or in vitro **zinc absorption tests** using radioisotopes (^{65}Zn or ^{69m}Zn) are valuable in puzzling cases of acrodermatitis enteropathica to demonstrate impaired zinc absorption. The lower values seen have less overlap with normal or disease states. In celiac disease the biologic half-life of zinc is decreased as a result of enhanced zinc loss.

    Anemia, increased serum copper, and decreased serum essential fatty acids also occur in 50% of patients. None is diagnostically significant. The immunologic status is variable, with depressed cellular immunity in some patients.

    Histologic changes in jejunal tissue are nonspecific. For example, inclusions seen in the jejunal Paneth cells, which gradually disappear with zinc therapy, are also seen in celiac disease.

7. The ultimate test is the clinical response to zinc (3 to 30 μmol zinc/kg/day for 5 days). When a favorable response occurs, diagnosis of a zinc-responsive dermatitis is assured.

8. The differential diagnosis centers on:

    cystic fibrosis (sweat test abnormal)
    celiac disease (responds to gluten withdrawal)
    Netherton's syndrome (ichthyosiform dermatitis, bamboo hairs, atopic diathesis, mental retardation)
    acrodermatitis enteropathica, non-zinc–dependent variant

Historically the thread of a zinc response was present, but not evident, for nearly 40 years after initial recognition of the specific disease. Mother's milk (rich in absorbable zinc), intramuscular insulin (rich in zinc), and Diodoquin (a promoter of intestinal absorption of zinc) were all effective treatments, but for an unrecognized reason. Not until Moynahan in 1973 serendipitously found that the simple zinc ion alone cleared his patients could anyone perceive the common metallic thread coursing through the earlier therapies.

Mack D, Koletzko B, Cunnane S, et al: **Acrodermatitis enteropathica** with normal serum zinc levels: Diagnostic value of small bowel biopsy and essential fatty acid determination. Gut 1989; 30:1426–1429.

A 2-month-old baby boy had the clinical constellation of acrodermatitis enteropathica. Since 2 weeks of age he had had 6 to 10 foul-smelling, pathogen-free, loose stools a day, despite multiple formula changes after the original cow's milk. He was irritable, hungry, underweight, and had multiple treatment-resistant **perianal erosions**, **sparse hair**, and ridging of the nails. Yet, three serum zinc level determinations were normal.

Evidence that this child had a normal zincemic variant of acrodermatitis enteropathica was obtained by:

1. Capillary gas-liquid chromatography determination of preprandial **plasma phospholipids**. Low values of linoleic, linolenic, and arachidonic acids resembled the poor absorption of essential unsaturated fatty acids seen in acrodermatitis enteropathica.
2. **Electron microscopy** of **small-bowel biopsy** specimens from the fourth part of the duodenum. This showed numerous characteristic pleomorphic filamentous inclusion bodies in Paneth cells.

The diagnosis was confirmed when oral zinc (30 mg daily) resulted in mood improvement in 4 days, increased serum phospholipids in 5 days, disappearance of the perianal rash in 2 weeks, and dramatic hair growth, weight gain, and normal bowel activity after 1 month. At that time a second diagnostic small-bowel biopsy showed normal secretory granules replacing the

Paneth cell inclusions. His alkaline phosphatase (one of 40 zinc-dependent metalloenzymes) originally in the normal range also climbed after zinc therapy.

It is concluded that serum zinc levels do not always reliably reflect tissue zinc levels. It is also noteworthy that this child had only a perianal dermatitis.

Graves K, Kestenbaum T, Kalivas J: **Hereditary acrodermatitis enteropathica** in an adult. Arch Dermatol 1980; 116:562–564.

A 33-year-old woman was thought to have epidermolysis bullosa, since she had been developing **blisters** at **points of trauma** from the time she was 1 year old until she reached menarche at age 19. She had **sparse hair** and occasionally experienced mild **diarrhea** associated with milk intake. Four siblings had had similar skin changes, with three dying in infancy. Her parents were related, but had no skin disease.

After age 19 her skin remained normal until age 31, when skin lesions returned with such severity that she had been depressed and bedridden for an entire year. Examination revealed a **psoriasiform eruption** of the trunk and extremities and an erythematous **vesiculobullous eruption** on the **palms** and **soles** with **paronychia** and nail dystrophy. A striking **pustular crusted eruption** involved the **perioral**, **perinasal**, and **eyelid** regions. She also had photophobia, **total alopecia**, and a peculiar **reticulated hyperpigmentation** on her torso.

A skin biopsy of a leg lesion showed intraepidermal vesicles and a marked dermal inflammatory infiltrate. Direct immunofluorescent microscopy was negative. *Staphylococcus aureus* was prominent in skin cultures and *Candida albicans* was cultured from her tongue. Despite atypical clinical and histologic findings, the diagnosis carried for the next 5 months was autosomal recessive **epidermolysis bullosa dystrophica**.

When numerous treatments continued to fail, the persistent perioral lesions raised the question, Could this be acrodermatitis enteropathica? Prompt confirmation came with the finding of dramatically low serum zinc levels of 10 μg/dl (normal 55 to 150) and 8 μg/dl.

All prior medications were stopped, and administration of oral zinc sulfate (220 mg tid) was initiated. Within 3 days the patient's longstanding profound depression lifted and the skin began to clear. After 5 months her hair had regrown and her skin had completely returned to normal except for marked postinflammatory hyperpigmentation.

When your diagnosis is a square peg in a round hole of clinical findings, get a zinc level.

Bronson DM, Barsky R, Barsky S: **Acrodermatitis enteropathica**. Recognition at long last during a recurrence in a pregnancy. J Am Acad Dermatol 1983; 9:140–144.

A 23-year-old woman in the ninth month of her third pregnancy had a widespread **pustular vesiculobullous** and **psoriasiform eruption**, with the elbows, knees, and distal extremities most severely affected. She also had an **erosive pustular dermatitis around the mouth** and **perineum**, **glossitis**, and **thinning** of **scalp hair**. The lesions had begun in the second trimester and were progressively worsening. Studies failed to confirm either herpes gestationis or impetigo herpetiformis, but the localization of lesions and their presence in childhood suggested acrodermatitis enteropathica. Her serum zinc level was 18 μg/dl (normal 55 to 150), and administration of oral zinc (220 mg tid) dramatically improved the skin lesions within 3 days. Following delivery she stopped the zinc therapy, and at 2 months post partum her skin was clear and her zinc level was 49 μg/dl.

Her "trail" of skin problems began at age 2 years with an undiagnosed widespread dermatitis. She had no gastrointestinal symptoms. Partial remissions occurred throughout childhood, and her skin remained normal from age 14 to 19 years, when she became pregnant. By the third month of pregnancy she had developed a weeping pustular dermatitis of the face, breast, abdomen, axillae, perineum, hands, and feet, thought to be impetigo herpetiformis. The skin lesions involuted within 48 hours of delivery and were completely gone at 1 month. The perioral dermatitis subsequently recurred whenever she took oral contraceptives. Her second pregnancy was terminated in the first trimester before any lesions appeared.

Her family history revealed that a sister died in early childhood from a generalized blistering disease.

This patient had lived a lifetime on and off the edge of unrecognized zinc deficiency and its associated dermatitis. During pregnancy or the administration of contraceptives, serum zinc levels fall, leading to the expression of latent acrodermatitis enteropathica. This was the connecting diagnostic thread that unraveled the mystery of 21 years.

Look for "zincopenia." It may explain inexplicable chronic dermatitis.

Shelley WB: Malignant melanoma and dermatofibrosarcoma in a 60-year-old patient with lifelong **acrodermatitis enteropathica**. J Am Acad Dermatol 1982; 6:63–66.

As one of the few survivors of acrodermatitis enteropathica into adulthood, this man at the age of 28 years was a "cutaneous cripple"—wizened, alopecic, hoarse, covered with **candidiasis**, and debilitated from diarrhea. At age 35 he was treated with the newly discovered diiodohydroxyquinoline, which cleared his candidiasis, **perinanal** and **acral dermatitis**, and much of the eczematous dermatitis except on his legs. The medication was discontinued after a few years when he was doing well.

At age 48 a large **dermatofibrosarcoma** was removed from his back, followed by a 10-cm recurrence and further wide excision. At age 57 a rapidly growing 10-cm fungating tumor, resembling a squamous cell carcinoma, was removed from his leg. It was a **malignant melanoma** with no obvious metastases.

Institution of zinc therapy at age 57 cleared the chronic dermatitis of his legs. Prior to this his skin had improved spontaneously, probably because of the ability of the gut to absorb more zinc as aging occurs. **Hypozincemia**, however, **impairs T-cell function**, lowering immunity against malignant growth. Presumably this accounted for the development of two rare malignant tumors in this patient.

Acrodermatitis enteropathica should be viewed as another immunodeficiency state leading to malignant disease.

West BL, Anderson PC: Alcohol and **acquired acrodermatitis enteropathica**. J Am Acad Dermatol 1986; 15:1305.

Cachexia and **alcohol abuse**, particularly in young women, may lead to zinc deficiency.

A 26-year-old disheveled, disordered, and cachectic woman, smelling of alcohol intake, had large florid, **eroded**, **crusted plaques around the mouth** and **anus**. Her palms and soles were fissured and peeling, while the **fingertips** were **desquamating** heavily. The mucosa was intact. She consumed almost nothing except juice, vodka, and soup. Her serum zinc level was approximately half normal. All skin lesions resolved within 5 days of the start of zinc therapy.

Weismann K, Hjorth N, Fischer A: **Zinc depletion syndrome** with acrodermatitis during longterm **intravenous feeding**. Clin Exp Dermatol 1976; 1: 237–242.

Seborrhea-like dermatitis of the face and loose scalp hair with patchy loss were the presenting complaints of a 49-year-old woman with **terminal ileitis** who had been receiving intravenous feeding for the past 2 months. A **hemorrhagic crusted eczema** then appeared about the **nostrils**, and a scaly pustular eruption developed at the **corners** of **her mouth** and **around the eyes**. Three days later large **hemorrhagic bullae** and erosions appeared on the **heels** and the palmar surface of the fingers. The paronychial areas of the fingers and toes were also affected. In addition, she had perianal erythema and minor erosion of the vulva.

The clinical diagnosis of acquired acrodermatitis due to zinc deficiency was confirmed by finding a serum zinc level of 3.8 μmol/liter (normal 10.6 to 17.7). Zinc sulfate (12 mg Zn^{2+}) was then given daily intravenously with dramatic clearing of facial lesions in a few days and rapid healing of erosions on the hands and feet. Moreover, a wound dehiscence site and a split-thickness skin donor site healed within 2 weeks, after having been static for 2 months. Noteworthy also was the rapid increase in serum alkaline phosphatase, a zinc-containing enzyme, which had been insidiously decreasing prior to zinc therapy.

A second hyperalimentation patient with a seborrheic dermatitis-like eruption of the forehead, hemorrhagic crusted erosions of the perianal area with secondary **candidiasis**, **blepharitis**, **perleche**, and hemorrhagic dermatitis of the ears and nasal orifices showed the same phenomenal recovery once oral zinc sulfate (135 mg/day) was started.

Tucker SB, Schroeter AL, Brown PW Jr, McCall JT: **Acquired zinc deficiency**. Cutaneous manifestations typical of acrodermatitis enteropathica. JAMA 1976; 235: 2399–2402.

A 20-year-old man with **ulcerative colitis** required **total parenteral nutrition** following subtotal colectomy, ileostomy, and development of multiple enterocutaneous abdominal fistulas. Approximately 5 months later he experienced abrupt **loss of scalp hair** and **psoriatic-like skin lesions**, which were erythematous plaques with fine scales located on the face (perioral, periorbital), neck, axillae, groin, elbows, antecubital fossae, knuckles, and perianal area. **Glossitis** and **stomatitis** were present, along with nonscarring scalp alopecia consisting of broken-off hairs. Mucocutaneous **candidiasis**, seborrheic dermatitis, and telogen effluvium were the initial diagnoses considered. However, low levels of serum zinc and copper were found, and when these two metals were supplemented, his alopecia and skin lesions dramatically improved. Unfortunately, he soon died of generalized candidiasis and septic shock.

Zinc deficiency leads to ulceration and **poor healing**. It probably developed in this patient as a result of chronic gastrointestinal disease and long-term total parenteral nutrition.

Heimburger DC, Tamura T, Marks RD: Rapid improvement in **dermatitis** after zinc supplementation in a patient with **Crohn's disease**. Am J Med 1990; 88:71–73.

A 58-year-old man with Crohn's disease for 4 years had a **generalized pruritic reticulated blanchable erythema** of 5 weeks' duration. There was prominent focal hyperpigmented scaling, as well as **necrolytic erosions** over pressure points. His nutritional status was poor, with an 18-kg weight loss over 4 months associated with marked diarrhea. A skin biopsy showed psoriasiform changes, with neutrophil infiltration of the epidermis. An ileum biopsy confirmed Crohn's disease.

Laboratory studies showed significantly decreased values for plasma zinc (3.7 μmol/liter), copper (6.9 μmol/liter), iron (6.4 μmol/liter), β-carotene, ascorbate, retinol-binding protein, and testosterone. A diagnosis of **kwashiorkor** and **zinc deficiency dermatitis** was made.

The rash improved within 4 days of therapy with intravenous zinc (16 mg/day), and after 2 weeks his skin was essentially normal. Noteworthy was the concomitant rise in plasma and erythrocyte zinc, retinol-binding protein, and testosterone levels.

Zinc deficiency is present in nearly half of patients with **Crohn's disease**. This probably reflects poor dietary intake, defects in absorption, and excessive loss due to diarrhea. If your Crohn's disease patient has cutaneous or mucosal lesions, think zinc.

Charles BM, Hosking G, Green A, et al: **Biotin-responsive alopecia** and developmental regression. Lancet 1979; 2:118–120.

A 10-month-old boy with generalized hypotonia, loss of head control, **blepharitis**, and inflamed nasal mucosa had profound **alopecia** and a "rash" resembling both **acrodermatitis enteropathica** and **anhidrotic ectodermal dysplasia**. Pilocarpine stimulation yielded only 8 mg of sweat, and no sweat pores were visible after staining with o-phthalaldehyde. His serum zinc was 12 μmol/liter and increased only slightly with zinc therapy. Screening for urinary organic acids revealed massively increased 3-hydroxyisovaleric acid, as well as increased β-methylcrotonyl glycine and 3-hydroxypropionate. Since the activities of several carboxylase enzymes were normal in cultured fibroblasts and the patient improved dramatically with oral biotin, a defect in biotin absorption or transport was postulated.

If you don't recognize it, you can call it cryptodermatitis.

Acrodynia

It's the hands that reach out to help you make this rare diagnosis caused by mercury poisoning. Red and swollen hands with peeling palms should arouse suspicion. The acral predilection includes the nose and feet. Once a common disease because of widespread use of mercury compounds (such as calomel in teething preparations), its rarity now makes it dip below the diagnostic horizon of most doctors.

The pediatrician may first see the infant child because of irritability, incessant crying, and weakness. The severe burning pain and itch result in excoriations and even self-mutilation, as the child frantically attempts to tear away the skin that hurts. The neurologist may also see the patient because of pain, polyneuropathy, unexplained weakness, and retarded motor growth. The dentist may see these patients because of profuse salivation, stomatitis, and loss of teeth. The ophthalmologist also may be consulted because of photophobia.

Look for an accidental spill of liquid mercury from a broken manometer or thermometer. Ask about possible exposure to latex paint, where mercury is used as a bacteriostat. To test your diagnosis, secure a 24-hour determination of the urinary mercury level, so that you won't be caught "red-handed."

Although the mercury atom is a powerful and universal poison, in acrodynia it is the sympathetic nerve damage that provides the cardinal diagnostic findings. The patient essentially develops algodystrophy (sympathetic reflex dysautonia) with pain and erythema, similar to that seen from electrical burns or gunshot wounds. It is truly an infant's causalgia.

Dinehart SM, Dillard R, Raimer SS, et al: Cutaneous manifestations of **acrodynia** (pink disease). Arch Dermatol 1988; 124:107–109.

A 14-month-old baby girl had irritability, depression, and muscle weakness for 10 weeks. Recently she had refused to walk, and developed marked personality changes with continual crying day and night, and had a tremor in her hands. Multiple skin and mucous membrane changes were present.

The **cutaneous clues** included:

a bright red tip of the nose
swollen erythematous gums with erosions
peeling of the palms and soles
loose teeth with three missing
profuse sweating with cold, moist skin
intense pruritus of the posterior thighs with constant scratching and eczematous changes
reticulate erythematous macular eruption of the hands and feet in a glove-and-stocking distribution
excessive salivation with drooling
photophobia
profuse clear nasal discharge

Ten days of extensive investigation, including skin, mucosal, bone, and muscle biopsies in another hospital had been to no avail, but a 24-hour urine screen for heavy metals quickly gave the answer, with a mercury level of 48 μg/24 hr (normal < 20 μg/24 hr). The levels for arsenic, bismuth, cadmium, copper, lead, and thallium were normal. Requestioning the mother disclosed that 2 months before the onset of the baby's symptoms an antique bottle of mercury (200 ml) had been spilled on the couch and carpet of the room where the child played. It had been cleaned up, but unacceptable mercury levels were still present in the home months later.

The infant thus had acrodynia (erythredema, pink disease). The common pathogenic thread in mercury poisoning is damage to the autonomic nervous system (sympathovasomotor dysfunction). Fortunately, sources of mercury exposure have been sharply reduced with recognition of its hazards. Nonetheless, a child with a red nose resembling Rudolph the red-nosed reindeer deserves urinary screening for mercury.

Mercury exposure from interior **latex paint**—Michigan. Arch Dermatol 1990; 126:577.

Redness, peeling, and **swelling** of the **hands, feet,** and **nose** as well as **hyperhidrosis** were the acute presenting signs in a previously healthy 4-year-old boy in August, 1989. He also had had intermittent fevers, rapid heartbeat, widespread **pruritus**, leg cramps, marked personality changes, and was unable to sleep. Weakness of the pectoral and pelvic girdles was evident, and nerve dysfunction was present in his legs. Acrodynia was confirmed by finding a mercury level of 65 μg/liter in the urine (24-hour collection). The urinary excretion level of mercury was increased 20-fold upon chelation therapy.

The parents and two siblings, although asymptomatic, also had mercury in their urine. The source was traced to inhalation of mercury-containing vapors from phenyl mercury acetate in latex paint applied to the inside walls of their home. The paint had 930 to 955 ppm mercury used as a preservative (permissible level 300 ppm). The 17 gallons of paint had been used in July in the air-conditioned home with the windows always closed. The poisoning might never have been recognized but for the 4-year-old. He was the canary in the mine. His acrodynia sounded the alarm.

Caution regarding the presence of mercury is not required on the label of water-based paints. It is routinely added as a fungicide and bactericide to interior water-based (latex) paints to prolong shelf life, while it is not permitted to be added to oil-based paints. Open the windows when you paint!

Open the windows of your mind to the thought that a hand eruption in a young patient might be due to mercury in the air or that the multiple complaints of an older patient might be due to a closed-up, freshly painted home. The patient who can't sleep, and has headache, insomnia, weakness, and tremor (and depresses you with his depression) may be a "crock," full of mercury. Order a determination of the urinary mercury level!

Foulds DM, Copeland KC, Franks RC: Mercury poisoning and **acrodynia**. Am J Dis Child 1987; 141:124–125.

A 30-month-old girl had progressive irritability and **pruritus** for 2 months, along with lethargy and hypertension (blood pressure 144/92). She was hypotonic and had multiple **excoriations** of the buttocks and thighs. Her **fingers** were **erythematous** and **swollen**. A urine toxicology screen was normal, and random urine specimens were negative twice for heavy metals (Reinsch's test). An EEG and abdominal CT were normal.

Review of the patient's history revealed that approximately 2 months previously her father had spilled mercury from a large manometer on a floor where the child frequently played and had cleaned it up with a vacuum cleaner. A 24-hour urine collection showed a mercury concentration of 214 μg/liter (normal < 20 μg/liter), as determined by atomic absorption. Treatment with D-penicillamine for 6 weeks gradually improved her symptoms, which took nearly 3 months to clear.

Accurate diagnosis of mercury poisoning requires analysis of 24-hour urine samples by atomic absorption. Reinsch's screening test for heavy metals is not sensitive enough for detecting mercury intoxication.

Aging

Youth is growth; age is atrophy. Old skin is thin, wrinkled, and appendageal poor. There is little sweat or sebum. The skin is dry and asteatotic with eczema but a hot bath away. The hair is sparse and white, even as the nails are thin and cracked. We all recognize aging skin and know it is a diagnosis we will sometime make in our own mirror. This old skin per se rarely came to pay the physician a call until the recent therapeutic measures that bring a degree of youthful growth back to both old atrophic skin and old retired hair follicles.

But the skin does more than merely age. It photoages. This **photoaging** accounts for many of the diagnoses we make in old skin. It is a photoaging from the cumulative lifelong exposure of the epidermis to ultraviolet rays of sunlight.

It is essentially limited to the face, neck, and hands, although the shirtless farmer, former professional lifeguard, or sun worshipper may exhibit larger areas of photoaging. To distinguish aging from photoaging, simply look at the unexposed areas of the body. Many a very photoaged individual will still show the very bloom of youth on his buttocks.

Photoaging is the pathology of an epidermis that has both a thinned stratum corneum and a poor melanin defense against UVL radiation, and which has slowed or stalled in its reparative function. As a consequence comes a constellation of changes. Patches of actinic keratosis appear as red scaling lesions. Given abstinence from excessive light, these keratoses may even reverse and disappear when the rate of damage is below the rate of repair. Actinic lentigines (liver spots) become the telltale sign of a gardener's hand. A defenseless site without DNA repair becomes an epithelioma, a melanoma, or simply an atrophic site of former destruction.

It is important to realize that the drama of both aging and photoaging may be played out in the skin of an infant, child, or young person. For aging there are the syndromes of progeria and for photoaging the syndrome of xeroderma pigmentosum.

It is hard to think of foreshortened life in the skin of a child, but it does occur. The first suspicion may come from an awareness that the infant has blotchy hyperpigmentation. Then as we stand back and see freckles, dryness, and atrophy, we sense the unimaginable. This skin is old. The child has **progeria**. In the case of the adult form of progeria (Werner's syndrome), the usual presentation to you will be an ulcer of the ankle or other bony prominence. The skin will be taut, atrophic, or sclerodermatous.

With **xeroderma pigmentosum**, the dawn of diagnosis is sensing the infant to be unduly photosensitive. It is the only baby at the picnic to be sunburned. Then come the freckles, the xerosis, and scaling, as well as telangiectasis. Finally, the perception comes of photoaging in baby skin. As the months and years pass, the tragedy of a profusion of sun-induced actinic keratosis, epitheliomas, even melanomas more than confirms your diagnosis of xeroderma pigmentosum. Your patient has the disease that has shown us in the research laboratory the DNA repair systems that permit us to live in a world of sunlight. It is this patient who cannot. He is without the enzymes and cofactors essential to remove and replace the ultraviolet light–damaged rings of DNA. The repair kit defects of these patients may vary. Today the laboratory not only can spot the defect, even prenatally, using fibroblast cultures, but can now recognize that xeroderma pigmentosum patients can be classified into eight different groups (A to H). This greatly adds to our diagnostic skill, because, for example, groups A, B, and D commonly exhibit neurologic abnormalities such as progressive mental deterioration.

Xeroderma pigmentosum has provided a remarkably productive juncture between molecular biology and disease.

Geronemus R: **Poikiloderma of Civatte**. Arch Dermatol 1990; 126:547–548.

Poikiloderma of Civatte is a chronic discoloration of the side of the neck, less commonly seen on the lateral aspects of the cheeks and chest. It is associated with some brown pigmentation and most commonly found in middle-aged and elderly women. In a few instances the patients may complain of hyperesthesia.

Pulsed-dye laser therapy in serial 5-mm spots produced 95% resolution of the redness in four sessions in three women studied.

Bauer EA, Uitto J, Tan EML, Holbrook KA: **Werner's syndrome**. Evidence for preferential regional expression of a generalized mesenchymal cell defect. Arch Dermatol 1988; 124:90–101.

For some people the arrow of time flies faster than for others, and for those with Werner's syndrome, the arrow flies extremely fast. These are the patients whose old age reaches them in their youth. Early on, they have the **white hair**, baldness, flatfeet, osteoporosis, cataracts, and calcified vessels of old age. They also have the thin, high-pitched voice, **thin skin**, **trophic ulcers**, degenerative joint disease, heart failure, and neoplasia we associate with aging.

Theirs is the autosomal recessive disease of foreshortened life.

Levy RS, Fisher M, Alter JN: **Penicillamine:** Review and cutaneous manifestations. J Am Acad Dermatol 1983; 8:548–558.

Penicillamine, a hydrolytic degradation product of penicillin, produced excessive **wrinkling** in a 38-year-old woman who had taken it for 17 years for the treatment of Wilson's disease.

Its use over many years has also been associated with the induction of **cutis laxa** and **elastosis perforans serpiginosa** as well as **purpura**.

The basic cause is interference with the synthesis of new collagen, and the long lag period reflects the very slow turnover of collagen.

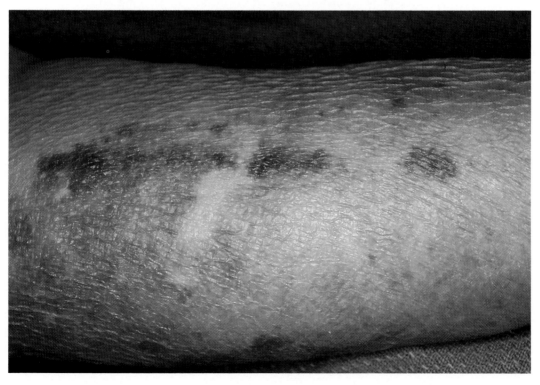

Premature Aging

Beauregard S, Gilchrest BA: **Syndromes** of **premature aging**. Dermatol Clin 1987; 5:109–121.

The classic presentation of premature aging is **progeria**. It begins within the first year, and diagnosis is usually made during the second year.

The earliest diagnostic sign is growth deficiency. It is this failure to thrive that brings most babies to the attention of the physician. As the months progress, the skin becomes aged, the **scalp** is **bald**, and the veins show through the **thin skin**. **Wrinkles** appear in some areas, and in others the skin is taut and shiny. **Scleroderma-like changes** may appear on the trunk. Later there are irregular patches of sunlight-induced pigmentation. The nails are atrophic or deformed.

The aging changes are proceeding elsewhere as well. Dentition is delayed and incomplete. The limbs soon become the spindly arthritic ones of aging. Perhaps the most striking is the disproportionately large head and prominent eyes unshielded by lashes. Meanwhile an inexorable progressive **arterio-sclerosis** evolves that foreshortens the patient's life from threescore and ten to ten or fifteen years.

There is an adult form of progeria known as **Werner's syndrome**. In this instance the aging does not develop until the late teens or twenties. First may come early **graying** and **thinning** of the **hair**, not only of the scalp, but elsewhere. The **skin** becomes **atrophic**, and subcutaneous fat is lost, especially on the face and distal areas of the extremities. The skin of the trunk has the aging changes of hyperpigmentation and telangiectasia.

Hyperkeratosis of the thinning skin of the bony prominences leads to deep, **indolent ulcers**. These are often the presenting complaint. Osteoporosis and arteriosclerosis become evident, and even early senile dementia may lead to early residence in a nursing home. Death comes as old age, often before the age of 50. Heart attacks, strokes, and malignant disease are in the cards for those with Werner's syndrome.

A special type of premature aging affects mainly the face and acral areas. It is called **acrogeria**. It is usually diagnosed before the age of 6 years by virtue of the **wrinkling atrophy** and dryness of the child's **face, hands,** and **feet**. The nails may present the **onychogryphosis** of the aged; the small stature and easy **bruising** as well as multiple fractures complete this acral caricature of aging.

The fourth and rarest form of premature aging is called **metageria**. Here the child is unusually tall and thin with **sclerodermatous hands** and **feet** but, again, with a **bird-like facies**.

Gilkes JJH, Sharvill DE, Wells RS: The **premature aging syndromes**. Report of eight cases and description of a new entity named **metageria**. Br J Dermatol 1974; 91:243–262.

This 24-year-old woman had developed areas of **telangiectasia** and **hyper-pigmentation** on her upper trunk and limbs when she was 12 years old. She had recurrent **ulceration** around both **ankles** and on her **feet** since age 7. This was the result of very poor peripheral circulation.

On examination, she was abnormally tall and thin, with a beaked nose, **bird-like facies**, and staring eyes. There was virtually **no subcutaneous fat**. Multiple telangiectatic lesions were scattered over the entire body, and areas of mottled hyperpigmentation gave a **poikilodermatous appearance**. No pulse could be felt below the femoral arteries.

The patient was viewed as representing a distinct separate new syndrome. It was given the name *metageria* to distinguish it from the three previously described premature aging syndromes.

She did not have the classic progeria that comes on in infancy and is associated with dwarfism. Nor did she exhibit the delayed adult onset so characteristic of the progeria known as Werner's syndrome. Finally, she was not an example of acrogeria in which the atrophic age changes are most evident on the limbs. Although this patient had virtually no subcutaneous fat, lipodystrophy was ruled out since her blood showed none of the characteristic findings of this disorder, i.e., elevated cholesterol and triglyceride levels.

Expert diagnosticians don't practice too fast or for too long a day.

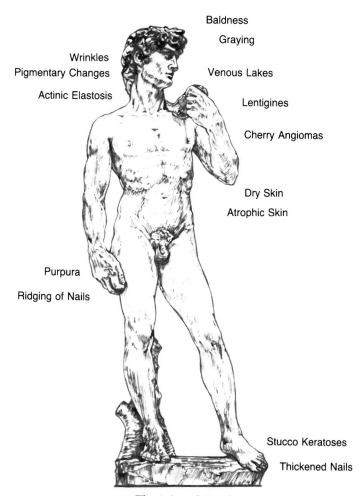

The Aging of David

Premature Photoaging

Kraemer KH, Lee MM, Scotto J: **Xeroderma pigmentosum:** Cutaneous, ocular, and neurologic abnormalities in 830 published cases. Arch Dermatol 1987; 123:241–250.

The signs of this rare autosomal recessive disease reflect an inability to repair DNA damaged by sunlight.

The first signs are generally observed between the age of 1 and 2 years when the infant shows sensitivity to sunlight. By 2 years the hallmark of protective **freckling** appears. Further damage becomes evident with the appearance of **telangiectasia, atrophy**, and the typical **actinic keratoses**.

By the time he is 10, the sun has produced a skin that is 50 years older than the child. **Neoplasms** appear usually on the face, head, and neck in the form of basal cell and squamous cell carcinomas. And these patients have 2000 times the risk the public has of developing malignant melanoma. An assortment of other neoplasms may develop, including keratoacanthoma, fibrosarcomas, and angiomas.

The eye is particularly vulnerable, with photophobia and conjunctival infection frequently a problem in early infancy. Keratitis with corneal clouding and vascularization may develop with neoplasms of the conjunctiva as well as the limbus and cornea. At least one in ten had impaired vision.

Again, one in five had neurologic disorders (**De Sanctis-Cacchione syndrome**):

> low intelligence
> ataxia and spasticity
> abnormal reflexes
> impaired hearing
> slow development
> microcephaly

The mouth may show contracture, and squamous cell carcinoma of the sun-exposed tip of the tongue is 20,000 times more frequent than in the normal individual.

An occasional patient may suffer from primary internal neoplasms, e.g., brain or lung tumors as well as leukemia.

Always the sun remains these patients' worse enemy, for it makes their skin dry, darkened, and diseased.

Cleaver JE, Kraemer KH: **Xeroderma pigmentosum**. *In* Scriver CR, Beaudet AL, Shy WS, Valle D (eds): The Metabolic Basis of Inherited Disease. New York, McGraw-Hill Book Co., 1989, vol 2, pp 2949–2971.

By **culturing fibroblasts** from patients with xeroderma pigmentosum, it is possible to show that the basic defect is inability of the cell to perform excision repair of DNA damaged by ultraviolet light.

Not all of these patients lack the same repair enzyme or cofactor. Indeed, it is now possible to identify and label eight distinct xeroderma pigmentosum patient groups (groups A to H) plus a variant. This is done by fusing fibroblasts (Sendai virus hybridization) from two different patients. If a repair-competent hybrid cell results, it implies that "complementation" has occurred and that the two patients represent two distinct groups. That numerous such complementation tests have demonstrated eight groups so far dramatically underscores the heterogenic nature of this genodermatosis.

Patterson JW, Jordan WP Jr: **Atypical fibroxanthoma** in a patient with **xeroderma pigmentosum**. Arch Dermatol 1987; 123:1066–1070.

In a 3-year-old boy who had unusual sun sensitivity, first noted at 5 months of age, xeroderma pigmentosum was diagnosed at age 19 months. By that time he had several pigmented keratotic and nodular lesions of the face.

On examination the skin of the head and neck was dry, freckled, and wrinkled with atrophy and telangiectasis. Since he had already had an actinic keratosis, a keratoacanthoma, and an invasive squamous cell carcinoma excised, the appearance of a **pink, dome-shaped papule** on the right ala nasi called for a histologic diagnosis. It proved to be an atypical fibroxanthoma.

The xeroderma pigmentosa patient has an inherited defect in repair of chromosomes damaged by sunlight. This favors the development of:

  actinic keratosis
  carcinomas
  malignant melanoma

as well as:

  endotheliomas
  fibromas
  sarcomas

The present case is an example of the mesodermal tumors that can be induced by ultraviolet light damaging the DNA.

If you commonly limit yourself to rare diagnoses, you'll rarely be right.

Alopecia

The diagnostic entrance points for alopecia are multiple. First, consider the patterning of the hair loss. The typical male and female **patterns** of androgenetic, i.e., hereditary, hair loss are as well known to the patient as to you.

Hair plucking is another diagnostic step. In the accelerated scalp hair loss known as telogen effluvium, numerous hairs come out with a simple pull. These hairs show the club-hair appearance of a hair that has stopped growing and is in a resting or telogen phase. It may be a temporary phase of loss, such as occurs months after the end of pregnancy or after a crash low-calorie diet. It is the type of loss seen following shock. In contrast, the anlagen hair, i.e., the growing hair with its attached root sheath, may be plucked out in the patient undergoing chemotherapy with antimetabolites and cytotoxic drugs.

Direct inspection of the hairs under the **microscope** provides another diagnostic entry point. The hair and scale should be examined for fungal elements indicative of tinea capitis. Too often there is failure to remember that adults also develop tinea capitis. The **Wood's light examination** for telltale fluorescence of ectothrix-infected hairs is valuable as well in making a diagnosis.

When the patient is a child or the hair loss has been present since birth or infancy, certain diagnostic possibilities arise. There are the patients in whom you may sense a familial or congenital anomaly. The hair may be abnormal. The skin may show focal nevoid change as in nevus sebaceous or a cyst, or aplasia may be present. More significantly, it is in these patients that the laboratory may be able to show a congenital correctable biochemical deficiency. These center on biotin, zinc, and calcium. In older patients, iron loss may be responsible as well.

Just as important a diagnostic entry point as age is the portal of race. Black patients in attempting to remove natural curl with hot combs and chemicals may damage the hair shaft to the point of **breakage** and consequent hair loss.

Look at the skin elsewhere for **keratinization defects:** milia, ichthyosis, or keratoderma allows greater diagnostic fractionation. Demonstration of sulfur deficiency in the hair shaft itself makes a diagnosis of trichothiodystrophy.

Scarring bespeaks of hair loss from destruction of the regenerative hair follicle. The cause may be radiation damage, lichen planus, or angiosarcoma.

You've looked and looked. Now you must seek a further diagnostic entrance point, i.e., the **history**. The child's fever may antedate hair loss. Prolonged pressure on the site during surgery may point to the cause. Neurologic change may antedate hair loss. **Drugs** such as beta-blockers are particularly potent in producing hair loss. Among the numerous drugs responsible for hair thinning, look for high-dosage vitamin A, topical selenium used in shampoos, and heparin.

The history may disclose **medical problems** that are responsible for hair loss. Thus, alopecia may reflect endocrine disease, amyloidosis, or malnutrition.

The ultimate diagnostic portal always remains the **biopsy**. Have your pathologist look for syringomas, myxomas, and granulomas. The pathologist can also confirm your diagnosis of trichotillomania.

Finally, there will always be a group of patients in whom the diagnosis is simply an act of faith. We look and look, but we cannot be certain there has been any hair loss despite the patient's avowal that hundreds of hairs are being lost every day. Until we have a method of doing a "hair count" as we do a blood count, the diagnosis of alopecia in some cases may be one we can neither confirm nor deny.

Happle R: Genetic defects involving the hair. *In* Orfanos CE, Happle R (eds): Hair and Hair Diseases. New York, Springer-Verlag, 1990, pp 325–362.

Although genetically determined **hypotrichosis** (hypotrichosis congenita simplex) is usually evident once the birthright of lanugo scalp hair is lost, the Marie Unna form does not become evident until puberty. At that time, hair loss appears on the crown and after years leads to almost complete alopecia. Prior to that, hair growth seems dense and strong, despite its coarse, unruly and uncombable nature that elicits a resemblance to an ill-fitting wig.

Additional examples of **autosomal dominant** forms of hypotrichosis are seen in association with such ectodermal defects as nail dystrophies, palmar and plantar hyperkeratosis, cleft palate, and hypohidrosis (Rapp-Hodgkin syndrome), EEC syndrome (ectrodactyly, ectodermal dysplasia, and cleft lip and palate). In the trichorhinophalangeal syndrome the pear-shaped nose, long philtrum, and phalangeal epiphyseal deformities are also present.

Interestingly, in the AEC syndrome (ankyloblepharon filiforme adnatum, ectodermal dysplasia,, and cleft lip and palate) the scalp hair is lost in infancy during periods of **scalp inflammation** unresponsive to antibiotics as well as steroids. The late loss of scalp hair during puberty favors a diagnosis of Basan syndrome, in which the dermatoglyphics are absent and a simian crease is present. Again, the ultimate hypotrichosis is heralded by **childhood hair** that is **wiry** and **coarse**. In some children the genetic nature of their thin hair becomes even more apparent when there is failure of eruption of permanent dentition.

Other examples of genetic hair loss are of **autosomal recessive** nature. Again, the child is born with normal intrauterine hair, only to experience failure in providing replacement terminal hairs. Other defects may be evident. Some patients may show a hamartomatous papular eruption of the face and neck. Others develop multiple hidrocystomas of the eyelids (Schöpf syndrome). Hypotrichosis is also seen in association with the poikiloderma of Rothmund-Thomson syndrome. There may also be concomitant mental retardation in some, dwarfism in others. It is a consistent trait of the premature aging syndromes of progeria and of Werner. Other examples occur in epidermolysis bullosa dystrophica and in autosomal recessive lamellar ichthyosis.

Turning to the **X-linked** genetic problems, **patchy** and **linear bands** of alopecia are seen. They exhibit the mosaic patterning that develops on the scalp of girls. It occurs in five conditions that are due to X-linked dominant genes lethal for hemizygous males. In the female, random inactivation of the X chromosome carrying the normal gene in some cells early in embryonic development leads to a swirl of hypotrichosis. This absence of hair reflects the presence of the mutant X gene. These five conditions of genetic mosaicism are incontinentia pigmenti, focal dermal hypoplasia, X-linked chondrodysplasia punctata, oral-facial-digital syndrome, and the CHILD syndrome (congenital hemidysplasia, ichthyosiform nevus, limb defects).

There are also X-linked nonlethal genes that interfere with hair growth. These include those of hypohidrotic ectodermal dysplasia, keratosis follicularis spinulosa decalvans, and nevoid basal cell syndrome with follicular atrophoderma (Bazex syndrome).

When the patient has little hair, look a little further for other ectodermal deficits or dysplasia.

Patterned

Orfanos CE: **Androgenetic alopecia:** Clinical aspects and treatment. *In* Orfanos CE, Happle R (eds): Hair and Hair Diseases. New York, Springer-Verlag, 1990, pp 485–527.

Androgenetic alopecia is diffuse hair loss resulting from circulating androgens acting on genetically predisposed hair follicles. The loss of scalp hair is associated with a shortened hair cycle with the result that the hair shaft becomes shorter and thinner with each consecutive cycle. The pigment content is also reduced. This terminal hair is slowly transformed into intermediate, then vellus or lanugo, hair.

This occurs in both men and women, but more prominently in men. Significantly, in women such loss reflects temporary peaks of heightened hormonal changes at puberty, post partum, and menopause. The post partum shedding appears 6 to 8 weeks after the end of pregnancy and spontaneously regresses after 4 months. If the loss persists for more than 8 months, the woman has passed into androgenetic alopecia.

The term **androgenic alopecia** is reserved to label **telogen effluvium** due to significant levels of circulating androgens. This is exhibited as a male pattern loss regardless of its neoplastic or non-neoplastic origin. In such circumstances look for non-neoplastic **hyperandrogenemia** to be of ovarian or adrenal origin in nearly half of the cases. By contrast, the androgen levels in androgenetic alopecia remain usually within normal range.

Androgenetic alopecia is the most frequent form of hair loss. It is a sign of sexual maturity, since it does not occur in children, in men with testicular insufficiency, or in early castrates. The genetic background is unknown but is probably polygenic. It progresses slowly, beginning in both men and women at age 18 to 25 years, but with acute phases of telogen effluvium occurring. These are followed by stable periods of several years.

The clinical picture is one of gradually diminishing hair density without any visible change in the skin itself. The frontal hairline is composed of shorter, less pigmented hairs. A fine fuzz of light vellus hairs appears at the temporal and crown areas. Eventually this is lost, with the sites being totally bald.

This **baldness pattern** may be characterized as male or female. The **male** pattern exhibits a triangular receding in the temple areas and an oval loss in the region of the vertex. These areas enlarge, linking together with only a fringe of hair remaining. The **female** pattern shows preservation of the frontal hairline, but diffuse hair loss becomes evident in the centroparietal area of the scalp. It can easily be confused with diffuse hair loss associated with other causes, e.g., thyroid disease, hepatic disease, drug-induced alopecia. This female pattern of androgenetic alopecia may be associated with varying features of **virilism** such as hypertrichosis of the upper lip, extremities, and linea alba. It is important to note that women may exhibit male as well as female patterned loss.

Endocrinologic surveys are indicated in progressive hair loss in women to rule out androgenital syndrome and Stein-Leventhal syndrome.

Other characteristics of androgenetic hair loss are **seborrhea**, reduced hair shaft diameter, and its episodic course. Nearly 80% of the patients note a marked increase in oiliness of the scalp. The decrease in hair diameter precedes the visible loss. Finally the fluctuant course brings showers of hair loss episodically every few years. Despite the subsequent periods of stability, the course is inexorably to a degree of baldness. Amidst all of this is the physiologic normal loss of aging. By age 60 at least half of the original complement of hair has been lost by everyone.

Although two thirds of all men and one third of all women have visible androgenetic hair loss, the number of men and women requesting physician help is equal.

The density of hair per square centimeter of scalp area can be a useful parameter for evaluating the progression of alopecia as well as evaluating the effect of cosmetic and therapeutic efforts. Any type of fenestrated instrument can be used for counting hairs during the course of a few months. A permanent stain of the scalp allows precise localization. The German group studied has a count of $340 \pm 76/cm^2$.

A small shaved area permits measurement of rate of hair growth at 4 and at 8 weeks. Normally in young adults the scalp hair grows 8 to 10 mm/month, with a maximum in the summer.

Counting hair loss is another valuable assessment. The normal median value is 56 hairs/day. During episodes of androgenetic loss, the number may climb to 120 to 200 hairs/day.

Finally, plucking a bunch of 60 to 80 hairs in a standard manner from a standard site (e.g., 2 cm behind anterior hairline in the trianguli) always 5 days after the last shampoo gives a **trichogram**. Normally, 60 to 70% of hairs will be anagen and 20% will be dysplastic anagen stage (without root sheaths). Only 12 to 15% will be telogen. An increase in the percentage of telogen hairs is consistent with a diagnosis of androgenetic hair loss.

All patients deserve a physician's attempt to exclude other causes. One of these is the **diffuse** form of **alopecia areata**. Here, follow-up weeks or months later will reveal the typical later circumscribed lesions. Otherwise, look for **hypothyroidism, drugs**, trauma, hepatic disease, and **syphilis** as possible causes.

The diagnosis of androgenetic alopecia ultimately rests on a family history of alopecia, progressive periodic course, increase in telogen and dysplastic hairs on pluck test, and typical patterning of loss.

The high forehead is always the high sign of androgenetic hair loss.

The longer your differential, the weaker your diagnostic clutch.

Infection

Grigoriu D, Delacrétaz J: Infection dermatophytique mixte du cuir chevelu. Dermatologica 1982; 164:407–409.

For 6 weeks a 10-year-old girl had noted a patch of scaling and diffuse hair thinning on her scalp, unresponsive to topical steroid and antibiotic therapy. Wood's light examination was positive, and plucked hairs showed both ectothrix and endothrix fungal spores (KOH examination). Dual growth of *Microsporum canis* and *Trichophyton tonsurans* occurred on culture.

Dual therapy with topical econazole and oral griseofulvin cured the infection within 2 months.

When you look for **fungus**, look for the **broken-off hairs**. And when you look at hair loss at any age, look for fungi.

Zoberman-Saltiel E: **Patchy alopecia** in a young girl. Arch Dermatol 1989; 125:113–118.

For the past year, this 6-year-old girl had noted a patch of hair loss on the vertex of the scalp. Examination showed five discrete irregular 1- to 2-cm patches of **scarring alopecia**. Each was **erythematous** and showed a **scale-crust**. Hairs were not easily lost to traction, nor were any exclamation hairs seen.

Wood's light examination was negative. Potassium hydroxide preparations were negative for hyphae. Furthermore, cultures of plucked hairs showed no growth.

The diagnosis was elusive, for a biopsy showed only a nonspecific dense granulomatous infiltrate. Not until silver methenamine demonstrated brown hypheal elements within a single hair follicle was the diagnosis of tinea capitis made.

It was presumed to be a *Trichophyton tonsurans* infection, since this organism induces a nonfluorescing endothrix infection with little to culture other than the sticks of intrafollicular hair marked at times by the black dots. Even the seborrheic scaling of *T. tonsurans* provides little material of value in culture.

But for the special biopsy stains, chronic **discoid lupus erythematosus** would probably have been diagnosed. As it was, an 8-week course of griseofulvin led to complete cure.

Hair loss in a child is **tinea capitis** until proven otherwise.

Barlow D, Saxe N: **Tinea capitis in adults**. Int J Dermatol 1988; 27:388–390.

For 2 years this 42-year-old woman had the clinical picture of the **frontal band** of **scarring alopecia**. It was diagnosed as **traction alopecia** until scrapings showed an endothrix present on microscopy and *Trichophyton violaceum* on culture.

Other forms of adult tinea capitis producing alopecia include **favus**. This is recognized by its scarring and its typical yellowish cuplike scale (scutulum). This is endemic in certain parts of Scotland, Eastern Europe, the Middle East, and Africa.

Moberg S: **Tinea capitis** in the **elderly**. A report on two cases caused by *Trichophyton tonsurans*. Dermatologica 1984; 169:36–40.

For 2 years a 69-year-old diabetic woman in a geriatric ward complained of loss of scalp hair associated with minimal erythema and scaling over the vertex. **Seborrheic dermatitis** was suspected, but closer examination disclosed numerous short hair stubs and **black dots** in an area of noncicatricial alopecia. Cultures grew out *Trichophyton tonsurans*.

A 59-year-old woman noted moderate hair loss for 3 years. Scalp examination revealed a diffuse, erythematous, slightly atrophic patch of hair loss with black dots mimicking follicular plugging at the periphery. No fluorescence was noted with Wood's light. **Discoid lupus erythematosus** was suspected, but a skin biopsy showed dilated follicles filled with arthrospores. *T. tonsurans* was isolated.

Neither of these patients had lesions elsewhere, and the sources of infection were never identified.

Burkhart CG: **Tinea incognito**. Arch Dermatol 1981; 117:606–607.

Localized patches of alopecia of the legs and trunk had been slowly enlarging for the past 6 years. The patient, who was 36 years old, stated that the hair loss sites were asymptomatic, and more recently they had appeared on the arms as well. There had been no change despite systemic and topical steroid therapy.

On examination, numerous round to **oval patches** of **alopecia** 1 to 10 cm in diameter were noted on the **trunk** and **extremities**. The patches showed no scale and were yellow with a degree of erythema. Although the loss mimics alopecia areata, exclamation point hairs were not seen.

The diagnosis came when a punch biopsy revealed numerous hyphae and spores in the stratum corneum. Confirmation of the diagnosis of alopecia due to occult **tinea corporis** came with a griseofulvin cure.

Winchell SA, Tschen JA, McGavran MH: **Follicular secondary syphilis**. Cutis 1985; 35:259–261.

This 36-year-old black man gave a history of 6 weeks of pruritic follicular papules of the beard and upper torso. On examination he was found to have erythematous hyperpigmented papules also on his palms, soles, and penis.

The initial clinical diagnosis was **alopecia mucinosa**, and on biopsy there was evidence of mild perifollicular mucin deposits. However, a Warthin-Starry stain showing spirochetes and a positive serologic test for syphilis made the diagnosis of secondary syphilis. He responded well to systemic benzathine penicillin.

Syphilis remains the great imitator.

The right diagnosis lets you turn to the right page of therapy.

Children

Weismann K, Hagdrup HK: Hair changes due to **zinc deficiency** in a case of sucrose **malabsorption**. Acta Derm Venereol 1981; 61:444–447.

A 7-year-old girl had developed **thinning** of her **scalp hair** in recent months. The scalp hair was **brittle** and very slow growing, as were her nails. The hair was also **colorless**, unkempt, and had a mohair appearance, especially in the occiput where it was loose, short, and thin. On microscopic examination, the hairs showed marked variation in shaft diameter, spearhead-like broken ends, and multiple cross-ridges with slight trichonodosis and short longitudinal splits. Her medical history disclosed **chronic diarrhea** resulting from congenital sucrase deficiency.

Her skin was dry and pale with superficial scaling on the dorsal aspect of the hands, but there was no evidence of acute or chronic zinc deficiency dermatitis. However, the history of chronic malabsorption raised suspicion of zinc deficiency, and a low plasma zinc level of 7.9 μmol/liter (normal 10.6 to 18.9 μmol/liter) was found. The thinning and microscopic changes of the hair are characteristic of those seen in acrodermatitis enteropathica.

Within 4 weeks of starting oral zinc sulfate therapy (100 mg bid), new scalp hair with dark-blond pigmentation was seen growing out. The old hair shafts also showed distinct pigmentation at the proximal ends, and her eyebrows and eyelashes became more pigmented and thicker. After 8 weeks Beau's lines appeared in the thumbnails. All this was associated with a climb of plasma zinc to normal levels.

A single ray from the spectrum of a disease may be all that is necessary to make the diagnosis and spotlight the therapy.

Swick HM, Kein CL: **Biotin deficiency** with neurologic and cutaneous manifestations but without organic aciduria. J Pediatr 1983; 103:265–267.

A 24-month-old boy developed chronic mucoid rhinitis without fever followed by alopecia progressing to **complete baldness** over a few weeks. Six weeks later a rough, dry, scaly, erythematous **maculopapular rash** appeared on the extensor surfaces of the knees and elbows, spreading to the face and trunk. **Blepharitis** and **keratoconjunctivitis** were present, along with ataxia. A few thin, sparse hairs remained on his scalp and eyebrows.

Serum immunoglobulins and amino acid screens were normal, as was urine organic acid excretion. Serum biotin was 13 pg/ml (normal 200 to 500 pg/ml), and treatment with biotin was curative.

Hochberg Z, Gilhar A, Haim S, et al: Calcitriol-resistant **rickets** with **alopecia**. Arch Dermatol 1985; 121:646–647.

Insidious progressive hair loss began in a little girl at age 6 months. By age 5 years she was **totally bald**, except for sparse eyebrows and normal eyelashes. She had concomitant rickets, first noted at 9 months of age, with low levels of serum calcium (6.8 mg/dl) and serum phosphorus (2.8 mg/dl) and an elevated alkaline phosphatase level (2200 IU). Rachitic bone changes on x-rays became gradually severe, and neither the hair loss nor the rickets responded to 1,25-dihydroxyvitamin D_3 (calcitriol) therapy.

Look for **hypocalcemia** in young patients with unexplained hair loss.

Barth JH, Dawber RPR: Focal naevoid hypotrichosis. Acta Derm Venereol 1987; 67:178–179.

Symmetrical well-defined patches of **hair loss**, one on each side of the parietal scalp in a 4-year-old black boy, represented a nevoid anomaly. Although there was total absence of hair in these sites at birth, some terminal hairs later appeared. No forceps or scalp electrodes had been used at birth.

Focal nonscarring hypotrichosis or alopecia in **infancy** is uncommon and is usually nevoid (epidermal nevus, organoid nevus). Congenital triangular aplasia is present at birth, but hairs do not grow. Occipital alopecia of the newborn due to a physiologic delay of hair fall after telogen conversion occurs at about 3 months of age. Other nonscarring alopecias considered were alopecia areata, tick-bite alopecia, and trichotillomania.

Monk BE, Vollum DI: **Familial naevus sebaceus**. J Roy Soc Med 1982; 75:660–661.

A 33-year-old woman had a bald patch on her left parietal scalp since birth. It was a 3- by 2-cm area of **alopecia** with a **yellow verrucous surface**, surmounted by a **red nodule** 1 cm in diameter. Excision confirmed a nevus sebaceus with a **syringocystadenoma papilliferum**.

Her 12-year-old daughter had a 2- by 1-cm nevus sebaceous at the occiput, present since birth as a bald patch. This is the first reported case of familial nevus sebaceous and raises the question of it being an inherited precursor of malignant disease.

Tosti A: **Congenital triangular alopecia**. Report of fourteen cases. J Am Acad Dermatol 1987; 16:991–993.

Unilateral or bilateral asymptomatic triangular bald patches may occur in the **frontotemporal** region of the scalp. Often overlooked by patient and physician alike until the age of 3 to 6 years, they are presumed to be a congenital defect in hair formation. Skin biopsy reveals vellus-like hair follicles.

Headington JT, Astle N: **Familial focal alopecia**. A new disorder of hair growth clinically resembling pseudopelade. Arch Dermatol 1987; 123:234–237.

Distinct patches of hair loss present since early childhood occurred in both a 14-year-old girl and her mother, causing "thin hair." Aplasia cutis congenita and congenital triangular alopecia were ruled out, since the condition was not congenital.

The patches of decreased hair density (up to 50% or more) had occasional short hairs, but no inflammation, follicular hyperkeratosis, or scarring characteristic of lichen planopilaris or discoid lupus erythematosus. The focal loss was not total, as in alopecia areata. It most closely resembled **pseudopelade** in its noninflammatory state but lacked characteristic isolated hairs centered in atrophic-appearing areas. Its focal nature distinguished it from early-onset androgenetic alopecia.

Biopsy showed no loss of follicles, but rather a distinctive arrest of hairs in the telogen phase. Unlike alopecia areata, there was no lymphocytic infiltrate to account for the telogen arrest.

Laub D, Horan RF, Yaffe H, et al: A child with hair loss. Arch Dermatol 1987; 123:1071–1074.

Distinct **patchy hair loss** over the **parietal** and **occipital** scalp had been present in this 2-year-old boy since age 2 months. The **hairs** were **short** in these areas, only millimeters in length. The hair elsewhere on the scalp was **dry** and **lusterless**, but with a **spangled** appearance in reflected light. There was a suggestion of beading.

A diagnosis of **pili torti** was made by microscopic observation of focal flattening and 180-degree rotations along the long shaft of the hair at regular intervals. The hair loss thus resulted from mechanical trauma to these fragile hairs. One can anticipate that puberty will bring increased diameter of the hairs and consequently less loss.

Any patient with this type of **twisted hair** needs assessment for:

1. Menkes' kinky-hair syndrome
    pili torti
    progressive cerebral deterioration
    seizures
    hypothermia
    arterial disease
    scorbutic bone changes
    characteristic facies
    early death
2. Björnstad's syndrome
    pili torti
    sensorineural hearing loss
3. Crandall's syndrome
    pili torti
    sensorineural hearing loss
    hypogonadism
4. Pseudomonilethrix
    pili torti—forme fruste (irregular twists)
    apparently beaded hair
    trichorrhexis nodosa (indented, not nodal)
5. Bazex syndrome
    (hypotrichosis, basal cell epitheliomas,
    atrophoderma)
6. Inflammation or infection of scalp
7. Other ectodermal abnormalities

Kersey PJW: **Tricho-dental syndrome**: A disorder with a **short hair cycle**. Br J Dermatol 1987; 116:259–263.

Persistently short hair may be due either to slow growth or to a short hair cycle.

A 13-year-old girl had the problem of "short hair and short teeth." She had never had a haircut, yet her scalp hair was but a few inches long. The hair diameter was about 50% of normal. The teeth were small conical pegs requiring crown restoration. Eleven teeth were absent. Five other members of her family had similar problems, and the inheritance appeared to be dominant.

The **short, fine hair** had always been assumed to result from slow hair growth, but when an area was shaved, the growth rate was found to be normal (0.4 mm/day). By calculation, her hairs remained in anagen only one fourth of the normal time. As a result, she proved to have 50% of hairs in telogen phase rather than the normal 10%. Her hair was short because it was genetically programmed to be short. In brief, she had "short anagen hair," leading to the barber's chair being replaced by the dentist's chair.

Hamm H, Traupe H: **Loose anagen hair of childhood**: The phenomenon of easily pluckable hair. J Am Acad Dermatol 1989; 20:242–248.

A 4-year-old boy with shoulder length hair was referred because of a 5-month history of diffuse hair loss. His parents' concern was the fact that he was losing about 300 hairs a day and that tufts of hair could be easily and painlessly plucked. The child was not taking any medication.

On examination there was, indeed, **diffuse alopecia** of the entire scalp. There was no sign of inflammation or scarring. Nearly all of the hairs plucked were anagen hairs with root sheaths. On lateral illumination the hairs showed **alternating dark and bright zones**. Light microscopy of the shafts revealed the presence of longitudinal grooves and twisting along the axis. There was a resemblance of the hairs to pili trianguli et canaliculi. A shaved area showed retarded growth with hair only 4 cm long one year later.

Biopsy showed a marked cleft formation between the hair shafts and inner root sheath, which was degenerating. There was no inflammatory change. For precise study of the cross section of the hairs, hair tufts were placed in small-caliber plastic tubes and heated to shrink tubes and fix hairs. Razor blade cross sections at room temperature were then mounted on a glass slide. This "shrinking-tube" technique showed that 20% of the hairs were abnormal, with triangular, quadrangular, trapezoid, kidney, heart, and drop patterns.

A diagnosis of **easily pluckable hair** was made. The role of the inner root sheath is critical not only in shaping but in holding the hair shaft in place. In this syndrome the inner root sheath shows premature homogenization and hence loss of its critical functions.

This condition involves no areas totally devoid of hair, no exclamation mark hairs, and no nail changes, and thus is distinguished from alopecia areata. It is also distinguished from trichotillomania, in which the hairs are difficult to pluck. Likewise, it differs from telogen effluvium, in which the hairs lost are in the telogen, not anagen, phase. Finally, although the hair shaft cross sections remind one of the uncombable hair syndrome, in that condition there is no hair loss.

Ormerod AD, Main RA, Ryder ML, Gregory DW: A family with diffuse partial **wooly hair**. Br J Dermatol 1987; 116:401–405.

A 19-year-old girl complained of **diffuse thinning** of her scalp hair over the past year. Examination revealed that a third of her hairs were short (5 cm), **fine, curly,** and **hypopigmented**. It was these **short kinky hairs** intimately interspersed with her normal long hair that produced the effect of "thinning."

Five other members of her family were found to have the same type of clinically unsuspected hair abnormality. Only one complained of thinning. The wavy hairs in each proved on scanning electron microscopy to show irregular angular kinks that produced changes in shaft direction. The cuticle showed splintering and weathering as well as trichorrhexis, suggesting a weakness of these abnormal hairs.

This dominantly inherited wooly hair must be distinguished from the autosomal dominant and recessive forms of wooly hair in which tight curling is present in *all* hairs of the scalp. It should also be differentiated from the **wooly hair nevus** in which abnormal hairs are found only within a well-demarcated area. Furthermore, the wooly hair nevus shows three signs not seen in this family: curvature of the follicles on biopsy, oval hair shafts, and conversion of a hair into a tight spiral in boiling water.

This family reminds us of the fact that many mammals have a double coat in which long straight hairs obscure a finer wavy and less pigmented "underhair." Look for this kinky undercoat in the next patient you see complaining of thinning of the hair.

Commens C, Rogers M, Kan A: **Heterotopic brain tissue** presenting as bald cysts with a collar of hypertrophic hair: The hair collar sign. Arch Dermatol 1989; 125:1253–1256.

A **cystic bald nodule** had been present since birth on the right side of the scalp of this baby boy. There was a striking band of rapid hair growth surrounding its base. The mother regularly shaved this collar of hair. A pediatrician had repeatedly aspirated yellow fluid from the cyst, only to see it refill in 24 hours.

At this point the "**hair collar sign**" pointed to a diagnosis of a heterotopic brain tissue mass, an encephalocele, or a cutaneous meningioma. Skull roentgenography, ultrasound, and computed tomography showed the cyst had no connection with the brain, nor was there any skull defect.

The 9-mm cyst was excised and proved to contain glial tissue, neuronal cells, and a cyst lined by ependymalike columnar epithelium. A diagnosis of heterotopic brain tissue was made.

It is assumed that an embryonic rest was caught in the ectoderm during the third to fifth week of embryonic life. It is at this time that the ectoderm separates from the neuroectoderm. Teratogens may be responsible.

The major diagnostic step in approaching any **congenital cystic mass** on the **scalp** is to rule out an encephalocele. Here brain tissue actually herniates and appears in the midline, unlike this patient's presentation.

Meningoceles as well as intracranial dermal sinus tracts also enter into the differential diagnosis. **Hypertrophic hairs**, a dimple, a vascular nevus, or a lipoma may be the only diagnostic clue. But awareness is critical, since needle aspiration or inept surgery can lead to retrograde infection. Each example requires **neurosurgical consultation, ultrasound**, and **computed tomography**.

When you see a cystic mass on the scalp of an infant, the connection in your brain should be "Is there a connection to his brain?"

If the laboratory doesn't support your clinical diagnosis, remember that the laboratory has never seen your patient.

Halder RM: Hair and **scalp disorders** in **blacks**. Cutis 1983; 32:378–380.

The trauma of hair care accounts for much of the hair loss in black patients. The art of diagnosis is the art of the history.

Hot comb (heat pressing) **alopecia**
    Cause: after heating the hair with a metal comb kept at temperatures of up to 500°C, not only the hydrogen bonds but the hairs are broken.
    Characteristics: **stubble** of fractured hairs protruding an inch or two from the scalp

Traction alopecia
    Causes:

tight braiding	tight rollers
decorative corn rowing	picking out with hard comb

    Characteristics: **symmetrical** areas of **hair loss** within the **hair margin**, anterior to ears and extending forward in a band an inch wide. Continued over long term, alopecia may become irreversible.

Permanent and **straightener alopecia**
    Cause: strong alkalies used beyond tolerance point of hair.
    Characteristics: hairs break off leaving 1 to 2 inches of normal hair.

Two additional problems are almost unique to black skin.

Keloidal folliculitis
    Characteristics: smooth, firm, skin-colored papules on nape extending into occipital region. Process may become confluent and exhibit pustules.

Dissecting cellulitis of the scalp (**perifolliculitis capitis** abscedens et suffodiens)
    Characteristics: painful **boggy abscesses** with burrows and sinus tracts; may exhibit permanent hair loss

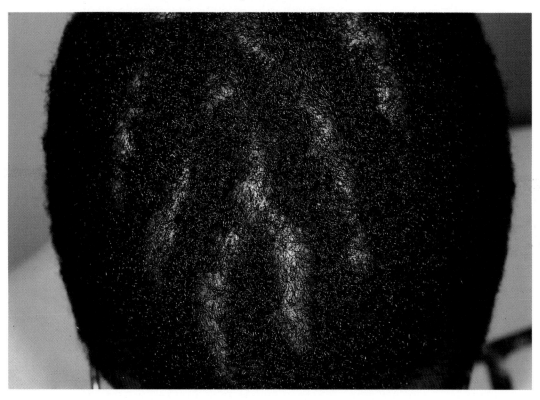

Keratinization Defects

Kanzler MH, Rasmussen JE: **Atrichia** with papular lesions. Arch Dermatol 1986; 122:565–567.

An 11-year-old boy had lost all of his hair except the eyelashes when he was 2 years old. Recently, multiple small, white, **cystic papules resembling milia** had appeared on his posterior scalp, neck, and extremities. Skin biopsy showed keratinous follicular cysts (milia) with foreign body granulomas. He also had atopic dermatitis, asthma, and common variable immunodeficiency with **hypogammaglobulinemia**, decreased IgG and IgA; he had had numerous hospitalizations for **pneumonia, otitis media**, and chronic **diarrhea**. His father, who also had alopecia starting at age 2 years and common variable immunodeficiency, died at age 26 of *Staphylococcus aureus* sepsis.

The diagnoses considered in this child were:

atrichia with papular lesions
alopecia universalis
eruptive vellus hair cysts (multiple small red or brown papules on the chest, arms, and legs of children)

Histologic study defined this as atrichia with papular lesions, a rare form of **ectodermal dysplasia**. In most cases, the fetal hair is normal at birth but is shed within 3 months and never replaced. Some patients, however, are hairless at birth. The mode of inheritance is uncertain, with autosomal recessive being postulated.

Eramo LR, Esterly NB, Zieserl EJ, et al: **Ichthyosis follicularis** with alopecia and photophobia. Arch Dermatol 1985; 121:1167–1174.

A 5-year-old boy had **skin** that felt **like sandpaper**, a scalp with **no hair**, and eyes that avoided light since birth. He had no problems with sweating, hearing, dentition, nail formation, or growth and development. However, the skin over his **knees** and **elbows** was very **hyperkeratotic**. His family history disclosed relatives similarly afflicted. A biopsy of the rough skin on his leg showed **keratosis pilaris**. The triad of spiny projections of the skin, dramatic generalized noncicatricial alopecia, and severe **photophobia** fit the diagnostic category of ichthyosis follicularis.

Thornlike projections coming out of subverted hair follicles make the skin feel like a nutmeg grater or the prickly surface of a rose leaf. At birth the skin may only appear dry, but keratotic spines emerge as greater follicular activity occurs. The persistent alopecia cannot be missed, and photophobia over the years leaves the child with a head always tilting away from the sun.

To assure the diagnosis, some diagnostic brambles must be cut away, but photophobia eliminates most of the keratotic syndromes other than these two:

Keratosis follicularis spinulosa decalvans (KFSD)
thorny spines, limited distribution (scalp, eyebrows, dorsal, hands, fingers)
alopecia, patchy or slight
photophobia, marked
Keratitis, ichthyosis, deafness (**KID**) **syndrome**
thorny spines, widespread
alopecia, striking
photophobia, marked
keratitis
deafness

Poulin Y, Perry HO, Muller SA: Olmstead syndrome: Congenital **palmoplantar** and **periorificial keratoderma**. J Am Acad Dermatol 1984; 10:600–610.

This 2-year-old child had universal alopecia and thick, brown-black, sharply marginated **hyperkeratotic plaques** around all of the body orifices as well as the palms and soles. Not only were the mouth, nostrils, and ears involved, but yellowish-brown plaques were present in the groin and on the anterior area of the neck. The fingers showed **paronychia**, and there was a history of **cradle cap**.

After careful study, a diagnosis of **acrodermatitis enteropathica** was made, and indeed the case was duly reported in the *Archives of Dermatology*. As the years passed, permitting further study and observation, the diagnosis of acrodermatitis enteropathica proved to be wrong. The patient had shown no response to zinc therapy. The hyperkeratosis of the palms and soles took center stage, becoming thicker, deeply fissured, and extending as linear starfishlike streaks up the wrists. When the patient was 17, the hyperkeratotic verrucous plaques appeared in the axillae. Meanwhile, the perioral lesions became much less evident. The joints became lax, but the fingers fixed in flexion because of the keratoderma.

With attention focused on the keratoderma, the correct diagnosis of Olmstead syndrome or congenital palmoplantar and periorificial keratoderma was made. The hallmark of this rare entity is the plaque of warty, hyperkeratotic change around the mouth. It is not seen in the other palmoplantar keratodermas.

Price VH, Odom RB, Ward WH, Jones FT: **Trichothiodystrophy**. Sulfur-deficient **brittle hair** as a marker for a neuroectodermal symptom complex. Arch Dermatol 1980; 116:1375–1384.

This 8-year-old mentally retarded boy had partial alopecia and extensive hair breakage along the scalp margins. The hair was easily broken off on light tugging. His skin showed marked atopic dermatitis as well as **ichthyosis**.

Examination of the brittle hair showed striking light and dark bands under polarizing microscopy. Chemical analysis showed the hair to have but half the usual amount of sulfur and a notably low content of the sulfur-containing amino acid cystine. It is this defect that apparently accounts for the structural weakness of this hair as well as a variety of associated findings, i.e., mental retardation, hypoplastic nails, dental caries, ichthyosiform changes in the skin, and ocular dysplasia.

To be safe, always carry a spare diagnosis.

Scarring

Goerz G, Kind R, Lehmann P: **Cicatricial alopecias**. *In* Orfanos C and Happle R (eds): Hair and Hair Diseases. New York, Springer-Verlag, 1990, pp 611–639.

Any irreversible damage to the scalp may destroy the hair follicles, with resultant cicatricial alopecia. Such focal alopecia may be diagnosable on the basis of history, appearance, or concomitant findings.

History:

aplasia cutis	drug-overdose immobility
alopecia triangularis	varicella, zoster
burns, thermal, electrical, radiation, chemical	furuncles
	kerion
trauma	tick bite
pressure-prolonged surgery	alopecia parvimaculata

Appearance:

ulerythema ophyrogenes; atrophoderma vermicularis

sarcoidosis	scleroderma; en coup de sabre
necrobiosis lipoidica	vasculitis
pseudopelade	temporal arteritis
ulcerative lichen planus	primary and metastatic tumors
lupus erythematosus	keratinous cyst

Concomitant findings:

incontinentia pigmenti
epidermolysis bullosa, dystrophic form
porokeratosis of Mibelli
chondrodysplasia punctata congenital malformation
ichthyosis
keratosis follicularis
lupus vulgaris
pemphigus vulgaris
bullous pemphigoid

Prendiville JS, Esterly NB: **Halo scalp ring**: A cause of **scarring alopecia**. Arch Dermatol 1987; 123:992–993.

A 9-month-old girl was seen for evaluation of a large, eccentric, incomplete circle of cicatricial alopecia over the vertex and occipital scalp. It had been present since birth.

Her history was of a large necrotizing hematoma present at the time of delivery. This healed slowly with areas of ulceration persisting until the patient was 4 months old.

The edematous swelling of the scalp occurring after a difficult vertex delivery is known as **caput succedaneum**. It results from prolonged pressure and may proceed to necrosis and a distinctive "halo" alopecia.

It is to be distinguished from aplasia cutis congenita and from the alopecia associated with the trauma of intrauterine pressure transducers, or fetal scalp monitoring.

Plastic surgical repair of the defect is possible at an early age. Such repair is facilitated by using tissue expanders.

Crotty CP, Su WPD, Winkelmann RK: **Ulcerative lichen planus**. Follow-up of surgical excision and grafting. Arch Dermatol 1980; 116:1252–1256.

For 12 years a 44-year-old woman had painful disabling **blisters** of her **soles**, which evolved into **chronic ulcers**. She also had **lost** her **toenails**, with atrophy of the nail matrix. In the past 3 years she had developed **diffuse cicatricial alopecia** of the **occipital scalp**. Her mouth and tongue had painful **erosions**, with a reticulate pattern of white papules on the **buccal mucosa**. Also noted were typical lichen planus papules of the right arm. A biopsy of the sole showed lichen planus.

Crippling ulcers and blisters of the feet are characteristic of this special form of lichen planus. Although its inflammatory elements suggest a clinical diagnosis of lupus erythematosus, the histologic findings clearly confirm it as a severe form of lichen planus. Excision with grafting is the preferable treatment because of the possible development of squamous cell carcinoma.

Knight TE, Robinson HM, Sina B: **Angiosarcoma** (angioendothelioma) of the **scalp**. An unusual case of **scarring alopecia**. Arch Dermatol 1980; 116:683–686.

A week after being given a permanent by a beautician, a 77-year-old woman noted **itching, burning**, and patchy hair loss. **Swelling** of her **forehead** ensued. On examination 4 months later, the entire vertex of the scalp was devoid of hair, and all **follicular orifices** were **obliterated**, giving the picture of scarring alopecia with scattered adherent serous crusts. The infraocular areas were **red** and **edematous**, and **vascular dilatation** was present on the **nose** and **cheeks**.

The histologic diagnosis on three biopsies proved to be angiosarcoma. This presentation was unusual, as it lacked the typical ill-defined indurated bluish or skin-colored plaques with alopecia limited to these sites. Ulceration may occur, as well as underlying bone invasion. The scalp, face, and neck of the aged remain the preferential sites. The prognosis is poor, although this woman's scalp lesions resolved after electron-beam radiation. However, the lesions recurred 7 months later, and she soon died of metastatic angiosarcoma.

If you're not comfortable with your diagnosis, you probably don't have the right one.

Distinctive History

Wasserteil V, Bruce S: **Fever** and **hypotrichosis** in a **newborn**. Arch Dermatol 1986; 122:1325–1328.

Recurrent fevers that on two occasions reached a temperature of 107°F appeared during the second week of this male infant's life. Antibiotic therapy had had no effect on the fevers. He appeared healthy but for the total absence of scalp and body hair.

The **facies** was **distinctive**, with a prominent forehead, central depression of the face, a saddle nose, and thick lips. His ears were large and low set, giving him an elfin appearance. The skin was dry, wrinkled, and thin, and showed eczematous changes on the arms, legs, and face.

A biopsy showed complete absence of sweat glands, which accounted for the fevers and confirmed the diagnosis of **anhidrotic ectodermal dysplasia**.

Recognizing this at once not only can save a life but can save a brain. Without environmental temperature control these infants can develop convulsions and die. Even one episode of very high fever can permanently damage the brain. Here is a dermatologic diagnosis that must not be missed. It is the absence of something rather than the presence of something that explains this "disease."

Although unexplained fever is the hallmark of this syndrome, the **absence** of **scalp** and **eyebrow hair** as well as **eyelashes** is a diagnostic tip. Furthermore, the facies is characteristic, with a square forehead, frontal bossing, a sunken face, saddle nose, satyr ear, thick lower lip, and pointed chin.

Typically there is **periorbital hyperpigmentation** with multiple palpebral lines. The lacrimal glands are usually inadequate, with resultant **conjunctivitis**.

Look to the eyes for corneal opacities and dysplasia as well as congenital cataracts and subluxation of the lens. Look to the mouth for absence of teeth or **malformed teeth**. Look to the skin for an **atopic**-type **eczema**. This is on a setting of dry, thin, wrinkled skin. Look to the chest for asthma and laryngitis because the mucous secretions are greatly reduced. This also accounts for recurrent rhinitis and pharyngitis.

Diagnostic maneuvers include biopsy as well as evaluation of sweating response by such noninvasive techniques as starch-iodine tests.

The differential list includes:

familial simple anhidrosis
pachyonychia congenita
Rothmund-Thomson syndrome
dyskeratosis congenita
congenital syphilis
hidrotic ectodermal dysplasia

Although anhidrotic ectodermal defect is usually diagnosed in infancy, we recall a 6-year-old girl whose problem went unrecognized until she collapsed of hyperthermia at a fourth of July parade.

The diagnois of anhidrosis is hard to make in cool weather or in an air-conditioned office.

Wiles JC, Hansen RC: **Postoperative (pressure) alopecia**. J Am Acad Dermatol 1985; 12:195–198.

This 54-year-old man was seen because of a 4-cm patch of alopecia with a central **boggy, scaling, crusted erythematous plaque** in the back of the scalp. It appeared to be a fungal infection, but neither KOH nor fungal culture yielded organisms. The presence of **pus** suggested a bacterial infection, but neither cultures of the pus nor the biopsy specimen itself grew pathogens. Treatment with erythromycin did not have any effect.

The history revealed the cause. This man had had **open heart surgery** the month before and had been under anesthesia for 4½ hours and under intubation for 84 hours. A diagnosis of pressure alopecia was made. Three months after surgery the hair had completely regrown and the scalp was normal.

The cause of this postoperative alopecia is **pressure ischemia** of the area during the long period of immobility. Usually the hair loss is reversible, but it can be permanent in some instances. Soon after surgery the patients complain of **scalp pain**, and within a day or two one will see erythema, oozing, and crusting at the pain site. Biopsies show a sequence of intravascular thrombosis, and later obliterative vasculitis.

Coma blisters arise from the same pressure ischemia but occur in areas other than the scalp, where the mooring hair follicles prevent bulla formation.

Aranoff SM, Levy HB, Tuchman AJ, Daras M: **Alopecia** in **meralgia paresthetica**. J Am Acad Dermatol 1985; 12:176–178.

Alopecia developed on the left anterolateral area of the thigh exactly in the distribution of the lateral femoral cutaneous nerve in a 50-year-old male. It was preceded by an 8-year history of underlying numbness, tingling, and dysesthesia in the area (meralgia paresthetica). The **alopecia** was **permanent**, nonscarring, and not caused by any conscious rubbing or stroking of the area by the patient. No pathologic features were noted on skin biopsy.

Herpes zoster and leprosy can also produce localized neuropathy, sensory changes, and alopecia. The role of **neuropathy** in hair loss remains an intriguing question.

Taylor JS: The pilosebaceous unit. *In* Maibach HI (ed): Occupational and Industrial Dermatology, 2nd ed. Chicago, Year Book Medical Publishers, Inc., 1987, pp 105–120.

Occupationally, **hair loss** can develop from exposure to **thallium, sodium borate**, or **chloroprene dimers** found in the manufacture of neoprene. These dimers are structurally related to vitamin A.

The skin gives you more diagnostic clues than other organs of the body.

Drug Induced

Merk HF: **Drugs** affecting **hair growth**. In Orfanos C, Happle R (eds): Hair and Hair Diseases. New York, Springer-Verlag, 1990, pp 601–609.

Any patient taking any one of the following **drugs** is at risk for **hair loss**:

vitamin A, 13-*cis*-retinoic acid or etretinate
oral contraceptives
beta-blockers
antidepressants, anticonvulsants
   (doxepin, lithium, haloperidol, valproic
   acid)

allopurinol
cimetidine
heparin, coumarin
cytotoxic agents
gentamicin
L-dopa

Teach your patients that hair loss induced by drugs usually **begins suddenly**, weeks to months after they start taking the drug. It commonly affects only the scalp hairs, and especially at the part line. It may lead to diffuse alopecia but is reversible and, in fact, may reverse even while the patient is taking the drug. And finally, only the cytotoxic agents produce total baldness.

Doubt your diagnosis of drug-induced hair thinning when you see inflammation or scarring.

Most drug-induced alopecia is noted by neither the patient nor the physician.

Ellis JK, Russell RM, Makrauer FL, Schaefer EJ: Increased risk for **vitamin A toxicity** in severe **hypertriglyceridemia**. Ann Intern Med 1986; 105:877–879.

Hyperlipoproteinemia appears to be a predisposing factor for hypervitaminosis A.

A 48-year-old woman with chronic relapsing pancreatitis, malabsorption, anorexia, weakness, and decreasing mental acuity had **thin hair, no eyebrows**, scales over her fingertips, slight exophthalmus, 3+ pedal edema, **red tongue, cheilosis**, severe periodontal disease, and an **enlarged liver**. Plasma triglycerides were 1495 mg/dl, plasma cholesterol was 390 mg/dl, and total plasma vitamin A was 871 µg/dl. She had been taking 60,000 IU daily of vitamin A as treatment for malabsorption.

Patients with type V hyperlipoproteinemia without vitamin A supplementation also had large increases in plasma retinol and retinyl ester.

Scott MJ Jr, Scott MJ III: Dermatologists and anabolic-androgenic drug abuse. Cutis 1989; 44:30–35.

In **athletes** and **body builders**, the possibility of **anabolic steroid misuse** must be considered when you see:

androgenic alopecia of scalp,
   especially in young women
hirsutism
seborrhea
cystic acne

extensive straie distensae
gynecomastia
cutis verticis gyrata
abscesses (sites of injection)

Fraunfelder FT, Meyer SM, Menacker SJ: **Alopecia** possibly secondary to topical ophthalmic **β-blockers**. JAMA 1990; 263:1493–1494.

Although it is well known that systemic administration of β-adrenergic blockers such as propranolol may induce a reversible **telogen effluvium** hair loss, this report suggests that the use of ocular beta-blockers (timolol) may have the same effects.

Ask your patients with hair loss not only what goes into their mouth, but also into their conjunctival sacs and other mucosal areas.

Escamilla RF, Lisser H: **Simmonds' disease**. J Clin Endocrinol Metab 1942; 2:65–96.

In 1914 Morris Simmonds, a pathologist at the University of Hamburg, described *hypophyseal cachexia*. Typically, a 30-year-old woman has severe **weight loss, amenorrhea**, and low thyroid tests dating from a **postpartum hemorrhage**. She will have **generalized alopecia** (axillary, pubic, scalp, eyebrows), pale, dry, **yellowish-brown skin** with premature aging, **breast** and genital **atrophy**, dental caries, bradycardia, and hypothermia with cold intolerance.

Laboratory

sella turcica x-ray (enlarged, destroyed, calcified)
glucose (decreased)
CBC (anemia, eosinophilia)

Kepler EJ, Nichols DR, Mills JH: The diagnostic value of regression of secondary sexual characteristics in cases of **hemochromatosis**. Ann Intern Med 1940; 14:810–816.

In two cases of hemochromatosis with only slight **pigmentation** of **sun-exposed areas**, the diagnosis was made with a skin biopsy showing hemosiderin deposition around sweat glands and increased melanin in the deep layers of the corium.

Regression of secondary sexual characteristics is an early finding in the disease, due to hypogonadism from either pigment deposition or anterior pituitary insufficiency. Findings include pallor; **loss of beard, pubic**, and **axillary hair**; atrophic testes; and changes in body habitus toward feminine. These changes occur prior to the development of skin bronzing, liver enlargement, and diabetes.

Snyder RA, Crain WR, McNutt NS: **Alopecia mucinosa**: Report of a case with diffuse alopecia and normal-appearing scalp skin. Arch Dermatol 1984; 120:496–498.

For 3 months a 69-year-old man had noticed **sudden, diffuse thinning** of his entire scalp hair, similar to early, diffuse alopecia areata. The follicular orifices appeared normal. A gentle pull removed many clubbed and unclubbed hairs of normal microscopic appearance. KOH examination and fungal culture were negative. However, a biopsy revealed **follicular mucinosis**. His acute alopecia mucinosa resolved gradually without treatment, and hair density was essentially normal 9 months later. He had no sign of lymphoma.

Primary follicular mucinosis usually involves the head and neck, with well-defined areas of inflammatory alopecia that usually resolve within a year. Occasionally, lesions persist and become widespread over several years. Early lesions appear as groups of **skin-colored follicular papules** or erythematous plaques with follicular accentuation and slight scaling.

Chronic lesions are usually **erythematous plaques** with variable induration and scaling, but may also be gelatinous-appearing nodules and tumors. In black patients, hypopigmentation may occur.

All such patients **need evaluation for lymphoma**, especially mycosis fungoides, since alopecia mucinosa may precede this disease. Rarely, it may also occur with lupus erythematosus, lichen simplex chronicus, and angiolymphoid hyperplasia with eosinophilia. Presumably, alopecia mucinosa is a nonspecific **reaction pattern** to several unrelated stimuli.

Wheeler GE, Barrows GH: **Alopecia universalis**. A manifestation of occult **amyloidosis** and **multiple myeloma**. Arch Dermatol 1981; 117:815–816.

A striking **generalized hair loss** involving the scalp, eyelashes, eyebrows, axillae, vulva, and extremities gradually afflicted a 65-year-old woman over

221

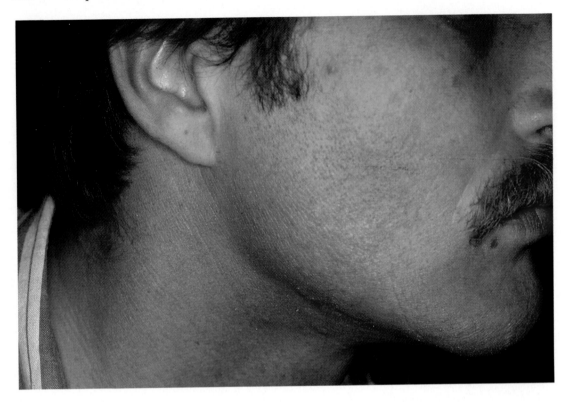

a 3-year period. Scalp biopsy revealed extensive amyloid deposits around hair follicles. Her **fingernails** were **absent**, and she had onycholysis of the toenails. Her **tongue** was **enlarged**, with dental indentations on the lateral margins. The external auditory canals were narrowed, and there was thickening of the skin of the chin and neck.

Laboratory study showed monoclonal λ light chains in the urine, an IgG-λ monoclonal protein on immunoelectrophoresis, and more than 30% plasma cells in the bone marrow, confirming the diagnosis of multiple myeloma.

It's more important to see the patient at a clinical meeting than to hear the discussion.

Neuman KM, Burnett JW: **Alopecia** associated with **syringomas**. J Am Acad Dermatol 1985; 13:528–529.

Five years of asymptomatic, generalized progressive loss of scalp hair in this 58-year-old woman was viewed as idiopathic hair loss until a biopsy was done. There was no familial history of hair loss, no intake of medication, no dermatitis, no scarring, and no stress factor.

The cause proved to be the presence of numerous syringomas seen in each of two scalp biopsies.

Once again, the **need for scalp biopsies** in patients with clinically unexplained loss of scalp hair is underscored. Other patients with biopsy "surprises" to explain their innocent looking hair loss proved to have angiosarcoma, follicular hamartoma, or eccrine sweat hamartomas. We have also personally seen occult pemphigus revealed by a scalp biopsy in a patient with unexplained alopecia.

Burket JM: **Alopecia** associated with **underlying nerve sheath myxoma**. J Am Acad Dermatol 1987; 16:209–211.

A 16-year-old girl had a puzzling 2.5-cm **localized patch** of **hair loss** of the midposterior scalp, present for 2 months. There was no evidence of fungal infection or alopecia areata, but she had felt a deep, mildly tender lump in the area for 3 to 4 years, interpreted as a lymph node.

The answer came when the skin was incised and the underlying mass was dissected out. It proved to be a rare nerve sheath myxoma. Within 4 weeks good hair growth had returned to the alopecic area.

MacDonald DM, Sarkany I: Lymphomatoid granulomatosis. Clin Exp Dermatol 1976; 1:163–173.

Loss of sweating, loss of potency, painful ulcers of the right heel, and **circumscribed patches** of **hair loss** on the **chest, arms, hands**, and **scalp** led a 54-year-old laborer to seek help. The patches of alopecia had prominent follicular markings and complete **absence of sweating**, even following thermal stimulation and introduction of pilocarpine by intradermal or electrophoretic means. Neurologic examination was normal, and blood studies were normal except for a bilirubin level of 1.4 mg/100 ml.

A skin biopsy from the chest revealed a dense dermal infiltrate sleeving the sweat coils, composed of lymphocytes, histiocytes, plasma cells, and epithelioid cells. The sweat glands were hypertrophied. Histologic examination of the **foot ulcer** showed **vasculitis** of large vessels associated with granuloma formation, leading to a diagnosis of lymphomatoid granulomatosis with possible lymphoma.

Two years later he had an episode of cellulitis of the left leg, followed by deep-vein thrombosis in the same leg. One year after this he developed hepatomegaly, generalized lymphadenopathy, and a pleural effusion, leading to a diagnosis of **Hodgkin's disease**.

A 75-year-old man had a 2-year history of **bluish-red nodules** and red, scaly patches arising on generalized ichthyosis and follicular hyperkeratosis. Small palpable nodules were present in the axillae and groin. Later he developed **circumscribed patches** of **alopecia** of the **scalp** and **body hair**. He had also had two episodes of thrombophlebitis. Chest x-ray and tomography showed intrapulmonary masses, but blood studies were normal.

Skin biopsies showed hypertrophied sweat glands and a dense focal granulomatous infiltrate with multinucleate giant cells centered partly on sweat glands and extending into the adjacent fat. Many small blood vessels were occluded. Improvement occurred with prednisone and cyclophosphamide before he died of pneumonia.

Alopecia Areata

The sudden appearance of a bald spot, whether it be beard or scalp, makes for an easy diagnosis of alopecia areata. The smooth, totally hairless skin is perfectly normal. There is no scarring. Around the edge is a fringe or sampling of diagnostic "exclamation-point" hairs. These are very short stub hairs tapering down to the skin. The "point" is within the follicle. They represent the sputtering attempt of the follicle to form a hair shaft while it is being shut down by a perifollicular infiltrate of T cells.

Additional diagnostic clues center on progressive loss of pigment near the base of affected hairs, appearance of new hairs without pigment, and failure to lose unpigmented white hairs. The nails may show patterned pitting, leukonychia, a friable surface, or even spotted lunulae. Vitiligo is a sometime association as well. The patient may also give a history of prior attacks, of others in the family having had the same problem, or autoimmune endocrine disease. On occasion you may be able to elicit a history of the atopic status. More dramatic are the rare stories of a shocking episode just prior to the hair loss.

The alopecic areas may enlarge and coalesce. New sites can be recognized by the pluck test in which innumerable club hairs come out in specific areas. Indeed, all of the hair may be shed (alopecia universalis), and in this case the history is the definitive guide to diagnosis. In a few individuals all of the dark hairs are shed rapidly, leaving only white hairs. These are the rarities of folklore in which someone "turned white overnight from fright."

The laboratory provides scant evidence at times for diagnostic support. More important is the frayed-rope appearance of the end of the hair as seen under the microscope. Organ-specific autoantibodies (e.g., thyroid) are present in a small percentage of these patients. Immunoglobulin studies may reveal the high IgE of the atopic state.

The diagnosis of alopecia areata is not always easy. When the alopecia areata is diffuse there are no loci of baldness, and the picture is one of telogen effluvium. Likewise, when there is loss of but a few eyelashes, it is hard to distinguish alopecia areata from trichotillomania. However, in the scalp, trichotillomania leaves a recognizable stubble of broken hair in the bald spots, unlike the smooth complete shedding of alopecia areata.

Pelade is the French term for alopecia areata. Hence, it is not surprising that pseudopelade enters into the differential list. However, here the process is a scarring one in which scalp hair loss occurs in circumscribed, slightly depressed patches. The patches progress, crossing the scalp as "footprints in the snow." In such patients look for evidence of lupus erythematosus, lichen planus, or scleroderma.

Since alopecia areata is completely symptomless, it is easy to miss examples of it in areas of the body where the hair is sparse and lightly pigmented. What neither we nor the patient sees must remain "alopecia inconsequentia."

Gollnick H, Orfanos CE: **Alopecia areata**: Pathogenesis and clinical picture. *In* Orfanos C, Happle R (eds): Hair and Hair Diseases. New York, Springer-Verlag, 1990, pp 529–569.

The symptomless loss of hair in sharply circumscribed areas is known as alopecia areata. Although usually occurring on the scalp, it may be present in the beard, eyebrows, eyelashes, or genital area. The patient suddenly becomes aware of an ivory-colored, slowly enlarging bald spot. It feels like a velvet-soft area of edema. There may be some vague itching or tingling, or slight tenderness may be noted, as well as erythema.

As the lesion becomes older, this vanishes and the area slowly enlarges, with

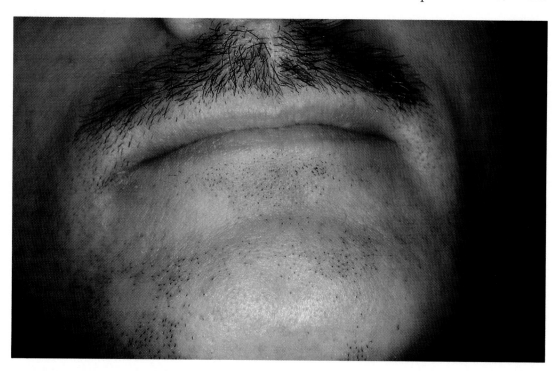

exclamation-point hairs becoming evident. These diagnostic markers are short hairs in which the shaft tapers toward the proximal part in evidence of follicular failure. The skin may show a phase of follicular hyperkeratosis, but the end point after several years is a taut, shiny skin site. It may seem slightly atrophic, but never is there evidence of scarring. Rarely, alopecia areata may pursue a fulminant course, with spreading within weeks to alopecia totalis.

Some unusual associations with alopecia areata are telogen effluvium, lymphadenopathy, **pitting** and **grooving** of the **nail plates**, punctate leukonychia, red spotted lunulae, and even onychomadesis. A few patients have associated **autoimmune disorders**, e.g., vitiligo, ulcerative colitis, pernicious anemia, Addison's disease, autoimmune gastritis, autoimmune thyroiditis, lupus erythematosus, rheumatoid arthritis, or scleroderma.

Regrowth occurs in the center of the lesions, expanding in a ringlike pattern. The hairs are unpigmented at first. Gradually the shaft becomes thicker and shows pigment. Sudden relapses may occur, and all that was regained, lost once again.

The diagnosis of alopecia areata is often made with ease at the beauty shop. However, certain examples pose a challenge:

   diffuse type
   alopecia areata in the elderly
   simultaneous presence of another type of hair loss

The differential diagnosis must include:

alopecia mucinosa	discoid lupus erythematosus
lichen planus	incontinentia pigmenti
pseudopelade	cicatricial pemphigoid
folliculitis decalvans	porokeratosis
syphilitic alopecia	necrobiosis lipoidica
morphea	lichen sclerosus et atrophicus

To which we would add trichotillomania.

Wooldridge WE: In defense of the anecdotal article. J Am Acad Dermatol 1979; 1:451–453.

Personal experiences of physician–patient medical encounters are often dismissed as an "anecdote" (a short entertaining personal or biographic account of some happening). But what is wrong with them? Is not the entire field of medicine based upon the personal exchange of information between patient and physician? Sometimes a properly observed and recorded case report may be worth reams of laboratory data.

A 71-year-old woman had had four episodes of **alopecia universalis**. At age 21, hair loss began within 48 hours after her infant son died suddenly. When she was 24, her husband died, and she completely lost her hair over the next 2 weeks, with regrowth over 3 months. When she was 70, after a quiet, uneventful life, her remaining son underwent coronary artery bypass surgery, and 4 days later her hair loss began, becoming total in 48 hours. At age 71, after learning that her son might need further surgery, her hair fell out again, only to regrow when surgery was postponed indefinitely.

For 2 months a 14-year-old girl had random attacks of **generalized urticaria**. Prednisone (20 to 40 mg/day) produced prompt involution, but lower doses of prednisone and antihistamines were ineffective. No clues were evident as to a cause, including foods, activities, medications, or stress, nor was there any association with recent occasional mild, poorly defined abdominal pains. However, the evening following a severe attack of hives, she described right lower quadrant abdominal tenderness. A diagnosis of **appendicitis** was made and an acutely inflamed appendix removed. By the following morning her hives were gone, never to return. (Sometimes the cause of urticaria comes only to those who watch and wait.)

Dear friends, I plead that you may vote
In favor of the anecdote.
For life itself, in part or total,
Is little more than anecdotal.

Shuster S: "Coudability": A new physical sign of **alopecia areata**. Br J Dermatol 1984; 111:629.

Affected but normal looking hairs in alopecia areata can be made to kink when bent or pushed inward. This **diagnostic kink** is about 5 to 10 mm above the scalp and is at the point where the alopecia areata hair shaft defect would later break, leaving dark dots of exclamation-mark stumps. The defect represents a short period of poor hair growth in which the hair shaft is narrowed, partly depigmented, and splayed. Sometimes a single hair may have several such areas, indicating episodic disease and recovery.

The "kinky" designation *coudability* refers to the similarity of these diagnostically induced hair kinks to the shape of the coudé catheter.

Dotz WI, Lieber CD, Vogt PJ: **Leukonychia punctata** and pitted nails in **alopecia areata**. Arch Dermatol 1985; 121:1452–1454.

A 36-year-old man developed patchy alopecia areata of the occipital area and leukonychia punctata of his fingernails and toenails. By the time he was 50, he lost all the hair on his scalp, and he noted **shallow pits** precisely in the sharply aligned rows of leukonychia.

Histologic examination of the plate showed multiple discrete parakeratotic foci, accounting for the white spots. The pits, in turn, resulted from shedding of these partially developed, poorly adherent cells, much as is seen in pit formation in the nails of the psoriatic. Only here the leukonychia and pitting are geometric, producing changes regularly appearing in a grid pattern. By contrast, in psoriasis the pits have a random distribution.

These **nail changes** may precede the **alopecia areata** and often persist long after the alopecia has resolved. Nor are the nail changes of alopecia areata limited to white spots and pits. The following have been observed:

roughening
ridging, longitudinal or transverse
red or moth-eaten lunula

thinning or thickening of the plate
koilonychia
onychomadesis

Alopecia areata is not just a disease of hair.

Oranje AP, Peereboom-Wynia JDR, De Raeymaecker DMJ: **Trichotillomania** in childhood. J Am Acad Dermatol 1986; 15:614–619.

Trichotillomania is seven times more common in children than adults, and it is much more common in girls. It presents as **irregular patches** of **hair loss** with linear or **bizarre patterns** resulting from the patient pulling the hair out. The hairs are broken and of different lengths. There are no club hairs. Hairs may be found in the mouth, and nail biting (**onychophagia**) may be present. A scalp biopsy shows empty follicles and disfigured follicles (trichomalacia), with keratinous material and clumped melanin. Extravasated erythrocytes are sometimes visible in the epidermis around the follicle. The main differential diagnosis is **alopecia areata**. If only the eyelashes are involved, it is impossible to make a diagnosis.

Trigger factors:

hospitalization of child or parent
moving to new house
sibling rivalry
school problems

In this study of 21 children under 15 years of age with trichotillomania, psychiatric consultation was necessary in 11, and 4 required intensive psychiatric care. Mental retardation was present in 4 girls, and 4 patients also had extremely aggressive behavior.

Braun-Falco O, Imai S, Schmoeckel C, et al: **Pseudopelade** of Brocq. Dermatologica 1986; 172:18–23.

Careful study of 41 cases of **scarring alopecia** revealed the following diagnostic distribution:

pseudopelade of Brocq	26
lichen planopilaris	7
discoid lupus erythematosus	5
scleroderma	2
folliculitis decalvans	1

The patients with pseudopelade showed irregularly defined and confluent patches of **alopecia** with mild **perifollicular erythema** (early stage) and moderate **atrophy** (later stage). Spontaneous arrest of progression occurred after 2 to 18 years, with total loss of hair in only one patient.

Skin biopsy of early lesions showed scattered foci of lymphocytes in the reticular dermis and around hair follicles, which were dystrophic. Later lesions lacked hair follicles and sebaceous glands and had fibrous streams extending into adipose tissue. Direct immunofluorescence was negative except for occasional cases with IgM deposited at the basal membrane.

Sometimes the scarring is so subtle as to fool you into making a diagnosis of alopecia areata.

Some diagnoses are easy to make but hard to keep.

Amyloidosis

Here, it is the pathologist's turn to make the diagnosis. Your duty is to think of the diagnosis and secure a biopsy. And when should you think of it? In our experience, the localized cutaneous form has come to us as a **pruritic papular eruption** of the shins or a **macular hyperpigmented area** of the midback. However, it may also present as nodules or poikiloderma. Since scratching or rubbing favors the deposition of amyloid, many chronic pruritic eruptions show some amyloid when stained appropriately.

The systemic form has come to us as "**pinch purpura**" (Hurley's sign). Amyloid infiltrates of blood vessel walls render them fragile, with leakage demonstrable by a firm pinch. Unexplained ecchymoses of the eyelids may result from wiping any tears or having a massive cough. Plaques, papules, tumors, and even bullae may evolve. Amyloid infiltrates may be so extensive as to suggest scleroderma and myxedema.

In all instances, localized and systemic, a search must be made for multiple myeloma with its plasma cell source of amyloid paraprotein. Study the urine for Bence Jones protein, and obtain an immunoelectrophoretic study of both serum and a urine concentrate, as well as a bone marrow biopsy.

The word *amyloid* was coined by the pathologist Virchow 150 years ago to indicate a tissue deposit found in many organs that stained with iodine, just like starch, i.e., amylum. Today, we recognize it as a focal response, often due to scratching, or as a sign of multiple myeloma. When amyloid appears in the central nervous system, we have the "starch brain" of senile dementia and Alzheimer's disease.

Breathnach SM: **Amyloid** and **amyloidosis**. J Am Acad Dermatol 1988; 18:1–16.

Amyloidosis results from the tissue deposition of immunoglobulin light-chain material derived from a circulating paraprotein. The diagnosis of amyloidosis is a histologic one dependent on staining with methyl and cresyl violet (metachromasia), PAS, Congo red and Sirius red with or without fluorescence, and thioflavine T with fluorescence. Electron microscopy reveals a loose meshwork of rigid linear nonbranching aggregated paired fibers.

Localized cutaneous amyloidosis

1. **Nodular** amyloidosis: papules or nodules on the trunk, limbs, face, or genitalia
2. **Macular** amyloidosis: pruritic brown or gray macules on the upper back and limbs, often with rippled hyperpigmentation
3. **Lichen** amyloidosis: pruritic hyperkeratotic papules of the shins, spreading to the calves, feet, thighs, and trunk
4. Unusual forms:

   periocular hyperpigmentation
   poikiloderma
   simulator of nevoid pigmentation
   anosacral type with pigmented macules and glossy hyperkeratotic lesions radiating out from the anus (elderly Japanese men)

Systemic amyloidosis

1. **Tongue.** **Enlarged** and **firm** with **dentate impressions** on the lateral borders. The surface may be smooth and dry or studded with waxy papules, nodules, plaques, bullae, fissures, ulcers, and hemorrhage.
2. **Purpura.** This results from amyloid infiltration of blood vessel walls and develops upon pinching the skin. Petechiae and ecchymoses occur

especially on the eyelids, nasolabial folds, mouth, neck, axillae, umbilicus, and anogenital area. **Periorbital purpura** follows coughing, vomiting, the Valsalva maneuver, and proctoscopy. Transient **purpuric halos around de Morgan spots** give targetlike lesions. The purpura leads to posthemorrhagic hyperpigmentation.

3. **Papules, nodules, and plaques.** These characteristic smooth waxy shiny nonpruritic lesions may be skin colored, amber, or yellow, often with hemorrhagic changes. Occasionally, translucent lesions suggest vesicles. Flexural sites are favored, including the eyelids, retroauricular areas, neck, axillae, umbilicus, and inguinal and anogenital areas. The central area of the face, the lips, tongue, and buccal mucosa are also common locations. These lesions may resemble xanthomas or condylomata lata on vulvar and perianal skin.

4. **Tumefactive** plaques. Plaques may coalesce to give a leonine facies, occlusion of the auditory meatus, or cutis verticis gyrata.

5. Diffuse infiltration. This may mimic **scleroderma** on the face, hands, and feet, with loss of mobility and contractures of the fingers. Myxedema may also be suggested by rigidity of the face, rigid thick drooping eyelids, pendulous lips, and projecting ears. Patchy or universal alopecia may also result.

6. **Bullae.** These involve the skin or mucous membranes and are due to shearing within thermal amyloid deposits. They may be confused with **porphyria cutanea tarda.**

7. **Dystrophic nails.** Brittle, crumbly nails with subungual striations and partial or complete anonychia can be the first sign of amyloidosis.

8. **Cords.** These represent amyloid deposits in the walls of larger vessels.

9. **Cutis laxa.** This has been present in a few cases of familial neuropathic amyloidosis (Finland) and in one patient with plasma cell dyscrasia and amyloidosis.

10. **Urticaria.** In the autosomal dominant **Muckle-Wells syndrome,** periodic urticaria, fever, and limb pains are associated with progressive perceptive nerve deafness and renal amyloidosis.

11. **Erysipelaslike** lesions. These occur on the legs along with urticaria in the autosomal recessive disease familial Mediterranean fever. **Henoch-Schönlein purpura** and vasculitic nodules are also seen, along with renal amyloidosis, peritonitis, pleurisy, and synovitis.

12. Trophic changes. These occur in heredofamilial amyloid polyneuropathy.

13. Xerophthalmia and xerostomia. The **sicca syndrome** occurs because of amyloid deposits in the lacrimal and parotid glands.

14. **Carpal tunnel syndrome.** Amyloid infiltration and entrapment of nerves results in paresthesias, peripheral neuropathy, and muscle weakness.

15. Systemic findings:

> peripheral neuropathy
> plasma cell dyscrasia (myeloma)
> hepatomegaly
> edema (cardiac failure, nephrotic syndrome)
> cardiac symptoms
> claudication
> ulcerative colitis-like symptoms
> hematologic complications:
>> factor X deficiency
>> disseminated intravascular coagulation
>> fibrinolysis with severe bleeding

To distinguish between "primary" and **myeloma-associated amyloidosis,** the following studies should be done:

immunoelectrophoresis of serum
immunoelectrophoresis of concentrated urine
Bence Jones protein
bone marrow biopsy

To know amyloidosis is to know medicine.

Wang W-J: Clinical features of cutaneous amyloidosis. Clin Dermatol 1990; 8:13–19.

Cutaneous amyloidosis comes in **many disguises**. Watch it fool you into mistaking it for:

lichen simplex chronicus	tinea cruris
prurigo simplex	pruritus ani
prurigo nodularis	bullous pemphigoid
lichen planus	pemphigus
keratosis pilaris	bullous drug eruption
colloid milium	porphyria cutanea tarda
papular mucinosis	poikiloderma
solar elastosis	**vitiligo**
postinflammatory hyperpigmentation	

Only by biopsy can you remove the mask and perceive the true identity of lichen amyloidosis, macular amyloidosis, and nodular amyloidosis. What you thought to be vitiligo, a bullous disease, or poikiloderma may actually be amyloidosis.

Ratz JL, Bailin PL: Cutaneous amyloidosis. A case report of the tumefactive variant and a review of the spectrum of clinical presentations. J Am Acad Dermatol 1981; 4:21–26.

A 72-year-old woman was referred for treatment of multiple basal cell carcinomas of the scalp. She also had recently developed atrophic lesions of the chest and back, read on biopsy as **lichen sclerosus et atrophicus**. The growths on the scalp were multiple **waxy** infiltrated **nodules** with **superficial telangiectasia**. Biopsy showed marked deposition of pale eosinophilic material, but no epithelioma. Crystal violet staining was positive for amyloid. Once the diagnosis of primary localized cutaneous amyloidosis had been made, the biopsy material from the atrophic chest lesion was stained with crystal violet and proved to be amyloidosis.

This nodular form of amyloidosis presents as **waxy nodules** easily mistaken for bullae. Patients must be examined carefully and followed for evidence of systemic amyloidosis. Plaques on the hands may also herald systemic amyloidosis, with the hands being taut, shiny, and waxy with decreased range of motion, all suggesting **scleroderma** until a biopsy and special stains are done.

"**Pinch purpura**," which develops instantly after trauma (e.g., a diagnostic pinch by the examiner), is another diagnostic sign of systemic amyloidosis. It occurs because the periadventitial deposition of amyloid results in a vessel wall that is easily ruptured. This does not occur in primary amyloidosis. The deposition of amyloid in systemic amyloidosis also may result in **alopecia**, enlarged tongue, **vocal changes**, and difficulty in swallowing. Such changes may suggest **lipoid proteinosis, hypothyroidism**, and senile purpura.

Should systemic amyloidosis be found, a search for multiple myeloma or plasma cell dyscrasia is indicated. However, longstanding chronic inflammatory or infectious disease more commonly is responsible, such as rheumatoid arthritis, osteomyelitis, or ulcerative colitis. In all, deposits of amyloid in the kidney and liver may be massive and disruptive.

But this patient showed only the nodules of the primary cutaneous form and an unusual atrophic form. Her atrophic lesions remind us that there is a poikilodermalike type of amyloidosis that may be diffuse, localized, or part of a syndrome that includes photosensitivity, palmoplantar keratoses, blisters, and short stature. She did not show evidence of the other two major forms: oval hyperpigmented patches (macular amyloidosis) or hyperkeratotic papules (**lichen amyloidosis**).

Amyloidosis can slip out of your diagnostic net if you fail to do a biopsy and stain for amyloid.

Wong C-K: Mucocutaneous manifestations in systemic amyloidosis. Clin Dermatol 1990; 8:7–12.

The mouth is an excellent entrance into the diagnosis of systemic amyloidosis. The **tongue** is enlarged with dental indentations, and it may also have yellowish nodules, **hemorrhagic bullae**, and sequential erosions. Firmness and induration indicate an amyloid infiltrate. In advanced cases macroglossia leads to difficulty in swallowing and speaking.

As you look at the mucosa, there may be petechiae and ecchymoses indicative of fragile amyloid-infiltrated blood vessels. The infiltrates may also cause swellings of the mucosa, **xerostomia**, and pain. Surprisingly the gingivae appear normal, although amyloid is present.

Intraoral biopsy is indicated and may be more instructive than the classically recommended rectal biopsy for diagnosing systemic amyloidosis.

Look for skin pallor due to the vascular infiltrates and also for the **palms** and **fingertips** to be **smooth** and **waxy**. Another valuable clue is periorbital purpura. Infiltrates in the skin may cause papules, nodules, and tumors. In the scalp or axilla, there may be a spot of alopecia or even diffuse hair loss. Again, the biopsy provides the diagnosis.

Wong C-K, Lin C-S: **Friction amyloidosis**. Int J Dermatol 1988; 27:302–307.

A 62-year-old man had markedly pruritic, hyperpigmented macules over his upper back, arms, shoulders, and shins for 10 years. The unique feature was the **rippled** patterning to the **pigmentation**. He often used a plastic "back scratcher" to relieve his itch.

Biopsy provided the diagnosis of **macular amyloidosis**. Staining was done with Congo red, pagoda red, and crystal violet. The globular deposits of amyloid seen in the papillary dermis, as well as the increase in melanin, were viewed as the result of a long period of friction.

If you don't know what else to do, palpate the lesion.

Angiomas

I. ANGIOMAS

The physician's diagnostic role in evaluating vascular growths in infancy is to distinguish the hemangiomas from the vascular malformations. The **hemangioma** is usually **inapparent** on the **day of birth**, whereas a vascular malformation may be present at birth. The single most important feature of a hemangioma is its **rapid growth**. In contrast, the malformation enlarges in a manner commensurate with the child's growth. The hemangioma is programmed to disappear, the malformation to persist. Thus the hemangioma will begin to show ulceration, bleeding, and the grayish areas of infarctive involution in the first few years. Look for this. Not all hemangiomas are superficial and bright red. Some are deep and have the subdued hue of the deeper venous, arterial, or lymphatic malformations. It is important not to make a fast diagnosis on the first visit but to observe the child at regular intervals during the early months.

Palpation is valuable. The **hemangioma** has a **firm** feel, whereas the **malformation** is **soft** and can be completely **emptied of blood by compression**. The hemangioma cannot.

The rapid growth of the bright red hemangioma does not signal malignancy. These growths are benign, but on very rare occasions a rapidly growing subcutaneous mass may be a sarcoma. Firmness of the mass is one indicator pointing to the need for computed tomography and biopsy. Computed tomography with dye injection is necessary, at times, to distinguish the heterogeneous density of a malformation from the homogeneity of a hemangioma.

The vascular malformation in its minor form presents as the **nevus flammeus**. Unlike the hemangioma it shows no growth spurt, only a steady lifetime enlargement commensurate with the child's growth. The more serious malformations lead to throbbing pain, local **hyperhidrosis, hypertrichosis**, pulsations, and functional impairment. The altered blood flow can lead to ulcers mimicking the stasis ulcer. More alarming, an arteriovenous aneurysm can present in an infant as congestive heart failure.

With all vascular malformations one has to ask:

    Could it be a hemangioma?
    Is there systemic involvement?
    Is the lesion malignant?
    Is the skeletal growth normal?
    Is the circulation compromised?
    Is the origin venous, arterial, or lymphatic, or a combination?

Consultation with the peripheral vascular specialist or the vascular surgeon is essential. In many instances of extensive complex vascular malformations, the problem rises above the level of medical competence.

II. KAPOSI'S SARCOMA

For over 100 years Kaposi's sarcoma was an entity that languished in the backwaters of medical diagnosis. It was a strange acquired angioma occasionally seen in elderly men from Middle Eastern Europe, where Kaposi first observed it in 1872. All this changed in the last decade. Kaposi's sarcoma suddenly became headline news when it was found to be the scarlet letter of AIDS. The purple or red macules of Kaposi were appearing in young men with AIDS and indeed could be the presenting diagnostic sign. At first, every new red spot became the object of biopsy.

Awareness grew of the fact that Kaposi lesions could appear in patients in whom **immunosuppression** was induced by chemotherapy or lymphoma. Also, an endemic form in tropical Africa received increasing attention.

The skin had become a window not only to the diagnosis of acquired immuno-deficiency but also to visceral disease. In the classic Kaposi's sarcoma, any internal organ or lymph node may show these angiomatous tumors. However, the small bowel is the most common site. In the **AIDS-related Kaposi's**, half of the patients have bowel or lymph node involvement and a third have the growths in their lungs. Kaposi's sarcoma is an internal disease that in some instances may skip the skin itself. However, whenever it is suspected, an HIV test is indicated.

Watch for it with **purple macules** that progress and coalesce to form dark red **plaques** and **nodules**, and even tumors. In the classic form the legs and feet will be involved. There eventually is associated local **brawny edema** as well as lymphedema that results from circulatory interference. In the AIDS form there is a predilection for lesions to appear on the face, the oral mucosa, and the trunk.

III. ANGIOSARCOMA

Think angiosarcoma when you see:

1. A patch of dilated vessels or erythema on the face or scalp of an elderly person
2. A growth on a limb with chronic lymphedema (the Stewart-Treves syndrome)
3. A papule, a thickening, or an ulcer in an area of prior irradiation

And don't just think. Do a biopsy.

IV. VASCULAR MISCELLANY

Blue and red are the colors of the flag of the blood vessel country; remember, they may fade when pressed. Likewise, they are darker with a tourniquet placed upstream. The colors are usually solid but, on occasion, may be linear wave forms. Such is **telangiectasia**. Its distinctiveness merits its own special heading elsewhere as another diagnostic entry point.

Without question, the most common growth of blood vessels is the **cherry angioma** or De Morgan spot. These small **bright-red papules** dot the trunk and speak of age, pregnancy, or liver disease. Occasionally a biopsy is necessary to distinguish them from the vascular papules of **Fabry's disease** (angiokeratoma corporis diffusum). Ordinarily the presence of the hyperkeratotic caps of Fabry's papules makes the distinction easy. Similarly the **angiokeratomas of Mibelli** coming as they do on the hands and feet are recognizable. More common are the **angiokeratomas** of the **scrotum** (Fordyce).

Of the vascular rarities, **angioma serpiginosum** is an intriguing example. Coming on as bright-red angiomatous puncta, it may become papular, form new lesions, and fade in the center. This progressive course leaves rings and serpiginous patterns on a background of erythema.

Dark-blue, easily compressed blebs on the lips, face, ears, or elsewhere are called **venous lakes**; they are the venous analogue of the cherry angioma.

Interest in the **pyogenic granuloma** has been enhanced by the fact that in **cat scratch disease** the pyogenic granulomas that appear can be shown on biopsy to be studded with small gram-negative bacilli. This common example of proud flesh may also appear in cystic acne patients receiving Accutane. The role of bacteria seems assured.

But whatever their names, their shades of red or blue, or their causes, everything in this section is an angioma.

Examples

Leung AKC, Feingold M: Picture of the month: **Salmon patches**. Am J Dis Child 1985; 139:1231–1232.

Bright-red "**angel kisses**" on the forehead and eyelids of newborns start to fade at about 6 months as skin translucency decreases. Occipital and nuchal "**stork bites**" often persist after 12 months, and these **nevus flammeus** lesions may still flush in adulthood with anger or extreme cold.

Bean WB, Walsh JR: **Venous lakes**. Arch Dermatol 1956; 74:459–463.

These dark-blue–purple papules resemble simple blood blisters until compression with a finger or glass slide evacuates the blood and fades the lesion to a red-claret color. When pressure is released, a 1- to 2-mm saucerlike depression remains, which refills slowly with venous blood flowing into this "stagnant venous estuary." After 10 to 20 seconds the crumpled surface is puffed out again. Lesions occur most commonly on the **ears, face**, and **lips** of men over 60 years of age and probably result from a combination of aging and outdoor exposure.

Mihara M, Kambe N, Shimao S: **Superficial spreading capillary hemangioma**. A peculiar type of capillary hemangioma. Dermatologica 1986; 172:116–119.

A dark-red, nonpulsatile, irregular 5- by 10-mm plaque on the right sole of a 57-year-old Japanese woman had been asymptomatic for several years but was slowly enlarging. Biopsy showed a capillary hemangioma.

The histologic **differential diagnosis** includes:

> eruptive senile angioma (red papule)
> granuloma pyogenicum (rapid growth)
> angioblastoma (painful, dark-violet plaque with black-brown nodules, slowly growing)
> gemmangioma (capillary hemangioma with mucinous stroma)
> strawberry mark (infancy)
> verrucous hemangioma (warty hyperkeratotic surface)
> tufted angioma (dark-red plaque on neck and trunk of adults; balloon pattern on biopsy)

Burge SM, Baran R, Dawber RPR, Verret JL: Periungual and subungual arteriovenous tumours. Br J Dermatol 1986; 115:361–366.

Four examples of tender, **painful** acquired **bluish nodules** under the fingernail were proven to be **arteriovenous tumors** (cirsoid aneurysms). The differential diagnosis included glomus tumor, pyogenic granuloma, and angiomatous nevus.

Each **subungual vascular tumor** presented as a **longitudinal red line** with distal fissuring of the nail plate. They could be distinguished from the glomus tumor clinically, since they were not exquisitely tender. Unlike a granuloma pyogenicum, they neither bled nor showed progressive enlargement.

Davies MG, Greaves MW, Coutts A, Black AK: Nevus oligemicus. A variant of nevus anemicus. Arch Dermatol 1981; 117:111–113.

A large irregular area of **persistent, fixed, livid erythema** had been present for 14 years on the right flank of a 46-year-old man. It appeared to be either a simple superficial angioma or inflammatory erythema. He had never been aware of any abnormality of sensation or sweating in the area.

Skin biopsy revealed normal morphology with no sign of hemangioma, but capillary microscopy revealed dilated capillaries. Photoelectric plethysmography showed a lower surface temperature than normal skin, indicative of reduced thermal skin blood flow. The lesion showed normal responses to vasodilator and vasoconstrictor stimuli. Incomplete autonomic sympathetic

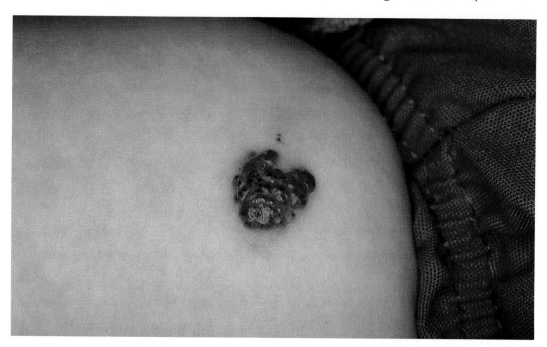

neural blockade, achieved with infiltration of local anesthetic, abolished parts of the nevus, suggesting that increased adrenergic activity played a major role in the genesis of this nevus.

vasodilator tests
> intradermal histamine phosphate (1.0 μg/0.1 ml phosphate buffered saline)
> topical thurfyl nicotinate (Trafuril)

vasoconstrictor tests
> topical scopolamine hydrobromide (9% in 0.154 M phosphate-buffered saline)
> intradermal norepinephrine bitartrate (0.05 ml of 0.00005 to 0.5 μg in 0.154 M phosphate-buffered saline)
> topical clobetasol propionate (0.05% ointment, 10 hr under occlusion)

Pharmacologic study indicated that the redness resulted from stasis of the superficial nutritional vasculature due to increased vasoconstrictor tone of thermoregulatory vessels in the involved skin. Like **nevus anemicus**, it is a **pharmacologic nevus**, with an underlying abnormality of sympathetic adrenergic activity with reduced cutaneous blood flow. By contrast, in nevus anemicus there is shutdown in both the nutritional and thermoregulatory vessel flow, producing a blanch rather than a flush.

Wilson Jones E, Orkin M: **Tufted angioma (angioblastoma)**: A benign progressive angioma not to be confused with Kaposi's sarcoma or low-grade angiosarcoma. J Am Acad Dermatol 1989; 20:214–225.

A slowly progressive angioma, often on the neck or trunk, may appear at any time in life. Histologic examination is indicated to rule out Dabska's malignant endovascular angioendothelioma in children as well, and angiosarcoma in the elderly, or Kaposi's sarcoma at any age.

The unique feature of this form of angioma is the presence of **multiple small vascular tufts** of vessels in the dermis.

Clinical diagnosis entertained before biopsy included:

lymphoma	lipogranuloma	birthmark
sarcoidosis	connective tissue nevus	morphea

Systemic Involvement

Meijer P, Hasper MF, Bijleveld CMA, et al: **Infantile hemangiomatosis** with involvement of skin, liver and placenta. Br J Dermatol 1988; 118:838–839.

A 2-month-old infant with multiple 1- to 4-mm **papular hemangiomas** developed **neonatal jaundice** that could not be controlled by phototherapy. Liver function tests indicated obstructive icterus. Fearing extrahepatic bile duct atresia, the surgeons performed a laparotomy and liver biopsy. Multiple hemangiomas (not seen on laparoscopy) were present in the liver, and the jaundice was attributed to hemangioma-induced cholestasis.

Following several months of systemic corticosteroid therapy given to reduce the risk of cirrhosis, the cutaneous hemangiomas totally regressed. Liver function tests returned to normal after 1 year.

The presence of multiple hemangiomas in the skin alerts the physician to their possible presence elsewhere in the body, with implications for causing bleeding, obstruction, and complications after invasive procedures.

Vase P, Grove O: Gastrointestinal lesions in **hereditary hemorrhagic telangiectasia**. Gastroenterology 1986; 91:1079–1083.

Gastrointestinal bleeding is the most frequent form of bleeding after **epistaxis** in patients with hereditary hemorrhagic telangiectasia. Endoscopic study of 28 patients with the disease revealed that the telangiectases were usually located in the upper gastrointestinal tract, predominately the stomach and duodenum. In this Danish study of affected persons in one county (several islands), there was a significantly higher frequency of blood group O among patients with hereditary hemorrhagic telangiectasia than in the background population, as it occurred in nearly 70% of the patients compared with 41% of controls.

Nakamura T, Kaneko H, Nishino I: **Angiokeratoma corporis diffusum** (Fabry disease): Ultrastructural studies of the skin. Acta Derm Venereol 1981; 61:37–41.

A 34-year-old man first noted a dark-red punctate eruption of the lower abdomen at age 20, which gradually spread over his chest, back, inguinal region, and scrotum. **Clusters** of symmetrical **pinhead-size punctate telangiectases** were seen over much of the body. From age 5 to 13 years he had experienced episodes of recurrent fever, myalgia, and fatigue several times a year. At age 23 he developed persistent edema of the legs and was found to have proteinuria and nephritis. His family history revealed that a 27-year-old male cousin had the same condition.

A skin biopsy showed dilated capillaries and fine PAS-positive granules in the sweat gland cells. Electron microscopy proved these granules to be the myelinlike concentric lamellar structures characteristic of **Fabry's disease**. They were also present in endothelial cells, fibroblasts, and myoepithelium. A low serum α-galactosidase level confirmed the diagnosis of Fabry's disease.

This inherited enzyme deficiency leads to damaging deposits of ceramide trihexoside in vascular walls, with resulting **renal failure**, cardiomegaly, hypertension, and **neurologic changes**. Gradually, endothelial cells are replaced by thrombi, which probably account for the telangiectatic lesions (angiokeratoma corporis diffusum).

This is another example of telangiectasis dilating our awareness of what is going on inside the body.

Viljoen D, Saxe N, Pearn J, Beighton P: The cutaneous manifestations of **Klippel-Trenaunay-Weber syndrome**. Clin Exp Dermatol 1987; 12:12–17.

A comprehensive survey of 20 patients with angio-osteohypertrophy.

The "big three" essentials for a diagnosis of Klippel-Trenaunay-Weber syndrome include: limb overgrowth, cutaneous angiomas, and varicose veins.

The types of angiomas include the **nevus flammeus** and **cavernous hemangiomas**. The nevi flammei are present at birth and may be located over all areas of the body, especially the involved limbs. They are sharply demarcated, rarely cross the midline, and are large dark-brown, purple, or erythematous macules that blanch on pressure. In early adulthood they develop nodular vascular excrescences. Cavernous hemangiomas are uncommon and not noted at birth. These raised bluish lesions blanch on pressure and vary in size from 1 cm to large tumors.

Varicose veins are sometimes not seen until late childhood. They are due to hypoplasia or atresia of deep venous channels and the absence of valves in superficial veins. High venous pressure leads to fluid leakage and **brawny, nonpitting edema**, with fibrosis of lymphatic vessels. Severe gravitational (**stasis**) **ulcers** result, as well as sepsis.

A common skin finding often necessitating hospitalization is **recurrent aseptic cellulitis**, with acute fever and painful erythematous indurated cutaneous plaques in the affected limb. Cultures are always sterile, leading to speculation that thrombotic episodes in small arteriovenous channels and capillaries are the cause, akin to sickle cell disease.

Miscellaneous unusual skin findings include:

> dark, sharply demarcated, **pigmented streaks** over the skin in a random distribution, seldom crossing the midline and not related to limb hypertrophy
> telangiectasia
> **polypoid fibromas**
> peau d'orange (prominent follicular openings)
> **cutis marmorata** (may reflect increased blood flow to underlying tissues of the affected limb)

Nielsen JR, Tschen EH: **Klippel-Trenaunay-Weber syndrome**. Cutis 1987; 40:51–53.

Superficial varicose veins and **port-wine stain** hemangiomas on an enlarged leg make up the triad of Klippel-Trenaunay-Weber. It may also occur on an arm or involve both legs. The varicose veins lead to compromised venous return, with resulting ulcers, dyskeratosis, and edema. Although many veins are filled with thrombi, pulmonary embolism is not a feature. The arterial system is generally normal except for arteriovenous fistulas, but lymphatic vessels may be hypoplastic or hyperplastic with **lymphangiomas**.

The angiomas are present at birth, whereas varicosities become evident as the child begins to walk, and **limb hypertrophy appears later**. All tissue layers are enlarged, presumably from heightened arterial perfusion. The prognosis is generally favorable, although limb amputation may be necessary if heart failure develops.

Björkholm M, Aschberg S: Functional aspects of the **Klippel-Trenaunay** and related **syndromes**. Acta Derm Venereol 1980; 60:409–413.

The simultaneous presence of varicose veins, hemangiomas, and **osteohypertrophy** of **one limb** is known as the Klippel-Trenaunay syndrome, described in 1900. A similar enlargement of one limb was described by Parkes Weber in patients with **arteriovenous fistulas**. Similarly, agenesis of the deep veins results in osteohypertrophy.

The present study of eight patients links these entities by pointing out that increased venous pressure in the epiphyseal zone is the common pathogenic denominator of osteohypertrophy. Thus, in essence, the hemangiomas of the Klippel-Trenaunay patients are acting functionally as arteriovenous fistulas with high venous pressures. Furthermore, the child with venous agenesis or deep-venous phlebitis has elevated venous pressure, again driving increased bone growth.

Tilsley DA, Burden PW: A case of **Maffucci's syndrome**. Br J Dermatol 1981; 105:331–336.

In 1881, Maffucci described a 40-year-old woman, mother of four healthy sons, who had frequent severe hemorrhage from an ulcerated tumor on her left middle finger. Her forearm was amputated in an effort to save her life, but a few days later she died of sepsis (probably acquired from cases of erysipelas on the ward). Maffucci undertook a thorough investigation at autopsy.

A 24-year-old man with Maffucci's syndrome had short stature, scoliosis, and innumerable hemangiomas hanging in grapelike clusters on the right hand, legs, and feet. His greatest handicap was inadequate footwear, necessitating bedroom slippers, which rotted in wet weather. When he tried to wear leather boots, friction caused skin breakage and infection. His big toenails became ingrown and infected, with resulting **recurrent cellulitis** and **lymphedema** of the right buttock. He walked with a waddle and tired easily.

History revealed the onset of hemangiomas at age 5 years on his right middle finger. No other siblings were affected. At age 12 he had a **pathologic fracture** of the left tibia, which was slow to heal and left a deformity. Later he had pain and swelling of the left knee joint.

X-rays revealed involvement of almost every bone with **enchondromatosis**, which resulted in growth impairment and asymmetrical shortening of long bones. The soft tissue swellings contained calcification, representing hemangiomas with phleboliths.

Over all this hangs the cloud that some day one of the enchondromas will transform into a malignant **chondrosarcoma**.

Esterly NB: **Kasabach-Merritt syndrome** in infants. J Am Acad Dermatol 1983; 8:504–513.

A 14-day-old baby boy was hospitalized with pallor and a **rapidly enlarging cavernous hemangioma** of the left axilla. Present since birth, the 8-cm mass was red, firm, nontender, and without bruits. Laboratory studies revealed hemoglobin 6.4, platelet count 19,000/mm^3, fragmented red blood cells on blood smear, prolonged prothrombin time (PT) and partial thromboplastin time (PTT), decreased fibrinogen, and elevated fibrin split products.

The diagnosis was Kasabach-Merritt syndrome: rapidly enlarging hemangioma with microangiopathic **hemolytic anemia** and **thrombocytopenia**.

Within days **petechiae** and **purpura** appeared, particularly concentrated over the hemangioma, as platelets fell to 1900/mm^3. Prednisone therapy (4 mg/kg/day) and heparin (75 mg/kg IV every 4 h) reversed the process.

Three other similar cases are presented. Immediate hematologic evaluation is indicated if the syndrome is suspected. Warning signs include rapidly **enlarging hemangioma**, sometimes **simulating cellulitis** (tense woody texture, taut, shiny, color change); petechiae and ecchymoses; pallor; and **prolonged bleeding** (from punctures and abrasions, the umbilicus, circumcision site, epistaxis, hematuria, hematochezia).

These infants come frighteningly close to death as platelets are trapped and destroyed in the hemangioma. **Disseminated intravascular coagulation** may also result.

Diagnosis can be facilitated by mentally transposing the lesion to other sites.

Hruza GJ, Snow SN: Cutaneous **Mycobacterium bovis infection** of 40 years' duration. Arch Dermatol 1990; 126:123–124.

An Asymptomatic red plaque had been on the right upper arm for 40 of this man's 57 years. It had been diagnosed by several of his physicians as a hemangioma. At this time, it was noted only incidentally in the course of therapy for actinic keratoses elsewhere.

On examination the 5- by 4-cm **red plaque** actually exhibited **numerous small red-brown nodules** over a few depressed white areas. The biopsy showed a **granulomatous inflammation**, but without well-formed granulomas. No hemangioma was present. Ziehl-Nielsen staining was negative. The mycobacterial culture, however, yielded *M. bovis*, and on repeat biopsy a solitary acid-fast bacillus was seen. Roentgenograms revealed a few calcified hilar lymph nodes and some calcified mesenteric lymph nodes.

A diagnosis of **lupus vulgaris** due to *M. bovis* infection was made. Noteworthy then was a long history of **positive tuberculin skin tests**, although his serial chest roentgenograms had been essentially negative, and he had no fever, night sweats, weight loss, cough, or dyspnea.

Years ago, *M. bovis* accounted for up to 50% of tuberculosis in man. Now the organism is a rarity. This patient's problem probably began in childhood as a result of drinking **unpasteurized milk**. Forty years later it took a high index of suspicion, two biopsies, and a mycobacterial culture to make the diagnosis.

Aso M, Kawaguchi T, Mihara M, et al: **Pseudotail** associated with spinal dysraphism. Dermatologica 1987; 174:45–48.

Human tails are caudal appendages of the sacrococcygeal or lumbar region and are usually associated with underlying bony defects such as **spina bifida** or spinal dysraphism. Overlying cutaneous signs of spinal dysraphism may include **hairy tuft, dimple, sinus, pigmented macule**, and **vascular nevus**.

A 5-year-old Japanese girl had a 1-cm pedunculated fatty mass with sparse terminal hairs protruding from the upper medial aspect of the enlarged left buttock. Present since birth, it was surrounded by a 4.5-cm area of **erythema with telangiectasia**. X-ray showed spina bifida of L-5 and sacrum, and expansion of the spinal canal lower than L-4. **Computed tomography** disclosed a bony defect in the left sacrum and confirmed that the mass had the same density as subcutaneous fat. The diagnosis was pseudotail with hairy vascular nevus.

Since there was no movement or contraction of this tail, and it did not contain striated muscle, it was not a true tail. This example contained a **lipoma**, but others may represent vertebral extension, chondrodystrophy, teratoma, or parasitic fetus.

Cotterill JA: **Lupus vulgaris simulating** a **port-wine stain**. Br J Dermatol 1988; 119:127–128.

A 67-year-old woman was referred for consideration of laser therapy for a presumed **port-wine stain**. She stated that she had been born with a small birthmark on the right ear lobe that had been unsuccessfully treated with cautery as well as with x-rays. Subsequently the lesion spread to her face and over the past 10 years had covered most of her right cheek. Biopsy of the vascular-looking violaceous eruption confirmed the clinical diagnosis of lupus vulgaris. Response to treatment with rifampin and isoniazid was excellent.

The diagnostic clue here was the **progression of the lesion**, not seen in port-wine stains.

Olsen TG, Helwig EB: **Angiolymphoid hyperplasia** with **eosinophilia**. A clinicopathologic study of 116 patients. J Am Acad Dermatol 1985; 12:781–796.

Angiomalike, **smooth, dome-shaped pink** to **red-brown papules** or plaques on the **face, scalp**, and **neck** suggest angiolymphoid hyperplasia with eosinophilia. Subcutaneous cystlike masses without distinguishing surface features also occur. Multiple lesions tend to merge into "**grapelike" plaques**, and some lesions are painful when compressed.

Skin biopsy reveals anomalous vascular proliferation with varying degrees of inflammatory infiltrates (lymphocytes and eosinophils). Arteriovenous shunts and intravascular endothelial proliferation are common features.

The **histologic spectrum** includes the following entities:

> inflammatory angiomatous nodules
> pseudo (atypical) pyogenic granuloma
> histiocytoid hemangioma
> epithelioid hemangioma
> Kimura's disease

Only once in 116 cases did the clinician make the diagnosis before biopsy.

Handfield-Jones SE, Kennedy CTC, Bradfield JB: Angiosarcoma arising in an **angiomatous naevus** following **irradiation** in childhood. Br J Dermatol 1988; 118:109–112.

A young woman had a vascular nodule below the right eyebrow. It had been flat at birth but gradually enlarged, causing displacement of the right eye by 7 months of age. She then received cobalt 60 irradiation over 6 months, followed by administration of grenz rays to a residual nodule. A small nodule remained at the inner canthus, and when she was age 20 it began to grow. Excisions then and again 2 years later failed to show malignancy, but at age 24 the recurring tumor was recognized as an angiosarcoma, requiring wide excision and grafting.

This **radiation-induced angiosarcoma** of early adulthood stands in contrast to the angiosarcoma of the face and scalp of the aged. Angiosarcoma may also occur in a limb with chronic lymphedema (Stewart-Treves syndrome).

Bondi EE, Clark WH Jr: Clinical differentiation of adult-onset cavernous angioma from nodular malignant melanoma. Arch Dermatol 1980; 116:299–300.

Thirty seconds of firm **thumb pressure on** a **nodule** of malignant melanoma has no effect, whereas the same maneuver virtually converts the nodule of an angioma into a macule.

The validity of the test proved biopsy-verifiable in all 16 patients studied. Interestingly, the **angiomas** were **blue-black** and **mimicked malignant melanoma** on simple visual inspection without compression.

*To learn how to recognize somebody's grandmother there's nothing
like meeting her.*

Alessi E, Sala F: **Bluefarb-Stewart syndrome**—Report of a new case. Dermatologica 1984; 169:93–96.

For 5 years a 25-year-old man watched a small violaceous patch on the medial surface of his right second toe become infiltrated with five smooth nodules. The lesions appeared to be **Kaposi's sarcoma**, clinically and histologically. However, the true diagnosis came with the demonstration of **arteriovenous fistulas** at the base of the toe, using Doppler flowmetry and right femoral arteriography.

The vascular growths were a pseudo-Kaposi sarcoma arising as a result of the acral arteriovenous malformation. This syndrome was independently described in 1967 by both Bluefarb and Stewart. It occurs on the **toes** in **young men** and is unilateral. It may also **mimic stasis dermatitis**.

Look beneath stasis dermatitis not only for venous incompetence but also for a venous fistula, using Doppler flowmetry.

Landthaler M, Stolz W, Eckert F, et al: **Pseudo-Kaposi's sarcoma** occurring after placement of arteriovenous shunt: A case report with DNA content analysis. J Am Acad Dermatol 1989; 21:499–505.

A **brown-to deep-purple plaque** covering the dorsum of the left hand of this 51-year-old man appeared 2 years after an **arteriovenous shunt** was placed in the left antecubital fossa for **hemodialysis**. The hand was painful and swollen.

Histologically the lesion showed dense proliferation of endothelial and spindle cells as well as slitlike vascular lumina. Although this is the picture of Kaposi's sarcoma, a diagnosis of pseudo-Kaposi's sarcoma was made in recognition of the pathogenesis of the lesion.

The patient had had a side-to-side anastomosis of the radial artery and the cephalic vein. This vein originates from a network on the dorsum of the hand but courses to the volar site of the anastomosis. The consequent retrograde blood flow resulted in elevated venous and capillary pressures with subsequent edema and a proliferative vascular response.

The same clinical picture may be seen in patients' with:

> chronic venous insufficiency
> congenital arteriovenous malformations
> Klippel-Trenaunay syndrome
> paralyzed limbs

And, oh yes, the DNA analysis of the spindle cells distinguished this patient's pseudoform from authentic Kaposi's.

Marshall ME, Hatfield ST, Hatfield DR: **Arteriovenous malformation** simulating Kaposi's sarcoma (**pseudo-Kaposi's sarcoma**). Arch Dermatol 1985; 121:99–101.

Based on observations of nodules on the first two toes of the left foot, a clinical and histologic diagnosis of Kaposi's sarcoma had been made 2 years previously in this 22-year-old man. Radiation therapy had been without effect.

The skin of the distal third of the foot had a mild purple hue. The foot itself was swollen, boggy, and considerably larger than the right foot. At times the area was painful. Auscultation disclosed a loud bruit over the nodule on the plantar surface.

Arteriography demonstrated a large arteriovenous malformation and thus the correct diagnosis of pseudo-Kaposi's sarcoma. The changes produced by such vascular malformations have also been called acroangiodermatitis or simply **angiodermatitis**. However, in this instance it closely simulated Kaposi's sarcoma and made for diagnostic error until arteriography was done.

Arteriovenous malformations are not difficult to suspect if one but remembers to:

> feel for the warmth and the diagnostic thrill of increased arterial blood supply
> listen for the bruit and the patient's complaint of pain and paresthesias
> look for edema and enlarged foot varices

Kolde G, Wörheide J, Baumgartner R, Bröcker E-B: Kaposi-like **acroangiodermatitis** in an above-knee **amputation stump**. Br J Dermatol 1989; 120:575–580.

A 31-year-old amputee was referred for treatment of **painful purple-blue** skin **lesions of the stump** of his left thigh. They were interpreted as Kaposi's sarcoma, and they had been present for a number of years. Tests had been negative for the presence of human immunodeficiency viruses.

Biopsy showed vascular channels lined by pleomorphic endothelial cells, but no atypical cells or vascular slits were seen. Antibody stains for endothelial proliferation were positive.

A femoral arteriogram showed numerous vascular collaterals, but no arteriovenous fistulas. A diagnosis of acroangiodermatitis was made.

The cause was demonstrated to be insufficient padding of the amputated leg stump. Both clinically and radiologically one could note absence of soft tissue and muscle on the lateral side of the stump. The end of the bone was literally adherent to the skin.

Following surgical revision of the stump and fitting of a new prosthesis, the patient had no dermatologic or orthopedic problems.

In all instances of **pseudo-Kaposi's sarcoma** it is necessary to **rule out** the common cause of underlying **arteriovenous malformation**, either of congenital or traumatic origin. Sometimes such a hemodynamic shunt can be identified by a palpable thrill, a bruit, or simply increased warmth of the area. A deep biopsy can disclose abnormal shunts, but the best approach is **percutaneous arteriography**.

Some patients have "shotgun symptoms" that they spray all over you, much to your discomfort.

Goette DK, Detlefs RL: **Postirradiation angiosarcoma**. J Am Acad Dermatol 1985; 12:922–926.

A chronically **eroded, deep-purplish nodular tumor** had gradually developed on the left abdominal wall of a 61-year-old woman during the past 6 months. Her history revealed that 23 years earlier she had received 3000 rads of radiation to the abdomen for treatment of squamous cell carcinoma of the cervix.

Biopsy showed the nodule to be an angiosarcoma, a rare late complication of radiation. Other forms noted in the literature were diffusely infiltrative, or ulcerated. Most were asymptomatic, purplish-red, and some felt spongy. They all appeared within the radiation site, but diagnosis was delayed months to years. This is regrettable, since the lesion is an aggressive one best treated by immediate total excision.

The **skin memory** for radiation injury is phenomenal, some postirradiation angiosarcomas appearing after an interval of 40 years.

Tyring SK, Lee PC, Omura EF, et al: Recurrent and metastatic cutaneous neuro-endocrine (**Merkel cell**) **carcinoma mimicking angiosarcoma**. Arch Dermatol 1987; 123:1368–1370.

Bright **red-to-purple confluent nodules** and plaques extending over the top of the scalp and over the left eyebrow were the presenting problems of a 79-year-old man. They were clinically consistent with a diagnosis of angiosarcoma.

Routine histologic examination was not sufficient for a diagnosis. Immuno-histochemistry (neuron-specific enolase) and electron microscopy were necessary to show the neurosecretory granules in the malignant APUD (*a*mino *p*recursor *u*ptake and *d*ecarboxylation) cells and thus make a diagnosis of **Merkel cell carcinoma**.

Systemic chemotherapy led only to temporary remissions. The patient's reactive depression was followed by suicide.

Bencini PL, Sala F, Valeriani D, et al: Self-healing **pseudoangiosarcoma**. Unusual **vascular proliferation** resembling a vascular malignancy of the skin. Arch Dermatol 1988; 124:692–694.

Hundreds of **soft purplish translucent, vascular papules** and **nodules** (3 to 5 mm) graced the left inguinal area of an **extremely obese** (145 kg) 58-year-old woman. They covered an area 25 by 20 cm, forming an **oval vegetating plaque** between an adipose mass and the medial aspect of the thigh. Biopsy revealed malignant lymphatic vascular proliferation, similar to Kaposi's sarcoma. It was elected to watch and wait. Four months of dieting resulted in a loss of 13 kg and complete disappearance of the "malignant" lesions.

This patient thus had pseudomalignancy (histologically malignant, clinically benign). Other examples of **vascular pseudomalignant conditions** include:

pseudo-Kaposi's sarcoma secondary to arteriovenous malformation	angiolymphoid hyperplasia histiocytoid hemangioma cellular angioma of childhood
iatrogenic arteriovenous fistula	acquired progressive lymphangiomas
acroangiodermatitis of the foot	inflammatory angiomatoses
reactive proliferating angioendotheliomatosis	papillary endothelial hyperplasia vascular proliferation in nevus flammeus
granuloma pyogenicum	

When it comes to blood vessels, it would seem that all that multiplies is not malignant.

Vascular Miscellany

Campbell JP, Grekin RC, Ellis CN, et al: **Retinoid therapy** is associated with excess **granulation tissue responses**. J Am Acad Dermatol 1983; 9:708–713.

Both isotretinoin (Accutane) and etretinate (Tegison) favor a pathologic increase in granulation tissue around **acne cysts** and **ingrown toenails**. The response is idiosyncratic and not predictable.

Marcsco WA, Lester S, Parsonnet J: Unusual presentation of **cat scratch disease** in a patient positive for antibody to the **human immunodeficiency virus**. Rev Infect Dis 1989; 11:793–803.

A 26-year-old homosexual florist removed a hangnail from his right index finger and 1 week later developed redness and tenderness of the finger with a red streak up the arm. Despite treatment with dicloxacillin, he became febrile (temperature 102°F) and had right axillary adenopathy. Cephalexin also did not help. A 1.5-cm **mushroomlike pedunculated nodule** then appeared on the thigh (thought to be a giant molluscum), along with a 5-mm **nodule** of **granulation tissue** on the tip of the infected index finger (thought to be a pyogenic granuloma). Removal of the lesions and treatment with ciprofloxacin caused marked improvement, but there was recurrence of fever and lymphadenopathy. A 1.0-cm brown crusted growth appeared on the medial nail bed of the index finger, with swelling, erythema, pain, and a red streak 23 cm up the arm. He was found to be HIV antibody positive.

The finger lesion was a **pyogenic granuloma** (lobular capillary hemangioma). Numerous special bacterial stains were negative, but the **Warthin-Starry silver stain** revealed numerous small **coccobacilli** with occasional branched forms in clusters surrounding blood vessels, typical of **cat scratch disease**. The bacilli were gram negative (Brown-Hopps Gram technique).

Warthin-Starry stains should be obtained on all pyogenic granulomas, even if the patient is not sick. **Involution** of **widespread vascular lesions** has been observed with erythromycin, doxycycline, and antituberculous drugs (isoniazid, rifampin, ethambutol).

Once again, AIDS has provided us with a magnifying glass for seeing both the lesion and the causative organism, which presumably came from the patient's declawed cat.

Cockerell CJ, LeBoit PE: **Bacillary angiomatosis**: A newly characterized pseudoneoplastic, infectious, cutaneous vascular disorder. J Am Acad Dermatol 1990; 22:501–512.

This is a disease of the **immunocompromised** or **HIV-infected patient** that requires recognition and treatment with erythromycin to prevent death from visceral and mucosal involvement. Caused by a weakly reactive gram-negative bacillus easily demonstrated in biopsy by the Warthin-Starry stain, it manifests itself by widespread **vascular papules resembling Kaposi's sarcoma**.

The patient may literally have thousands of **pinpoint red papules** looking **like florid De Morgan spots** or but a few that fool the clinician into thinking of them as **pyogenic granulomas**. Others are subcutaneous. They feel rubbery and at times are fixed to underlying structures. When they are punctured the diagnostic sign of spirited bleeding appears. Any of the lesions may ulcerate with crusting or may simply have a normal-colored smooth surface. The oral mucosa and the gastrointestinal tract are other common sites. They may also arise in the conjunctival sac.

In the differential diagnosis, one finds bartonellosis due to infection by *Bartonella bacilliformis*, but this is limited to Peru. It does emphasize, however, the point that **bacteria can induce vascular growths**. Any disseminated pyogenic granulomata are bacillary angiomatosis until proven otherwise by a negative Warthin-Starry stain.

Think of bacillary angiomatosis in any subcutaneous tumor or a crusted ulcer in an AIDS patient.

Trau H, Fisher BK, Schewach-Millet M: Multiple clear cell acanthomas. Arch Dermatol 1980; 116:433–434.

Clear cell acanthomas have

> the vascular look of a pyogenic granuloma
> the stuck-on appearance of a seborrheic keratosis
> the exudate and scale of eczema
> the advancing rounded border of an epithelioma

Surprise your pathologist and recognize one before he does.

Hasegawa Y, Yasuhara M: **Phakomatosis pigmentovascularis type IVa**. Arch Dermatol 1985; 121:651–655.

The concurrent presence of large pigmentary and vascular nevi in an infant merits the label of phakomatosis pigmentovascularis. It may be further characterized as:

> Type I (Adamson-Best)—nevus flammeus and nevus pigmentosus et verrucosus
>   II (Takano-Krüger-Doi)—nevus flammeus and aberrant mongolian spots
>   III (Kobori-Toda)—nevus flammeus and nevus spilus
>   IV (Toda-Ono)—nevus flammeus, nevus spilus, and blue spots

Further subdivision of each type is made on the basis of systemic findings being absent (type a) or present (type b).

Never ask a new patient a question without notebook and pencil in hand.

WILLIAM OSLER

Anhidrosis

Anhidrosis and its lesser form, **hypohidrosis**, are easily overlooked. Sweating disorders may be **patchy** (psoriasis, atopic dermatitis), **diffuse** (miliaria rubra), or **segmental** (diabetic neuropathy, sympathectomy). In Horner's syndrome, unilateral anhidrosis of the face indicates sympathetic disruption, as from lung cancer.

The anhidrosis that must not be overlooked is the **generalized** form. With total inability to sweat, the patient in very hot environments becomes febrile and collapses. If the anhidrosis is unrecognized, the fever may be viewed as infectious and the collapse of vagal origin. The most **common cause** of a generalized inability to sweat is the congenital absence of sweat glands, seen in many ectodermal dysplasias. Other causes include Fabry's disease, multiple myeloma, diabetes mellitus, and atropine poisoning. Acquired anhidrosis also follows miliaria, as seen in military troops in the tropics. This may produce the **tropical asthenia syndrome**, with victims often accused of malingering. Even though the head and neck are drenched in sweat, the rest of the body is bone dry. Finally, **erythroderma** may be followed by permanent total inability to sweat because of destruction of sweat glands, as is seen with atabrine sensitivity.

In the patient suspected of having "**sweat gland insufficiency**" there is need for challenge by exposure and exercise in a hot room, as well as injection intradermally of pilocarpine or mecholyl. Once hypohidrosis is confirmed, the eccrine sweat glands should be searched for and studied histologically. Assessment of central nervous system and sympathetic nerve function is also indicated.

Challenge the sweat gland or you will miss the diagnosis of anhidrosis.

Etiology

Sato K, Kang WH, Saga K, Sato KT: Biology of sweat glands and their disorders: II. Disorders of sweat gland function. J Am Acad Dermatol 1989; 20:713–726.

Anhidrosis

Anhidrotic **ectodermal dysplasia** (Christ-Siemens-Touraine), usually X linked:

- hypotrichosis
- conical teeth
- saddle nose
- prominent forehead
- hyperkeratosis of palms and soles
- nail dystrophy
- congenital absence of sweat glands

Anhidrosis with **sensory neuropathy**, generalized anhidrosis, insensitivity to pain, mental retardation

- self-mutilation, painless ulcers, high fevers
- absence of myelinated nerves but normal numbers of sweat glands

Segmental anhidrosis

- heat intolerance
- may have tonic pupil (Ross syndrome)

Generalized idiopathic anhidrosis

Acquired generalized anhidrosis

- after sunstroke
- postmiliaria
- Guillain-Barré syndrome
- diabetic neuropathy
- Fabry's disease
- Sjögren's syndrome
- congenital ichthyosiform erythroderma

Localized hypohidrosis

- incontinentia pigmenti
- vitiligo in dermatomal distribution
- carbon monoxide poisoning
- any area of damage, e.g., scar, tumor, irradiation, infection, granuloma
- scleroderma
- vasculitis

Discerning an absence of sweating is much more challenging than simply observing hyperhidrosis.

Grice K, Verbov J: Sweat glands and their disorders. Recent Adv Dermatol 1977; 4:155–198.

Look for anhidrosis:

skin diseases

miliaria	atopic dermatitis
erythroderma	ichthyosis
psoriasis	ectodermal dysplasia

neurologic disorders

sympathetic section or injury	quadriplegia
Adie's syndrome	idiopathic orthostatic hypotension
Horner's syndrome	peripheral nerve lesion
multiple sclerosis	diabetic neuropathy

Cockayne's syndrome

247

multiple myeloma

Hodgkin's disease

Shelley WB, Horvath PN, Pillsbury DM: **Anhidrosis**: An etiologic interpretation. Medicine 1950; 29:195–224.

The diagnosis of anhidrosis is not made by simply looking at the patient. As **a diagnosis of function** it must be elicited by history or by observation of the skin under thermal or pharmacologic challenge (**sweat function tests**).

Most examples of anhidrosis are trivial, localized, inapparent, and of little concern to the patient or doctor. In fact, localized anhidrosis is produced daily with antiperspirants, which block the sweat ducts.

Numerous dermatitides likewise induce poral blockade, as witnessed in dyshidrosis with its sweat entrapment. The sweat gland may also be destroyed, as in radiodermatitis or a thermal burn, or may undergo a temporary **fatigue hypohidrosis**. Immune reactions may damage the gland, or drugs may inhibit its function. Usually the patient couldn't care less (a "no-sweat" situation).

Sometimes even extensive medically significant anhidrosis is inapparent unless tested for. Most subtle and serious is the congenital absence of sweat glands seen in hypohidrotic **ectodermal dysplasias**. This may adversely affect an individual for years before the absence of sweat function is sensed by the physician, particularly in temperate climates where sweating is usually not obvious even in normal persons.

A second major anhidrotic state is seen in the tropics as tropical asthenia. Here, **compensatory hyperhidrosis** of the **face** may deceive both the patient and the physician into thinking that sweating is normal, while over 90% of the body surface is totally anhidrotic.

Serious **widespread anhidrosis** is also associated with **extensive skin diseases** such as atopic dermatitis, psoriasis, or exfoliative dermatitis. This often persists for months after the primary skin lesions have cleared and accounts for **heat intolerance** and **summer lassitude**. Other examples include scleroderma, ichthyosis, Sjögren's syndrome, and senile skin. Such silent anhidrosis is also common in premature infants and other newborns, necessitating avoidance of the "too-hot" tropical environment some mothers favor.

Since the sweat gland is under the control of the sympathetic nervous system and the hypothalamus, look for anhidrosis in **diabetic neuropathy**, after sympathectomy, and in **atropine poisoning**. Hypothalamic lesions may shut down the entire eccrine homeostasis unit, and even hysteria may induce total anhidrosis.

It is well to think of causes of anhidrosis but remember that the diagnosis rests on demonstrating a **failure of the skin to sweat when challenged**. No challenge, no diagnosis.

Low PA, Fealey RD, Sheps SG, et al: Chronic **idiopathic anhidrosis**. Ann Neurol 1985; 18:344–348.

Chronic idiopathic anhidrosis comes in the guise of **heat intolerance**. Eight examples are described in which the presenting signs were vertigo, weakness, dyspnea, and **flushing** when exposed to a hot environment or upon protracted exercise.

In each patient it was possible to rule out the following peripheral **autonomic neuropathies** known to produce hypohidrosis or sudomotor failure:

acute panautonomic neuropathy   familial dysautonomia

diabetic neuropathy   Tangier disease

Guillain-Barré syndrome

Furthermore, none exhibited nervous system degeneration as seen in the anhidrosis of the Shy-Drager syndrome. Nor was there any evidence of disabling somatic motor or sensory failure or of destructive lesions of the brain or spinal cord that could cause widespread anhidrosis by interruption of sympathetic pathways. None had signs of autonomic failure as evidenced by orthostatic hypotension or changes in bowel and bladder control.

Each of the eight patients had anhidrosis as an essentially isolated finding. Orthostatic hypotension was ruled out (no diagnostic changes in blood pressure or heart rate when recorded with the patient supine and after standing for 1 min). However, three of seven patients showed abnormal vasoconstrictor responses to the Valsalva maneuver, as well as to contralateral cold stimulus. Three patients also had **Raynaud's phenomenon**, and one had **flushing** of the cheeks. Plasma norepinephrine and epinephrine values were normal in all.

Acetylcholine iontophoresis (10%, 5 mA min) revealed that four of the eight patients had postganglionic sudomotor lesions. The others had preganglionic defects.

Five of the patients had **unilateral anhidrosis**. In the others it was limited in extent. In one patient, sweat function returned to normal. The prognosis for chronic idiopathic anhidrosis is better than for other autonomic neuropathies, since none of these cases progressed to generalized autonomic failure.

Low PA, Walsh JC, Huang CY, McLeod JG: The sympathetic nervous system in **diabetic neuropathy**. Brain 1975; 98:341–356.

Symptoms that indicate disordered **autonomic function** include:

orthostatic hypotension
disturbed bowel function
abnormal sweating
impotence

In ten patients with diabetes mellitus and peripheral neuropathy, **sweat tests** were performed by dusting the patient with a modified Guttmann's powder in which alizarin red replaced quinizarin. The patient was warmed by raising the ambient temperature until either the sublingual temperature rose 1°C or brisk sweating had occurred over the forehead. Areas of sweating became a deep violet color.

All ten diabetic patients had abnormal sweat patterns. **Sweating** was either **absent** or reduced in a **glove-and-stocking pattern**, with occasional small patches of anhidrosis also noted on the trunk.

Bilous RW: **Diabetic autonomic neuropathy**. A common complication which rarely causes symptoms. Br Med J 1990; 301:565–566.

Autonomic damage in diabetics begins with loss of sweating in the feet and progresses to sweat disturbances of the upper body.

Other early signs include impotence and bladder dysfunction. Next come abnormalities in the cardiovascular reflexes, and finally symptomatic postural hypotension, gastroparesis, diarrhea, and bladder atony.

The best diagnosticians take the best history.

Congenital

Clarke A: **Hypohidrotic ectodermal dysplasia**. J Med Genet 1987; 24:659–663.

Hypohidrotic ectodermal dysplasia is an uncommon X-linked condition appearing in about 1 in 100,000 births. Very rarely there is an autosomal recessive form. The affected infant may have a puzzling **dry peeling skin** at birth. Many have crusts of nasal secretion obstructing the nose and interfering with feeding. The **absence of mucous glands** may result in recurrent chest infections, as well as gastrointestinal problems. They are uniquely susceptible to dusty or smoke-filled environments. Asthma and eczema are frequent fellow travelers. The inability to sweat accounts for **fevers** and associated convulsions. It may even explain some cot deaths. **Lacrimal and salivary secretion** are also **deficient**.

As the child becomes older, the **sparse hair** and **dental dysplasia** become evident. The conical teeth and oligodontia interfere with nutrition. In association with the **distinctive facies** (prominent forehead, depressed nasal bridge, prominent lips) and absence of body fat, the wolflike teeth may cripple the child socially.

There were at least 117 varieties of ectodermal dysplasia in 1984, but only a few are likely to cause confusion in diagnosis.

In the **differential diagnosis**, recessive problems include:

autosomal recessive hypohidrotic ectodermal dysplasia (look for female carrier: dental problems), absence of sweat pores (patterned anhidrosis of back in lines of Blaschko)
Fried's tooth and nail syndrome (severe nail dystrophy, normal sweating)
Hypohidrotic ectodermal dysplasia with hypothyroidism (normal teeth)
Berlin's syndrome (mottled pigmentation, mental retardation, normal sweating)
Rosselli-Gulienetti syndrome (facial clefts, popliteal pterygia)

In the differential diagnosis, also consider dominant ectodermal disorders:

Rapp-Hodgkin syndrome (facial clefts)
Clouston's dysplasia (severe nail dystrophy, normal sweating)
Basan syndrome (simian creases, absent fingerprints)
Zanier-Roubicek syndrome (transverse streaks in dental enamel)
Koshiba's tricho-onychodental dysplasia (distinctive dental malformation)
Lenz-Passarge dysplasia (X-linked dominant)

Finally, from the genetic standpoint, the appearance of these X-linked dysplasias in women was puzzling until Mary Lyon recognized that random inactivation of one X chromosome in each female cell may take place in early embryogenesis. As a result, affected women have dysplasia that is not universal but rather patterned. Whole-back sweat tests reveal **swirling bands of hypohidrosis** that follow the lines of Blaschko.

Sybert VP: Early diagnosis in the **ectodermal dysplasias**. Birth Defects 1988; 24:277–278.

While it is easy to diagnose ectodermal dysplasia in a child or adult who has abnormalities of hair, teeth, or nails, the infant with ectodermal dysplasia masquerades as normal. He passes review as a normal toothless, sparse-haired being with indistinct fingerprints.

Look to the early diagnosis of this dysplasia. It permits avoidance of life-threatening complications in infancy and allows planning for long-term management. It also provides accurate recurrence risks for couples who have not completed their families.

The first step is for the obstetrician to **take a family history**. Although some infants with hypohidrosis result from a new mutation, others may have affected maternal male relatives. Indeed, the astute obstetrician may recognize the subtle physical findings of the **carrier female**, i.e., moderate heat intolerance, patchy, thin hair, hypodontia. Likewise, a history of a previous child with an ectodermal defect alerts the obstetrician to the possibility that the next child may have the same problem.

The physician also must be alert to the possibility of ectodermal dysplasia being present in any infant with a **lobster-claw hand** or **foot**, or a **cleft palate** or **cleft lip**. Watch for persistence of thin, sparse, fragile hair in the scalp, eyebrows, and eyelashes. Watch the nail growth for hypoplasia, and remember that absence or **hypoplasia of the nipples** suggests ectodermal dysplasia. Use a magnifying glass to look for absence of palmar sweat pores and **disturbances in the fingerprint** regularity.

Periorbital pigmentation is another common early sign of ectodermal dysplasia. Scaling, peeling skin may also be an index sign.

Later, think of the diagnosis in the baby who cries **without tears**, has recurrent **conjunctivitis** or repeated respiratory infections, and whose teething never seems to occur. The diagnosis may come to you as you realize that the baby tolerates heat poorly, doesn't develop replacement of baby hair, develops puzzling fevers, and is **asthmatic with atopic dermatitis**.

Much later in childhood, one perceives the obvious facies, the **monstrous nails** of the Clouston type of ectodermal dysplasia, or the **bulbous nose** of the trichorhinophalangeal syndrome. Always the screening test for ectodermal defect is the clinician's eye ("the eye does not see what the mind does not know"), until rapid gene analysis is available from a microdot of blood.

Next time a mother brings in a baby for evaluation of thin hair, dry skin, or eczema, think ectodermal defect. More than that, look at the palm with a **hand lens for absence of sweat pores** and irregular dermatoglyphs. Look at the hair under the microscope for monilethrix or trichorrhexis. Consider dental x-rays if the child is **toothless at 1 year of age**. Check the family history. Search for these diagnostic clues—if you don't, the family and the patient will have to wait until some other doctor does.

Pike MG, Baraitser M, Dinwiddie R, Atherton J: A distinctive type of hypohidrotic **ectodermal dysplasia** featuring **hypothyroidism**. J Pediatr 1986; 108:109–111.

A 3-week-old baby girl failed to thrive and had recurrent chest infections and abnormally loose stools. A diagnosis of **cystic fibrosis** was made when high sweat sodium levels were found. The chest infections continued and were notable for high fever and the absence of sputum. The hair, which had been normal in infancy, was progressively lost after age 6 months, and the skin became dry and the nails ridged and deformed. A **lacy freckling** appeared on the trunk.

Review at age $3\frac{1}{2}$ years revealed hypothyroidism (T_4 12 μmol/liter, normal 70 to 180). Thyroxine produced a marked increase in growth rate but no effect on the ectodermal abnormalities.

When the girl was 9 years of age, extensive studies revealed hypohidrotic ectodermal dysplasia, with no eccrine glands or hair follicles present on biopsy. There was no palmar sweating. The variety of associated problems made her an example of **ANOTHER** syndrome (*a*lopecia, *n*ail dystrophy, *o*phthalmic complications, *t*hyroid dysfunction, *h*ypohidrosis, *e*phelides, enteropathy, *r*espiratory tract infections).

The lesson to learn is that ectodermal dysplasia can result in **high sweat sodium** concentrations. As a result, a diagnosis of cystic fibrosis is very suspect in the presence of ectodermal defects.

Pinheiro M, Penna FJ, Freire-Maia N: Two other cases of **ANOTHER** syndrome? Family report and update. Clin Genet 1989; 35:237–242.

Ectodermal dysplasia centers diagnostically on the presence of two or more of the following four signs:

Trichodysplasia
Dental defects
Onychodysplasia
Sweat gland dysplasia

The resulting groupings now manifest themselves as 135 clinical conditions.

A young Brazilian girl is described in whom ectodermal dysplasia was recognized very early to be associated with hypothyroidism. Further assessment revealed that she had the ANOTHER syndrome. Her younger sister had a similar syndrome of ectodermal dysplasia without thyroid deficiency.

Juhlin L: **Absence of eccrine sweat glands** without other ectodermal defects. Acta Derma Venereol 1980; 60:73.

A healthy 26-year-old woman had been totally unable to sweat since birth, which became evident in warm environments. Her skin would become red, and her hands, feet, and **eyelids** would **swell**. Her temperature also climbed to about 38°C, and she developed **headache** and **nausea** and **felt sick**. Her nails, hair, teeth, and facial features were entirely normal.

Demonstration of the inability to sweat was done by exercise, using starch iodine visualization. She also failed to show a response to intradermal mecholyl (10^{-4}). **No sweat pores** could be demonstrated with o-phthaldialdehyde staining of the skin surface or with cyanoacrylate replicates. Biopsies of the abdomen and arms showed no sweat units, leading to a diagnosis of congenital aplasia of the eccrine sweat glands. Her mother, but not her siblings, had the same **anhidrosis**.

Significantly, she did have apocrine sweat glands, as shown by intradermal skin testing in the axilla with epinephrine (10^{-4}).

This patient's monoglandular skin problem has compromised her homeostasis, rendering her **an invalid every summer**.

Verbov J: Hypohidrotic (or anhidrotic) ectodermal dysplasia—an appraisal of **diagnostic methods**. Br J Dermatol 1970; 83:341–348.

Hypohidrotic ectodermal dysplasia is characterized by hypohidrosis, hypotrichosis, and absence of or defective (conical) teeth. The affected males show a distinctive prominence of the forehead and a depressed nasal bridge. Usually this developmental failure of the sweat gland, hair, and teeth is transmitted by an X-linked recessive gene, with males being the only ones affected.

Female carriers can be detected by finding a reduction in the number of sweat pores (o-phthaldialdehyde stain) and flattening of the ridges of the palmar skin (silicone imprints). Abnormalities in the **dermatoglyphic patterns** also serve to confirm the carrier state.

Detection of these heterozygous **carriers of recessive traits** is valuable for genetic counseling.

Deceptive patients give deceptive histories.

Okuno T, Inoue A, Izumo S: **Congenital insensitivity to pain with anhidrosis**: A case report. J Bone Joint Surg 1990; 72A:279–282.

A 17-year-old girl was seen repeatedly in orthopedic surgery for **fractures**, which strangely were always **painless**. On testing she failed to sense the pain of a pinprick, although her sensations of touch, cold, heat, and vibration were normal. She also had multiple **ulcers on the fingertips** and around the nails.

The second major finding was the **inability to perspire**, even in summer. She frequently had **high fevers**. A subcutaneous injection of pilocarpine (0.13 mg/kg body weight) failed to induce any sweating, although it did result in 200 ml of saliva pouring out in the next 2 hours.

A biopsy revealed normal sweat glands except for a complete lack of unmyelinated fibers around them. Furthermore, a sural nerve biopsy revealed a dramatic **reduction in** both small myelinated and unmyelinated **nerve fibers**. These observations explain the indifference to pain as well as inability to perspire.

Morris JGL, Lee J, Lim CL: **Facial sweating in Horner's syndrome**. Brain 1984; 107:751–758.

Knowing the facial sweating pattern can be useful in localizing the site of the lesion responsible for Horner's syndrome.

Horner's syndrome, first described in 1869, consists of **partial ptosis, miosis** with normal pupillary constriction in response to light, and **loss of sweating on the face**.

Other signs may include elevation of the lower lid, loss of the ciliospinal reflex, **heterochromia iridis**, and loss of the lid fold. Facial flushing and ocular hypotony may occur transiently. The **anisocoria** of Horner's syndrome increases in dim light, being much more marked after 5 seconds in dim light than after 15 seconds. The presence of these signs signifies a lesion of the sympathetic pathway but does not help to determine whether the lesion is proximal or distal to the superior cervical ganglion. **Pharmacologic testing** with cocaine eye drops (5%) may be used to confirm the diagnosis of Horner's syndrome. Phenylephrine and hydroxyamphetamine eye drops are also widely used to help determine whether the lesion in Horner's syndrome is preganglionic or postganglionic.

Assessment of the ability to sweat on the face was made by wrapping the patient in a body bag through which hot air was blown from two commercial hair dryers for 20 to 30 minutes. Alizarin powder, a yellow dye that becomes purple when wet, was applied to the face with a cotton ball. Heating was continued until sweating occurred on the forehead and around the mouth on the normal side of the face.

Of 31 patients with Horner's syndrome, 12 showed little or no sweating on the entire side of the face with Horner's syndrome. However, in six patients the **loss of sweating** was selective, occurring only on the medial aspect of the forehead and the side of the nose, indicative of a lesion in the sympathetic pathway distal to the bifurcation of the common carotid artery. This is in contrast to the classic Horner's syndrome finding of **hemifacial anhidrosis** seen in the group of 12. In these patients the lesion, such as a Pancoast tumor of the lung apex, had damaged the sudomotor as well as the oculosympathetic fibers at a lower level.

Another six patients showed the miosis and ptosis of Horner's syndrome, but no anhidrosis. Most of these patients had suffered avulsion of the brachial plexus, usually from **motorcycle accidents**.

Maloney WF, Younge BR, Moyer NJ: Evaluation of the causes and accuracy of pharmacologic localization in **Horner's syndrome**. Am J Ophthalmol 1980; 90:394–402.

Horner's syndrome derives from an **interruption of the sympathetic pathway** in its course between the hypothalamus and the orbit. There are three types of neurons involved:

preganglionic
> first (central) neurons—arise in the hypothalamus and end in the ciliospinal center between C-8 and T-1
> second (intermediate) neurons—ascend over the pulmonary apex and end high in the neck in the superior cervical ganglion

postganglionic
> third (peripheral) neurons—arise in the superior cervical ganglion and distribute to the head and neck

The neural fibers responsible for facial sweating travel with the external branches of the carotid artery to the face.

Horner's syndrome was confirmed in 450 patients by means of electronic infrared pupillography to demonstrate three **pupillary characteristics**:

> anisocoria
> delay of redilatation
> absence of dilatation to a psychosensory stimulus

Pharmacologic pupillary testing was then done with eye drops containing various drugs, including 4% cocaine, 1% epinephrine, and 1% hydroxyamphetamine (Paredrine) in an attempt to localize the lesion in the sympathetic pathway. Hydroxyamphetamine is now the drug of choice, which can often distinguish between preganglionic and postganglionic lesions.

Heterochromia of the **iris** is often associated with **congenital** Horner's syndrome and indicates a long duration of sympathetic denervation. Further search for other causes is unnecessary. In children without heterochromia, Horner's syndrome is usually due to a **malignant tumor**.

In adults with Horner's syndrome of undetermined cause, there is also a significant risk of underlying malignant tumor, almost always in the preganglionic neurons. If the hydroxyamphetamine test indicates a peripheral location, the lesion is probably benign. In this study, 10 of 13 patients with Horner's syndrome due to previously undiagnosed malignant disease had tumors involving the pulmonary apex, resulting in **Pancoast's syndrome** (Horner's syndrome and characteristic arm pain).

Kang WH, Chun SI, Lee S. **Generalized anhidrosis** associated with **Fabry's disease**. J Am Acad Dermatol 1987; 17:883–887.

In the course of treating a 28-year-old man for recurrent **erythema and edema of both feet** and ankles, thought to be **cellulitis**, it was learned that the patient had noted an inability to sweat since the age of 16 years. His heat intolerance greatly limited his daily activities.

When the nature of the anhidrosis was explored, it was found that exposure to heat for 1 hour induced palpitations, flushing, paresthesias, and **severe burning of the hands and feet**, with almost no visible sweating. Skin biopsy showed that he had a decreased number of sweat glands. The glands present showed PAS-positive granular inclusions, which on electron microscopy proved to be regular laminated structures diagnostic of Fabry's disease. A **deficiency of α-galactosidase in the leukocytes** confirmed the diagnosis. The accumulation of nonmetabolized ceramide trihexoside in the sweat glands explained their failure.

The **clinical signs** of Fabry's disease in this man included severe paroxysmal pain of the lower extremities with fever, leg edema, and generalized anhidrosis. Interestingly, he did not have the corneal opacities, periorbital puffiness, or angiokeratoma corporis diffusum characteristic of Fabry's disease.

Examination of his 6-year-old daughter revealed no skin or eye involvement. However, a skin biopsy showed the characteristic lamellar granules in blood vessel endothelium.

Mitchell J, Greenspan J, Daniels T, et al: **Anhidrosis** (hypohidrosis) in **Sjögren's syndrome**. J Am Acad Dermatol 1987; 16:233–235.

The **dry mouth** and **dry eyes** of Sjögren's syndrome may be accompanied by the **dry skin** of anhidrosis. A 55-year-old man who complained of failure to sweat for the past 6 months revealed a lack of response to **intradermal methacholine** (0.1 ml, 1:500) in several locations. Visualization with bromophenol blue powder revealed very few scattered dots of eccrine sweating. A skin biopsy showed a moderate number of sweat glands surrounded by a dense plasma cell and lymphocyte infiltrate.

He had already been proven to have Sjögren's syndrome of several years' duration. Tear flow was reduced (positive Schirmer's test), and stimulated parotid gland output showed a flow rate one tenth of normal. He had a dry mouth, with erythema, fissuring, and **papillary atrophy of the tongue** as well as right angular cheilitis. Ophthalmologic examination revealed keratoconjunctivitis sicca.

Chronic inflammatory atrophy of the sweat glands thus explains the **heat intolerance** noted by some patients with Sjögren's syndrome.

Psoriasis is an acronym for a Pitting, Scaling, Ongoing, Red, Inflammatory, Anguishing, Symmetrical, Inherited, Skin disease.

Test Procedures

Juhlin L, Shelley WB: **A stain for sweat pores**. Nature 1967; 213:408.

A 5% solution of *o*-phthaldialdehyde in xylene selectively stains the sweat gland orifices. Within 2 to 3 minutes, black puncta appear at each pore and remain for 5 to 8 days until surface desquamation occurs.

Staining does not occur if sweating is completely absent. With gross sweating, diffuse staining of the stratum corneum develops.

The black nonfluorescent pigment results from the reaction of *o*-phthaldialdehyde with ammonia in the sweat. The pigment cannot be dissolved but can be removed mechanically with Scotch tape strippings or abrasive rubbing.

The healed plaques of psoriasis fail to show any staining, demonstrating that no functional sweat pores exist in these areas.

O'Leary E, Slaney J, Bryant DG, Fraser FC: A simple technique for recording and **counting sweat pores** on the dermal ridges. Clin Genet 1986; 29:122–128.

The palm is rubbed vigorously with alcohol pads and then lightly with pencil **carbon paper** in all directions. Four-inch-wide **cellulose tape** (3M Scotch tape) is then firmly applied to the carbon-coated skin of the palm, with $\frac{3}{4}$-inch-wide tape applied to the fingertips. The tape is gently removed and transferred to glossy white paper for an easily mailed or filed permanent record. Sweat pores appear as white dots along the dark ridges, and counts per linear millimeter can be made under a dissecting scope at $12\times$ power.

Individuals affected with **X-linked hypohidrotic dysplasia** will show no pores. The obligate female heterozygotes show a reduction in the pores, with patchy absence. By use of 4-inch-wide tape the palmar **dermatoglyphics** can be visualized; again, abnormalities speak for the carrier state.

The **value** of the procedure is greatest for recognizing hypohidrotic X-linked ectodermal dysplasia at an early age. The diagnosis is frequently overlooked in infants, since sparse hair and absence of teeth are normal at this age. This may lead to unnecessary hospital admissions for study of fevers of unknown origin. By early recognition, bouts of hyperthermia can be prevented and hence brain damage or even death.

Finally, when this simple carbon paper–tape technique shows a normal pore pattern, reassurance can be given to apprehensive parents who are known carriers or have a family history of ectodermal defect.

Low PA, Caskey PE, Tuck RR, et al: Quantitative **sudomotor axon reflex test** in normal and neuropathic subjects. Ann Neurol 1983; 14:573–580.

By **iontophoresis of acetylcholine** (10% solution) into a focal area of skin, a normal response of axon reflex sweating will be observed. Loss of postganglionic sympathetic function, and hence an impaired axon reflex, results in reduction or absence of sweating. The accuracy of this diagnostic test is enhanced by quantifying the sweat excretion. This can be achieved by metering the humidity of nitrogen passed through a plastic chamber covering the skin test site.

A study of 20 patients with peripheral neuropathies, 4 patients with surgical sympathectomies, and 62 control subjects demonstrated the value of this quantitative sudomotor axon reflex test (Q-SART) in the **detection of postganglionic autonomic neuropathy**.

Rosenberg ML: The **friction sweat test** as a new method for detecting facial anhidrosis in patients with Horner's syndrome. Am J Ophthalmol 1989; 108:443–447.

To instantly detect the unilateral anhidrosis of Horner's syndrome, simply draw an office **prism bar** down the alcohol-cleansed forehead of the patient. The amount of friction against movement will be appreciably greater on the normal side (often preventing movement at all), since even the inapparent sweating increases friction. When the bar is drawn down on the **anhidrotic** side, the bar moves in an almost **frictionless** manner.

This simple physical test will detect anhidrosis that may not even be made evident by the **starch iodine test**. (To perform the starch iodine test, apply an iodine solution to an area of the body and let it dry. Then apply starch and induce the patient to sweat. Anhidrotic areas remain white, while sweating areas turn purple.)

Causes of **Horner's syndrome** include:

migraine
tumor
infarction
aneurysm
trauma

The sympathetic fibers controlling sweating on the face are located in the brainstem associated with the fibers controlling Müller's muscles in the eyelids and the pupillary dilator. The cause of Horner's syndrome is usually not readily discernible. Paredrine (1% hydroxyamphetamine) is often used to distinguish a preganglionic from a postganglionic problem.

Doss LL: The "**hatband**" sign in **Horner's syndrome**. JAMA 1986; 255:3115–3116.

A case of ptosis of the left eyelid eluded the diagnosis of Horner's syndrome until it was realized that the narcotics the patient was taking had constricted the pupils, eliminating evidence of diagnostic miosis on the left. Although there was no direct evidence of **anhidrosis** at the time of examination, inspection of his hatband revealed it to be stained only on the right.

The narcotics were taken for relief of left shoulder pain, subsequently demonstrated to be due to **carcinoma of the lung** in the left superior sulcus (Pancoast tumor). This tumor had compromised the patient's cervical sympathetic pathway and produced the classic triad of Horner's syndrome, but with only the **ptosis** being evident on direct inspection.

Gebhart W: What is new on sweat glands. Dermatologica 1989; 178:121–122.

The patient with generalized anhidrosis is denied the protective effect of secretory immunoglobulins, particularly **IgA**, which are normally secreted **in sweat**. Thus, he has one less defense against viral, bacterial, fungal, and antigenic assaults on the stratum corneum.

Cross lighting may reveal the invisible dermatosis.

Annular Erythemas

The patient comes to you with a diagnosis of **ringworm**. But is it? A KOH study can at once call into question the diagnosis and assure the patient that you will study the problem seriously. A second major group of annular lesions can be instantly recognized by their morphology. Thus the annularity of lesions of urticaria, psoriasis, and lichen planus is not of diagnostic aid. You would recognize them even if they were star-shaped.

Again, the patterning of the annular (ellipsoid) lesions of **pityriasis rosea** in the lines of cleavage as well as the herald patch are the diagnostic determinants. The location of the annular lesions of **seborrheic dermatitis**, the pustules of **subcorneal pustular dermatosis**, and the denudation of the necrolytic migratory erythema deserve your attention more than any annularity. Again, the target circles of **erythema multiforme**, the crusts of **impetigo**, and the thread border of **porokeratosis** catch your diagnostic eye more than any ring conformation.

Still, for some diseases the annular or arciform configuration does indeed light a diagnostic lamp. We think of **granuloma annulare**, **sarcoidosis**, and **mycosis fungoides** when the raised ringed lesion comes in view. **Leprosy** and **syphilis** should also come to mind.

Above all, however, annularity is the diagnostic entry point into the group of annular erythemas. The index example is **erythema annulare centrifugum** with its expanding ring of erythema and its trailing edge of scale. The **gyrate erythemas** with their waves of erythema are a distinctive group, alerting one to the possibility of internal malignant disease. Another example of an ever-expanding ring of erythema is the cutaneous sign of Lyme disease, i.e., **erythema chronicum migrans**. Less obvious in its circular geometry is the **necrolytic migratory erythema** in which the rings of damaged epidermis slough off.

Finally, recurrent fleeting arcs of erythema may signal the **erythema marginatum** rheumaticum associated with acute rheumatic fever or simply a response to recurrent group A β-hemolytic streptococcal pharyngitis. Also, among the miscellany of annular lesions are those of **lupus**, whether neonatal, discoid, or systemic. With pigmented expanding rings, one must think of **erythema dyschromicum perstans**, also known as **ashy dermatosis**.

However, amid all these possibilities, ringworm is still the most commonly seen annular lesion.

Erythema Annulare Centrifugum

Mahood JM: **Erythema annulare centrifugum:** A review of 24 cases with special reference to its association with underlying disease. Clin Exp Dermatol 1983; 8:383–387.

Annular erythemas are best divided into three groups:

Erythema annulare centrifugum
Erythema gyratum repens
Erythema chronicum migrans

Erythema annulare centrifugum is characterized clinically by persistent erythema comprising annular, circinate, gyrate, or serpiginous lesions. Initially a papule, the lesion **enlarges slowly** with **central clearing**. There may be a slight scale on the inner aspect of the advancing **palpable border**. At times vesicles may develop, but blisters are unusual.

Erythema annulare centrifugum is to be distinguished from **erythema gyratum repens**, which **extends rapidly in days**, is **not palpable**, has more scale, and presents a bizarre overall pattern. It is also to be distinguished from **erythema chronicum migrans**, in which there are but few lesions, these being regular in contour and associated with insect bites. Also in the differential diagnosis is **necrolytic migratory erythema**, which presents as erosions, bullae, and post inflammatory hyperpigmentation.

Erythema annulare centrifugum in this study of 24 cases did not prove to be a sign of internal malignant disease, drug eruption, or systemic disease. With a case incidence of 1/100,000 population/year, it is a rare disease that has spawned an uncommonly large synonymy in lieu of an etiology or diagnostic test. Witness its **synonyms** and wince:

erythema perstans
erythema gyratum perstans
erythema microgyratum perstans
erythema figuratum perstans
erythema marginatum perstans
erythema exudativum perstans
erythema simplex gyratum

Confronted with the erythema group we order determination of:

CEA and full **neoplasm survey** if it is erythema gyratum repens
Borrelia **antibody** titer if it is erythema chronicum migrans
glucagon level if it is migratory necrolytic erythema

Tsuji T, Kadova A: **Erythema annulare centrifugum** associated with **liver disease**. Arch Dermatol 1986; 122:1239–1240.

For the past month, this 70-year-old man had erythema annulare centrifugum lesions on the legs and arms. Immediately preceding the eruption he had suffered **abdominal pain and jaundice**. Within 3 days of operative removal of gallstones obstructing the bile duct, the erythema annulare centrifugum had resolved completely.

Erythema annulare centrifugum is a **reaction pattern** that calls for a search to eliminate causal factors such as:

infection (bacterial, fungal, viral)
drugs (salicylate, antimalarials)
malignant tumor
parasitic infection
hormones affecting the menstrual cycle
food (blue cheese)

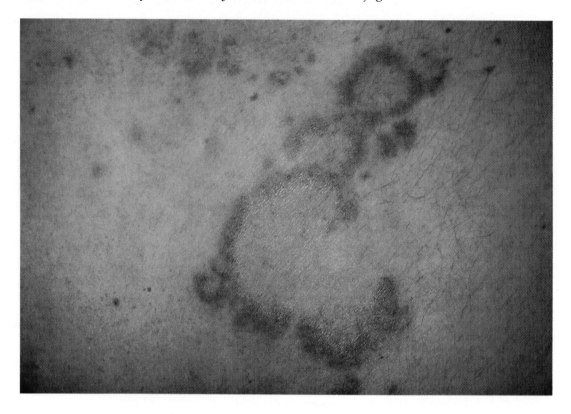

Differential diagnosis:

erythema gyratum repens
    lesions move in days
familial annular erythema
    appears in early childhood
erythema chronicum migrans
    history of insect bites, fewer lesions
necrolytic migratory erythema
    bullae, erosions
subacute cutaneous lupus erythematosus
    lesions coalesce, producing gyrate patterns
    look for grayish hypopigmentation and telangiectasia

Hendricks AA, Lu C, Effenbein GJ, Hussain R: **Erythema annulare centrifugum** associated with **ascariasis**. Arch Dermatol 1981; 117:582–585.

Erythematous, **arcuate, annular, and gyrate lesions** with scaly borders had been appearing over much of the body of this 10-year-old girl for the past 6 months.

The **eosinophil count** was 23% (total WBC 7900/mm³), and **stool examination** revealed *Ascaris lumbricoides* ova. Otherwise, extensive testing was negative. This included blood counts; chemical profile; fungal cultures of vagina and stool; x-rays of chest, sinus, and teeth; complement; immunoglobulins; and skin tests for yeast, fungi, and PPD.

Although two 48-hour treatments with piperazine citrate were followed by appearance of worms in the stool and lessening of the eruption, within a few months the lesions became prominent again. *Ascaris lumbricoides* ova were once again seen in the stool. Again, comprehensive **diagnostic studies** were noncontributory. These included liver/spleen scan, complete gastrointestinal series of x-rays, intravenous pyelography, lymphocyte stimulation tests, screening for *Mycoplasma* febrile agglutinins, heterophil antibody, helminth serum antibodies, and hemagglutinin tests for ascariasis.

Repeat treatment was followed a month later by resolution of all of the lesions. A diagnosis was made of erythema annulare centrifugum due to ascariasis. At this time the **drinking water** was finally studied and shown to be **fecally contaminated**, coming as it did from an open-ditch well near the family privy. Closure of the well by the state health department resulted in permanent elimination of the patient's skin problem.

Infestation by *Ascaris* always requires a careful search for the **source** of the infective eggs, viz., **food, drink, contaminated soil**. In this patient's case, one had only to look in the back yard.

Hudson LD: **Erythema annulare centrifugum:** An unusual case **due to hydroxychloroquine sulfate.** Cutis 1985; 36:129–130.

Widespread **annular erythematous patches** with trailing scale covered the arms, legs, back, and face of a 56-year-old woman. Present for 10 months, they followed the initiation of hydroxychloroquine therapy for possible lupus erythematosus. Blood studies and immunofluorescent microscopy failed to show any evidence of lupus erythematosus, but skin biopsy showed a dense perivascular lymphohistiocytic infiltrate of the upper dermis, suggestive of erythema annulare centrifugum. No occult dermatophyte or yeast infection was found, and internal malignant disease and intestinal parasitosis were ruled out.

Elimination of hydroxychloroquine resulted in slow improvement in the eruption, but complete disappearance took 1 year. Hydroxychloroquine was presumed to be the cause, as other examples of chloroquine-induced erythema annulare centrifugum have been reported. The high degree of tissue retention of chloroquine may account for the prolonged course. **Chloroquine has been found in the urine** as long as **5 years after** the last known ingestion of the drug!

In this case, stopping the drug did not immediately remove the antigen.

Ormerod AD, Daly BM, Main RA, Horne CHW: **Bullous pemphigoid resembling erythema annulare centrifugum.** Br J Dermatol 1984; 110:378–379.

Widespread pruritic, large, circular erythematous lesions with raised palpable borders provided a diagnostic challenge in a 60-year-old man. They had been present for 3 months, beginning in the umbilicus, and had the geographic pattern of erythema annulare centrifugum. Biopsies of **tense blisters** appearing in the largest patches proved the eruption to be bullous pemphigoid.

In another report, **pemphigus** had a similar presentation of erythema annulare centrifugum. Likewise, **bullous pemphigoid** may also appear as **erythema gyratum repens**.

It is apparent that only the pathologist can distinguish among the bullous variant of erythema annulare centrifugum, pemphigus, and bullous pemphigoid.

If you don't question your diagnosis, others will.

Erythema Gyratum Repens

Levine LE, Morgan NE, Fretzin D, Rubenstein D: **Erythema gyratum repens**. Arch Dermatol 1985; 121:170–171.

This 69-year-old man had had progressive gyrate bands of erythema and scaling appearing first on the feet and legs for the past 8 months. They had become generalized and showed a "**wood-grain" patterning** of concentric rings in the axillae and groin.

A diagnosis of erythema gyratum repens was made. The underlying cause was found to be a squamous cell **carcinoma of the lung**.

All such patients deserve exhaustive **search for underlying malignant disease**. In at least 40% of the examples reported, the wood-grain pattern has been the veneer for **bronchogenic carcinoma**.

Langlois JC, Shaw JM, Odland GF: **Erythema gyratum repens** unassociated with internal malignancy. J Am Acad Dermatol 1985; 12:911–913.

Erythematous concentric palpable bands with a **trailing edge of scale** resembling wood grain covered the entire body of this 67-year-old man. Only the face and scalp were exempt. The eruption would wax and wane within a 24-hour period but never disappear. All studies of fungus infection, systemic disease, or drug eruption were negative.

A diagnosis of erythema gyratum repens was made. Because this condition is classically associated with malignant disease, a **full search for tumors** was made, including full-body computed tomography. None was found, nor was any tumor found on careful, detailed autopsy when the patient died of a myocardial infarction 39 months later.

Neumann R, Schmidt JB, Niebauer G: **Subacute lupus erythematosus-like gyrate erythema**. Report of a case associated with a breast cancer. Dermatologica 1986; 173:146–149.

Gyrate polycyclic erythematous lesions on the back of a 40-year-old woman were clinically diagnosed as lupus erythematosus, and some improvement was achieved with chloroquine and topical steroids. The eruption persisted for 3 years before **ductal breast cancer** was discovered. Radical mastectomy was followed by immediate disappearance of all lesions.

The eruption **reappeared** 2 years later as widespread gyrate erythematous lesions with palpable scaly borders and mild atrophy and depigmentation in the center. Lupus erythematosus was ruled out with lupus antibody tests and the absence of the lupus band on biopsy. Further examination revealed two enlarged lymph nodes in the left supraclavicular region, which on biopsy showed **metastatic breast cancer**. Three weeks after excision of the nodes the skin was totally clear and has remained so.

All patients with skin lesions resembling gyrate erythemas should be carefully **screened for internal malignant tumors**. Such investigations should be repeated at frequent intervals.

Delfino M, Suppa F, Piccirillo A, et al: **Erythema gyratum perstans:** Association with a familial **neurologic disease**. Dermatologica 1986; 172:268–271.

Slightly raised, **slowly enlarging polycyclic lesions** appeared in a 3-day-old baby girl. The centers had a purplish livid tint. Within a few weeks all had faded away to be replaced by a new group. These annular lesions continued to plague the patient **for 20 years with no true remission**. She had an associated hypertrophic type of **Charcot-Marie-Tooth disease**, with enlarged nerves, muscle wasting, and clubfeet, and she also complained of **cold feet** and **plantar hyperhidrosis**.

Her 18-year-old brother also had a lifelong history of identical lesions, which had appeared when he was 2 years old. Their father had hypertrophic neuritis but no skin lesions.

The skin changes represent a **familial** form of erythema gyratum perstans. Distinctive features include onset in the first few days of life, relentless crops of lesions for many years, and an association at times with hereditary motor sensory neuropathy (type 1 Charcot-Marie-Tooth disease). **Its early onset and familial history** make it a distinctive form not to be confused with gyrate erythemas associated with drugs, infection, and malignant disease.

Monti M, Cavicchini S, de Bitonto A, Caputo R: **Gyrate erythema** in a patient with **dental** radicular **cyst**. Dermatologica 1987; 174:30–33.

A 55-year-old man had symmetrical **scaling erythematous figurate plaques** of the genitocrural folds, buttocks, and deltoid areas. They began in the groin and spread to other sites over 8 months. **Tinea corporis** was **suspected**, but there was no response to oral griseofulvin and clotrimazole cream given for 1 month. Further tests led to the diagnosis of gyrate erythema.

In addition, many teeth were lacking, and he had dental caries and mild periodontitis; treatment with ampicillin (2 gm/day IM for 20 days) did not affect the skin lesions. **Surgical excision of a dental cyst** found on routine dental x-rays led to improvement in 3 weeks and **cure** by 6 weeks.

Differential diagnosis of gyrate erythema:

> bullous erythema multiforme
> lupus erythematosus, subacute
> parapsoriasis en plaque
> pustular psoriasis
> tinea corporis

Moral: **Look for focal infection** in all gyrate erythemas.

You'll never get the big picture without looking at the little details.

Erythema Chronicum Migrans

Berger BW: **Erythema chronicum migrans** of **Lyme disease**. Arch Dermatol 1984; 120:1017–1021.

A study of 51 patients with erythema chronicum migrans showed that usually there is but one lesion. However, **25% showed multiple lesions**. The lesions began as red macules that expand centrifugally. In some, the central patch of red was surrounded by normal skin that, in turn, was surrounded by a band of redness. This produced a **targetlike lesion** or red circle with a halo. As the lesion enlarged, shape distortions occurred. The palms and soles as well as the mucous membranes were lesion free.

The lesions did show, at times, slightly elevated centers or edges. Scaling was rare, as was a central papulopustule. Some patients described burning and itch. An occasional patient experienced localized or generalized urticaria. Infrequently the eruption became a generalized erythematous macular eruption. Such variable patterns gave rise to a **differential diagnosis** in selected cases:

> spider bite
> erysipelas
> fixed drug eruption

In the majority of patients, **other symptoms** developed. Many had fatigue, fever, arthralgia, myalgia, and headache.

Burke WA, Steinbaugh JR, O'Keefe EJ: **Lyme disease mimicking secondary syphilis**. J Am Acad Dermatol 1986; 14:137–139.

Multiple **annular papulosquamous lesions** with marked peripheral scaling had been present for 2 months on the arms, legs, hands, and feet of this 27-year-old black man. The lesions had begun several days after a **tick bite**, although he denied any lesions such as erythema chronicum migrans surrounding the bite.

The involvement of the **palms** and **soles** strongly **suggested** a diagnosis of **secondary syphilis**. However, on biopsy no spirochetes could be found on a Warthin-Starry stain and the VDRL test was negative.

The diagnosis of Lyme disease was supported by the clear history of a tick bite and an *Ixodes dammini* **serum antibody test** positive to a dilution of 1:512.

Fishing for a diagnosis is mostly baiting and waiting. But you can get hooked on it.

Necrolytic Migratory Erythema

Sigg C, Schneider BV, Schnyder UW: **Glucagonoma syndrome** with necrolytic migratory erythema. Report of 2 cases of metastasizing glucagonoma without overt diabetes. Dermatologica 1988; 177:37–40.

A glucagon-secreting tumor of the pancreatic alpha islet cells causes recurrent episodes of **gyrate, red, edematous** and **eroded skin patches**, diarrhea, weight loss, and abdominal pain. The patient may also have **vulvitis, stomatitis**, atrophic glossitis, angular cheilitis, diffuse hair loss, paronychia, and onychodystrophy.

Look to the laboratory for confirmatory blood studies:

elevated	decreased
glucagon	protein
sugar	hemoglobin
zinc	amino acids

Differential diagnosis:

zinc deficiency syndrome	pemphigus foliaceus
acrodermatitis enteropathica	acrodermatitis continua of Hallopeau
pellagra	psoriasis
subcorneal pustulosis	staphylococcal scalded skin syndrome

In both cases presented here, the erythematous skin lesions contained *Staphylococcus aureus*, *Trichophyton rubrum*, and *Candida albicans*, but antibacterial and antimycotic treatment did not alter the skin lesions. Treatment with **somatostatin** cleared the lesions but did not alter the tumor masses or elevated glucagon levels.

Glucagonomas may produce polypeptide hormones other than glucagon, including **gastrin, neurotensin, pancreatic polypeptide**, and **vasoactive intestinal polypeptide**. These hormones may also produce necrolytic migratory erythema (pseudoglucagonoma).

Hashizume T, Kiryu H, Noda K, et al: **Glucagonoma syndrome.** J Am Acad Dermatol 1988; 19:377–383.

This 53-year-old diabetic sought help for a **vesicular, erosive dermatitis** of his lower extremities and trunk of 2 months' duration. A diagnosis of **subcorneal pustular dermatosis** was made on biopsy; however, despite an initial response to steroids, the dermatitis extended and worsened.

After 6 years of such care, he was admitted to a hospital on two occasions for study, dapsone therapy, and subsequently a blood transfusion. Three years later, another hospitalization found him profoundly anemic and cachectic, and the skin showed **annular, gyrate, erythematous macules** and patches with central clearing and peripheral crusting. The dorsum of the left foot as well as the anterior aspect of the leg showed a **bright-red erosion** with a well-defined irregular edge.

A year later, 10 years after his initial visit, the diagnosis of glucagonoma was finally made. He was found to have a **plasma glucagon level** ranging from 820 to 1100 pg/ml (normal 40 to 180). Although computed tomography and ultrasonography revealed no pancreatic tumor, celiac angiography demonstrated a hypervascular mass in the tail of the pancreas.

At laparotomy, a 4-cm tumor was found in the tail of the pancreas with metastases to the adjacent lymph node. Partial **pancreatectomy** and lymphadenectomy were done; the tumor was an alpha-cell tumor of the pancreas. Within 10 days of its removal, the patient's **skin was clear**.

Walker NPJ: Atypical **necrolytic migratory erythema** in association with a **jejunal adenocarcinoma**. J Roy Soc Med 1982; 75:134–135.

Necrolytic migratory erythema has three main features:

Waves of extending annular or circinate erythema
Superficial necrosis with shedding of skin
Complete resolution of an involved area within 2 weeks

A 69-year-old farmworker with subacute small-bowel obstruction developed five areas of **vesiculation and crusting** up to 3 cm in diameter on the ankle, forearms, cheek, and back, as well as a gradually extending area of **annular erythema** on one thigh. There also was florid **oral ulceration**, but a normal tongue. Over 8 weeks, new lesions appeared, and older lesions enlarged with some central healing, with no response to topical or systemic steroids. Bilateral **conjunctivitis** also developed. Six months previously a **jejunal adenocarcinoma** had been resected.

Skin biopsies showed focal dyskeratosis and parakeratosis, scattered foci of necrotic keratinocytes, and areas of confluent eosinophilic coagulative necrosis of the superficial layer. A chronic inflammatory cell infiltrate was present in the upper dermis. Direct immunofluorescence was negative.

Soon thereafter he died of pneumonia, and postmortem examination showed no evidence of metastases or other neoplasia. Skin lesions were histologically but not clinically typical of necrolytic migratory erythema. Individual lesions extended slowly and showed little tendency to heal.

Wilkinson SM, Cartwright PH, Allen C, et al: **Necrolytic migratory erythema:** Association with **neuroendocrine tumour** with predominant insulin secretion. Br J Dermatol 1990; 123:801–805.

This 80-year-old woman was admitted unconscious with a low blood glucose level and a rash. The rash was a **scaling figurate erythema** most marked in the **perianal area** and on the lower legs.

Examination revealed hepatomegaly. The glucagon levels were somewhat elevated but not at the level seen with glucagonomas. Insulin, proinsulin, and C-peptide levels were all elevated. Measurements of blood levels of gastrin, vasoactive intestinal polypeptide, and neurotensin were normal, but the pancreatic polypeptide values were elevated.

The skin biopsy showed superficial necrolysis. Immunofluorescence was normal, apart from linear fibrin deposits in the peaks of the dermal papillae. A diagnosis of necrolytic migratory erythema was made.

Abdominal ultrasound showed **hepatomegaly** with target lesions suggestive of **metastases**. CT showed enlargement of the proximal end of the pancreas. Liver biopsy showed an infiltrating neoplasm consistent with a **metastatic neuroendocrine carcinoma**. Immunostains for gastrin, glucagon, and somatostatin were negative, but some cells were positive for insulin.

After her death, postmortem examination confirmed the presence of a pancreatic tumor with metastases to the liver and regional lymph nodes. It was this tumor that was responsible for the **elevated insulin levels**.

As to the exact cause of the rash, there is less certainty. Necrolytic migratory erythema does occur in association with **increased plasma glucagon**, as in **glucagonoma**, **cirrhosis**, and **angioplasia**, but it is also seen when the glucagon level is normal as in chronic pancreatitis and small-bowel disease. Nonetheless, necrolytic migratory erythema can be induced by glucagon.

In this patient, diazoxide therapy restored the glucose level to normal with a concomitant drop in the glucagon levels. The skin improved, but the view is held that this actually resulted from the **oral zinc** that was prescribed in view of marginally low serum zinc levels.

Grant JM: **Annular vesicular lupus erythematosus.** Cutis 1981; 28:90–92.

Ringlike erythematous lesions on the neck and dorsal forearms of this 91-year-old white woman suggested a diagnosis of **tinea circinata**. However, scrapings and cultures for fungi were negative. The edges were vesicular and crusted, with centrifugal spread and central clearing.

Biopsies suggested a diagnosis of **lupus erythematosus**. Although leukopenia (leukocytes 3000/mm^3) was present, general laboratory studies were negative, including antinuclear antibodies.

The findings were neither those of systemic lupus erythematosus nor those of discoid lupus erythematosus. The lesions were nonscarring and did not show follicular plugging. At times, flaccid bullae were seen.

The final diagnosis was subacute cutaneous lupus erythematosus. It is of note that **Hailey-Hailey disease**, **bullous pemphigoid**, and **pemphigus erythematosus** had been eliminated in the early diagnostic jousting.

Subacute lupus erythematosus must be considered in the differential diagnosis of any **migratory erythema** with or without vesiculation.

Callaway JL: A leper's victory over VA red tape. Cutis 1987; 39:111.

A 46-year-old man had a pruritic erythematous eruption of the right hip, thought to be lymphoma but read as nonspecific dermatitis on biopsy. After 2 years of second, third, and fourth opinions, he had **generalized gyrate,** serpentine, **annular lesions that were anesthetic**. His face was slightly erythematous and the **ear lobes were thickened**. A biopsy showed tuberculoid leprosy, complete with acid-fast bacilli. Attention was then paid to his 4 years of army service in the South Pacific where at times he was housed in native huts.

It was evident that the **leprosy** was indeed service acquired, but because it had not appeared until long after the approved 3-year period, it could not be legally acknowledged as "service connected." Special appeals to county, regional, state, and national agencies were to no avail. Finally recognition of the government's responsibility came in the form of a specific bill in the House of Representatives (HR 11631). The patient and his family now receive compensation for a disease that may measure its latent period in decades. His was a victory over both legal and diagnostic red tape.

Kay MH, Duvic M: **Reactive annular erythema** after **intramuscular vitamin K**. Cutis 1986 37:445–448.

This 70-year-old woman complained of **tender, erythematous, annular plaques** of the lower abdomen and upper arms. They were bilaterally symmetrical and enlarged to a final diameter of 20 cm. The centers were purpuric with a collarette of scale and an outer erythematous border. A skin scraping and culture were negative, and a biopsy showed only a nonspecific perivascular infiltrate. Careful review of the history disclosed that a month ago she had received **injections of vitamin K** at each of the four **sites** involved. Such a **reactive erythema** is common after the injection of a variety of agents. These include:

corticosteroids	heparin
collagen	anticancer agents (doxorubicin, vincristine)

It always helps to ask the patient what he or she thinks the cause is.

Warin RP: The role of **trauma** in the **spreading wheals** of **hereditary angioedema**. Br J Dermatol 1983; 108:189–194.

Trauma often initiates the swellings of hereditary angioedema, which once formed may continue to spread. Indeed, a simple pinprick may initiate a **spreading annular wheal**.

Patients with a **reticulate erythema** or **erythema marginatum** should be tested for **C1 esterase inhibitor levels**. A low value may thus indicate that these expanding rings of fading urticaria are indeed the prodrome of hereditary angioedema.

Starzycki Z: **Ringworm-like late syphilides**. Acta Derm Venereol 1989; 69:173–174.

An irregular **ring** of densely grouped **rose-colored papules** covered an area on the right side of this 54-year-old woman's neck. It had been present for 5 months and had been diagnosed as **ringworm**.

The woman's suspicions of a misdiagnosis were raised when en masse screening in her town revealed she tested positive for syphilis.

Examination revealed not only the original ring, but a second one within the center. She also had small similar ringwormlike lesions in the left preauricular region and on the left arm. There were no mucosal lesions.

Darkfield examinations, repeated five times, were negative, but the serologic tests for syphilis were strongly positive, including a treponema pallidum immobilization test. On biopsy, staining with silver showed many spiral **treponemes in the dermal infiltrate** but not in the epidermis. A diagnosis of **late nonulcerative syphilid** was made.

Smith NP, Sanderson KV, Crow KD: **Reticular erythematous mucinosis syndrome**. Clin Exp Dermatol 1976; 1:99–103.

A 37-year-old woman had an asymptomatic, slowly extending rash over the center of her back for 3 years that did not improve with topical steroids or sun exposure. She was well, except for chronic uveitis of the left eye. Examination revealed an **erythematous reticular maculopapular rash** over the thoracic and lumbar spine. The borders of erythema were indistinct, but in some places formed thin spurs that projected into the normal surrounding skin. The eruption was slightly infiltrated, and a few comedolike lesions were present. Skin biopsy showed a dense perivascular and perifollicular lymphocytic infiltrate throughout the dermis. Alcian blue and mucicarmine stains were **positive for mucin**, but staining was negative with toluidine blue and azure A. She was treated with mepacrine (200 mg bid), and after 8 weeks the rash had disappeared.

There appears to be a spectrum of **cutaneous mucinosis diseases** in which mucin has variable staining characteristics with alcian blue, toluidine blue, mucicarmine, and azure A. Clinical lesions vary from plaques to **reticulate erythema**.

Prior therapy may remove not the disease, but all its diagnostic clues.

Aphthous Ulcers

The patient comes with the self-diagnosis of canker sores. His recurrent prodromal pain and subsequent tender superficial ulcers of the oral mucosa with a short course of a few days support the diagnosis. Such aphthous ulcers are very common and still remain mysterious as to etiology.

Severe oral ulcerations may herald **Behçet's syndrome**. Others that localize on the palate and gums may represent recurrent **herpes simplex** virus infections. A particularly recalcitrant type is Sutton's **periadenitis mucosa necrotica recurrens**.

Always, oral ulcerations bring into the **differential diagnosis** such diseases as pemphigus vulgaris, drug eruption, lichen planus, and lupus erythematosus. Always search for inflammatory bowel disease as well.

Although the primary lesion may be bullous, the presenting lesion is usually erosive. A biopsy with immunofluorescent studies is often valuable in cases that appear not to be run-of-the-mill aphthae.

Definition

Scully C, Porter S: **Recurrent aphthous stomatitis:** Current concepts of etiology, pathogenesis and management. J Oral Pathol Med 1989; 18:21–27.

There are three types of lesions:

1. **Minor ulcers:** round or oval shallow ulcers with a gray-white pseudomembrane and thin red halo, usually less than 5 mm in diameter and located on the labial and buccal mucosa. They heal in 10 to 14 days without scarring and are very common, beginning in childhood or adolescence.
2. **Major ulcers** (periadenitis mucosa necrotica recurrens): oval deep ulcers 1 to 3 cm in diameter, usually located on the lips, soft palate, or fauces. They persist up to 6 weeks and often heal with scarring. The onset is after puberty, and the course is chronic.
3. **Herpetiform ulcers:** multiple recurrent crops of 2- to 3-mm painful ulcers that are widespread throughout the mouth. As many as 100 ulcers may be present, and they tend to fuse into large irregular ulcers. The age of onset is later than that of other aphthous ulcers, and they affect mainly women.

Most patients with recurrent aphthous ulcers are otherwise well. However, similar lesions are seen in various **systemic disorders**, including:

Behçet's disease
Sweet's syndrome
cyclic neutropenia
periodic fever and pharyngitis
various nutritional deficiencies (with or without gastrointestinal disorders)
immunodeficiencies such as AIDS

Hematinic deficiencies are sometimes related to small-intestinal disease, particularly celiac disease. Gluten-sensitive enteropathy has been demonstrated in about 5% of outpatients with recurrent aphthous ulcers. They may be asymptomatic, but patients usually have **folate deficiency** and sometimes IgA-class reticulin antibodies. Gluten withdrawal may be helpful. In some patients, ulcer formation may also be related to **atopy**, exposure to certain **foods**, and the phase of the **menstrual cycle**.

Trauma may initiate ulcers in susceptible people, but ulcers are uncommon when there is mucosal keratinization. Ulcers are uncommon in smokers.

It seems likely that in **genetically predisposed** people, immunopathologic reactions lead to the ulcers. In the preulcerative phase, large granular lymphocytes with antibody-dependent cellular cytotoxic (ADCC) abilities are present in the mucosa, along with T4 (CD4) helper-inducer lymphocytes. The ulcerative phase is associated with T8 cells during healing. Local immune complexes may also be involved, since circulating immune complexes have been found in some patients. There are immune deposits in some lesions, especially in the stratum spinosum, and vasculitis (leukocytoclastic or immune complex) may lead to nonspecific deposition of immunoglobulins and complement.

The **precipitating factors** remain unknown. Oral streptococci, either as direct pathogens or as antigenic stimuli leading to antibodies that cross-react with keratinocyte antigenic determinants, have been extensively investigated. The initial L-form isolate from aphthous ulcers was typed as *S. sanguis*, later found to be a strain of *S. mitis*. However, lymphocyte mitogenic responses to these organisms in patients with aphthous stomatitis do not differ significantly from those in controls. Some patients have elevated serum antibody titers to viridans streptococci, but data are contradictory.

Viruses may also play a role in aphthous stomatitis, with adenoviruses and

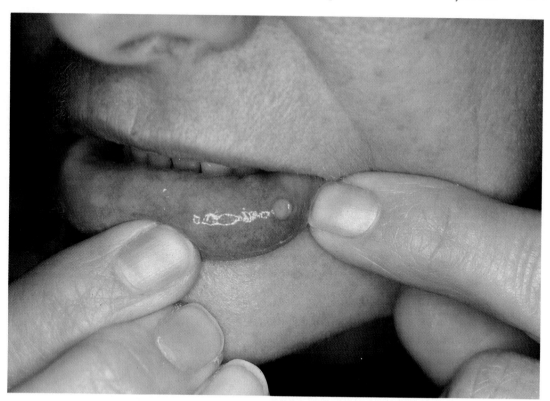

herpes simplex virus (HSV) being variously implicated. RNA complementary to HSV has been detected in circulating mononuclear cells in some patients, and HSV-1 DNA has been found in Behçet's syndrome and circulating immune complexes. In Behçet's syndrome there is also impaired T-cell response to HSV-1, as well as circumstantial evidence that mononuclear cells are virally infected.

Drinnan AJ, Fischman SL: Controversies in oral medicine. Dent Clin North Am 1990; 34:159–169.

Oral ulcers are a frequent complaint of patients seeking dental treatment. They may arise primarily in the oral cavity as an ulcer, result from a systemic disease, or represent a ruptured blister of a vesiculobullous disease. Approximately 20 to 50% of the population is affected by aphthous ulcers (canker sores, dyspeptic ulcerations).

The term *aphthous* means ulcerous, and the ulcer is a deep crater extending through the entire thickness of the epithelium into the underlying connective tissue. As soon as an ulcer forms, it is subjected to irritating oral fluids and flora, which induce acute and chronic inflammation. Therefore, many ulcers of diverse causes show similar histologic changes.

Aphthous ulcers are round or oval with yellowish necrotic bases surrounded by inflamed mucosa. "Minor" ulcers are less than 1 cm in diameter, while "major" ulcers are larger than 1 cm. Lesions are multiple and painful, occurring most frequently on the labial or buccal mucosa, floor of the mouth, and soft palate. Recurrent attacks last about 10 days, although major aphthous ulcers may persist for months. Secondary lymphadenitis may accompany each episode.

Many **precipitating factors** have been suggested, including trauma, stress, allergy, poor nutrition, endocrinopathies, and subclinical systemic disease. Minor local trauma, including dental treatment and cheek biting, is often implicated. Since **stress** produces gastric ulcerations in animals, the joint occurrence of oral and gastric ulcers in humans suggests that **psychological** and **physiological stress** may play a role in oral ulceration. Nutritional deficiencies of iron, zinc, vitamin B_{12}, and folic acid have also been implicated, but they have not been supported in controlled clinical studies. It is likely that more than one cause is involved, possibly a broad spectrum of causes.

Graykowski EA, Barile MF, Lee WB, Stanley HR Jr: Recurrent **aphthous stomatitis.** Clinical, therapeutic, histopathologic, and hypersensitivity aspects. JAMA 1966; 196:637–644.

All 62 patients complained of **severe localized pain.** In 50%, the first symptom noticed was a nodule. Generalized edema of the oral cavity (tongue and oral mucosa), paresthesia, low-grade fever, lymphadenopathy, and vesicle-like formations containing mucus were other findings.

Ten patients had **periadenitis aphthae**, large single or multiple deep erosive ulcerations with elevated margins surrounded by diffuse erythema, extensive localized edema, and scar formation. Patients with periadenitis aphthae usually have typical smaller aphthae initially, which gradually increase in severity. Periadenitis aphthae involves deeper mucosal tissues with cellular infiltration of the periglandular submucosa (periadenitis).

Early aphthous lesions are associated with and possibly the result of epithelial disturbances of **ducts of minor salivary glands**, associated with lymphocytic infiltration. Disruption of marginal and ductal epithelium starts at the basal layer and progresses superficially.

Microorganisms morphologically resembling the pleomorphic streptococcus are almost always present in histopathologic sections of aphthous ulcers. Intradermal skin tests with this organism induced a delayed hypersensitivity reaction of 2 to 4 cm in 30 patients with aphthous ulcers. In four patients with periadenitis aphthae, necrosis developed, followed by scar formation. Most controls had no reaction.

In earlier work, this pleomorphic **streptococcus**, isolated from a patient with periadenitis aphthae, induced aphthouslike lesions in the skin and oral mucosa of guinea pigs and rabbits.

It is difficult to name a flower after it has been run over by a truckload of therapy.

Wray D, Graykowski EA, Notkins AL: Role of **mucosa injury** in initiating recurrent aphthous stomatitis. Br Med J 1981; 283:1569–1570.

Recurrent aphthous stomatitis is the most common disease of oral mucous membranes.

In 30 patients with recurrent aphthous stomatitis and 15 control patients, the buccal mucosa was injured by three **different methods**: injection of local anesthesia, insertion of a suture left in for 24 hours, and piercing with a towel tenaculum. Each method produced two puncture wounds, with only one side of the mouth being used. None of the 15 controls developed ulcers, but 13 of the 30 patients tested developed a total of 26 lesions at one or more of the puncture sites. Sutures induced the most lesions, with 15 ulcers having diameters of 2 to 3 mm and lasting 2 to 7 days. Only two 1-mm painless lesions developed at injection sites.

The mechanically induced ulcers were indistinguishable clinically and histologically from spontaneous ulcers except that they were smaller and healed more quickly. The same phenomenon of **lesions being induced by injury** is seen in **Behçet's disease** and in the **Ehlers-Danlos syndrome**. Possible mechanisms include impaired wound repair, more rapid mobilization of mast cells, and detrimental effects of histamine release.

Thomas HC, Ferguson A, McLennan JG, Mason DK: **Food antibodies** in oral disease: A study of serum antibodies to food proteins in aphthous ulceration and other oral diseases. J Clin Pathol 1973; 26:371–374.

Patients with recurrent minor aphthous ulcerations have a **greater incidence** of antibodies to food antigens than do controls. However, there was no evidence to suggest that the aphthae were due to hypersensitivity to food antigens.

Ulcerations of various types in the mouth presumably lead to **increased absorption of antigenic molecules** and an increased immune response. Similar changes occur in **inflammatory bowel disease** (celiac disease and ulcerative colitis) because of large areas of mucosal breakdown. Defective IgA secretion may also contribute to increased absorption of food antigens through an otherwise normal mucosa.

Wilson CWM: **Food sensitivities**, taste changes, **aphthous ulcers** and atopic symptoms in allergic disease. Ann Allergy 1980; 44:302–307.

Food sensitivity analysis in 61 atopic patients showed that all had abnormalities in buccal sensation and taste when they ate the offending foods. Offending allergens were detected by asking which foods patients dislike and/or do not ingest.

Aphthous ulcers occurred in 56% of the patients, and **food** was **associated** with their appearance in **18%**. These patients reported a burning and tangy sensation in their mouths when they ate the offending foods. Three patients developed aphthous ulcers 12 to 48 hours after taking the specific food allergen that produced a burning sensation in the buccal mucosa. The same foods produced burning and pain within 30 seconds of application to the exposed ulcer base in six patients. The **responsible food allergens** included cabbage, tomatoes, cheese, apple, chocolate, eggs, and milk.

Subjective buccal sensations in food allergy should be accepted as valid **diagnostic criteria**. These include rough and tangy feelings, creamy, slimy, soggy, and coated sensations, and wet and dry sensations. Abdominal symptoms, nausea, upper or lower abdominal pain, distension, belching, flatulence, and diarrhea alternating with constipation occur within 30 minutes to   273

2 hours after consumption of specific foods. Disliked foods often are described as horrible or tasteless and cause difficulty in swallowing, deep pain in the chest, and regurgitation. Other signs and symptoms include debilitating tiredness, inability to concentrate, sweating, palpitations, and excess wakefulness and excitement. Some patients also had rhinitis, asthmatic symptoms, migraine, or **skin burning** (eczema) aggravated by certain foods.

The most common foods giving symptoms were **cow's milk** protein, **eggs**, cabbage, turnips, parsnips, **pork**, **fish**, wheat germ, tea, and coffee.

Skin prick tests to food give the most accurate diagnosis of food sensitivity. Food challenge is a less sensitive method for diagnosis, and radioallergosorbent tests (RAST) are not a dependable method for diagnosis of some food sensitivities.

Eversole LR, Shopper TP, Chambers DW: Effects of suspected **foodstuff challenging** agents in the etiology of recurrent aphthous stomatitis. Oral Surg 1982; 54:33–38.

Patients with recurrent aphthous ulcers often relate the appearance of lesions to certain foods, particularly tomatoes, berries, and nuts.

Direct-food challenges with 4-ounce portions of black walnuts, cherry tomatoes, and fresh whole strawberries failed to document any causal role in the majority of 58 subjects tested. However, **7%** of these patients did **develop aphthae** after the food challenges, suggesting that the foods may be important in precipitating lesions in some patients.

Possibly the acidic or astringent nature of certain foods helps cause enough discomfort to focus awareness on lesions that were already present.

Taylor KB, Truelove SC, Wright R: **Serologic reactions** to gluten and cow's milk proteins in gastrointestinal disease. Gastroenterology 1964; 45:99–108.

Of 36 patients with multiple recurrent "major" **aphthous ulcerations**, 35 had sera with high titer reactions (1:20 to 1:20,000) to the milk protein **casein**. Many patients also reacted to **wheat gluten** and the other chief proteins of cow's milk, α-lactalbumin and β-lactoglobulin. Findings were similar in celiac disease, idiopathic steatorrhea, and ulcerative colitis but not in pernicious anemia, duodenal ulcer, and regional enteritis.

High-titer serologic reactions may represent increased absorption of whole proteins with antigenic moieties or may reflect a state of hypersensitivity to the particular dietary antigens. Their connection to diseases of the gastrointestinal tract is uncertain.

Veloso FT, Saleiro JV: **Small-bowel changes** in recurrent ulceration of the mouth. Hepato-gastroenterol 1987; 34:36–37.

This study suggests that a significant number of patients with recurrent aphthous stomatitis may have a mild form of **gluten enteropathy**.

Jejunal biopsies were done on 24 patients with recurrent aphthous stomatitis, but no evidence of malnutrition, either by clinical or laboratory evaluation (including D-xylose excretion and the Schilling test). Subtotal **villous atrophy** was found in four patients (16%). These changes reversed after 1 year on a gluten-free diet. The **mouth ulcerations** also disappeared in three of the four patients after **gluten** withdrawal, but promptly reappeared with the reintroduction of gluten.

In addition to villous atrophy, lymphocyte infiltration of the small-intestine epithelium is a reliable sign of gluten sensitivity. In this study, all patients with aphthous stomatitis had significantly increased intraepithelial lymphocytes when compared with controls.

Field EA, Speechley JA, Tyldesley WR: Clinical and haematological assessment of children with **recurrent aphthous ulceration**. Br Dent J 1987; 163:19–22.

Hematologic screening for deficiencies of **vitamin B₁₂**, **folate**, and **iron** is recommended in children with recurrent aphthous ulcers.

In 100 children (7 to 16 years), such **deficiencies** were found in **21%**. Iron deficiency was found in 18 children, including 5 with anemia. Two children also had folate deficiency, confirmed by low red cell folate levels. No vitamin B₁₂ deficiency was found. In most of these patients there was improvement of the ulcers with iron and folate supplementation.

Jejunal biopsies were performed in seven patients with abnormal blood results. Celiac disease was found in one patient who was deficient in both iron and folate. With such a low yield, it was concluded that jejunal biopsies should *not* be done in children with aphthous ulcers unless there is also failure to thrive, coupled with diarrhea.

Palopoli J, Waxman J: Recurrent aphthous stomatitis and **vitamin B₁₂ deficiency**. South Med J 1990; 83:475–477.

A 31-year-old woman developed **recurrent aphthous stomatitis**, with four to five ulcers appearing every few weeks on her lips, cheeks, and sides of the tongue. Gradually she developed diffuse **swelling of the tongue** with generalized pain. When a small **genital ulcer** was discovered, she was believed to have early Behçet's disease, and colchicine therapy was started. Over the next 4 years the dosage of colchicine was increased several times, always with temporary improvement of the mouth ulcers but eventually culminating in intolerable diarrhea and discontinuation of the drug.

Evaluation at age 37 years revealed **anemia** (hemoglobin 8.9 gm/dl and serum B₁₂ < 50 pg/ml [normal 200 to 1000]). Bone marrow aspiration revealed megaloblastic erythroid hyperplasia. A Schilling test showed less than 1% intestinal absorption of vitamin B₁₂ with intrinsic factor, leading to a presumptive diagnosis of **pernicious anemia**. **Vitamin B₁₂ therapy** was initiated (1000 μg/day IM daily for 1 week, then twice weekly for 1 month, then monthly); there was dramatic improvement within a day, followed by complete and lasting remission of oral ulcerations, glossitis, and anemia.

A repeat Schilling test after 1 week of treatment showed only 4.1% intestinal absorption of vitamin B₁₂, confirming the diagnosis of pernicious anemia.

Colchicine is helpful in relieving aphthous ulcers, probably by inhibiting leukocyte chemotaxis. Simultaneously, however, it interferes with vitamin B₁₂ absorption, probably by reducing the quantity of intrinsic factor–vitamin B₁₂ receptors in the intestinal mucosa. Serum vitamin B₁₂ levels should be monitored in patients receiving long-term colchicine therapy.

Behçet's disease may also lead to vitamin B₁₂ deficiency, through poor dietary intake due to the stomatitis and poor absorption of vitamin B₁₂ due to terminal-ileum ulcers.

Glossitis is found in only about one half of patients with pernicious anemia. Recurrent aphthous stomatitis can be another oral sign of vitamin B₁₂ deficiency, perhaps the earliest symptom in the absence of anemia.

Challacombe SJ, Scully C, Keevil B, Lehner T: Serum ferritin in **recurrent oral ulceration**. J Oral Pathol 1983; 12:290–299.

Iron deficiency can be assessed fairly accurately by estimation of the serum **ferritin level**, which is reduced if iron stores are low. Serum ferritin can distinguish between patients with true iron deficiency (with or without anemia) and secondary sideropenia (low serum iron level with normal or decreased iron-binding capacity).

Mean serum ferritin levels were **reduced** in patients suffering from recurrent oral ulceration, Behçet's syndrome, and other erosive oral lesions.

Approximately 8% of 105 patients with recurrent oral ulcers and 15% of 41 patients with Behçet's syndrome were found to have iron deficiency. Treatment with ferrous gluconate (300 mg/day) for 2 months greatly improved the mouth ulcers in five of six patients but did not stop recurrences in most patients.

In addition to recurrent oral ulcerations, iron deficiency anemia may also be associated with **atrophic glossitis** and **oral candidiasis**.

Grant SCD, Harrington CI, Harris SC: **Aphthous ulceration** as a presentation of *Giardia lamblia* infection. Br Dent J 1989; 166:457.

A 36-year-old English steelworker described occasional **aphthous ulcers** over 20 years, which became troublesome in the preceding 12 months. He had also noted **periodic epigastric pain**, precipitated by food, over the past year. Bowel action and motion were normal. Foreign travel had included trips to Germany, Ireland, and Spain. Examination revealed two small aphthous ulcers, the liver palpable 1 cm below the costal margin, and glove-and-stocking diminution of pinprick sensation.

Laboratory evaluation was normal except for a reduced serum B_{12} of 125 mg/liter (normal 170 to 900), but duodenal biopsies revealed abundant *Giardia lamblia*, and **G.** *lamblia* **cysts** were subsequently found **in the feces**. Treatment with metronidazole for 3 days had cleared the infection as well as the oral ulcerations, abdominal pain, and peripheral neuropathy at a 6-week follow-up.

Infection with the protozoan *G. lamblia* occurs through ingestion of cysts in contaminated food and water, particularly in the tropics, subtropics, and Eastern Europe. It usually causes acute or chronic **diarrhea** and may lead to significant **malabsorption**.

There are other known associations of aphthous ulcerations with gastrointestinal diseases, including **celiac disease** and **Crohn's disease**. Therefore, when malabsorption is suggested through disturbances of bowel habits, abnormal serum B_{12} and folate levels, or increased fecal fat, a jejunal biopsy is useful. In this case, the reduced B_{12} level provided an indication for jejunal biopsy, which led to the diagnosis of an unsuspected *G. lamblia* infection.

Tyldesley WR: Recurrent **oral ulceration** and **coeliac disease**. Br Dent J 1981; 151:81–83.

During 1979 in Liverpool, **97 patients** with recurrent aphthous ulcers were **screened for celiac disease**. Initial **screening tests** included complete blood count, erythrocyte sedimentation rates, serum folate, vitamin B_{12}, iron, and total iron-binding capacity. Abnormalities were found in 20 patients.

Jejunal biopsies were done in 15 of the 20 patients. Biopsies consistent with celiac disease were found in six (6.2% of patient pool). All six had low folate levels, while two had low hemoglobin levels with low iron saturation, and one had slight B_{12} deficiency.

Most of the patients with celiac disease had **herpetiform ulcerations** with many small painful ulcers on the margins of the tongue, floor of the mouth, and lips.

Treatment with a **gluten-free diet** (elimination of wheat and rye flour) resulted in clearing of the oral ulcers, as well as a general subjective feeling of improved health and desirable gain of weight. Several also had subjective improvement in "irritable skin," although none had dermatitis herpetiformis. A few patients had recurrence of oral ulcers after knowingly deviating from the gluten-free diet. Overall, patients believed that the diet was well worth while.

Ferguson MM, Wray D, Carmichael HA, et al: **Coeliac disease** associated with recurrent **aphthae**. Gut 1980; 21:223–226.

If a patient with recurrent aphthae is found to have depression of the whole-**blood folate** value, a **jejunal biopsy** should be done to search for celiac disease.

In Glasgow, 50 consecutive patients with recurrent aphthae were investigated for evidence of nutritional deficiency and celiac disease.

Two females, ages 48 and 26 years, with minor aphthae for 6 months and 6 years, respectively, were found to have celiac disease. Neither had a history of skin disease, but one had chronic constipation with large foul-smelling stools. Jejunal biopsies, which initially showed subtotal villous atrophy, returned to normal after 4 months of a gluten-free diet along with individual nutritional replacement therapy. One patient received iron, while both received folic acid.

Biochemical evidence of **nutritional deficiency** was found in 28% of the patients, although only 10% had abnormal hemoglobins. Blood tests included hemoglobin, mean corpuscular volume, blood smear, whole-blood folate, serum vitamin B_{12}, serum iron, and total iron-binding capacity. A low blood folate value was found in 8 patients (16%).

Antibodies to an aqueous extract with wheat flour, oatmeal, or gluten were not detected in any of the patients. Patients with celiac disease often have circulating antibodies to wheat or gluten, as well as several other dietary antigens, presumably because of increased permeability of the inflamed intestinal mucosa to macromolecules. **Testing for antibodies to food** antigens in patients with recurrent aphthae **does not appear to be useful**.

Feder HM Jr, Bialecki CA: **Periodic fever** associated with aphthous stomatitis, pharyngitis and cervical adenitis. Pediatr Infect Dis J 1989; 8:186–187.

A 15-year-old boy had a temperature of 103°F (39.5°C), **aphthous ulcers** under the tongue and on the buccal mucosa, erythema of the posterior pharynx, and prominent tender anterior cervical adenopathy. Extensive immunologic tests were normal except for elevated **Epstein-Barr virus** serologic values resulting from infectious mononucleosis 1 year before.

By history he had been having recurrent aphthous stomatitis since age 2 years, and since age 10 had experienced fever (temperature up to 105°F), malaise, pharyngitis, and cervical adenitis along with the mouth ulcers. The episodes recurred every 6 to 8 weeks but became more frequent after the **infectious mononucleosis** and resulted in about 40% absenteeism from school. Each episode lasted 5 days, and between attacks he thrived.

Treatment with **cimetidine** was given because H_2 antagonists can modulate immune response. No further attacks occurred, and it was discontinued after 6 months. Perhaps breaking the cycle for 6 months corrected the underlying defect.

The **differential diagnosis** of **periodic fevers** includes:

cyclic neutropenia
periodic fever with hyperimmunoglobulinemia D
familial Mediterranean fever

In this case the first two were ruled out by normal neutrophil counts and immunoglobulins, while the latter was ruled out by a negative family history and lack of serosal involvement. **Behçet's disease** rarely has fever, and also includes genital ulcers, uveitis, and erythema nodosum—like lesions.

Marshall GS, Edwards KM: **PFAPA syndrome**. Pediatr Infect Dis J 1989; 8:658–659.

Periodic	*Pharyngitis*
Fever	*Adenitis, cervical*
Aphthous stomatitis	

The PFAPA syndrome may not be rare and is not geographically restricted. Patients may also manifest some, but not all, of the features.

Diagnostic criteria:

Onset prior to age 5 years

Regularly recurring abrupt episodes of fever lasting about 5 days, with constitutional symptoms, aphthous stomatitis and/or pharyngitis, leukocytosis or elevated erythrocyte sedimentation rate

Asymptomatic intervals (usually less than 10 weeks), normal growth, and absence of sequelae

Exclusion of cyclic neutropenia with serial neutrophil counts before, during, and after episodes

Exclusion of other **episodic syndromes**:

familial Mediterranean fever	hyper-IgD syndrome
familial Hibernian fever	Behçet's disease

Absence of clinical and laboratory evidence of:

immunodeficiency	autoimmune disease	chronic infection

Marshall GS, Edwards KM, Butler J, Lawton AR: Syndrome of **periodic fever, pharyngitis**, and **aphthous stomatitis**. J Pediatr 1987; 110:43–46.

Periodic disease encompasses a heterogeneous group of diseases with uniform limited periods of illness that recur regularly for many years in otherwise healthy individuals.

This report describes 12 children with a syndrome of periodic fever associated with symptoms strikingly similar to those seen during neutropenic episodes in **cyclic neutropenia**. Laboratory tests remained normal except for mild leukocytosis and elevation of erythrocyte sedimentation rates during attacks.

Attacks are characterized by abrupt onset of fever, malaise, chills, **aphthous stomatitis**, pharyngitis, headache, and tender **cervical adenopathy** that occur at 4- to 6-week intervals. Episodes resolve after 4 to 5 days with no long-term sequelae and may be aborted by short courses of prednisone. Antibiotics and nonsteroidal anti-inflammatory agents were ineffective.

Blignant E: Cefaclor associated with **intra-oral ulceration**. S Afr Med J 1990; 77:426–427.

In three young children, **mouth ulcers** of varying sizes covered with thick pseudomembranes persisted after cefaclor was discontinued. All children had also had **vesicular lesions** on the **skin** resembling a primary herpes virus infection, chickenpox, or a coxsackievirus infection, which cleared when the cefaclor was stopped.

Despite lack of confirmative evidence, it was thought that the mouth ulcers represented an **allergic response to cefaclor**, which has been reported to cause erythema multiforme, particularly in children. This drug shares a β-lactam ring with penicillin.

Lehner T: Recurrent **aphthous ulceration** and **autoimmunity**. Lancet 1964; 2:1154–1155.

Recurrent crops of one to four aphthous ulcers of the nonkeratinized mucosa lasting 7 to 14 days were studied in 60 patients. An immunologic reaction to nonspecific mucosal damage was suggested, as serum from 75% of the patients caused specific **hemagglutination of cells** coated with an extract of fetal buccal mucosa. The titers were higher and in much greater proportion than in controls. The reaction could be autoimmune or due to an antibody cross-reacting with an infective agent.

Bishop PMF, Harris PWR, Trafford JAP: **Oestrogen treatment** of recurrent **aphthous** mouth **ulcers**. Lancet 1967; 1:1345–1347.

Since estrogen produces hyperkeratinization and hyperplasia of oral and vaginal epithelium, the premenstrual withdrawal of estrogen may lead to failure of **keratinization** and a tendency for aphthous ulcers to develop.

In 33 of 43 women, recurrent aphthous ulcers were clearly related to the **menstrual cycle**, becoming more numerous and painful in the **premenstrual** week and during menstruation. Eleven patients also had **vaginal** or **vulval ulceration** along with the mouth ulcers.

Treatment with **estrogen** (0.2, 3.0, or 5.0 mg) for up to 3 years effectively stopped the aphthous ulcers in 30 of 33 patients with premenstrual aphthae and 5 of 10 patients with aphthae unrelated to the menstrual cycle.

Chellemi SJ, Olson DL, Shapiro S: The association between **smoking** and **aphthous** ulcers. Oral Surg 1970; 29:832–836.

In previous studies the incidence of aphthous ulcers was found to be 20% among hospital outpatients and 55% in professional-school student populations. The **greater incidence** among professional students has been postulated to be due to psychosomatic factors or possibly the trend toward **non-smoking** to promote good health.

In this study at the University of Maryland Dental School, 36 medical center employees with active aphthous ulcers 1 to 4 mm in diameter were examined. They reported painful distress 2 to 3 days after formation of the ulcer, and most had ulcers on the labial and buccal mucosa.

Psychosomatic factors were not examined, but a **smoking history** revealed that 30 of the 36 did not have any experience as smokers. Only two patients were "smokers" (one pack of cigarettes a day or three pipefuls of tobacco a day), while four had two to four cigarettes a day, and one had stopped smoking 8 months previously.

Does smoking play a significant role in inhibiting the formation of aphthous lesions?

Bookman R: **Relief** of **canker sores** on **resumption** of cigarette **smoking**. Calif Med 1960; 93:235–236.

In four men with painful recurrent aphthous stomatitis, **resumption of smoking** dramatically **relieved** the condition within a few days. In two of the patients it required about five cigarettes a day to prevent recurrence of the ulcers. The type and brand of cigarette made no difference.

All four patients had multiple large confluent ulcerations that were very painful and made eating and speaking difficult. In all patients, **cessation of smoking** was associated with **recurrence of ulcers** within 2 to 3 days. Initial symptoms had begun in two of the patients 1 to 2 weeks after cessation of smoking.

Dorsey C: More observations on relief of **aphthous stomatitis** on resumption of **cigarette smoking**. Calif Med 1964; 101:377–378.

The **cessation of smoking** may **precipitate** severe prolonged **attacks** of oral aphthae, as well as herpes simplex on the lips.

A 27-year-old man had stopped smoking 6 months previously and within 2 days developed a severe attack of **herpes simplex** on the **lips**. A few days later, deep painful aphthae appeared inside the mouth and gradually increased in number and severity until he was never without at least half a dozen lesions. He had daily fever and constant painful swelling of cervical lymph nodes. He was advised to **start smoking** again, and within 1 week was free of symptoms. He remained free of aphthae during a 3-month follow-up period.

A 40-year-old woman who had been a moderately heavy smoker for years stopped smoking abruptly. The next day she noted an **inflamed sore throat** with multiple small ulcerations throughout the mouth and throat. She also developed a low-grade fever, malaise, and cervical lymphadenopathy. One week later she also experienced a severe attack of herpes simplex of the lips. Her lips cleared, but she continued to have multiple tiny ulcers of the oropharynx. Treatment with Dexamyl to combat weight gain stopped the ulcers, but they recurred several times in a milder form after she stopped the medication. She did not wish to resume smoking, and the ulcers eventually disappeared.

A 40-year-old woman abruptly cut her smoking to six cigarettes a day, having been a moderate smoker for years. Within 2 days she developed severe **herpes simplex** of the lips and aphthae of the mouth. She also had a low-grade fever every afternoon, felt weak and tired, and had difficulty talking and concentrating on her work. Six weeks later she had 10 to 15 tiny white ulcers on the oropharynx and also had moderate cervical lymphadenopathy. Two months after the onset of her illness she resumed smoking her usual number of cigarettes, and within 2 days the throat soreness was relieved.

Gordon N, Gordon S: **Aphthous stomatitis and foreign bodies**. Lancet 1974; 1:565.

A 22-year-old woman developed aphthous stomatitis shortly after insertion of an **intrauterine contraceptive device**. The stomatitis gradually worsened over 2 years until the IUD was removed, when the ulcers disappeared.

Months later she began to wear **contact lenses** and the aphthous stomatitis returned. She stopped wearing them after 1 year, and the stomatitis cleared. As a trial, the lenses were replaced for 2 months, during which time the ulcers recurred. Removal of the lenses correlated with relief of the stomatitis.

This provocative case suggests an association between aphthous ulcers and foreign bodies.

Sallay K, Kulcsar G, Nasz I, et al: **Adenovirus isolation** from **recurrent oral ulcers**. J Periodontol 1973; 44:712–714.

In two patients with recurrent oral **ulcerations** of the **herpetiform** type, two strains of adenovirus type 1 were isolated from scrapings of the ulcers.

By means of an immunofluorescent technique, adenovirus antigens were also demonstrated in the cell nuclei of scrapings from four of seven aphthous ulcer cases.

Although there is no proof for a direct etiologic role of the adenoviruses in the ulcers, it is possible that **adenovirus type 1** exists in a latent form and causes clinical manifestations similar to those of herpes simplex virus from time to time.

Pedersen A: **Varicella zoster virus** and recurrent **aphthous ulceration**. Lancet 1989; 1:1203.

Aphthous ulcerations may be caused by reactivation of locally latent varicella zoster virus (VZV).

In five patients with recurrent aphthous ulcers, specific antibody titers to several viruses (cytomegalovirus, VZV, adenovirus, influenza A and B, para-influenza, respiratory syncytial) were measured in the ulcerative stage and 10 to 14 days later.

All five patients had at least a fourfold difference in **VZV antibody level** between the two samples. A fourfold difference in titers is usually interpreted as current infection (reinfection).

Eglin RP, Lehner T, Subak-Sharpe JH: Detection of **RNA** complementary to **herpes simplex virus** in mononuclear cells from patients with **Behçet's syndrome** and recurrent **oral ulcers**. Lancet 1982; 2:1356–1361.

Viral agents may be searched for using **labeled viral DNA probes** to hybridize specifically with complementary RNA in the cells (in situ hybridization).

Such methods used in this study strongly support an **association of HSV-1** with arthritic and ocular Behçet's disease (8 of 10 cases) and with minor aphthous ulcers (4 of 8 patients). The HSV-2 DNA probes also gave twice-higher hybridization than control viral DNA probes.

At least part of the HSV genome may be present and transcribed in peripheral blood mononuclear cells (probably **lymphocytes**) of these patients.

In diagnosis:
   The "splitters" can't see the forest for the trees.
   The "lumpers" can't see the trees for the forest.

Differential Diagnosis

Grattan CEH, Scully C: **Oral ulceration:** a **diagnostic problem**. Br Med J 1986; 292: 1093–1094.

The term *mouth ulcers* should not be used as a final diagnosis.

Most mouth ulcers are caused by **trauma** or are aphthous. Mucosal irritation develops from prostheses or appliances or trauma such as a blow, bite, or dental treatment. Such an ulcer usually heals rapidly in the absence of further trauma. Aphthous ulcers heal in 7 to 10 days.

Failure of a mouth ulcer to heal within 3 weeks raises the possibility of **malignancy** and calls for a biopsy. About 90% of malignant oral growths are **squamous cell carcinomas**, often presenting as a persistent fissure or ulcer with induration and a rolled edge. They are often associated with white lesions (**leukoplakia**) or red lesions (**erythroplasia**).

Aphthous ulcers may be associated with **deficiency** of the essential hematinics (**iron, folic acid**, and **vitamin B$_{12}$**), possibly due to chronic blood loss or malabsorption secondary to disease in the small intestine. The ulcers also may be related to the menstrual cycle or to giving up smoking.

Most infective mouth ulcers are caused by **viral infections** and are nonrecurrent, scattered, small round ulcers in a febrile child or young adult. Primary herpetic stomatitis is the most common form, with scattered vesicles and ulcers and diffuse gingivitis. Other causes include chickenpox, infectious mononucleosis, herpes zoster, and enterovirus infections (herpangina; hand, foot, and mouth disease).

Autoimmune blistering diseases and **lichen planus** must also be considered in chronic oral ulcerations, a biopsy often being required for diagnosis.

Baikie AG, Amerena VC, Morley AA: **Recurring ulcers** of the **mouth**. Lancet 1967; 1:45.

Patients with recurring mouth ulcers should be checked for **cyclic neutropenia** with twice-weekly white counts (total and differential) for 3 to 4 weeks.

Among 20 patients with cyclic neutropenia, 9 had recurring oral ulcers. In 4 patients, oral ulceration was the only symptom of the neutropenia. Ulcers appear at the time of most severe neutropenia and then heal spontaneously. In 8 of 9 patients the cyclic neutropenia was **familial**. In the other patient it was associated with lymphosarcoma.

If cyclic neutropenia is found, family members should be studied, since the disease is often familial. **Lymphosarcoma** and **agammaglobulinemia** are less common associations.

Gorlin RJ, Chaudhry AP: The oral manifestations of **cyclic (periodic) neutropenia**. Arch Dermatol 1960; 82:344–348.

An 8-year-old somewhat frail white girl had been having gum infection and mouth sores since the age of 4. Every 3 to 4 weeks the gingiva would bleed for 7 to 10 days, and she would have mouth ulcers consisting of a soft white core that dropped out. The glands would be tender and "swelled like mumps," and she would have fever for the first few days. Any **skin abrasion** while she had mouth trouble would become **infected**. Examination revealed a 1-cm ragged **ulcer on the lower lip**, several enlarged firm, swollen, tender submandibular nodes, and **redness**, swelling, and tenderness of the marginal gingiva. Her father had a similar history and at age 18 had had extraction of teeth because of severe periodontal breakdown and loose teeth.

During 6 weeks of hospitalization, frequent blood counts revealed a 21-day periodicity of neutropenia. Both circulating and bone marrow **neutrophils** would **disappear completely** for 3 to 4 days of each cycle. The oral lesions preceded the complete neutropenia by a day. Total WBC fluctuated from 3000 to 9000 with 0% to 60% neutrophils.

Cyclic neutropenia causes scarring oral ulcerations and **periodontal disease** at a young age. The ulcers are probably the same as Sutton's periadenitis mucosa necrotica recurrens, with large painful ulcers that healed with scarring and recurred at regular intervals. **Prepubertal gingivitis** is very rare and should suggest a search for cyclic neutropenia. In addition to gingivitis, periodontitis, and mouth ulcers, other symptoms may include malaise, fever, sialorrhea, abdominal pain, headache, arthralgia, conjunctivitis, and cutaneous infections.

Kay MH, Rapini RP, Fritz KA: Oral lesions in **pityriasis rosea**. Arch Dermatol 1985; 121:1449–1451.

Aphthous-like ulcers 1 to 4 mm in diameter appeared on the buccal mucosa, palate, lower lip, and underside of the tongue in a 19-year-old woman who was developing hundreds of **round to oval plaques** with an inner collarette of scale. The numerous shallow mucosal ulcerations were coated with a yellow-gray membrane and presented a regular border with an erythematous margin. Eating, drinking, and talking were difficult.

The patient denied any previous history of oral ulcerations, herpes simplex, dental work, trauma, cigarette smoking, aspirin or other drugs, diabetes, blood dyscrasias, allergies, or vesiculobullous disease. Cultures of the oral lesions showed no herpesvirus. **Blood tests** showed no evidence of folate or vitamin B_{12} deficiency. A rapid plasma reagin test was negative, and scrapings of the scaling eruptions were negative for dermatophytes.

A diagnosis of **mucocutaneous pityriasis rosea** was made. Such mucosal lesions are well known, but rarely looked for. They come in five forms:

punctate hemorrhages   erythematous annular lesions
erosions—ulcerations   erythematous plaques
erythematous macules

All are self-limited, fading with the skin lesions in 4 to 12 weeks.

Graykowski EA, Barile MF, Stanley HR: **Periadenitis aphthae:** Clinical and histopathologic aspects of lesions in a patient and of lesions produced in rabbit skin. J Am Dent Assoc 1964; 69:118–126.

A 23-year-old man was admitted to National Institutes of Health with a 15-year history of periadenitis aphthae. On admission he had a 1-cm erythematous nodule on the upper left labial mucosa that began 12 hours before.

A biopsy taken immediately yielded a pure culture of a transitional **L-form of bacteria**, thought to be an **alpha-hemolytic streptococcus**. This organism was identical to previous isolates from several other patients with periadenitis aphthae, obtained from the ulcers, from blood during exacerbation of lesions, and from biopsy tissue of early lesions. To recover the organism the pseudomembrane of the ulcer must be removed and the base of the ulcer abraded with a cotton-tipped applicator. The lesion should be less than 2 days old or L-forms are difficult to recover.

Inoculation of 0.1 ml of tissue culture suspension of the bacteria into rabbit skin led to erythematous nodules within 12 hours, followed by central softening of the nodules, crust formation, and 6-mm ulcer craters. Biopsies were similar to the periadenitis aphthae, and the same bacteria were recovered from the rabbit lesions, satisfying Koch's postulates.

Redmond AD: A potentially **life-threatening aphthous ulcer**. Br Dent J 1987; 162:136.

A 16-year-old girl had suffered with recurrent aphthous ulcerations for several years. In recent months a single ulcer had bled on several occasions, but the bleeding had stopped quickly and spontaneously.

On one occasion she developed uncontrolled **arterial hemorrhage** from a discrete ulcer on the mucosal surface of the left upper lip. She was pale and sweaty with tachycardia (100 beats/min) and blood pressure 100/60 mm Hg. Hemostasis could be achieved only by oversewing the ulcer with silk. The lesion resolved following a course of prednisolone.

Shortly thereafter the lesion recurred, with less severe hemorrhage controllable by pressure. The role of accidental or self-inflicted trauma remains unclear. Aphthous ulcers have been reported in **dermatitis artefacta**.

Hasler JF, Schultz WF: **Factitial gingival traumatism**. J Periodontol 1968; 39:362–363.

A 10-year-old boy had a 2-month history of **chronic ulceration** of the maxillary **buccal gingiva**. He was otherwise healthy. Examination revealed bilateral thin white plaques covering ulcers of the gingiva, extending from the canines to the second molars. The plaque stripped off easily, revealing extensive gingival tissue destruction. Smears were negative for *Candida*, a biopsy was nonspecific, and x-rays showed no pathologic condition. A complete blood count (CBC) and blood sugar were normal. Despite treatment with oral mycostatin and evaluation by a periodontist, the ulcers fluctuated, sometimes causing loss of the interdental papillae and exposure of the buccal roots of the deciduous molars.

Four months later he developed **infection of the thumbnails** with partial nail loss. ***Candida albicans*** was cultured from these lesions. A CBC showed leukocytosis (19,500) with a normal differential. A bone marrow biopsy was normal, but immunoelectrophoresis demonstrated a low gamma globulin fraction. Treatment with gamma globulin injections caused no improvement.

Careful interrogation in the oral diagnosis clinic at the University of Indiana finally led to the answer. Two months prior to the development of the ulcers he had noted "bumps on the upper gums that itched" (apparently associated with the erupting permanent second molars and exfoliating deciduous molars). He scratched these areas with his thumbnails to relieve the itching, with the formation of a pleasant habit. He further admitted that he was unhappy at school, citing unduly harsh treatment by his teacher and inability to match the academic performance of his peers. He also described frequent daydreams and fantasies. Apparently he received gratification from the attention received during frequent professional interviews. When asked about the cause of the problem and what might be done to correct it, he immediately stated that he was causing the tissue damage with his thumbnails and that it would heal if he cut his **fingernails shorter**. Within 2 weeks the gingival ulcerations had completely healed.

A professor is one who knows exactly what the diagnosis is but isn't quite sure.

Atopic Dermatitis

The portrait of atopic dermatitis is a recognizable one. It is one of skin thickened and red from months, years, even **decades of scratching**. It is a portrait of papules, oozing and crusted, on the face of infants. It is a portrait of lichenified eczema of the antecubital and popliteal spaces of the neck, wrists, and ankles of the child. And it is a portrait that extends to include the hands in the adult.

The atopic patient is **born to itch**. He has the genes for **pruritus** as well as for asthma and hay fever. You well know him for this constellation of drip, wheeze, and itch. Although there are no reliable laboratory tests for discerning the allergens of atopy, measuring the level of IgE gives an index of the severity of the atopic state.

Your diagnostic challenge is less in recognizing the atopic dermatitis than in discerning the trigger factors. These center on **inhalants** and **foods**. But irritants and sensitizers may figure prominently. Look for them on an empiric basis. Suspect any food the atopic child dislikes. Suspect inhalants that produce respiratory symptoms. Be alert to the hazards of contactants at home and at work. Overbathing or simply the use of lanolin-containing preparations may spell further itch.

Finally, remember that atopic dermatitic skin is commonly colonized by **bacteria**, on occasion by **dermatophyte fungi** and **yeasts**, and rarely by **herpes simplex virus**. Cultures and scrapings are often appropriate in making the "second diagnosis" for the atopic patient.

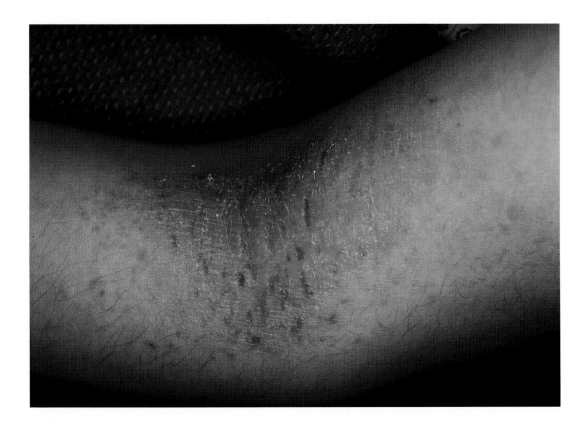

The Disease

Costa C, Rilliet A, Nicolet M, Saurat J-H: **Scoring atopic dermatitis:** The simpler the better? Acta Derm Venereol 1989; 69:41–45.

Objective assessment of the severity of atopic dermatitis can be provided by a combined score for intensity of dermatitis and for topography.

Intensity—Each of the following items scored from 0 (no lesion) to 7 (extremely severe):

erythema	scales
edema	lichenification
vesicles	pigmentation-depigmentation
crusts	pruritus
excoriations	loss of sleep

Topography—Each of ten areas scored 0 to 3 according to extent of involvement:

Symmetrical	Nonsymmetrical
hands	face
arms	scalp
feet	anterior trunk
knees	posterior trunk
legs	buttock

The **cumulative intensity and extent score** gives one number expressing the current status of the atopic patient. *E pluribus unum.*

Carrel CF, Mevorah B, Frenk E: Diagnostic value of 10 minor **clinical signs** in **atopic dermatitis**. Dermatologica 1988; 177:29.

Signs that point to atopic dermatitis:

cheilitis	**wool intolerance**
pityriasis alba	**nipple eczema**
white dermatographism	**fissure under ear**

Signs that do not point to atopic dermatitis:

infraorbital eyelid folds (Dennie, Morgan)
anterior neck folds
follicular keratoses
hyperlinear palms and soles

These conclusions are based on a statistical study in Switzerland of 105 patients with atopic dermatitis and 113 controls.

Colver GB, Mortimer PS, Millard PR, et al: The '**Dirty Neck**'—a reticulate pigmentation in atopics. Clin Exp Dermatol 1987; 12:1–4.

Reticulate pigmentation of the anterior or anterolateral aspect of the **neck** was observed in 13 atopic patients out of 500 screened. The skin appears unwashed, and hence the designation *dirty neck*. It can be distinguished from the dirty neck commonly seen in **X-linked ichthyosis**, since it does not scale, is not limited to males, and is not associated with ichthyotic scaling elsewhere.

Skin biopsies revealed mild acanthosis, abundant melanin in the epidermis, mild focal spongiosis, and a slight to moderate perivascular mononuclear cell infiltrate, including macrophages containing melanin (pigmentary incontinence).

Other **causes of blotchy pigmentation**:

allergic contact dermatitis
berloque dermatitis
Dowling-Degos disease
dyskeratosis congenita
Fanconi's syndrome
fixed drug eruption

incontinentia pigmenti
lichen planus
macular amyloidosis
nutritional deficiency
poikiloderma of Civatte
secondary syphilis

Fredriksson T, Faergemann J: The **atopic thigh**: A starting-school symptom? Acta Derm Venereol 1981; 61:452–453.

The incidence of atopic dermatitis localized to the lower gluteal and posterior thigh areas is highest in **children 6 to 8 years of age**. This age of onset may be related to sweat retention caused by prolonged sitting in atopics beginning their first years in school. For the first time in their lives, these children have to remain seated for prolonged periods.

One might view it as an **occupational disease** that remits as hardening occurs during the years that follow.

Kristmundsdottir F, David TJ: **Growth impairment** in children with **atopic eczema**. J Roy Soc Med 1987; 80:9–12.

Short stature is sometimes seen in children with atopic eczema. In 89 children (ages 1–16 years) with atopic eczema, 10% had a standing height below the 3rd percentile. Both sexes had significantly delayed skeletal maturity scores. Impaired growth was **associated with widespread eczema, asthma**, and use of **potent topical steroids**. Malabsorption, dietary restrictions, and sleeping badly (which interferes with growth hormone release) may be contributing factors.

Listen to what the patient says, more than to what other doctors have said.

The Triggers

Kemmett D, Tidman MJ: **Premenstrual exacerbation** of atopic dermatitis. Br J Dermatol 1989; 121 (suppl 34):38.

Of 150 women surveyed, **one in three** reported deterioration in atopic dermatitis during the week prior to menstruation.

Likewise, **pregnancy** had had an **adverse effect** in 62% and a beneficial effect in 22% of 50 women studied.

Sampson HA: Role of **ingested allergens** in **atopic dermatitis**. *In* Chandra RK (ed): *Food Allergy*. St. John's, Newfoundland, Nutrition Research Education Foundation, 1987, pp 203–216.

The best method for **diagnosing food hypersensitivity** in children is a **positive prick test** followed by **food challenge**. A negative prick skin test virtually excludes immediate food hypersensitivity.

Evaluation of atopic dermatitis in 160 patients using double-blind placebo-controlled oral food challenges showed that six antigens caused nearly 90% of 181 positive **clinical reactions: eggs** (38%), **peanuts** (24%), **milk** (11%), **fish** (7%), **soy** (5%), **wheat** (4%). Chicken, pork, beef, and potatoes caused another 5% of positive reactions.

Reactions consisted of pruritic erythematous macular or morbilliform eruptions over more than 5% of the body surface, with scratching and superficial excoriations. Urticaria was rare and consisted of only two to three lesions. Gastrointestinal symptoms were seen in 43% and respiratory symptoms in 28% of positive food challenges. All reactions occurred within 2 hours of challenge, often within 10 to 15 minutes, and plasma histamine was increased.

There was almost **no evidence of species cross-reactivity** in the food challenges, so that the practice of avoiding all foods within a certain botanical family is probably unnecessary.

Food challenges were performed in the hospital with a heparin lock in place. Two challenges were performed daily, using placebo and one test food given in the form of a dehydrated powder in either an opaque capsule or 100 cc of juice over a 1-hour period. The initial dose of 500 mg was increased stepwise every 10 to 15 minutes until a reaction occurred or 8 gm was consumed. After a negative challenge, the food was fed openly prior to discharge to ensure accuracy and provide reassurance.

Prior to food challenge, each patient was **prick tested** with 20 foods. A positive test was a wheal 3 mm larger than the negative control. Among 575 positive tests, six antigens accounted for 56%: eggs, peanuts, milk, wheat, soy, and fish—the same antigens that caused most of the positive food challenges. Foods often thought to exacerbate eczema (tomatoes, corn, chocolate, strawberries) rarely induced positive immediate skin tests.

Most children reacted to approximately three skin tests (range 0 to 8), but to only one or two foods on challenge. This suggests that children with atopic dermatitis are not allergic to a wide variety of foods.

Following appropriate elimination diets, in one third of 99 cases reevaluated with oral food challenge, patients **lost** their **hypersensitivity after 1 to 2 years**.

Wüthrich B, Hofer T: Food allergy: The **celery-mugwort-spice syndrome**—associated with **mango allergy**? Dtsch Med Wochenschr 1984; 109:981–986. (JAMA 1985; 253:285.)

Celery allergy, confirmable with a scratch or prick test using a fresh celery bulb, was associated with multiple **cross-sensitizations** in the umbelliferous family:

mugwort pollen—87%	fennel—13%
carrot—52%	green pepper—10%
caraway—26%	aniseed—3%
parsley—16%	

It may also be associated with mango allergy (an unrelated botanical family).

Wüthrich B: **Atopic dermatitis** flare provoked by **inhalant allergens**. Dermatologica 1989; 178:51–53.

Atopic dermatitis of the face, antecubital fossae, and abdomen appeared for the first time 6 months ago in this 31-year-old man with a family history of atopy.

Patch tests to contact allergens as well as prick and intradermal skin tests to numerous inhalants (house dust, molds, pollens) were negative. A history of the patient's having had an **aquarium** for the past 3 years and of his noting a degree of rhinitis after feeding his fish led to a scratch test with the pet-**fish food**. It was 4$^+$ positive. This was followed by a class 4 radioallergosorbent test to the main allergen in most pet-fish food, the nonbiting **red midges** (*Chironomus thummi*).

Removal of the aquarium resulted in complete clearing of the atopic dermatitis. A diagnosis of atopic dermatitis due to **fish food inhalation** was made.

It is important to recognize that 60% of patients with atopic dermatitis have **associated respiratory allergies**. However, skin tests so valuable in ascertaining the cause of allergic asthma or rhinitis are seldom of use in finding inhalant allergens of significance in atopic dermatitis. Nonetheless, a seasonal occurrence or exacerbation in spring with **periocular localization** is a good clinical index of the importance of **pollen allergens**.

In this case, knowledge of the aquarium allowed one to fish for the correct cause of the patient's atopic dermatitis.

Troilius A, Möller H: **Unilateral** eruption of endogenous **eczema** after **hemiparesis**. Acta Derm Venereol 1989; 69:256–258.

Five patients who suffered cerebrovascular **hemiplegia** noted that their **dermatidides** expressed themselves largely **on the healthy innervated side**. The specific diseases were nummular eczema, atopic dermatitis, an id reaction, and dyshidrosis.

A consultant is one who doesn't need to take a biopsy.

Differential Diagnosis

Guin JD, Skidmore G: **Compositae dermatitis** in childhood. Arch Dermatol 1987; 123:500–502.

A 9-year-old boy who had suffered for 7 years with an eczematous eruption of the face, palms, and antecubital areas was considered to have atopic dermatitis. Indeed, there was a family history of atopy. Yet **two findings** spoke to the **need for further analysis:**

The process was much more prominent in the summer.
The feet were entirely clear.

Patch testing with the standard scout tray of contactants did not provide the answer, but patch testing with the Hollister-Stier tray did. The boy had 2+ reactions to dandelion, ragweed, and sagebrush, as well as several other members of the Compositae plants. Thirty other plant allergens were negative.

Once the boy avoided contact with the sesquiterpene lactones of **dandelion** and the other **weeds**, his skin cleared. Wind and dust have not proven hazardous for him.

No longer are commercial **plant antigens** available. It is now necessary to prepare one's own: dip plant in ether, evaporate, reconstitute residue in petrolatum in a 1% concentration.

This type of weed contact dermatitis can mimic **photosensitivity**, but a look at this boy's palmar dermatitis eliminated that possibility.

Kaidbey KH, Messenger JL: The clinical spectrum of the **persistent light reactor**. Arch Dermatol 1984; 120:1441–1448.

Lichenification is the hallmark of **chronic photodermatitis**, and in the persistent light reactor it may persist 5 to 19 years after the last known contact with the photosensitizer.

A key diagnostic test is a **photopatch** test to **musk ambrette** (1% in petrolatum), a common photosensitizer in cosmetics and toiletries.

The differential diagnosis includes **atopic dermatitis**, **lichenoid drug eruption**, and **airborne contact dermatitis**.

Fisch RO, Tsai MY, Gentry WC Jr: Studies of **phenylketonurics with dermatitis**. J Am Acad Dermatol 1981; 4:284–290.

Check for phenylketonuria (PKU) in patients with "**atopic dermatitis**" who have no family history of atopy and a **normal IgE level**. As many as 46% of untreated PKU patients have an atopiclike dermatitis that shows a predilection for flexural creases. It is worse in younger patients and improves on dietary restriction of phenylalanine. Patients have elevated serum phenylalanine and tyrosine levels and urinary orthohydroxyphenylacetic acid and phenylketones.

Not all PKU is diagnosed in infancy. An example is cited of an 18-year-old man with **persistent eczema since infancy**, whose **phenylketonuric state** had not been diagnosed until he was 14.

PKU is an autosomal recessive disease caused by a deficiency of phenylalanine hydroxylase, the enzyme that converts phenylalanine to tyrosine. Mental retardation, **seizures**, dermatitis, and pigment dilution result.

Gupta AK, Love P, Rasmussen JE: **Hair abnormalities** and a **rash** with a **double-edged scale**. Arch Dermatol 1986; 122:1201–1204.

290

This 3½-year-old girl had a generalized **erythematous scaly rash** that was diagnosed and treated by others as an eczema. She also had sparse scalp hair that broke easily on combing.

The eruption that had been present since birth consisted of erythematous papules that coalesced to form **generalized migratory annular lesions** with a distinctive double-edge scale. The hairs showed bamboo-like junctures characteristic of **trichorrhexis invaginata**.

A diagnosis of **Netherton's syndrome** was made because of the conjoint ichthyosiform dermatitis and hair defect. In this case the ichthyosis presented as **ichthyosis linearis circumflexa**, but others may exhibit nonbullous congenital **ichthyosiform erythroderma** (lamellar ichthyosis).

One also expects to find an **atopic diathesis**. In this child the IgE level was 7050 IU/ml (normal 17 IU/ml). This may explain the angioedema some of these patients experience on eating nuts.

Patients with this autosomal recessive disorder of Netherton's syndrome may show mental retardation, delayed growth, recurrent infections, hypergammaglobulinemia or hypogammaglobulinemia as well as **aminoaciduria**. The latter bring an accompaniment of hair shaft disorders.

The **differential diagnosis** includes atopic dermatitis, seborrheic dermatitis, and acrodermatitis enteropathica.

Carter RL: **Majocchi's granuloma**. J Am Acad Dermatol 1980; 2:75.

For 2 years a 4-year-old boy suffered from an unidentified erythematous, eczematous dermatitis of the back of the right thigh acquired in Ethiopia. There were scattered 1- to 2-mm firm papules and residual areas of hyperpigmentation. Repeated KOH examinations and cultures of skin scrapings were negative. A biopsy showed nonspecific inflammatory change, and PAS, Giemsa, and acid-fast stains were negative. Two months of low-dose griseofulvin therapy (125 mg/day) was without effect. **Atopic dermatitis** with secondary infection was favored until **fungal culture** of a **biopsy revealed *Trichophyton rubrum***. The lesions then cleared with further griseofulvin therapy.

The **biopsy culture** can be wondrously diagnostic in cases of Majocchi's granuloma, where a penny's worth of fungus produces a pound of inflammation.

Wilkel CS, Grant-Kels JM: **Cutaneous B-cell lymphoma**. An unusual presentation. Arch Dermatol 1987; 123:1362–1367.

Nummular eczema was the initial diagnosis for an eruption a 72-year-old man had had for 18 months. Once it progressed to large indurated erythematous plaques that were pruritic, scaly, and crusted with focal ulcers and small nodules, the diagnosis of **mycosis fungoides** was made.

However, immunoperoxidase staining of the lymphomatous infiltrate proved it to be a **B-cell lymphoma** and not the T-cell lymphoma one would have anticipated from the clinical picture of mycosis fungoides.

Unlike this example, B-cell lymphomas ordinarily present as a few uniform, nonpruritic, nonscaling, nonulcerative plaques or nodules of 6 to 24 months' duration. Systemic involvement ensues in 6 months to 5 years with a poor prognosis despite early systemic chemotherapy. The diagnostic significance of **immunophenotyping** is thus clearly apparent in prognosis and therapeutic planning.

A single diagnosis may bespeak a dozen causes.

Atrophy

Today when the clinician is confronted with an idiopathic-atrophic change in the skin, the first thought is **Lyme disease**. Even when the biopsy fails to show *Borrelia* organisms on silver stain and the *Borrelia* antibody test is negative, a response to intensive penicillin therapy may confirm the view that, indeed, the atrophy has been produced by microorganisms.

Far more frightening are the **genetic hypoplasia syndromes**. Here the collagen fails to form rather than being destroyed by inflammatory disease. By contrast, many **diseases** have an **atrophic end stage**. These include acne, lichen planus, sarcoidosis, syphilis, lichen sclerosus et atrophicus, drug eruptions, the atrophoderma of Pasini and Pierini, and acrodermatitis chronica atrophicans.

Anetoderma has a special niche in the cathedral of morphology. Here are gathered the examples of a special form of atrophy, the unexplained focal loss of elastic tissue. They may or may not have been preceded by obvious inflammatory change that destroyed the elastic fibers, critical in holding the dermis in shape. Sequels to an anonymous disease, they are the permanent sign of irreversible elastolysis. They present as soft circumscribed cutaneous hernias or as foci of easily indented skin.

The biopsy will confirm your diagnosis, and it places anetoderma in a niche next to wrinkles in which photodamage has destroyed the elastic tissue. *Anetos* is the Greek word for slack. Thus, the slack skin of **cutis laxa** with its pendulous folds is but another example. It may be inherited or acquired. The slackness is widespread or acral, whereas anetoderma is strictly focal. A subset of anetoderma is the perifollicular form seen following folliculitis, as is acne.

As in so many instances, the changes in the skin are but visible examples of similar internal pathologic changes. Thus, these patients may have loci of lost elastic tissue in **other organs**, accounting for mitral valve prolapse, emphysema, and hip dislocation.

Perhaps the most difficult distinction to be made diagnostically is that between anetoderma and **neurofibromatosis**. In the latter, the soft papules or easily indented skin represents areas in which nerve fibers have largely replaced the collagen.

Wrinkles was a diagnosis so commonplace as never to have reached the diagnostic lexicon of dermatology. Few textbooks even allow the word to enter their index. Yet they deserve attention. Smokers as well as sunbathers acquire these wrinkles earlier in life than the rest of us. Their response to Retin-A has launched many a research project to learn more about them. They are actually a diminutive form of the widely known entity cutis laxa. Their presence, whether from photoaging or from inflammatory disease, indicates a loss or impairment of elastic tissue.

Cutis laxa itself may be genetically determined or acquired. Always, the histologist finds fragmented elastic fibers or absence of elastic fibers to account for the sagging skin. In the event of granulomatous change (**granulomatous slack skin**), the possibility of a T-cell lymphoma is real. The differential diagnosis for cutis laxa centers on the **Ehlers-Danlos syndromes**, in which the skin is hyperextensible as a result of abnormal collagen.

Our dermis is the connective sheath that holds us all together. We know when it is thin. We know when it is thick. And we know when it is sick. And everyone else knows when it is wrinkled.

Brownstein MH, Rabinowitz AD: The **invisible dermatoses**. J Am Acad Dermatol 1983; 8:579–588.

More than 90% of routine skin biopsies can be correctly diagnosed at low magnification. When the dermatopathologist encounters what looks like essentially normal skin, the invisible dermatoses must be considered.

A strategy for uncovering invisible dermatoses includes:

Examine the epidermis for:

fungi
cornoid lamellae (disseminated superficial actinic porokeratosis)
absence of the granular layer (dominant ichthyosis vulgaris)

Study the dermis for:

hyaline deposition (macular amyloidosis)
mast cells (telangiectasia macularis eruptiva perstans—six or more mast cells per high-power field)
microfilaria
dermal melanocytosis
silver granules
absence of sweat glands (anhidrotic ectodermal dysplasia)

Obtain special stains:

periodic acid-Schiff (PAS)—fungi	azure A—mast cells
Gomori's methenamine silver—fungi	DOPA—melanocytes
crystal violet—amyloid	Perls' iron—hemosiderin
Congo red—amyloid	Verhoeff's—elastic fibers
Giemsa—mast cells	acid orcein—elastic fibers
toluidine blue—mast cells	aldehyde fuchsin—elastic fibers

Use darkfield microscopy—silver granules

Compare with normal skin:

best, a full-thickness specimen taken perpendicular to edge of lesion, including normal or abnormal skin
must include deep dermis and subcutis
adjacent specimens from abnormal and normal skin acceptable

Look for:

connective tissue nevus	lipoatrophy
atrophoderma	pigmentation changes

If you don't **extend the biopsy to include normal skin** for comparison, your pathologist may miss:

anetoderma	connective tissue nevus
atrophoderma of Pasini and Pierini	hypopigmentation
lipoatrophy	hyperpigmentation
anhidrotic ectodermal dysplasia	urticaria

And **let him know if you are looking for**:

tinea	macular amyloidosis
porokeratosis	mastocytosis
ichthyosis	onchocerciasis

Otherwise, your patient's dermatosis may remain histologically invisible.

McConkey B, Fraser GM, Bligh AS, Whiteley H: **Transparent skin and osteoporosis**. Lancet 1963; 1:693–695.

Extremely thin skin on the dorsal aspect of the hands revealing the underlying fine veins was seen in 14 of 100 consecutive women over 60 years of

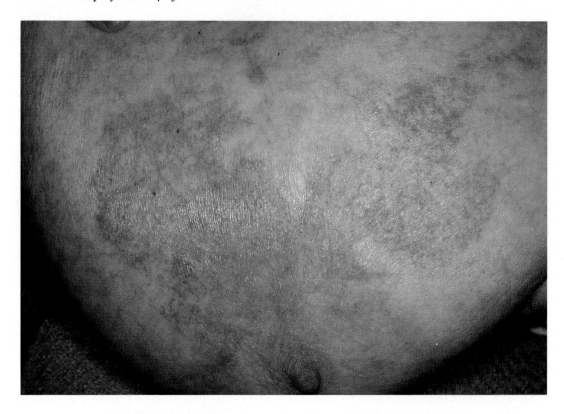

age. Such skin is smooth, loose, inelastic, and often hypopigmented. Histology showed thinning of both epidermis and dermis. **Osteoporosis** was present **in 83% of women** with "transparent" skin, compared with 12.5% of controls with opaque skin. Transparent skin was also seen in 12 men, 42% of whom had osteoporosis.

Since **bone matrix and dermis** are both connective tissues, a common underlying disorder is postulated for osteoporosis and transparent skin.

Hall EH, Terezhalmy GT: **Focal dermal hypoplasia syndrome:** Case report and literature review. J Am Acad Dermatol 1983; 9:443–451.

Here are the details on the more than **130 defects**, anomalies, and hypoplasias of skin, soft tissue, and oral and ocular tissue that have been observed in the 125 patients known to have the focal dermal hypoplasia **syndrome of Goltz and Gorlin**. The case of a 23-year-old man is presented, which illustrates many of the anomalies.

This serious **developmental defect**, almost always seen only in **females**, produces a **grotesque caricature** of the normal body. Small in stature as well as cranium, these patients may show **asymmetrical growth** with a distorted face, scoliosis, and kyphosis. The hands may be three-fingered **claws** or a web of **syndactyly**, bearing no nails.

The most evident **aplasia** is in the skin, where the skin is totally absent at various sites or thin in a linear, reticular, vermiform, or cribriform pattern. **Telangiectases** are common. The **nails** are often absent or **dystrophic** in a spooned or grooved fashion. The **hair** may be **sparse** and brittle or totally lacking in focal areas, or show patches without pigment (poliosis). **Pigmentary disturbances** are common, with linear bands or reticular areas of too little or too much pigmentation. **Fat tumors** or lipomatous lesions are also common.

The **mouth** is ringed with **papillomatous** and **verrucous growths**, which also affect the tongue, buccal mucosa, high-arched palate, anus, vulva, inguinal, and periumbilical areas. Impacted, missing, malformed, and carious teeth arise from a hemihypoplastic mandible or maxilla. In some patients, the **eye** shows its **hypoplasia** with microphthalmia and colobomas. Strabismus and nystagmus may add to the burden these patients carry. The ears may signal the syndrome by their **protrusion** and asymmetry. **Mental deficiency** and cardiac and renal anomalies are to be searched for. No mesoectodermal structures escape.

The list of defects goes on and on, and as we examine such a patient we cannot but stand in awe of a DNA that faltered.

Imamura S, Yamada M, Yamamoto K: **Lipodystrophia centrifugalis abdominalis infantilis:** A followup study. J Am Acad Dermatol 1984; 11:203–209.

The parents of a Japanese girl first noted an **ecchymosis**-like macule on the left groin at the age of 4 years. Within months it progressed to a well-defined 2.0- by 1.5-cm **depressed lesion** surrounded by slight scaly erythema. The left labium majus was atrophic, and the left inguinal lymph nodes were swollen. Skin biopsy showed an intense mononuclear cell inflammatory infiltrate in the subcutaneous fat, and a diagnosis of lipodystrophia centrifugalis abdominalis infantilis was made. The lesion gradually enlarged, and about 1 year later a second **violaceous atrophic lesion** appeared in the right groin associated with inguinal lymph node enlargement. By age 7 the lesion enlargement stopped, and the depressed areas became less evident, with disappearance of the lymph nodes. By age 11 the skin was essentially normal.

A survey of 86 Japanese cases of this disease showed it to be distinctive and **recognizable**:

> onset by the age of 3 years
> development in groin or axillary areas
> slightly inflamed edges with erythema, scaling, and induration
> loss of fat in depressed areas with panniculitis in surrounding areas
> enlargement of lesions centrifugally for several years to involve large parts
>   of the abdominal or chest wall
> **spontaneous cessation** by age 13, with restoration of normal skin contours

The **differential diagnosis** centers on the **inflammatory lipoatrophies**:

> Weber-Christian disease
> Rothmann-Makai syndrome
> morphea
> connective tissue panniculitis of Winkelmann and Padilha-Goncalves
> lupus erythematosus profundus

But the **noninflammatory lipoatrophies** also must be considered in the later stages of the disease:

> panatrophy of Gowers   annular atrophy of the ankles
> lipoatrophia annularis   lipoatrophia semicircularis

The cause of lipodystrophia centrifugalis abdominalis infantilis remains unknown, but the long-term prognosis is good.

Trevisan G, Cinco M: **Lyme disease:** A general survey. Int J Dermatol 1990; 29:1–8.

Clinical patterns

Erythema chronicum migrans:
> An expanding papuloerythematous lesion arising within 4 to 25 days at site of introduction of *Borrelia burgdorferi* by a tick bite. Shows partial central clearing. May be accompanied by other annular lesions. May be

faint and not noted. Patient may have lymphadenopathy and myalgias, arthralgias, testicular swelling, neck stiffness, and headaches.

Lymphadenosis benigna cutis:

Erythematous cyanotic nodules appearing like lymphomas 2 months to $1\frac{1}{2}$ years later. Develops near bite site or on ear lobe or areola. May remain for years. Patient may have major problems in nervous system, muscles, and joints.

Acrodermatitis chronica atrophicans:

Asymptomatic acral atrophy resulting in thin glistening skin with visible veins in later years. Arthritis becomes prominent. Patient may have **multiple sclerosis–like syndrome**.

Morphea: patches of sclerodermatous skin evolve.

Laboratory diagnosis

Direct:

culture *Borrelia*

Sample skin lesion, blood, CSF. Grow in BSK medium, but infrequently successful because of paucity of organisms.

silver stain biopsy for *Borrelia* (erythema chronicum migrans)

monoclonal antibodies to demonstrate spirochetes in tissue

Indirect:

serologic tests for IgM: may not peak for 3 to 6 weeks

serologic tests for IgG: peak months later

(Both utilize immunofluorescence assays or ELISA, and are not standardized at present.)

Abele DC, Bedingfield RB, Chandler FW, Given KS: **Progressive facial hemiatrophy (Parry-Romberg syndrome)** and borreliosis. J Am Acad Dermatol 1990; 22:531–533.

The **failure** of a 5-year-old girl **to tan** on the left side of her face along with subsequent **asymmetry of her smile** led her parents to seek medical advice. One year before she had been struck under the left eye by a swing. The skin was undergoing progressive thinning and tightening on the left side of her face, associated with mottled discoloration that extended to the left side of the chin and neck. The left side of her face appeared shrunken because of **loss of both the dermis and subcutaneous** fat.

Neurologic studies, skull x-rays, and computed tomography showed no abnormalities. However, a *Borrelia* **titer was positive**, and the child had a **history of a bite** on the left arm several months before the onset of the facial changes. The bite had produced a red swollen area with red streaks up the arm, which was treated for several days with amoxicillin.

A skin biopsy showed mild dermal sclerosis with mild lymphocytic infiltration. Rare elongated, loosely coiled microorganisms were seen in the dermis on silver stain. They fluoresced when stained with indirect immunofluorescent **monoclonal antibody** specific for *Borrelia* spp. A diagnosis was made of progressive facial hemiatrophy, presumably due to *Borrelia* **infection**. Within a month of penicillin therapy, the pigment had returned to normal, and the skin lost much of its atrophic nature.

Note that in progressive facial hemiatrophy the skin is not truly sclerotic. Instead, the **atrophic skin is soft and pliable**, similar to acrodermatitis chronica atrophicans, which is a well-recognized complication of borreliosis (Lyme disease). It is interesting that this child had a false-positive serologic **test for syphilis**, which is also seen in borreliosis.

Borreliosis also may be responsible for **morphea, lichen sclerosus et atrophicus**, and **linear scleroderma**. Cutaneous sclerosis may be viewed as a reaction pattern with many possible causes. **Sclerotic changes** are seen in scleroderma, morphea, porphyria cutanea tarda, lichen sclerosus et atrophicus, acrodermatitis chronica atrophicans, and polyvinyl chloride toxicity.

Hruza GJ, Kerdel FA: Generalized **atrophic sarcoidosis with ulcerations**. Arch Dermatol 1986; 122:320–322.

A 52-year-old man had persistent **violaceous atrophic skin lesions** covering much of the trunk, upper arms, and thighs, present for over 20 years and associated with nonhealing leg ulcers. The diagnosis of sarcoidosis was made on **biopsy** of an atrophic lesion; it explained his other problems of diabetes insipidus, hypogonadism, and anterior uveitis with corneal opacity and blindness of the left eye.

Atrophic sarcoidal lesions are very unusual, as are these other **rare forms of sarcoidosis**:

hypopigmentation	cicatricial alopecia
ichthyosiform	nonscarring alopecia
erythroderma	follicular
psoriasiform	verrucous
subcutaneous	ulcerative
lupus erythematosus–like	mutilating

In all of these the sarcoid granuloma will be found on biopsy. The one nonspecific signal of sarcoidosis is **erythema nodosum**, which should alert one to look elsewhere for sarcoidal infiltrates.

In this patient, **looking "beyond"** the atrophic lesions resulted in finding sarcoidosis in the pituitary gland, gonads, bones, joints, and liver, as well as in the skin, lungs, and eyes.

Arrieta E, Milgram-Sternberg Y: **Honeycomb atrophy of the right cheek**. Arch Dermatol 1988; 124:1101–1104.

The right side of a 10-year-old girl's face showed extensive honeycomblike depressed **scarring** present since the age of 3 years. The scars were irregular in shape, 1 to 3 mm in depth, and up to 5 mm in size. They were separated by ridges of normal skin. There had been no prior inflammatory change, and the biopsy showed fibroblast proliferation, focal calcification, and follicular plugging.

A diagnosis of **folliculitis ulerythematosa reticulata** (honeycomb atrophy) was made. Basically this is one subset of **keratosis pilaris atrophicans**, the other variant being **keratosis follicularis spinulosa decalvans**.

Ulerythema is a simple **Greek hybrid** of the words *scar* (ul) and *redness* (erythema). It vies with *reticulatum* (reticulate) and *vermiculatum* (worm-eaten) for pride of place in the litany of this atrophy. Thus we have:

ulerythema ophryogenes (eyebrows)
ulerythema acneiforme
atrophoderma reticulatum
atrophoderma reticulata symmetrica
atrophoderma vermiculée
acne vermoulante

With or without diagnostic euphony, it remains a chaotic patterned scarring of the face of unknown origin.

Look for the reticulate atrophy, follicular horny plugs, milia, and the waxy look with telangiectasia. It can be associated with various forms of congenital problems, including cardiac abnormalities (**Noonan's syndrome**).

Distinguish it from acne scarring and from nevus comedonicus (and from factitial scarring!).

Michaëlsson G, Olsson E, Westermark P: The **Rombo syndrome**: A familial disorder with **vermiculate atrophoderma**, milia, hypotrichosis, **trichoepitheliomas**, **basal cell carcinomas** and peripheral vasodilation with **cyanosis**. Acta Derm Venereol 1981; 61:497–503.

This syndrome is **named for the family** that has exhibited it for over four generations. Beginning around age 7 years, it gradually becomes more pronounced. Look for these **three characteristics**:

Coarse grainy **facial skin** with a **worm-eaten** appearance, reddish-yellow tone, and interplay between follicular atrophy and yellowish papules

Absence of **eyelashes** on the lower eyelids and partial absence on the upper eyelids. Beard scanty, slow growing, and irregular

Cyanotic redness on the lips, hands, and feet

This is the first report of this syndrome, which closely resembles the **Bazex syndrome** of follicular atrophoderma, hypotrichosis, and basal cell carcinoma appearing in early childhood. It is also similar to the syndrome of trichoepitheliomas, cylindromas, and milia described by Rasmussen.

The findings in the Rombo syndrome are essentially triggered by years of **sunlight exposure**, with basal cell carcinomas eventually being the climactic development.

Schifferli JA, Blanc E: **Partial lipodystrophy**, meningococcal meningitis and nephritis. Dermatologica 1986; 173:9–12.

In a 12-year-old girl, **measles** was followed by partial lipodystrophy with insidious loss of fat from the face, arms, and trunk. At age 17 she had *Neisseria meningitidis* **meningitis**, and at age 23 she developed glomerulonephritis and hypocomplementemia (C3).

Measles has often been associated with the onset of partial lipodystrophy and was probably the **triggering event**. The *Neisseria* meningitis reflects loss of the protective role of complement and has been reported previously in five other cases of partial lipodystrophy. Any patient with an inherited or acquired **C3 complement deficiency** is at similar risk. Hypocomplementemia in this patient resulted from a circulating autoantibody called the nephritic factor (Nef), which is associated with membranoproliferative glomerulonephritis.

It is strongly recommended that all patients with partial lipodystrophy have a **complement determination**, so that life-threatening infections can be anticipated by patients and physicians alike.

The best bird watchers use binoculars. The best diagnosticians use loupes.

Anetoderma

Venencie PY, Winkelmann RK, Moore BA: **Anetoderma:** Clinical findings, associations, and long-term follow-up evaluations. Arch Dermatol 1984; 120:1032–1039.

The **diagnosis** of anetoderma is based on:

circumscribed areas of slack skin
palpable loss of dermal substance
characteristic herniation on palpation
histologic loss of elastic tissue in the mid-dermis

Long-term follow-up of 16 patients with anetoderma seen at the Mayo Clinic indicated that the disease was still active 15 or more years after its onset. The older lesions did not heal, despite many therapeutic trials. New lesions continued to develop in seven patients, with some enlarging peripherally and coalescing into larger areas.

There was no correlation between the **mode of onset** (inflammatory or non-inflammatory) and the course of anetoderma. Some patients had both types of lesions at the same time. The original color (flesh, gray, red, or light violet) usually faded with time. The loose, shiny, wrinkled overlying skin showed characteristic herniation when palpated by a finger, and was either saclike or depressed below the level of normal skin. The arms, neck, chest, and upper back are most commonly involved.

Anetoderma is synonymous with **macular atrophy** and is a clinical and histologic syndrome. **Primary anetoderma**, whether of the **inflammatory (Jadassohn) type** or **noninflammatory (Schweninger-Buzzi) type**, occurs in clinically normal skin, although it may be associated with another dermatologic or systemic disease. **Secondary anetoderma** occurs at the site of another skin lesion, including these skin tumors: urticaria pigmentosa, pilomatrixomas, nodular amyloidosis, xanthomas, and lymphocytoma cutis.

Anetoderma and acquired cutis laxa may be parts of the same disease spectrum. Typical lesions of anetoderma may be associated with chalazodermia (cutis laxa) of the face or with **blepharochalasis**. Anetoderma lesions may also coalesce into larger lesions resembling acquired cutis laxa. In both conditions there is a **dermal defect of elastic tissue**.

Systemic associations in isolated cases of anetoderma include:

systemic lupus erythematosus
   (must be ruled out in every patient)
cataract, blue sclerae
congenital hip dislocation

diverticulum of esophagus
mitral valve prolapse
emphysema

The **differential diagnosis of anetoderma** includes focal dermal atrophies without anetoderma:

scars (discoid lupus erythematosus,
   chickenpox, cowpox)
lichen sclerosus et atrophicus
morphea
atrophia maculosa varioliformis cutis
atrophoderma of Pasini and Pierini
perifollicular atrophoderma

perifollicular macular atrophy
atrophoderma vermicularis
striae distensae
focal dermal hypoplasia
nevus lipomatosis
connective tissue nevus
neurofibroma

Friedman SJ, Venencie PY, Bradley RR, Winkelmann RK: **Familial anetoderma**. J Am Acad Dermatol 1987; 16:341–345.

Anetoderma consists of **flaccid, herniated, often saclike skin** resulting from an **absence of elastic tissue** in the mid-dermis. If there is local inflammatory change visible at the time of onset, the anetoderma is classified as the Jadassohn type. The noninflammatory form, by contrast, is labeled the Schweninger-Buzzi type.

Patients with a familial history of anetoderma deserve examination for associated **systemic abnormalities**. Case examples of the following have been observed:

optic atrophy	brachydactyly	dysosteosclerosis
sixth nerve palsy	osteogenesis imperfecta	metaphyseal dysplasia

Familial anetoderma is uncommon. Two families reported here included a 31-year-old Korean woman and her 10-year-old Korean-Caucasian daughter, both of whom had numerous **atrophic mildly hypopigmented lesions** on the chest, abdomen, and back. The lesions were longer (3 to 16 mm) and more saclike with a herniation phenomenon on palpation in the mother, who had had the lesions for 17 years. The daughter developed lesions 4 months after having a **group A streptococcal pharyngitis** with a papular exanthem. Skin biopsy in the daughter revealed a sparse perivascular round cell infiltrate and loss of elastic tissue in the mid-dermis. Granular IgM deposits were seen at the dermoepidermal junction, dermal blood vessels, and coating the elastic fibers. Abnormal laboratory results included ANA 1:160 (homogeneous), ASO 333 Todd units (normal < 166), and WBC 4300.

In two sisters, ages 5 and 3 years, anetoderma developed simultaneously, 1 year after each girl had **chickenpox**. The hypopigmented atrophic depressed herniated lesions on the trunk did not correspond to the varicella scars. ANA results were negative, but ASO titers were not tested.

Infections have been suggested in the **pathogenesis of anetoderma**, including tuberculosis, leprosy, and syphilis. An upper respiratory tract infection also preceded the anetoderma in one report. Perhaps infection could trigger a cell-mediated immune reaction against abnormal antigenic elastic fibers.

Venencie PY, Winkelmann RK: **Monoclonal antibody studies** in the skin lesions of patients with anetoderma. Arch Dermatol 1985; 121:742–749.

In five patients with anetoderma lesions present for 13 to 48 years, monoclonal antibody studies revealed substantial numbers of T cells, with a predominance of helper T cells. The majority of inflammatory cells reacted with anti-Leu-1, pan-T-cell, and anti-Leu-3a antibodies.

Inflammatory perivascular infiltrates were seen in all biopsy specimens, confirming that anetoderma is **inflammatory**. A cell-mediated immunity phenomenon directed against abnormal antigenic elastic fibers seems likely.

The **six monoclonal antibodies** studied and their specificities included:

anti-Leu-1—pan-T-cell
anti-Leu-2a—cytoxic/suppressor T cell
anti-Leu-3a—helper/inducer T cell
anti-HLA-DR—β lymphocytes, monocytes, macrophages, activated T cells, Langerhans' cells
anti-OKM$_1$—peripheral blood monocytes
anti-OKT$_6$—Langerhans' cells

Marks VJ, Miller OF: **Atrophia maculosa varioliformis cutis.** Br J Dermatol 1986; 115:105–109.

Discrete **linear** and **rectangular facial depressions** appeared on the cheeks of a 22-year-old student. They resembled scars of a factitial dermatitis, but there was no preceding inflammation. His 18-year-old brother and 19-year-old sister had recently developed similar changes. Histologically there was only a slight depression of the stratum corneum and epidermis, with no loss of elastic tissue. The problem was considered to be a rare form of **idiopathic facial macular atrophy** first described in 1918 as atrophia maculosa varioliformis cutis. It **differs from anetoderma** in that the elastic tissue is normal, the skin is not slack, and herniation is not present.

Rae V, Falanga V: **Wrinkling** due to **middermal elastolysis**. Arch Dermatol 1989; 125:950–951.

Progressive wrinkling of the **abdomen, back,** and **upper arms** for 8 months was the presenting complaint of a 33-year-old white woman. There had been no antecedent urticaria, trauma, or other skin disease, and there were no signs of inflammation or atrophy. **Plaques of rippled wrinkled skin** were seen, with wrinkles closely spaced in parallel patterning. The face, breasts, and buttocks were spared.

A **biopsy** showed mid-dermal elastolysis, with complete loss of elastic tissue in the middle dermis (revealed by an elastic tissue stain). No other changes were seen.

Elastic tissue staining should be done in all cases of acquired fine wrinkling. Without it the diagnosis cannot be made, but even with it, the cause cannot be seen.

Randle HW, Muller S: Generalized **elastolysis associated with systemic lupus erythematosus**. J Am Acad Dermatol 1983; 8:869–873.

For 2 years a 41-year-old woman had noted **progressive wrinkling** of her skin, beginning as **fine wrinkling on the face, extremities,** and **upper trunk,** with subsequent loss of tone and sagging. **Red, annular, macular lesions** preceded the wrinkling. Seven years before the onset of the wrinkling she had developed polyarthralgias and a positive ANA, and **systemic lupus erythematosus** had been diagnosed. Later she had had lupus nephritis, requiring steroids intermittently.

A **skin biopsy** showed a marked decrease in the number of elastic fibers. Direct immunofluorescence revealed granular IgM at the basement membrane and also in the papillary dermis deposited on the elastic fibers. A diagnosis of **acquired elastolysis** was made, and the autoimmune reactivity of the lupus was considered responsible.

Any patient with an inflammatory eruption is at risk of developing **elastolysis** and the consequent looseness or wrinkling of skin. **Examples** have been seen following insect bites, urticaria, and erythema multiforme. Other patients with widespread elastolysis know of no antecedent inflammation and exhibit an idiopathic form of wrinkling.

Infants may also develop elastolysis. In the autosomal recessive type, early death occurs because of internal organ involvement. In contrast, the autosomal dominant form is usually limited to the skin and has a good prognosis. If the history discloses an X-linkage inheritance, look for skeletal defects. In one case an infant exhibited a reversible acquired form that was due to the mother's taking **penicillamine,** which chelated copper and probably produced low enough copper levels in the fetus to interfere with elastic tissue synthesis.

Localized elastolysis is classically seen in **anetoderma**. Again, there is a preceding change: red papules in the Jadassohn type, **urticaria** in the **Pellizari type,** and inapparent or slight erythema in the Schweninger-Buzzi type. Anetodermas also may be the end stage of inflammatory diseases such as sarcoidosis, syphilis, and tuberculosis.

A dramatic form of localized elastolysis is the baggy eyelid of **blepharochalasis**. Examples with wrinkled spots several centimeters in diameter on the breast and eyelids with fine telangiectasias have been termed **dermatochalasis circumscripta**. Another type of localized elastolysis may follow positive **skin tests,** resulting in hanging-bag–like folds (dermohypodermitis).

Mere laxity of the skin does not signify elastolysis. **Pseudoelastolysis** occurs in senile or actinic skin and in conditions such as Ehlers-Danlos syndrome, neurofibromatosis, and pseudoxanthoma elasticum. The folded loose skin of **leprechaunism** is thickened, not lax, and the facies makes the diagnosis. The atrophic skin of acrodermatitis chronica atrophicans represents a loss of both collagen and elastic tissue and follows early inflammation.

When elastolysis is found histologically, **direct immunofluorescence** should also be done in an effort to determine a cause. It is evident that wrinkles don't always mean old age.

Crivellato E: Disseminated **nevus anelasticus**. Int J Dermatol 1986; 25:171–173.

A 23-year-old Italian man had **diffuse fine wrinkling** of the skin of the **back** and **trunk**. The lesions first appeared 5 years earlier as multiple solitary or bridged **pinkish-red soft papules** around the umbilicus. The papules were oval, slightly raised, and often had a central umbilication pierced by a lanugo hair. Size varied from a few millimeters to 1 cm. They became dark red with trauma. He was in good health and had a negative family history of skin lesions.

On the back and anterior aspect of the chest the individual lesions had coalesced to form thin wrinkled skin, with the wrinkles arranged parallel along the cutaneous lines of cleavage on the upper back. On the upper chest and interscapular region there were multiple **sharp pits** related to **pilosebaceous orifices**, resembling a **hammered-iron sheet**.

Skin **biopsies** were normal except for the elastic tissue in the subpapillary and mid-dermis. Elastic fibers were either sparse or absent and showed clumping with focal fragmentation. There was no inflammation, and the dermal collagen appeared normal. Changes were consistent with an elastic tissue nevus.

Bordas X, Ferrandiz C, Ribera M, Galofre E: **Papular elastorrhexis:** A variety of nevus anelasticus? Arch Dermatol 1987; 123:433–434.

Flat, firm, **yellowish**, isolated asymptomatic 2- to 5-mm oval **papules** kept appearing since puberty on the abdomen of a 17-year-old Spanish boy. They were solid and showed no bladderlike soft protuberances as seen in anetoderma.

Biopsy revealed only a decrease in elastic tissue. Elastic stains showed remarkable fragmentation of elastic fibers, giving a speckled appearance to the middle and deep dermis. It was distinguished from perifollicular elastolysis by its location away from perifollicular areas. X-ray examination ruled out osteopoikilosis, which at times is associated with connective tissue nevi.

A **nevus elasticus** is a **connective tissue nevus** in which elastic fibers are predominantly affected. There may be an excess of elastic tissue, or the elastic fibers may be reduced, fragmented, or absent (nevus anelasticus).

Dootson G, Sarkany I: **D-Penicillamine** induced **dermopathy** in **Wilson's disease**. Clin Exp Dermatol 1987; 12:66–68.

A 44-year-old woman was seen because of striking **wrinkling and loose folds** of her **face, neck,** and **axillae,** present for about 6 years. Her skin was very fragile, as shown by hemorrhages and milia on the knees, elbows, and knuckles. The cause was **D-penicillamine,** which she had been taking for 26 years as treatment for **Wilson's disease**. This compound interferes with collagen and elastin metabolism, with a resulting picture of cutis laxa, wrinkling, and **elastosis perforans serpiginosa**. Other unwanted side effects include urticarial and maculopapular eruptions, aphthous stomatitis, and hypertrichosis.

Penicillamine may also induce lichen planus, pemphigus, benign mucous membrane pemphigoid, lupus erythematosus, and dermatomyositis. In other words, it is an all-round heavy-duty **drug-eruption inducer**.

Cooke AM: **Osteoporosis**. Lancet 1985; 1:877–882, 929–937.

Osteoporosis commonly leads to shortening of the trunk with a rounded kyphosis and **transverse fold of skin across the upper abdomen**. The infolded skin is keratinized, showing that the fold is longstanding and not just due to a temporary postural phenomenon.

The symptoms of osteoporosis vary from none at all to total incapacity from severe **pains in the back** radiating around the trunk and to the buttocks and legs. Pains are aggravated by movement, jarring, coughing, sneezing, and straining at stool. Spinal cord compression does not occur.

Knowing the diagnosis is good.
Knowing the cause is better.
Knowing the cure is best.

Cutis Laxa

Ting HC, Foo MH, Wang F: **Acquired cutis laxa and multiple myeloma**. Br J Dermatol 1984; 110:363–367.

A 45-year-old Malay woman noted **progressive drooping** of her **skin** for 5 years, beginning insidiously with the eyelids. The **skin laxity** progressed over the face, neck, trunk, and perineum, resulting in loose folds and sagging skin befitting someone twice her age. **Biopsy** showed complete absence of elastic fibers in the upper dermis and marked reduction in the lower dermis, consistent with acquired cutis laxa. The absence of elastic tissue was not limited to the skin. She also had a large rectocele, bladder diverticulum, and abnormal respiratory function.

Further study revealed **multiple myeloma**, with an IgG paraproteinemia, Bence Jones protein in the urine, and 57% plasma cells in the bone marrow. The question arises of an association between the two diseases, as two similar cases have been reported.

Could this patient's immunoglobulin possess antielastin activity?

Lewis PG, Hood AF, Barnett NK, Holbrook KA: **Postinflammatory elastolysis** and **cutis laxa**: A case report. J Am Acad Dermatol 1990; 22:40–48.

Six days after surgical arthrodesis with allograft bone for trauma-induced arthritis, a 5-year-old boy developed a fever (temperature 40°C) and widespread erythematous 6- to 10-cm **urticarial-like lesions** that blanched on mild pressure. His hands and feet were mildly swollen. Over the next 2 months the lesions gradually faded, leaving severely **atrophic wrinkled areas**. The pronounced wrinkling of the face produced a **bloodhound-like appearance**. During this period crops of 5- to 10-mm **papules** continued to develop, which cleared with antihistamines.

Major laboratory abnormalities included very high levels of SGOT, SGPT, and creatinine phosphokinase. Serum copper and ceruloplasm levels, ECG, chest x-ray, and pulmonary function tests were normal. A **skin biopsy** showed marked diminution of elastic fibers in the reticular dermis. A diagnosis of postinflammatory elastolysis and cutis laxa was made. This rare form of cutis laxa has previously been reported only in African and South American children.

The initial lesions suggested **erythema chronicum migrans**, but this entity clears without atrophy. **Anetoderma** was ruled out by the large size of the lesions, the lack of progression of the lesions, and his young age (much younger than patients with Schweninger-Buzzi anetoderma). **Granulomatous slack skin** was ruled out by the absence of granulomas in the biopsy. Similarly, this was not a form of Ehlers-Danlos syndrome, since no collagen changes were present on light and electron microscopy. The absence of collagen changes as well as a negative family history also eliminated **Marfan's syndrome** and **pseudoxanthoma elasticum**.

It is assumed that this disfiguring dermatosis results from the massive release of **elastase** from neutrophils in the urticarial lesions early in the febrile stage of the disease. Like some other patients with cutis laxa, these patients may have decreased levels of elastase inhibitor, sufficient enough under normal circumstances to prevent elastic tissue damage. In the event of a massive hypersensitivity reaction with a marked neutrophilic response and release of elastase, the elastase inhibitor may be overwhelmed, with subsequent loss of elastic fibers. A disturbance in copper metabolism may modulate the serum elastase inhibitor in some patients with cutis laxa, but that was not found in this patient.

Fisher BK, Page E, Hanna W: **Acral** localized **acquired cutis laxa**. J Am Acad Dermatol 1989; 21:33–40.

304

Episodic swelling of the hands and feet had been experienced by a 27-year-old woman since age 13. As the years passed, the volar skin of the finger pads became loose and redundant, giving them a flat saucer appearance. **Wrinkled atrophic patches** were also seen dorsally over the phalangeal joints and elbows. Less marked changes were seen on the undersurface of the toes. Dapsone (100 mg/day) was effective in controlling the episodes of **urticaria**, but its effect on the progression of cutis laxa is unknown.

Skin **biopsies** of the fingertip and elbows showed absence of elastic fibers with only a few clumped fragments and fibers, leading to a diagnosis of acral acquired cutis laxa. An urticarial biopsy specimen showed a diffuse neutrophilic infiltrate in the reticular dermis with abundant nuclear dust. The **neutrophils** were **lined up along elastic fibers**.

Presumably, **elastin destruction** comes from the elastase-containing neutrophils of the preceding urticaria. The role of neutrophils is further shown by the fact that dapsone, of known benefit in neutrophilic disease, had a protective effect.

Two inherited types of **cutis laxa** appear **at birth** or soon thereafter. The absence of elastic fibers results in an aged appearance due to loose folds of skin hanging down. If transmitted as an autosomal dominant, it is fairly benign except for **inguinal hernias** and **bronchiectasis**. The recessive form is far more serious, with marked systemic involvement and possible early death from **emphysema**. The facies in both types is notable, with a hooked nose, everted nostrils, and large upper lip. A third inherited form is sex-linked cutis laxa, associated with **low serum copper values** and abnormalities of the genitourinary tract and skeletal system. It affects males, causing characteristic facies and mild skin laxity.

In this patient the cutis laxa was acquired, with no family history of the disorder. Such acquired forms begin later than inherited forms and are either generalized or localized:

Type 1: Generalized, beginning with loose skin on the face and neck in adulthood after an antecedent erythematous, urticarial, or papulovesicular eruption. Systemic involvement may include inguinal and hiatal hernias, emphysema, aortic dilatation, and gastrointestinal and genitourinary diverticula.

Type 2: Marshall's syndrome. Localized, in black infants and young children, mainly girls in South Africa, with preceding acute inflammation. Acute lesions are usually well-defined plaques that enlarge peripherally but may be quite diffuse. These are soon followed by localized areas of skin laxity, which always involve the face.

Acquired **postinflammatory elastolysis** has also been reported following urticarial reactions to penicillin and penicillamine, chronic acrodermatitis, syphilis, sarcoidosis, necrobiosis lipoidica, and multiple myeloma.

Yedomon HG, Ango-Padonou FD: **Cutis laxa acquise** post-inflammatoire. Ann Dermatol Venereol 1990; 117:547–548.

A 30-year-old black woman from Africa had had an erythematous plaque-type eruption with fever at age 5, which persisted several months. It was followed by **plaques of loose skin** and striking folds; these stabilized after about 2 years. The axillae were most severely affected, with lesser changes on the neck, chest, abdomen, and sacral area.

When the loose folds of skin were distended they relaxed with slow return to the initial position, characteristic of **cutis laxa**. Histopathology showed fragmentation of the collagen and elastic fibers in the mid-dermis.

She suffered from severe emotional problems because of the extreme cosmetic problem of looking old at a very young age.

Postinflammatory cutis laxa usually affects female children between 18 months and 6 years of age, following an urticarial or other inflammatory rash. Insect bites and drug reactions have been suspected triggering factors.

Tsuji T, Imajo Y, Sawabe M, et al: **Acquired cutis laxa** concomitant with **nephrotic syndrome**. Arch Dermatol 1987; 123:1211–1216.

A 41-year-old Japanese woman noted marked **facial wrinkling and skin laxity** extending down from the angles of her mouth. Within 6 months the wrinkling involved the neck, back, and chest. There had been no antecedent skin disease. On examination the eyelids, legs, and feet were edematous. The skin showed marked laxity and greatly diminished elasticity over the entire body, with many loose folds and much sagging, most marked over the face, neck, axillae, and trunk. However, the skin of the distal extremities appeared normal.

A diagnosis of acquired cutis laxa was confirmed with a skin **biopsy** by finding virtual absence of elastic fibers in all layers of the dermis. Only a few remnants of fragmented elastic fibers remained. Direct immunofluorescence studies were negative for IgG, IgM, IgA, and C3.

Laboratory study also disclosed low complement levels (C3, C50) and proteinuria, but negative tests for systemic lupus erythematosus. **A renal biopsy** showed membranoproliferative **glomerulonephritis** (type 2) with C3 and IgG deposits. She also had a goiter (negative immunofluorescence) and iron deficiency anemia.

There have been only 26 reported cases of acquired cutis laxa; 11 of the patients had a prior erythematous rash, and 18 had associated problems from **elastic tissue deficits elsewhere** (emphysema, diverticula, hernias).

Although no circulating antibodies to elastic fibers were detected in this patient, it is interesting to speculate that there may be a common immunoglobulin that caused both the acquired cutis laxa and the membranoproliferative glomerulonephritis.

Muster AJ, Herman JJ, Esterly NB, et al: Fatal cardiovascular disease and cutis laxa following **acute febrile neutrophilic dermatosis**. J Pediatr 1983; 102:243–248.

A 16-month-old black girl with asthma and a right middle lobe infiltrate developed symmetrical annular facial plaques associated with temperature spikes to 40°C. New papules and nodules then appeared rapidly on the trunk and limbs and evolved into **annular plaques** with heaped-up indurated margins and depressed centers. The WBC was 26,000/mm^3 with 52% polymorphonuclear leukocytes and 10% eosinophils, and platelet counts averaged 862,000/mm^3. A skin biopsy was consistent with **Sweet's syndrome**.

Treatment with prednisone for 13 months calmed the fever and skin lesions, but postinflammatory cutis laxa was noted.

At age 30 months she was hospitalized with recurrent fever, lethargy, and a newly developed grade 3/6 systolic ejection murmur and grade 2/6 blowing diastolic murmur. An ECG showed left ventricular hypertrophy, and an echocardiogram showed a dilated ascending aorta and thickened aortic leaflets. **Angiocardiography** also revealed a diverticulum-like aneurysm on the aorta. She died suddenly 9 days after cardiac catheterization.

Necropsy revealed patches of wrinkled hyperpigmented skin interspersed with areas of normal skin on the face, trunk, and limbs. In areas of cutis laxa there were no perceptible elastic fibers in the papillary dermis and no normal elastic fibers in the deeper dermis. Electron microscopy revealed only abnormal elastic fibers composed almost exclusively of elastin and lacking an internal microfibrillar framework.

Histologic findings in the ascending **aorta** showed a recent neutrophilic infiltrate within the aortic wall with almost total elastolysis of the elastic layer. Older lesions showed myxomatous degeneration. Coronary artery disease was also present, with intimal fibrosis and total occlusion of the right coronary artery ostium.

Postinflammatory **cutis laxa following Sweet's syndrome** has been documented in two other young black girls. It has not been noted in adults with Sweet's syndrome.

Turner-Stokes L, Turton C, Pope FM, Green M: **Emphysema and cutis laxa**. Thorax 1983; 38:790–792.

Emphysema presenting in **teenagers** is unusual, even in homozygous alpha$_1$-antitrypsin deficiency. In two cases presented here it was associated with cutis laxa that began around the age of 10 years. Chronic asthma may have been a factor.

A 14-year-old boy had an attack of **severe breathlessness** that led to hospitalization. He had a history of infantile eczema and asthma, but had been active in sports until recent years. In addition to a supraumbilical hernia, **skin laxity** was noted, with infraorbital sagging and loose skin around the eyelids and earlobes. A chest x-ray showed severe bilateral basal emphysema, and pulmonary function tests showed a severe obstructive defect. A **skin biopsy** showed short thick elastic fibers with fragmentation, characteristic of cutis laxa.

A 13-year-old girl who had previously enjoyed sports began to lose weight and develop progressive dyspnea at age 10 and eventually could barely climb one flight of stairs. She was thin and breathless, with **pendulous earlobes** and **lax skin on the genitalia**. Skin biopsy was unrevealing, but chest x-ray showed severe bullous emphysema. She died at age 14 years of respiratory failure.

When the patient returns "no better," question your diagnosis as well as your treatment.

Axilla

When the patient's arm goes up for inspection of the axilla, what awaits us? It may vary from the commonplace odor of soured apocrine sweat to the rarity of colored apocrine sweat. It may range from the commonplace contact dermatitis to the rarity of Hailey-Hailey disease.

Of course, the axilla may play host to almost any condition. However, the unique anatomy of the axillary vault provides two localizing factors—**moisture** and **friction**. Moreover, it is the home of the apocrine sweat gland.

The moisture and maceration of the axilla favor infection. The most dramatic example is **hidradenitis suppurativa**. It may present as **apocrinitis**, which is often mistaken for **folliculitis**. Chronic and recalcitrant, these apocrine infections may then progress from the gland itself to involve the entire subcutaneous apocrine organ. As a consequence, tender, boggy, tumorlike masses appear. These are scarred and may drain pus for years.

More superficial bacterial infections involving the axilla are **bullous impetigo** and the impetiginization of an **axillary dermatitis**. The moisture and warmth of the axilla allow a variety of bacterial, yeast, fungal, and viral organisms to thrive. Look for the gross colonies of corynebacteria on the hair shaft seen in **trichomycosis axillaris** of the axilla that is never bathed. Suspect the marginated darkened patches of **erythrasma** and confirm the diagnosis by seeing them glow coral-red under your Wood's light. Entertain the diagnosis of **candidiasis** and affirm it by noting satellite pustules.

Not only is infection favored in the axilla and other such intertriginous areas, but superinfection is as well. Any chronic eczematous eruption—especially **Hailey-Hailey disease**—can support bacterial, yeast, or viral colonization. A culture is your only entry to knowledge of this.

The second major localizing factor for axillary dermatoses is friction. It is this friction accentuated by the wetness of the area that gives rise to a Koebner form of **psoriasis**. Its red sharply circumscribed plaques may resemble **seborrheic dermatitis**, but recall that the typical scale of psoriasis is rubbed off by movement of the arm.

And it is friction, sweat, and use of harsh antiperspirants that localize Hailey-Hailey disease in the axillae. These patients have the inborn defect of epidermal adherence; the area often cannot withstand the shearing forces of friction.

Again, the profuse axillary eccrine sweat washes out dyes and other contactants from clothing. This can lead to a **contact dermatitis** remarkably restricted to the armpits.

The axilla remains a secret garden where many dermatoses may grow.

Mali-Gerrits MMG, van de Kerkhof PCM, Mier PD, Happle R: Axillary apocrine chromhidrosis. Arch Dermatol 1988; 124:494–496.

> A 35-year-old woman had a 10-month history of **black stains** appearing in the **armpits** of her blouses during periods of emotional excitement or stress. The diagnosis of apocrine chromhidrosis was made by simple manual expression of **brownish-black droplets** from a fold of axillary skin. Skin biopsy showed prominent brown granules in the secretory cells of the apocrine glands. The granules were PAS positive and showed yellow autofluorescence in ultraviolet light. Further spectroscopic studies indicated that the color was due to a lipopigment, but not lipofuscin.

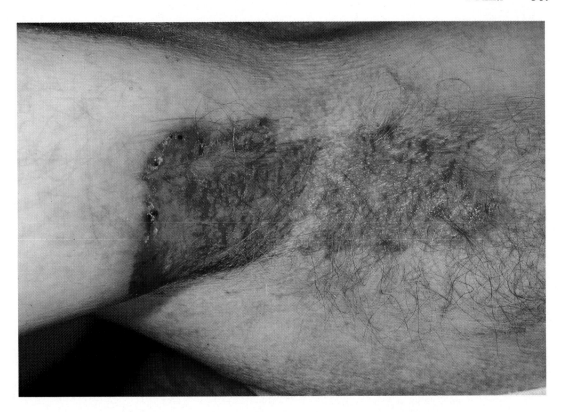

The condition must be distinguished from **pseudochromhidrosis** in which either **chromogenic bacteria** or a **clothing dye** causes the colored sweat. Also, **ochronosis** must be ruled out, since it can cause brown axillary sweating. In this patient urinalysis showed no homogentisic acid.

Poh-Fitzpatrick MB: "**Red sweat.**" J Am Acad Dermatol 1981; 4:481–482.

Cherry-red droplets and **dots** were observed appearing on the faces, arms, and hands of **flight attendants** en route between New York and Florida. No passengers or pilots were affected. Occupational chromhidrosis was suspected, and the possible role of fumes or leaks in the fluid containment systems was explored.

The mystery was solved when it was observed that a fine red powder came off labels of **life vests** during demonstrations by the flight attendant. Later, when the dye was solubilized by sweat or sebum, the strange "red sweat" appeared. Removal of the marked vests resulted in instant cure.

Brenner DE, Lookingbill DP: Anaerobic micro-organisms in chronic **suppurative hidradenitis**. Lancet 1980; 2:921–922.

In five patients with severe hidradenitis, **anaerobic cultures** revealed heavy growths of *Bacteroides fragilis* and *Bacteroides melaninogenicus*. These **gram-negative rods** could be seen in smears of pus from the sinus tracts, from which aerobic cultures were either negative or showed *Staphylococcus epidermidis*, *S. aureus*, or beta-hemolytic streptococcus. Successful anaerobic cultures were obtained by deep needle aspiration within sinus tracts. *B. fragilis* is sensitive to clindamycin, chloramphenicol, cefoxitin, and metronidazole.

Zaim MT, Bickers DR: **Herpes simplex associated with Hailey-Hailey disease**. J Am Acad Dermatol 1987; 17:701–702.

Superinfection of the lesions of Hailey-Hailey disease occurs not only with **staphylococci** and **candida** but also with the **herpes simplex virus**.

Almeida L, Grossman ME: **Benign familial pemphigus** complicated by **herpes simplex virus**. Cutis 1989; 44:261–262.

This 64-year-old woman developed **erosions** of her neck, **axillae**, inframammary area, perineum, and gluteal cleft. The history indicated that she had had a recurring blistering dermatosis of the axillae. Her **mother and brother** had a similar problem. A diagnosis of benign familial pemphigus had been made histologically, and negative immunofluorescence tests confirmed this. She had had no lesions for 5 years.

A **culture** of the erosions showed a growth of **group A streptococci**. However, despite oral antibiotic therapy the lesions continued to expand, and primary umbilicated vesicles were seen. A **Tzanck smear** was positive for multinucleated giant cells. Herpes simplex virus type 2 was then cultured from an inframammary vesicle.

A diagnosis of herpes simplex was made, and complete healing occurred promptly upon the institution of **acyclovir therapy**.

Recall that the intertriginous sites of familial benign chronic pemphigus provide wonderfully favorable soil for the growth of pathogenic bacteria and yeast, as well as the herpes simplex virus.

Engesser L, Broekmans AW, Briët E, et al: **Hereditary protein S deficiency:** Clinical manifestations. Ann Intern Med 1987; 106:677–682.

A hereditary clotting defect may be present when **superficial thrombophlebitis, deep venous thrombosis** in unusual locations (**axilla**, mesentery, cerebral veins), or pulmonary embolism occurs without a predisposing cause (surgery, trauma, childbirth, old age, or disease).

Protein C and protein S are vitamin K–dependent proteins that work together as **anticoagulants** to stimulate fibrinolysis. **Deficiencies** of either one of these proteins may lead to **venous thrombotic events**, starting around age 28 years. Both defects are autosomal dominant traits.

Protein C deficiency may lead to **coumarin-induced hemorrhagic skin necrosis** in the early phase of oral anticoagulant treatment, but this has not been seen in protein S deficiency.

Hughes DG, Dixon PM: **Poolplayers' thrombosis**. Br Med J 1987; 295:1652.

Phlebographic-proven **thrombosis** of the **subclavian** and **axillary veins** in two young men accounted for **pain and swelling of the right arm** that appeared the day after they had played pool. The pathogenesis is related to extension and rotation of the right shoulder with subsequent stretching and compression of the subclavian vein. **Spontaneous thrombosis of the arm veins** *is usually related to strenuous or unaccustomed activity.*

Light N, Meyrick Thomas RH, Stephens A, et al: Collagen and elastin changes in **D-penicillamine–induced pseudoxanthoma elasticum-like skin**. Br J Dermatol 1986; 114:381–388.

In a 59-year-old man, **yellowish elastotic papules** of the neck and face, a "**plucked-chicken skin**" appearance in the **axillae**, and large loose redundant folds of skin on the chest, abdomen, and back were the result of 19 years of large-dose D-penicillamine used to treat cystinuria. **D-Penicillamine** inhibits urinary calculus formation in **cystinuria** by lowering urinary cystine excretion. It also interferes with collagen and elastin cross-linking, which was believed to be the cause of his skin problems.

Other **adverse cutaneous effects** of D-penicillamine therapy include hemorrhagic bullae, elastosis perforans serpiginosa, and **cutis hyperelastica**.

Cochran RJ, Wilkin JK: An unusual case of **calcinosis cutis**. J Am Acad Dermatol 1983; 8:103–106.

This 22-year-old man had a 3-week-old **red-brown rash** of the axillae, crural areas, and upper inner thighs. The axillary involvement **spared the vault** and had a **reticulated** appearance. Its clinical appearance suggested the "**chicken skin**" morphology of pseudoxanthoma elasticum, yet funduscopic examination was normal. On palpation the lesions had a **woody-hard indurated** feel.

A **biopsy** showed dense basophilic deposits in the dermis that were calcium (von Kossa stain). A technetium 99m bone scan revealed plaques of uptake in the axillary and inguinal areas.

The presence of elevated serum calcium levels supported a diagnosis of **metastatic calcinosis cutis**. It was presumed that inapparent frictional damage to the elastic tissue in these sites accounted for the selective deposition of calcium and for the clinical **resemblance** of the rash to **pseudoxanthoma elasticum**.

All that feels hard is not scleroderma.

'Tis better to have a working diagnosis than no diagnosis at all.

Basal Cell Carcinoma

Watch out for the pitfalls. Sure, it is easy to recognize the nodule with rolled waxy edging, telangiectasia, and central ulceration as a basal cell epithelioma. But recall there may be as many as a score of clinical versions and settings. Some may mislead you. Here are examples we have seen:

- a basal cell carcinoma hidden within the furrows of rhinophyma
- a slightly raised, slowly enlarging plaque that over 7 years enlarged to cover most of the right cheek of a physician's wife. He thought it was not a basal cell carcinoma because it did not ulcerate.
- a scarring basal cell epithelioma camouflaged among acne scars
- a pigmented basal cell carcinoma that mimicked a malignant melanoma
- a pure ulcer within normal skin. It looked like a trephine biopsy site
- a basal cell carcinoma that looked like actinic keratosis

Although the face is the primary site for basal cell epitheliomas, they can occur elsewhere. On the leg they may pass as a stasis ulcer. Your only diagnostic chance may be a biopsy.

A cluster of basal cell epitheliomas or numerous ones raise the possibility of either the basal cell nevus syndrome or the Bazex syndrome. A little palm reading for pits—as well as an x-ray for bone cysts and a search for atrophoderma—is helpful. A few examples may still be the result of arsenic, e.g., exposure to Paris green or Fowler's solution.

Remember, your index of suspicion for basal cell epitheliomas must increase in the sun worshipper, the patient who has had radiation, and the immunosuppressed patient. Look for them to develop in nevus sebaceus, porokeratosis, and linear epithelial nevi. And never stop looking for these lesions in the PUVA-treated patient, the tar-and-light–treated psoriatic, and the xeroderma pigmentosum patient.

Be suspicious of basal cell epithelioma in any unexplained ulcer, no matter what its depth. They can bore down through cartilage and bone, even though they rarely metastasize. They can be serpiginous, and they can be large. We once saw one neglected for 20 years that presented as a fungating foul-smelling mass covering half of the man's back.

Biopsy anything strange that grows and enlarges, no matter how slowly. Don't be surprised if the report is sebaceous hyperplasia, Bowen's disease, Paget's disease, Spitz nevus, seborrheic keratosis, or even an amelanotic melanoma. Recently we had one turn out to be an angioma.

You serve the patient best when you biopsy and let the pathologist be the ultimate diagnostician.

Kuflik EG: Clinical **variants** of basal cell carcinoma. Cutis 1981; 28:403–408.

papular	cystic
nodular	morpheiform
ulcerative	superficial
pigmented	

Pratt MD, Jackson R: **Nevoid basal cell carcinoma syndrome**: A 15-year follow-up of cases in Ottawa and the Ottawa Valley. J Am Acad Dermatol 1987; 16:964–970.

Major findings:

multiple basal cell carcinomas	pits on palms, soles
odontogenic keratocysts of jaw	ectopic calcification—falx cerebri

Associations:

facies—bossing, hypertelorism
skin—cysts, milia, confluent eyebrows, supernumerary nipples
skeletal—prognathism, cleft palate, poly-syn-arachnodactyly, deformed clavicle, scapula, pes planus, hallux valgus
CNS—hydrocephalus, deafness, retardation
eye—congenital blindness (cataract, glaucoma)
misc.—hypogonadism, fibromas, fibrosarcoma, squamous cell carcinoma
autopsy—brain cysts, atrophy, leiomyomas, kidney malformation, adrenal adenomas

Plosila M, Kiistala R, Niemi K-M: The **Bazex syndrome**: Follicular atrophoderma with multiple basal cell carcinoma, hypotrichosis and hypohidrosis. Clin Exp Dermatol 1981; 6:31–41.

Numerous **small sharp pits** on the **backs** of the **hands, elbows,** and **knees** were of concern to this 13-year-old boy. His history revealed a severe atopic dermatitis at age 3, at which time congenital scarcity of hair and the presence of facial **milia** were noted. By age 11 he was found to have developed basal cell epitheliomas of the face.

On the dorsa of both hands was seen a sharply outlined island of abnormally deep and wide follicles. This **orange-peel pattern** of **follicular atrophoderma** covered the elbows, knees, and back. No palmar or plantar pits were seen. There was diffuse **alopecia** of the scalp, eyebrows, and eyelashes. The scalp hair was short and under the microscope showed features of pilus tortus.

Biopsies showed small keratin plugs at the openings of atrophic disfigured follicles. No sweat glands were discerned, and this correlated with sweat secretion studies, which confirmed the patient's **hypohidrosis**.

Four family members showed the same pitted skin; this revealed the hereditary nature of this problem.

A diagnosis of Bazex syndrome was made on the basis of the tetrad of findings: follicular atrophoderma, hypotrichosis, multiple basal cell epitheliomas, hypohidrosis. It is a dominantly inherited disorder in which follicular abnormalities are the centerpiece.

Pits on the palms and pits on the backs of the hands, both bespeak nevoid basal cell epitheliomas, present or future.

Monihan JM, Nguyen TU, Guill MA: **Brunsting-Perry pemphigoid** simulating basal cell carcinoma. J Am Acad Dermatol 1989; 21:331–334.

A 66-year-old woman was referred for removal of two suspected basal cell carcinomas of her forehead and chest. Both lesions were **crusted erythematous**, slowly enlarging **plaques**. Trauma from washing caused bleeding.

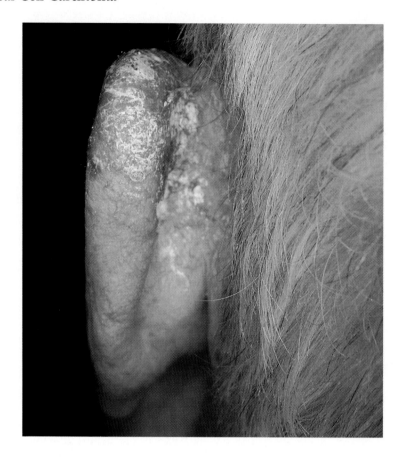

On initial examination the lesions appeared to be superficial multicentric basal cell carcinomas. Close examination, however, revealed the diagnostic presence of rare, small, flaccid **vesicles** in the lesions. Immunofluorescent study of the biopsy revealed a prominent continuous granular band of IgG at the dermoepidermal junction. No tumor could be found, and a diagnosis of Brunsting-Perry pemphigoid was made.

A few weeks of topical steroid therapy proved to be just as curative and much less traumatic than the scalpel proposed.

Brodkin RH, Rickert RR, Fuller FW, Saporito C: **Malignant disseminated porokeratosis**. Arch Dermatol 1987; 123:1521–1526.

Numerous symmetrical, **atrophic, pink macules** with thin or thick whitish-gray **flaky scale** covered the entire body of a 56-year-old man. Although these had been present for over 25 years, in the last 3 years inflammatory red plaques and large moist bright-red granulation-tissue–like **fungating draining masses** had appeared on one arm and one thigh. Clinical diagnoses included multiple superficial basal cell carcinomas and parapsoriasis with mycosis fungoides.

Excisional biopsies of the two fungating tumors showed **squamous cell carcinoma** arising from lesions of porokeratosis with definite cornoid lamellae. Several nodular **basal cell carcinomas** were also removed from the face and legs. In the ensuing years, additional squamous cell carcinomas were excised, but 8 years later he developed widespread metastases and died of *Escherichia coli* sepsis.

This unique variant of porokeratosis was nonfamilial, not related to excessive sunlight exposure, and highly premalignant. It is quite different from the three other **types of porokeratosis**:

1. **Porokeratosis of Mibelli:** simple dominant heredity, rare, more common in males; begins in childhood; characterized by one or several lesions up to 10 cm in size and visible furrow in border; may evolve into Bowen's disease or squamous cell carcinoma
2. **Porokeratosis palmaris et plantaris disseminata:** familial, very rare, more common in males; onset in early adulthood; affects palms and soles; lesions up to 5 cm in size, often tender, no visible furrow; patient may develop squamous cell carcinoma
3. **Disseminated superficial actinic porokeratosis:** the most common form; sun-exposed areas; multiple small lesions 0.5 to 1.0 cm in size, distinct border but no visible furrow; patient may develop squamous cell carcinoma

Poyzer KG, deLauney WE: **Pseudorecidivism** of **irradiated basal cell carcinoma**. Aust J Dermatol 1974; 15:77–83.

A lesion resembling **keratoacanthoma** or **seborrheic keratosis** may arise at the site of a previously irradiated basal cell epithelioma. It appears 2 to 4 weeks postradiation and then spontaneously disappears within 2 months.

You can get arrested for speeding through a history.

Behçet's Syndrome

The diagnostic entry point for Behçet's syndrome is the history of **recurrent aphthous ulcers**. Given the association of **genital ulcers** and **inflammatory eye changes**, the circle is complete for recognition of the triple symptom complex first described in 1937 by the Turkish dermatologist Hulusi Behçet. These lesions form only the tip of the iceberg, as beneath the skin there is an all-pervading **vasculitis** that may trouble almost any organ. This diagnostically tantalizing syndrome has bits and parts that may be separated by years. First may come malaise, unexplained fevers, arthralgias, and myalgias, so destructive to the diagnostician's ego. But eventually the appearance of aphthous stomatitis brings the thought of Behçet's, strengthened later by the appearance of genital ulcers and the eye changes of uveitis, iritis, and iridocyclitis. The diagnostician then has a handle on all of the gastrointestinal, cardiac, renal, central nervous system, and musculoskeletal pathology that may ensue.

One of the most intriguing diagnostic maneuvers that one can undertake is a simple **needle prick**, which in Behçet's syndrome leads to a positive tuberculin-like reaction within 24 to 40 hours. This pathergic response to simple injury occurs in both the skin and mucosa, putting these patients at grave risk. The cause of the vasculitic changes in Behçet's syndrome remains unknown, but a viral agent or an L-form of streptococcus is the leading contender.

Patients with chronic recurrent aphthous ulcers, especially the severe forms, must be considered candidates for the diagnosis of Behçet's syndrome and deserve long-term consultation with the ophthalmologist, internist, and gynecologist. Behçet's disease is very serious, being the leading cause of **blindness** in Japan. It is within the clinician's grasp to make the diagnosis, once it is recognized that the whole syndrome may not be present at one time.

Teter MS, Hochberg MC: **Diagnostic criteria** and epidemiology. *In* Plotkin GR, Calabro JJ, O'Duffy JD (eds): Behçet's Disease: A Contemporary Synopsis. Mount Kisco, New York, Futura Publishing Co., Inc., 1988, pp 9–27.

The **major criteria** for making a diagnosis of Behçet's syndrome are:

1. Recurrent aphthous ulcerations in the mouth
2. Skin lesions, e.g., erythema nodosum, thrombophlebitis, positive reaction to needle stick
3. Eye lesions: iritis, iridocyclitis, chorioretinitis
4. Genital ulcerations

The **minor criteria** are:

1. Arthralgia
2. Abdominal pain, melena
3. Epididymitis
4. Central nervous system syndromes
5. Vascular lesions, occluded blood vessels, aneurysms

International Study Group for Behçet's Disease: **Criteria for diagnosis** of Behçet's disease. Lancet 1990; 335:1078–1080.

Experts from seven countries took the five complicated sets of diagnostic criteria presently in use and condensed them into one set of diagnostic criteria that are simpler to use.

Recurrent oral ulceration *must* be present, with **three recurrences in one 12-month period**; may include minor aphthous, major aphthous, or herpetiform ulceration.

Two of the following must also be present:

recurrent **genital ulceration** (aphthous ulceration or scarring)
eye lesions:
    anterior uveitis
    posterior uveitis
    cells in vitreous (slit-lamp examination)
    retinal vasculitis
skin lesions:
    erythema nodosum
    pseudofolliculitis
    papulopustules
    acneiform nodules (postadolescent—not receiving steroid therapy)
    positive pathergy test—read by physician at 24 to 48 hours

Lakhanpal S, O'Duffy JD, Lie JT: Pathology. *In* Plotkin GR, Calabro JJ, O'Duffy JD (eds): **Behçet's Disease**: A Contemporary Synopsis. Mount Kisco, New York, Futura Publishing Co., Inc., 1988, pp 101–142.

The sine qua non of Behçet's syndrome is recurrent **aphthous stomatitis**. It occurs in virtually all patients with this disorder and often is the first sign. The ulcers are located on the lips, gingiva, buccal mucosa, tongue, and less commonly on the palate, tonsils, and pharynx. They may be single or multiple and may cluster, beginning as erythematous, slightly raised areas that ulcerate in 1 or 2 days. The **ulcer** size ranges from 2 to 10 mm with a **central yellow base** surrounded by a discrete **erythematous halo**. Healing usually occurs without scarring but may be delayed up to 30 days. Recurrence is the rule. Glossitis also occurs. A biopsy reveals only the monocytic inflammatory infiltrate common to all aphthae.

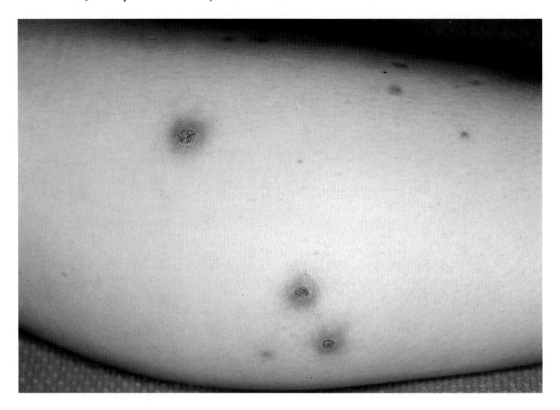

Genital ulcers are similar to the oral lesions, but are fewer, larger, deeper, and less recurrent than their oral counterparts. In females, they occur on the vulva, vagina, cervix, perineum, and perianal area. In the vagina they may be asymptomatic, with the patient being unaware of them. In males, ulcers appear at the urethral orifice and on the penis, scrotum, and perianal area and are very painful. Biopsy may show **necrotizing vasculitis** in the subcutaneous tissue in addition to the same changes as seen in oral aphthae.

Most patients also have cutaneous lesions that reflect vasculitis. Nodular lesions similar to **erythema nodosum** occur on the legs as well as the face, neck, trunk, and buttocks. They may ulcerate and heal with hyperpigmentation. **Vesicles**, sterile **pustules**, and **purpuric areas** may evolve into deep punched-out ulcers. Folliculitis, abscesses, acne, pyodermas, erythema multiforme, and figurate erythemas join the parade of skin findings. Also look and palpate for **thrombosed veins**.

Most significant is the erythematous tuberculin-like reaction or sterile pustule that appears a day or two after a simple needle prick or injection of sterile saline. This is the diagnostic pathergy of Behçet's syndrome.

O'Duffy JD: **Behçet's syndrome**. N Engl J Med 1989; 322:326–328.

The characteristic **oral lesions** are discrete round or oval, **white ulcerations** 3 to 15 mm in diameter with a **red rim**. They recur in crops and heal without scars.

In some patients, cutaneous **nodular pustules** develop **at** the site of simple **needle sticks** during exacerbations. They are similar to the aneurysmal arteriovenous communications that sometimes result from angiographic procedures.

Behçet's syndrome shares features with other autoimmune disorders such as rheumatoid arthritis. The earliest infiltrates in the dermis and basal layers of the epidermis preceding the epidermal slough are mostly immunocompetent **T lymphocytes** and **plasma cells**. Elsewhere, including the retina, brain, and subcutaneous tissue, **vasculitis** is a key feature.

Behçet's syndrome is most common in countries of the eastern Mediterranean and eastern rim of Asia, where it is a leading cause of **blindness** most often seen in young men. In North American and British patients it is less severe, affects women twice as frequently as men, and is not a leading cause of blindness.

Plotkin GR: **Triple symptom complex** (classic triad). *In* Plotkin GR, Calabro JJ, O'Duffy JD (eds): Behçet's Disease: A Contemporary Synopsis. Mount Kisco, New York, Futura Publishing Co., Inc., 1988, pp 143–178.

Behçet's syndrome may appear at any age. The earliest appearance was in an 8-day-old infant whose mother had Behçet's disease for 8 years.

Patients with Behçet's syndrome experience **generalized symptoms** just prior to the onset of the acute attack. These include malaise, weakness, headache, sweating, lymphadenopathy, and substernal or facial pain. Often there is a history of **repeated sore throats**, tonsillitis, myalgias, and migratory arthralgias, followed by erythema nodosum lesions. Exacerbations may occur in the premenstrual phase of the menstrual cycle. This may reflect a reduction in mucosal keratinization and, hence, vulnerability to trauma as a result of increasing progesterone and decreasing estrogen plasma levels. The symptoms may subside during pregnancy and the immediate postpartum period.

The average interval between **recurrences** is **2 months**. The intervals become longer with time, and eventual resolution results. But a permanent sequel may be blindness. Most importantly, the full complex may take many years to evolve after the onset of the oral ulcerations. Only one facet of the triad may be evident at a given time.

The oral lesions may bleed readily, and since they are painful the patient may have difficulty in speaking, chewing, or swallowing, with resultant dehydration and weight loss. Major aphthous ulcers (**periadenitis mucosa necrotica recurrens, Sutton**) may occur as well as the common minor aphthae. They are intractable and indolent, and as they persist for months and recur at the same site the mucosa becomes thickened and necrotic, and slough may develop, leaving deep ulcers and finally scars. The **scarring** of the pharyngeal area may be so severe as to produce dysphagia, even dyspnea. Perforation of the soft palate has also occurred. However, a larger percentage of patients shows the herpetiform ulcers that are characteristically grouped and not as severe.

Coexisting **relapsing polychondritis** and Behçet's syndrome have been reported as the **MAGIC syndrome** (*m*outh *a*nd *g*enital ulcers with *i*nflamed *c*artilage).

In addition to the ulcers, Behçet patients may show leukoplakia, **furred tongue**, and **absence of fungiform papillae** due to replacement by filiform papillae. The latter finding is seen also in the Riley-Day syndrome (familial dysautonomia). Those patients with **atrophic glossitis** also may have low serum iron levels.

The **genital ulcers** in women may require routine pelvic examination for detection. They may be responsible for discharge, bleeding, and **dyspareunia**. Even destruction of the vulva, fenestration of the labia minora, and labial perforation may occur. The severity of the ulceration has been so great in the male as to necessitate penile amputation.

Morgan ED, Laszlo JD, Stumpf PG: **Incomplete Behçet's syndrome** in the differential diagnosis of genital ulceration and postcoital bleeding. A case report. J Reprod Med 1988; 33:844–846.

The genital ulcers of Behçet's syndrome can be exposed to trauma during **coitus**, leading to significant **bleeding**.

A 30-year-old woman had had recurrent **aphthous ulcers** of the tongue and buccal mucosa since age 5. Three years previously, in the seventh month of her third pregnancy, she had also developed recurrent painful genital ulcers in the labia, cervix, and vagina, **thought to be genital herpes**. The oral and genital ulcers lasted 1 to 2 weeks and seemed independent of each other. All three children were healthy, but two of them had also developed painful oral ulcers.

A diagnosis of Behçet's syndrome had been made the previous year following an episode of postcoital vaginal bleeding that required surgery and transfusion with 2 units of blood. Since that time she had been taking colchicine. She came to the emergency room again with painless heavy vaginal bleeding for 3 hours after coitus. There were multiple ulcerations on her vulva and introitus, and several **vaginal ulcers** had active bleeding. She also had several aphthous ulcers on the tip of her tongue and buccal mucosa. Under general anesthesia the larger vaginal ulcer was sutured and the smaller ones were cauterized with silver nitrate. A vulvar biopsy 1 month later revealed vasculitis, with C3 in blood vessel walls.

Behçet's syndrome should be considered in the differential diagnosis of genital herpes, especially when oral or ocular lesions are evident. In this case there was no evidence of eye disease.

The diagnosis made in the laboratory usually costs more than the one made in the office.

Kaneko F, Takahashi Y, Muramatsu Y, Miura Y: Immunological studies on **aphthous ulcer** and **erythema nodosum-like eruptions** in Behçet's disease. Br J Dermatol 1985; 113:303–312.

Evidence pointing to a **role for streptococci** in Behçet's disease includes:

Chronic infectious foci containing streptococci, such as tonsillitis and dental diseases, often precede the onset of symptoms in Behçet's disease.
Streptococcal antigens injected intracutaneously cause intense delayed hypersensitivity skin responses.
Deposits of IgM with streptococcal-related antigen have been found in vessel walls and sites infiltrated by inflammatory cells.
Lymphoid cells infiltrating the epithelia of aphthous ulcers bear immunoglobulins and streptococcal-related antigen.

Hamza M: Behçet's disease and **dental treatment**. J Rheumatol 1989; 16:12–13.

In Tunisia, a 29-year-old woman underwent a **dental extraction** for an **abscess**. Two months later she developed buccal aphthous and subcutaneous **phlebitis**, followed by **erythema nodosum**. One year later she again underwent dental treatment, and 1 week later developed iliac **vein thrombosis**.

A 23-year-old man with oral and scrotal aphthosis, necrotic pseudofolliculitis, erythema nodosum, and left **iliac vein thrombosis** present for 1 year underwent dental treatment. The next day he developed right leg thrombosis and retinal vasculitis with hyalitis.

Are bacterial antigens responsible?

Cooper C, Pippard EC, Sharp H, et al: Is Behçet's disease triggered by **childhood infection**? Ann Rheum Dis 1989; 48:421–423.

In Leeds an epidemiologic study of 30 patients with Behçet's disease suggested triggering of the disease by infection during childhood or adolescence in an immunogenetically predisposed host.

Risk factors appeared to be tonsillectomy, a history of cold sores, large sibship size, late birth order, sexual intercourse before age 16, and travel to countries with a high incidence of the disease.

Type 1 **herpes simplex virus** may be one of a number of pathogens that trigger Behçet's disease singly or in combination.

Panush RS: Nutritional therapy for rheumatic diseases. Ann Intern Med 1987; 106:619–621.

A concept of **delayed reactions to foods** (a few hours to several days) is emerging, reactions which are not mediated through IgE–mast-cell events, but through other immunologic mechanisms. Symptoms may include **headache**, behavioral or **gastrointestinal disorders**, and **arthritis**.

Foods induce immune responses in humans that are similar to other environmental antigens. Food antigens, food antibodies, complexes of food antigens and antibodies, and sensitized lymphocytes are found in the circulation. Most **food allergies** recognized are **immediate**, causing anaphylactic, cutaneous, respiratory, or gastrointestinal symptoms.

Foods have been associated with rheumatic diseases in several case reports:

Behçet's syndrome with: **black walnuts**
systemic lupus erythematosus with:
    L-canavanine (in alfalfa)
    hydrazine

321

rheumatoid-like arthritis with:
sodium nitrate
dairy products
dust and molds
petrochemicals
tartrazine

Woodrow JC, Graham DR, Evans CC: Case report. Behçet's syndrome in **HLA-identical siblings**. Br J Rheumatol 1990; 29:225–227.

HLA-linked genes appear to be only part of a complex pathogenesis of Behçet's syndrome.

In Liverpool, two HLA-identical brothers had severe forms of Behçet's syndrome, one brother with severe ocular involvement and the other with severe pulmonary involvement.

One brother, now aged 35 years, first developed recurrent oral and pharyngeal ulcers at age 14. The ulcers were painful, often larger than 1 cm, and occurred two or three at a time at monthly intervals. He also experienced erythema nodosum of the legs, penile ulcers, and pain in the ankles and right wrist. At age 19 he developed **blurred vision**, with posterior uveitis and hypopyon developing first in one eye, then in the other eye, leading to almost total **blindness**.

His brother began having painful mouth ulcers at age 20, along with erythema nodosum. At age 23 he developed **recurrent hemoptysis**. Despite prednisolone therapy he died 5 years later of hemoptysis, induced by vasculitis in the large pulmonary arteries and multiple pulmonary infarcts.

In Japan, Turkey, Israel, Italy, and France there is a strong association between HLA-B5 and Behçet's syndrome. The association is much weaker in the United Kingdom and the United States. In patients in the United Kingdom, HLA-B12 is particularly associated with the mucocutaneous form and HLA-B5 and HLA-DR7 with ocular involvement.

Dündar SV, Gencalp U, Simsek H: **Familial cases** of Behçet's disease. Br J Dermatol 1985; 113:319–321.

Seven families in Turkey had two or more people afflicted with Behçet's disease. Two siblings were involved in five families, while three siblings (including fraternal twins) were involved in one family. A father and son were affected in one family.

Tissue typing of seven patients in three of the families revealed **HLA-B5**. This tissue type has been predominant in several other studies of Behçet's disease, suggesting that genetic factors are important in the pathogenesis of the disease.

Fellner MJ, Kantor I: Behçet's syndrome: **Skin puncture test** as guide to therapy. NY State J Med 1964; 64:1760–1761.

The appearance of a **pustule** within 24 hours after **pricking the skin** with a sterile needle may be specific for Behçet's syndrome. The same phenomenon occurs after intradermal injection of 0.1 cc saline or water.

In a 25-year-old woman with ulcerations of the mouth, genitalia, and conjunctiva and migratory polyarthritis, the prick test became negative as her lesions healed with **systemic steroids**. The proper maintenance dose of steroid was thought to be near the point at which the prick test was only slightly reactive or else negative.

Freidman-Birnbaum R, Bergman R, Aizen E: Sensitivity and specificity of **pathergy test** results in Israeli patients with Behçet's disease. Cutis 1990; 45:261–264.

In Haifa, 46 Jewish and Arab Israeli patients (from different countries) with active Behçet's disease were tested for skin hyperreactivity. Forty-six control patients with vasculitis (rheumatoid, cutaneous, systemic lupus erythematosus, cryoglobulinemia) were also tested.

The pathergy test consisted of an intradermal injection of 0.2 ml normal saline on the flexor forearm, as well as **pricking the skin** 6 to 7 cm away with a sterile, disposable 25-gauge needle. A positive test at 24 hours was either 0.5 cm palpable erythematous induration or a sterile pustule with an erythematous halo that did not disappear after 48 hours at the needle-prick site.

The pathergy test was positive in 45 of 46 patients with Behçet's disease, but negative in all of the controls. It therefore seems to be a **highly sensitive** and **specific test** for Behçet's disease in Israel, as well as in Turkey and Japan. It may be used to confirm the diagnosis in patients with the incomplete syndrome.

Yazici H, Chamberlain MA, Tüzün Y, et al: A comparative study of the **pathergy reaction** among Turkish and British patients with Behçet's disease. Ann Rheum Dis 1984; 43:74–75.

The lack of positivity of the pathergy phenomenon in British and American patients with Behçet's disease has led to **skepticism** about its usefulness.

In this study, 48 patients with Behçet's disease from Istanbul and 12 patients from Leeds were tested for the pathergy phenomenon. Tests were also done in 24 healthy Turkish and 7 healthy British controls. All patients except one were Caucasian. Readings were done blindly from photographs, which made it difficult to judge papules and decreased the sensitivity of the test.

The pathergy phenomenon was present only among the Turkish patients, being found in 28 of 48. All **British patients** and controls had **negative tests**. The absence of the pathergy test in British patients suggests that it does not have an important role in the pathogenesis of the disease.

Haim S, Sobel JD, Friedman-Birnbaum R, Lichtig C: **Histological and direct immunofluorescence study** of cutaneous hyper-reactivity in Behçet's disease. Br J Dermatol 1976; 95:631–636.

To test for pathergy (skin hyperreactivity) in Behçet's disease, inject 0.2 ml normal saline intracutaneously into the forearm and perform a simultaneous needle prick nearby.

In 18 such patients in Israel, all had positive reactions at both sites after 24 hours, consisting of a 1- to 2-cm erythematous zone with a central pustule.

Skin biopsies at 24 hours showed **increased mast cells** and mild to intense perivascular lymphocytic and plasma cell infiltration in the upper dermis and around skin adnexa. Direct immunofluorescence was negative for IgA, IgG, IgM, IgE, C3, C4, fibrinogen, and albumin. This suggests that local humoral factors are not relevant in the pathogenesis of cutaneous hyperreactivity. Perhaps mast cells play a role. The time sequence for this reaction (12 to 48 hr) is somewhat late for an early hypersensitivity type of reaction, but early for a delayed type of hypersensitivity response.

Mizushima Y, Matsuda T, Hoshi K, Ohno S: **Induction** of Behçet's disease symptoms **after dental treatment** and **streptococcal antigen skin test**. J Rheumatol 1988; 15:1029–1030.

A 45-year-old Japanese woman with Behçet's disease that had been nearly inactive for several months underwent **dental extraction** because of periodontitis. The following day she had an oral aphthous ulcer, followed for a week by severe acne-like eruptions, ocular attacks, and **erythema nodosum** (which she had not experienced for 3 years).

A 57-year-old Japanese woman with incomplete Behçet's disease stabilized by treatment with colchicine had six gum incisions at an interval of several days for dental treatment. **Each time** after surgery she experienced many **oral aphthae** and **erythema nodosum** on both legs. After completion of dental treatments, she had only a few aphthous ulcers.

Investigation of other patients with Behçet's disease, using intradermal skin tests with bacterial antigens, showed strong **positive reactions to Streptococcus pyogenes**, followed the next day by ocular attacks in two patients and aphthous ulcers in two other patients. Prick tests to *Staphylococcus aureus* and *Escherichia coli* were also positive in some cases but did not precipitate any flares of Behçet's disease.

Compared with healthy persons, patients with Behçet's disease have a high incidence of history of **tonsillitis and dental caries**. The role of streptococci may be important, as lymphocytes from patients with recurrent aphthous stomatitis and Behçet's disease have been found to be sensitized to streptococcal antigens. Streptococcus-related antigen has also been found in the lesions of Behçet's disease.

Possibly the **streptococcus-related antigens** used in skin tests, as well as microbial antigens that enter the blood stream during dental surgery, trigger Behçet's disease in genetically predisposed individuals.

Ranzi T, Campanini M, Bianchi PA: Successful **treatment** of genital and oral ulceration in Behçet's disease with topical 5-aminosalicylic acid (5-ASA). Br J Dermatol 1989; 120:471.

A 24-year-old woman had suffered with aphthous stomatitis, genital ulcers, small blisters, and cutaneous and subcutaneous erythematous nodules for 4 years. They became progressively worse, and she lost 4 kg in weight over 2 months. A 2-cm ulcer on the inside of the lower lip destroyed the frenulum, and another similar ulcer in the right inferior retromolar area made eating difficult. An irregular extensive **ulcer** on the right labium minus of the **vulva** caused an **underlying abscess** and loss of tissue, with half of the labium minus disappearing. The lesion was extremely painful, making walking difficult. A biopsy of this lesion showed acute and chronic inflammation with vasculitis and occasional multinucleate giant cells. Other skin lesions included intensely itchy erythematous nodules on the buttocks and forearms. Routine blood studies and immunologic tests (C3, C4, ANA, antimitochondrial and anti-smooth muscle antibodies) were normal.

Topical applications twice daily of gauze impregnated with a suspension of **5-ASA** (1.5 gm) in water led to complete healing of the ulcers within 50 days. With continuing treatments, the ulcers did not recur.

Behçet's disease. Lancet 1989; 1:761–762.

Although vasculitis is the pathologic hallmark of Behçet's disease, its etiology remains unknown, despite tantalizing glimpses of viral and streptococcal infection in some patients. **Pesticides** have been proposed as a cause, since a Behçet's-like disease occurs in immature swine fed organophosphates. However, this association has not been sustained.

The hallmark of **diagnosis is pattern recognition**, which must include anterior and posterior uveitis as well as a conglomeration of clotting abnormalities and a bizarre distribution of vascular lesions.

The array of clinical features was first **described by Hippocrates**: "Many had their mouths affected with aphthous ulcerations. There were also many defluxations about the genital parts and ulcerations, boils (phymata), externally and internally about the groins."

Tasdemir I, Sivri B, Turgan C, et al: The expanding spectrum of a disease. Behçet's disease associated with **amyloidosis**. Nephron 1989; 52:154–157.

Renal involvement in Behçet's disease is rather uncommon despite its being a systemic vasculitis.

If **proteinuria and nephrotic syndrome** develop in a patient with Behçet's disease, amyloidosis should be suspected. Renal biopsy confirms the diagnosis and rules out other causes of proteinuria seen in Behçet's disease (glomerulonephritis, interstitial nephritis, renal vein thrombosis, and a nephritis-like condition).

Amyloidosis may be an intrinsic feature of Behçet's disease, as it sometimes occurs without any evidence of suppuration or inflammation. In most cases, however, it is probably **secondary to chronic suppuration** (skin, eyes, joints) and thrombophlebitis.

An exact diagnosis is important, as colchicine rather than steroids should be used in treatment. **Colchicine inhibits** characteristic **activity of polymorphonuclear leukocytes** and may inhibit amyloid formation, while long-term steroids may accelerate amyloid deposition.

Dilsen N, Konice M, Aral O, et al: Behçet's disease associated with **amyloidosis** in Turkey and in the world. Ann Rheum Dis 1988; 47:157–163.

In a review of 24 cases it appears that patients with Behçet's disease who develop amyloidosis are usually middle-aged men with disease of extremely long duration. Outstanding symptoms in this group included genital ulceration, eye involvement, thrombophlebitis, peripheral **arthritis, neuropsychiatric problems**, and a positive skin pathergy test.

Renal biopsy was performed in 13 patients having massive proteinuria and nephrotic syndrome (5), uremia (5), and hypertension (3). **Renal amyloidosis** was found in 8 patients and was of the secondary AA amyloid protein type.

Treatment with **colchicine** appeared to slow down the progression of amyloidosis in two cases. In addition to being a useful treatment in Behçet's disease, colchicine is helpful in **familial Mediterranean fever**, another disease that leads to secondary amyloidosis.

Bang D, Honma T, Saito T, et al: Ultrastructure of **vascular changes** in cutaneous manifestations of Behçet's disease. Acta Derm Venereol 1988; 68:33–40.

Needle-prick stimulation of the skin in Behçet's disease induces endothelial cell proliferation and **thrombus formation** with secondary lymphocytic vasculitis and obliteration of the vascular lumen.

Similar changes occur in the erythema nodosum–like lesions of Behçet's disease.

Kaneko F, Takahashi Y, Muramatsu R, et al: **Natural killer cell** numbers and function in peripheral lymphoid cells in Behçet's disease. Br J Dermatol 1985; 113:313–318.

Patients with active Behçet's disease lack a factor—possibly interferon—that activates peripheral blood NK cells. The NK cells apparently are not functionally impaired.

In 18 patients with Behçet's disease, a **reduction of the T cell** population was found in the clinically active stage of the disease, considered to be due to a decrease of the helper T cell population.

Cengiz K: Serum **IgE concentrations** in complete Behçet's disease. J Clin Pathol 1990; 43:262.

In 18 patients with Behçet's disease, the serum **IgE levels** were three times **higher** than in 12 controls. The patients had no personal or family history of atopy. Total eosinophil counts were approximately the same in the two groups.

It is postulated that an IgE-mediated antigenic response, probably by action on mast cells or basophils, can induce platelet activation and aggregation. **Platelet aggregates** could then lead to the thrombosis in the great veins and arteries seen in Behçet's disease. An **immune complex vasculitis** is thought to be the basic pathologic process in Behçet's disease.

Aitchison R, Chu P, Cater DR, et al: **Defective fibrinolysis** in Behçet's syndrome: Significance and possible mechanisms. Ann Rheum Dis 1989; 48:590–593.

Behçet's syndrome is an uncommon systemic vasculitic disorder complicated by **venous thrombosis** in about one third of cases. Thrombotic events may be related to abnormal fibrinolysis and reduced fibrinolytic activity.

This study demonstrates decreased production of tissue plasminogen activator.

Chun SI, Su WPD, Lee S, Rogers RS III: **Erythema nodosum–like lesions** in Behçet's syndrome: A histopathologic study of 30 cases. J Cutan Pathol 1989; 16:259–265.

In a study of 30 patients with Behçet's syndrome and erythema nodosum–like lesions, the authors could not distinguish the lesions from erythema nodosum in other systemic disorders.

The histologic changes consisted of lymphocytic vasculitis (40%), septal panniculitis (40%), lobular panniculitis (33%), and nonspecific inflammation in the fat (27%). Neutrophilic, lymphohistiocytic, and **granulomatous infiltrates** were observed in different patients with Behçet's syndrome.

Bang D, Honma T, Saito T, et al: The pathogenesis of **vascular changes** in erythema **nodosum–like lesions** of Behçet's syndrome: An electron microscopic study. Hum Pathol 1987; 18:1172–1179.

Perivascular lymphocytic cuffs and blood vessels with endothelial cell hypertrophy and necrosis suggest a **delayed-type hypersensitivity** reaction in these lesions.

Montalban J, Codina A, Alijotas J, et al: **Magnetic resonance imaging** in Behçet's disease. J Clin Pathol 1990; 43:442.

A 28-year-old man with recurrent oral and genital ulcers, arthritis, and uveitis developed **occipital cephalgia**, mild lethargy, and gait disturbance. Neurologic examination showed slight right hemiparesis with right patellar and ankle clonus and the right plantar response being extensor. He also had evidence of dysmetria and ataxia.

Magnetic resonance imaging showed a large **pathologic area in the pons** extending upward to the cerebral peduncles and **downward to the medulla oblongata**. Treatment with steroids cleared the symptoms, and 2 months later a repeat MRI showed that the pathologic area in the brain had disappeared. This suggests that the lesion was *not* due to ischemic necrosis from vasculitis but was more likely caused by an immunologically mediated demyelinating process.

MRI could be the **method of choice** for diagnosing neurologic involvement in Behçet's disease.

Rakover Y, Adar H, Tal I, et al: Behçet disease: **Long-term follow-up of three children** and review of the literature. Pediatrics 1989; 83:986–992.

Behçet's disease is **rare in children** and difficult to diagnose. Active disease attacks involve many systems and last a few weeks each, with intervals of months to years between them.

In the three patients described here, symptoms began at the ages of 7, 11, and 12 years. Eventually all three had **aphthous stomatitis** and **arthritis**, while two also had genital ulcers, iridocyclitis, erythema nodosum, and CNS involvement. Other manifestations included fever of unknown origin, testicular pain, and a Stevens-Johnson–like eruption.

All patients required long-term treatment with steroids. In two of the children followed for more than 10 years, the course was benign, with complete cure in one patient.

The **differential diagnosis** of Behçet's disease in children includes:

systemic lupus erythematosus
Reiter's disease
inflammatory bowel disease
herpetic infection

Neonatal Behçet's disease has also been described in three infants born to mothers with the disease. The neonates had aphthous stomatitis and skin phenomena that disappeared spontaneously within 6 months.

Lang BA, Laxer RM, Thorner P, et al: Pediatric onset of **Behçet's syndrome with myositis**: Case report and literature review illustrating unusual features. Arthritis Rheum 1990; 33:418–425.

A 15-year-old girl of Mediterranean descent had been hospitalized three times during a 16-month period for unilateral or bilateral **calf swelling, redness**, and **pain**, without preceding trauma. Venograms had always been negative. Now she was hospitalized again with fever (temperature 38.2°C) and left calf tenderness, slight erythema, and swelling (circumference 3 cm greater than the right calf). There was a positive Homans' sign, as well as a 2-cm cutaneous ulcer above the right medial malleolus. She also had an **aphthous ulcer** on the buccal mucosa and a small ulcer on the right pinna.

Whereas a Doppler flow study of the left calf showed normal venous flow, 327 ultrasound scan suggested **myositis**. A biopsy of the left gastrocnemius muscle showed a multifocal inflammatory infiltrate (lymphocytes and macrophages) in the interstitial and perivascular regions, vasculitis, and **focal necrosis of myocytes**. A biopsy of the ulcer of the right leg also showed marked vasculitis in the deep dermis. Blood tests revealed neutropenia, anemia, ESR 120, creatine phosphokinase 503, and elevated immunoglobulin levels.

Despite treatment with antibiotics and colchicine, the patient developed new areas of skin ulceration on the right thigh and at the muscle biopsy site. Repeat biopsies showed vasculitis, and treatment with prednisone resulted in rapid clearing of the ulcers.

The past history revealed recurrent erythema multiforme–like rashes since age 7, splenomegaly, neutropenia, migratory arthralgias, painful mouth ulcers, genital ulcers, and acute pericarditis. She had no evidence of ocular disease.

Behçet's syndrome is quite uncommon in children, with only about 40 cases reported in the past 25 years. Aphthous ulcers, skin lesions, and joint symptoms are similar to those in adults, but **eye disease** is **uncommon**. Unusual manifestations include neutropenia and splenomegaly.

Myositis should be considered in the differential diagnosis of painful swelling of an extremity. In Behçet's syndrome, however, ultrasound or MRI studies are preferable to muscle biopsy because of the tendency for pathergy and **poor wound healing**.

Firestein GS, Gruber HE, Weisman MH, et al: Mouth and genital **ulcers with inflamed cartilage**: **MAGIC syndrome**. Am J Med 1985; 79:65–72.

Relapsing polychondritis and Behçet's disease have many clinical features in common and may reflect a **common pathogenic mechanism**.

Autoimmunity to components of cartilage other than type 2 collagen, such as proteoglycans or **elastic tissue**, could be the common mechanism. Elastic tissue is present in high concentrations in large arteries, skin, and cartilage. Particularly striking is the similar histologic picture in abdominal aortic lesions in relapsing polychondritis and Behçet's disease, with **arteritis**, degeneration of elastic fibers, and aneurysms. Large-artery thrombosis is also common in both diseases.

Skin lesions shared by both diseases include:

oral and genital ulcers
erythema nodosum
sterile pustules
migratory thrombophlebitis
swollen red ears and nose

The **arthropathy** seen in both diseases affects mainly **large joints** and is asymmetrical, migratory, and nonerosive. Nonspecific synovial inflammatory changes are seen in both. Inflammatory eye disease, audiovestibular disease, inflammatory bowel disease, and renal disease also may occur in both diseases.

Eisenbud L, Horowitz I, Kay B: **Recurrent aphthous stomatitis** of the Behçet's type: Successful treatment with thalidomide. Oral Surg 1987; 64:289–292.

A 48-year-old man had a 27-year history of **continuous debilitating mouth ulcers** of the major type, which began after military service in Panama. Each lesion started as a painful palpable submucosal nodule, which broke down within 24 hours to form a round or oval necrotic ulcer. He would develop six or seven lesions at one time in different areas of the oral cavity or oropharynx, with successive crops of lesions arising as the old ones were healing.

Concurrent with each episode of oral lesions he developed **widespread necrotic pustular nodules**.

Treatment with thalidomide (25 to 50 mg/day) immediately stopped all of the lesions and enabled him to discontinue prednisone, which had caused profound side effects over the years. Within the first 2 weeks of taking thalidomide he developed an erythematous butterfly rash, which subsided when the drug dose was lowered.

Viraben R, Dupré A: **Erythema nodosum** following thalidomide therapy for Behçet's disease. Dermatologica 1988; 176:107.

A 25-year-old Algerian man had **recurrent thrombophlebitis** for 4 years, along with oral and genital ulcers, pustules on the buttocks, and arthritis of the knees and ankles. Five days after thalidomide (100 mg/day) therapy was started, he developed numerous **painful erythematous nodules** on the legs. The thalidomide was then stopped, and the nodules cleared, but when thalidomide was readministered 3 months later for painful aphthae, profuse nodules occurred after 2 days and involved the arms and legs. The thalidomide was then stopped, and the nodules resolved over the next month.

Paradoxically, thalidomide is a very effective treatment of erythema nodosum leprosum.

Making a diagnosis brings calm after the turmoil of confusion.

Bites and Stings

The smaller the bites the bigger the diagnostic problem. Patients bitten by an alligator scarcely need see a diagnostician, yet we have seen patients hospitalized for diagnostic surveys when the bites were those of mites from their household pet. If the patient has not seen or felt the bites, and the reactions are allergic in nature, he will reject any suggestion that a creature outside the visual range is responsible. Far more acceptable is the idea that the itch is caused by something several orders of magnitude smaller, a virus perhaps? Meanwhile, his fingernails ply continuously to remove any evidence of ectoparasitism.

In this atmosphere of patient disbelief, and in the presence of totally nonspecific **punctate excoriations**, you must spend time with the **history**. A hayride, dried-flower arranging, a family member who also itches, contact with a dog, cat, or bird—each raises the possibility that the patient is or has been bitten by mites. The bites, as well as the consequent itch, are invisible, but clearly the search for mites must begin. The most common example, scabies, has its own entry in this book. Scrape, scrape, scrape, and look for the mite, its eggs, or even its scybala.

A wide swatch of **cellophane tape** applied to the patient or to his pet may trap an offending mite, allowing visualization on inspection with a head loupe. Instruct the patient as to what the search is all about. Have him participate by taking his pet to a veterinarian for a diagnostic look. Examine and cross-examine your patient for clues. One of our practice mysteries was solved by finding out that our patient had been a guest staying in a guest bedroom that had previously been used but a single night many weeks before by another guest and her dog with fleas. Another puzzle in a pruritic patient was solved by finding myriads of mites in a brand new recently purchased horsehair mattress. A diagnostic lindane treatment can do much to strengthen or weaken your diagnostic hand, as can an intradermal mite antigen skin test.

With the larger arthropods, such as fleas and carpet beetles, **careful inspection** must be made of **bedding**, bird cages, and air conditioners. Bedbugs are as large as 5 mm and can be seen sometimes when the bedding is whipped off at 2 AM to reveal them on the white sheet background.

Look for lice on the patient, including the scalp, pubic area, and perianal hairs. Don't forget to look in the patient's clothing for "seam squirrels." Secondary findings of nits are equally significant and can account for chronic pyoderma. And always look with a fresh spirit of confidence. Doubt blinds one's ability to see. Thus, we have seen pubic lice dismissed as freckles. On the other hand, we have seen school nurses confuse dandruff and hair casts with nits.

Awareness of an antecedent bite, or the possibility of such, is particularly valuable when the bite is the **vector of disease**. We have seen insect bites acquired in Israel evolve into the lesions of leishmaniasis. And we have seen the bite of a spider produce gangrene and subsequent disseminated intravascular coagulation. Today the tick bite has the potential of producing borreliosis with its hallmark of erythema chronicum migrans and the devastation of multisystem Lyme disease.

You must know where your patient has traveled. The beaches of Cancun may spell jellyfish stings. The hunter may come back with chigger bites, and the barefoot swimmer with leech bites.

Think bites for unexplained pruritus, pyoderma, bullae, unexplained fevers, and even gangrene. In that way you won't get stung.

Fleas, Mites, Bedbugs, Thrips

Burns DA: The investigation and management of **arthropod bite reactions acquired in the home**. Clin Exp Dermatol 1987; 12:114–120.

Patients with insect bite reactions are by and large "**diagnosis doubters.**" After all, others in the house don't have problems, and their animals are regularly dusted or sprayed with insecticide or wear flea collars. They must be instructed that they are unique because of their allergic state and that the insects live in the home, carpet, and bedding, and not just on the animal.

There are necessary **steps for converting the doubters**:

Fleas:

Examine the **animal** or combings for concretions of flea feces and flea eggs adhering to fur. Examine the animal **bedding** for feces, eggs, and larvae by having the patient place the bedding in a large plastic bag and vigorously shake it. After removing the bedding, examine the residual debris in the bag for the "pepper-and-salt" appearance of feces and eggs. The larvae are 5 to 6 mm long and look like maggots, with 13 body segments, antennae but no eyes, and peglike anal struts. If there is no animal bed, have the patient bring in brushings or a **vacuum bag specimen from the carpet** where the animal often lies (e.g., in front of the fireplace). If no evidence of cat fleas (*Ctenocephalides felis*) or dog fleas (*Ctenocephalides canis*) is to be had, look for the common bird flea (*Ceratophyllus gallinae gallinae*). They winter over in the bird nest in a pupal stage, emerging to bite in the spring and early summer. **Look for nests in the eaves**, ventilator pipes, and air conditioners. The gardener is at risk near outdoor birdhouses or nests within the garage. The bites will be more generalized when the fleas gain access to the bedroom and its disrobed occupants. Recall that dog and cat flea bites are usually **grouped papular urticaria** on the **lower legs**, especially in women with exposed legs. Men tend to be protected by socks and trousers (within a flea leap).

To identify fleas, leave them in 10% potassium hydroxide for 48 hours to remove interfering pigment and then look at the combs (ctenidia) on the head and thorax. There are no spines on the genal (anterior) comb of the bird flea, and the first spine of the genal comb of the dog flea is much shorter than the next. The cat flea has spines of equal length.

Mites:

The bites of **dog mites (Cheyletiella *yasguri*)** are small erythematous papules with a central vesicle or pustule that may become necrotic. **Unlike fleas,** these **mites penetrate clothing easily**, so that if the owner holds the infected animal, lesions will be on the **thighs** and **abdomen**. To confirm the diagnosis, look at the dog and place it on a large black paper. Then vigorously comb the center of the back for "**walking scale,**" which should be placed in 50 to 100% lactic acid as a temporary mounting medium. Combings by the patient are not adequate, as you must get scale.

Cat mites (*Cheyletiella blakei*) and **rabbit mites** (*C. parasitovorax*) are equally suspect, but morphologic distinction is difficult, resting on the shape of a sense organ on the first pair of legs.

The **itch mite**, *Sarcoptes scabiei* var. *canis*, produces severe pruritus and **mange in the dog**, with scaling and denuded areas on the face, ears, and elbows. In turn, the owners develop severe pruritus with multiple **tiny inflammatory papules** but no burrows on the trunk and limbs. The dog must be seen and scraped for mites on any affected areas.

If the patient has no dog, cat, or bird, **ask if he has recently moved** into a   331

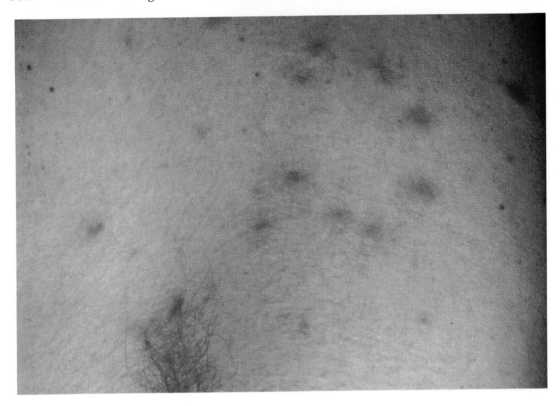

house previously occupied by pets or if he regularly visits family or friends with pets. The lesions may not have been acquired in his own home.

BEDBUGS:

Lesions may be papular, urticarial, or bullous and are extensively distributed. Yet a patient is described with bullae only on the left arm. These resulted from her habit of sleeping with her left arm under the headboard, the home of a colony of bedbugs (*Cimex lectularius*) that came with her recently acquired secondhand bed. **Bedbugs live in the walls of old houses as well as in furniture and emerge about an hour before dawn.** Indeed, the patient may see one (5 mm in size) and bring it in to you. If not, it may be necessary to visit the home for a definitive search.

Shelley WB, Shelley ED, Welbourn WC: Polypodium fern wreaths (Hagnaya)—a new source of **occupational mite dermatitis**. JAMA 1985; 253:3137–3138.

A 21-year-old man suddenly developed a pruritic eruption of **red papules** within hours of returning to work after a vacation. The lesions involved the volar surface of the **forearms**, lower part of the legs, and eyelids, with a few vesicles seen on the fingers. He worked as a wholesale florist, and occupational contact dermatitis was suspected.

He denied exposure to solvents, harsh soaps, fiber glass, or epoxy resins but did have contact with a wide variety of plant material. He also had a dog at work and a cat at home, but neither animal was itching. He had had one prior attack of dermatitis 4 months previously.

When first seen he had been off work for 6 days because of severe pruritus. After returning to work he noted no problem on the first day, but developed pruritus and a punctate dermatitis of the dorsal aspect of the hands on the second day. He then developed **severe itching of the finger webs** and was noted to have linear excoriations of the volar surface of the forearms and vesicles on the fingers. Scrapings were negative for scabies, but an intradermal skin test to house-dust mite antigen (0.02 ml) was strongly positive with a 1.2-cm wheal and 5 cm of erythema after 15 minutes. Application of lindane lotion to the entire body gave complete relief from pruritus.

One month later he had a third attack of itching and dermatitis, which appeared on the day he began unwrapping and **unpacking dried Hagnaya wreaths** from the Philippines. Skin scrapings were again negative for mites. By avoiding contact with the Hagnaya wreaths, he had no further attacks during a 1-year follow-up period.

He brought in two Hagnaya **wreaths for examination**. These were placed in a plastic bag and shaken vigorously for 30 seconds. The collected debris (3 to 5 gm each) was placed on top of three nested sieves (1.0, 0.25, and 0.125 mm) and tapped for 30 seconds. The contents of the lower two sieves were placed in alcohol, poured into ridged plastic dishes, and examined under a dissecting microscope for mites. Permanent slide mounts were made of the mites and sent off for identification to the Acarology Laboratory, Ohio State University, Columbus. Seven genera of mites in six families were identified, including two *Cheyletiella* family mites, probably responsible for the bites.

A persistent puzzling pruritic eruption in a healthy individual calls for a search for mites as a cause. In contrast to scabies, mites that "bite and run" never remain on the skin surface. Success in diagnosis may rest on microscopic **study of materials with which the patient works**. Such sources of mites have included cheese, evaporated milk, copra, bean paste, mammals, chickens, birds' nests, stored food, dried fruit, crude sugar, grains, hay, straw, oatmeal, fish food, feather pillows, and vegetation. Grocers, florists, farmers, sportsmen, orchard workers, and veterinarians are at particular risk.

Shelley ED, Shelley WB, Pula JF, McDonald SG: The diagnostic challenge of **non-burrowing mite bites. *Cheyletiella yasguri.*** JAMA 1984; 251:2690–2691.

A 6-year-old girl had an unexplained **recurrent pruritic rash** for 4 months. Her mother and brother had had similar episodes of itching, but her father was not affected. **Scabies** had been **suspected**, and treatment with lindane lotion had temporarily cleared the eruption. The family had a dog that scratched incessantly, but it received regular treatments for fleas.

One day she had streptococcal pharyngitis and stayed home from school, curling up on a quilt in the dog's box. She then broke out acutely with **hundreds of 5-mm pruritic urticarial papules** over her torso and legs. Each urticarial papule had a large halo of erythema. No lesions were present on the hands or intertriginous areas, and scrapings were negative for mites.

As canine scabies was a possibility, the family dog was taken to a veterinarian. Combings of the **dog's hair showed numerous mites**, identified as *Cheyletiella yasguri*. Subsequent fumigation of the dog's box and treatment of the dog and family with lindane lotion were curative.

If no veterinarian is available, combings from family pets may be examined using double-stick cellophane tape. Look for mites when:

> the patient has unexplained pruritus
> lesions are distinct separate excoriations
> family members or work colleagues have pruritus
> bedbugs, lice, mosquitoes, fleas, and spiders have been excluded
> primary lesions have no central puncta
> the mite antigen skin test (Hollister-Stier) is strongly positive

the eruption resembles atypical scabies, dermatitis herpetiformis, or neurotic excoriations

lesions occur mostly at sites of direct contact with a pet (abdomen, thighs, forearms)

COMMON NONBURROWING ITCH MITES	SOURCE
Cheyletiella yasguri	dogs
Cheyletiella blakei	cats
Cheyletiella parasitovorax	rabbits
Pyemotes ventricosus	straw, oatmeal, puffed wheat, wheat
Tyrophagus putrescentiae	grains, cereals, dried fruit, cheese,
Glycyphagus destructor	dried fish, red peppers,
Acarus siro	evaporated milk
Ornithonyssus bacoti	rats, chickens, pigeons, house
Dermanyssus gallinae	mouse
Liponyssodes sanguineus	
Ornithonyssus sylviarum	poultry

Aylesworth R, Baldridge D: *Dermatophagoides scheremetewskyi* and **feather pillow dermatitis**. Minnesota Med 1983; 66:42–43.

A 21-year-old man had a 3-week history of **pruritus of the scalp and forearm**. A few urticarial papules were present on the left wrist and scalp. He brought along a piece of clear **plastic tape that contained several mites**, identified as *Dermatophagoides scheremetewskyi*.

A search of the patient's home uncovered three **feather pillows** containing large numbers of the **mites**. After removal of the pillows, the pruritus abated, but it recurred in a few days. The dermatitis finally cleared after application of 0.5% Diazinon solution to cracks and corners and 3% malathion solution to areas of human contact.

This mite has rarely been reported to cause dermatitis of the scalp and upper trunk. It has been found in pillows, a bed, monkey food, a sparrow's nest, and on rats, muskrats, bats, and mice.

Maurice PDL, Schofield O, Griffiths WAD: *Cheyletiella* **dermatitis**: A case report and the role of specific immunological hypersensitivity in its pathogenesis. Clin Exp Dermatol 1987; 12:381–384.

A 36-year-old truck driver had **unrelenting pruritus** for 5 months along with tiny punctate erythematous papules and pustules and excoriated crusted lesions of the trunk, limbs, and face. His hands showed a patchy eczematoid dermatitis. All studies and scrapings were negative, until finally a biopsy of a new group of papules showed an upper dermal perivascular lymphocytic infiltrate suggestive of insect bite reaction. Mite bites were suspected.

Attention was turned to a **boxer dog** the patient had acquired 3 months before the eruption began. **Brushings** from the scruff of the dog revealed numerous **nonburrowing mites**, *Cheyletiella yasguri*. The game appeared over when the dog was treated with three applications of a lindane preparation. However, the patient, whose lesions had cleared when in the hospital away from his dog, developed new lesions within a few days of being back home. The diagnosis of *Cheyletiella* dermatitis remained steadfast when reexamination of the dog showed it still harbored mites. The happy ending, with a cure of the patient (and his best friend), was found in the successful use of a more potent miticide, Bromocyclen, on the dog.

One of the "red herrings" in this case was the fact that the patient was atopic and had had pompholyx, hay fever, multiple positive prick test reactions, and an elevated IgE level (716 U/ml). **Atopic dermatitis was ruled out** by demonstration of a remarkably strong specific delayed intradermal test reaction to a *Cheyletiella* mite extract prepared from dog hair infested with *Cheyletiella*. Another red herring was the putative role of a rat the patient also kept as a pet.

Evans J, Clarke T, Mattacks CA, Pond CM: **Dermatofibromas and arthropod bites**: Is there any evidence to link the two? Lancet 1989; 2:36–37.

Examination of 100 dermatofibromas revealed **no traces** of arthropod mouthparts and no histologic evidence of a foreign body giant cell reaction.

Thirty patients with dermatofibromas were also questioned closely about contact with stinging or blood-sucking arthropods before the development of lesions. Their responses did not differ significantly from matched controls.

Despite these data, it remains possible that some ingredients of saliva or venom, or introduced pathogens, may resist macrophage digestion and thus account for histiocytic reactions characteristic of dermatofibromas.

Fishman HC: **Thrips**. Arch Dermatol 1987; 123:993–994.

A 43-year-old woman in Southern California complained of a **rash of the left side of the neck**. Examination showed grouped red puncta in a palm-sized area, resembling insect bites. But it was examination of the patient's dress, not the lesions, that revealed the cause. On the neckline was a tiny brownish insect, identified by an entomologist as a **flower thrips** (*Frankliniella californica*). They feed on flowers and blossoms of citrus trees and may be hard to differentiate from the citrus thrips.

Many species of **plant-feeding thrips may bite and suck the blood of man**, including onion thrips, pear thrips, and cotton thrips. Immature forms often feed on the heads of grasses, oats, or rye and then go into a winged state as the grasses and grains dry up. Migrations of winged thrips are especially threatening, since the minute insects (about 1 mm long) **easily pass through window screens** and attack man.

Options for counterattacks include:

Burn infested fields before migrations occur.
Place fine cloth over the screens.
Treat the screens with lethal DDT or lindane.
Scratch.

Diagnosis is the art of letting others see what you see.

Lice

Fisher I, Morton RS: *Phthirus pubis* infestation. Br J Vener Dis 1970; 46:326–329.

The rising incidence of pubic lice infestation parallels the increase in other sexually transmitted diseases, particularly gonorrhea and nongonococcal urethritis.

Pubic irritation is the main complaint, along with "VD lice." The average incubation period is 30 days from exposure to onset of symptoms. The lice feed continuously and live less than 20 hours when away from the nest. The lice favor pubic hair because of the wide 2-mm spacing of hairs, which matches the hind-leg span of the lice. They also commonly infest perianal hairs and hair on the abdomen and thighs.

Eggs continue to hatch for 1 week after treatment, so that more than a single treatment is usually required. Shaving of the pubic area is discouraged because of resulting irritation and folliculitis.

Elgart ML: **Pediculosis**. Dermatol Clin 1990; 8:219–228.

Head lice and body lice are identical morphologically, although the body louse tends to be longer. Head lice grown on the body take on the characteristics of body lice and vice versa. Pubic lice are shorter, with claws on the second and third pairs of legs. Lice **die of starvation after 10 days** away from a host.

"While the crab louse festers under the skirts of propriety, the head louse shelters beneath the cloak of secrecy."

Head lice are much more common in girls and women, and much less common in blacks. A female louse lays three eggs (nits) daily and cements them to the base of the hair. The **duration of the infestation** can be determined by measuring the length of the hair to the highest nit from the scalp surface, assuming that hair grows 1 cm per month. In developed nits, an eye spot is visible. A nit with an air bubble is nonviable, and brown nits become white when the louse hatches (white nits are empty). The nit is not movable along the hair shaft, in contrast to pilar casts and seborrheic scale.

Living lice may be hard to find. Look under the hair near the ear and under long hair at the back of the neck (warm areas) to find large numbers of nits. Itching and prickling of the scalp are the common symptoms, although scratching and poor hygiene may produce pyoderma. The head louse does not transmit any other diseases. The spread of lice is through direct contact and fomites.

Body lice are the **only lice that transmit diseases**, including epidemic typhus, louse-borne relapsing fever, and trench fever. Uninfected bites are small papules or puncta on a red base. Usually, however, the patient with "**vagabond's disease**" is covered with ulcerations, infections, and excoriations, especially on the trunk, axillae, and groin. The **diagnosis** is made not from the patient but **from his clothing**. Lice remain in clothing seams, where they complete their life cycle (a single gravid pair may produce 3000 eggs). Most commonly involved are the trouser waist, inside shirt, and skirt seams.

Typhus is suggested by the presence of many red dead lice (due to the rupture of the louse guts filled with typhus rickettsiae).

Pubic lice infest only short hairs (pubic, body, axillary, beard, neck, eyebrows, eyelashes, occasionally occiput). Acquired by sexual contact or fomites, there may be no symptoms for 30 days. Itching then develops, and small brown lice may be seen at the base of hairs, **resembling freckles**. Adult lice hold onto two hairs, and **blue macules** (maculae ceruleae) due to the action of saliva on blood products, may occur nearby.

Weinstein RA: The case of the **spotted underwear**. Lancet 1989; 2:1154.

A 40-year-old man had a 3-month history of "**blood spots**" on his **underpants**. The reddish-brown spots were weakly positive for occult blood. Examination revealed a few erythematous plaques on the glans penis and several 2- to 3-mm varicosities on the scrotum. Adherent ova of **pubic lice** were seen on several pubic hairs.

When he refused to believe the **diagnosis** of pubic lice, he was given a loose-fitting condom with a cotton ball at its end. After 8 hours the cotton ball remained clean, while the underpants had multiple reddish-brown spots. He was then convinced, and after treatment with lindane shampoo he had no further problems.

It was thought that the underwear spots represented lice excrement or bleeding at sites of lice bites, which appeared as varicosities on the scrotum.

Slonka HF, Fleissner ML, Berlin J, et al: An **epidemic of pediculosis capitis**. J Parasitol 1977; 63:377–383.

During 1972 to 1973 in Buffalo, New York, the overall incidence of head lice in school children reached 7.2%. As in other epidemics, black children were spared.

The method of closeting garments appeared to be a major factor in the distribution of lice. Students who hung their clothes in cloakrooms with individually assigned hooks had a significantly lower attack rate, as did students with individual lockers. **Sharing lockers** led to a higher attack rate, and a previous study had observed that when lockers were shared, the locker partner became infested 2 to 3 days after the first person developed head lice.

Slonka GF, McKinley TW, McCroan JE, et al: Epidemiology of an outbreak of **head lice** in Georgia. Am J Trop Med Hyg 1976; 25:739–743.

An outbreak of pediculosis in Barrow County, Georgia, increased to unmanageable proportions in January 1974. It was confined to elementary school children (kindergarten through grade 6) in six schools and necessitated **examination of all children** enrolled in these schools (approximately **2300** students).

Examinations were made by 50 volunteer citizens who inspected for lice and nits in the hair and scalp, particularly on the nape and behind the ears. The hair was parted with wooden applicator sticks as investigators looked for nits and crawling forms visible to the naked eye, sometimes with the help of a flashlight and hand lens. In questionable cases, hair specimens were taken for microscopic examination. Each student also filled out a questionnaire.

Among 1783 white pupils, 54 (3%) were infested, whereas none of the 500 black pupils had head lice. Special education students had the highest attack rate (17.3%), probably reflecting a greater degree of interpersonal contact. **Infestation** was not affected by either hair length or sex but was related to **bed sharing**, **lower socioeconomic status**, **home crowding**, large family size, and **infestation of other family members**.

Initiation of control measures effectively stopped the epidemic. These included **education** of school officials and parents about head lice and treatment, distribution of free medications for families unable to afford treatment, and sending infested children home immediately from school and not allowing them to return to class until they were free of lice.

The right diagnosis ages with grace.

Ticks

Hovmark A, Asbrink E, Olsson I: The spirochetal etiology of **lymphadenosis benigna cutis** solitaris. Acta Derm Venereol 1986; 66:479–484.

A 28-year-old man removed a **tick** from his back in the summer of 1984. The bite was followed by a **migrating erythema** of 6 months' duration, which reached the right side of the chest and then disappeared. After another 6 months, a **painful swelling** developed in the right breast area. Serologic tests for **Borrelia antibody** were positive (IgG ELISA titer 570), and a biopsy confirmed the diagnosis of lymphadenosis benigna cutis. Penicillin therapy (phenoxymethyl penicillin, 3 gm/day for 3 weeks) produced clearing of the tumor within 5 weeks.

An additional nine patients with lymphadenosis benigna are reported. In one, spirochetes were cultivated from the biopsy of the lymphadenosis lesion. Among the ten patients, four knew of a prior tick bite within the year, five had experienced **erythema chronicum migrans** near the site of the lymphadenosis, and six had elevated levels of antibodies to the *Borrelia* spirochete. One patient also had **facial palsy** with meningitis. All patients responded promptly to penicillin therapy (phenoxymethyl penicillin 2 to 3 gm/day for 10 to 20 days).

It is concluded that the *Ixodes ricinus*–transmitted **Borrelia spirochetes can cause lymphadenosis benigna**.

Walker DH, Gay RM, Valdes-Dapena M: The occurrence of eschars in **Rocky Mountain spotted fever**. J Am Acad Dermatol 1981; 4:571–576.

Eschars are typical of many rickettsial infections, including rickettsialpox, scrub typhus, boutonneuse fever, Queensland tick typhus, and North Asian tick typhus. However, an eschar is not anticipated in Rocky Mountain spotted fever, epidemic typhus, or scrub typhus.

The inoculation of *Rickettsia rickettsii* by a **tick bite** may result in a necrotic lesion with **eschar** prior to the fever, chills, and rash of the systemic disease of Rocky Mountain spotted fever. Early excision of the eschar, together with frozen sections for direct immunofluorescence of *R. rickettsii*, may enable an early diagnosis.

Two cases are presented:

A 31-year-old house painter developed **fever, chills, nausea, and vomiting. Three days later** a necrotic, round, crusted **eschar** on the left lower leg was noted where he had been bitten by an unidentified arthropod 1 to 2 weeks previously. No other skin lesions were present until 2 days later when he developed a diffuse petechial macular rash on the chest and upper arms and a palpable spleen. He **died 36 hours later**, despite hospital treatment with antibiotics. At necropsy the eschar above the medial malleolus was 8 by 10 mm and surrounded by a red ring. Microscopic sections revealed coagulative necrosis, vasculitis with thrombosis, and blood vessels containing *R. rickettsii*.

A 13-year-old girl was **bitten by three ticks** on her right leg while camping in Tennessee. She became ill with fever (temperature 40°C) and headache 10 days later and after 2 more days developed the **generalized rash of Rocky Mountain spotted fever**. One tick bite site developed an ulcer surrounded by purple induration. She died despite intensive treatment, 8 days after becoming ill. Frozen sections of the 8- by 10-mm **eschar on her leg revealed numerous R. rickettsii** within dermal blood vessels.

Jones BE: Human 'seed tick' infestation: *Amblyomma americanum* larvae. Arch Dermatol 1981; 117:812–814.

A 5-year-old boy had 12 pinhead-sized **gray-brown tiny** "bugs" attached to the scrotum and lower abdomen the day after he had been **sitting in tall grass** in eastern North Carolina. He was asymptomatic, and no inflammatory changes were present.

Removal of a bug with forceps was difficult and ruptured the body. Microscopic examination revealed the **larval form of the Lone star tick** (*Amblyomma americanum*). Its common name stems from a single white spot on the dorsal plate of the adult female. Since the larvae look like tiny seeds, they are known as seed ticks. After hatching, they have three pairs of legs and crawl up the nearest blades of grass lying in wait (for months) to grab onto a passing animal or human host for a blood meal. After feeding for 1 to 2 weeks they drop back to the ground to molt into nymphs with four pairs of legs.

As the most common tick infecting man in the south-central states from Missouri to the Atlantic coast, it can be a **vector for spotted fever and probably tularemia.** Both adults and the transovarially infested larvae are a hazard. Since the mouth pieces are long, simple plucking off of the tick may leave the mouthparts in the skin. Rupture of the tick during removal can also liberate rickettsial organisms, which are capable of entering intact skin.

In this case, application of lindane shampoo successfully removed the ticks by the next morning—an elegant maneuver for "deticking."

Ross MS, Friede H: **Alopecia due to tick bite.** Arch Dermatol 1955; 71:524–525.

Moth-eaten alopecia in children from March to August should suggest the possibility of tick infestation. This was seen in two siblings, ages 8 and 11 years, and **resembled secondary syphilis.**

The **children** stated that their itching and scalp trouble came when they played **in the woods** near their home. Examination revealed a **tick** attached to the scalp of the younger child, later identified as *Dermacentor variabilis*. Removal of the tick revealed an underlying area of alopecia about $\frac{1}{4}$ inch long (about the size of the tick).

Both children had areas of alopecia about $\frac{1}{2}$ inch in the long axis, particularly over the occiput. Each area was completely devoid of hair with no obvious hair follicles. There was no inflammation or scale.

All diagnoses must pass the test of time.

Spiders

Wong RC, Hughes SE, Voorhees JJ: **Spider bites**. Arch Dermatol 1987; 123:98–104.

Most diagnoses of spider bites are "misdiagnoses" since:

spiders are shy and avoid humans
spider bite jaws (chelicerae) are usually too weak to penetrate human skin
most bites seen are of insect origin

Avoid making an outright diagnosis of spider bite unless the spider was recovered or positive results have been obtained by hemagglutination tests or in vitro lymphocyte transformation tests on fluid expressed from the bite site. Nonetheless, **think of a spider bite in unusual pustular or necrotic lesions** of uncertain origin. Although nearly all of the 100,000 species of spiders are venomous and can bite, only a few account for most documented bites.

1. Tarantulas:

Its fright is worse than its bite (we once saw a grocer break his leg trying to escape a tarantula, which emerged from a shipment of bananas). Pet shops now sell them as fearsome creatures the size of your fist, with a guarantee to enliven any cocktail party. The tarantula is a wandering night hunter, while its natural daytime habitat is a burrow under a rock in the American Southwest. It has poor eyesight and bites only if cornered. The bite may be almost symptomless or cause deep throbbing pain lasting no more than an hour. **Urticaria and pruritus** develop from **contact with its abdominal hairs**, which it shoots out as a defensive maneuver (leaving bald spots on its abdomen). These hairs contain chemicals that produce hives that can last several weeks and require oral steroid therapy.

2. The brown recluse spider (*Loxosceles*):

This **potentially lethal** brown to gray spider has a **dark brown violin on the dorsal thorax** (to play at your funeral). The venom of the *Loxosceles* spider is more potent than that of a rattlesnake and potentially more lethal than that of the black widow spider. Its web is in dry, dark, undisturbed places such as attics, closets, garages, and storage areas. The spider is shy and avoids light, but it may be encountered in stored clothing and bedding (watch out for sleeping bags and children playing "dress-up" in old clothes). The initial bite is often painless but can lead to a stinging or burning sensation and at times severe systemic shock and death. The **bite site** remains painful for hours and sometimes develops an ominous **blue-gray macular** halo indicating local hemolysis and arterial spasm. This can be followed by a **cyanotic bulla** or pustule with an oblong, **irregular area of erythema**, edema, and purpura, which may extend over a whole limb or most of the torso. Subsequent **necrosis** evolves into **deep stellate ulceration** and eschar formation, followed by deep scarring after 6 months.

The severity of the bite depends on the size of the spider, amount of venom injected, age and health of the victim, and the location of the bite. Fatty areas such as the thigh and buttocks show more cutaneous reaction and extensive involvement of the entire subcutaneous layer.

The diagnosis of necrotic arachnidism due to *L. reclusa* is easily made, with a typical clinical picture of an **increasingly painful solitary plaque** with a **central white ischemic area** surrounded by erythema, and identification of the spider.

If the bite is mild or atypical, or the spider has not been retrieved, one can test for venom during the first 24 hours by expressing fluid from the site of the bite and using it in a passive hemagglutination inhibition test. For older lesions, the in vitro lymphocyte transformation test is helpful (Toxicon 1973; 11:465–470).

Early histologic examination of a bite reveals dermoepidermal separation, full-thickness dermal edema, thrombosis of small arterioles, an inflammatory infiltrate of neutrophils and eosinophils, and marked extravasation of red blood cells. Later there is marked necrosis of the epidermis and dermis.

As the lesion progresses, **systemic signs** become evident within 72 hours. These include malaise, restlessness, jaundice, generalized urticaria, arthralgias, myalgias, headache, convulsions, hemolysis, disseminated intravascular coagulation, high fevers, vomiting, diarrhea, hemoglobinuria, hematuria, proteinuria, anemia, delirium, shock, and coma. Death often comes from massive intravascular hemolysis.

The **differential diagnosis** of spider bites includes:

other arthropod bites (ants, fleas, bedbugs, ticks, mites, mosquitoes, biting flies)

bee stings	pyoderma
lepidopteran blisters	pyoderma gangrenosum
erysipelas	ophthalmic zoster
cellulitis	urticaria
ecthyma	angioedema
vasculitis	burns

3. The **black**, **brown**, and **red widow spiders** (*Latrodectus*):
The first victim of the female spider after copulation is supposed to be her male partner, hence the popular name of widow. (Actually, he usually escapes by spinning a web around her when she is still in a somnolent state of ecstasy.) The jet-black females resemble an old-fashioned shoe button with a **red death mark of X on the abdomen**, although immature females may not have the hourglass mark. The males are much smaller (<6 mm in size) and brightly colored. They carry a heavy load of neurotoxic venom, and once their web—in a garage, barn, or privy—is disturbed, they bite vigorously. Although the victim may feel only a **sharp pinprick**, inspection shows two tiny red marks at the entrance point of the fangs. Within 10 to 60 minutes a dull to **severe pain** spreads from the bite to the abdomen and legs. Abdominal pain may mimic an acute abdominal condition, leading to fruitless exploratory surgery. As the neurotoxin continues to act, the patient experiences **extreme anxiety**, headaches, dizziness, weakness, fever, diaphoresis, salivation, nausea, vomiting, speech disturbance, chest tightness, backache, respiratory distress, priapism, urinary retention, tremors, hyperactive deep tendon reflexes, muscle fasciculations, and peripheral paresthesias. **Burning of the soles** is very suggestive of latrodectism. Without *L. mactans* antivenin (Lyovac) treatment, 50% of young children will die from the bite.

There are five species of widow spiders in the United States:

southern black widow (southern New England to the South)
northern black widow (East coast to eastern Texas)
western black widow (Midwest to the Southwest)
red widow (Florida)
brown widow (southern Florida)

4. **Miscellaneous spiders:**

running spiders (*Chiracanthium*)	black jumping spiders
black and yellow garden spiders	broad-faced sack spiders
wolf spiders	parson spiders
green lynx spiders	

Think of any of these spiders with an episode of pain, pruritus, ecchymotic whealing, and/or necrosis.

Oppenheim BA, Taggart I: More in **spider venom** than venom? Lancet 1990; 335:228.

A 40-year-old guitarist spent the night in a London hotel frequented by

Australian students. The next morning he noted a small bite on the dorsum of the web space of the right hand, which then became swollen and painful. Despite antibiotics, he developed **severe cellulitis** and skin breakdown.

Two months later, blisters developed over the elbow. Experts from Australia were consulted and suggested that similar cases following spider bites were due to acid-fast bacilli. Aspiration of a blister then did reveal **acid-fast bacilli**, but no organisms were isolated despite prolonged cultures. Treatment with clofazimine and rifabutin was curative after 3 months.

Campbell DS, Rees RS, King LE: **Wolf spider bites**. Cutis 1987; 39:113–114.

The dangerous brown recluse spider (*Loxosceles reclusa*) bite is rarely felt but produces local necrosis and systemic symptoms. In contrast, the bite of another dark spider, the wolf spider (Lycosidae), produces an **immediate severe pain** (like a Hymenoptera sting) **but very little aftermath**. The spider is large (up to 3.5 cm) and powerful, and its bite may puncture the skin, causing bleeding.

Parents can thus be assured that the painful dark spider bite is far safer than the painless bite. It is the venom and not the bite that causes trouble.

Hoover EL, Williams W, Koger L, et al: Pseudo-epitheliomatous hyperplasia and **pyoderma gangrenosum after a brown recluse spider bite**. South Med J 1990; 83:243–246.

A 54-year-old man was bitten by an insect, presumably a spider, in the bathroom of a halfway house. Six hours later he had pain and swelling in his left leg, and three weeks later he had a 3-cm **ulcer** crater with raised edges and surrounding induration and erythema on the medial aspect of the left lower leg. Biopsy showed necrotizing dermatitis and acute inflammation.

Despite skin grafts on three occasions, extensive **satellite lesions** progressed to involve the entire left leg with circumferential granulation tissue. Repeat biopsies showed pseudoepitheliomatous hyperplasia and extensive liquefactive necrosis of the epidermis and dermis (consistent with pyoderma gangrenosum).

Presumably this man was bitten by a **brown recluse spider**. The spider venom contains collagenase, protease, phospholipase, and hyaluronidase, which promote tissue destruction as the venom spreads. The bite itself may have precipitated the **pyoderma gangrenosum**.

Some diagnoses can't be made—until somebody describes the disease.

Elgart ML: **Flies and myiasis**. Dermatol Clin 1990; 8:237–244.

Flies cause disease by **biting**, living on decayed matter in wounds (**maggots**), and **burrowing** into the skin (**myiasis**).

Biting flies (*Diptera*)
mosquitoes:
   transmit filariasis, yellow fever, malaria, *Dermatobia hominis* eggs (carrier)
sandflies:
   Phlebotomus—transmit Old World leishmaniasis (Asia, Africa)
   Lutzomyia—transmit New World leishmaniasis, bartonellosis (South America)
   bites resemble papular urticaria
Simulium flies (black fly, buffalo fly):
   transmit onchocerciasis
   bites are slashing or tearing, with bleeding, local itching, and sometimes great swelling
biting midges:
   tiny 1- to 3-mm flies attacking in swarms, leaving punctures that become small erythematous papules in sensitized individuals
Tabanidae flies (deerfly, horsefly):
   deep, immediately painful bite that becomes secondarily infected
   transmit anthrax, tularemia, loiasis
Muscidae (housefly, stable fly):
   stable fly bite painful, the fly persistent, trying to complete feeding
tsetse flies:
   transmit trypanosomiasis
   minimal bite with small punctum

Myiasis can occur on any exposed surface. An open wound attracts the fly, which rapidly deposits eggs. They hatch into voracious maggots, most of which feed on the surface and may help to debride wounds (black blowfly larvae were available from Lederle Laboratories from 1920 to 1940). Screwworm fly larvae can penetrate normal tissue after necrotic tissue is completely removed and destroy large quantities of tissue in man and livestock.

Furuncular myiasis (lesions resembling acne cysts)
Dermatobia hominis (Central, North, and South America)
botflies (North America)
tumbu fly (Africa)

Kubba R, Al-Gindan Y, El-Hassan AM, Omer AHS: Clinical **diagnosis of cutaneous leishmaniasis** (oriental sore). J Am Acad Dermatol 1987; 16:1183–1189.

Cutaneous leishmaniasis is endemic in Saudi Arabia, where it is **transmitted by the sandfly** *Phlebotomus papatasii*. The fly may bite several times in an area because of the difficulty of sucking blood through a proboscis congested with promastigotes of the parasite. The principal animal reservoir of *Leishmania major* is the gerbil.

Leishmaniasis begins with one or more insect-bite–like **erythematous papules at the bite site**, after an incubation period of 1 week to 3 months. The papule slowly **enlarges into a nodule** and turns darker. The nodule then softens, oozes seropurulent discharge, and **becomes crusted** over a shallow ulcer crater with a spongy base. Lesions are usually asymptomatic unless secondary bacterial infection makes them painful.

Typical lesions are on **exposed sites**; they are often paired or clustered and elongated in alignment with skin creases. The "**volcanic**" **nodule** is the most distinctive lesion, with sloping smooth sides and a shallow crater covered with a crust. Some nodules have rolled borders, while others have subcutaneous components ("iceberg" nodules) that radiate evenly or have tongue-like proximal extensions. Routine palpation may also disclose lymphatic dissemination in the form of **beaded cords** or 0.5- to 1.0-cm smooth, mobile, nontender subcutaneous nodules proximal to the skin lesions. About 20% of patients have multiple 2- to 5-mm smooth inflammatory **satellite papules** within 2 cm of the primary lesion. These erupt late, often following anti-leishmanial treatment with pentavalent antimony, ketoconazole, and cryo-surgery. Healing occurs after several weeks, starting in the center, and results in an atrophic hyperpigmented irregular **cribriform scar**.

In addition to typical cutaneous findings in "oriental sore," the **diagnosis** of leishmaniasis may depend on the typical natural history and the successful response to antileishmanial treatment. The parasite could not be found in 10 to 20% of cases. Leishman-Donovan bodies (amastigotes) were found in tissue smears (50 to 80%, depending on investigator and technique) and skin biopsies (70%), while promastigotes were found in parasite cultures (50%—research procedure). Serologic testing lacks specificity, and the leishmanin skin test is of no diagnostic value in endemic areas (and not readily available elsewhere).

Differential diagnosis of *acute* cutaneous leishmaniasis:

insect bite	kerion
impetigo	myiasis
furuncle	dracunculosis
carbuncle	molluscum
ecthyma	warts
anthrax	pyogenic granuloma
orf	tropical ulcer
milker's nodule	foreign body granuloma
tularemia	keratoacanthoma
swimming pool granuloma	basal cell carcinoma
tuberculosis cutis	squamous cell carcinoma
yaws	metastases
sporotrichosis	lymphoma
blastomycosis	leukemia

Differential diagnosis of *chronic* cutaneous leishmaniasis:

lupus vulgaris	acne
leprosy	rosacea
sarcoidosis	cellulitis
granuloma faciale	erysipelas
Jessner's lymphocytic infiltrate	keloids
lymphocytoma cutis	Wegener's granulomatosis
discoid lupus erythematosus	syphilitic gumma
psoriasis	

Cochran R, Rosen T: **African trypanosomiasis** in the United States. Arch Dermatol 1983; 119:670–674.

A month after hunting wild game in a rain forest in Tanzania, a 72-year-old man became very weak, delirious, and **bedridden with shaking chills**. He had been **bitten dozens of times by tsetse flies** during the hunt. A 10-cm edematous, **indurated, crusted, fluctuant plaque** was present on the upper right arm, and oval erythematous macules that blanched on pressure were seen on the legs. A biopsy of the arm lesion showed a perivascular infiltrate of lymphocytic and plasma cells.

A diagnosis of African trypanosomiasis was made, with the arm lesion being considered the trypanosomal chancre. This was confirmed by finding numerous **hemoflagellates in thick blood smears**. A trypanosomiasis fluorescent antibody titer was positive at 1:4096. He responded well to intravenous suramin therapy.

The typical **trypanosomal chancre** of African sleeping sickness due to the protozoon *Trypanosoma brucei*, *T. gambiense*, or *T. rhodesiense* appears within hours or days of the tsetse fly bite. It is a tender, violaceous area of induration that subsides in a few weeks. At times, the bite site remains inapparent. More common in whites is a generalized **fleeting erythematous macular rash**, usually **on the trunk**. Lymphadenopathy is often present, being known as Winterbottom's sign when it appears in the posterior cervical triangle.

In the rain forests of Africa, you are the big game the tsetse fly hunts, and just one of its shots can put you to "sleep."

Lane RP, Lovell CR, Griffiths WAD, Sonnex TS: Human **cutaneous myiasis**—a review and report of three cases due to *Dermatobia hominis*. Clin Exp Dermatol 1987; 12:40–45.

While in the rain forests of Belize, a 30-year-old entomologist experienced more than 300 **insect bites**, which had cleared 2 weeks later except for four painful inflammatory papules over the right scapula. **Each papule** had a central hole **revealing movement within**, which could be induced by touching the lesion. Excision of one papule confirmed the presence of a human **botfly larva** (*Dermatobia hominis*), with an overlying sinus tract and heavy mixed cellular infiltrate rich in eosinophils in the deep dermis.

This large bluish-gray fly catches another insect, such as a mosquito, and sticks 15 to 30 eggs onto its abdomen. When mosquito bites man, the larva senses human warmth, rapidly hatches, and within minutes painlessly penetrates the skin or colonizes a wound. Positioned head down, it feeds on the dermis using sickle-like mouth hooks. Its oxygen demands are met by its posterior end spiracles located at the skin opening in the patient. Spines on the surface of the larva, as well as its shape, make removal difficult, so that it usually **remains in the skin for a couple of months**. It then climbs out and drops to the ground to pupate in hospitable soil. Within a month it arises as an adult fly, sexually active after 3 hours. In its brief life of 8 to 9 days as a fly, the female must lay and transfer about 400 new eggs. Meanwhile, the patient's "larval" lesion has healed completely. To abort the cycle, larvae are best removed surgically by probe and forceps following a cruciate incision.

This review gives extensive documentation for other worldwide examples of myiasis, which is the invasion of mammalian tissue by the larvae of *Diptera* (two-winged flies). Infestation may involve the skin surface, dermis, subcutaneous tissue, nasopharynx, eyes, intestines, and urogenital system. Some interesting examples include:

Wohlfahrtia vigil. Larvae of this North American fly will penetrate only infant's skin, causing **impetigo-like lesions**.

Cordylobia anthropophaga (**tumbu fly**). This large yellow-brown fly of Africa lays eggs on grass, soil contaminated with urine or perspiration, or bed linen hung out to dry. As soon as skin contact occurs, the larvae hatch and penetrate the skin within minutes, preferring the feet, forearms, scrotum, and back where they cause a pustule. They **remain in the skin for only 8 to 10 days**, so that they are seen only in *recent visitors* to endemic countries. The larvae can be expelled by gentle pressure (their shape is inverse to that of botfly larvae) or the application of petrolatum to cut off their air supply.

Elgart GW: **Ant, bee, and wasp stings.** Dermatol Clin 1990; 8:229–236.

Most patients who die from insect stings are adult men who have had late onset of symptoms and have delayed seeking treatment. Respiratory failure causes most deaths. Large doses of venom from **multiple stings** may cause **anaphylaxis-like symptoms** or other toxic reactions. Children, and possibly also adults, are very unlikely to react to subsequent envenomation even with positive RAST tests. In general, however, sensitive individuals should avoid outdoor dining and the wearing of perfumes and white, blue, or brightly colored clothing.

Honeybees are fuzzy with broad wings and no sharp division between the width of the thorax and abdomen. **Stings can be identified by the presence of the stinger and venom sac**, which are left in the skin because of the barb on the stinger. Most bee stings occur when the victim walks barefoot in clover.

Hornets, including yellow jackets, have slender tapered bodies and smooth shiny exoskeletons. They are commonly encountered around trash receptacles and are easily provoked to sting. Although they leave no stinger, multiple stings are uncommon unless their hives are threatened.

Wasps may sting multiple times, but usually sting only when hunting or provoked. The wasp abdomen is the most tapered and connects by a narrow tube to the thorax. Wasps are brown or black (less colorful than hornets) and shiny. The paper wasp is probably most common, as it builds a paperlike hive under the eaves of houses.

Fire ants are either red or black and live in large mounds interconnected by tunnels a few inches underground. Multiple stings are common, since ants are social insects. The method of stinging is unique among *Hymenoptera*, being a two-part process. The ant bites with its jaws, which leave two hemorrhagic puncta. While its head is attached, it swivels its body around in a circle, stinging multiple times. A circle of erythematous papules results, with vesicles and then sterile pustules evolving. Therefore, sterile **pustules in an annular array around two hemorrhagic puncta are diagnostic**.

Borochowitz Z, Hardoff D: Severe late clinical manifestations after **hornet (*Vespa orientalis*) stings**—in a young child. Eur J Pediatr 1982; 139:91–92.

A 3-year-old boy in Israel sustained 109 **Oriental hornet stings** while rushing into a hornet nest in the bushes. One hour later he had generalized edema and severe irritability, which gradually subsided as the lesions started healing. On the sixth day the **skin lesions became necrotic** and he had mild jaundice and decreased urinary output. Immunofluorescence of a skin biopsy showed no immunologic involvement. Following peritoneal dialysis given over 3 weeks, the skin lesions **healed with scars** at each sting site.

Schwartz HJ: Skin sensitivity in **insect allergy**. JAMA 1965; 194:113–115.

The clinical history, rather than the results of **skin tests** to a mixture of whole-body extracts of bees, wasps, and yellow jackets, remains the keystone to diagnosis in *Hymenoptera* allergy. There was no significant difference in reactivity to serial dilutions (1:10,000, 1:1000, and 1:100) among patients with known insect sensitivity, atopics with rhinitis or asthma but no insect sensitivity, and nonatopic subjects. **Skin sensitivity did not correlate with clinical reactivity.** Skin tests are valuable mainly as a general guide for the starting dose of hyposensitization therapy.

Rosen T: **Caterpillar dermatitis.** Dermatol Clin 1990; 8:245–252.

Lepidopterism refers to the adverse effects caused by contact with butterflies, moths, or their caterpillars. Members of 12 families of moths and one family of butterflies may induce localized inflammatory lesions of the eye (conjunctivitis, keratitis, iridocyclitis), respiratory tract (rhinitis, wheezing), and skin (dermatitis). More serious, but rarely seen problems include tachycardia, arrhythmia, chest pain, dyspnea, bleeding diathesis, peripheral neuropathy, paralysis, shock, and convulsions.

Caterpillar dermatitis presents as localized or widespread erythematous macules that rapidly evolve into urticarial wheals, often followed by small papules or papulovesicles. The onset of itching or burning may be instantaneous or delayed 2 to 10 hours after contact. Swelling of an affected extremity may also occur. Symptoms subside within a few hours to 7 to 10 days, depending on the species of caterpillar.

Caterpillars have specialized toxic hairs or spines that comprise only a minority of the total number. These hairs are straight and sharp ended and retain an irritant potential for years. Presumably, toxic hairs penetrate the skin and transmit a toxin with enzymatic and proteolytic activity but usually no histamine. Toxins appear to vary between species, and there appears to be no "universal" toxin. The caterpillar **hairs may be encountered on vegetation or dog or cat fur or may become airborne**, causing epidemics of dermatitis.

The **puss caterpillar** ("wooly worm") *Megalopyge opercularis* is common in the eastern and southern United States, including Texas, and eats a wide variety of trees, corn, and flowers. It is 20 to 35 mm long, 10 to 20 mm wide, and covered with thick pale yellow to gray-brown hairs, with a tuft of hair at the posterior end. It causes **painful stings** that result in a characteristic **gridlike pattern** of **hemorrhagic papules**. Cardiovascular and neurologic symptoms may result.

The **Io moth** (corn emperor moth, *Autumeris io*) caterpillar is pale green with distinctive lateral maroon over white stripes and clumps of bristles. Contact with it produces a pronounced short-lived wheal with a wide flare. It eats almost any leafy plant and ranges from Canada to the Gulf Coast along the Atlantic seaboard.

The **gypsy moth** (*Lymantria dispar*) caterpillar escaped from a laboratory in Massachusetts in 1889 and quickly spread over New England. In 1981 an explosive increase in the moth population caused an **epidemic** of **pruritic dermatitis**. The 20- to 30-mm-long larva has lateral tufts of buff to yellow hairs and two dorsal white stripes. The caterpillar defoliates deciduous trees, particularly oaks.

The **brown-tail moth** (*Euproctis chrysorrhoea*) is the most common cause of lepidopterism in England. It came to the United States on roses imported from Holland and spread in the Northeast and adjacent areas of Canada. The 40- to 50-mm-long light brown caterpillar has two dorsolateral white stripes and eats fruit trees, elms, oaks, hawthorns, and blackthorns. Related species include the various Tussock moths: Oriental, Mulberry, and Douglas fir. The latter causes dermatitis in forestry workers in the Pacific Northwest and Western Canada.

The **saddle-back caterpillar** (*Sibine stimulea*) feeds on oleanders, croton bushes, and palm trees in the Southeast United States. The 20- to 30-mm-long brown caterpillar has a green back and flank and causes urticarial stings of short duration.

Processionary caterpillars (*Thaumetopoea* genera) are endemic to Israel and the Mediterranean coast. They thrive on pine trees and induce a short-lived intense dermatitis.

Hylesia family moths in Central and South America are nocturnal and swarm **aboard ships** anchored in port. Contact with venomous hairs on the abdomen of the adult female moth causes a dermatitis known as The "**Caripito itch**" (after Caripito, Venezuela).

Beetles, Centipedes, Scorpions

Ahmed AR, Moy R, Barr AR, Price Z: **Carpet beetle dermatitis**. J Am Acad Dermatol 1981; 5:428–432.

For **5 years** a 22-year-old man had **pruritic papules** on the extremities and other hairy areas. Lesions began as 4- to 5-mm urticarial papules that in a few hours became **papulovesicles** and later scabbed. The clinical diagnosis was papular urticaria, but repeated visits to specialists in several cities provided no relief. Patch tests done by three different physicians as well as intradermal and prick tests for common allergens were all negative.

The denouement came by focusing on the fact that his **pruritus began when he moved into a new home with a bedroom furnished with two wool carpets**. He further realized that he never developed new lesions when sleeping elsewhere. Careful examination of the bedroom **carpets disclosed a horde of carpet beetle larvae**. Professional fumigation of the home with sulfuryl fluoride provided a permanent cure.

Injection of 0.02 ml of a 1:500 w/v **ad hoc prepared antigen** of whole beetle larvae (directions given) confirmed the diagnosis of carpet beetle dermatitis by eliciting a wheal with pseudopodia within 20 minutes. Control subjects showed no reaction. Patch tests to the same beetle extract were negative.

The cure came in this case by treating not the patient, but his room.

Rustin MHA, Munro DD: **Papular urticaria** caused by *Dermestes maculatus Degeer*. Clin Exp Dermatol 1984; 9:317–321.

Numerous excoriated and secondarily infected papules covered the face, trunk, limbs, and penis of a 2-year-old West Indian boy. He had had the problem for 9 months, but no other family member was affected, and no scabies mites were found. Despite treatment with topical gamma benzene, topical steroids, and systemic antibiotics, hospitalization was required.

The cause of the eruption was discovered by a visit to his home, where **beetles and larvae were found in his bed and bedroom** and throughout the house (even in the food in the kitchen). The beetles were identified as *Dermestes* ("skin eater") *maculatus*. Their eradication led to a prompt cure of the **boy's papular urticaria**.

The larvae of these beetles are covered with protective hairs, to which he probably became sensitized. They are voracious (having to meet the metabolic demands of seven molts) and eat anything from dried fish to woolen sweaters during this stage, which lasts for 1 month to 1 year. These "super beetles" have been known to bore through lead sheaths of cables and honeycomb the hull of a ship, almost sinking it.

This little boy's story demonstrates once again the diagnostic value of making a **house call**.

Nicholls DSH, Christmas TI, Greig DE: Oedemerid **blister beetle dermatosis**: A review. J Am Acad Dermatol 1990; 22:815–819.

This distinctive seasonal **vesiculobullous disorder** occurs several hours after unknown contact with a blister beetle. Tense vesicles or bullae without erythema or symptoms appear suddenly, usually on the neck, arms, or upper trunk. Sometimes in linear or kissing patterns on opposing surfaces, they rupture spontaneously in a day and heal in a week.

Oedemerid beetles neither bite nor sting but **contain a vesicant** (either cantharidin or pederin) which is released when a beetle is brushed against, pressed, or crushed on the skin. Pederin causes an inflammatory reaction, with urticaria and dermatitis preceding the blisters.

There are more than 200 species of blister beetles, with the most famous being **Spanish fly** (*Lytta vesicatoria*) found in southern Europe in the summer. The beetles are world wide.

Mumcuoglu KY, Leibovici V: **Centipede (Scolopendra) bite:** A case report. Israel J Med Sci 1989; 25:47–49.

A 71-year-old woman in Jerusalem was standing near a bonfire at night when a 10-cm-long **centipede** fell from a tree and **bit her on the neck.** She immediately removed it and took it in with her to the hospital, where it was identified as a species of *Scolopendra*. The bite site was swollen and mildly erythematous, with pruritus and local pain. She was unable to move her head for several hours and also had nausea. By the next day the symptoms had almost disappeared.

Centipede bites are common in Israel and other Mediterranean countries. There is local **burning pain, redness, and edema** or a wheal. An **erysipelas-like** state may follow, with lymphangitis and lymphadenitis, as well as fever and nausea. Symptoms last for a few hours to a few days.

Centipedes are fast-moving nocturnal predators with one pair of legs per body segment and two long antennae. They are 3 to 250 mm long, with 15 to 181 pairs of legs. The first pair of legs has evolved into a biting apparatus through which the neurotoxic and hemolytic poison is injected. During daylight hours centipedes hide under stones and tree bark or in leaf litter or holes in the ground. Sometimes they find their way into houses; most **bites occur when the victim is in bed or putting on clothes** in which the centipede lodged during the night.

Centipedes usually leave the skin immediately after biting, but occasionally have to be anesthetized with ether or alcohol to facilitate removal.

Binder LS: Acute **arthropod envenomation**. Incidence, clinical features and management. Med Toxicol Adverse Drug Exp 1989; 4:163–173.

More than 650 species of **scorpions** are known, largely in arid and tropical areas. Their long crustaceous body may be up to 8 cm long, with a pair of pincers for grasping prey and a segmented **tail with a stinger** (telson). They sting by arching their tails over their heads and injecting venom that is inflammatory and vasotoxic.

The **sting** results in local edema, inflammation, and a sharp burning sensation that develops over several minutes. **Ecchymosis** and **lymphangitis** may ensue. Symptoms usually resolve over several days. Infrequently, an allergic reaction and anaphylaxis occur.

Severe **cholinergic toxicity** may result from the sting of *Centruroides sculpturatus* (striped scorpion), found particularly in the southwestern United States. Symptoms include salivation, lacrimation, urinary incontinence, diarrhea, tenesmus, bronchospasm, bradycardia, fever, muscle fasciculations and spasm, hyperactivity, and convulsions. A specific antivenin for this scorpion is available through seven laboratories worldwide (in the United States: Arizona State University, Tempe, Arizona).

Scorpions are nocturnal and hide in damp cool areas under rocks and logs or in cracks and crevices of homes. They may **get into shoes, clothing**, and **sleeping bags**, where they become trapped against bodies. Children under 10 years old sustain 80% of the stings. In the United States scorpions cause three to four deaths per year.

Never underestimate the diagnostic value of a house call.

Burnett JW, Calton GJ, Burnett HW: **Jellyfish envenomation syndromes**. J Am Acad Dermatol 1986; 14:100–106.

The common finding is a **painful linear urticarial eruption** at the site of **contact with the jellyfish tentacle**. The responsible polypeptides and enzymes are both toxic and antigenic. The lesions may rapidly become vesicular, hemorrhagic, necrotizing, or ulcerative. Lesions may also appear at sites distant from the locus of contact. Subsequent fat atrophy, limb necrosis, gangrene, keloids, and contractures can occur.

Delayed reactions may present as granulomatous lesions persisting for many months.

Urticaria may result **from eating jellyfish**, or even from contact with powdered jellyfish used in cooking.

Fatal reactions may occur if at least 50 feet of box jellyfish tentacles touch the skin of an adult. Anaphylaxis, central respiratory failure, and acute renal failure with intravascular hemolysis have been reported. Interestingly, serum sickness after jellyfish envenomation has not been observed. The application of local heat may be advantageous in many instances, as all jellyfish venoms are heat labile.

Barnes JH: Cause and effect of **Irukandji stingings**. Med J Aust 1964; 897–904. (Irukandji stings. Lancet 1964; 2:190.)

For a few days each summer, when the **winds blow** northward instead of southeasterly off the northeastern coast of **Australia**, sunbathers are at risk for **stings from "invisible" jellyfish**. Within minutes the victim develops violent generalized pains, vomiting, and prostration, lasting a few days before recovery. Slight erythema appears at the sting site, but no wheals. Despite water movement that casts jellyfish onto the beach, no culprits were found.

Careful underwater searching of surface waters with a black object and oblique lighting led to discovery of two transparent mobile tiny "box" jellyfish with 1-cm bullet-shaped bodies speckled with tiny reddish "warts," each having four tentacles 3 to 18 cm long. The jellyfish pulsed rapidly and traveled at about 2 knots.

Three **volunteers** who exposed their wet arms to the jellyfish for 3 to 10 seconds developed symptoms of Irukandji stings within 10 to 20 minutes, requiring intravenous pethidine and oral acetylsalicylic acid for relief.

The entire tropical coastline of Australia and Indonesia may be subject to occasional visitations of noxious jellyfish and a metereologic warning system could be helpful.

Ohtaki N, Satoh A, Azuma H, Nakajima T: Delayed **flare-up reactions caused by jellyfish**. Dermatologica 1986; 172:98–103.

Bizarre linear vesicular erythema developed in four women 1 week after exposure to jellyfish while ocean swimming. Biopsy revealed allergic contact dermatitis. The residual hyperpigmentation was an intriguing scribble-like tracing of the exact lines of contact with the tentacles.

Coelenterate envenomation may induce both immediate and delayed hypersensitivity reactions, as well as cause immediate toxicity from toxins, enzymes, and polypeptides located within nematocysts on the jellyfish tentacles.

Burnett JW, Hepper KP, Aurelian L, et al: **Recurrent eruptions** following unusual solitary **coelenterate envenomations**. J Am Acad Dermatol 1987; 17:86–92.

Recurrent linear eruptions, separated by 1 to 4 weeks, may follow a single episode of a **jellyfish sting**.

A 32-year-old woman, stung while diving off Cancun, initially developed patchy **linear erythematous pruritic lesions that lasted 4 weeks**. She then had four more less severe attacks of shorter duration over the next 5 months.

Rosson CL, Tolle SW: Management of **marine stings and scrapes**. West J Med 1989; 150:97–100.

Jellyfish, **sea anemone**, and **Portuguese man-of-war tentacles** have similar stinging **nematocysts** with venom containing many polypeptides, quaternary ammonium compounds, histamine, 5-hydroxytryptamine, and catecholamines. Mild stings produce local burning and paresthesias, with pain radiating throughout the limb and into the groin or axilla. Wheals and a papular dermatitis may erupt and remain for as long as a week. Skin necrosis with ulcerations may also develop. Neurologic, cardiopulmonary, musculoskeletal, and gastrointestinal reactions also occur. **Tentacles of dead men-of-war** can retain live nematocysts **able to sting for several days**. Following a sting, the site should be immediately bathed in seawater or vinegar (5% aetic acid) to inactivate nematocyst discharge. Baking soda paste may also be applied and then scraped off with a knife. Tentacle fragments should be removed with a razor.

Box jellyfish stings occur mainly off the coast of Queensland, Australia, and are fatal in 15 to 20% because of a cardiotoxin. Antivenom is available in Australia.

Corals do not sting but produce knifelike **sharp cuts with pruritus**, erythema, and urticaria at the wound site. **Cellulitis** and ulceration may follow. Healing may be very slow with prolonged discomfort, possibly due to infection or microparticles of coral or sediment in the wound. Antibiotics are often recommended.

Sponges contain **spicules** that become embedded in the skin of snorkelers and divers and cause both irritant and allergic contact dermatitis. The symptoms, erythema, pruritus, vesicles, and weeping, resemble those of poison oak. Joint swelling, erythema multiforme, and anaphylaxis are rare complications. Spicules should be removed with adhesive tape and the area bathed in vinegar.

Sea urchin spines contain a purple dye that may discolor the skin. Some spines are quite sharp and hollow and contain a toxin with serotonin, steroid glycosides, and acetylcholine-like agents. The spines can rapidly embed, producing severe burning dysesthesia and swelling. Some species have venomous triple-jawed pincers that cause edema and hemorrhage at the wound site followed by paresthesias, paralysis, respiratory failure, and, rarely, death. The spines and pincer-like organs should be removed if possible, as they may produce infection and foreign body granulomas. X-rays may help locate the calcium carbonate spines. Antibiotic therapy may be advisable.

Stingrays inhabit shallow warm coastal waters and are frequently stepped on by unwitting bathers. The stingray lashes out its tail, which carries a stinging spine with retroserrate teeth and grooves holding venomous glands. The resulting puncture or **jagged laceration** contains the stinger, so that secondary infection is common. The sting site has swelling and bleeding and localized burning pain that peaks in a few hours and resolves over 2 days. The area becomes red and hemorrhagic. Serotonin, phosphodiesterase, and 5′-nucleotidase in the venom may cause severe muscle cramps, nausea, vomiting, diaphoresis, tachycardia, cardiac arrhythmias, hypotension, and loss of consciousness. Immersion in hot water for 90 minutes, evaluation in a health care center, and antibiotics are recommended.

Catfish stings occur in both fresh and salt water of North America and cause immediate intense pain through the entire length of the involved extremity. Most stings involve the upper extremity when the fish is handled without protective gloves or a towel. Hot water immersion is recommended.

The **lionfish**, **scorpionfish**, and **stonefish** are noted for camouflage and are popular for tropical aquariums. They inhabit the Florida Keys, Gulf of Mexico, Hawaii, and the southern California coast. They sting with the spines of their dorsal, pectoral, and anal fins, with the stonefish being the most venomous. Stings cause intense throbbing pain and pallor at the puncture wound site, followed by cyanosis and swelling. Gastrointestinal, neurologic, and cardiovascular effects may occur, along with secondary infection. Hot-water immersion and tetanus prophylaxis are recommended. Antivenom is manufactured in Australia and is available through Sea World (San Diego and Ohio) and the Steinhart Aquarium (San Francisco).

Asada M, Komura J, Hosokawa H, et al: A case of delayed **hypersensitivity reaction** following a **sea urchin sting**. Dermatologica 1990; 180:99–101.

A 28-year-old woman, who had been **snorkeling** 2 months before, had pruritic erythema on her knees and right ankle where she had been stung by a *Diadema* species of **sea urchin** with long sharp fragile **spines**. Initially she noted painful redness and tenderness of the wounded areas, which healed over several days. Then, 10 days after the sting, the penetration sites became red and pruritic. Skin biopsy showed a perivascular mononuclear cell infiltrate. An x-ray of the area was negative for radiopaque foreign materials.

Patch tests were performed with extracts made from ground *Diadema* spines and were positive at 48 hours. It was therefore concluded that she had a delayed hypersensitivity reaction to residual sea urchin antigens at the wound sites.

Immediate reactions to sea urchin stings occur within a few hours and cause burning pain, redness, edema, and often profuse bleeding. Delayed reactions usually appear 2 to 4 months later and consist of either foreign body or sarcoidal granulomas. A delayed vesicular reaction has also been reported. Sometimes a portion of spine left in the skin can be detected by x-ray.

Zeman MG: **Catfish stings**. A report of three cases. Ann Emerg Med 1989; 18:211–213.

Catfish stings and envenomations can occur when the fish is carelessly handled or trod on by an innocent wader. The stinging apparatus consists of venom glands attached to the bony dorsal and pectoral fin spines, which extend when the fish is frightened or excited. Venom is released when the victim's skin is punctured. The spines have sharp retrorse teeth that act like barbs and make removal difficult. The spines commonly break off and may become buried in the wound, sometimes penetrating a joint. X-ray visualization of the bony spines is extremely helpful.

The catfish sting causes an **immediate stinging** or throbbing sensation that radiates up the limb and may be associated with **muscle fasciculations**. The wound area becomes cyanotic and edematous. Peripheral neuropathy, local wound necrosis, and persistent lymphedema may result.

Catfish venom is heat labile, so that immersion of the affected part in **hot water** gives **dramatic relief of pain**. Catfish fishermen often carry a thermos of hot water or use water from the boat's engine to treat envenomations. Since the venom is unaffected by freezing, injury may occur from handling a recently frozen catfish.

Infection of the deep puncture wound with *Aeromonas* (*Proteus*) species is probably common, and treatment with a broad-spectrum antibiotic is recommended. Infection with *Mycobacterium terrae* has also been reported.

Grenza TE: **Catfish spine envenomation** of the hand. J Hand Surg 1989; 14:1035–1036.

A 43-year-old fisherman was stung on the left thenar eminence through a rubber glove while handling a freshwater catfish. Following immediate pain, which increased over 24 hours, he developed a sharply demarcated **erythematous plaque** of the palm and wrists. There were no lymphangitic streaks or enlarged nodes, and x-rays were negative for an embedded spine. Despite intravenous antibiotics, the erythema had progressed to 35 cm above the wrist crease by the fourth day after the sting. Gradual resolution of the swelling, erythema, and tenderness then occurred over the next 2 weeks.

Catfish toxin, yet to be identified, produces immediate intense local pain, described as stinging, throbbing, and scalding. This is followed by erythema and swelling that **resemble streptococcal cellulitis**.

Adams SL: The emergency management of medicinal **leech bite**. Ann Emerg Med 1989; 18:316–319.

The medicinal leech (*Hirudo medicinalis*) causes a **triradiate bite**, resembling the corporate logo of Mercedes-Benz.

This freshwater leech is approximately 10 cm long and has two suckers, one at either end. The mouth lies in the anterior sucker and contains three jaws with teeth. The leech can suck 5 to 15 ml of blood (10 times its own weight), and will not feed again for almost a year. Blood is digested in the gut with the assistance of *Aeromonas hydrophila*, which may cause infection of the site of the leech bite. Before attaching, the leech may move around, sometimes crawling into a body orifice, where it may cause obstruction as it feeds.

The salivary glands of the leech secrete the anticoagulant hirudin, which inhibits thrombin and prevents coagulation of ingested blood. Also secreted are hyaluronidase, proteolytic enzymes, fibrinase, and collagenase. These cause **continued oozing of blood after removal of the leech**, sometimes up to 24 hours. Ecchymosis and scarring are common sequelae. Local allergic reactions and even anaphylaxis may occur.

In 1866 leeches were reported to transmit syphilis, erysipelas, and puerperal fever by cross-use in patients. Recent studies point to leeches as a reservoir for viruses and *Trypanosoma cruzi*.

Burnett JW, Cargo DG: Cutaneous irritation induced by **crab larvae**. J Am Acad Dermatol 1979; 1:42–43.

Calcified spines on the tiny millimeter-sized larvae of crabs account for **pricking sensations** in swimmers and crab fishermen when encountering them en masse. These **larvae**, described as **floating sand particles**, do not produce allergic reactions or inject any venom. There are no skin lesions, and removal of the larvae from the exposed skin brings rapid relief.

When the patient says he is bothered by "crabs," you have to find out which kind.

Flandry F, Lisecki EJ, Dominigue GJ, et al: Initial antibiotic therapy for **alligator bites**. South Med J 1989; 82:262–266.

A 22-year-old man was assisting in the transport of a 4-foot alligator in a burlap sack when he lost his grip on the animal and was bitten through the sack. The alligator held his thumb clenched with its teeth until a bystander struck the animal on the head with a blunt object and forced it to release its grip.

Examination revealed a crush injury of the distal phalanx of the thumb with puncture wounds at the base of the eponychium and at the distal dorsal interphalangeal joint crease. Digital Allen's test was negative, and sensation was intact distally. X-rays revealed a fracture of the distal phalanx. Two days after surgical debridement and jet lavage irrigation, cultures showed a heavy growth of *Aeromonas hydrophila* (sensitive to first-generation cephalosporin) as well as four other types of bacteria, including *Clostridium* species. All organisms were sensitive to trimethoprim-sulfamethoxazole, which was then given and resulted in wound healing in 2 weeks and healing of the fracture in 2 months.

A study of the oral flora and dental plaque from ten alligators and their environmental water samples yielded mainly gram-negative species, both aerobic and anaerobic. **Aeromonas hydrophila** was the most consistent isolate from both the water and the alligators. This organism accounts for most of the reported **infections from alligator bites** and causes **bullae** or **cellulitis** within 24 to 48 hours, followed by necrosis and drainage of **foul-smelling** purulent material.

The frequency of encounters between humans and alligators is increasing as a result of alligator farming and hunting and their encroachment in areas frequented by man. "Domestication" may produce nuisance alligators, particularly large males that become much more aggressive when hungry and may attack humans in an attempt to feed.

An inadequate biopsy specimen can be more misleading than no specimen at all.

Animals and Snakes

Galloway RE: **Mammalian bites**. J Emerg Med 1988; 6:325–331.

Cat bites:
high risk (30 to 50%) of infection with *Pasteurella multocida*, particularly
for puncture wounds
watch out for cat scratch disease

Dog bites:
low risk (2 to 5%) of infection with *Staphylococcus aureus* or *P. multocida*

Rat bites:
10% infection rate
usually occur in laboratory workers or poor children
rat-bite fever is an unusual complication (look for petechiae on the palms
and soles)
rabies prophylaxis not indicated

Monkey bites:
15% infection rate

Skunk bites:
frequent carrier of rabies
musk expulsion is accurate up to 13 feet and may result in burns, temporary blindness, nausea, seizures, and syncope

Herbivore (cow, horse) bites:
rarely seen, but have a high infection rate
do not require rabies prophylaxis

Human bites:
high risk (15 to 50%) of infection with *Streptococcus viridans*, *Staphylococcus aureus*, and *Eikenella corrodens* (a slow-growing gram-negative
anaerobe)
most bites involve the scalp in children and the dorsal surface of the hand
in adults ("fight bite")
clenched fist injury: a laceration of the dorsal aspect of the hand may
result in infection of the metacarpophalangeal joint (not covered by the
dorsal expansion hood in the clenched position). Teeth gain ready access
into the joint space, which is then sealed when the fingers are reex-
tended. An x-ray is recommended to rule out fractures, osteomyelitis,
and retained teeth. Cellulitis, abscesses, osteomyelitis, and tenosynovitis are common complications.

Local wound infections account for 95% of complications following an animal
bite. *Pasteurella multocida* infections develop within the first 2 days after a
bite, whereas *Staphylococcus* or *Streptococcus* infections occur 2 days after
the bite. Tetanus is a rare but possible complication. Rabies must be considered in any unprovoked attack by a bizarrely acting animal. **Rabies prophylaxis** is usually given for bites by skunks, bats, foxes, raccoons, and bob-
cats. Domestic animals should be **quarantined** and observed for evidence of
rabies.

Wiley JF II: **Mammalian bites**. Review of evaluation and management. Clin Pediatr
1990; 29:283–287.

Dog bites affect boys twice as often as girls, and in 90% of cases the dog is
known by the victim (15%, family dog). Apparently dogs bite children who
either tease them or unknowingly threaten them. School-aged children are
bitten most often on the hand or arm, while children under 4 years are
bitten more often on the face and neck. Other than scarring, **infection with
Pasteurella multocida** (a gram-negative facultative anaerobe) is the main

problem. Augmentin (amoxicillin and clavulanic acid) is the treatment of choice. Dog bites may also transmit rabies.

Cat bites and scratches affect girls more often than boys. Infection with *P. multocida* is the primary danger, although cat bites may also transmit tularemia and plague. **Cat scratch disease**, caused by a gram-negative coccobacillus, may begin after 7 to 12 days of incubation, with low-grade fever, localized lymphadenopathy, and sometimes a papule or pustule at the original site.

Human bites occur most often in teenagers and young adults, particularly as a clenched-fist laceration during a fight. Toddlers and schoolchildren may suffer accidental superficial bites, especially on the face, during sports and play. **Infection is common** with streptococcus and *Eikenella corrodens*, a facultative gram-negative rod. Treatment with a combination of Augmentin and a penicillinase-resistant penicillin is recommended. The human bites may also transmit syphilis, hepatitis B, and tuberculosis, but so far not AIDS.

Overall, dogs account for the majority of mammalian bites and almost all of the fatalities. Human bites and cat bites account for the majority of infected wounds.

Barnham M: **Pig bite** injuries and infection: Report of seven human cases. Epidem Inf 1988; 101:641–645.

In North Yorkshire and Humberside there is a high level of pig farming. Although farmers say that pigs are usually indifferent or playful with their owners, these strong animals occasionally inflict serious, deep injuries that usually become infected.

The sow can bite away pieces of skin and subcutaneous tissue in humans, usually on the posterior aspect of the thigh because of the height of the animal and its unseen approach from behind. The boar has very sharp tusks that can inflict slicing or tearing injuries down into the muscle, with nerve and blood vessel damage.

There is a **high risk of infection** from a variety of organisms in the mouths of the pigs, including streptococci, pasteurellae, *Bacteroides* spp, *Proteus* spp, and *Escherichi coli*. Infections vary from cellutitis to abscess formation and septicemia. Prophylactic broad-spectrum antibiotics are recommended, and tetanus immunity must be assessed.

Gold MH, Roenigk HH Jr, Smith ES, Pierce LJ: **Human bite** marks: Differential diagnosis. Clin Pediatr 1989; 28:329–331.

Human bites cause **oval or annular erythematous lesions** that are nonscaly. Individual tooth marks may be present early but then become confluent. They mimic annular or arciform dermatoses.

In a 30-month-old girl, annular erythematous lesions on the arms, trunk, and face were first noted after she returned from a day-care facility. Two small abrasions with crust formation were present on the left side of the forehead. They resembled ringworm but did not respond to a topical antifungal medication. Over the next 4 days the lesions became more erythematous, and a dermatologist suspected human bites. Referral to forensic odontologists confirmed bites, but dental impressions of family members and day-care workers failed to identify the source. The lesions healed uneventfully within 1 week. She refused to say that she was bitten.

In addition to **tinea corporis**, other **annular lesions** that may be confused with human bites include fixed drug eruption, subacute cutaneous lupus erythematosus, pityriasis rosea, and granuloma annulare.

Most human bites are superficial abrasions on the arm, hand, face, or neck.

Children are usually bitten by other children. In teenagers, fist injuries are common from fighting, with other bites occurring during lovemaking or sports activities.

Human bites are common findings in physical and sexual abuse, homicides, fights, and among institutionalized persons.

Kizer KW, Constantine DG: **Pet ferrets**—A hazard to the public health and wildlife. West J Med 1989; 150:446.

Although European ferrets (relatives of the polecat) are cute and playful, they sometimes unleash frenzied rapid-fire **bite and slash attacks**. They may inflict hundreds of bites, especially on the heads and throats of infants. They may then "drink the victim's blood and eat the shredded tissues." Several near-fatal attacks have been reported as well as at least one fatality.

Most attacks were inflicted by pet ferrets belonging to households other than that of the victim. Infants are apparently viewed as prey by the ferrets. Ferret play frequently assumes the form of mock attacks.

Ferrets have a great propensity for escaping and developing feral populations. In the wild they are destructive of poultry and wild animals such as rabbits, and also may develop rabies. Because of this, the keeping of ferrets as pets has been outlawed in California. Many medical and public health organizations oppose keeping pet ferrets because of the hazard to infants.

Al-Boukai AA, Hawass NE-D, Patel PJ, Kolawole TM: **Camel bites**: Report of severe **osteolysis** as late bone complications. Postgrad Med J 1989; 65:900–904.

Camel bites are usually a sudden **vengeance** for offenses committed previously and forgotten by the handler. They occur on the arm as the handler raises his arms to pull on the reins of the camel's head to make it kneel for mounting. Most bites occur during the winter months when the camel becomes wild during the breeding season.

The **bites are deep and often cause fractures**, which have delayed union or nonunion. Post-traumatic osteolysis, with concentric shrinkage of the diaphyses with tapering ends (sucked-candy appearance), is probably a common complication. Infection and traumatic vascular ischemia are also contributing factors to the osteolysis.

Acro-osteolysis has also been reported after snakebites and scorpion stings.

Conant R: Some rambling notes on **rattlesnakes**. Arch Environ Health 1969; 19:768–769.

Poisonous snakebites cause three recognizable symptoms that develop within 30 minutes: **swelling**, **intense pain**, and **marked discoloration** at the bite site.

Rattlesnakes, copperheads, cottonmouths, and some other poisonous snakes have a deep facial pit on each side of the head, located midway between the eye and nostril but at a lower level. The pit serves as a heat detector and assists in guiding strikes at warm-blooded animals.

Assistance in identification of snakes is readily available from herpetologists in zoos and natural history museums and can be obtained rapidly by phone.

The fourth dimension in diagnosis is intuition.

Black Skin

For those who rarely see black patients, dermatologic diagnosis can be difficult. Here are some of the diagnostic blocks.

The **color** characteristics of skin disease are largely obscured. You don't see the erythema of contact dermatitis or the salmon patch of pityriasis rubra pilaris.

The **localization** clues are different. Atopic dermatitis is more likely to occur on the extensor surface than the flexural. Pityriasis rosea occurs on the extremities rather than the trunk.

Morphology of lesions is different. Seborrheic dermatitis may be granulomatous. Pityriasis rosea is often papular with a blue-black necrotic-looking center.

The **postinflammatory hyperpigmentation** or **hypopigmentation** is more dramatic and persistent than in white skin, and the patient may be more concerned about this than the disease itself.

Some problems may be **unique** or unusually common in black skin. These include dermatosis papulosa nigra, pseudofolliculitis barbae, acne keloidalis, keratotic papules of the palms, and sarcoidosis.

Special **cosmetic habits** in blacks account for, at times, puzzling pomade acne, traction alopecia, hot-comb alopecia, and hair-straightener trichorrhexis nodosa.

Finally, the **reaction patterns** of black skin are accentuated and may be confusing. Follicular, papular, and granulomatous lesions are seen with regularity never observed in white skin.

Black dermatology is indeed a specialty.

McLaurin CI: Unusual patterns of **common dermatoses in blacks**. Cutis 1983; 32:352–360.

In black skin, **gray, black,** or **purple lesions** will be seen instead of the tan or red lesions of white skin.

In black skin an increased tendency to **fibroplasia** leads to more **annular, follicular, papular,** granulomatous, keloidal, and fibromatous skin lesions. **Look for more papules, plaques, lichenification, nodules, and tumors in black skin.**

Black skin **pigments and depigments more dramatically** than white skin. The changes may be more prolonged and severe. **Vitiligo** in blacks may have a **trichrome** appearance of normal, hypopigmented, and hyperpigmented skin in the same area. Initially, vitiligo may be missed, being mistaken for the secondary hypopigmentation of a variety of diseases. Corticosteroids will depigment black skin to a degree not seen in white skin.

Pityriasis rosea in blacks occurs in an **inverse** distribution, appearing on the face, neck, axillae, lower abdomen, or as papules of the palms and soles. The lesions are purple or gray, not fawn as in whites. Severe hyperpigmentation that ensues justifies systemic steroid therapy.

Lichen planus also induces prolonged **hyperpigmentation**.

Atopic **eczema** produces **follicular lesions** in blacks.

In blacks a **perioral dermatitis suggests a diagnosis of sarcoidosis.**

An **annular lesion** in blacks suggests secondary syphilis, but it may just as well be seborrheic dermatitis, lichen planus, or lupus erythematosus.

Fibroplasia in blacks accounts for acne keloidalis, keloids, and keloidal folliculitis.

Black skin favors the development of **granulomas** such as sarcoidosis. Expect it in hypopigmented as well as hyperpigmented sites and in ichthyosiform

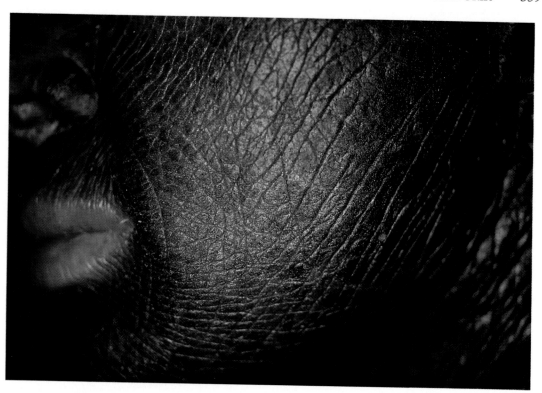

changes. Anticipate it in papular, nodular, and plaque lesions. These all call for a biopsy. The melanocyte and the fibroblast of black skin both enormously magnify our view of the inflammatory process in black skin. Awareness of this aids in the diagnosis of black skin disease. Look for the black and white footprints of disease that has been passing by.

Henderson AL: **Skin variations in blacks.** Cutis 1983; 32:376–377.

Voigt's or Futcher's lines mark the dermatomal border between the dark extensor skin and the lighter flexor skin of the **upper arm**. They can be striking in black skin and yet inapparent in white skin. **Midline hypopigmentation** seen on the **anterior chest** and at times on the neck, chin, and abdomen is another trait in black but not white skin. It has a hereditary basis.

Pigmentary contrast again is vivid in oral mucosa of black skin. Patches of pigment may be seen on the gums, palate, buccal mucosa, or even tongue. Its color can vary from light to dark brown or slightly bluish.

Minus HR, Grimes PE: Cutaneous manifestations of **sarcoidosis in blacks**. Cutis 1984; 32:361–363, 372.

Shiny, somewhat waxy, papular lesions are the most frequent cutaneous manifestations of sarcoidosis in blacks. But here are some of its **guises**:

lichenoid patches	nummular eczema
hypopigmented macules	erythema multiforme
shiny violaceous plaques	granulomas
angiolupoid (telangiectatic plaques)	ulcers
lupus pernio (nose, ears, malar)	erythroderma
psoriasiform plaques	

Sarcoidosis can have so many forms it is wisest to include it in the differential diagnosis of practically all skin eruptions in blacks.

Blastomycosis

When confronted with a **verrucous, pustular, infiltrative plaque**, or a **fungating mossy foot**, get a biopsy and culture or you won't get a diagnosis.

Barnes L: A case of **fungating skin tumors** in a young man. Arch Dermatol 1986; 122:713–717.

Digging a septic tank in a neighbor's yard was the prelude to a young man's year-long struggle with seven fungating masses on the abdomen, arms, and thighs. It began with a "sore" on the abdomen, which enlarged into a **4-cm foul-smelling mass**. Although it was followed by six sister lesions, he did not seek medical care because they were asymptomatic. The **edges** were **heaped** with friable tissue and studded with **debris, pustules**, and **hemorrhagic dots**. The **centers** were **clearing** with thin scar formation.

The **diagnosis** was made when a **KOH preparation** of minced skin biopsy tissue showed broad-based buds coming from thick-walled parent cells. The same yeast forms could be seen in neutrophilic abscesses on **histologic section**. A third portion of the **biopsy** specimen was **cultured**, and in 5 days *Blastomyces dermatitidis* became evident.

It is likely that this man's North American blastomycosis was acquired by **inhalation of the dimorphic fungus while digging the septic tank**.

The **clinical differential diagnosis** for blastomycosis includes:

histoplasmosis	leprosy
actinomycosis	granuloma inguinale
mycetoma	halogen eruption
tuberculosis	pyoderma gangrenosum
syphilis (gumma)	mycosis fungoides

But a peek under the microscope provides the best differentiation.

Dolezal JF: **Blastomycoid sporotrichosis**. Response to low-dose amphotericin B. J Am Acad Dermatol 1981; 4:523–527.

For 5 years a 21-year-old Iowa man had a 10- by 6-cm crescent-shaped **verrucous violaceous plaque** below the right armpit. Although diagnosed as ringworm, it had failed to respond to therapy. It began as a sore on the right elbow followed by lymphadenopathy, after he had spent a summer on a Kansas farm. As these resolved 4 months later, the chronic verrucous lesion appeared and slowly enlarged, with **healing** and **scarring** in some areas. Similar small lesions also developed in the inguinal creases.

Blastomycosis was suspected, but no organisms were found on histologic study (including PAS stains). However, a **culture** of the **biopsy specimen** revealed *Sporotrichum schenckii*.

Molecular biologists can take a trace of DNA and harvest large quantities, using the polymerase chain reaction. Similarly, you can take an invisible amount of fungal pathogen and harvest large quantities by the "polymerase chain reaction" of a culture.

A diagnosis that cannot be confirmed is a diagnosis in doubt.

Blood Count

In searching for the cause of what you see, look at what you can't see. Do a blood count. Patients appreciate it. Look what you can find:

Anemia can account for many of your patient's complaints. Here are some:

ridged, brittle, misshapened nails, atrophic glossitis, beefy-red sore tongue, angular cheilitis, darkened skin of the face, alopecia, premature gray hair, vitiligo, thromboses, ankle ulcers, jaundice, purpura

Polycythemia may account for plethoric facies, flushing, erythematous eruptions.

Leukocytosis appears in infection.

Lymphocytosis supports a diagnosis of infectious mononucleosis.

Eosinophilia appears in allergic states, hypereosinophilic syndrome.

Basophilia comes with chickenpox, ulcerative colitis, drug eruptions.

Neutropenia is noted in ulcers of the tongue, cellulitis, extensive purpura.

Acute leukemia leads to *Pseudomonas* infections, infections, purpura, mouth ulcers.

Chronic leukemia appears in herpes zoster, herpes simplex.

As you see, a blood count can count.

Hoffbrand AV, Pettit JE: Clinical Hematology Illustrated—An Integrated Text and Color Atlas. Philadelphia, W.B. Saunders Company, 1987, p 282.

Methemoglobinemia

I. **Hypochromic Anemias**
   A. **Iron deficiency anemia**

      pallor: lips, conjunctivae, nail beds, palmar creases, and skin— becomes evident when the hemoglobin is about 9.0 gm/dl.

      nails: ridged, brittle, koilonychia

      angular cheilosis

      glossitis: atrophic, with flattening and loss of filiform papillae giving a bold fissured appearance

      dysphagia

      retinal hemorrhages

      look for hemorrhage, pregnancy, poor diet, malabsorption, and hemosiderinuria

   B. **Sideroblastic anemia**

      In this congenital or acquired anemia, the need for numerous blood transfusions results in **iron overload** with resulting **melanin skin pigmentation.**

   C. **Lead poisoning**

      Look for a **lead line** (dark gray) in the **gums** in a person with anemia, abdominal colic, constipation, and peripheral neuropathy. Marked **punctate basophilia** of **red blood cells** will be seen in the peripheral blood.

II. **Megaloblastic Anemias**
   A. **Vitamin B$_{12}$ deficiency**

      Lemon yellow color results from pallor and jaundice (increased unconjugated bilirubin results from excessive red blood cell and hemoglobin breakdown)

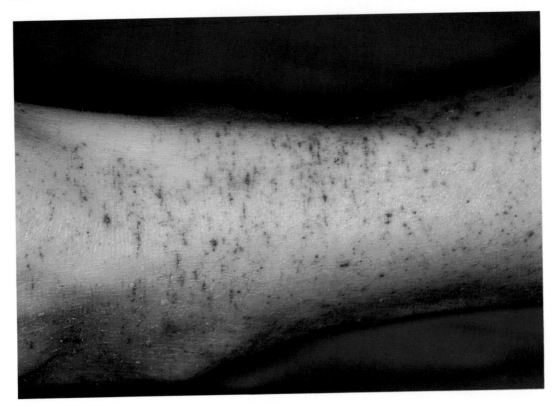

glossitis
    beefy **red sore tongue**, particularly with hot or acidic foods
    results from disordered proliferation of epithelial surface
angular cheilosis
melanin pigmentation of face, nail beds, skin creases, **peri-orbital** and **perioral** areas
peripheral neuropathy, especially in legs, bilaterally symmetrical, tingling, gait unsteadiness, decreased strength, altered sensation, falling over in the dark
purpura secondary to thrombocytopenia
look for:
    inadequate diet
    gastric malabsorption due to gastrectomy or pernicious anemia
intestinal malabsorption: stagnant loop ileal resection, Crohn's disease syndrome, jejunal diverticulosis, ileocolic fistula
associations:
    premature graying of hair
    blue eyes
    vitiligo
    thyroid disorders
    Addison's disease
    autoimmune diseases
    hypoparathyroidism
    gastric atrophy with achlorhydria
        parietal cell antibodies—90%
        intrinsic factor antibodies—50%
        gastric carcinoma (increased to 2 to 3 times)

B. **Folate deficiency**
    look for:
        inadequate diet
            poverty
            institutions
            goat's milk
            special diets
        excess losses
            dialysis
            congestive heart failure
        drugs
            anticonvulsants
            barbiturates
        alcohol
        liver disease
        malabsorption
            gluten enteropathy
            dermatitis herpetiformis
            tropical sprue (celiac disease)
        ↑ utilization
            pregnancy
            prematurity
            hemolytic anemia (excess marrow turnover)
            malignant disease—myeloma, cancer
            inflammatory diseases
                Crohn's disease
                rheumatoid arthritis
                widespread eczema
C. **Abnormalities of vitamin B$_{12}$ metabolism**
    congenital
        transcobalamin II deficiency
        homocystinuria with methylmalonic aciduria
    acquired
        nitrous oxide anesthesia (prolonged)
    folate metabolism
        congenital
        acquired—drugs
            methotrexate
            pyrimethamine
    DNA synthesis
        congenital
            orotic aciduria
            Lesch-Nyhan syndrome
            thiamine responsive
        acquired—drugs
            hydroxyurea
            cytosine arabinoside
            6-mercaptopurine
            5-azacytidine

III. **Hemolytic Anemias**
        pallor
        fluctuating jaundice
        splenomegaly
A. **Autoimmune hemolytic anemia**
        (+) direct Coombs' (antiglobulin test) (red cells agglutinate)
            "warm" type—37°C
            "cold" type—40°C

        IgM antibody
        intravascular hemolysis
        Raynaud's phenomenon

B. **Drug induced**
    penicillin
    phenacetin
    methyldopa

C. **Paroxysmal nocturnal hemoglobinuria** → recurrent venous thromboses

D. **Drug overdose** with oxidizing drugs
    dapsone
    sulfasalazine

IV. **Thalassemia**
excessive bone marrow activity and **extramedullary hemopoiesis** → expansion of flat bones of face and skull
    prominent maxillae
    widening of nasal bridge
    frontal bossing
    splaying teeth (widening of maxilla and mandible)
iron overload → ↑ melanin **pigmentation**
delayed puberty and small stature
ankle ulcers (anoxia and stasis)

V. **Sickle Cell Anemia**
    asthenic build
    mild jaundice
    ankle ulcers
    bone deformities (due to infarcts)
    hand-foot syndrome—unequal growth of fingers and toes

VI. **Aplastic Anemia:** pancytopenia due to hypoplasia of bone marrow
A. Acquired
    drugs
        sulfonamides
        chloramphenicol
        phenylbutazone
        gold
    radiation
    infection—**viral hepatitis**
    skin findings:
        mucosal hemorrhages (spontaneous)
        purpura (petechiae, ecchymosis)
        infections secondary to neutropenia
            purple macules and blisters
            Pseudomonas infection
            herpes simplex ulcers (mouth)
            Candida—red nodules

B. Congenital
  1. **Fanconi**
      hyperpigmentation
      small stature
      hypogonadism
  2. **Dyskeratosis congenita**
      teeth and gums, irregular
      thick nails
      telangiectasia

alopecia
abnormal sweating

VII. **Bone Marrow Transplantation:** complications
widespread **herpes simplex** infection of skin
nails—horizontal ridges and atrophy of nail bed secondary to whole-body radiation

VIII. **Graft-Versus-Host Disease**
Acute
<100 days—**widespread erythematous rash**
most severe on hands and feet—red, maculopapular rash, may have bullae and ulceration and widespread exfoliation
Chronic
patchy red plaques
scleroderma-like hands (contractures, ulcers, pigmentation)
erythema and exfoliation of palms and soles
mucous membranes—**lichen planus–like** and denudation

IX. Evaluation of white blood cell count and differential:
Leukocytosis: increase in WBC > 12×10^9/liter
Neutrophil leukocytosis
bacterial infections
vasculitis
uremia
gout
corticosteroid therapy
malignancy
leukemia

Eosinophilia: increase in blood eosinophils above 0.400×10^9/liter
asthma, hayfever
urticaria
intestinal parasites
dermatitis herpetiformis
erythema multiforme
hypereosinophilia syndrome
leukemia

Monocytosis
infections
ulcerative colitis
systemic lupus erythematosus
Hodgkin's disease
leukemia

Basophil (**basophilia**) leukocytosis
chronic granulocytic leukemia
polycythemia vera
myxedema
chickenpox
smallpox
ulcerative colitis

Neutropenia: blood neutrophil count <2.5×10^9/liter
<1×10^9/liter → recurrent infections
<0.2×10^9/liter → very grave risks
drug induced
cyclic
familial
infections
autoimmunity

painful intractable infections (**ulcers**) of **tongue** and buccal mucosa
skin infection: extensive **cellulitis**—staphylococcus, pseudomonas
anal infection
Felty's syndrome
rheumatoid arthritis + splenomegaly + neutropenia
skin **ulcers** on **anterior tibia**

Lymphocytosis
viral infections
chronic infections
thyrotoxicosis
leukemia

Infectious mononucleosis (glandular fever)
sore throat, fever, malaise, lethargy
lymphadenopathy
gross swelling and erythema of oropharynx—tonsils have purulent
exudate
palatal petechiae
periorbital and **facial edema**
erythematous **morbilliform eruption**
splenomegaly >50% of patients
Diagnosis
lymphocytosis 10 to 20 $\times$ 10^9/liter—many atypical
Paul-Bunnell test—heterophil antibodies at high titer
Differential diagnosis
acute leukemia
toxoplasmosis
infectious hepatitis
follicular tonsillitis

Acute Leukemia: accumulation of early myeloid or lymphoid precursors
(blasts) in bone marrow, blood, and other tissues
bone marrow failure
anemia
infections
easy bruising
hemorrhage
organ infiltration by leukemic cells (lymph nodes, spleen, liver,
meninges, CNS, testes, skin)
skin, especially in M_5 type of acute myeloblastic leukemia
(**monocytic**)
testicular infiltration—acute lymphoblastic leukemia
ulcers, cellulitis, purplish-black bullae with **red haloes**
(**pseudomonas**)
bacterial infections of skin, perianal and perineal areas, pharynx
fungal infections of skin with prolonged neutropenia
candida cellulitis and streptococcal cellulitis
candidiasis of mouth
herpes simplex—mouth ulcer
petechial hemorrhage
infiltration of skin (M_5 type)
widespread nonitchy, **raised, hemorrhagic rash**
nodules
swelling of gums

Chronic Leukemia
Chronic lymphocytic leukemia (CLL)

disease of the elderly
immature B lymphocytes
symmetrical node enlargement
bruising, **purpura** ($\downarrow$ platelets)
tonsils possibly enlarged
    Infections
        herpes zoster
        herpes simplex
        oral candidiasis
        hepatosplenomegaly (advanced disease)

Chronic granulocytic leukemia (CGL)

disease of the middle-aged
splenomegaly—massive
anemia
bleeding disorder
gout—acute inflammation and swelling of finger
visual disturbance
neurologic symptoms
infiltration of **skin**—**red nodules**
    hypermetabolism symptoms
        anorexia
        lassitude
        weight loss
        night sweats
Philadelphia chromosome (Ph) positive

Juvenile CGL

Philadelphia chromosome—negative
marked lymphadenopathy
eczematoid rash

Myeloid dysplastic syndromes

elderly with refractory anemia—may progress to chronic myelo-
    monocytic leukemia (CMML)
infections
    herpes simplex
    cellulitis
thrombocytopenia—**purpura**

New facts may demand a new diagnosis.

Breasts

The patient with cancer of the breast may come to you not with a lump but with eczema—**eczema of the nipple** on one side. The patient may delay coming for months, thinking the nipple has simply been chafed by the bra or irritated by scratching. But there must be no delay in sending a biopsy, including not only the dermatitic areola but also part of the nipple. It is a search for adenocarcinoma cells of **Paget's disease** that have come up from the duct to invade and destroy the epidermis.

Classically the process is sharply circumscribed, unlike a contact dermatitis. Far more common in women than in men, it is inflammatory, pruritic, and often crusted—at times keratotic. Although it may **resemble atopic dermatitis**, its unilateral nature is a strong differential point. Only by early biopsy diagnosis and mastectomy can the inexorable progress to lymph node involvement and metastasis of this adenocarcinoma be averted.

Recall that other apocrine areas such as the axilla, ear canal, groin, and perianal region are subject to extramammary Paget's disease. Here again, the major warning signal is a chronic eczematous patch. Too often it is ignored for years by the patient and then initially misdiagnosed by the physician as a **fungal infection** of the groin or **lichen simplex chronicus**. Such genital Paget's disease can even be the tip of the iceberg of an underlying malignant condition in the rectum or urinary tract.

The nipples are indeed a common site of benign eczema, whether in the nursing mother, atopic individual, or person with scabies. The breast itself may exhibit any dermatosis, but most commonly it is the site of inframammary intertrigo, candidiasis, or psoriasis. Most alarming is the **erysipelas-like** scirrhous skin of breast cancer extension through the skin.

The breast is a cancer-bearing organ, and even the most banal dermatitis must be viewed with diagnostic distrust. When in doubt, do a biopsy and order a mammogram!

Harris JR, Hellman S, Henderson IC, Kinne DW: **Breast Diseases.** Philadelphia, JB Lippincott Co, 1987, 751 pp.

Physical examination of the breast should include the following:

With the patient sitting:

1. Look for **asymmetry, bulging** of the skin, skin or **nipple retraction**, or **nipple ulceration**.
2. Have the patient put her hands on her hips to contract the pectoralis major muscles to accentuate skin retraction.
3. Have the patient raise her arms to see changes in the lower half of the breast, including retraction, **edema** of **periareolar skin**, and changes in the inframammary folds.
4. With talc on the fingers to reduce friction and enhance deeper palpation, palpate the breast with and without her arm raised. Include the supraclavicular areas and both sides of the neck to detect lymphadenopathy.
5. Examine the axilla with the patient's right arm flexed at the elbow and supported by the physician's right arm to allow relaxation of the chest wall musculature. Palpation is done with the left hand and should include the upper, middle, and lower portions of the axilla.

    Benign nodes are soft, small (less than 1 cm), mobile, and secondary to lymphadenitis from low-grade inflammatory skin problems on the hands and arms.

    Metastatic nodes are firm, large (≥1 cm), irregular, multiple, or matted together, possibly fixed to the underlying chest wall.

6. Closely inspect the skin and nipple—look for:

     edema (**peau d'orange**) caused by lymphatic obstruction in the breast
     or axilla

     erythema—an ominous sign, especially with warmth and an **erysipe-
     loid edge** (inflammatory carcinoma, periductal mastitis, or abscess
     formation)

     retraction and **ulceration** of the **nipple**, discharge, and eczematous
     changes with crusting, scaling, and erosions

With the patient lying supine (arm raised above head, folded sheet or small
pillow under ipsilateral shoulder to splay the breast over the chest wall):

1. Palpate the entire breast with finger pulps (rather than fingertips) from
    the sternum to the midaxillary line and clavicle to the lower rib cage.

     Premenstrual engorgement of glandular elements may be impossible
     to assess, so that examination should be repeated 1 to 2 weeks after
     menstrual period.

     Benign lesions: soft, smooth, regular borders, not fixed to underlying
     tissue

         fibroadenoma—feels like marbles in young women

         cyst—soft, circumscribed, fluid may be ballottable

         sclerosing adenosis—firm, small (<1 cm), peripherally located
         nodules close to the skin

     Malignant lesions:

         firm irregular thickenings or masses fixed to the skin or under-
         lying fascia (typical of carcinoma).

2. Ask about physiologic cyclic swelling and breast tenderness.

3. Determine nodularity (persistent lumpiness):

     diffuse bilateral finely granular or nodular pattern

     pseudolumps, "**fibrocystic disease**"

4. Ask about breast pain (**mastalgia**):

     diffuse or localized, often cyclic

     may have trigger spot

     look for costochondritis and cervical radiculopathy

         ask about old trauma—scar and fat necrosis or hematoma

         rule out cancer with mammogram

5. Search for dominant lumps:

     distinct, persistent, unchanging

     first diagnostic step: aspirate with 22-gauge needle and syringe

         collapse of cyst

         fluid—straw colored, brown, green, black

     three types

         gross cyst—not grossly bloody

         galactocele—milk-filled cyst, firm, nontender, in upper quadrants

         fibroadenoma— ↑ with menses

             painless, well circumscribed

             movable, lobulated

             rounded

             rubbery and firm unless calcified (very hard)

6. **Nipple discharge:** very common

     galactorrhea

         spontaneous secretion of milky discharge

         controlled by pituitary secretion of prolactin

         hyperprolactinemia occurs in menstrual disorders ± galactorrhea

         Evaluation of increased discharge

             thyroid tests

             serum prolactin—visual fields, CT of pituitary fossa

     abnormal discharge:

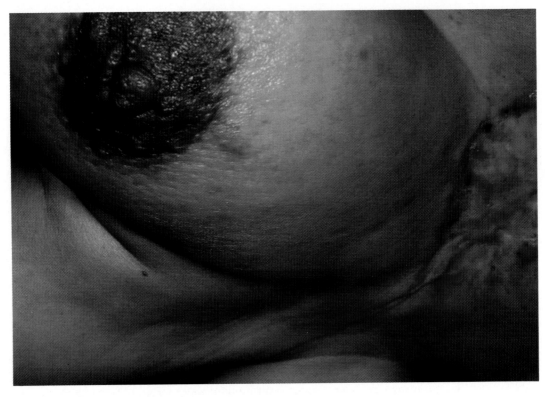

types
grossly bloody or guaiac (+)
sticky and clear fluid
elevation: smear on glass slide for cytology
causes of bloody discharge:
intraductal papilloma
duct ectasia
fibrocystic disease
carcinoma

7. **Breast infections**—may be intrinsic or extrinsic, rare except puerperal period
intrinsic mastitis, *lactational*—inflammatory
chronic recurrent **subareolar abscess**
squamous metaplasia of lactiferous ducts: extrude keratin into breast stroma, causing severe inflammation and obstructive mastopathy
acute mastitis
localized redness, swelling, pain, and fever
due to internal rupture of cyst with inflammatory reaction
extrinsic infections
can come from thoracic cavity through chest wall (via communicating internal mammary vessels)
abscess of Montgomery glands
primary syphilis: chancre of nipple
Wegener's granulomatosis

Neville EM, Freeman AH, Adiseshiah M: Clinical significance of recent **inversion of the nipple:** A reappraisal. J Roy Soc Med 1982; 75:111–113.

In the absence of a palpable mass, recent nipple inversion is only **rarely associated with breast carcinoma**, particularly in women under the age of 50. Mammography is important and should be repeated after 1 year. Nipple inversion is commonly seen with mammary duct ectasia (plasma cell mastitis) and fibroadenosis.

In this study of 63 cases of inverted nipple in 62 patients, unaccompanied by a palpable mass, three carcinomas were found on combined clinical and mammographic examination—an incidence of 5%.

Kleinberg DL, Noel GL, Frantz AG: **Galactorrhea:** A study of 235 cases, including 48 with pituitary tumors. N Engl J Med 1977; 296:589–600.

One of every three women with galactorrhea and associated amenorrhea had a radiologically evident **pituitary tumor**. Their prolactin levels were the highest observed.

In another one of three, no cause could be discerned.

One of every ten patients noted a relationship of the galactorrhea to the taking of **oral contraceptives**. Either it began when the patient started taking the contraceptive or it developed when the contraceptive was stopped.

Sixteen patients had galactorrhea associated with **drug therapy**, e.g., tranquilizers. Another 18 had the **Chiari-Frommel syndrome** of persistent galactorrhea and amenorrhea following pregnancy.

Signer SF: **Nipple priapism**. JAMA 1987; 258:3122.

Persistent nipple firmness may be similar to Peyronie's disease, with vasculitis inducing fibrosis of the covering sheaths of erectile tissue. Eosinophilia may play a role. Look for possible drug causes, including beta-adrenergic blockers, neuroleptics, alpha-adrenergic blockers, antihypertensives, and antidepressants.

Ten suspect drugs:

> propranolol hydrochloride (Inderal)
> labetalol hydrochloride (Normodyne, Trandate)
> chlorpromazine (Thorazine)
> mesoridazine besylate (Serentil)
> molindone hydrochloride (Moban)
> thioridazine (Mellaril)
> thiothixene (Navane)
> prazosin hydrochloride (Minipress)
> hydralazine hydrochloride (Alazine, Apresoline)
> trazodone hydrochloride (Desyrel)

Harris JR, Hellman S, Henderson IC, Kinne OW: Breast Diseases. Philadelphia, JB Lippincott Co, 1987, p 23.

Increased prolactin from the pituitary is fairly common and causes menstrual disorders and galactorrhea.

Causes of increased prolactin include:

thyroid disorders	brain tumors
breast or chest stimulation	craniopharyngioma
surgical scars	benign pituitary adenoma
oral contraceptives	prolactinoma
drugs (CNS tranquilizers)	pregnancy and lactation

Madlon-Kay DJ: **"Witch's Milk":** Galactorrhea in the newborn. Am J Dis Child 1986; 140:252–253.

Galactorrhea is **diagnosed by firm palpation** on the breast nodule to express secretion from the nipple. It was associated with larger breast nodules in 4.6% of 640 children followed from birth to 2 months of age. Neither sex predominated, and the condition commonly persisted up to 10 weeks. No hypothyroidism was found (mandatory state screening).

Midwives and grandmothers used to express "witch's milk" to prevent stagnation as well as the stealing of the secretion by witches and goblins for special brews. Inflammation and breast abscesses were the result.

Paslin D: **Staphylococcus aureus** **induration** of inflammatory plaques of nipples and areolae. J Am Acad Dermatol 1989; 20:932–934.

A 30-year-old woman noticed the onset of **painful rawness, cracking,** and **weeping of the nipples** and areolae during the **fourth month of nursing** her second child. She discontinued nursing, but serous seepage continued, and inflammatory plaques developed in the area.

Staphylococcus aureus was isolated by her physician when the condition had persisted for 4 months; however, a variety of topical and systemic antibiotics produced no improvement.

An areolar biopsy showed a heavy infiltrate of eosinophils and plasma cells in the dermis, as well as dilated capillaries and extravasated red cells. A diagnosis of an **eczematous psoriasiform dermatitis** was made. Resolution and cure came 3 months later after the conjoint use of a steroid cream and a 1% silver sulfadiazine cream.

The unusual nature of this reaction to staphylococci probably reflects the unique anatomy of the site of infection.

Smith NP, Wilson Jones E: **Erosive adenomatosis** of the **nipple.** Clin Exp Dermatol 1977; 2:79–84.

In a 44-year-old woman, a **warty, eczematous change** and enlargement of the left nipple over a 2-year period, with bleeding on two occasions following trauma, proved not to be Paget's disease but rather a benign process—erosive adenomatosis.

Described in more than 200 patients, this problem is **usually diagnosed** clinically as **Paget's disease,** since it presents as an eczematous eroded or crusted nipple showing blood-stained or serous discharge. It occurs in both men and women, may be bilateral, and sometimes is so **asymptomatic** that it is noted only on histologic study of mastectomy specimens. Mammography may show thickening behind the affected nipple.

Simple local excision of the nipple and plastic reconstruction is the treatment of choice.

Oldfield M: **Mondor's disease**—a **superficial phlebitis** of the **breast**. Lancet 1962; 1:994–996.

Sudden mild aching pain in the breast of a middle-aged woman often begins after overhead activity that has repeatedly stretched the pectoralis major muscle. This is followed by appearance in the breast of a **hard tender cord** that **radiates from the areola** in one of three directions: upward and outward toward the axilla (lateral thoracic vein); downward and inward toward the epigastrium (superior epigastric vein); or directly downward toward the abdominal wall (thoracoepigastric vein). There is **redness** of the skin over the **linear** or **spindle-shaped swelling,** with the long axis radiating from the areola.

After 7 to 10 days a linear hard tender cord is present, and there may be either a **groove in the skin** where it is adherent to the underlying cord or a ridge stretched like a bowstring across the inframammary sulcus. Visualization is easier if the patient's arm is raised above her head. Histologic findings reveal **thrombophlebitis** and periphlebitis. Early carcinoma, breast abscess, and boil are in the **differential diagnosis**. Resolution occurs spontaneously in 3 to 6 weeks.

Abramson DJ: **Mondor's disease** and **string phlebitis**. JAMA 1966; 196:1087–1089.

In ten cases, the subcutaneous fibrous cords were 2 to 5 mm wide and up to $8\frac{1}{2}$ inches in length. They were most commonly located on the anterolateral aspect of the chest or breast and could be seen either as a **deep groove or cord** resembling a bowstring under tension.

Ascensao AC, Marques MSJ, Capitao-Mor M: **Paget's disease of the nipple**. Clinical and pathological review of 109 female patients. Dermatologica 1985; 170:170–179.

Paget's disease is the progressive marginated eczematoid change of the nipple or areola that heralds the spread of an underlying carcinoma of the breast into the epidermis.

Look for breast cancer when there is:

> ulceration
> erythematous scaling papules or plaques
> nipple destruction
> exudative crusting lesions
> nipple retraction
> nipple invagination

Only one in four had a palpable breast mass in association with these Paget's lesions, but one in three had palpable **axillary adenopathy**.

Stephenson TJ, Cotton DWK: **Paget's disease in an epidermal cyst**. Dermatologica 1987; 174:186–190.

A painless 50-mm **firm mobile lump** without skin tethering developed over 6 weeks in the breast of a 52-year-old woman. On biopsy it was an epidermal cyst lined with Paget's disease. Mastectomy revealed an **underlying ductal adenocarcinoma and Paget's cells infiltrating the nipple**. These cells stained positive for mucin, EMA (epithelial membrane antigen), and CEA (carcinoembryonic antigen).

Epidermal cysts may also contain evidence of:

> basal cell carcinoma   mycosis fungoides
> Bowen's disease   pseudoepitheliomatous hyperplasia
> lichen planus   squamous cell carcinoma

Dabski K, Stoll HL Jr: **Paget's disease** of the breast presenting as a **cutaneous horn**. J Surg Oncol 1985; 29:237–239.

A 67-year-old white woman noted crusting and oozing of the right nipple that progressed into thick accumulation of a **hard, compact, keratinized cutaneous horn**. Over a 3-month period it regrew and fell off several times, leaving a nonulcerated erythematous shiny base. The underlying breast tissue was not indurated or nodular, and no mass was palpable. A shave excision of the entire tip of the nipple revealed Paget's cells, and subsequent mastectomy revealed an **intraductal carcinoma**.

Paget's disease usually presents as a nipple erosion or unilateral eczematoid patch covering the nipple and part of the areola with oozing, crusting, and erosions. In most cases a ductal carcinoma is found, although Paget's cells may arise as an independent focus.

Cutaneous horns are conical hyperkeratotic growths usually smaller than

1 cm. Although many are benign, **histologic examination** is warranted in all cases and should include the entire epidermis.

Skin tumors forming cutaneous horns include:

actinic keratosis	Keratoacanthoma
angioma	Paget's disease
basal cell carcinoma	Papilloma
Bowen's disease	Seborrheic keratosis
histiocytoma	Squamous cell carcinoma
Kaposi's sarcoma	

Kuhlman DS, Hodge S, Owen LG: **Hyperkeratosis of the nipple and areola**. J Am Acad Dermatol 1985; 13:596–598.

Two months of progressive thickening and hyperpigmentation of the nipples and areolae in this 67-year-old man **suggested a diagnosis of seborrheic keratosis or acanthosis nigricans**. However, the biopsy showed only the nonspecific picture of hyperkeratosis.

The lesions promptly resolved after a week of applications of Keralyt gel (6% salicylic acid).

If unilateral, such areolar hyperkeratosis suggests a diagnosis of **epidermal nevus**. When it is bilateral, think of **ichthyosis**, endocrinopathy, or **acanthosis nigricans**. Several examples have been associated with **diethylstilbestrol** therapy, and in some women of childbearing age it appears as a nevoid growth.

Soden CE: **Hyperkeratosis of the nipple and areola**. Cutis 1983; 32:69–74.

Malodorous, thickened nipples and areolae had been this 33-year-old woman's problem for 4 years. She denied usage of birth control pills, breastfeeding, ill health, or familial history of skin disease.

Both nipples and areolae showed thickening and brown pigmentation. The possibility of acanthosis nigricans or of an epidermal nevus was considered, but the **biopsy** showed no evidence of either. The finding of papillomatosis and keratin plugging placed her problem into the rare entity of **hyperkeratosis of the nipples and areolae**. The odor resulted from inability to regularly cleanse and rid the numerous crevices of bacteria.

Lancer HA, Moschella SL: **Paget's disease of the male breast**. J Am Acad Dermatol 1982; 7:393–396.

A 2- by 3-cm patch of **red, scaling, dry skin around the right nipple** of this **85-year-old man** excited little interest until about **1 year later** when it had become a tender, red, exudative process involving the nipple and areola. At that time an **underlying dermal mass** could be felt.

A clinical diagnosis of **Paget's disease** was made and confirmed by biopsy.

A high index of suspicion and early biopsy of unilateral nipple areolar dermatitis is warranted in *both* men and women.

Gold RH, Montgomery CK, Minagi H, Annes GP: The significance of **mammary skin thickening** in disorders other than primary carcinoma: A roentgenologic-pathologic correlation. Am J Roentgenol Radium Ther Nucl Med 1971; 112:613–621.

The thickness of the skin of the normal breast seldom exceeds 1.5 mm except for the inframammary crease. Pronounced thickening of mammary skin **suggests lymphatic permeation by metastases** from an underlying primary carcinoma, and it is an important sign in mammography.

In several cases, mammography studies with skin thickening are displayed beside skin biopsies of the same breasts. **Breast abscesses, fat necrosis**, and **lymphoma** could not be **distinguished** from carcinoma except **on deep breast biopsy**. Skin biopsies in these conditions showed nonspecific chronic inflammation with perivascular mononuclear cell infiltrates.

Kokal WA, Hill LR, Porudominsky D, et al: **Inflammatory breast carcinoma:** A distinct entity? J Surg Oncol 1985; 30:152–155.

Erythema, tenderness, induration, and increased local warmth extending over at least one third of the breast **point to inflammatory breast carcinoma.** Edema of the skin and breast enlargement are also often present. A skin biopsy will confirm the diagnosis, showing tumor emboli in the dermal lymphatics.

Drovlias CA, Sewell CW, McSweeny MB, Powell RW: **Inflammatory carcinoma of the breast:** A correlation of clinical, radiologic and pathologic findings. Ann Surg 1976; 184:217–222.

In a review of 75 cases of inflammatory breast carcinoma, it was found that the breast was usually **diffusely involved with tumor, edema, and redness** and was **painful** in more than 50% of patients.

On **mammography**, generalized skin thickening and increase in the overall density of the breast should alert the radiologist to the possibility of inflammatory carcinoma and may precede inflammatory signs by several weeks.

Skin biopsy taken from an area of erythema not overlying a mass **may show only edema** of the dermis and vascular dilatation without carcinoma, although often it will show the dermal lymphatics plugged with tumor cells and tumor cell infiltrates in the deep dermis.

Photographs show two cases of inflammatory carcinoma: patchy erythema with nipple retraction, central edema, and a mass of the upper central left breast; and diffuse involvement of both breasts with marked edema, dilated lymphatics, and **purplish-red discoloration**.

Deininger HK: **Wegener granulomatosis** of the breast. Radiology 1985; 154:59–60.

Two women had unsuspected Wegener granulomatosis that **mimicked breast carcinoma** clinically and on mammography. Fine-needle aspiration biopsy showed severe inflammation with eosinophils, lymphocytes, plasma cells, fibroblasts, histiocytes, and multinuclear giant cells. Findings disappeared with treatment.

Case 1. A 48-year-old woman had a mild cough, loss of strength, and exhaustion. She consulted a physician because of **induration** of the right **breast**, nipple retraction, and peau d'orange thickening of the skin.

Case 2. A 57-year-old woman had coryza and bronchitis for a few weeks before noting induration of both breasts.

Papioannou AN: Hypothesis: Increasingly intensive locoregional treatment of **breast cancer** may promote **recurrence**. J Surg Oncol 1985; 30:33–41.

A dramatic full-page color photograph shows **gyrate erythematous thickening** of skin over the anterior and posterior chest wall and supraclavicular fossa **surrounding a mastectomy scar and radiation portal**. The scalloped border has crept beyond the midline to the opposite breast, up the neck, and below the radiation portal of the anterior chest. Biopsies of the border showed breast carcinoma. Nodules around the scar were rapidly growing and ulcerating, suggesting "**in transit metastases**" caused by lymph stasis resulting from tissue damage.

Sauven P: **Musculo-aponeurotic fibromatosis** treated by surgery and testosterone. J Roy Soc Med 1982; 75:281–283.

A 19-year-old girl had a 9- by 7-cm mass fixed to the lateral chest wall and spreading anteriorly into the axillary tail of the left breast. It began as a pea-sized nodule in the left breast. There was no lymphadenopathy, and the breast was otherwise normal. Histopathologically an incisional breast biopsy specimen showed **fibromatosis**, which **deeply infiltrated the intercostal muscles** but preserved the breast. Following radiation and excision the lesion recurred deep to the scar. Treatment with testolactone, a 17-oxosteroid, kept the lesion in check.

Hawk JLM: **Dermatofibrosarcoma protuberans**. Clin Exp Dermatol 1977; 2:85–89.

A **firm area over the right breast** had been present since childhood in a 46-year-old woman. After her first pregnancy, she had noted nodules that would come and go within the indurated area every few months, but in the past 10 years about 20 partially **confluent sessile nodules** had persisted, the largest being about 1 cm. An indurated variegated **yellowish-brown nodular plaque**, 14 by 10 cm with an irregular well-demarcated outline, covered the upper right breast, including the nipple and areola and extending toward the axilla.

Histologically the distinctive cartwheel appearance of the tumor cells of dermatofibrosarcoma protuberans was seen.

Such tumors usually begin as **bluish-red flat thickening of the skin**. They also may be yellow, brown, or flesh colored. The skin thickening may **persist for decades** before irregularly shaped protuberant nodules suddenly appear. In some cases, erythema, mild pain, and tenderness are associated. **Telangiectasia** and **epidermal atrophy** are frequent. The masses are firm but freely mobile over the deeper tissues.

The treatment of choice is wide excision.

Haupt HM, Hood AF, Cohen MH: **Inflammatory melanoma**. J Am Acad Dermatol 1984; 10:52–55.

Pain, tenderness, erythema, edema, and a **nodule of the left breast** prompted this 59-year-old woman to seek help. Her physician suspected she had inflammatory carcinoma of the breast, but a **biopsy** from an area of indurated erythema demonstrated **metastatic melanoma**. The primary source was a malignant melanoma excised from the left scapula the year before.

Cellulitis-like reactions are the hallmark of patients with inflammatory carcinoma (carcinoma erysipelas). The same picture occurs with **metastatic** tumors of bronchogenic, pelvic, or pancreatic origin. To this we must now add melanoma.

It is a picture of awesome portent. This patient survived a scant 6 months after the diagnosis was made.

Yates VM, King CM, Dave VK: **Lichen sclerosus et atrophicus** following radiation therapy. Arch Dermatol 1985; 121:1044–1047.

This 54-year-old woman developed **indurated ivory-white papules** and **plaques** of the right **breast 2 years after radiotherapy** for carcinoma of that breast. The initial radiation dermatitis had not been unusual and healed in 6 weeks.

The new lesions had an atrophic wrinkled surface with some follicular plugging. The clinical impression of lichen sclerosus et atrophicus was confirmed histologically.

It was the characteristic ivory-white papules and plaques and the homogenized collagen band seen on **biopsy** that **distinguished this from chronic radiodermatitis**. Certainly the sclerosis, atrophy, and telangiectasia are shared by both.

It is assumed that the lichen sclerosus et atrophicus was an isomorphic Köbner response to the trauma of radiation therapy.

It is also known that **lichen sclerosus et atrophicus may appear in a vaccination site, scratch marks, excision scars**, and even **bruises**.

Beard DB, Haskell CM: **Carcinoembryonic antigen** in breast cancer: Clinical review. Am J Med 1986; 80:241–245.

In addition to being a marker for gastrointestinal neoplasms, **CEA may be increased in patients having advanced breast cancer** with **bony metastases**.

If it looks like something you think you should know, the pathologist will know.

Bullous Diseases

Blisters call for an immediate assessment. Does the patient have a classic blistering skin disease? Do you see the **erosions** of pemphigus vulgaris, the intact blisters of bullous pemphigoid, or the **pruritic** vesicles of dermatitis herpetiformis? Do the blisters conform to the areas of a contact dermatitis or burn or the **frictional sites** of epidermolysis bullosa? Are the blisters of a fixed or widespread drug eruption or the target blisters of erythema multiforme?

If not, first look for the uncommon presentation of blisters in diseases such as lichen planus, pityriasis rosea, or lupus erythematosus. Recall that **metabolic** diseases may present as bullae, including diabetes and porphyria cutanea tarda, or that an **internal malignant disease** may be responsible. Think of **infections** such as bullous impetigo and varicella, particularly with cloudy vesicles. Even the lowly mosquito or other **insect bite** may account for blisters on the legs. Blisters may also simply be evidence that the adherence of baby epidermis to dermis is poor, as seen with the blisters of urticaria pigmentosa.

Unexplained blisters are always a happy hunting ground. Therein the diagnostician will find lots of small, as well as big, game at which to shoot. Of all this game, the most vicious is pemphigus. It may appear not as a "blister beast" but as the raw red meat of erosions or simply the hoarse cry of a denuded larynx. The immunofluorescent laboratory will serve you well in identification of this once-fatal disease, for it is an autoimmune-mediated cell-by-cell separation of the epidermal sheath itself.

The unexplained appearance of **large tense blisters** always suggests bullous pemphigoid. This is true whether or not the surrounding skin is erythematous and the blisters are hemorrhagic or pruritic. Although considered to be a disease of old age, it may appear at any age. Typically the Nikolsky sign is absent, and healing is without scars. The diagnostic blisters appear at sites of an autoimmune inflammatory reaction in the epidermal basement membrane that causes the epidermis to detach in toto, with fluid flowing in to form an intact bulla or vesicle. Direct immunofluorescence showing the deposition of antibasement membrane zone antibodies and complement permit a precise diagnosis. Blood studies may reveal eosinophilia and an elevated IgE level as well as circulating antibodies to the basement membrane.

The tense, tough, intact blister distinguishes bullous pemphigoid from its fellow autoimmune disease pemphigus vulgaris. In pemphigus the blister is often more conceptual than real, since the epidermis crumbles, leaving a **moist red erosion** rather than a blister, especially in the oral mucosa. Likewise, in pemphigus foliaceus and pemphigus vegetans the true blister is usually not evident. Nor is the blister always evident in the early stages of bullous pemphigoid; puzzling urticarial or eczematous plaques months later may evolve into bullae. Rare forms include vesicular pemphigoid, pemphigoid nodularis, and pemphigoid vegetans.

Korman N: Pemphigus. J Am Acad Dermatol 1988; 18:1219–1238.

Until the early 20th century, all blistering diseases were grouped under the name *pemphigus*, derived from the Greek *pemphix* (meaning bubble) and first used by Hippocrates.

Pemphigus vulgaris. Flaccid bullae arise on normal or erythematous skin. They break easily, leaving denuded areas as they rub off.

> ***Nikolsky sign.*** Lateral pressure on the edge of a blister results in detachment of the epidermis. It is not specific, since it also occurs in toxic epidermal necrolysis, epidermolysis bullosa, and bullous pemphigoid.
>
> ***Asboe-Hansen sign.*** Pressure on the center of any intact bulla produces lateral enlargement.
>
> Pruritus is present as the blister forms; pain results from open erosions. The distribution favors the face, scalp, axilla, and oral cavity and correlates with the high level of pemphigus antigen found in those sites.
> In the majority of patients, **onset** is in the **oral cavity**.
> **Eosinophilia** is present in 45% of patients.

Pemphigus foliaceus. There are no blisters, only crops of superficial erosions that show erythema, crust, and scale.

> mimics seborrheic dermatitis
> location: chest, back, face, scalp, not mucosa
> Brazilian form (fogo selvagem)
> > in rural areas in Brazil
> > usually in children, young adults
> > distinguished by epidemiology

Pemphigus erythematosus (**Senear-Usher**)

> hyperkeratotic, erythematous, scaly lesions involving the nose, malar area, upper back, chest, and intertriginous areas
> mucosa clear

Pemphigus vegetans

> hypertrophic granulation tissue
> pustules evolving from blisters
> involves axillae, groin, flexural surfaces, vermilion border of lips
> cerebriform tongue lesions

Pemphigus herpetiformis

> clinically, dermatitis herpetiformis
> immunofluorescent findings of pemphigus; a nonclinician's hybrid

Pemphigus due to drugs

> penicillamine, penicillin, captopril, phenobarbital, rifampin, piroxicam, thiopronine, and a-mercaptopropionyl glycine have all been associated

Stanley JR: Pemphigus. Skin failure mediated by **autoantibodies**. JAMA 1990; 264:1714–1717.

There are two major clinical types of pemphigus: pemphigus vulgaris and pemphigus foliaceus. Pemphigus vegetans is a form of pemphigus vulgaris, and pemphigus erythematosus is a form of pemphigus foliaceus.

Pemphigus vulgaris usually begins with painful mouth erosions, eventually followed by skin erosions and blisters. The fragile flaccid blisters break and then expand at the edges, leaving large erosions.

Pemphigus vegetans is a form of pemphigus vulgaris in which crusted papillomatous (vegetating) lesions are limited to the scalp and intertriginous

379

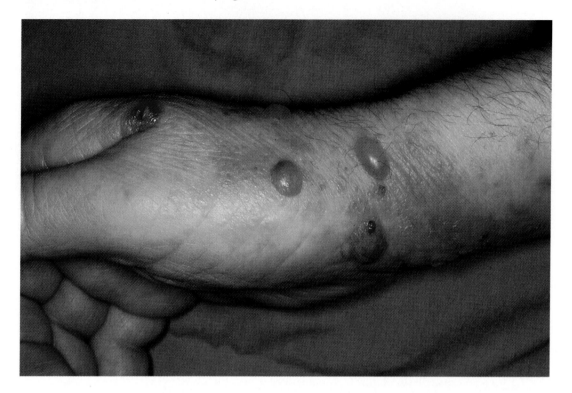

areas. Eventually, over time, more generalized pemphigus vulgaris develops in these patients.

Pemphigus foliaceus presents with scaly, crusted, well-demarcated lesions on the face and upper trunk. Mucous membrane involvement is uncommon. It may be localized or result in generalized erythroderma.

Pemphigus erythematosus represents the most localized form of pemphigus foliaceus, with lesions limited to the face, often in a malar distribution. It may have serologic and clinical overlap with systemic lupus erythematosus.

Fogo selvagem is a form of pemphigus foliaceus endemic to rural areas along inland rivers in Brazil. The **skin looks burned**, hence the Portuguese name *fogo selvagem*, meaning "wild fire." The bite of a certain type of black fly may be the precipitating factor.

Patients with both types of pemphigus have **IgG autoantibodies** directed against the cell surface of keratinocytes. The disease severity generally correlates with the serum antibody titer, as determined by indirect immunofluorescence. In general, the immunofluorescence patterns of the two types of pemphigus are indistinguishable, even though the blisters develop at different levels in the epidermis.

In pemphigus foliaceus the blister is more superficial, with the deeper epidermis remaining intact. This probably accounts for its more favorable prognosis, as the barrier function of the skin is not totally destroyed by the autoantibody.

Autoantibodies in the **pemphigus group** of diseases mediate a loss of cell-to-cell adhesion, resulting in blister formation and ultimate failure of the barrier function of the skin. They are directed against polypeptide complexes in the adhering junctions, particularly desmoglea (the intracellular "glue" of the desmosome) and plakoglobin (in the dense plaque of both the desmosome and the adherens junction). Exactly how the autoantibodies mediate **loss of cell adhesion** is unknown.

Both pemphigus vulgaris and pemphigus foliaceus may rarely be **drug induced**. The most common offending drugs are penicillamine and captopril.

Pemphigus of both types may be associated with **myasthenia gravis** and **thymoma**.

Beutner EH, Chorzelski TP, Wilson RM, et al: **IgA pemphigus foliaceus**. Report of two cases and a review of the literature. J Am Acad Dermatol 1989; 20:89–97.

A 33-year-old woman developed a **vesiculobullous eruption** on the pretibial surfaces, anterior aspect of the thighs, and axillae. The blisters were 0.2 to 1.2 cm in size and were initially tense, but quickly became flaccid and evolved into dry, scaly, superficial crusts. Pemphigus foliaceus, subcorneal pustular dermatosis, and impetigo were the **diagnoses considered**. Treatment with antibiotics and steroids did not help, but dapsone stabilized the disease.

A skin biopsy showed a subcorneal blister with acantholytic cells and polymorphonuclear leukocytes, which formed "rosettes" around some of the acantholytic cells. The pronounced **acantholysis** led to a diagnosis of pemphigus foliaceus. Direct immunofluorescence revealed widespread uniform deposits of IgA in the intercellular substance of the subcorneal region of the epidermis. Indirect immunofluorescence was negative.

IgA pemphigus foliaceus **looks like pemphigus foliaceus** both clinically and histologically, but has its own niche because immunofluorescence shows **intercellular IgA** and not the expected IgG in the upper epidermis. Most cases show some **overlap** clinically and histologically with **subcorneal pustular dermatosis** (Sneddon-Wilkinson disease). However, intercellular IgA deposits will distinguish between them. Pemphigus, in general, can now be divided into **IgG pemphigus** and **IgA pemphigus**.

The pathologist continues to assail the diagnostic high ground of the clinician.

Anhalt GJ, Kim SC, Stanley JR, et al: **Paraneoplastic pemphigus**. N Engl J Med 1990; 323:1729–1735.

A 62-year-old man with malignant follicular large-cell lymphoma developed a **pruritic urticarial** skin eruption resembling a **drug eruption**. Over 4 months it progressed to numerous confluent vesicles and erosions of the trunk, extremities, conjunctivae, oropharynx, and esophagus. The lips, palate, and conjunctivae were covered with bleeding erosions, and the upper trunk had confluent crusted and denuded areas. He also was febrile and debilitated and had generalized lymphadenopathy. Severe **erythema multiforme** and **toxic epidermal necrolysis** were suspected.

An initial biopsy showed focal acantholysis with granular complement deposition at the epidermal basement membrane zone and weak deposition of intercellular IgG within the epidermis. Indirect immunofluorescence showed pemphigus-like antibodies at a titer of 1:80. Later biopsies showed epidermal necrosis, and the serum pemphigus-like antibody titer was 1:160.

Two weeks after hospitalization he developed new pruritic vesiculobullous lesions on the trunk, extremities, mouth, and conjunctivae. A skin biopsy revealed an **acantholytic intraepidermal blister** consistent with pemphigus vulgaris. Circulating pemphigus-like antibodies were present at a titer of 1:2560. The lesions responded poorly to treatment, and he died of lymphoma about 7 months later.

Four other patients are presented with a similar syndrome, called **paraneoplastic pemphigus**. Unique clinical features include:

painful persistent treatment-resistant erosions of the oral mucosa, lips, and conjunctivae (pseudomembranous conjunctivitis) polymorphous pruritic erythematous scaly papules evolving into **target lesions** with central blister formation, **resembling erythema multiforme** confluent erythema in the V area of the upper chest and back becoming eroded and extensively denuded, **resembling toxic epidermal necrolysis**

Histologic studies in paraneoplastic pemphigus show three predominant features:

suprabasilar intraepithelial acantholysis
necrosis of individual keratinocytes
vacuolar-interface change

Immunofluorescence testing shows faint and focal IgG deposition in the intercellular spaces of skin and mucosal epithelial cells. There is often high background cytoplasmic staining in the epidermis. Granular-linear complement is found along the basement membrane zone as well as in the intercellular spaces. The antibodies contain a unique complex of four polypeptides and bind to tissues containing desmosomes.

The **autoantibodies** in paraneoplastic pemphigus **are pathogenic**. Injection of autoantibody into newborn mice produces cutaneous blisters, esophageal and epidermal acantholysis, and a positive Nikolsky's sign.

Ahmed AR, Rosen GB: Viruses in pemphigus. Int J Dermatol 1989; 28:209–217.

What stimulates the formation of IgG autoantibodies that react with the intercellular cement substance of stratified squamous epithelium in pemphigus and induces acantholysis?

A **viral etiology** of **pemphigus** has been postulated by many authors, but data are conflicting. Injection of sterile blister fluid from pemphigus patients into rabbits, mice, and chick embryos has caused emaciation, paralysis, and death, but **no virus has been consistently isolated**.

Various sizes and shapes of elementary bodies and particles suggestive of virus have been seen in pemphigus blister fluid, roofs of bullae, inoculated rabbit corneas, and inoculated chorioallantoic membranes.

Viruses are postulated to cause autoimmune disease by several **mechanisms**. Dissolution of virus-infected cells could release "sequestered" antigens that could stimulate cellular and humoral responses. Host cell membrane antigens also could be altered by virus, or immunologic cross-reactivity between viral and host antigens might develop. Autoantibody production also might be initiated by viral alteration of immune regulator cells (T and B lymphocytes).

Further viral studies need to be done in pemphigus utilizing the newer tools of virology, including specialized methods of tissue culture with cell fusion, enzyme immunoassays, and nucleic acid hybridization.

Hacham-Zadeh S, Even-Paz Z: A modified technique for eliciting **Nikolsky's sign**. Arch Dermatol 1980; 116:160.

Using moderate pressure, slide the rounded end of a **paper clip** along the skin in the direction of the clip's narrow axis. The resultant shearing force tests epidermal integrity and adherence just as Nikolsky did in 1895 using only his thumb.

A positive test is classically seen in various forms of pemphigus as well as epidermolysis bullosa.

Barr RJ, Herten RJ, Graham JH: Rapid method for **Tzanck preparations**. JAMA 1977; 237:1119–1120.

The Paragon Multiple Stain (PMS), used mainly for frozen sections, provides a rapid, simple, inexpensive method for Tzanck preparations. It results in hematoxylin-eosin–like staining.

Here's **how to do it**:

Swab an intact vesicle with 70% isopropyl alcohol, then open the vesicle with a blade and gently scrape the base to avoid hemorrhage. Smear the material on a clean dry slide.

Fix immediately in 70% isopropyl alcohol for 3 minutes.

Dip five times in a mixture of 50% alcohol and 50% tap water (by volume), then dip five times in 100% tap water.

Add 2 to 3 drops of PMS stain for 5 seconds, then rinse with tap water and blot dry.

Add a drop of water and a coverslip for immediate examination, or use clear nail polish for semipermanent mounting.

Look for:

acantholytic squamous cells (pemphigus family)
multinucleated syncytial giant cells (herpes infection)
eosinophilic ground–glass intranuclear inclusions (herpes infection)

You can be sued for making the wrong diagnosis or for even making no diagnosis at all.

Bullous Pemphigoid

Korman N: Bullous pemphigoid. J Am Acad Dermatol 1987; 16:907–924.

Differential points:

Bullous pemphigoid:
Bullae involve the flexural areas of the arms, legs, trunk, and groin.
Immunoreactants are deposited in the lamina lucida.
It may be exacerbated by PUVA, UVB, and furosemide (Lasix).

Epidermolysis bullosa acquisita:
Bullae with scars and milia occur on the extensor and acral surfaces.
Immunoreactants are located in and below the lamina densa.
Increased skin fragility is present, and blisters are induced by trauma.
Look for diabetes mellitus and inflammatory bowel disease.

Cicatricial pemphigoid:
Bullae with scars involve the oral mucosa, skin, conjunctivae, larynx, genitalia, and esophagus.
Immunoreactants are present in the lamina lucida.

Dermatitis herpetiformis:
Papules, vesicles, and small bullae are symmetrically distributed over the extensor surfaces, back, and neck. Itching is severe.
Immunoreactants are located in the sublamina densa.
Look for gluten-sensitive enteropathy and thyroid disease.

Herpes gestationis:
Urticarial plaques, vesicles, and bullae involve the abdomen and extremities and cause severe pruritus.
Immunoreactants are in the lamina lucida.
It occurs in pregnancy, but may be exacerbated by birth control pills.

Clinical variants of pemphigoid include:

childhood pemphigoid (immunofluorescence diagnosis—IgG at basement membrane zone)
veiscular pemphigoid (small grouped blisters)
polymorphic pemphigoid (resembles dermatitis herpetiformis; may represent linear IgA disease)
vegetating pemphigoid (purulent verrucous vegetating intertriginous lesions; resembles pemphigus vegetans)
hyperkeratotic scarring pemphigoid (biopsy diagnosis)
pemphigoid nodularis (mimics prurigo nodularis)
erythrodermic pemphigoid (blisters precede erythroderma)

Weigand DA, Clements MK: **Direct immunofluorescence** in **bullous pemphigoid**: effects of extent and location of lesions. J Am Acad Dermatol 1989; 20:437–440.

Direct immunofluorescence is generally accepted to be the **principal diagnostic test** for bullous pemphigoid.

The intensity of the direct immunofluorescence reaction correlates roughly with the extent of the disease, rather than with the specific anatomic region. Duplicate tests from the trunk and legs are generally of equal intensity.

In **localized bullous pemphigoid** there is a tendency for weak or possibly negative direct immunofluorescence. In these cases, light microscopy may be more reliable than immunofluorescence.

Hodge L, Marsden RA, Black MM, et al: **Bullous pemphigoid**: The frequency of mucosal involvement and concurrent malignancy related to indirect immunofluorescence findings. Br J Dermatol 1981; 105:65–69.

A review of 124 cases of bullous pemphigoid revealed that:

In 72% there was a **circulating IgG basement membrane zone antibody**.

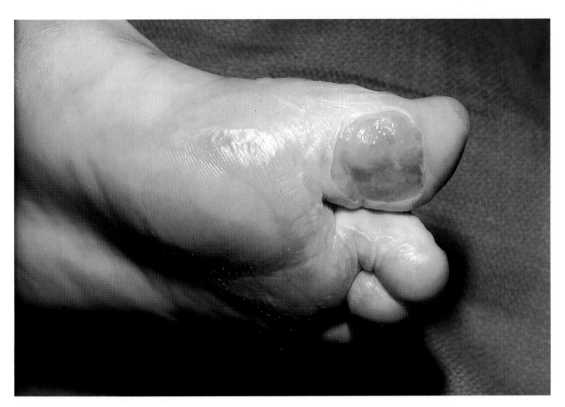

The antibody titers did not correlate with the extent of the disease or the presence of mucous membrane lesions.

In 23% of the **seronegative group**, **malignant disease** occurred within 6 months of the pemphigoid, compared with only 4% of the seropositive group (the difference was significant).

While only 12% had mucosal lesions, they were more common (17%) in the seronegative group.

Overall, it appears that malignancy is more common in bullous pemphigoid with negative indirect immunofluorescence findings. This is the second study that shows a **malignancy rate** of **about 25%**.

Gammon WR, Kowalewski G, Chorzelski TP, et al: **Direct immunofluorescence studies** of **sodium chloride–separated skin** in the differential diagnosis of bullous pemphigoid and epidermolysis bullosa acquisita. J Am Acad Dermatol 1990; 22:664–670.

Bullous pemphigoid and **epidermolysis bullosa acquisita** may be indistinguishable on the basis of clinical, histologic, and routine immunohistologic features. They can be readily distinguished by immunoelectron microscopy and immunochemical methods, but these tests are expensive and not readily available.

A new method has been devised to distinguish the two diseases using direct immunofluorescence. The biopsy specimen is incubated in 10 to 20 ml NaCl (1.0 mol/liter) for 72 to 96 hours at 4°C. After the specimen is blotted on filter paper, the epidermis is gently displaced laterally 1 mm across the dermis, which is left adherent. The specimen is then snap-frozen in liquid nitrogen and sectioned for direct immunofluorescence.

This technique separates the basement membrane zone through the lamina lucida, leaving keratinocyte plasma membrane and hemidesmosomes on the epidermal side and the lamina densa and sublamina densa zone on the dermal side of the separation.

Results:

> In **bullous pemphigoid**, IgG deposits are located only on the epidermal side or on both the epidermal and dermal sides of separation.
> In **epidermolysis bullosa acquisita**, IgG deposits are located only on the dermal side of separation.

Shimizu H, Hayakawa K, Nishikawa T: A comparative **immunoelectron** microscopic **study** of **typical and atypical cases of pemphigoid**. Br J Dermatol 1988; 119:717–722.

By means of immunoelectron microscopy, three Japanese patients with typical bullous pemphigoid were compared with three patients with atypical pemphigoid with the following characteristics:

> a 50-year-old woman with prurigo nodularis–like lesions on the legs and trunk (**nodular pemphigoid**)
> a 72-year-old woman with pruritic vesicles and erythema similar to dermatitis herpetiformis (**polymorphic pemphigoid**)
> an 80-year-old woman with recurrent blisters on a localized area of the back, resulting in a circumscribed plaque with pigmentation and erythema (**localized pemphigoid**)

There was no significant difference in the in vivo ultrastructural localization of IgG and C3 in the basement membrane zone between the two groups. In all cases, IgG and C3 were detected between the basilar surface of the basal keratinocytes and the basal lamina. The immunoreactants were not deposited beneath melanocytes.

Liu H-N, Su WPD, Rogers RS III: **Clinical variants of pemphigoid.** Int J Dermatol 1986; 25:17–27.

Direct immunofluorescence enables recognition of nonbullous as well as bullous variants of pemphigoid.

Surprisingly, some examples of **prurigo nodularis** are actually **nodular pemphigoid**. The pruritic, hypertrophic, scarring plaques with excoriations are the only residue of subclinical or clinical bulla formation.

Likewise, except for immunofluorescent studies, **pemphigoid vegetans** would be misdiagnosed as pemphigus vegetans. The massive purulent, verrucous, vegetative plaques of the groin, axilla, scalp, and hands are clinically identical in both diseases.

Immunofluorescence studies also must be done to distinguish **vesicular pemphigoid** from dermatitis herpetiformis. The only clinical clues are that the tense pruritic vesicles of pemphigoid are not herpetiform in grouping and have a **random distribution** rather than favoring the sacral and elbow areas.

Another "clinical fooler" is **dyshidrosiform pemphigoid of the palms** and/or **soles**, with subepidermal blisters clinically identical to dyshidrosiform dermatitis and **bullous tinea pedis**. Immunofluorescent studies are the only diagnostic guide post.

Immunofluorescent analysis has also taught us that bullous pemphigoid is not a disease limited to the elderly. It is seen in children, and also in pregnant women under the label of herpes gestationis.

Pemphigoid is not necessarily a generalized disease. It may be **localized** in the mouth or pretibial area. It can simulate **bullous fixed drug eruption** or the **bullous disease of diabetes**. It may also come to you as scarring, crusted, atrophic lesions of the face and neck. Only the history alerts you to the bullous element, and only the immunofluorescence tells you this is the **Brunsting-Perry type of pemphigoid**.

The **cicatricial scarring form of pemphigoid** that affects ocular mucous membranes and leads to blindness is well known and recognized. However, this same type of pemphigoid may scar the oral mucosa, esophagus, larynx, ear, penis, vagina, and arms, leading to strictures of the affected sites and deafness.

The **differential diagnosis** centers clinically on:

epidermolysis bullosa acquisita (triggered by trauma)
linear IgA bullous dermatosis (linear IgA at basement membrane in uninvolved skin)
chronic bullous dermatosis of childhood (rosette jewel-like blisters in pelvic region with linear IgA deposits—represents linear IgA dermatosis of the child)

Immunofluorescence may humble you as a clinician, but it will exalt you as a diagnostician. Use it.

Amato DA, Silverstein J, Zitelli J: The **prodrome of bullous pemphigoid**. Int J Dermatol 1988; 27:560–563.

Bullous pemphigoid should be considered in any person of the appropriate age who has a persistent and **recalcitrant dermatitis**, **papulovesicular**, or **urticarial eruption** with intense pruritus.

Indirect immunofluorescence can be a **valuable screen** for prodromal bullous pemphigoid, particularly with sensations of pruritus and burning. Direct immunofluorescence may remain negative for months to years.

This report includes two women, ages 70 and 58 years, who had prodromal periods of 18 months and 6 years, respectively. In both cases, direct immunofluorescence showed weak linear staining of the dermal-epidermal junction with C3 prior to conversion to bullous pemphigoid. Eosinophilic spongiosis also developed in both patients as the disease progressed.

In one case, PUVA treatments ended the prodromal period by precipitating blisters and erythema only in the light-exposed areas.

Asbrink E, Hovmark A: **Clinical variations in bullous pemphigoid** with respect to early symptoms. Acta Derm Venereol 1981; 61:417–421.

Although the blister is the hallmark of bullous pemphigoid, many patients suffering from this disease have a **puzzling nonspecific prodromal rash** for weeks to years. Sometimes the prodromal eruption is papular or urticarial, **simulating** a **drug eruption**. It may also be eczematous, appearing as small vesicles of the palms and soles. The clinical impression may be **tinea pedis** with an **id eruption** of the **palms**.

Horizontal rather than vertical study of such a patient is necessary to yield the correct diagnosis. Bullous pemphigoid should be considered in all middle-aged and elderly patients with eczematous, papular, or urticarial eruptions. These patients should be studied with repeated immunofluorescence examinations.

Bean SF, Michel B, Furey N, et al: **Vesicular pemphigoid**. Arch Dermatol 1976; 112:1402–1404.

A 23-year-old woman had a **pruritic vesicular eruption** that initially involved only the face but later spread to the chest, back, and arms. A skin biopsy showed a subepidermal blister, and direct immunofluorescence revealed IgG and C3 at the basement membrane zone. Later, she also had circulating antibodies to the basement membrane zone. Treatment with sulfapyridine and **dapsone** was **unsuccessful**, and prednisone (160 mg daily) was required to control the eruption.

Six other similar cases are described, each resembling atypical dermatitis herpetiformis but all except one unresponsive to sulfones. The lesions were **small tense vesicles**, often **grouped**. Only one patient eventually developed bullae.

Honeyman JF, Honeyman AR, De la Parra MA, et al: **Polymorphic pemphigoid**. Arch Dermatol 1979; 115:423–427.

Is there an **overlap between bullous pemphigoid and dermatitis herpetiformis**? When it is difficult to decide which one the patient has, suspect polymorphic pemphigoid.

A review of 20 patients with a chronic **pruritic**, **burning**, **polymorphic eruption** (vesicles, bullae, crusted erythematous plaques, urticarial plaques, residual pigmentation) showed that a diagnosis could be made only with direct and indirect immunofluorescence. In 14 cases the immunofluorescence corresponded to bullous pemphigoid, while the other 6 cases showed linear IgA in the basement membrane zone. In one patient there was conversion from a linear IgA pattern with negative serologic studies to a linear IgG pattern with a positive reaction for IgG pemphigoid antibodies.

Skin biopsies showed subepidermal bullae and microabscesses in the dermal papillae. Eosinophils were prominent in blister fluid, especially in nine patients with **eosinophilia** ($>$10% in peripheral blood).

Therapeutically, many patients responded initially to sulfapyridine or dapsone but later required steroids.

Gawkrodger DJ, O'Doherty C StJ: **Pemphigoid en cocarde**. J Am Acad Dermatol 1989; 20:1125.

A 74-year-old woman had a 10-week history of bullae on her arms and the backs of her hands. The resultant clinical picture was striking. She had **rosette-like** (en cocarde) ulcers with hyperkeratotic islands in the center. Immunofluorescent studies confirmed the diagnosis of pemphigoid.

It is proposed that this variant be called pemphigoid en cocarde (rosette-like pemphigoid). Other distinctive types of pemphigoid to be recognized include pemphigoid vegetans, pemphigoid nodularis, and **seborrheic pemphigoid**.

Trattner A, Hodak E, Ingber A, Sandbank M: **'Jewel-like' blisters in bullous pemphigoid**. J Am Acad Dermatol 1989; 21:583–584.

Jewel-like blisters and rosettes refer to clusters of **new blisters that appear around resolving lesions**. It is highly characteristic of chronic bullous dermatosis of childhood and has been described in bullous pemphigoid in childhood, but is rare in adults.

A 76-year-old man had several months' history of an itchy bullous eruption. Tense blisters on an erythematous base were located mainly on the flexural aspects of the right arm, but a few scattered lesions were also present. There were no scars. Despite treatment with prednisone, new blisters continued to appear around the edges of subsiding lesions, forming **rosettes**.

A skin biopsy revealed a subepidermal blister with eosinophils and polymorphonuclear leukocytes. Direct immunofluorescence showed linear C3 in the basement membrane zone, typical of bullous pemphigoid.

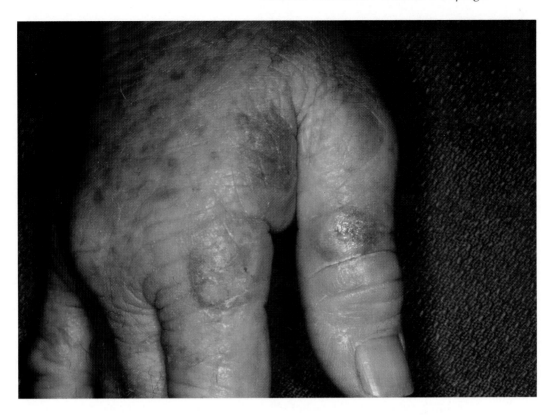

Hadi SM, Barnetson RStC, Gawkrodger DJ, et al: Clinical, histological, and immunological studies in 50 patients with **bullous pemphigoid.** Dermatologica 1988; 176:6–17.

Patients with pemphigoid often have **high IgE levels** and peripheral blood **eosinophilia,** features not commonly associated with autoimmune diseases.

The majority of patients in this study observed over a 2-year period were able to discontinue steroid therapy without further blistering. This confirms that pemphigoid is a self-limiting disease and not a marker for malignancy. However, 3 of the 50 patients had **figurate erythema** and **pemphigoid.** All 3 died of **neoplastic disease,** suggesting that extensive screening for cancer could be rewarding for this subset of patients.

Moral: If pemphigoid is associated with figurate erythema, look for malignant disease.

Leibovici V, Noemi R, Goldenhersh M, Holubar K: **Coexistence of pemphigus and bullous pemphigoid.** Int J Dermatol 1989; 28:259–260.

A 92-year-old woman had a widespread pruritic eruption of **tense and flaccid bullae** on both normal and inflamed skin. Some bullae were hemorrhagic. The Nikolsky sign was positive.

Skin biopsies variously showed subepidermal bullae and suprabasal acantholytic splits. Direct immunofluorescence showed IgG in the intracellular spaces, as well as IgG and C3 along the basement membrane zone. Indirect immunofluorescence showed circulating antibodies to both junctional and intercellular antigens. Antigen mapping revealed a split within the lamina lucida.

Clinicians continue to observe that the presence of one autoimmune disease increases the likelihood of developing an additional one.

Sander HM, Utz MMP, Peters MS: **Bullous pemphigoid and dermatitis herpetiformis:** Mixed bullous disease or coexistence of two separate entities? J Cutan Pathol 1989; 16:370–374.

For 5 years a 73-year-old man had experienced a **pruritic vesicular eruption** of the **elbows and knees**. The clinical diagnosis of dermatitis herpetiformis had been confirmed by histologic and immunopathologic evaluations, and the lesions were well controlled with dapsone.

Four months after the dapsone was discontinued because of anemia, he developed **large flaccid bullae** on the hips, thighs, lower back, right shoulder, elbows, knees, and palate. He also lost 35 pounds in a 3-month period. Recurrent adenocarcinoma of the prostate was diagnosed, and he died 2 months after the bullae appeared.

A skin biopsy of a bulla revealed a subepidermal blister without eosinophils or neutrophils. Direct immunofluorescence revealed linear IgG, IgM, and C3 at the basement membrane zone, as well as heavy granular and clumped IgA in the papillary bodies and along the basement membrane zone. Indirect immunofluorescence was negative.

This case emphasizes that the **subepidermal bullous disorders may overlap**. Even after a specific diagnosis has been established, if the clinical morphology of the blisters or response to therapy changes, repeat histologic and immunofluorescence studies should be performed.

Provost TT, Maize JC, Ahmed AR, et al: **Unusual subepidermal bullous diseases** with immunologic features of bullous pemphigoid. Arch Dermatol 1979; 115:156–160.

Acute localized subepidermal bullae, particularly on the legs, were seen in 11 patients, **suggesting a diagnosis of insect bites or bullous fixed drug eruption**. However, direct immunofluorescence confirmed bullous pemphigoid. The lesions healed quickly with topical steroids.

A chronic **disfiguring, bullous, hyperkeratotic, scarring eruption** was seen in two women, ages 24 and 52 years. The lesions were nonpruritic and involved mainly the **arms** and **legs**. In one case a **factitial dermatitis**, resembling cigarette burns, was suggested. Each patient had had lesions for more than 5 years. Skin biopsies showed acanthosis, hyperkeratosis, and subepidermal bullae with mixed inflammatory cell infiltrates. Direct immunofluorescence showed basement membrane deposition of IgM, IgG, and C3, and, in one case, IgA. Both patients had positive indirect titers to IgG basement membrane zone antibodies.

Bart BJ, Bean SF: **Bullous pemphigoid following** the topical use of **fluorouracil**. Arch Dermatol 1970; 102:457–460.

An 84-year-old man had multiple actinic keratoses on his bald scalp, face, neck, chest, back, and dorsal aspect of the hands. Treatment with fluorouracil solution (1% in propylene glycol) applied daily for 4 weeks led to blistering of all treated lesions, as well as a few bullae on untreated normal skin. Despite discontinuation of the fluorouracil solution, the bullous eruption became generalized, requiring hospitalization. The **bullae** were both **tense and flaccid**, with little underlying inflammation. Some bullae were hemorrhagic, and most were 1 to 3 cm in diameter. A complete blood count revealed **28% eosinophils**. Treatment with prednisone (60 mg/day) was required to suppress the lesions, with gradual tapering over 9 months required for complete cure.

Skin biopsies revealed subepidermal blisters containing mainly eosinophils and a mixed inflammatory cell infiltrate in the dermis. Direct immunofluorescence revealed basement membrane antibodies, which were present in a serum dilution of 1:640 on indirect immunofluorescence. Bullous pemphigoid was diagnosed.

Interestingly, no trace of the actinic keratoses could be found after the skin cleared!

Bean SF, Good RA, Windhorst DB: **Bullous pemphigoid in an 11 year old boy.** Arch Dermatol 1970; 102:205–208.

In an 11-year-old black boy, ulcerative colitis was diagnosed after barium enema examination and sigmoidoscopy. Ten days after starting **salicylazo-sulfapyridine** (Azulfidine) treatment, he developed **blistering** of the skin and mucous membranes, thought to be erythema multiforme. A generalized vesiculobullous eruption with large bullae, erosions of skin and mucous membranes, and target lesions still persisted a few weeks later, despite treatment with prednisone (80 to 120 mg/day). After 4 months of hospitalization the eruption was finally controlled with prednisone (60 mg/day) and azathioprine (200 mg/day). Over a 3-year period the azathioprine was gradually discontinued, while the prednisone dose was tapered (12.5 mg/day). A trial of dapsone resulted in fever, hemolysis, and increased eosinophilia, but no increase in bullae.

A skin biopsy showed a subepidermal blister filled with eosinophils and a perivascular inflammatory infiltrate. These findings were compatible with bullous pemphigoid, dermatitis herpetiformis, and erythema multiforme. Indirect immunofluorescence revealed **basement membrane antibody** at a titer of 1:1280. The leukocyte count was around 16,000/cu mm, with eosinophilia up to 40%. Although the disease started like erythema multiforme and appeared to be sulfonamide induced, the persistence of basement membrane antibodies confirms bullous pemphigoid. Presumably the drug acted as an antigenic haptene to stimulate an immune reaction.

Kardaun SH, De Jong MCJM, Tupker RA: **Localized bullous pemphigoid.** Br J Dermatol 1988; 118:835–836.

Problem: Blisters on the **amputation stump** of a 70-year-old man.

Solution: To distinguish between bullous pemphigoid and epidermolysis bullosa acquisita, a double immunofluorescence technique was used. This showed continuous linear IgG and C3 deposition in the base of the blister, as well as laminin and collagen type IV, indicative of bullous pemphigoid. In epidermolysis bullosa, the IgG and laminin are found in the roof of the blister, not the base.

Viraben R, Dupre A: **Scabies mimicking bullous pemphigoid.** J Am Acad Dermatol 1989; 20:134–136.

For **5 months** a 34-year-old woman with a past history of atopic dermatitis had had a **bullous eruption.** The histologic finding of subepidermal blisters with a sparse inflammatory infiltrate and intact dermal papillae and the presence of **eosinophilia** led to a diagnosis of bullous pemphigoid. Despite prednisone and azathioprine therapy, the eruption progressed to **erythroderma**, with the entire skin covered with papules and an ichthyosiform scale. The palms and soles were hyperkeratotic. Blood tests revealed eosinophilia (1100/mm^3) and an increased serum IgE (1000 IU). Culture of the bullae was negative, and immunofluorescent study of the biopsy specimen revealed no bullous pemphigoid antibodies, immunoglobulin, or complement.

The diagnosis came with **examination of the scales**, which harbored numerous *Sarcoptes scabiei* mites. Antiscabiectic therapy (20% precipitated sulfur for 4 days, 25% benzyl benzoate for 3 days) led to a prompt cure, and the eosinophils and serum IgE returned to normal.

Remember scabies can:

blossom as the blisters of pemphigoid and dermatitis herpetiformis
be confused with contact dermatitis
be diagnosed as Darier's disease by mistake
explain an erythroderma
be the unrecognized cause of urticaria and dermographism

Beware of the rare—look for the common presenting as the uncommon.

Alcalay J, David M, Ingber A, et al: **Bullous pemphigoid mimicking bullous erythema multiforme:** An untoward side effect of penicillins. J Am Acad Dermatol 1988; 18:345–349.

Discrete tense bullae of the face, trunk, and extremities in a 16-year-old boy with fever followed a half dozen penicillin injections given 2 weeks before. Mucosal lesions were present on the mouth, nose, and penis. **Classic target lesions** on the **palms** and **soles** suggested erythema multiforme, but histologic and immunofluorescence studies proved that the diagnosis was bullous pemphigoid. A mast cell degranulation test to procaine penicillin G was strongly positive.

This type of bullous pemphigoid is distinctive, occurring at a younger age than classic bullous pemphigoid and also involving mucous membranes. The patients have erythematous target lesions on the palms and soles, **severe erosions** of all **mucous membranes**, high temperature, and prostration. In all cases presented here, it was **associated with penicillin sensitivity**.

Fleming MG, Bergfeld WF, Tomecki KJ, et al: **Bullous systemic lupus erythematosus.** Int J Dermatol 1989; 28:321–326.

Bullous systemic lupus erythematosus (SLE) is rare and **histologically resembles dermatitis herpetiformis**. Occasionally it may be drug induced.

Direct immunofluorescence shows either granular or linear staining at the dermoepidermal junction, with combinations of IgG, IgM, IgA, and complement. The immunoreactants are located in the upper dermis, just below the lamina densa.

Bullous SLE must be distinguished from bullous pemphigoid in a patient with SLE and also from epidermolysis bullosa acquisita. Negative indirect immunofluorescence for anti–basement-membrane-zone antibodies is no longer considered to be a distinguishing factor.

A 65-year-old woman developed a generalized rash of **papules** and **small vesicles** on a background of erythema, involving mainly the **extensor surfaces** of the arms and legs. Some lesions had an **annular** configuration. Skin biopsy revealed a subepidermal bulla containing neutrophils and a dense dermal infiltrate of neutrophils, interpreted as dermatitis herpetiformis. Later she developed violaceous plaques on the back and extremities, which showed a bandlike infiltrate of histiocytes. Direct immunofluorescence on both types of lesions revealed granular IgM at the dermoepidermal junction. The ANA titer was 1:160, homogeneous pattern. She had been taking **hydralazine** for 5 years, and after this was stopped the rash cleared up in 1 month.

Hydralazine produces a **positive ANA** titer in 24 to 50% of patients and overt SLE in 8 to 13%. Drug-induced lupus usually begins in later life and is a milder disease with a homogeneous-pattern ANA. **Antihistone antibodies** are usually present, but are less frequent in hydralazine-induced lupus than in **procainamide-induced lupus**.

Kettler AH, Bean SF, Duffy JO, Gammon WR: **Systemic lupus erythematosus presenting as a bullous eruption** in a **child**. Arch Dermatol 1988; 124:1083–1087.

In an 8-year-old Texas girl, bullous pemphigoid and chronic bullous disease of childhood were the two working diagnoses to best explain a mildly pruritic, painful blistering eruption on the face, neck, axillae, and groin. The lesions were **confluent tense bullae** on **erythematous annular urticarial plaques**, sometimes in a serpiginous **string-of-pearls** arrangement. The mucous membranes were extensively involved (lips, tongue, buccal mucosa, nasal mucosa, labia). Temperature was 101°F at her first visit (2 months after the blisters first appeared on the face). Immunopathologic findings on biopsy were consistent with either **epidermolysis bullosa acquisita** or bullous systemic lupus erythematosus. Despite an ANA titer of 1:2560, there was insufficient evidence to make a diagnosis of systemic lupus erythematosus.

One year later she developed **proteinuria** as a result of membranous glomerulopathy, thereby fulfilling the American Rheumatism Association's strict criteria for systemic lupus erythematosus. The renal disease has continued despite complete control of the bullous disease with dapsone and sulfapyridine.

It is important to recognize that **bullous disease** may be the **presenting sign** of **systemic lupus erythematosus**. In particular, the early immunologic characteristics may resemble epidermolysis bullosa acquisita, with identical circulating anti–basement-membrane-zone antibodies.

Duschet P, Schwarz T, Gschnait F: **Bullous pemphigoid after radiation therapy.** J Am Acad Dermatol 1988; 18:441–444.

Generalized cutaneous **reactions after radiation therapy** usually center on **erythema multiforme**, which includes a potpourri of macular, maculopapular, urticarial, purpuric, and bullous eruptions.

Bullous pemphigoid, with its distinctive immunofluorescent patterning, must now be added to this list, as seen in a 75-year-old man undergoing radiotherapy to the right inguinal area for metastatic squamous cell carcinoma. Initially, sharply defined **erythema** and **tense bullae** were exactly confined to the irradiation area, but 1 week later the eruption disseminated over the entire body. **Eosinophils** were **20%** (absolute number, 2150/mm^3). Treatment with niacinamide (500 mg tid) and tetracycline (300 mg tid) suppressed the lesions, but could not be withdrawn without relapse.

Localized cutaneous reactions induced by radiation therapy include radiodermatitis, lichen sclerosus et atrophicus, and graft-versus-host disease.

Scaparro E, Borghi S, Rebora A: **Kaposi's sarcoma after immunosuppressive therapy** for bullous pemphigoid. Dermatologica 1984; 169:156–159.

A generalized bullous eruption of 1 month's duration in an 86-year-old man proved to be bullous pemphigoid. The bullae cleared following prednisone therapy (75 mg/day), but during the fourth week of treatment numerous **red-violaceous painless nodules** appeared on the right lower leg and left foot. Skin biopsy revealed Kaposi's sarcoma.

Presumably, **steroid-induced** immunosuppression reduced the immunologic control of a previously latent angiogenic virus. The same immunosuppression is seen with drugs, diseases, and AIDS and has long been associated with the appearance of Kaposi's sarcoma.

Masouyé I, Schmied E, Didierjean L, et al: **Bullous pemphigoid and multiple sclerosis:** More than a coincidence? Report of three cases. J Am Acad Dermatol 1989; 21:63–68.

There are now reports of six patients who developed bullous pemphigoid on top of advanced multiple sclerosis. This probably represents the coexistence of **autoimmune phenomena**.

Multiple sclerosis is thought to be a **cell–mediated autoimmune disease**

triggered by a **viral infection**. Immunologic abnormalities include autoimmunization against several constituents of the central nervous system white matter, as well as reduction of peripheral blood suppressor T lymphocytes. Possibly this immunologic imbalance could lead to production of autoantibodies, such as those in bullous pemphigoid.

Multiple sclerosis has sporadically been reported in other autoimmune disorders, including rheumatoid arthritis, thyrotoxicosis, Hashimoto's thyroiditis, systemic lupus erythematosus, pemphigus vulgaris, and systemic scleroderma.

Bullous pemphigoid has also been **associated with** several **autoimmune diseases**:

rheumatoid arthritis
systemic lupus erythematosus
myasthenia gravis
pernicious anemia
primary biliary cirrhosis
alopecia universalis
Hashimoto's thyroiditis
immune nephritis

Stone SP, Schroeter AL: **Bullous pemphigoid and associated malignant neoplasms.** Arch Dermatol 1975; 111:991–994.

In an age-controlled study of 219 patients, the incidence of systemic malignant disease was **no higher in patients with bullous pemphigoid** (8 in 73) than in patients with psoriasis (10 in 73) or in patients with contact dermatitis (11 in 73). Extensive diagnostic studies for malignant neoplasms should be based on consideration of age, condition of the patient, and clinical findings rather than on the presence of bullous pemphigoid.

Telegdy E, Schneider I: Association of cutaneous **T cell lymphoma and bullous pemphigoid**. Dermatologica 1989; 179:220.

A 61-year-old woman in Hungary with **plaque-type mycosis fungoides** developed lentil-sized **tense vesicles** on the left flexor forearm, abdomen, waist, and edges of the tongue 6 days after receiving a single dose of oral methotrexate (25 mg). She was also taking prednisone (90 mg/day). After 1 month the bullae had cleared, and methotrexate could be repeated without recurrence.

Skin biopsies revealed **mycosis fungoides and bullous pemphigoid**. Direct immunofluorescence showed a linear band of IgG along the basement membrane zone. Indirect immunofluorescence testing was negative.

Previous work has shown that **seronegative bullous pemphigoid** may be a **paraneoplastic symptom**. Perhaps antigen binding by the tumor is responsible for the inability to detect circulating antibody in the serum.

Graham-Brown RAC: **Bullous pemphigoid with figurate erythema** associated with carcinoma of the bronchus. Br J Dermatol 1987; 117:385–388.

The presence of a **figurate erythema in bullous pemphigoid merits search for an underlying neoplasm**, particularly if the indirect immunofluorescence is negative.

A 74-year-old healthy man developed an acute widespread eruption of small **annular erythematous lesions** of the extensor surfaces of the limbs and dorsal aspect of the hands, which appeared initially to be **erythema multiforme**.

However, 5 days later, tense clear bullae arose, leading to the diagnosis of bullous pemphigoid, which was confirmed by direct immunofluorescence (linear IgG, C3, and C4 in the basement membrane zone). Indirect immunofluorescence was negative. New figurate annular areas of erythema spreading in waves began to appear on the abdomen and thighs, consistent with **erythema gyratum repens**.

Further study revealed shadowing of the right midzone of the lung, which on bronchoscopy proved to be **squamous cell carcinoma of the bronchus**. Radical radiotherapy of the tumor was followed by involution of the skin lesions.

Slazinski L, Degefu S: **Herpes gestationis associated with choriocarcinoma.** Arch Dermatol 1982; 118:425–428.

A **generalized, pruritic bullous eruption** had been present for 3 weeks when a 36-year-old woman was admitted to the hospital. There were erythematous, **gyriform, edematous papules and plaques** with **grouped vesicles**, bullae, and occasional erosions.

History revealed that 4 weeks before she had had uterine suction curettage for an episode of **heavy vaginal bleeding**, which occurred approximately 3 months into a "pregnancy" in which the uterus was too large for the estimated dates. The pathologic diagnosis was a **hydatid mole** with malignant features (**choriocarcinoma**). Serum and urinary human chorionic gonadotropin levels were elevated. Chest x-ray showed four metastatic nodules in the middle lung fields. CBC was abnormal with **20% eosinophils** and 480,000 to 865,000 platelets.

Skin biopsy showed a subepidermal bulla with a pleomorphic infiltrate containing many eosinophils. Direct immunofluorescence showed IgG and C3 deposition at the basement membrane zone, establishing the diagnosis of **herpes gestationis**. Several courses of methotrexate over the next 2 months resulted in complete clearing of the skin lesions, as well as disappearance of the choriocarcinoma.

Herpes gestationis and bullous pemphigoid may be **difficult to differentiate** because of identical histopathology and direct immunofluorescence on skin biopsy. In this case, factors favoring herpes gestationis included the pruritus, eosinophilia, and childbearing age. Herpes gestationis has previously been reported in only two other cases of hydatid mole and in two cases of choriocarcinoma. Blistering eruptions have also occurred occasionally with uterine carcinoma.

Goodnough LT, Muir WA: **Bullous pemphigoid as a manifestation of chronic lymphocytic leukemia.** Arch Intern Med 1980; 140:1526–1527.

An 81-year-old woman with rheumatoid arthritis had pruritus for 6 weeks, along with a progressive **papulovesicular eruption** that spread diffusely over the trunk, head, and extremities. She was hospitalized with numerous blisters and tense bullae, along with palpable axillary nodes.

A skin biopsy showed subepidermal bullae with polymorphonuclear leukocytes and eosinophils in the blister cavity. Direct immunofluorescence was positive for anti-IgG and C3 at the basement membrane, confirming bullous pemphigoid. Indirect immunofluorescence was negative for basement membrane zone antibody, but positive 1:40 for antibody against basal cells. The WBC count was 26,200/cu mm with 35% lymphocytes and 10% atypical lymphocytes. Chronic lymphocytic leukemia (**CLL**) was **confirmed on bone marrow aspirate** and biopsy.

Despite treatment with prednisone (60 mg/day), the WBC count rose to

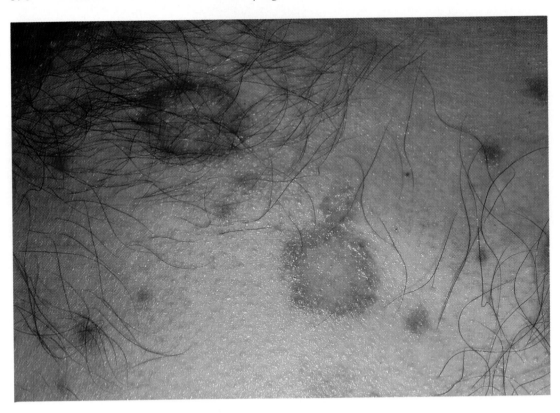

65,000/mm^3, and new bullae continued to appear. Chlorambucil (6 mg/day) was then added and the prednisone dose was tapered over 3 months, with clearing of the blisters and control of the leukemia. This clinical course suggests an association between the **coexisting bullous pemphigoid and CLL**.

Hsu VM, Krey PR, Schwartz RA: **Bullous pemphigoid and rheumatoid arthritis.** Cutis 1989; 43:30–32.

The coexistence of rheumatoid arthritis and bullous pemphigoid may not be coincidental, since **both are autoimmune diseases**. Both involve immune-complex–mediated inflammation with influx of activated leukocytes into either the synovium or the basement membrane of the skin. Sporadic cases of association of the two diseases have been reported.

A 57-year-old woman had deforming **arthritis** for 4 years and generalized subepidermal **vesiculobullous lesions** for 7 months. The rheumatoid factor was 1:5120 and ANA was 1:80 with a speckled pattern. Direct immuno-fluorescent studies were negative.

She had been receiving **furosemide** for 3 months, which may have contributed to the pemphigoid. However, drug-induced pemphigoid is usually transient, localized, and disappears upon discontinuation of the provoking agent.

Barth JH, Kelley SE, Wojnarowska F, et al: **Pemphigoid and ulcerative colitis.** J Am Acad Dermatol 1988; 19:303.

Autoimmunity is not thought to be the main pathogenic mechanism in ulcerative colitis. However, ulcerative colitis may be associated with other autoimmune diseases, including bullous pemphigoid.

There are now 15 **reported cases of** patients with **ulcerative colitis** who **subsequently developed pemphigoid**, counting the eight cases from Great Britain in this report. Four of the eight cases also had other autoimmune disorders, including thyroid disease, hemolytic anemia, and glomerulonephritis.

Perhaps the diseased colon, which is extremely permeable, acts as an entry site for antigenic material that cross-reacts with skin antigens.

Kubba R, Champion RH: **Nickel sensitivity resembling bullous pemphigoid.** Br J Dermatol 1975; 93:(Suppl 11):41–43.

A 55-year-old woman developed multiple tense **blisters on the left lower leg**. Although they resembled bullous pemphigoid clinically and on light microscopy, no immunofluorescent antibodies could be found on direct and indirect studies.

Past history revealed that 14 years prior she had a Pott's fracture of her **left ankle** that was fixed with a **vitallium screw**. She had also had hand eczema that took several months to clear. She had also reacted to metals many years ago. Patch tests to nickel sulfate and cobalt chloride both showed 2+ eczematous responses. An **intradermal test to nickel** sulfate (0.05 ml, 0.01%) reproduced a tense bulla by 48 hours, while intradermal tests to chrome, cobalt, and molybdenum were negative.

A diagnosis was made of a pemphigoid-like eruption due to sensitivity to the nickel that leaked out of the vitallium screw, which was subsequently removed.

Gammon WR, Briggaman RA, Woodley DT, et al: **Epidermolysis bullosa acquisita—a pemphigoid-like disease.** J Am Acad Dermatol 1984; 11:820–832.

As many as 50% of cases of epidermolysis bullosa acquisita are misdiagnosed as bullous pemphigoid.

Here is a disease truly **recognized only by the immunoelectron microscopist**. Although its blisters and erosions are induced by trauma, it can completely mimic bullous pemphigoid and cicatricial pemphigoid clinically, histologically, and immunohistologically. Only by immunoelectron microscopy of perilesional skin, which demonstrates IgG deposits beneath the lamina densa of the basement membrane, can the definitive diagnosis be made of this dermolytic form of pemphigoid.

Until such studies are done, many examples of **epidermolysis bullosa acquisita will be called bullous pemphigoid or cicatricial pemphigoid**. Even ocular and oral mucous membrane inflammation and scarring may be immunologically mediated examples of epidermolysis bullosa acquisita, not cicatricial pemphigoid.

There is still a role for the clinician to separate out a clinical set of EBA characterized by:

> tense blisters and vesicles occurring in older individuals on extensor skin surfaces, under wrist bands, or on the back where bed sheets rub
> erosions in the mouth at sites of dental trauma
> associated erythematous plaques, hemorrhagic blisters, sequential erosions, and pruritus
> Nikolsky sign, scarring, or milia variably present

If on seeing a patient you think of bullous pemphigoid, think next of epidermolysis bullosa acquisita.

Wojnarowska F, Marsden RA, Bhogal B, Black MM: **Chronic bullous disease of childhood, childhood cicatricial pemphigoid, and linear IgA disease of adults:** A comparative study demonstrating clinical and immunopathologic overlap. J Am Acad Dermatol 1988; 19:792–805.

Long-term study of 25 cases of **chronic bullous eruption of children**, 25 cases of **adult linear IgA disease**, and four cases of **childhood cicatricial pemphigoid** suggest that they are **the same disease**, with childhood cicatricial pemphigoid being a more severe scarring form. They are not variants of dermatitis herpetiformis because of the lack of association with gluten-sensitive enteropathy and the high incidence of mucosal involvement.

While **pruritus or stinging** is an invariable finding, the skin lesions are quite variable, including urticaria and annular polycyclic and target lesions. The most common finding is large bullae, occasionally hemorrhagic, developing in three of four patients. In children the perineum, limbs, and trunk are usually involved, with grouped lesions forming a "**cluster of jewels" sign**. Another important finding is the "**string of beads" sign**, referring to vesicles and bullae that appear at the edge of annular lesions.

Mucous membrane involvement is common, and nearly half of the children with chronic bullous eruption have ocular symptoms with redness, pain, grittiness, and discharge. Two of these patients showed fine scarring in the eyes, strengthening the view that chronic bullous eruption and scarring pemphigoid are the same disease. Mouth ulcers were recurrent, as were mucosal lesions in the genital area.

Childhood cicatricial pemphigoid began with a generalized eruption and later proceeded to involve the eye. The four children with childhood cicatricial pemphigoid showed the changes of symblepharon and ectropion. In one case blindness developed. All had oral ulcers, with one having scarring of the lower lip. Another had hoarseness. Involvement of the vulvar mucosa was noted in one patient complaining of dysuria.

In adults, **linear IgA disease** may cause similar ocular and mucous membrane involvement. Signs may include painful oral ulceration, gingivitis, hoarseness, nasal stuffiness, crusting, and bleeding. Erosions and blisters may also be on the genitals. **Associated problems** in some patients included atopic symptoms, autoimmune disease, carcinoma, lymphoma, and myeloma.

In **adult linear IgA disease** the trunk and limbs were most commonly affected. All patients showed deposition of IgA anti–basement membrane zone antibodies. Combinations of IgM, IgG, and C3 deposition were also found in some cases. The serum IgA was normal in all but four patients. All patients responded rapidly to dapsone therapy.

The major diagnostic problem is to recognize linear IgA disease and not be fooled when it comes in the **guise** of:

pruritus (can precede lesions by a year)	erythema multiforme
dyshidrosis	bullous pemphigoid
urticaria	

IgA autoantibody is also found in dermatitis herpetiformis, IgA nephropathy, and Henoch-Schönlein purpura. The reason for an IgA response to a normal basement membrane antigen is unclear. Possibly it reflects a mucosal route of entry of a cross-reacting antigen, either dietary or infectious. **Prodromal events** in both children and adults with linear IgA disease often include a preceding infection or the taking of either antibiotics or nonsteroidal antiinflammatory drugs.

Burge S, Wojnarowska F, Marsden A: Chronic **bullous dermatosis of childhood persisting** into adulthood. Pediatr Dermatol 1988; 5:246–249.

An 18-year-old white woman had suffered with a chronic pruritic bullous eruption since age 2 years. Originally, **crusted excoriations** were surrounded by clusters of bullae on the **perineum, buttocks, legs, and abdomen**. Perioral skin and scalp were less severely affected. The original diagnosis was **chronic bullous dermatosis of childhood**.

As **years went by** the disease fluctuated and was difficult to control. It included **episodes of oral ulceration**, intermittent nonscarring **conjunctivitis**, and **dysuria**. Blistering was exacerbated by sunlight. At age 18 she was still getting tense uncomfortable vesicles predominantly on perioral skin, suppressed by dapsone (50 mg/day).

A skin biopsy showed **dermatitis herpetiformis–like histology**, with papillary microabscesses and subepidermal bullae containing neutrophils and eosinophils. Direct immunoelectron microscopy demonstrated that the **linear band** of IgA was localized below the lamina densa. Indirect immunofluorescence also demonstrated a **circulating IgA anti–basement membrane zone antibody** that bound to both the epidermal and dermal sides of the cleavage plane in skin that was mechanically separated.

Most cases of chronic bullous disease of childhood remit within a few years. The disease rarely persists into adult life. Mucosal involvement occurs in about 75% of cases, but improved in this patient with the onset of puberty. The disease appeared to **convert to the adult form of linear IgA disease**.

Don't overlook looking over the patient.

Bullae with Other Skin Diseases

Walker GB, Harrison PV: Seasonal **bullous eruption due to mosquitoes**. Clin Exp Dermatol 1985; 10:127–132.

Bullae that recur each summer on the **knees** and **lower legs** of women are probably **due to mosquito bites**. In three volunteer patients, bites from *Aedes detritus* mosquitoes (collected from small ponds and water containers), reproduced the lesions. Skin biopsies showed subepidermal bullae with a chronic inflammatory infiltrate in the upper dermis and a mild perivascular infiltrate.

Patients are often unaware of the bite or its source. The low flight pattern of this mosquito accounts for most lesions being on the lower legs. **Gravitational forces** apparently **lead to blister formation**, as bites elsewhere on the body produced only papules or small vesicles. Other species of mosquitoes also show regional preferences, such as the head or nose.

The seasonal timing favors the diagnosis of bullous mosquito bites, but the **differential diagnosis** also includes:

> phytophototoxic plant dermatitis
> horsefly bites
> blister beetle dermatitis
> localized bullous pemphigoid

Brenner S, Yust I: Bullous eruption in a case of **bullous pediculid**. Cutis 1988; 41:281.

For several months a 79-year-old woman had a severely pruritic eruption of large 1- to 2-cm tense **bullae on erythematous plaques** on the legs and abdomen. Skin biopsy showed a subepidermal bulla and mixed perivascular infiltrate with many eosinophils, with negative immunofluorescence. The cause became apparent only by examination of the pubic area, which revealed **countless pubic lice**. Treatment with lindane solution and prednisone produced a cure in 1 week.

Other skin reactions caused by lice include:

> **pediculid**—skin-colored papules 2 to 3 mm in diameter seen in children with pediculosis capitis
> **maculae ceruleae**—sky blue or slate-colored macules on the sides of the trunk or medial thighs, which persist many weeks

Moral: Don't forget to **peep at the pubic area** in puzzling cases, even in the elderly.

Jones SK, Strong L, Burton JL: **Perioral blisters in a bug-biting baby**. Br J Dermatol 1988; 119:121–125.

A 6-month-old baby boy's perioral blisters resulted not from a bug biting him but from his biting the bug.

The **baby had bitten** a 1.5-cm green shield "stink" bug (*Palomena prasina*) that had crawled up to him on the lawn. His mother found a crushed green "beetle" with a pungent smell next to him, just after he suddenly started crying. The perioral erosions were apparently due to irritant aldehydes released at the time the baby attacked. They healed without scarring.

The stink bug is just one of a host of beetles, ants, and bugs that release toxic chemicals as a defensive measure. **Contact with insects** should be considered as a **cause of blistering eruptions**, especially in children who are more likely to handle insects.

It behooves us not only to think of what bug bit the child but also what bug the child bit.

400

Weber PJ, Salazar JE: **Bullous eruption in a psoriatic patient.** Arch Dermatol 1989; 125:689–694.

A 72-year-old man with psoriasis for 10 years developed vesicles and bullae on the legs, arms, and groin 1 week after undergoing a liver biopsy for evaluation of possible methotrexate therapy. He was taking propranolol and hydrochlorothiazide for mild hypertension and sulfonylureas for diabetes mellitus. **Numerous tense bullae** were present on the anterior surface of the legs, along with occasional hemorrhagic periungual vesicles.

A skin biopsy, direct immunofluorescence, and indirect immunofluorescence all confirmed **bullous pemphigoid.**

The relationship between psoriasis and bullous pemphigoid is unknown, but the two diseases occur together more often than would be randomly expected.

Hori Y, Tsuru N, Niimura M: **Bullous Darier's disease.** Arch Dermatol 1982; 118:278–279.

A 50-year-old woman had had many **pruritic vesicles and bullae** of the medial **lower extremities** and flexor aspects of the **arms** each summer since early childhood. The blisters subsided in the autumn, leaving hyperpigmentation. When she was 20 years old she first noted **brown keratotic papules** on the face, neck and chest (**seborrheic areas**). Her **palms** and **soles** also developed small punctate hyperkeratotic papules.

The family history revealed similar papules without bullae in her father, brother, and daughter. A skin biopsy on her daughter showed Darier's disease.

Biopsies of the keratotic papules as well as the bullae showed suprabasilar clefts (lacunae), acantholysis in the upper epidermis, corps ronds in the granular layer, and grains in the horny layer. Direct immunofluorescence was negative. A diagnosis of bullous Darier's disease was made.

Ultraviolet light, heat, high humidity, and stress appeared to be precipitating factors of bullae in this patient. Possibly, **hydrostatic forces** in her legs were also important in blister formation.

It is interesting to speculate on the relationship between Darier's disease and familial benign chronic pemphigus, which may closely resemble each other clinically and histologically. Could familial benign chronic pemphigus be a bullous variant of Darier's disease? To date, however, they appear to occur independently in involved families.

Telfer NR, Burge SM, Ryan TJ: **Vesiculo-bullous Darier's disease.** Br J Dermatol 1990; 122:831–834.

Drainage of a right submandibular **abscess** in a 49-year-old man with Darier's disease was **followed by** the development of generalized **tense blisters** within 48 hours. The patient became erythrodermic, and sheets of epidermis were shed as a result of friction. The Nikolsky sign was positive.

Staphylococcus aureus was cultured from the abscess and from the initial blisters of the hands. However, blood cultures were negative, and no virus or bacteria could be found in the vesicles. **A biopsy confirmed the diagnosis of Darier's disease with blistering.** Frozen sections of a vesicle roof were negative for either the necrotic epidermis of a drug–induced toxic epidermal necrolysis or the granular layer split diagnostic of staphylococcal scalded skin syndrome.

It is likely that the **etretinate** the patient was receiving for Darier's disease had predisposed him to circulating bacterial antigen–induced bulla formation. Etretinate is well known to produce epidermal erosions and skin fragility by inhibiting desmosome production and interfering with epidermal cell adhesion.

Kwee DJ, Dufresne RG, Ellis DL: **Childhood bullous lichen planus.** Pediatr Dermatol 1987; 4:325–327.

A 7-year-old black boy with generalized xerosis developed a generalized eruption of **violaceous papules and plaques.** **Bullae and erosions** were present on the legs and arms. Cultures of blister fluid yielded only *Staphylococcus epidermidis*, and treatment with antibiotics for presumed bullous impetigo superimposed on lichen planus did not help. Dapsone, however, was curative in 1 month.

A skin biopsy showed bullous lichen planus. Direct immunofluorescence revealed **IgM-staining cytoid bodies.**

Indirect immunofluorescence demonstrated IgG and IgA in the stratum granulosum and stratum spinosum. These areas contain a **lichen planus–specific antigen (LPSA)**, which is found in 80% of adults with lichen planus.

The LPSA may be a useful diagnostic tool in childhood bullous diseases in which bullous lichen planus is a serious consideration.

Camisa C, Neff JC, Rossana C, Barrett JL: Bullous lichen planus: **Diagnosis by indirect immunofluorescence** and treatment with dapsone. J Am Acad Dermatol 1986; 14:464–469.

In a 42-year-old man, multiple **small tense blisters** on normal to **erythematous violaceous skin** of the neck and lower abdomen had been diagnosed histologically as bullous pemphigoid over a $2\frac{1}{2}$-year period. The patient reported that new lesions began with pruritus, followed in 1 hour by a red area that began to blister. Rupture of the blister led to healing.

Evaluation with direct immunofluorescence revealed only fibrinogen at the dermoepidermal junction. However, further immunofluorescent study with the autologous indirect assay revealed IgG and IgA in the stratum granulosum, but no anti–basement membrane zone antibodies.

The identity of bullae has become an exercise in immunofluorescence, not in "clinical fluorescence."

Kobayasi T, Willeberg A, Serup J, Ullman S: **Generalized morphea** with **blisters.** A case report. Acta Derm Venereol 1990; 70:454–456.

Bullae appeared across **sclerotic areas** of the **buttocks** and gluteal cleft of a 70-year-old woman who had carried the diagnosis of generalized morphea for 5 years. Her treatment had consisted of **D-penicillamine**, 750 mg/day. The blister content was yellowish, gelatinous, and sterile.

The appearance of the blisters suggested a D-penicillamine drug eruption or was consistent with the idea that the correct diagnosis was not morphea but was **lichen sclerosus et atrophicus**. This is in keeping with the fact that bullae appear more commonly in lichen sclerosus et atrophicus than in morphea.

A biopsy reconfirmed the diagnosis of morphea and showed the blisters to be the acantholytic ones of a penicillamine reaction rather than blistering in the dermis itself. This was the result of mechanical shearing forces on damaged collagen fibers.

Johnson TM, Rapini RP, Hebert AA, et al: **Bullous amyloidosis.** Cutis 1989; 43:346–352.

A 56-year-old black man with hypertension for 17 years developed **pruritic bullae** of the **trunk** and proximal aspect of the extremities. The bullae were serum filled and nonhemorrhagic, and occurred mainly in **frictional areas** of the groin, medial surface of the thighs, and axillae. Three weeks later he developed **nephrotic syndrome**.

Skin biopsies revealed subepidermal blisters with eosinophils, consistent with **bullous pemphigoid**. Direct immunofluorescence showed linear deposition of IgG at the basement membrane zone.

Despite treatment with prednisone and azathioprine the skin lesions failed to improve. He then started developing **hemorrhagic blisters** induced by minimal trauma. Marked **skin fragility** was also noted on the trunk, extremities, and dorsal surface of the hands.

Worsening renal function and fatigue led to a **renal biopsy**, which revealed **amyloid deposition**. Repeat skin biopsy of a bulla for electron microscopy also revealed amyloid. **Reexamination** of the original **skin biopsy** specimen showed very subtle **amyloid deposits** in the dermal papillae.

Bullous amyloidosis usually indicates systemic involvement, and is most often associated with **myeloma**. The blisters may be intraepidermal or subepidermal. Direct immunofluorescent findings may mimic pemphigoid, epidermolysis bullosa acquisita, or linear IgA disease. Bullae may be confined to the extensor aspect of the arms, hands, and fingers, **mimicking porphyria cutanea tarda**.

Amyloid may bind clotting factors from the blood, particularly X and IX, leading to bleeding.

If a bullous eruption looks like pemphigoid, doesn't respond to treatment, and becomes hemorrhagic, suspect amyloidosis.

Breathnach SM: **Bullous amyloidosis**. *In* Wojnarowska F, Briggaman RA (eds): Management of Blistering Diseases. New York, Raven Press, 1990, pp 289–294.

Bullae and erosions may appear in patients with primary or myeloma-associated amyloidosis. These may be widespread or localized, as on the hands or feet. Even the tongue and buccal mucosa may be involved. On the hands, the lesions resemble **porphyria cutanea tarda**, and in some patients healing results in extensive **milia formation**.

Trauma induces the bullae, as in the purpura and ecchymoses of amyloidosis. An aid to clinical diagnosis also is the presence of **waxy smooth amber-colored papules**, nodules, and plaques in the flexural areas. **Other amyloid-induced skin changes** are macroglossia, scleroderma-like plaques, alopecia, and **cutis verticis gyrata**.

Bullous amyloidosis is **another example of diagnosis by biopsy**. Ask for a special stain for amyloid to be sure you won't miss it. The **differential diagnosis** includes bullous pemphigoid, bullous drug eruption, porphyria cutanea tarda, and epidermolysis bullosa acquisita.

Maeda K, Jimbow K, Takahashi M: Association of **vesiculobullous eruptions** with mycosis fungoides. Dermatologica 1987; 174:34–38.

A generalized pruritic erythematous eruption for 2 years in a 51-year-old Japanese woman consisted of several thin-walled vesicles and bullae on erythematous and nonerythematous bases, **resembling pemphigus vulgaris**.

Numerous skin biopsies revealed:

1. 4 months: parapsoriasis.
2. 16 months: subcorneal bulla with acantholytic cells, leukocytes, and large atypical lymphocytes
   Bullous impetigo was ruled out by Gram stain. Pautrier microabscesses were present in the epidermis.

3. 22 months: intraepidermal bulla with large atypical mononuclear cells and a dense dermal infiltrate of lymphocytes, histiocytes, and atypical lymphocytes. Frozen sections revealed Ia$^+$–activated T cells with helper/inducer phenotype (Leu 1$^+$, Leu 2$^-$, Leu 3$^+$). The diagnosis was **mycosis fungoides.**

Lee SH, Chung KY, Lee WS, Lee S: **Behçet's syndrome** associated **with bullous necrotizing vasculitis.** J Am Acad Dermatol 1989; 21:327–330.

An 11-year-old Korean boy had been sick for 2 months with high spiking fever, oral and genital ulcerations, and ulcers with thick purulent crusts on the legs. The ulcers were preceded by tense, fingertip-sized bullae, which continued to form at the margins of the necrotic areas. Purple maculopapular lesions were also seen around the ulcers and on the dorsal aspect of the feet. **Necrotic ulcers** with white coatings were present on the prepuce, left cheek, and left earlobe, and conjunctival infection was visible in the right eye. Behçet's syndrome was diagnosed.

A skin biopsy was negative for direct immunofluorescence, but showed epidermal necrosis with subepidermal vesicles. Thrombi and necrosis occurred in all dermal blood vessels, with perivascular lymphohistiocytes and eosinophils. Lymphocytic vasculitis in the subcutaneous fat resulted in septal and lobular **panniculitis.** The WBC was 12,200 cells/mm^3 with 60% neutrophils and 20% eosinophils.

Eventually he developed a left pleural effusion, finally proven to contain acid-fast bacilli. **Antituberculosis therapy** was added to the other treatments of dapsone and prednisone and resulted in **healing** of the skin lesions.

Chern L-C, Lin C-S, Wong C-K: **Cutaneous chylous reflux.** Br J Dermatol 1989; 120:695–700.

For 5 years a 22-year-old woman in China had episodes of creamy fluid weeping from the left upper thigh. The milklike fluid would exude for as long as 5 days and then stop. Examination revealed multiple pinhead-sized white **vesicles that released a milky fluid** when ruptured. There was no edema of the leg, and the patient was in excellent health.

Biopsy showed dilated lymphatic channels in the upper dermis. A lymphangiogram showed dilatation and tortuosity of the left iliac lymphatics with a dermal backflow onto the upper medial left aspect of the thigh. The milky fluid was sampled and had the same composition of cholesterol and triglyceride as chyle (lymphatic fluid that originates in the bowel lacteals and passes through the cisterna chyli and thoracic duct into the blood stream). A diagnosis of **cutaneous chylous reflux** was made.

Skin lesions usually appear on the external genitalia, thighs, abdominal wall, feet, and knee joints. They may appear as **white vesicles**, representing dilated cutaneous lymphatics, or solid white lesions containing creamy chyle mixed with macrophages and histiocytes. There is usually **associated lymphedema** of a limb. It is likely this rarity reflects a malformation of the cisterna chyli or the mesenteric lymph nodes. Surgery to date has been associated only with recurrences, which reflect the extensive nature of this anatomic defect.

Bennion SD: **Annular vesiculation.** Arch Dermatol 1989; 125:1569–1574.

Three **ring-shaped vesiculobullous lesions** appeared on the forearm of a 20-year-old woman. Present for only a week, they were pruritic and had enlarged from small vesicles to 1 to 5 cm in size and were now showing central regression. **Diagnoses considered** included herpes simplex, bullous impetigo, bullous fixed drug eruption, insect bite reaction, and allergic contact dermatitis.

A Tzanck preparation revealed **fungal hyphae** intermixed with clumps of epidermal and acute inflammatory cells. A biopsy showed spongiotic vesicles in the epidermis and an edematous dermis. By silver methenamine stain it was possible to demonstrate fungal hyphae, shown to be ***Trichophyton rubrum*** on culture.

Although bullae on the soles or palms make one think of tinea, those on glabrous skin do not. If you proceed directly to biopsy of that isolated blister, having skipped a KOH preparation and culture, be sure to ask the pathologist for a PAS or silver methenamine stain.

Most cases of bullous tinea on glabrous skin have been caused by *T. rubrum* infection. Presumably, epidermal spongiosis (similar to acute contact dermatitis) is caused by a delayed hypersensitivity reaction to *T. rubrum* antigen in a previously sensitized individual.

Every blister should have a **Tzanck smear** and a **Gram stain** as part of the initial work-up (as well as a **KOH** preparation).

Many dermatoses remain invisible as long as you don't look for them.

Metabolic Bullous Diseases

Venning VA: **Bullous dermatoses associated with renal disease.** *In* Wojnarowska F, Briggaman RA (eds): Management of Blistering Diseases. New York, Raven Press, 1990, pp 295–301.

Patients undergoing **hemodialysis** may develop a bullous eruption that is clinically and histologically indistinguishable from **porphyria cutanea tarda**.

Patients with chronic renal failure have a predilection for developing bullae on sun-exposed areas when receiving furosemide (Lasix).

Patients with immune complex glomerulonephritis may have a variety of blistering diseases, including bullous pemphigoid, dermatitis herpetiformis, and linear IgA disease.

Toonstra J: **Bullosis diabeticorum.** Report of a case with a review of the literature. J Am Acad Dermatol 1985; 13:799–805.

A 57-year-old **diabetic man** had experienced **recurrent blisters of his fingers** for no apparent reason for the past year. Usually located on the palmar surfaces, the bullae were preceded a few hours before by a localized burning sensation. The surrounding skin was not influenced, and the blister fluid was clear and sterile. Healing required several weeks; there was no scar formation. Biopsy showed a subepidermal blister with separation in the lamina lucida. No immunoreactants were found. Suction blister threshold tests on his forearm revealed that he formed blisters in 13 minutes compared to 23 minutes in healthy controls.

A diagnosis of **bullosis diabeticorum** was made. This condition usually is confined to the feet and lower legs, but even the trunk may exhibit such blistering. The cause remains unknown.

Mochizuki T, Tanaka S, Watanabe S: A case of **hypothyroidism with bulla formation.** Dermatologica 1984; 169:146–149.

Bullae, at times hemorrhagic, kept appearing on the **hands and feet** of a 73-year-old Japanese woman for the past year, leading to shallow ulcers and atrophy. The elbows and knees were similarly involved, and the Nikolsky sign was positive. For 5 years she had also had **hyperkeratosis and erythema** on the **palms** and **soles,** with fissures in winter, and for 6 months she had experienced cold intolerance.

Examination revealed cold extremities and a scaly **ichthyosis-like eruption** of the trunk, arms, and legs. The eyelids were swollen, and the hair of the eyebrows and scalp was sparse. **Hypothyroidism** was confirmed, and skin biopsy showed blister formation above the basement membrane. The blisters no longer formed after she started thyroid therapy.

The **differential diagnosis** included:

    bullosis diabeticorum
    friction blister
    epidermolysis bullosa acquisita
    epidermolysis bullosa simplex
    pellagra
    autoimmune disease (pemphigus, dermatitis herpetiformis, bullous
        pemphigoid)

If the patient's thyroid is working slowly, you may have to work fast to make the diagnosis.

Murphy GM, Wright J, Nicholls DSH, et al: **Sunbed-induced pseudoporphyria.** Br J Dermatol 1989; 120:555–562.

A 28-year-old woman with red hair, numerous freckles, and an orange-brown tan had a 3-year history of **recurrent blistering and erosions.** For the same period she had used **UVA sunbeds repeatedly,** having been exposed to an estimated total dose of 10 kJ/cm^2. On examination she had groups of blisters on the limbs as well as linear purpuric streaks and skin fragility. There was evidence of atopic dermatitis on the sides of the neck, and she had dry aged skin with numerous excoriations.

The **possibilities** of porphyria, drug eruption, epidermolysis bullosa acquisita, and cutaneous amyloidosis were excluded. A toxicology screen was negative for the following **drugs known to produce pseudoporphyria**: tetracycline, naproxen, furosemide, dapsone, and pyridoxine. Quantitative **porphyrin studies** on blood, urine, and stool were **normal**. General laboratory studies, including immunoglobulins, were also normal.

A skin biopsy showed a noninflammatory subepidermal split with marked solar elastosis. There was no evidence of amyloid on special Congo red staining. Immunofluorescent studies ruled out antibodies to intercellular or basement membrane antigens, but revealed marked upper dermal perivascular deposits of IgG and fibrin. Monoclonal type IV collagen antibody studies also showed marked perivascular fluorescence.

A **diagnosis of sun-bed induced pseudoporphyria** was made, thus revealing a new hazard for fair-skinned individuals who visit tanning salons.

Cripps DJ, Peters HA, Gocmen A, Dogramici I: **Porphyria turcica due to hexachlorobenzene:** A 20 to 30 year follow-up study on 204 patients. Br J Dermatol 1984; 111:413–422.

Thirty years after 3000 individuals in Turkey developed **porphyria** as a result of eating wheat contaminated with the **fungicide** hexachlorobenzene (C_6Cl_6), the victims are still recognizable. They have large scars (resulting from bullae) on their cheeks, arms, and dorsal surface of hands. They can be recognized by their **pinched**, **scarred faces**, **hyperpigmentation** in sun-exposed areas, and **hypertrichosis**. Years before, they were the "**monkey children**" born of the 1955 tragedy. Small, arthritically deformed, yet pain-free hands add to the picture. Nearly all will tell you of their weakness and paresthesias.

The possibility of avoiding such massive lifelong episodes of food poisoning justifies every penny spent by the United States FDA.

Long SA, Argenyi ZB, Piette WW: **Arciform blistering** in an elderly woman. Arch Dermatol 1988; 124:1705–1708.

A mildly pruritic vesiculobullous eruption of the abdomen, sacral region, and extensor surfaces of the extremities had persisted for 3 months in a 60-year-old woman. Examination revealed several annular erythematous plaques with peripheral tense blisters, as well as coalescing **annular lesions with peripheral vesicles**.

A diagnosis of bullous pemphigoid had been made on the basis of a subepidermal split in the biopsy. However, direct immunofluorescence of perilesional skin showed bright linear **deposits of IgA** at the basement membrane zone and provided the diagnosis of linear IgA dermatosis. This is a histologic diagnosis that distinguishes it from bullous pemphigoid and dermatitis herpetiformis, which are remarkably similar on clinical grounds.

A diagnosis of **linear IgA dermatosis** can be confirmed by doing a **biopsy** on **perilesional skin** for direct immunofluorescence. Linear deposits of IgA at the basement membrane distinguish it from bullous pemphigoid (with IgG and C3 at the basement membrane) and dermatitis herpetiformis (with granular IgA and C3 in the papillary dermal tips).

Immunofluorescent and **immunoelectron microscopy** are allowing us to discern new pigeonholes within the old pigeonholes of classification. In this case, however, we wonder about the possible role of chlorothiazide (a sulfonamide) in inducing the eruption.

Infectious Bullous Diseases

Naides SJ, Piette W, Veach LA, Argenyi Z: **Human parvovirus B19-induced vesiculopustular skin eruption.** Am J Med 1988; 84:968–972.

A 27-year-old black woman developed pruritus of the left antecubital fossa and left palm, as well as headache, anorexia, chills, fever, and a pruritic rash of the left arm. On day 3 the rash became painful and spread, and she also experienced arthralgias, nausea, and tender lymphadenopathy. On day 5 she was hospitalized. The rash consisted of **fine erythematous papules with petechiae** and small tense **pustules** and confluent pseudopustules. Petechiae were present on the palms and hard and soft palates, and tender papules were seen on the lower lip. The WBC was 3200/mm^3 with a depressed neutrophil count.

Biopsy of a vesiculopustule showed ballooning degeneration with keratinocyte necrosis and mixed inflammatory infiltrate with eosinophils, dilated vessels, extravasated erythrocytes, and a dense perivascular lymphohistiocytic infiltrate with large atypical cells. It combined features of morbilliform and vesiculopustular viral lesions. Because her community was involved in an outbreak of **fifth disease**, **serologic testing for human parvovirus B19** was performed, showing both anti-B19 IgM and anti-B19 IgG antibodies. Since IgM antibodies are present for only 2 to 3 months following acute infection, they are diagnostic of acute infection.

Viral infections previously known to **induce pustule formation** include herpes simplex, varicella-zoster, smallpox, and vaccinia. Human parvovirus B19 must now be added to the list.

Human parvovirus B19 causes **erythema infectiosum** (fifth disease) in children, with the "**slapped-cheek**" appearance. In adults, however, the infection often spares the face and is much harder to recognize. A faint transient rash occurs on the torso and extremities, along with a flu-like illness, arthralgias, synovitis, and lymphadenopathy. Long-term consequences may include a **rheumatoid arthritis–like synovitis** and chronic bone marrow suppression. Exposure during pregnancy may result in fetal infection and fetal death.

Pattishall EG III, Feingold M: Picture of the month: **Varicella.** Am J Dis Child 1985; 139:795–796.

Large umbilicated vesicles and small bullae occurred in a boy receiving steroids for poison ivy dermatitis. The lesions were asymmetrical and probably **localized in areas of poison ivy dermatitis**.

Yoshida M, Kusuda S, Tezuka T: **Varicella bullosa** in an adult. Br J Dermatol 1990; 123:846–848.

Four days before admission a 33-year-old woman developed papules and vesicles on the face. Within 2 days **giant bullae** (2 to 6 cm) appeared on the upper half of the body, and the entire skin exhibited 2- to 3-mm **vesicles and pustules**.

Positive cultures for the varicella-zoster virus were obtained from the vesicles, but not the giant pustules. *Staphylococcus aureus* was isolated from the pustules, and smears showed a few varicella-zoster virus-specific–antigen-positive epidermal cells. Skin biopsy of a giant pustular lesion showed a split in the granular layer with intracellular edema and acantholytic cells below, as seen in impetigo and the staphylococcal scalded skin syndrome. A diagnosis of varicella bullosa was made.

This variant of varicella, complicated by giant bullae, is **caused by superinfection with S. aureus** producing an exfoliative toxin. It is rare and usually affects infants and children.

Dawson TAJ, Dermott E, Connolly JH: **Unusual herpes** viral disease. Lancet 1980; 2:852.

In Northern Ireland 12 cases of a unique type of herpes-induced skin disease were seen in 1979–1980 from November to August. A **single vesicle** (0.5 to 2 cm) or zosteriform group of vesicles appeared on the scalp or foot (reminiscent of herpes simplex, herpes zoster, or orf), followed in a few days to several weeks by a **widespread varicelliform eruption of deeply seated pustules**. Headache, malaise, rigors, and diarrhea for a few days accompanied the pustules, which were most numerous on the **face**, **palms**, and **soles**. The mouth was usually spared. Varicelliform lesions sometimes clustered around the initial lesion, which was slow to heal and often lasted several weeks, causing local lymphadenopathy. The varicelliform eruption lasted about 2 weeks, but **debility** and **malaise** sometimes **lingered** another month.

Smears from bases of both initial and varicelliform lesions revealed **herpes-group virus on electron microscopy**. Acute and convalescent antibody titers showed no change for herpes simplex, varicella-zoster, cytomegalovirus, or Epstein-Barr virus. Attempts to isolate the virus were unsuccessful.

Kahn D, Hutchinson EA: **Generalized bullous orf.** Int J Dermatol 1980; 19:340–341.

A 65-year-old **sheep rancher** sustained a minor laceration of the left index finger while loading a truck. It produced an **open sore** that would not heal and became progressively more inflamed. After 1 month he sought treatment, which consisted of oral ampicillin and topical silver nitrate. About 3 weeks later he developed itching in the axilla and groin, followed by erythematous papules that evolved into tense vesicles and bullae, also involving the face.

Examination revealed **tense bullae** with **erythematous borders** on the trunk and arms. **Heavy serous crusts** were present on the face. The Nikolsky sign was absent. The finger was healing, but was still red and tender. He was afebrile. **Many hemorrhagic bullae** continued to develop on the scalp, trunk, extremities, and groin over the next 10 days, along with painful oral erosions. Spontaneous healing then occurred.

Cultures of vesicle fluid were negative for bacteria. A skin biopsy showed a V-shaped subepidermal bulla containing numerous polymorphonuclears and eosinophils, as well as a mild perivascular lymphocytic infiltrate. Crusts and bullous fluid were negative for virus on electron microscopy, but the **orf virus was isolated in viral culture**. The orf titer was originally 1:16, but became negative 2½ months later.

This man **acquired orf** through direct contact with sheep **while vaccinating** the entire flock for orf. Two ewes had been noted to have crusted lesions of sheep-pox of the lips and teats, and one lamb had had a sore on the nose.

A few cases of **erythema multiforme** associated with orf have been reported, as well as orf associated with a generalized varicelliform papulovesicular eruption. No virus was found in the secondary lesions.

In this case the generalized eruption began a full month after the presumed initial lesion of orf and was not associated with any systemic symptoms. It required more than a month to resolve. For the first time, orf virus was cultured from the disseminated lesions.

Bhawan J, Gellis S, Ucci A, Chang T-W: **Vesiculobullous lesions caused by cytomegalovirus infection** in an immunocompromised adult. J Am Acad Dermatol 1984; 11:743–747.

A 54-year-old **immunocompromised man** with progressive glomerulonephritis, cytomegalovirus infection, and pulmonary infection due to *Pneumocys-*

tis carinii developed isolated vesicles and bullae on an erythematous or hemorrhagic base on the arms, legs, and scalp. The **vesicles**, which were clear at first, rapidly became cloudy, and vasculitis or disseminated viral infection was suspected.

A **Tzanck smear** showed numerous **multinucleated giant cells** in the base of the vesicles. **Culture of fluid** from the vesicles, grown on **human lung fibroblasts**, showed refractile, enlarged cells at the end of 3 weeks. During the following week, these cells developed satellite foci. Culture on human amnion cells was negative. **Cytomegalovirus infection** was diagnosed, since this virus grows only on human fibroblasts. In contrast, herpes simplex and herpes zoster viruses grow rapidly in both types of cell cultures.

This study shows that a **positive Tzanck test** may indicate cytomegalovirus infection as well as herpes simplex, herpes zoster, and varicella. In the proper setting (immunocompromised patients), **precision in diagnosis** is attained only **by culture**. This patient, who had been taking prednisone and cyclophosphamide for glomerulonephritis, had previously had esophagitis; biopsy showed cytomegalovirus (large intracytoplasmic and intranuclear inclusions in squamous epithelium). In the skin, however, it was not possible to make the diagnosis on biopsy, which showed an intraepidermal vesicle with epidermal multinucleate giant cells and leukocytoclastic vasculitis.

Keane JT, James K, Blankenship ML, Pearson RW: **Progressive vaccinia associated with** combined **variable immunodeficiency**. Arch Dermatol 1983; 119:404–408.

A healthy 56-year-old woman preparing for a trip had a routine **smallpox vaccination**. Unlike the one she had had as a child, this one became a progressively enlarging **6-cm necrotic area**, surrounded by a ring of vesicles and a 15-cm diameter area of erythema and edema. Within 2 weeks she had a large white plaque on the side of the tongue, as well as multiple umbilicated white vesicles of the intergluteal fold, groin, and vulva. A biopsy of the primary lesion showed changes consistent with **vaccinia**, including focal epidermal necrosis with eosinophilic intracytoplasmic inclusions in epidermal cells.

A diagnosis of **progressive vaccinia** was made. Immunologic studies revealed anergy to the common skin test antigens, a very low B cell count, and diminished responsiveness of lymphocytes to phytohemagglutin, pokeweed antigen, and concanavalin A. Further studies confirmed that she had a combined variable immunodeficiency, which was unmasked by the progressive vaccinia. **Viral infection can modulate cell-mediated immune responses.**

Bronstein SW, Bickers DR, Lamkin BC: **Bullous dermatosis caused by** *Staphylococcus aureus* in locus minoris resistentiae. J Am Acad Dermatol 1984; 10:259–263.

High-dose dexamethasone therapy for an inoperable brain stem glioma resulted in numerous large pink striae on the arms, axillae, abdomen, and thighs of a 9-year-old girl. The subsequent development of terminal *Staphylococcus aureus* septicemia was associated with **S. *aureus*–induced bullae limited precisely to the striae atrophicae** of the left thigh.

The striae were viewed as a locus minoris resistentiae, permitting colonization and penetration by the bacteria and their toxins. *Locus minoris resistentiae* refers to a localized area of skin with diminished resistance to disease.

Fleming MG, Milburn PB, Prose NS: *Pseudomonas* **septicemia with nodules and bullae**. Pediatr Dermatol 1987; 4:18–20.

A 12-year-old girl with **systemic lupus erythematosus** was hospitalized with a temperature of 41°C while taking prednisone (60 mg daily). A chest x-ray revealed a cavity in the right middle lobe, which soon developed a fluid level.

Five days after admission, clear and **hemorrhagic bullae**, some with **erythematous rims**, appeared on the trunk and extremities. They were intermixed with **erythematous indurated nodules**. Gram's stain of bulla fluid revealed gram-negative rods, and ***Pseudomonas aeruginosa* grew on culture**. The same organism was cultured from the sputum, confirming cavitating pseudomonal pneumonia. Despite antibiotic treatment, she died 6 days after the onset of skin lesions.

A skin biopsy from the margin of a bulla showed an abscess cavity filled with neutrophils. Although no organisms were found, the tissue necrosis presumably occurred after **hematogenous dissemination** of *P. aeruginosa*.

Case records of the Massachusetts General Hospital. (Case 46-1990). N Engl J Med 1990; 323:1406–1412.

A 63-year-old woman was well until 1 month earlier when she noted intermittent constipation and diarrhea with occasional fecal incontinence. Two days prior to hospitalization she **had fallen** and was unable to rise. She then developed fever, bullae surmounting a 40- by 40-cm **purple indurated area of the right buttock**, and **subcutaneous crepitus** extending over both legs to the feet and also up the right side of the trunk to the neck. Admission studies revealed WBC 28,800, **gram-negative bacteremia**, and an extremely high creatine kinase level (24,225 U), indicating muscle destruction. **Aspiration of the bullae** released a large amount of **gas** and disclosed **gram-positive rods**.

The massive subcutaneous emphysema as well as the enzymatic evidence of muscle necrosis led to a diagnosis of **gas gangrene with myonecrosis**. A muscle biopsy of the gluteus maximus revealed gram-positive bacilli, identified as *Clostridium septicum*.

The **spreading purplish bullae** and crepitus alerted the staff to the possibility of clostridial sepsis, but it was the **muscle necrosis** that underscored this. Other bacterial organisms (*Proteus, Enterococcus, Escherichia coli, Staphylococcus, Streptococcus, Enterobacter, Klebsiella, Pseudomonas*, and *Bacteroides*) can induce similar bullae, but not muscle necrosis under ordinary conditions.

The **source** of clostridia was suspected to be a **carcinoma of the colon** undergoing necrosis. In turn, *C. septicum* was suspected as the most likely one of more than 60 species of clostridia known to produce gas gangrene. Although rare, it is the one seen in cases exhibiting both myonecrosis and colonic cancer.

The patient died shortly after admission, and autopsy totally confirmed the clinician's great insight.

Tyring SK, Lee PC: **Hemorrhagic bullae associated with *Vibrio vulnificus* septicemia.** Arch Dermatol 1986; 122:818–820.

Small gram-negative rods found in a smear of serosanguineous bulla aspirate explained why a 40-year-old woman suddenly developed fever, widespread leg pain and swelling, **purpura**, and **bullae**. They also explained why she died a day later. The patient had been **salt water fishing** a few days before in the Gulf of Mexico and received several **scratches** on the legs, which presumably were the portal of entry for the **lethal infection**.

This bacterium is well known on our Southern shores. It can produce septicemia in a patient who has waded into salt water or who has waded into a meal of uncooked oysters. Indeed, anyone who eats **uncooked seafood**, whether in the North or South, plays Russian roulette with these bacteria.

At particular risk are patients who have cirrhosis, renal insufficiency, chronic alcoholism, or immunosuppression, as their chemotactic, phagocytic, and complement defense systems often prove inadequate. The **bullae result** from **bacterial exotoxins** that cause dermal necrosis and subepidermal separation. Clusters of bacteria may be seen in dermal vessels, without surrounding inflammation. The **spectrum of other skin changes includes** macules, papules, pustules, petechiae, purpura, urticaria, erythema multiforme, cellulitis, and gangrene.

Vibrio vulnificus **septicemia** is not a diagosis to be made at leisure, or the patient will die in haste.

Grossman ME, Fithian EC, Behrens C, et al: Primary **cutaneous aspergillosis in six leukemic children**. J Am Acad Dermatol 1985; 12:313–318.

Hemorrhagic bullae appeared at the **sites of intravenous cannulas** and arm board taping in six children with acute leukemia receiving chemotherapy. All were neutropenic. A rapid presumptive diagnosis of cutaneous aspergillosis was made by doing **KOH** testing of the **blister roof**, which revealed broad septate hyphae. **Fungal cultures** were positive, and **biopsies** also revealed fungal hyphae in the dermis.

Lesions typically appeared on the palm or foot where the tape or arm boards made contact, beginning as erythematous papules or plaques. They then progressed through a hemorrhagic bullous phase to a **purpuric ulcer** with a central necrotic eschar. **Initial diagnoses included cellulitis and an irritant contact dermatitis to the tape.**

The most common organism isolated was *Aspergillus flavus* (three cases), but *A. fumigatus* and *A. niger* were also grown from some bullae tops.

The remarkable clustering of these patients—five in one hospital—called for **epidemiologic investigation**. The source of these contaminant molds, which grasped the opportunity to grow on immunosuppressed children, was tracked down to the **false ceiling of the hospital storage room**. It had been **recently flooded by a leak** from the bathroom above. Cultures of adhesive tape in the intravenous therapy cart and other supplies in the room resulted in isolation of the same three species of aspergillus as found in the patients. After the storeroom was closed and all supplies were discarded, the hospital did not see another case of cutaneous aspergillosis in the subsequent 3 years. Another source of *Aspergillus* infection in immunosuppressed patients in hospitals has been hospital reconstruction or renovation, when false ceilings are disturbed, liberating spores into ventilation systems.

Good detective work in both the roof of the blister and the roof of the storage room was required to solve these cases.

Betz TG, Davis BL, Fournier PV, et al: **Occupational dermatitis associated with straw itch mites** *(Pyemotes ventricosus)*. JAMA 1982; 247:2821–2823.

A 32-year-old woman manager of an import store developed a **chickenpox-like pruritic rash** on the torso and extremities. The lesions were thin-walled vesicles with erythematous areolae and 10 days later they had spread to the face and the rest of the body. She also complained of chills, fever, anorexia, diarrhea, and malaise.

Her two children, who visited the store frequently, and all four other employees had skin lesions similar to hers. One employee had a chigger-bite–like rash covering the antecubital spaces. Lesions were noted to appear only after the individual entered the storeroom. The onset of skin lesions coincided with the arrival of a shipment of **dried natural wheat** sold for decorative purposes.

The wheat and assorted dried flowers and grains were shaken over Petri dishes, and their contents were then examined under a dissecting microscope. A large number of **straw itch mites**, *Pyemotes ventricosus*, and a few larval ticks were isolated from the wheat. All other materials were negative for mites. An investigator who held the wheat developed numerous lesions, starting $1\frac{1}{2}$ hours after exposure. The central vesicle ruptured in 1 to 2 days, leaving granulomatous-like areas that healed in 7 to 10 days and residual hypopigmented areas that lasted more than 6 weeks.

The **wheat** harboring the mites had been imported from Spain 3 years earlier and stored in a warehouse in Los Angeles where there had been rodent infestations. The exact source of the mites was never determined, but 82 of 92 stores in Texas that received the wheat reported problems with bites.

This mite has apparently caused several epidemics of dermatitis in Europe and the United States related to infested straw or grain. Sources have included straw mattresses, straw used for animal bedding, puffed wheat, and oatmeal-containing fish food. Harvesters in Ohio and Indiana have been affected with "**grain itch**," which seems to parallel mild winters and a concomitant increase in the insect hosts of the mite.

The **mites are barely visible** with the naked eye as moving white specks on a dark background. Gravid females increase drastically in size, up to 2 mm in diameter, and are easily visible as pearly spheres.

Development of a **varicelliform or chigger-bite–like dermatitis** without a good history of outdoor exposure should suggest a search for products brought into homes or places of employment.

P. ventricosus can cause fever, malaise, anorexia, diarrhea, and other constitutional symptoms.

The need to reexamine, rethink, and retest your diagnosis continues throughout every visit.

Drug-induced Bullous Diseases

Fellner MJ, Katz JM: Occurrence of **bullous pemphigoid after furosemide therapy**. Arch Dermatol 1976; 112:75–77.

A 78-year-old woman with Parkinson's disease developed congestive heart failure and a urinary tract infection simultaneously. Therapy was started with several medications, including ampicillin for 1 week and furosemide (Lasix, 40 mg) daily. About 3 weeks after finishing the ampicillin, she developed a generalized pruritic maculopapular eruption. Furosemide was discontinued, and hydrochlorothiazide was substituted for diuresis. Four days later she returned with a **severe bullous eruption**, with tense bullae on erythematous bases, located in the same areas as the previous eruption.

A skin biopsy showed a subepidermal bulla with numerous eosinophils. Direct immunofluorescence confirmed the **diagnosis of bullous pemphigoid**, with IgG and C3 in a linear band at the basement membrane.

Her skin **cleared when the furosemide was discontinued**, but a fresh bulla appeared 10 days after furosemide therapy was begun again for diuresis. The skin then remained clear after furosemide was again withdrawn.

Other cases of drug-induced bullous pemphigoid have been reported with the following drugs:

penicillin V	topical fluorouracil
salicylazosulfapyridine	furosemide

In one similar case due to furosemide the bullous reaction developed after a maculopapular eruption in the antecubital fossae. The eruption was called **erythema multiforme**, but no histologic or immunofluorescence findings were reported.

Poh-Fitzpatrick MB, Ellis DL: **Porphyria like bullous dermatosis after chronic intense tanning bed and/or sunlight exposure**. Arch Dermatol 1989; 125:1236–1238.

Five patients had porphyria-like blisters and **mechanical fragility of skin after** long-term exposure to either the **sun or tanning-bed devices**.

Skin findings included vesicles and erosions variously involving the hands, face, arms, and legs, heavy freckling, and coarse wrinkling of thickened leathery skin. Milia, hypertrichosis, and sclerodermoid changes were generally absent. **All studies for porphyrins were normal** (red blood cell, plasma, urine, stool). Four of the patients used systemic photosensitizers either prior or during the development of vesiculation.

There is now a growing list of **drugs associated with photo-induced porphyria cutanea tarda–like lesions**. These include:

sulfonamides	naproxen
dapsone	pyridoxine
furosemide	tetracycline
nalidixic acid	

Porphyria cutanea tarda–like lesions **also occur in** patients with chronic renal failure undergoing **hemodialysis**.

Varma AJ, Fisher BK, Sarin MK: **Diazepam-induced coma with bullae and eccrine sweat gland necrosis**. Arch Intern Med 1977; 137:1207–1210.

Blisters that became eroded were the presenting sign in a semicomatose 27-year-old male nurse who had tried to commit **suicide** 36 hours previously **by taking 40 Valium** (10 mg) tablets. Most of the blisters were over bony prominences. Notable also was the presence of dark-brown crusts on the

414

penis, as well as ulcerations and swelling of the uvula. The **blisters were angular, geometric, circinate,** and surrounded by red borders.

Biopsies of the lesions showed a large subepidermal vesicle with an eosinophilic necrotic epidermal roof. The dermis was edematous with a sparse inflammatory infiltrate and necrotic sweat glands. A diagnosis was made of **bullous lesions associated with poison-induced coma.** He came out of the coma 2 days later, and after 2 weeks the skin lesions had healed.

It is believed that the bullae **result from pressure hypoxia,** hyperthermia with excessive sweating, and an associated toxic drug effect. The condition has been commonly known to occur in a variety of drug-coma states, particularly those induced by barbiturates and carbon monoxide poisoning. Other incriminated **drugs have included** methadone, hydrocodone, meprobamate, imipramine hydrochloride (Tofranil), acetyl-bromo-diethylacetyl-carbamide (Acetylcarbromal), glutethimide, and methyprylon (Noludar). **Hypoglycemic coma, cranial trauma, cerebrovascular accident, brain tumor,** and **viral encephalitis** have **also** been associated with bullous eruptions.

Bullae occur in approximately 5% of drug-induced comas. The bullae are irregular with maplike erythematous lesions having eroded centers. The lesions begin as distinct circumscribed **red patches over pressure areas** and then become cyanotic and develop blisters.

Reed KM, Sober AJ: **Methotrexate-induced necrolysis.** J Am Acad Dermatol 1983; 8:677–679.

A 72-year-old woman receiving daily **ultraviolet light treatments** for severe widespread psoriasis was given 15 mg of **methotrexate** intramuscularly. Five days later her back, chest, and intertriginous areas showed erythema, maceration, and **skin breakdown.** The UVB therapy was discontinued, and the patient made an uneventful recovery. However, she had numerous other major medical problems, including congestive heart failure, hypothyroidism, anemia, and renal insufficiency.

Six months later when she was receiving no UVL, methotrexate was again tried in low oral dosage (2.5 mg every 12 hr, 3 doses). Within 7 days the psoriatic plaques developed marked redness and tenderness, followed by **bullae and necrotic** areas of denuded epithelium on the back, buttocks, legs, and intertriginous areas, as well as in the mucosa. Clearing required 6 weeks. A positive Nikolsky sign was present.

Skin biopsies showed numerous dyskeratotic cells in the epidermis (maturation defect consistent with a **toxic antimetabolic effect**) and a subepidermal bulla with a slight perivascular lymphocytic infiltrate. This toxic epidermal necrolysis–like reaction suggests a sensitization phenomenon rather than a direct toxic effect of the methotrexate.

Chang JC: **Acute bullous dermatosis and onycholysis due to high-dose methotrexate and leucovorin calcium.** Arch Dermatol 1987; 123:990–992.

Multiple, variably sized, subepidermal unilocular **bullae** without inflammation appeared on the **palms, soles,** and dorsal aspect of the **hands and feet** of a 74-year-old man receiving a complex chemotherapy program for lymphocytic lymphoma. Analysis revealed that the bullae **appeared about 1 week after each dose of methotrexate** (1 gm IV) followed the next day by leucovorin calcium (100 mg IV every 6 hr × 5). The lesions became more numerous and larger with each methotrexate administration and eventually ulcerated. After cessation of methotrexate treatment there was no further cutaneous toxicity. Two other patients also had the same strange drug-related bullae. In one patient there was also extensive onycholysis, with eventual shedding of several fingernails and toenails and severe desquamation of the skin.

The principal **toxicities of methotrexate** are myelosuppression, oral and gastrointestinal mucositis, and hepatitis. Uncommon toxicities include alopecia, liver cirrhosis, interstitial pneumonitis, osteoporosis, and immune dysfunction. Rare cutaneous side effects include reactivation of solar dermatitis, acute desquamative dermatitis, papular skin rashes, **acute paronychia**, and blistering reactions.

Tomecki KJ, Wikas SM: **Cocaine-related bullous** disease. J Am Acad Dermatol 1985; 12:585–586.

For 2 years a 26-year-old man had bullae on the trunk and extremities, some with an iris appearance and others on an erythematous base. Spots of macular hyperpigmentation gave evidence of prior lesions. **Erythema multiforme** of unknown cause had been **diagnosed 1 year previously**. He denied any episodes of infection (herpetic, pulmonary, or other) and denied taking any drugs (prescribed, proprietary, or recreational). Biopsy revealed only a subepidermal bulla with a nonspecific perivascular infiltrate.

Innumerable tests ranging from fungal serology to examination of stools for ova and parasites were negative. The break in the case came with the finding of **cocaine in a urinary toxicology assay**.

When confronted with this objective observation, he admitted to the regular use of cocaine and also to the knowledge of an association between its use and the appearance of blisters. A diagnosis of **cocaine bullous disease** was made, and the patient (if not the bullae) disappeared forthwith.

Cocaine mix ("street cocaine") is an ill-defined mixture of one or more foreign diluent substances such as quinine, sugar, procaine, and amphetamines. Cocaine is a **potent topical vasoconstrictor** and local anesthetic that when sniffed can produce prolonged nasal vasoconstriction and ischemic necrosis with **perforation of the nasal septum**. It may also produce **acral vasospasm** and **laboratory evidence** of **connective tissue disease**.

Korenberg RJ, Landau-Price D, Penneys NS: **Vasopressin-induced bullous disease** and cutaneous necrosis. J Am Acad Dermatol 1986; 15:393–398.

A 70-year-old diabetic Hispanic woman, a member of Jehovah's Witnesses, having declined a blood transfusion, was given **intravenous vasopressin** to control bleeding from esophageal varices. The next day she developed flat purpuric **plaques with flaccid bullae on the anterior surface of the left thigh** and hip (nonpressure areas). No other areas were involved. The vasopressin, which was being given continuously through a central venous catheter at a rate of 0.2 U/minute was then discontinued. The bullae opened, leaving hemorrhagic ulcerations that slowly healed.

Rechallenge 3 days later with vasopressin (given continuously [0.6 U/minute] through a vein in the upper arm) for renewed gastrointestinal bleeding and impending shock resulted within 24 hours in **more extensive blistering** of the lower legs and feet with purpura and a small amount of ulceration and necrosis. There was no gangrene of the toes or fingers. Biopsy showed an intraepidermal bulla but no underlying vasculitis or thrombus formation. The vasopressin was gradually discontinued, and the patient was discharged with extensive ulceration of the lower legs but no new bullae.

Extravasation of intravenously administered vasopressin is well known to produce local ischemic necrosis with bulla formation and gangrene, as well as bullae at distant areas subject to pressure. This patient, by contrast, is the **first to develop bullae at a distance** from the intravenous site in areas not subject to compression.

Miscellaneous Causes of Bullae

Barnadas MA, Moreno A, Brunet S, et al: **Linear IgA bullous dermatosis associated with Hodgkin's disease.** J Am Acad Dermatol 1988; 19:1122–1124.

A 68-year-old man developed severe tonsillitis and dysphagia. **Excision of the right tonsil** revealed Hodgkin's disease. A **week later a pruritic bullous eruption** appeared, with some bullae reaching 10 cm in diameter. Some of the vesicles and bullae were hemorrhagic. He also had fever (temperature 38°C), malaise, lymphadenopathy, hepatosplenomegaly, and marked edema of the legs.

A skin biopsy showed a subepidermal blister containing fibrin, with an inflammatory infiltrate of mononuclear cells and eosinophils beneath the bullae. Microabscesses of polymorphonuclear neutrophils were present adjacent to subepidermal bullae. **Direct immunofluorescence revealed IgA** in a homogeneous linear pattern at the dermoepidermal junction, with IgG, C3, and IgM in lesser quantities in the same area.

Linear IgA disease was further confirmed with immunoelectron microscopy, which showed that the IgA **deposits were located below the lamina densa.** This pattern may be unique to patients who also have malignant disease associated with linear IgA bullous dermatosis. Other patients without known malignant disease have had the IgA deposits either at the lamina lucida (same location as bullous pemphigoid) or at the lamina lucida very close to the lamina densa.

Other bullous diseases that have been seen **with Hodgkin's disease** include erythema multiforme, pemphigus vulgaris, and pemphigus foliaceus. This is the third reported case of linear IgA bullous dermatosis associated with Hodgkin's disease.

In this case, five courses of chemotherapy over 5 months cleared the symptoms and the skin lesions. A few months later, however, the bullae reappeared. No recurrence of Hodgkin's disease was detected, but chemotherapy was restarted. The patient suddenly died of pancytopenia with gastrointestinal hemorrhage, and Hodgkin's disease was found in the spleen at autopsy. The parallel course of the cutaneous lesions and Hodgkin's disease in this case suggest that the two diseases were related.

McEvoy MT, Connolly SM: **Linear IgA dermatosis: Association with malignancy.** J Am Acad Dermatol 1990; 22:59–63.

Although there are documented cases of malignant disease reported in association with linear IgA dermatosis, **only two of ten** successive cases with this dermatosis at the Mayo Clinic were found to have a malignant disease. A 61-year-old-woman had chronic lymphatic leukemia, while a 65-year old man had a plasmacytoma that caused a T-8 compression fracture.

A review of ten other case reports of linear IgA dermatosis and malignant disease shows that most of the patients are over 60 years of age. **Hodgkin's disease**, other lymphomas, and **bladder cancer** were the most commonly seen malignant diseases.

The bullae of linear IgA dermatosis thus join those of bullous pemphigoid and epidermolysis bullosa acquisita in raising the **warning signal** of possible internal malignant disease.

Leigh G, Marsden RA, Wojnarowska F: **Linear IgA dermatosis with severe arthralgia.** Br J Dermatol 1988; 119:789–792.

An 8-year-old farm boy had been bottle-feeding lambs, two of which had recently suffered from "joint ill," a suppurative arthritis often linked to strep-   417

tococci of Lancefield groups C and D. Shortly thereafter he had a sore throat, fever, and abdominal pain, followed 5 days later by **myalgia and arthralgia**. Three days after the onset of joint pains he developed a vesicular eruption on the nose.

The joints were never swollen, but the ankles, wrists, and elbows were the sites of sharp pains, along with the muscles of the forearms and calves. Symptoms persisted for 2 months, along with low-grade progressive anemia (hemoglobin 9.4 gm/dl) and intermittent fever. The spleen tip became palpable, and he was found to have **tonsillitis (beta-hemolytic streptococcus** Lancefield group A) with an ASO titer greater than 800 U/ml. He was then treated with high-dose penicillin. The ESR was 130 mm/hour and slowly fell to 40 mm/hour by the fourth month.

By the **11th week** he had thin-roofed, friable, mildly **pruritic vesicles** on the arms, neck, ears, and face. In the 17th week he developed the "**cluster of jewels**" **sign** with a circle of new lesions surrounding a central healing area. Treatment with sulfapyridine gave immediate relief of blisters and joint pains but had to be continued for 14 months.

A skin biopsy showed a dermoepidermal junction split with neutrophils in the epidermis and superficial dermis and a scanty perivascular lymphocytic infiltrate. **Direct immunofluorescence** showed a linear band of IgA at the dermoepidermal junction. Indirect immunofluorescence was negative.

In the authors' experience with 29 children with **linear IgA dermatosis**, the eruption was **preceded by an upper respiratory tract infection or viral exanthem** (such as chickenpox) in 11 cases. Many of the children had received antibiotics. Likewise, 6 of 24 adult patients with linear IgA dermatosis had a preceding infection, ranging from an upper respiratory tract infection to brucellosis and tetanus. Twenty percent of the adults had taken **nonsteroidal anti-inflammatory drugs** before the onset of the eruption.

Green ST, Natarajan S: **Linear IgA disease and oesophageal carcinoma.** J Roy Soc Med 1987; 80:48–49.

A 68-year-old woman had numerous **pruritic small, tense, fluid-filled bullae** on the upper arms, shoulders, and back. The rash had been intermittent for **4 years.** Skin biopsy showed subepidermal bullae with a few eosinophils and lymphocytes, and direct immunofluorescence showed a fine linear band of IgA and patchy C3 at the dermo-epidermal junction. **Treatment with dapsone kept the skin clear for 15 months,** but she then developed dysphagia and weight loss, leading to discovery of a **squamous cell carcinoma of the esophagus,** which caused her death 9 months later.

Linear IgA disease **may be a cutaneous marker of malignant disease**.

Watsky KL, Orlow SJ, Bolognia JL: **Figurate** and **bullous eruption** in association with **breast carcinoma.** Arch Dermatol 1990; 126:649–652.

Blisters of the **hands, feet,** and **waist** of a 70-year-old woman were clearly discerned as due to trauma. A biopsy showed a subepidermal split and, on immunofluorescence, linear deposits of IgG and C_3 at the dermoepidermal junction. At this point, the diagnostic options were bullous pemphigoid and epidermolysis bullosa acquisita.

Within 3 month, and despite prednisone and azathioprine therapy, the patient developed **multiple concentric arcuate plaques** on the trunk and extremities. Numerous **erosions** were also seen on the dorsum of the hands and feet as well as the elbows. Further studies included porphyrin assays that ruled out porphyria cutanea tarda and variegate porphyria. No tumors were shown on tomography of the head, chest, and abdomen. However, the cause was finally revealed in a mammogram. This showed an asymmetric density in the medial aspect of the left breast that, on biopsy, proved to be an infiltrating ductal carcinoma.

Radiation therapy of the breast cancer was followed by complete disappearance of the patient's eruption. There has been no recurrence.

Shehade SA, Joyce HJ, Kumararatne DS, et al: Transitional cell **carcinoma of the bladder** associated with **generalized bullous eruption**. Clin Exp Dermatol 1988; 13:28–30.

A 65-year-old man, who had worked as a roof asphalter for 51 years, developed **hematuria** as a result of bladder carcinoma. Prior to his receiving radiotherapy, an extensive **erythematous vesiculobullous eruption** appeared on the trunk and limbs, along with erosions of the pharynx and glans penis. **Erythema multiforme was suspected**.

Results of a **skin biopsy** more closely resembled **bullous pemphigoid**, with a subepidermal blister containing leukocytes and eosinophils, and a similar upper dermal perivascular infiltrate. No antibodies to intercellular cement or basement membrane were detected, but indirect immunofluorescence revealed binding of **IgG3 autoantibodies** to the **cytoplasm** of **basal cells** of the epidermis. IgG3 antibodies are complement fixing and hence could be expected to damage the basal layer and induce blisters.

Autoantibodies to epidermal antigens, detected by indirect immunofluorescence, show three cytoplasmic staining patterns: general cytoplasmic (G-CYT), upper epidermal cytoplasmic (U-CYT), and basal cell cytoplasmic (BCL). Antibodies specific to the basal cell layer of the epidermis are very uncommon. They are seen mainly with **drug reactions** and **burns**, but have been reported in one patient with adenocarcinoma of the rectum.

Weismann K, Høyer H, Christensen E: Acquired **zinc deficiency** in **alcoholic liver cirrhosis**: Report of two cases. Acta Derm Venereol 1980; 60:447–449.

Bullae and later **erosions** developed on the **soles** of a 52-year-old man with a long history of alcohol abuse. On examination, he showed erosions of his heels as well as a **desquamating dermatitis** of the **palms** and **soles**. He also had a region of **alopecia** on the occiput.

Because of his alcoholic cirrhosis, a serum zinc level was obtained. It was low (7.7 µmol/liter, normal 11.4 to 18.9), and a diagnosis of **zinc deficiency dermatitis** was made.

Within 2 weeks of zinc therapy (220 mg zinc sulfate bid) his skin became normal and his mental status improved. Subsequently, hair regrew in the occipital area and Beau's lines appeared in his nails.

Anh **alcoholic** with a **treatment-resistant dermatitis** or **ulcer** deserves a zinc level determination.

Groff JW, White JW: **Vesiculobullous cutaneous lymphatic reflux**. Cutis 1988; 42:31–32.

A 70-year-old woman who weighed more than 300 pounds had received radiotherapy for adenocarcinoma of the cervix 2 months prior to admission for respiratory distress. In the hospital she developed multiple clear vesicles and **bullae** on the lower abdomen and entire right leg. These were tense to flaccid, thin roofed, and fragile, and **once ruptured, clear watery fluid continued to exude from the base**. A Tzanck smear, Nikolsky sign, and exudate smear were all negative, but biopsy showed a large lymphatic vessel opening directly in the subepidermal bulla.

Lymphedema due to radiation or tumor occlusion of the lymphatic flow causes this type of vesiculobullous eruption. The **steady seepage** after a bulla is broken will continue until the vessel is either resected or spontaneously repairs itself.

Lymphedema also can be **responsible** for many other skin problems, including cellulitis, elephantiasis, ulceration, and lymphangiosarcoma.

Di Leonardo M, Jacoby RA: **Acquired cutaneous lymphangiectasias** secondary to scarring **from scrofuloderma**. J Am Acad Dermatol 1986; 14:688–690.

Translucent **thick-walled vesicles** arranged in a **linear pattern** on the right side of the trunk in a 68-year-old black woman proved to be dilated lymphatic spaces. The vesicles were up to 5 mm in diameter and had developed years before in an area of scrofuloderma that had healed with an underlying scar. Since the scarring was superficial and did not involve the main lymphatic channels, there was no associated lymphedema.

Such **lymphatic vesicles result from lymphatic obstruction**. They may appear following surgical scarring, trauma, radiation therapy, recurrent infection, scleroderma, and anomalies of the deep lymphatics.

Ziv R,, Schewach-Millet M, Trau H: **Lymphangiectasia. A complication of thoracotomy** for bronchial carcinoid. Int J Dermatol 1988; 27:123.

Six years after a left upper lobectomy a 68-year-old man noted **grayish-brown** "bumps" appearing in the **incisional scar**. They gradually increased in size and number, accompanied by mild pruritus. Close examination revealed translucent, thick-walled, fluid-filled vesicles and grayish-brown warty growths in a zosteriform pattern on the left chest wall. **Histologic study confirmed lymphangiectasis.** Any interference with lymphatic drainage may produce this type of lesion. It has been reported with keloids, scleroderma, mastectomy scars, scrofuloderma scars, and radiation therapy.

Burges GE, Walls CT, Maize JC: **Subcutaneous phaeohyphomycosis** caused by *Exserohilum rostratum* **in an immunocompetent host**. Arch Dermatol 1987; 123:1346–1350.

Brown jelly-filled blisters and systemic symptoms of nausea, dizziness, and chills **followed a probable jellyfish sting** of the right leg in a 55-year-old healthy woman. Hemorrhagic blisters and nodules persisted on the area of the sting for 3 months despite antibiotics. At that time a biopsy disclosed a **dermal abscess** containing **golden-brown** spherical and cylindrical mycelial elements. **Culture** (brain-heart infusion agar) of a 6-mm punch biopsy of another purpuric nodule resulted in a **green-black colony of *Exserohilum rostratum***. Conjoint excision and ketoconazole therapy proved curative.

Three other examples of similar cutaneous abscesses due to these dematiaceous fungi are cited. **Phaeohyphomycosis** refers to infection caused by fungi with **dark septate mycelial elements** in tissue. Specific causative organisms are in the genera *Bipolaris* and *Exserohilum*, previously classified as *Helminthosporium* and *Drechslera*.

Seligman PJ, Mathias CGT, O'Malley MA, et al: **Phytophotodermatitis from celery** among grocery store workers. Arch Dermatol 1987; 123:1478–1482.

Red blotchy streaks and **blisters** followed by hyperpigmentation were found to be **due to sun exposure** or tanning salon use in 19 grocery **workers who** handled celery. The cause was the photosensitizer psoralen present in healthy celery. In these celery samples the leafy ends showed levels of 5-methoxypsoralen and 8-methoxypsoralen of more than 20 parts/million, which is sufficient to photosensitize the skin. Cutaneous provocation tests with trimmed surfaces of the celery samples produced phototoxic reactions.

Noteworthy is the implication of "healthy" celery, since the usual problem with phytophotodermatitis comes from celery infected with **pink rot fungus** (*Sclerotinia sclerotiorum*). This fungus, as well as other environmental stresses such as herbicide exposure, **cause the celery plant to produce greater amounts of psoralen**, thus posing greater risks to those who harvest and handle celery.

Parsnips, limes, lemons, figs, dill, carrots, and parsley are the **other psoralen-containing plants** that lurk in the grocery store, waiting to afflict those who would "touch and tan." Packaging untrimmed celery and parsnips in large-enough plastic bags should help reduce the problem of phytophotodermatitis, as most contact with psoralen occurs from cut or abraded plant surfaces.

Friedmann PS, Coburn P, Dahl GC, et al: **PUVA-induced blisters**, complement deposition, and damage to the dermoepidermal junction. Arch Dermatol 1987; 123:1471–1477.

Nonhemorrhagic, **tense blisters** 0.5 to 2 cm in diameter developed on normal skin in 7 of 56 **patients receiving psoralen plus long-wave ultraviolet light** therapy. They appeared after 6 to 14 exposures and were related to friction and trauma, appearing on the feet, shin, hand, and elbow.

Skin biopsies revealed mainly epidermal changes, with intracellular edema, vacuolization, and keratinocyte destruction. Suprabasal blistering and dermoepidermal separation were also seen. Direct immunofluorescence showed **C3 in granular deposits at the dermoepidermal junction** and/or around upper dermal vessels. Spontaneous PUVA blisters showed separation above the basal layer, while suction PUVA blisters separated through the lamina lucida of the dermoepidermal junction.

It was demonstrated that during PUVA treatment patients are more susceptible to experimental blistering by suction, because of **light-induced damage to the dermoepidermal junction**. This explains their susceptibility to the commonplace friction blister, which occurred on acral sites or over bony prominences. Blistering times were still reduced 3 weeks after completion of therapy.

Skill in taking a history calls for recognition of what part is true, what part relevant, and what part garbage.

Burns

Burns rise to the level of diagnostic challenge only in the patients who cannot or will not give you a history. We recall a patient with what appeared to be multiple cigarette burns. Although she quietly denied any knowledge of their origin or nature, she produced fresh burns on her wrists the day after we told her that we would know the diagnosis if the eruption involved the flexural surface of the wrists.

Burns are crudely classified, even by Boy Scouts, as:

first degree–erythema only, followed by peeling, as in the common sunburn
second degree–vesicles and bullae that, on healing, leave no scars
third degree–ulcer, which heals with a scar
fourth degree–complete destruction of skin and underlying tissue, followed by toxemia

Burns may become **infected** with bacteria, fungi, or viruses, with ensuing cellulitis, erysipelas, and sepsis. And recall that a chronic ulcer in a burn scar, the feared **Marjolin's ulcer**, may become malignant.

Kligman LH, Kligman AM: Reflections on **heat**. Br J Dermatol 1984; 110:369–375.

In the midst of our concern over harm to the skin from ultraviolet light, a plea is made to recognize the **hazards of infrared radiation** (heat). Infrared radiation causes increased synthesis of elastin and microfibrils by irradiated fibroblasts. It also greatly enhances elastic fiber proliferation induced by ultraviolet radiation, contributing to chronic sun damage.

Witness these **examples**:

kang cancer: sleeping on beds of hot bricks in China
Kashmir cancer: wearing pots of hot coals next to the skin in Kashmir, India.
Kairo cancer: contact with benzene-burning flasks to keep warm in Japan
turf or peat fire cancer: on the lower legs of women working before an open hearth in Ireland
eyeglass cancer: focused heat rays from rimless eyeglasses
erythema ab igne: fireplace, heating pad, space heater
premature aging of skin: glass blowers, bakers, kitchen workers
focal cutis laxa: hair dryer used 1.5 hours at high intensity daily for 7 years.

Stay cool and your skin will stay young.

Amy BW, McManus WF, Goodwin CW Jr, Pruitt BA Jr: **Lightning injury** with survival in five patients. JAMA 1985; 253:243–245.

Lightning causes **unique arborizing and serpiginous patterns** of superficial dermal burns due to the splash effect of an arcing lightning bolt. Includes two photographs.

Schuler G, Honigsmann H, Wolff K: The syndrome of **milker's nodules in burn injury**: Evidence for indirect viral transmission. J Am Acad Dermatol 1982; 6:334–339.

The appearance of solid, shiny, **red papules within a freshly reepithelialized burn site** in this 3-year-old girl posed a diagnostic problem. The burn had occurred 10 days prior when the little girl had stepped into a milker's bucket filled with hot water.

The biopsy showed vacuolized cells in the epidermal granular layer, as well as an edematous dermis filled with a diffuse lymphohistiocytic infiltrate and

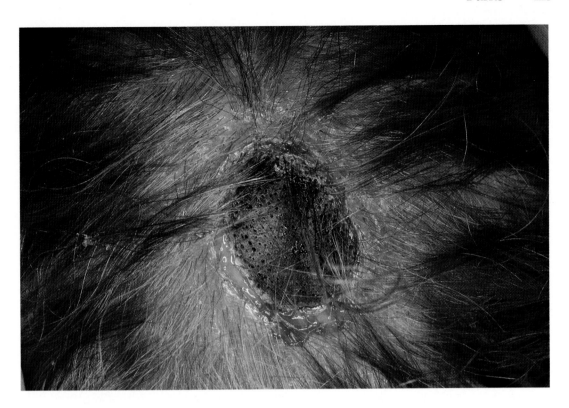

dilated capillaries. But the diagnostic answer came with **electron microscopy showing viral particles** typical for pox virus, subgroup II in the vacuolized cells.

Propagation of the virus in **tissue culture** established the **definitive diagnosis of paravaccinia infection**.

Interestingly, the lesions resembled the papules seen in the so-called vaccine rouge following smallpox vaccination with vaccine containing contaminant paravaccinia virus.

The burned skin provided optimal conditions for growth of traces of virus that could not induce disease in normal skin. Thus, like orf, milker's nodules can be transferred indirectly.

And the little girl—all of her ominous papules healed without treatment and without scarring, within the month.

Louis DS, Wilson MR, Hankin FM: '**Kissing lesions**' of the thorax and upper extremity. Arch Surg 1987; 122:821–822.

A 56-year-old man slept on his forearm while under the influence of drugs. At the time of admission the resultant **erythematous lesions on the forearm and ipsilateral chest wall** were **misinterpreted as thermal burn injuries**, since his disoriented state precluded an accurate history and examination.

After the patient was on the burn service for 2 days, a consultant identified the problem as the **skin necrosis of compartmental syndrome** seen in crush injury. Such kissing lesions may demand fasciotomy to avoid permanent functional loss.

These true pressure ulcers involve the muscle as well as the skin. They may **occur with relatively short periods of compression** of the arm by the weight of the body in any comatose patient.

Candidiasis

The secret for making a diagnosis of candidiasis is in the fold and in the pustule. Candidiasis is a disease of warm, moist, macerated intertriginous skin. This biosphere allows the yeast *Candida albicans* to grow in such quantity as to produce toxins injurious to the skin. As a result, the folds become tender, red, even erosive. There are no pustules in the fold. These distinctive signs of candidiasis are seen as satellite lesions in adjacent skin not subject to the shearing force of motion. Here the toxin is a chemoattractant for the myriads of intraepidermal leukocytes, visible as a pustule.

Consider the **folds** that may show candidiasis. The classic examples are inframammary, axillary, inguinal, gluteal, and perianal. These are the great folds, but the little folds of the angles of the mouth, the interdigital spaces and nail folds, the preputial fold, the labial folds, and retroauricular areas must be considered as candidiasis prone. We recall the diagnostic force majeure that we could summon years ago by telling a patient she had dermatitis erosiva interdigitalis blastomycetica. Today, it is plain candidiasis of the finger webs, an occupational hazard for anyone in wet work.

Once the clinical diagnosis is entertained, it can be confirmed by KOH examination, Gram stain, and culture on Sabouraud's agar.

If one looks **behind the diagnosis**, candidiasis suggests diabetes, a malnourished state, or the immunodeficiency of the elderly, a patient undergoing chemotherapy, or a patient with AIDS. It is a disease of the infant kept in wet diapers. And it is a disease of the newborn who acquires it passing through a vagina thick with yeast. In chronic mucocutaneous candidiasis, a heritable cell defect is present. This is the most intractable form and may herald a thymoma in an adult. It can persist for years, producing nail dystrophy as well as granulomas.

The **oral** and **vaginal orifices** are as common a site for candidiasis as the folds. Here, white leukoplakic plaques suggest the diagnosis. In the infant this has the special designation of **thrush**. It is a common accompaniment of cradle cap, the scalp seborrheic dermatitis of yeast origin. **Perleche** is the diagnosis for candidiasis at the angles of the mouth where drooling trapped by a labial overhang sets the stage. Again, candidal growth accounts for much of the paronychia seen.

Yeast remains a ferment for much cutaneous disease. Look for it.

Ro BI: **Chronic mucocutaneous candidosis**. Int J Dermatol 1988; 27:457–462.

onset:
   infancy
location:
   diaper area
   oral
   nails
morphology:
   red, raised, serpiginous, scaling, hyperkeratotic
   paronychia
   dystrophy—nails
associated endocrinopathy, autoimmune:
   hypothyroidism
   hypoparathyroidism
   hypoadrenalism
   diabetes mellitus
unusual:
   adult onset, suggests presence of thymoma, myasthenia gravis
course:
   decades

Perel Y, Taïeb A, Fontan I, et al: Candidose cutanée congenitale: Une observation avec revue de la littérature. Ann Dermatol Venereol 1986; 113:125–130.

A 9-day-old baby girl was seen in consultation concerning a **pustular eruption of the palms and soles** of 1 week's duration. Examination disclosed a **generalized erythematous** and **papular eruption** with many small superficial pustules. Papuloerosive lesions with peripheral desquamation were present on the buttocks.

A **smear** from a palmar pustule immediately confirmed the clinical diagnosis of **congenital cutaneous candidiasis**. Numerous hyphae admixed with polymorphonuclear leukocytes were present. Blood and urine cultures were sterile, as were vaginal cultures of the mother.

The **differential diagnosis** centered on impetigo, herpes, varicella, and syphilis, as well as postnatal acquired candidiasis. Most importantly, pustular erythema toxicum was ruled out by the smear.

This condition suggests an **intrauterine infection** due to candidal chorioamnionitis, since it often is present at birth. Amniocentesis could provide a portal of entry. Another source is an ascending infection of the birth canal.

Dons RF, Cashell AW: **A recurrent intertriginous rash** responsive to topical as well as surgical therapy. Arch Dermatol 1988; 124:431–434.

Intermittent **KOH-positive intertrigo** of the groin and intergluteal and inframammary areas was present for **5 years** in an obese 31-year-old woman, previously treated with an ileojejunal bypass. It failed to clear despite treatment with oral ketoconazole, topical antifungals, and topical steroids. Serum zinc levels were normal. Computed tomography revealed a **mass in the pancreas**, and serum **glucagon levels were elevated** (2600 to 4600 ng/liter [normal 50 to 200 ng/liter]). Serum amino acids were decreased to 11% of normal. A diagnosis of **necrolytic migratory erythema** was made, with skin biopsy showing hyperkeratosis, parakeratosis, and mild psoriasiform hyperplasia of the epidermis. After the glucagonoma was resected, the eruption cleared.

Note: **Hypoaminoacidemia** is a universal feature of the glucagonoma syndrome.

Beware of a casual approach to intertrigo, for delay in recognizing an underlying glucagonoma may result in metastasis.

Witkowski JA, Parish LC: **Candidiasis**: The **isomorphic response**. Acta Derm Venereol 1985; 65:355–358.

After 10 days of hospitalization, a 72-year-old diabetic man developed a **linear band of erythematous papules**, **pustules**, and scaling on the right chest wall. This band followed a dermatomal distribution corresponding to T-12. **Herpes zoster was suspected**, but microscopic examination showed the pseudohyphae and budding yeast cells of candidiasis. The **cause** was **scratching with nails badly infected with *Candida albicans***. Most of the fingernails were yellowish and hyperkeratotic, with erythema and edema of the surrounding nail folds (**chronic paronychia**).

An 82-year-old diabetic woman with generalized pruritus and right hemiparesis had a well-defined patch of **erythema** and **scaling** studded with **pustules** on her left hip and thigh. Discrete erythematous **linear streaks with papules and pustules** were present in the surrounding skin, only in **areas she could reach to scratch**. **Chronic paronychia** and yellow hyperkeratotic nails were present on three fingers of the left hand. **Candidiasis** was diagnosed in both the skin lesions and fingernails.

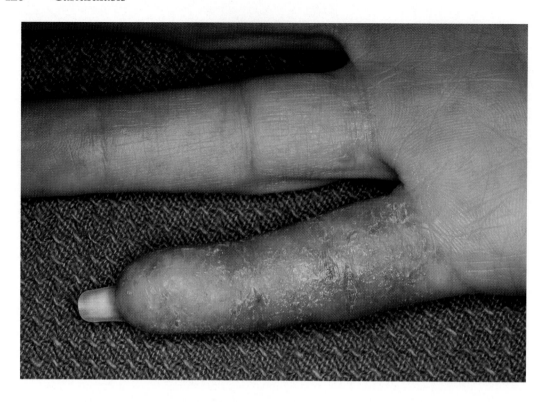

If pustules are present in erythematous scaly scratch marks, think of candidiasis.

Kien CL, Kohler E, Goodman SI, et al: **Biotin-responsive in vivo carboxylase deficiency** in two siblings with secretory diarrhea receiving total parenteral nutrition. J Pediatr 1981; 99:546–550.

Alopecia and mucocutaneous candidiasis occurred in two children, ages 7 and 5 years, with secretory diarrhea and seizures, only after they had been receiving **biotin–free total parenteral nutrition** for several months. Measurements of serum biotin levels were normal, but **urine biotin excretion** was **low**. Possibly they developed clinical signs of carboxylase deficiency (organic aciduria, metabolic acidosis) only when the serum biotin fell to the lower range of normal.

Cowan MJ, Wara DW, Packman S, Ammann AJ: Multiple **biotin–dependent carboxylase deficiencies** associated with defects in T-cell and B-cell immunity. Lancet 1979; 2:115–118.

A 3-month-old girl developed an **erythematous rash on the face** and **eyelids** and **cracks** in the **interdigital spaces**. At 6 months of age she had delayed motor milestones, mild nystagmus, and mild hypotonia, and at 16 months she had an acute viral illness followed by truncal ataxia, **alopecia, conjunctivitis,** bilateral **corneal ulcerations**, and **periorificial dermatitis** with cultures positive for *Candida albicans*. The rash cleared with the use of topical antifungal/steroid cream. At 18 months she was found to have **lactic acidosis**, and analysis of the urine revealed increased excretion of metabolites associated with the catabolic pathways for leucine, isoleucine, and valine, confirming **multiple carboxylase deficiency. Treatment with biotin** corrected these abnormalities, and she had no further problems with candida dermatitis, keratoconjunctivitis, alopecia, or corneal ulceration.

Ammann AJ: New insights into the causes of **immunodeficiency disorders**. J Am Acad Dermatol 1984; 11:653–660.

Late in the first year of life this patient developed **mucocutaneous candidiasis, dermatitis, keratoconjunctivitis**, and **alopecia**. He proved to be at risk for **recurrent infections**, both bacterial and viral, with otitis media and pneumonia prime possibilities. Not only were immunologic deficits present, but neurologic deterioration could be expected to occur with progressive ataxia.

He was found to have organic aciduria, **lactic acidosis**, hyperammonemia, and hyperglycinemia. A **diagnosis of multiple carboxylase enzyme deficiency** was made. Biotin in a dose of 5 to 40 mg/day was remarkably effective in clearing the problem.

Multiple carboxylase enzyme deficiency must be suspected in any infant or child with mucocutaneous candidiasis and recurrent infections. It must be distinguished from the **autoimmune endocrinopathy** state that also accounts for mucocutaneous candidiasis but in which there is no biotin metabolic error.

Biotin is the necessary cofactor for all of the carboxylases and hence is the sovereign remedy for these enzyme deficiencies. (It thus shares pride of therapeutic place with zinc, an essential component of other enzymes whose deficiency likewise results in mucocutaneous candidiasis.)

Samaranayake LP, MacFarlane TW (eds): Oral Candidiasis. London, Wright, 1990; 265 pp.

This is the ultimate reference source on candidiasis of the oral cavity, with special sections on clinical diagnosis and laboratory confirmation.

There's a little bit of factitial dermatitis in most everything you see.

Cellulitis

The diagnosis of cellulitis covers a spectrum as wide as that of sunburn. It extends from a simple tender area of erythema to a localized painful bullous eruption. It is often due to group A hemolytic streptococci. This is the *Streptococcus pyogenes* infection we recognize as a distinct form of cellulitis called **erysipelas**. Once a serious, frightening, at times fatal, disease, it has now been subdued by penicillin.

Recognition of the mild forms of erysipelas may be difficult, especially those that are a sequence of **dermatitis** or **lymphedema**. It is too easy to dismiss the redness as nonspecific inflammatory change. We recall a case of frostbite in which the shift to erysipelas was missed.

Cellulitis is a clinical diagnosis resting firmly on the history and clinical changes in the skin. Laboratory help comes in assessing possible systemic effects, in looking for bacterial or fungal origins, and in ruling out such specific forms as eosinophilic cellulitis (Wells' syndrome).

A blood count, biopsy, and culture are your three worthy helpers in searching for more than your eye can see. Use them. Culture that portal of entry as well as the throat and the nose for pathogens you can attack. Biopsy for the unsuspected. And take the history once more. The causes of cellulitis are as broad as they are long. Could it be a drug eruption or even a factitial burn?

Chartier C, Grosshans E: **Erysipelas**. Int J Dermatol 1990; 29:459–467.

Erysipelas is a special form of **cellulitis due to streptococcal infection**. It demands recognition because of its almost universal dramatic response to penicillin. When first sighted by the patient, it may be no more than a small area of tender erythema, but preceded by a day by acute onset of chills, fever, malaise, and nausea.

When seen by the physician, erysipelas is usually a **tense shiny erythematous plaque**. The area is edematous and has a sharp demarcation. **Lymphangitis** and **lymphadenopathy** may be present. **Purulent bullae** and small areas of necrosis are also seen at times. Attenuated examples occur in which the fever and attendant systemic signs are absent.

The most frequently involved sites are the **lower extremities**, although the classic photogenic examples are on the face. Erysipelas of the trunk may develop after surgery or appear in the **neonate** following infection of the umbilical stump or circumcision site. Other **portals of entry** are leg ulcers, pyodermas, insect bites, and fissures.

Complications include abscesses, necrosis or gangrene, and thrombophlebitis. The necrotic form often has a backdrop of arteriosclerosis or diabetes. Rarely, glomerulonephritis may develop, and septicemia as well as cachexia has been reported. Recurrent attacks of erysipelas may occur, and this leads to **chronic lymphedema**.

The **diagnosis** is made on the basis of the clinical findings. Although group A streptococci are the usual cause, culture of aspirates from the lesion are negative, and cultures from a presumed portal of entry, such as a cut, show these pyogenic streptococci in only 11%. The blood count will reveal polymorphonuclear leukocytosis. At times, a throat culture or a nasal swab will disclose the source of the invading streptococci. It is well also to look for **hematuria** and **proteinuria** at the first week and again at 3 weeks because of the possibility of streptococcal glomerulopathy.

Although erysipelas is usually a manifestation of group A or group B streptococcal infection, **other organisms may produce a clinically identical picture. Thus, rarely, one may see staphylococcal erysipelas, pneumococcal erysipelas, and *Yersinia* erysipelas.

Of major **immediate differential diagnostic concern** is **necrotizing fasciitis**. Here the infection is in the subcutaneous tissue and by closing major vessels leads to necrosis requiring surgical debridement. The clinical picture is that of erysipelas, but in a highly magnified, more serious form with overwhelming systemic signs.

Hook EW III: **Acute cellulitis**. Arch Dermatol 1987; 123:460–461.

Cellulitis:

erythema, edema, pain
due to bacterial infection, usually gram-positive organism: beta-hemolytic
    streptococci and/or *Staphylococcus aureus*
isolation successful in only one of four patients:
    swab of portal of entry, if seen
    needle aspiration
    biopsy
    blood culture
differential diagnosis:
    gram-negative cellulitis
    dermatophytic infection or id

Erysipelas:

a specific type of cellulitis in which **borders are sharp**, **lymphangitis** occurs due to group A beta-hemolytic streptococci—rarely group C or D

Hurwitz RM, Tisserand ME: **Streptococcal cellulitis proved by skin biopsy** in a coronary artery bypass patient. Arch Dermatol 1985; 121:908–909.

A warm erythematous edematous area of the left lower leg in a 53-year-old diabetic man was found on **biopsy** to be cellulitis with **chains of gram-positive organisms** present **in the dermis**. A diagnosis of streptococcal cellulitis was made, and his response to oral erythromycin was excellent.

Two important points deserve attention: The patient had had a saphenous vein harvested from that leg for coronary bypass surgery 2 years before. Secondly, he had an active scaling KOH-positive **tinea pedis** of the soles and interdigital spaces. Presumably the **fungal-induced fissures allowed streptococci to enter** and lodge in a **locus minoris resistentiae**.

Patients who have had **saphenous venectomy** deserve long-term foot care to eliminate interdigital maceration, tinea pedis, or any fissures that might serve as portals of entry for bacteria.

Tharakaram S, Keczkes K: **Necrotizing fasciitis**: A report of five patients. Int J Dermatol 1988; 27:585–588.

This is a **think-quick diagnosis**. Any delay can be fatal, since this is cellulitis that rapidly produces gangrene of the subcutaneous tissues. It is usually a malignant form of **streptococcal infection** and **requires surgical debridement**.

Heralded by chills and fever, this infection is evident in a day or two as the affected **skin becomes reddish-blue and develops vesicles and bullae**, followed by **infarction and eschar**. The gangrene rapidly extends to and below the skin, producing deep ulceration and thick black eschars.

Immediately **culture** the fluid from an unbroken bulla for identification of the responsible organism and its antibiotic sensitivity pattern. It is hard to be too aggressive medically or surgically in treating this condition, first described by Meleney in 1924 as **hemolytic streptococcal gangrene**.

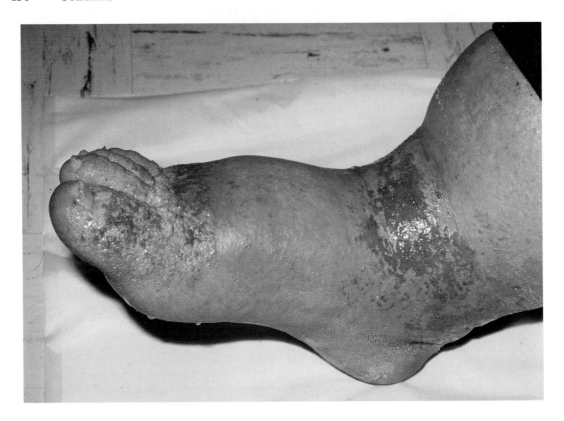

The **differential diagnosis** centers on:

> Fournier's gangrene of the genitalia
> synergistic necrotizing cellulitis with myonecrosis
> progressive synergistic gangrene

And don't forget to think of it next time you see erysipelas.

Feingold DS: **Gangrenous and crepitant cellulitis.** J Am Acad Dermatol 1982;
6:289–299.

Prompt diagnosis is urgently needed to expedite mandatory therapy and avoid unnecessary multilating surgery in any case of gangrenous or crepitant cellulitis. **First, secure blood cultures and soft tissue x-ray studies.**

If crepitus or gas is found in tissue by x-ray examination:

> Surgeon must lay open infected area to visualize subcutaneous tissue, fascia, muscle.
> Obtain exudate for odor, Gram stain, and aerobic and anaerobic cultures.

If progressive necrosis or rapidly spreading cellulitis, proceed as above, but in addition:

> **examination** of aspirate or **crushed tissue** for **fungus** (KOH, Wright stain, India ink)
> **punch biopsy edge of lesion** for **frozen section**, PAS, silver methenamine stain

If rate of spread of cellulitis is slow, necrosis minimal:

> treat with antibiotics and watch

The following **clinical entities of this subset** of pyodermas and cellulitis are recognized:

Clostridial cellulitis:

> usually due to *Clostridium perfringens*. Cardinal sign is **gas in tissue**, but recognize that gas may also occur after trauma or rupture of lung or viscera.
> no odor

Nonclostridial crepitant cellulitis: gas plus **putrid odor** due to growth of anaerobes.

Necrotizing fasciitis:

> on surgical exploration, no resistance met by blunt instrument to passage along fascial plane
> often due to streptococcal infection, but may be mixed infection
> painful
> overlying skin erythematous, anesthetic
> patient toxic
> Fournier's gangrene special form affecting genitalia and perineum

Progressive bacterial synergistic gangrene (Meleney's postoperative):

> **follows surgery**
> days to weeks later—tender, red, swollen area
> becomes shaggy ulcer with gangrenous purple margins and extensive undermining
> severe pain, no toxicity
> culture: **edge, streptococcus; center, *Staphylococcus aureus* or *Enterobacter***
> **resembles pyoderma gangrenosum**

Synergistic necrotizing cellulitis:

> usually in **perineum**
> usually in **diabetics**
> patchy necrosis and small ulcers
> foul-smelling pus
> crepitus in 25%
> on surgical exploration, muscle involved, but not fascia
> may isolate gram-negative enteric bacterium

Phycomycotic gangrenous cellulitis:

> in burn cases or wounds occluded with elasticized adhesive tape (Elastoplast), which may contain *Rhizopus* organisms not killed in sterilizing procedure
> watch for in compromised or diabetic patients and around ileostomy
> central **black anesthetic ulcer, purple edematous margins**
> may spread with excessive rapidity
> highly toxic
> diagnosis difficult
> best made by **biopsy**, stained by PAS, showing hyphae, invading tissue

Infected vascular gangrene:

> putrid odor, gas in area of prior gangrene
> due to **anaerobes**

Finally, in many cases of sepsis in the immunocompromised patient the skin lesion may afford the best chance for diagnosis.

Wickboldt LG, Sanders CV: *Vibrio vulnificus* infection: Case report and update since 1970. J Am Acad Dermatol 1983; 9:243–251.

Within hours after feasting on **raw oysters** in New Orleans, this 52-year-old woman awakened at 2 AM with nausea, vomiting, and abdominal cramping. She became febrile, and the following night awakened with severe pain over the left thigh as well as swelling of the left wrist. The skin over the **left thigh** became **erythematous, indurated, and dotted with islands of necrosis.**

Hospitalized with a diagnosis of cellulitis and septic shock, she continued to develop new areas of necrosis. The left hand and forearm continued to swell and develop **vesicles** and **bullae.**

Within 6 hours of admission, **cultures** of the necrotic skin and also the blood were growing a motile **curved gram-negative rod** compatible with marine *Vibrio*. This was definitively identified as *Vibrio vulnificus* and shown to be sensitive to a wide variety of antibiotics, including ampicillin. Despite intensive antibiotic therapy, on the tenth day full-thickness **gangrene** had developed on the left thigh, left hand, and right buttock. This necessitated debridement and grafting during a 2-month hospitalization.

This patient's *Vibrio vulnificus* infection was acquired as a result of eating uncooked oysters, which led to the gastroenteritis, septicemia, and ultimate skin infection. Less common modes of entry are through the lung (aspiration of sea water) and through an open skin wound, cut, or insect bite (exposed to sea water).

These **halophilic bacteria** are ubiquitous in coastal waters and may be present in fish, shrimp, prawns, oysters, lobsters, crabs, and tortoises. Only prolonged cooking at boiling temperatures kills these organisms; simple steaming of oysters for a minute or until their shells open is not enough. A full 5 minutes in boiling water is necessary.

Once the bacteria gain access to the blood stream, **no organ is safe**. Muscle, lung, and nerve are as vulnerable as skin. The skin lesions are striking in the pain and cellulitis that they cause, with a range including maculopapular, urticarial, and erythema multiforme lesions. Typically, as in this patient, **indurated tender plaques** evolve that show **blue-purple suffusion, vesicles,** and **bullae**. Those lead to necrosis, sloughing, and deep ulcers down to the fascia.

The **differential diagnosis** includes:

erysipelas   brown recluse spider bite
necrotizing fasciitis   thrombophlebitis
necrotizing cellulitis

Since *Vibrio vulnificus* **infections are often fatal**, anyone who eats uncooked seafood is playing a dietary form of Russian roulette.

Igelman JD, Smith BJ, Rosen T, Tschen JA: **Persistent facial plaque**. Arch Dermatol 1987; 123:937–940.

Cellulitis of the entire right cheek in a 31-year-old man developed from a deep pimple that had appeared 3 weeks previously. Although first seen in Houston, he had only recently moved there from northern California.

The tender, boggy, erythematous plaque did not respond to ampicillin or dicloxacillin, although **bacterial cultures** showed *Staphylococcus aureus* and *Acinetobacter anitratus*. Incision was nonproductive and was followed by shallow ulcer.

The diagnosis was then made by a **biopsy** 2 weeks after the initial visit. The characteristic 50- to 70-cm **thick-walled spores of *Coccidioides immitis*** were seen in the infiltrate.

After 5 months of ketoconazole therapy, 600 mg/day, there has been slow improvement; a year or more of such therapy is anticipated.

The **usual presentation of cutaneous coccidioidomycosis** is:

a verrucous granuloma

a nodule with or without ulcerations
a subcutaneous abscess

Hall JC, Brewer JH, Crouch TT, Watson KR: **Cryptococcal cellulitis** with multiple sites of involvement. J Am Acad Dermatol 1987; 17:329–332.

A 28-year-old woman had a fever and four areas of **tender, erythematous skin** of the right leg, buttock, and abdomen. A **diagnosis of bacterial cellulitis** was made, but systemic antibiotic therapy was without effect.

A **biopsy** on the fourth day revealed the cause: **yeast organism** in the dermis. **Culture was positive for *Cryptococcus neoformans***. The serum cryptococcal antigen titer was 1:4096.

Cryptococcosis of the skin is virtually always a **sign of disseminate disease**, with the respiratory tract the usual portal of entry and the lungs and central nervous system the usual residence sites for the yeast.

Cryptococcal cellulitis **occurs only in markedly immunocompromised patients**, and such was the case with this patient. She had recently had a renal transplant and was receiving azathioprine and prednisone. Other patients at risk are those with systemic lupus erythematosus, leukemia, and myeloma.

Unless a high index of suspicion is maintained, the diagnosis of cryptococcal cellulitis will be missed. The following are the **incorrect diagnoses** made in other instances: staphylococcal cellulitis, erysipelas, contact dermatitis, herpes zoster, and herpes simplex.

A **biopsy, Tzanck smear**, and **aspirate stained with India ink or Gram stain** are three tools to hasten diagnosis and avoid life-threatening or fatal delay in initiating therapy.

Lebwohl M, Fleischmajer R, Janowitz H, et al: **Metastatic Crohn's disease**. J Am Acad Dermatol 1984; 10:33–38.

This 44-year-old woman was **admitted** to the hospital **with a diagnosis of erysipelas**. She had a well-demarcated erythematous plaque over the left upper lip and cheek. It did not respond to antibiotic therapy.

Her past history included 17 **years of Crohn's disease** and for the past 3 years episodes of swelling and tenderness of the left upper lip and cheek.

A **biopsy** showed extensive, noncaseating granulomatous inflammation throughout the skin and subcutaneous tissue. A **diagnosis of metastatic Crohn's disease** was made, since this label describes cutaneous granuloma formation remote from the gastrointestinal tract in patients with Crohn's disease of the bowel.

The following are **incorrect diagnoses made** on patients with metastatic Crohn's disease:

cellulitis
hidradenitis suppurativa
factitial dermatitis
cystic acne
severe seborrheic dermatitis
intertrigo ulceration in abdominal folds, under breast, base of penis, retroauricular
erythema nodosum

Also think of Crohn's disease in **perianal fistulas and ulcerations**, as well as pyoderma gangrenosum.

To miss Crohn's disease is to miss metastatic Crohn's disease.

Aberer W, Konrad K, Wolff K: **Wells' syndrome** is a distinctive disease entity and not a histologic diagnosis. J Am Acad Dermatol 1988; 18:105–114.

This **looks like a bacterial cellulitis** of the face, trunk, or limb with acute redness and edema that **may blister** and cause **burning pain.** The swelling subsides, leaving a **blue-gray** or **green-gray induration resembling morphea.** The skin returns to normal in 2 to 6 weeks. The patient usually is not sick but may be febrile. **Recurring attacks** are common, and some patients show **eosinophilia.** Skin biopsy reveals marked dermal edema with eosinophils and **flame figures** (masses of eosinophils and histiocytes on collagen). Subepidermal blisters rich in eosinophils are also seen. There is no vasculitis. This condition responds only to systemic steroids.

Differential diagnosis:

erysipelas	toxocariasis
cellulitis	sporotrichosis
arthropod bites	erythema chronicum migrans
drug eruption	lymphoma, hematologic disease

Three instructive cases are included:

1. A 59-year-old man had recurrent episodes of massive swelling and erythema on the trunk and extremities for 1 year. The eruptions **mimicked thrombosis, thrombophlebitis,** and **angioedema** with urticaria. Polycythemia vera was discovered, and treatment with phlebotomy, busulfan, and cyclophosphamide decreased the frequency of episodes. One year later he had massive swelling and skin infiltration of the right hand, arm, and shoulder, with sharp rosy borders, central involution with brownish and greenish discoloration, and aberrant urticarial lesions. He complained of itching and burning. Hemoglobin was 23.5 gm/dl, and WBC was 17,000/mm^3 with 3% eosinophils. A bone marrow examination confirmed polycythemia vera with early myelofibrosis. **Repeated skin biopsies showed Wells' syndrome,** with negative immunofluorescence and bacterial and fungal cultures. Treatment with corticosteroids led to rapid resolution of the monthly eruptions, but had to be discontinued because of progressive fibrosis of the bone marrow. Resumption of busulfan therapy stabilized both the hematologic condition and the skin eruption and was discontinued after 1 year. He never had eosinophilia.

2. A 40-year-old woman had recurrent swelling of the left cheek and neck. The ill-defined **stony-hard angioedema-like** swelling of the left cheek and submandibular regions had blotchy erythema and brownish and blanched areas. Although it was not painful, it caused burning sensations. There was eosinophilia (eosinophils 12%), and deep skin biopsy revealed **granulomatous dermatitis with eosinophilia and flame figures.** Treatment with alternate-day low-dose systemic steroids (6-methylprednisolone [10 mg]) and dapsone (100 mg/day) controlled the disease. No underlying precipitating factor was found.

3. A 46-year-old farmer had **acute purulent tonsillitis** with fever, treated with oral chloramphenicol. Two weeks later he developed an **urticaria-like eruption of the forearms, face,** and **neck,** with subsequent central blisters and arthralgias. The **feet** became **massively swollen,** and new lesions developed on the hands and feet, resolving centrally. Skin biopsy showed Wells' syndrome, but there was no eosinophilia. The lesions resolved with low-dose steroid treatment, but recurrences were common.

Clark DP, Anderson PC: **Eosinophilic cellulitis caused by arthropod bites.** Int J Dermatol 1988; 27:411–412.

A 16-year-old farm worker developed numerous **pruritic papules resembling mite bites** on his clothed areas. After 2 days they had faded, but then **annular**

erythematous plaques appeared on the forearms and right eyelid. During the next 3 days the right **forearm** became **massively swollen** and **indurated**. Skin **biopsy revealed eosinophilic cellulitis**. The complete blood count indicated white cells 6900/mm^3, with 41% polymorphonuclears, 40% lymphocytes, and **17% eosinophils**. Creatine phosphokinase was twice normal, but a urinalysis and chemistry profile were otherwise normal. During the next 6 weeks the edema slowly resolved, leaving a **morphea-like lesion** that faded over the next 2 months. Months later, while mowing grass on the farm, he was again bitten by insects and the clinical syndrome replayed. Intradermal scratch testing with crude mite extract induced a marked inflammatory response.

Think of **eosinophilic cellulitis** (**Wells' syndrome**) as a special type of hypersensitivity reaction. Your pathologist will diagnose it on the basis of dermal edema, granulomatous dermatitis, massive infiltration of eosinophils, and **flame figures** (**eosinophilic debris**). It is up to you to decide whether it was triggered by bites of spiders, ticks, or mites or by streptococcal infection, drug sensitivity, or fungous infection. The **clinical spectrum** may include subcutaneous panniculitis, **scarring alopecia**, and urticaria, in addition to the more usual fixed pruritic erythematous and edematous papules and plaques.

van den Hoogenband HM: **Eosinophilic cellulitis as a result of onchocerciasis.** Clin Exp Dermatol 1983; 8:405–408.

A 42-year-old man had a **pruritic papular eruption** of the right arm and shoulder of 3 months' duration. The eruption gradually extended over the trunk, becoming **more urticarial**. The right **arm** became **edematous**, and the axillary nodes were swollen.

A punch **biopsy** of the swollen arm **gave a clear diagnosis of eosinophilic cellulitis**. The cause remained unknown until **skin-snip biopsies** revealed the presence of the **microfilariae** of onchocerciasis.

It was the patient's history of having been **in Africa 2 years earlier**, and having had a period of diarrhea, that pushed for the ultimate studies of tropical parasitic diseases and thus the definitive diagnosis for a very nondiagnostic clinical picture of "itching and swelling."

Ferrier MC, Janin-Mercier A, Souteyrand P, et al: **Eosinophilic cellulitis (Wells' syndrome): Ultrastructural study of a case with circulating immune complexes.** Dermatologica 1988; 176:299–304.

Each of **three bouts** of biopsy-proven eosinophilic cellulitis in a 42-year-old woman appeared to be **triggered by a different medication** (lincomycin, Nesdonal, aspirin) taken 10 days before each attack. She had itchy erythematous infiltrated plaques on the legs and face, which spread over most of the body in 6 weeks. The **plaques** were fixed and **circinate**, with **greenish centers** and **red borders** and occasional **bullae**. Treatment consisted of short-term steroids and long-term dapsone.

Skin biopsy revealed a dense inflammatory infiltrate of eosinophils and macrophages in the dermis and subcutaneous fat, with **flame figures** in the deep dermis. There was no vessel-wall necrosis or vasculitis, but direct immunofluorescent studies revealed C3 and IgG around vessel walls. Blood studies revealed an elevated white blood cell count (18,300/mm^3), negative ANA, normal complement, and high **circulating immune complexes** (78 to 87%, normal 46%).

It is to be noted that **in 10 of the 46 cases in the literature, a drug** may have served to **trigger the attack**. The specific drugs included aspirin, penicillin, erythromycin, tetracyclines, bleomycin, chlorambucil, and local anesthesia.

King CM, Chalmers RJG: **Dermatitis simulata**—a hitherto unrecognized form of contrived disease. Br J Dermatol 1984; 111 (suppl 26):40.

Disease simulation as practiced by three young women (ages 10 to 25 years):

impetigo	induced by an antibiotic cream
cellulitis	induced by a cosmetic blusher
dermatitis with exfoliation	induced by a contact adhesive

Emotional problems were evident in two of the three patients. Dermatitis simulata is contrasted with **dermatitis artefacta**, in which more serious self-mutilation occurs.

Goldminz D, Barnhill R, McGuire J, Stenn KS: **Calcinosis cutis following extravasation of calcium chloride.** Arch Dermatol 1988; 124:922–925.

A 27-year-old woman with hypoparathyroidism received intravenous calcium chloride (1 gm/100 ml normal saline). **Extravasation** occurred with resulting edema, warmth, and tenderness, and the next day **multiple erythematous tender papules** appeared along the venous track of the left forearm. Within a week these papules became irregular, firm, and yellowish-white, measuring 0.5 to 2.0 cm.

Biopsy at 10 days showed a nonspecific urticarial reaction with negative calcium stains. At 25 days, granular calcific deposits could be visualized in the dermis with the von Kossa stain, and x-ray of the skin biopsy specimen showed multiple radiodensities. At 40 days, the calcium could be seen in the epidermis as well as the dermis. Over the course of 4 months there was gradual improvement with elimination of a whitish material from the centers of the papules.

Calcinosis cutis may be **misdiagnosed as hematoma, abscess, or cellulitis.** Although after a week it can be seen in soft tissue roentgenograms, **initially** the extravasated calcium solution is **radiolucent.**

Koch SE, Wintroub BU: **Pott's puffy tumor: A clinical marker for osteomyelitis** of the skull. Arch Dermatol 1985; 121:548–549.

Nontender bogginess of the **midforehead** of an afebrile 74-year-old man was **diagnosed as erysipelas.** Since it did not respond to penicillin, a needle aspirate was obtained. *Staphylococcus aureus*, coagulase positive, grew out, and in 2 weeks a red nodule formed at the aspiration site. Further systemic antibiotic therapy was without effect.

The skin biopsy then showed granulation tissue. **Although the skull roentgenogram showed no bony abnormality, computed tomography revealed multiple osteolytic lesions.**

On exploratory surgery, a **subgaleal abscess** was found. Subsequently, multiple draining sinuses developed, compatible with chronic osteomyelitis.

The diagnosis was thus **Pott's puffy tumor**, first described by Sir Percivall Pott of chimney sweep's fame. He recognized that it was a cutaneous sign of underlying osteomyelitis of the skull. **Antecedent** events are usually **trauma or frontal sinusitis.**

Differential diagnosis often includes **erysipelas**, cellulitis, subgaleal hematoma, and angiosarcoma. A technetium bone scan or computed tomography is a more valuable diagnostic aid than a skull plate.

The **complications** that may result from ignoring the patient's simple complaint of some swelling of the forehead are awesome. They include subdural abscess, meningitis, and sagittal sinus thrombosis with cerebral edema and death.

Some bumps are worse than others.

Contact Dermatitis

Nowhere in dermatologic diagnosis are suspicion and history more important. It is an axiom that the best history is taken by one who knows the diagnosis. In the case of contact dermatitis, the best history is taken by one who suspects the diagnosis. And what arouses suspicion? It is the **patient's itch**. The target organ in this disease is the epidermis, home of the itch receptors. Unless a contactant, such as an acid, destroys the epidermis and its nerves, contact dermatitis is pruritic. Listen to the patient for this cardinal sign. Then proceed to look for the contactant.

With potentially hundreds of thousands of chemicals in the patient's occupational, home, and hobby environment, the search is a daunting task; yet most patients have a limited number to consider. First, **eliminate primary irritants** as the cause. If it is hand dermatitis, immerse yourself in every detail of the patient's **hand-cleaning routine**. How often does he wash? We have seen the compulsive hand washer develop contact dermatitis from the cumulative damage of 20 scrubs a day. The degree of irritancy of a compound is always a function of the length of exposure. Does he use **solvents** or **turpentine** to remove grime and grease? Know his occupation and the contactant hazards. Does he deal with **alkaline** or **acidic compounds**? Does he work with organic solvents? Are other workers bothered?

If the dermatitis is not due to a contactant known to be universally damaging to the epidermis, the search moves to contact allergens. The agents are more invisible, more elusive. The patient is uniquely sensitive, and when he follows the wisdom of the herd, he does himself harm. With the exception of poison ivy, what others handle with impunity, he must avoid. His acquired sensitivity even deprives him of the wisdom of his own former exposure and experience. We recall one woman with contact sensitivity to her girdle, remarking indignantly, "It can't be that, I've worn it for 7 years." Thus, the first step is **education of the patient** to suspect even his "best friends" of years' standing. Without this suspicion arousal, the patient may fail to tell you the key exposure. No detective succeeds when the witnesses remain silent.

Examples of contact dermatitis are limitless. Some are so obvious the patient comes not for diagnosis but treatment. Such is the contact dermatitis in which the location and outline indicate the cause, as the contact dermatitis from a ring, a belt buckle, or surgical gloves. Others are easy once the patient realizes that that which was safe before has become pathogenic. Such is the contact dermatitis from eye shadow, hair dye, after-shave lotion, and perfume.

But the rest calls for advanced dermatologic diagnosis. It calls for elimination and, when possible, challenge tests. Avoidance of suspect contactants, even work, may be necessary. As to tests, the standard **patch test** is valuable but limited to only the more common allergens. Sources can direct you to preparation of non-irritating formulations of many other compounds, but generally this is done only by world-class patch test centers. Without question, the more patch tests that are done the more examples there will be of contact dermatitis causes identified.

But aside from failure to test, what blocks us from making the diagnosis of contact dermatitis? There are five blind spots:

1. **Mimicry.** Whenever the clinical signs of contact dermatitis are identical to another skin disease, a misdiagnosis may be made. We have seen contact dermatitis to hair tonic diagnosed as seborrheic dermatitis. Likewise, contact dermatitis to a sunscreen may be viewed as sunburn. And on the hands, contact dermatitis may mislead one by its mimicry of atopic dermatitis.
2. **Failure to make a second diagnosis.** We tend to make but a single diagnosis. This blinds us at times to the appearance of superimposed contact dermatitis. We may view contact dermatitis to topical medication simply as worsening of the primary skin problem, such as atopic dermatitis or rosacea.

437

We also see failures to recognize contact dermatitis as the cause of a Koebner induction of psoriasis.

3. **Occult exposure.**   There is real difficulty in remembering that something in the pants pocket such as a set of keys may cause contact dermatitis. Many exposures are occult, such as fingernail polish contamination of a jar of cold cream. We also have seen contact dermatitis in an executive whose secretary, unbeknownst to him, had been using a phenolic antiseptic to sterilize his phone and other objects. **Intermittent exposures** are especially misleading. We recall a woman with chronic idiopathic hand eczema that proved to be due to sensitivity to the red dye in her window curtains. Occasional washings of these kept the nature of the dermatitis unknown for more than a year. Even more inapparent are the **airborne contactants**—the bathroom sprays, perfumes, or chemicals in the air at work. Finally, the contactant that reaches the epidermis from within does so by **systemic absorption**. Here **foods** and **drugs** are the contact allergens missed so easily.

4. **Failure of patch testing.**   Sometimes the diagnosis of contact dermatitis is discarded when a critical patch test is negative. But recall the pitfalls. The patch test result may be falsely negative or positive. The wrong compound may have been applied, the tape may have come off, readings were not made later at 96 hours. The test may not duplicate actual clinical exposure in terms of time of exposure, area sensitized, and such cofactors as cleansing and ultraviolet light exposure.

   Moreover, the test concentrations of many allergens are unknown, and hence tests are not done.

5. **Inadequate or deceptive history.**   A major blind spot is in the history. Many patients fail to recognize or describe the many contactants to which they are exposed. For hand dermatitis, these vary from colored newsprint to treated copying paper. Other patients may practice deceit. They may secretly use Fels Naphtha soap as a contact irritant for secondary gain. We had one patient with multiple personalities who repeatedly applied the poison ivy plant under an Ace bandage to her left arm. Her presentation suggested vascular occlusion. Hospitalization was required to detect her deception.

Nethercott JR: **Practical problems** in the use of patch testing in the evaluation of patients with contact dermatitis. Curr Probl Dermatol 1990; 11:97–123.

Irritant contact dermatitis is five times as common as **allergic contact dermatitis**.

Patch testing for **allergic contact dermatitis** is based on the premise that if one applies the allergen to the skin at a subirritant concentration, only a subject allergic to the test chemical will show a positive response. The subirritant concentrations are determined by testing a group of volunteers. Hence there are data on only a limited number of compounds, and commercial test preparations are available for but a few.

Only if there is no clue as to a specific substance to which the patient may be allergic should one employ a **screening patch test series**. The more random tests being done, the greater the number of false positives. As a rule, anticipate one misleading **false-positive** reading for every 20 patches applied at the same time. The reason for this is that a fixed subirritant concentration as established for a group may be at irritant level for a specific individual.

Photopatch testing is not standardized, and the interpretation of test responses is difficult. Note that such testing may induce photoallergic contact dermatitis, even at times a persistent light reaction. Its use should be limited to the study of selected patients in whom photocontact dermatitis is the likely diagnosis.

The **Finn chamber** (aluminum well attached to tape) is the most widely used test appliance. Commercially prepackaged post-test systems will be available, such as Epiquick (Germany) and True Test (Sweden).

Although most readings are done at 48 hours, **10% of positive responses are evident only after 4 or 5 days**.

A positive test reaction or an area of dermatitis may induce a false-positive in an adjacent test. This is the **excited skin syndrome**.

Patch testing can be the initial exposure to a compound that acts as a **sensitizer**. The possibility of such active sensitization must be a recognized risk when deciding whether or not to patch test.

Möller H: **Intradermal testing** in doubtful cases of **contact allergy to metals**. Contact Dermatitis 1989; 20:120–123.

In Sweden, 350 of 1670 patch-tested patients had a **contact allergy to metal salts**. Of these patients, 49 had doubtful patch test results. In 24 of 78 instances of this, a true metal allergy (**chromate, cobalt,** or **nickel**) was confirmed by **intradermal testing** with **dilute solutions** (1 mM in saline).

The exact concentrations thus proved to be 0.029% for potassium dichromate, 0.013% for cobalt chloride, and 0.016% for nickel sulfate. A red, raised infiltrate greater than 4 mm as seen **72 hours** following the subepidermal injection of 0.1 ml was considered positive.

Bruynzeel DP, Maibach HI: **Excited skin syndrome** (angry back). Arch Dermatol 1986; 122:323–328.

Even a small area of dermatitis, such as hand eczema, adhesive-tape dermatitis, or a strong positive patch test reaction can produce a state of hyperirritability in normal-appearing skin (excited skin syndrome). Such a state of **nonspecific sensitivity** often leads to multiple false-positive patch test readings, which are nonreproducible. It may also be responsible for a **strange spreading of the dermatitis**. In the early phase of severe acute inflammation, skin reactivity may be depressed, whereas later it may be enhanced with chronic inflammation.

Other terms used to describe **hyperreactivity of the skin** include:

crazy back	multiple nonspecific reactions
angry back syndrome	rogue positive reactions
status eczematicus	metallergic and parallergic reactions
skin fatigue	conditioned hyperirritability
spillover	reflektorisches ekzem

Hezemans-Boer M, Toonstra J, Meulenbelt J, et al: Skin lesions due to exposure to **methyl bromide**. Arch Dermatol 1988; 124:917–921.

Methyl bromide (CH_3Br) fumigation of a beetle-ridden 13th century castle resulted in six workers rapidly developing **burning and redness of the axillae, groin,** and **scrotum**. Despite having been cleaned by showering, the skin began to swell and 8 hours later developed **vesicles** and **bullae**. Examination revealed sharply demarcated erythema with multiple vesicles and large clear bullae, as well as severe **edema** of the **penis** and **scrotum**. Skin biopsies showed subepidermal blisters and diffuse perivascular infiltrate of neutrophils and eosinophils.

The eruption, which healed within 2 weeks, was viewed as a **primary irritant** response to high concentrations in the air of the volatile methyl bromide. The localization of lesions resulted from **moist skin favoring** the **absorption** of methyl bromide. Standard protective clothing was not adequate, although systemic poisoning was prevented by adequate airway protection.

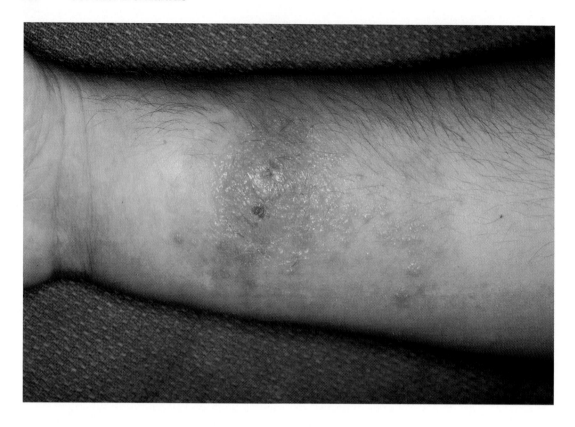

Two workers also developed an **urticarial rash** 1 week after exposure to the methyl bromide, with no evidence of an immunopathologic reaction.

This is another example of the **vulnerability of moist or wet skin**.

Tegner E: **Sheet dermatitis.** Acta Derm Venereol 1985; 65:254–257.

In 25 patients a characteristic **pruritic papular eruption** of discrete 1- to 3-mm skin-colored or slightly erythematous papules developed on the **ears, cheeks**, and **sides of the neck**. It began within 1 to 2 days of sleeping on new, unwashed, brightly colored, inexpensive, **permanent-press cotton sheets** and **pillow cases**. The textiles were hard, stiff, and uncomfortable to the touch. Discarding the sheets resulted in remission within 1 week, and the eruption did not recur when the washed sheets were used.

Some individuals never developed a rash despite sleeping on the new unwashed sheets. Others, who slept again on the unwashed sheets, failed to have a second attack. Patch tests with the unwashed sheet produced a positive reaction in only one of the six patients tested. Possibly, textile fibers hardened by the permanent press resin acted as an irritant. Indeed, an initial diagnosis of **fiber glass dermatitis** was favored.

In contrast, sheet dermatitis in Canada was caused by a true allergen that resulted from breakdown products of the permanent press polymer. The eruption was similar but appeared only after 10 days of contact with either washed or unwashed sheets and persisted for weeks after contact with the offending sheets was avoided.

A "**pillowcase history**" can give you a diagnostic advantage in patients with a puzzling pruritic papular eruption of the ears, cheeks, and neck.

Warin AP: **Contact dermatitis** to **partner's hair dye**. Clin Exp Dermatol 1976; 1:283–284.

Acute recurrent dermatitis of the inner aspect of the left arm of a 39-year-old man was traced to direct contact with his partner's hair, freshly dyed with **paraphenylenediamine**.

Another example in the literature presented as an axillary nummular eczema in a man, resulting from his wife's habit of reading in bed with her head of dyed hair nestled on the patient's armpit.

Romaguera C, Grimalt F, Vilaplana J: **Eczematous** and **purpuric allergic contact dermatitis** from **boots**. Contact Dermatitis 1989; 21:269.

A short time after beginning to wear a pair of apparently leather boots, black outside and white inside, a 49-year-old housewife began to itch on the dorsum and soles of both feet. This was followed by **papular-squamous lesions of the feet** that extended up the legs. Later the lesions became purpuric while still pruritic.

A diagnosis of **PPPP syndrome** (pruritus, petechiae, purpura, paraphenylenediamine sensitivity) was confirmed by a positive patch test (2+) to N-isopropyl-N'-phenyl-4 phenylenediamine. She also proved to be sensitive to dibutyl thiourea. Although both compounds may be present in boots, patch tests to her own footwear were negative.

This is another example of how testing with the material itself fails to reproduce the clinical condition of weeks of exposure in a hot, humid environment.

Johnson R, Nusbaum BP, Horwitz SN, Frost P: Transfer of topically applied tetracycline in various vehicles. Arch Dermatol 1983; 119:660–663.

By using the **fluorescence of tetracycline** as a **tracer**, it was possible to show that **ointments** and **creams** (but not lotions) applied only to the preauricular area were **rapidly transferred** to the entire face, neck, arms, hands, and genitalia.

It is evident that **topical medications do not stay put**. Nor do their allergenic and pharmacologic effects.

Wolf R, Wolf D, Viskoper RJ, Sandbank M: **Norwegian-type scabies** mimicking contact dermatitis in an immunosuppressed patient. Postgrad Med 1985; 78(1):228–230.

For 2 months a pruritic rash of the back, axillae, breasts, and genital area of this 26-year-old woman was **viewed as contact dermatitis**. The patient had had a renal transplant 4 years ago and was receiving high-dose **immunosuppressants**.

On examination there were **large erythematous scaly plaques sharply demarcated** and limited to the area covered by the bra, including the shoulder strap. Similar plaques were seen in the axilla and periumbilical, perianal, and inguinal regions. The hands were free of lesions.

Scrapings revealed **numerous** live **mites**, making the correct diagnosis scabies. A 25% benzyl benzoate lotion applied for 3 consecutive days cured this "contact (with mites) dermatitis."

Salomon RJ, Briggaman RA, Wernikoff SY, Kayne AL: **Localized bullous pemphigoid:** A mimic of acute contact dermatitis. Arch Dermatol 1987; 123:389–392.

Vesicular lesions and **bullae** on an **erythematous base** at and immediately

around a colostomy stoma in an 87-year-old woman **suggested acute contact dermatitis** due to a stomal "skin preparation" used.

However, **immunofluorescence** studies showed the lamina lucida staining pattern of **bullous pemphigoid**. Since it was localized to a site of trauma, such studies were necessary also to rule out epidermolysis bullosa acquisita.

One should recall that there are **four types of localized pemphigoid**:

pretibial	oral (desquamative gingivitis)
dyshidrosiform	Brunsting-Perry type

None are scarring, which distinguishes them from cicatricial pemphigoid, which is also localized.

Lacroix J, Morin CL, Collin P-P: **Nickel dermatitis from a foreign body in the stomach.** J Pediatr 1979; 95:428–429.

Within 18 hours of **swallowing a Canadian quarter** (which contains 98.5% nickel), an 8-year-old boy developed **generalized pruritus and urticaria**. This was followed by persistent erythema, edema, and a generalized **vesicular eruption** that had large exudative areas with crusting and scaling. He was febrile (temperature 39.5°C) with white blood cells 13,000/mm^3, including **20% eosinophils**. Only after the coin was surgically removed 2 weeks later from its entrapment within edematous gastric mucosa did the rash fade and disappear. Eosinophils dropped to 1% 18 hours after surgery. A patch test to the quarter produced a strongly positive vesicular reaction within a few hours.

Helping to confirm the diagnosis of systemically induced contact dermatitis was the history that ever since the age of 1 year he had developed vesicular dermatitis in areas touching nickel-containing devices. His mother and 2-year-old brother were also allergic to nickel.

Shelley WB: **Focal contact sensitivity** to **nitrogen mustard** in lesions of cutaneous T-cell lymphoma (mycosis fungoides). Acta Derm Venereol 1981; 61:161–164.

A 59-year-old man developed contact dermatitis to nitrogen mustard **only in the plaques of mycosis fungoides**. Open patch tests with nitrogen mustard (1/5,000 aqueous) were negative on normal skin but elicited a pruritic eczematous change on a plaque of mycosis fungoides. Treatment with nitrogen mustard was associated with high fever and shaking chills, which could be blocked by a preceding dose of prednisone (40 mg).

The phenomenon of focal contact sensitivity would appear to be the analogue of the **fixed drug eruption**. Perhaps patchy eczematoid dermatitis may sometimes represent a "**fixed contact dermatitis**."

Marks JG Jr, DeMelfi T, McCarthy MA, et al: **Dermatitis from cashew nuts.** J Am Acad Dermatol 1984; 10:627–631.

People who are sensitive to poison ivy shouldn't eat cashew nuts. Here is a report of 54 individuals who developed a very pruritic, erythematous, maculopapular eruption within a week of eating cashew nuts contaminated with oil from the **cashew shell**. The eruption favored the flexural sites.

This shell oil contains an antigen virtually identical to the pentadecylcatechol of poison ivy, so that these poison ivy–sensitive patients had an ingestant-induced contact dermatitis due to the cashews. Proper processing of the cashews should prevent this by eliminating the shell as a source of immunologic harm.

This is another example of the fact that **contact allergens can reach the epidermis by other than outside contact.**

Cysts

The most important consideration in the diagnosis of cysts is location. On the scalp we see the **wen**. This is the **pilar cyst** that is clinically indistinguishable from the epidermoid or keratinous cyst. Both are tense, at times fluctuant, swellings that are freely movable over the underlying tissue. A comedone or pore may be seen in the center as their point of origin, and in the case of the keratinous cyst there may be an odor. When there has been rupture of the cyst wall, a marked inflammatory reaction and, later, scar tissue may ensue. Diagnosis is confirmed by observing soft whitish material exude on pressure.

The face may exhibit such keratinous cysts as well as the cysts of acne. There also are the diminutive keratinous cysts we call **milia**. The eyelids and cheeks may be the sites of the clear **retention cysts** of apocrine or eccrine gland origin. The ears may be the site of a pseudocyst following cartilage damage. Within the mouth one finds the retention cysts of the mucous gland. In the anterior area of the neck, branchial cleft cysts and thyroglossal cysts are always under consideration. These developmental anomalies are usually soft tender lesions that, in the case of the **branchial cleft cyst**, lie on a line extending from a point anterior to the ears down to the sternocleidomastoid muscle insertion in the sternum. The **thyroglossal cysts** are over the thyroid and may be fluctuant and may transilluminate.

Again, the chest location favors the diagnosis of acne cyst and on rare occasion the cysts of steatocystoma multiplex. Commonly, keratinous cysts are seen on the scrotum, and the penis can be the locale for a median raphe cyst of "nature's mal-suture."

The best example of location as a diagnostic determinant for cysts is the **synovial cyst** of the fingers or toes. Here, taut, dome-shaped lesions show a thinned-skin window onto a local collection of mucin. The distal groove in the nail speaks to the pressure on the nail matrix. Incision permits diagnostic seepage of a gelatinous material.

Some caveats regarding cysts:

1. **Cysts on the scalp**, especially in **infants**, require careful preoperative evaluation. If they are pulsatile they may contain blood or cerebrospinal fluid. Some vascular tumors (sinus pericranii) connect with an intracranial vessel. There may be absence of underlying bone detectable by computed tomography. Beware of dermoid tumors that extend into the ventricle, as well as cephaloceles containing meninges or even brain. Leptomeningeal cysts may develop following skull fracture in a young child with herniation of brain. Meningitis, uncontrollable bleeding, and brain infarction await the unwary. A cyst on a baby's scalp may cry for a neurosurgeon.
2. **Multiple keratinous cysts** of the scalp call for consideration of **Gardner's syndrome** (multiple osteomas, fibromas, dermoid cysts, leiomyomas). These patients may have intestinal polyposis leading to carcinoma of the colon. Death before the age of 50 years is the penalty for ignorance and thus failure to have surgical prophylactic treatment.
3. **Multiple myxomatous cysts** call for thinking of the LAMB syndrome (NAME syndrome, Carney syndrome). Careful cardiac follow-up is necessary for these patients who are candidates for deadly atrial myxomas.

Ultimately the precise diagnosis for any cyst is in the province of the pathologist. All need histologic examination. Only then can one learn that the patient had a ciliated cyst or an eruptive vellus hair cyst. Only by histologic examination can squamous cell carcinoma and metastatic carcinoma be dismissed as possible diagnoses.

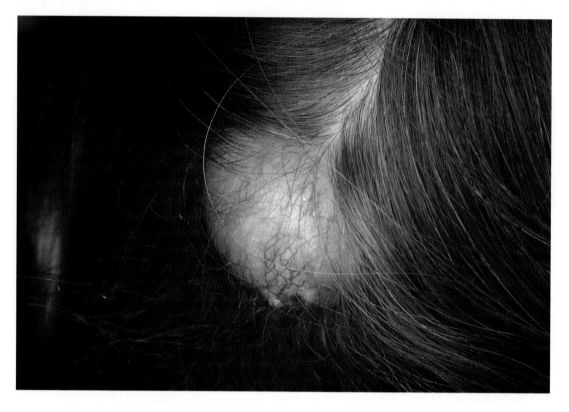

Sonnex TS: **Digital myxoid cysts:** A review. Cutis 1986; 37:89–94.

Synonymy: Mucous cyst, synovial cyst, myxomatous cyst, nail cyst, dorsal cyst, periungual ganglion, periarticular fibroma, cystic nodule, epidermal cyst

Clinical appearance: A soft to rubbery, round or oval, 3- to 13-mm dome-shaped **swelling of the dorsal aspect of a finger** between the nail fold and the distal interphalangeal joint. It is often painful and may rupture, leaking gelatinous material.

Predilection: Women of middle age, especially on the index and middle fingers. They occasionally occur on the toes and under the nail plate.

Diagnosis: **Transilluminate** the cyst to distinguish it from a periungual fibroma.

Associations: Nail deformity—a linear nail dystrophy with grooves, thinning, furrowing, or splits due to pressure of the cyst on the nail matrix. This often returns to normal after cyst removal.

    Osteoarthritis with Heberden's nodes of the associated distal interphalangeal joints

    Communicating tract or pedicle with the associated joint in many cases (demonstrable with methylene blue diluted with saline or lidocaine, mixed with hydrogen peroxide). The cyst contains hyaluronic acid, which suggests origin from herniation of tendon sheath or joint lining.

Differential diagnosis

    epidermoid cyst (usually on the flexor surface)

    ganglion (deep, not attached to skin, near wrist or flexor side of proximal phalanx)

    fibrous nodule (periarticular or juxta-articular, not attached to skin)

    leiomyoma (very tender, subcutaneous, noncystic, on extensor finger but not distal)

xanthoma (yellowish, not cystic, subcutaneous or deeper, flexor aspect)
knuckle pad (dorsal aspect of intermediate finger joints, round, fibrous, noncystic)

Gordon ML, Kest E, Phelps RG: **Flesh-colored nodule on the forearm.** Arch Dermatol 1988; 124:263–266.

Two asymptomatic flesh-colored nodules (1.0 to 1.5 cm) present for 2 months on the left forearm of a 62-year-old woman required biopsy for the diagnosis. They were slightly erythematous and felt cystic on palpation. No lymph nodes were palpable. Past history was remarkable for esophageal webs, aspergilloma, and advanced sarcoidosis. Clinically one could think of lipomas or epidermal inclusion cysts, but skin biopsy revealed endothelial hyperplasia with dilated vascular spaces and fronds of delicate connective tissue lined by a single layer of epithelium. A thick-walled medium-caliber vessel showed luminal occlusion.

The **diagnosis was intravascular papillary endothelial hyperplasia,** which usually presents as a solitary, slow-growing, compressible papule or nodule of flesh or bluish-red color. While many are asymptomatic, at least a third of them present with pain. At times they simulate a ganglion cyst or Kaposi's sarcoma, as well as lipomas and epidermal inclusion cysts. The entire pathology is intravascular, without invasion of surrounding tissue. Thrombi are usually present, and the endothelial cells may have mild nuclear atypia and occasional mitotic figures. The course is benign, and it is possible that it represents a reaction pattern to a thrombus rather than a primary vascular neoplasm.

Kelly JJ: **Blackthorn inflammation.** J Bone Joint Surg 1966; 48B:474–477.

The blackthorn or sloe is a perennial shrub in hedges and thickets all over the British Isles. It has narrow thorns up to $2\frac{1}{4}$ inches long, which can penetrate the skin and break off, leading to a foreign body nonsuppurative inflammatory reaction. Most injuries occur on the hand and forearm, causing a "cyst" with aching pain and tenderness but no signs of local inflammation. Arthritis and synovitis may result if the blackthorn penetrates a joint. The patient is often not aware of the blackthorn injury or else has pulled out the thorn and assumed that it was completely removed (difficult to do, as tip fragments often remain). Surgical removal is curative.

Gardner EJ: A genetic and clinical study of **intestinal polyposis,** a predisposing factor for carcinoma of the colon and rectum. Am J Hum Genet 1951; 3:167–176.

A study was made of 68 descendents of one couple in Utah. It was possible to do sigmoidoscopy on 39 of the 50 still living. Five had polyposis, and two of these had established carcinoma. All of these as well as all who had previously died of carcinoma of the digestive tract exhibited conspicuous surface lumps or **soft cystlike tumors** of the head and body. The family believed that there was a relationship between the surface tumors and the fatal cancers, but they would not allow removal or histologic examination of these surface growths, as one family member died of intestinal cancer shortly after removal of a benign skin tumor. It could be established, however, that the inheritance pattern for the surface tumors and **associated intestinal polyps** was that of a **simple dominant gene.**

Diagnosis is the art of converting the unknown into the known.

Delusions

Delusions of parasitosis is an easy diagnosis to make. Sometimes it is too easy. The constellation of symptoms, signs, and findings is so characteristic that physicians may fail to question if their own diagnosis is a "delusion." To do this, assume the patient may be right. Look at the material brought in. Really look for particles of glass or glass wool. Look for mites. Examine the skin and look for head lice as well as pediculi in the clothing. The patient may be misinterpreting and overreacting.

Carefully question. Could the patient be a **drug addict**? Do a urinary toxicologic screen. Could he be exposed to chemicals such as LSD that produce hallucinatory phenomena? We once identified a drug-induced "delusions of parasitosis" in a chemist working with a new compound that proved to be **hallucinogenic**.

Is the patient's symptom complex sharply focused or are there a multiplicity of symptoms that the **schizophrenic** patient brings to you? Does the patient need neurologic evaluation, computed tomography? Could positron emission tomography find the source of the problem? Patients accept these objective tests far more readily than a referral to a psychiatrist.

The ultimate therapeutic confirmation of a diagnosis of delusions of parasitosis comes with a response to pimozide.

Note: For further analysis of other types of delusions and hallucinations, see the section **Paresthesias**.

Koblenzer CS: Psychocutaneous Disease. New York, Grune & Stratton, 1987, pp 108–130.

Delusions are false beliefs, whereas **hallucinations are false perceptions**. The patient with **delusions of parasitosis** is typically anxious to the point of agitation. Totally immersed in symptoms, the patient, usually a woman, gives an unbelievably detailed descriptive account with scores of details. Her lifestyle reflects her attempts to eradicate the parasites attacking her. Within minutes, the shower of details reveals multiple visits to other doctors, repeated services of pest exterminators, and consultations with state entomologists. Her life revolves about escaping from the parasites and protecting her family. If you share her belief, her actions are entirely rational. Indeed, in all other areas, she is totally normal.

She will describe her skin as being **attacked by parasites** such as lice, mites, beetles, flies, cockroaches, and new ill-classified bugs, worms, or creatures. They may burrow into the skin, or they may be trapped in the skin, or they may descend as a cloudlike misery of mites. Parasitic worms may compete for the patient's food, their finicky eating habits forcing the patient into a diet that does not displease them.

The **sensations** experienced are not those of pruritus, an important distinction from the usual symptom of ectoparasitosis. These patients rather note crawling, tickling, biting, or stinging. The story is very convincing, including their explanation of pest control failure as due to egg resistance. Indeed, in one of three cases, one or more family members acquire the "parasites" and the diagnosis becomes *folie à deux* or *folie partagée*.

Failure of the physician to see, much less to eradicate, the pests leads the patient to search further for a doctor who has competence.

But before she leaves, the physician should run down the **differential** of alternative diagnoses. Is there

a true infestation
an underlying medical disorder
a vitamin deficiency

a toxic psychosis
an organic brain syndrome
evidence of schizophrenia?

Bishop ER Jr: Monosymptomatic **hypochondriacal syndromes in dermatology**. J Am Acad Dermatol 1983; 9:152–158.

With all scientific, clinical, and objective evidence to the contrary, some patients persist in maintaining the belief that they have a parasitic infection, a serious cosmetic defect, or an odor. Their **delusional beliefs** are best categorized:

    delusions of parasitosis
    delusions of dysmorphosis
    delusions of bromhidrosis

As a general statement, all reflect hypochondriasis channeled into a single complaint. All totally and completely shun psychiatric care. Even to suggest such a referral is to lose the patient.

Patients with delusions of parasitosis are remarkably successful in inducing the delusion in others (*folie à deux, folie à trois*) in the entire family (*folie à famille*) or even in the physician (*folie à médicin*). In evaluating these conditions, look for the **clinical context**. Here is a checklist:

psychiatric:

brief anxiety reaction	depression
obsessive disorder	paranoia
psychosis	schizophrenia

neurologic:

lesions of CNS	cerebral atrophy

toxic factors:

drug reaction	anticholinergic drugs
cocaine	delirium tremens
amphetamine	

medical factors:

hypothyroidism	polycythemia vera
diabetes mellitus	vitamin B_{12} deficiency
cardiovascular disease	

Patients with **delusions of dysmorphosis** are likely to want inappropriate cosmetic surgery. Moles become mountains that must be removed. A favorite site for dysmorphic concern is the nose: let the plastic surgeon beware.

The third group of patients have a pathologic conviction that they are emitting an **offensive odor**. Their delusion leads to social withdrawal, excessive body washing, frequent clothes changes, and a never-ending search for treatment. In rare instances the odor is perceived as arising outside of the individual's body and is recognized as a hallucinatory manifestation of temporal lobe epilepsy.

When these patients come to your office they have a problem, but it is not in the skin.

Elpern DJ: **Cocaine abuse and delusions of parasitosis.** Cutis 1988; 42:273–274.

Inhalation of 5 to 10 gm/day of cocaine for 8 days was clearly the cause of the "**little black bugs crawling out**" of a 39-year-old man's skin. He was also agitated, aggressive, and hostile. A week off cocaine and the "bugs" were gone (in search of more cocaine). His girlfriend shared the delusion (*folie à deux*), as well as the cocaine.

Fishman HC: **Rat mite dermatitis.** Cutis 1988; 42:414–416.

A 73-year-old woman with intense prolonged itching of the entire body misled her dermatologist into a **diagnosis of delusions of parasitosis** by bringing in sheets of cellophane tape speckled with "bugs" she had removed from her skin. Each bug, dutifully examined, proved to be keratin, crust, or blood. The skin itself was a battleground of excoriations, and her animated rambling about the bugs crawling over, around, and on her led the dermatologist to consider ways of getting psychiatric help. However, a **tiny tan object** was seen **moving over her shoulder**, which under the microscope proved to be the tropical rat mite *Ornithonyssus bacoti*, the cause of her pruritus. The source of these "bite-and-run" mites was traced to the **recent demolition of the house next door** and its two palm trees, which served as homes for rats. She was hanging out laundry on the day of demolition.

The dermatitis of rat mite bites varies from excoriations to linear erythematous pruritic papules or urticaria. The 1- to 2-mm papules may be in groups of three (breakfast, lunch, and dinner), with a 2-mm halo of erythema and no central punctum. Incidentally, the rats also get rat mite dermatitis.

The next time you see a patient bringing you a "bug collection," **ask yourself whether it is the patient or you who has the delusions**.

Sometimes the history brings out the diagnosis and other times the diagnosis brings out the history.

Dermatitis Herpetiformis

There are itches and there are itches, but the mother of all itches is dermatitis herpetiformis. When you have a patient whose itch is so severe that it is a burning itch, the diagnosis is dermatitis herpetiformis. Sure, atopic dermatitis, contact dermatitis, lichen planus, and scabies itch, but not with the intensity of dermatitis herpetiformis.

What will you see with this bonfire of itch? You will usually see only the embers of erosions and crusts of scratched-out primary lesions. They have a pattern of symmetry, grouping, and hyperpigmentation, even scarring. Large unaffected areas will be seen. Expect to find postlesional signs on the buttocks, sacral area, forearms, posterior axillary folds, and scalp and neck.

But will you see primary lesions? Yes, in acute attacks or flares such as induced by **iodine intake** from seafood. These lesions are polymorphous. As the name *herpetiform* indicates, they may be vesicular, but often you see only papules reminding you of prurigo. Some patients have urticaria, and a few have large bullae suggesting pemphigoid.

Always the patient's fingernail thwarts the diagnostician by removing the telltale vesicle or blister. Caution your patient to look for the vesicles and, if possible, get an immediate appointment so you can see their nature. There will be time to see an unscratched version of the disease, since it is a lifelong immune reaction associated with sensitivity to gluten. It may take time to make the diagnosis. Recall that Duhring, who first described this disease, took years to discern that it was not just another itchy eczema.

What looks just like dermatitis herpetiformis but isn't? **Scabies, neurotic excoriations**, and insect bites head the list. Patients with nummular eczema or contact dermatitis are less likely to fool you. In the bullous phase of dermatitis herpetiformis, all of the blistering diseases such as pemphigus, pemphigoid, chronic bullous eruption of childhood, and drug eruption come into the differential diagnosis.

If you can't make a clinical diagnosis, the pathologist can help. A fresh vesicle will show the subepidermal separation induced by the eosinophil-neutrophil infiltrate. Immunofluorescence will show a hallmark of **IgA deposits** in the papillae of clinically normal skin. He will also sort out linear IgA bullous dermatitis.

The ultimate confirmation of any diagnosis of dermatitis herpetiformis is the rapid, splendid relief provided by dapsone therapy.

Buckley DB, English J, Molloy W, et al: **Dermatitis herpetiformis:** A review of 119 cases. Clin Exp Dermatol 1983; 8:477–487.

    Clinical diagnosis:

        very itchy dermatosis
        polymorphic lesions
        tendency to group and appear in crops
        characteristic distribution:
                extensor surface of forearms
                intergluteal
        rapid response to dapsone therapy
        chronic

Hall RP: The pathogenesis of dermatitis herpetiformis: Recent advances. J Am Acad Dermatol 1987; 16:1129–1144.

    Clinical picture:

        burning, stinging prelude, severe

449

erythematous papule, urticarial plaque, vesicles
when patient is seen, crusted **excoriations** all that usually remains

Symmetrical localization:

elbows, knees	posterior aspect of neck, scalp
upper back	facial—hairline
buttocks	rare in mucosa

Pierce DK, Purcell SM, Spielvogel RL, Bergquist E: **Purpuric papules and vesicles of the palms** in dermatitis herpetiformis. J Am Acad Dermatol 1987; 16:1274–1276.

Tender, purpuric papules and vesicles of the palms and fingers recently appeared in a 27-year-old man with a 7-year history of dermatitis herpetiformis of the elbows, knees, sacral area, scalp, and face. These purpuric lesions proved on biopsy to be another manifestation of the dermatitis herpetiformis.

Bovenmyer DA: **Aggravation of dermatitis herpetiformis by dental fluoride treatments.** J Am Acad Dermatol 1985; 12:719–720.

Blisters appeared on the hands and forearms of this 83-year-old man several hours after he received a topical **sodium fluoride dental treatment**. His lips became swollen at the same time. The preparation used was 1.23% sodium fluoride gel, which was kept in place over the gums for 4 minutes.

For 8 years this man had had dermatitis herpetiformis under satisfactory control with a daily dose of 100 mg dapsone. The present attack was believed to be due to fluoride induction of a flare similar to those known to occur with iodide exposure.

Campbell-D'Hue G, Estes SA: A **Koebner phenomenon** in dermatitis herpetiformis. J Am Acad Dermatol 1983; 9:767–768.

A 57-year-old nurse with a 12-year history of dapsone–responsive dermatitis herpetiformis noted a dramatic **linear band of papulovesicles encircling the anterior surface of the waist** and also in the inframammary area just 3 weeks after stopping dapsone treatment.

She stated that similar lesions previously had appeared in these two sites after the wearing of tight-fitting underclothing. She denied intake of any drug or proprietary remedy. A Tzanck test was negative. A biopsy and direct immunofluorescence staining (positive for IgA) proved the diagnosis to be dermatitis herpetiformis.

Resumption of dapsone therapy led to prompt clearing. Other diseases showing this phenomenon of **isomorphic lesions in traumatized uninvolved skin (Koebner)** are typically psoriasis, lichen planus, lichen nitidus, vitiligo, or pityriasis rubra pilaris.

Leonard JN, Tucker WFG, Fry JS, et al: **Increased incidence of malignancy in dermatitis herpetiformis.** Br Med J 1983; 286:16–18.

Patients with dermatitis herpetiformis have a significantly increased risk of malignant growths, as do patients with celiac disease. Malignant disease was not seen, however, in patients with normal small-intestinal biopsies.

Among 109 patients with papillary IgA dermatitis herpetiformis, **seven (6.4%) had a malignant neoplasm** diagnosed 2 to 127 months (mean 41 months) following clinic presentation. There were three lymphomas, three lung carcinomas, and one somatostatinoma of the small intestine.

Malignant disease was also found in three of eight patients with linear IgA dermatitis herpetiformis, including bladder carcinoma, melanoma of the eye,

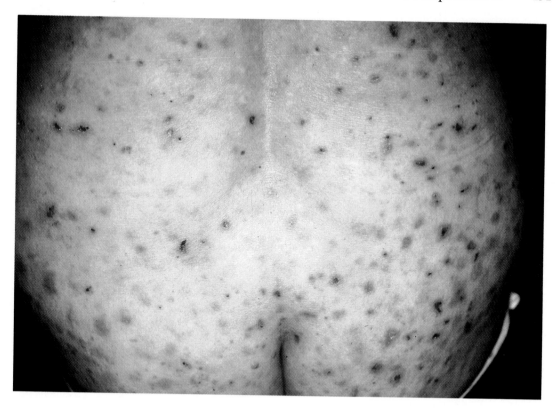

and lymphoma. The mean time from initial diagnosis to onset of malignant disease was 5 years (range 12 to 87 months).

Jenkins D, Lynde CW, Stewart WD: Histiocytic **lymphoma** occurring in a patient with dermatitis herpetiformis. J Am Acad Dermatol 1983; 9:252–256.

This 56-year-old woman with a 10-year history of dapsone-controlled dermatitis herpetiformis began to note pain in the left lower quadrant of the abdomen. Two months later she suddenly developed an "**acute abdomen**" requiring surgery. At that time she was found to have a diffuse histiocytic lymphoma, which had led to a perforation of the jejunum.

This is the 12th reported case of lymphoma in patients who have dermatitis herpetiformis. All had evidence of a gluten-sensitive enteropathy, and in eight the jejunum was the site of the lymphoma. It would appear to be analogous to the lymphomas reported in 9% of patients with celiac disease.

Noteworthy also is the fact that patients with dermatitis herpetiformis are not strangers to other malignant diseases. A wide variety of cancers, leukemia, and multiple myeloma has been reported.

With this **malignant diathesis of dermatitis herpetiformis** in mind, listen to more than your dermatitis herpetiformis patient's complaints of itch. He may need to be screened for malignant disease.

Ackerman AB, Stewart R, Stillman M: **Scabies masquerading as dermatitis herpetiformis.** JAMA 1975; 233:53–54.

A 79-year-old man had an extremely pruritic widespread dermatitis for 3 months. Examination showed papular dermatitis of the arms, legs, and thighs. Lichenified and excoriated papules were present on the buttocks. A single large bulla was present on one thigh. He was instructed to return if new vesicles appeared.

Two days later he returned with a **crop of papules and vesicles** on the inner aspects of the thighs and buttocks. Because of this grouping, a diagnosis of dermatitis herpetiformis was made.

A biopsy, however, showed the scabies mite in the cornified layer. All lesions disappeared within 2 weeks of lindane treatment for scabies.

Scabies and dermatitis herpetiformis have much in common creating diagnostic difficulty.

1. Widespread symmetrical lesions
2. Grouped wheal-like papules, vesicles, and crusted erosions
3. Extreme pruritus
4. Buttocks, a favored site
5. Bullous lesions possible

For contrast, scabies in adults spares the head and neck, whereas dermatitis herpetiformis involves scalp. Scabies has predilection for intertriginous areas, whereas dermatitis herpetiformis favors extensor surfaces.

Biopsy is an effective method of diagnosing scabies. Five examples are given in which the diagnosis of dermatitis herpetiformis was erroneously made until a biopsy was done showing the mite.

Ruzicka T, Schmoeckel C, Ring J, et al: **Bullous amyloidosis.** Br J Dermatol 1985; 113:85–95.

A 45-year-old woman suffered recurrent bouts of generalized pruritus followed by elevated, erythematous, urticarial, intensely pruritic plaques in rapidly changing locations. The buttocks and thighs were usually involved, with the head, palms, soles, and mucous membranes being spared. **Vesicles and bullae** appeared on erythematous skin only to be rapidly replaced by erosions, crusts, and hyperpigmented excoriated sites. Three hospitalizations and 12 years of observation had not yet led to a diagnosis, although atypical dermatitis herpetiformis was favored.

The **polymorphic picture** was puzzling, including diffuse pigmentation, extensive depigmented patches, and inapparent vesicles and flaccid bullae on darkly pigmented lichenified and ichthyosiform hyperkeratotic patches on the sides of the neck, antecubital fossae, knees, and dorsal surface of the feet. Add to this the distraction of mottled melanosis and scars and a tight doughy, firm, waxy feel to the skin, as if infiltrated. She also developed a very high IgE level (3660 U/ml) as the disease progressed; the erythrocyte sedimentation rate was 90 to 118 mm Westergren in the acute phases.

Six biopsies over the years did not reveal the diagnosis until a thioflavine T stain showed marked yellow fluorescence in the upper dermis and dermal papillae. In the same location, green birefringence was seen under polarized light with a Congo red stain. Bullous amyloidosis was diagnosed, and prednisone therapy gave prompt relief. Apparently the blisters resulted from shearing forces tearing the amyloid masses, producing subepidermal bullae.

No matter how many features a patient may have, the correct diagnosis may stem from a single observation. In cases of "atypical" dermatitis herpetiformis, look for amyloid!

Batista G, Santos ANC, Sampaio SAP: **Neutrophilic spongiosis.** A new entity? Br J Dermatol 1986; 114:131–134.

A **vesiculopustular eruption** of the face, axillae, and abdomen, as well as erosive denudation of the oral and vaginal mucosa led to 6 hospitalizations of a 22-year-old woman over a 3-year period. A burning sensation preceded the appearance of lesions, but they were not pruritic. The individual vesicles were 0.5 to 1.5 mm in size and symmetrically distributed. Early vesicles had a dewdrop appearance. The significant finding was spongiotic epidermis filled with neutrophils. Direct immunofluorescence was negative originally, but later showed granular deposition of IgA at the dermoepidermal junction.

A dozen treatments failed, but the 13th, **dapsone** (100 mg/day), **resulted in complete clearing** within 48 hours. Recurrence was rapid each time the dapsone was stopped. Clofazimine (100 mg/day) was also effective.

Hashimoto T, Inamoto N, Nahamura K, Nishikawa T: **Intercellular IgA dermatosis** with clinical features of subcorneal pustular dermatosis. Arch Dermatol 1987; 123:1062–1065.

Irregular erythematous areas with small pustules, crusts, and desquamation covered the trunk, upper arms, and thighs of this 31-year-old woman for 3 years. The lesions coalesced, forming **annular and serpiginous patterns** with scaly edges. As the lesions faded, many faintly pigmented areas remained.

Biopsy showed subcorneal bullae with neutrophils, and direct as well as indirect immunofluorescence studies showed clear staining of the upper epidermis with IgA. This **chronic, relapsing, pustular eruption** resembled subcorneal pustular eruption of Sneddon and Wilkinson, known to be associated with IgA gammopathy or IgA myeloma. It is not known whether this is a unique disease or a subset of Sneddon-Wilkinson's disease.

Impetigo can be easily distinguished by culture of pathogenic organisms. **Dermatitis herpetiformis** and linear IgA dermatosis have characteristic deposition of IgA at the basement membrane zone. **Pemphigus foliaceous** has its intercellular IgG autoantibodies as well as clear acontholytic changes. Hardest to distinguish is the annular centrifugal variant of **pustular psoriasis**. It, however, does not respond to dapsone as did this patient's problem, and usually there are recognizable psoriatic plaques, not seen in this patient.

Marsden RA, Dawber RPR, Millard PR, Mowat AG: **Herpetiform pemphigus** induced by penicillamine. Br J Dermatol 1977; 97:451–452.

A 56-year-old man with mild psoriasis since childhood and gout for 10 years developed seronegative polyarthritis with wasting of the quadriceps and shoulder muscles. He was treated with penicillamine (up to 1 gm daily). After 3 months he developed an intensely itchy widespread eruption consisting of **annular urticarial lesions and small tense vesicles**. Dermatitis herpetiformis was diagnosed clinically.

Skin biopsies showed intraepidermal vesicles containing neutrophils and eosinophils, adjacent spongiosis, and a moderate dermal perivascular infiltrate with lymphocytes, neutrophils, and eosinophils. Direct immunofluorescence was negative, but indirect immunofluorescence was positive for intercellular epidermal fluorescence at a titer of 1:160.

Pemphigus presenting like dermatitis herpetiformis usually shows eosinophilic spongiosis on histology rather than acantholysis.

Lewis GM: Trichophytosis (*T. rubrum*), with **dermatitis herpetiformis-like dermatophytid**. Arch Dermatol 1959; 79:736–737.

A 55-year-old man with tinea pedis for many years had noted a pruritic **vesicular and scaly eruption** on the buttocks and extensor surfaces of the arms and legs for 2 years. The lesions were irregularly spaced, but usually symmetrical. The feet were red and scaly, with porous yellow toenails.

A complete blood count showed 10% eosinophils. No skin biopsy was performed. Fungal cultures from the feet and buttock revealed *Trichophyton rubrum*. There are apparently other reports of *T. rubrum* causing a vesicular eruption simulating dermatitis herpetiformis.

Dermatomyositis

Swollen purplish eyelids, rough thickened knuckles, and **telangiectasia of the nail folds** form the diagnostic triad of skin manifestations of dermatomyositis. This is the heliotrope eyelids, the **Gottron papules**, and the paronychial redness symptom constellation. The myositis half of the syndrome may vary in degree from inability to readily arise from a chair to inability to lift even the lightest object such as a comb.

The skin changes are of the color purple. Look for scaly purplish patches over the hands, elbows, and knees. Look for the purplish discoloration of **Raynaud's phenomenon**. Telangiectasia is another sign. It may be a change in the eyelids with vessels so minute as to require a hand lens. Or it may be a progressive generalized telangiectasia as reported by us in a case of dermatomyositis. The diagnostic thread throughout all of this is a vascular one with changes induced by an inflammatory change within the skeletal muscles. Edema, urticaria, photosensitivity, even erythema multiforme may be fellow travelers with the myositis. In the childhood form of dermatomyositis, **calcinosis** of the skin over the bone prominences is a feature not ordinarily seen in adults unless they have a sclerodermatous element (sclerodermatomyositis).

Since dermatomyositis is a skin and muscle complex, evidence must be sought for the muscle component. This may manifest itself as weakness and muscle tenderness. Press on the eyelids to detect myositis of the *orbicularis oculi*. Ask if there is any difficulty swallowing. Is there dyspnea from chest wall muscle weakness? Watch as the patient arises from the chair. Does he exhibit weakness?

Order a serum creatine kinase determination. It will be elevated if there is widespread myositis. But note that exercise, hypothyroidism, and drugs also produce elevations in this enzyme. Arrange consultation for EMG studies and appropriate muscle biopsy. The electromyogram will show fibrillation potentials, and the biopsy, characteristic myopathic and inflammatory change.

Still, one thing remains: Adults—but not children—who have dermatomyositis deserve study for the presence of **underlying malignant disease**. Finding and removing an ovarian carcinoma spelled a cure for one of our dermatomyositis patients. Recurrence of the tumor was made evident by the reappearance of the dermatomyositis.

Bunch TW: Polymyositis: A case history approach to the differential diagnosis and treatment. Mayo Clin Proc 1990; 65:1480–1497.

Dermatomyositis is a special example of polymyositis in which there is a characteristic rash. The muscle problem is symmetrical **proximal muscle weakness** that is associated with increased muscle enzymes in the serum, characteristic electromyographic pattern, and inflammatory myopathic change seen in muscle biopsy.

The best-recognized sign of dermatomyositis is the **heliotrope (purplish) rash of the eyelids**. Often there is associated periorbital edema. A scaly violaceous rash of the bony pressure points of the hands, knees, and elbows as described by Gottron is also typical. These patients may have an erythematous eruption in sun-exposed areas. Capillary microscopy of the nail fold may reveal the bushy, branching pattern seen in scleroderma. In some patients the cutaneous manifestation proves to be a psoriasiform eruption or an aberrant type of pityriasis rosea or lichen planus.

Dupre A, Viraben R, Bonafe J-L, et al: **Zebra-like dermatomyositis**. Arch Dermatol 1981; 117:63–64.

Blotchy purple streaks appeared on the trunk and extremities of this 14-year-

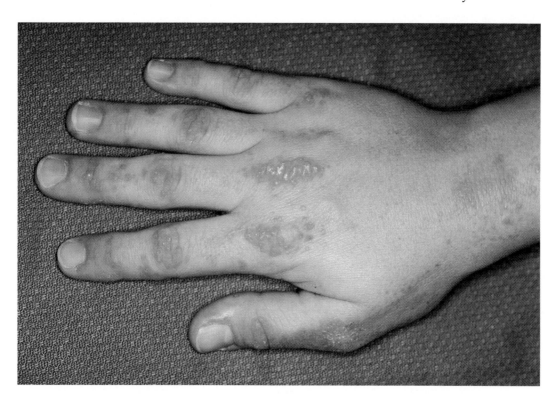

old girl, giving her a zebralike appearance. The streaks that ran in parallel were longitudinal on the limbs, vertical on the shoulders, and in a Christmas-tree arrangement on the back. The **child appeared to have been flogged,** but the concurrent presence of heliotrope erythema of the face, and Gottron's papules of the knuckles led to the diagnosis of dermatomyositis. This was confirmed by electromyographic study and by an elevated serum creatine phosphokinase level.

As to the pathogenesis, the stripes appeared to lie in same planes as the tensile strength lines. This "zebra sign" disappeared shortly after steroid therapy was initiated.

Malleson P: **Juvenile dermatomyositis:** A review. J Roy Soc Med 1982; 75:33–37.

The violaceous rash has a characteristic distribution beginning periorbitally with marked edema and spreading onto the nasal bridge and malar areas. **Scaly erythematous patches** also occur over the knuckles, elbows, knees, medial malleoli, and shawl areas. The rash fades in time, leaving postinflammatory hyperpigmentation and scarring. Photosensitivity causes the rash to wax and wane. Severe **skin ulcerations** may develop because of vasculitis.

The mean age of onset is 7 years, and girls are affected twice as frequently as boys. **Calcinosis** occurs in two forms: subcutaneous deposits on the elbows, knees, and fingers with extrusion through the skin or secondary abscess formation; and deposits in intermuscle fascial planes.

In addition to the rash, three or four other criteria must be met for a definite **diagnosis** of juvenile dermatomyositis:

1. Symmetrical limb girdle weakness (progressive tenderness and weakness)
2. Muscle biopsy showing myositis and necrosis

3. Elevated muscle enzyme levels—measure them all (aspartate amino-transferase (AST), aldolase, creatine phosphokinase), as any one may be normal while the others are abnormal

4. Electromyographic changes of myositis

Chamberlain MJ, Whittaker SRF: Hashimoto's disease, dermatomyositis and ovarian carcinoma. Lancet 1963; 1:1398–1399.

A 52-year-old woman with hypothyroidism and thyroglobulin antibodies (1:2,500,000) developed an **erythematous macular rash** that became generalized over her face, arms, and trunk. She also had weakness of her arms and legs, inability to sit up, difficulty swallowing, tender swollen legs, and generalized muscle wasting. The erythrocyte sedimentation rate was 52 mm/hour. She improved with steroids over a 3-month period, but suddenly developed ascites and gross edema of the legs and soon died.

Necropsy revealed undifferentiated **carcinoma of the ovary** with metastases, muscle atrophy with foci of muscle fiber degeneration, thyroid gland destruction with autoimmune thyroiditis, and normal skin. Despite a clinical diagnosis of dermatomyositis, the muscle changes were nonspecific and more consistent with **carcinomatous neuromyopathy**. This condition has been reported with carcinoma of the lung and breast and resembles dermatomyositis in many ways.

Fudman EJ, Schnitzer TJ: **Dermatomyositis without creatine kinase elevation:** A poor prognostic sign. Am J Med 1986; 80:329–332.

Among seven patients with dermatomyositis and normal creatine phosphokinase (CPK) values, three had malignant disease (apparent in only one patient at the time of diagnosis) and two had interstitial lung disease. The 1-year survival was 33%.

A normal CPK should *not* stop the diagnostic pursuit of suspected inflammatory myopathy. Electromyography and muscle biopsy should be carried out, and values of **other serum muscle enzymes**, including lactic dehydrogenase, serum glutamic oxaloacetic transaminase, and serum aldolase, should be obtained.

Missing the rare form of a common disease is more disturbing than missing the common form of a rare disease.

Drug Eruptions

Anything you can think of, anything you can see, and some things you don't even think of can be due to a drug. This is only to alert you to the need for knowing and being suspicious of any and all drugs taken by your patient.

Such knowledge is not easy to come by. It requires repeated cross-examining, naming specific medicines, asking again what treatment is given for each systemic complaint that surfaces. It demands educating the patient that medical molecules can cause as well as cure disease. It calls for instructing the patient that eye drops can be as hazardous as dental anesthesia, that laxatives cause pigment spots as well as cure constipation. Your patient must learn to distrust old friends such as aspirin, Motrin, and mouthwashes. If there is to be success in diagnosis, he must not hold back or repress information on use of anabolic steroids, recreational drugs, or vitamins. He must give the dates of starting, stopping, and changing brands as accurately as possible. He must be fully aware that a single tablet can trigger a drug eruption.

The actual employment of this repeatedly updated and, it is hoped, excellent drug history is in your hands. If you know the nature and cause of the problem, e.g., impetigo, the drug history may be irrelevant aside from its value in determining future therapy. If you don't know the cause of the patient's problem, consider the possibility that it is a drug eruption.

Now, while it is true that **any eruption can be caused by any drug**, in practice certain eruptions are more commonly due to drugs than others. The number 1 sign of drug sensitivity is circulatory in nature, for it is in the blood stream that the drug has its initial opportunity to damage. Looking through the epidermis, we commonly see a scarlatiniform, morbilliform, or diffuse erythema signaling drug intolerance. If the harm of the drug is more than endothelial vasodilatation, we will see the urticaria of fluid leakage, the petechiae and purpura of red cell leakage. Significantly, specific areas of reaction occur, depending on regional factors, blood flow, and past history. A unique form of localization is seen in the fixed nonpigmenting drug eruption that recurs at symmetrical intertriginous sites upon drug intake. Even more intense drug damage results in the vasculitis of erythema multiforme and systemic lupus. This may extend to actual skin necrosis.

The drug may leave the vessel and target the epidermis, where the intraepidermal nerves cry out in pruritus. More severe reactions appear as eczematous lesions, exfoliative dermatitis, bullae, even the total destruction of toxic epidermal necrolysis. A more specific target is the skin appendage. We sense the attack on the follicle most easily as the hair falls out. Sometimes the drug cannot wreak its havoc without a co-conspirator, viz., ultraviolet light. This is the case of photosensitivity drug eruptions, which may be phototoxic or photoallergic in nature. Most interesting is the drug eruption that expresses itself in a fixed site, i.e., an island of sensitive skin that becomes red and later hyperpigmented following each exposure to the offending drug.

Even as there are these common vascular and epidermal drug reactions, there is a commonality of drugs that produce the majority of drug disease in the skin. Our

457

suspicions run high when the following drugs are in the patient's medicine cabinet or history:

penicillin
sulfonamides
chlorothiazide
Zyloprim

For specific patterns of reaction we think of more specific drugs:

urticaria:
   aspirin
   ibuprofen

photosensitivity:
   chlorothiazide
   quinine

alopecia:
   beta-blockers
   chemotherapy

Always the number of drug eruptions you will see depends on both the total usage and incidence of sensitization.

The rarities of drug eruptions are the greatest challenge. In these instances, comparing your patient's problem and the drug list with the texts on drug reactions will greatly aid. You will find reactions ranging from the acne of patients taking lithium to mycosis fungoides type of growths due to cobalt sensitivity.

Testing for drug sensitivity is still the clinical art of elimination and challenge. The laboratory does provide the **radioallergosorbent test** for penicillin, and a blood count may show the **eosinophilia and basophilia** that precede and accompany drug allergies. **Drug elimination** is the most practical approach to identifying a cause. But the many drugs the older patient may be taking are so essential that elimination has to be done on a piecemeal basis. Insofar as substitution is concerned, care must be taken not to prescribe a molecularly similar compound. Challenge is rarely undertaken unless the drug is absolutely essential.

Next time you see a skin disease you don't quite know, greet it by asking, "Could your name be *Drug*?"

Wintroub BU, Stern R: **Cutaneous drug reactions:** Pathogenesis and clinical classification. J Am Acad Dermatol 1985; 13:167–179.

Think drugs when you see:

    morbilliform eruptions
    urticaria
    photosensitive eruptions
    erythema multiforme
    vasculitis
    lichen planus
    toxic epidermal necrolysis
    pigment change

Think these drugs when you see:

    granuloma–iodides
    erythema multiforme–diphenylhydantoin
    alopecia–Cytoxan
    hyperpigmentation–Minocin
    photosensitivity–hydrochlorothiazide
    urticaria–ibuprofen
    necrosis–Coumadin

Think of drugs when you see skin disease.

Shear NH: **Diagnosing cutaneous adverse reactions to drugs.** Arch Dermatol 1990; 126:94–97.

Stepwise approach:

1. Clinical diagnosis
    Confirm with laboratory tests and consultation.
2. Analysis of drug exposure
    Get details on timing; dose; past experiences from patient, physicians, pharmacists, family, nurses, and repeated questioning.
3. Differential diagnosis
    Look for causes other than drugs.
4. Literature search
    Correlate drugs taken by patient with eruptions recorded.
5. Confirmation
    Consider penicillin skin tests, in vitro lymphocyte toxicity assay and challenge.
6. Advice to patient
    avoidance of specific drugs
    cross-sensitivity list (congeners and classes)
7. Report results to aid others in diagnosis of drug eruptions.

Making a diagnosis can be as exhilarating as downhill skiing, but both require an uphill climb.

Eczematous Drug Eruptions

Guillet G, Delaire P, Plantin P, Guillet MH: **Eczema** as a complication of heparin therapy. J Am Acad Dermatol 1989; 20:1130–1132.

Subcutaneous injections of calcium heparinate were regularly followed 3 days later by a pruritic erythematous plaque overlying the injection site. Intradermal tests with this and another type of heparin produce a similar dermatitis.

Prior reports emphasized the ability of heparin injections to induce ecchymosis, hair loss, urticaria, necrosis, scleroderma-like change.

Ghadially R, Ramsay CA: Gentamicin: **Systemic exposure to a contact allergen.** J Am Acad Dermatol 1988; 19:428–430.

This 84-year-old woman had had stasis dermatitis with recurrent ulcerations for 3 years. Secondary bacterial infection with culture demonstrated *Pseudomonas aeruginosa* was recently treated with gentamicin cream. Shortly thereafter the dermatitis became more extensive. Crusted and weeping, it completely surrounded the right lower leg. By that time a few eczematous plaques had appeared on the arms.

She was admitted to the hospital, the local treatment changed, and intravenous gentamicin started. Within several hours she developed a **pruritic eczematous eruption** on both arms extending up onto the neck. The gentamicin was discontinued; steroid cream was applied with subsequent resolution.

Patch tests to gentamicin (20% in petrolatum) gave a strong 2+ reaction, but not until the fourth day. The other allergens in the standard tray produced no reaction except for neomycin, which gave a 2+ reaction at 48 hours.

It is significant that this patient had not only a contact dermatitis to gentamicin but also an erythematous drug eruption when it was given intravenously. Interestingly, the structurally related **neomycin** proved to be another hazard for this patient.

Gentamicin and neomycin are twin allergens inside or out. Also note that a patch test negative at 2 days may not be negative at 4 days!

460

Fixed Drug Eruptions

Kanwar AJ, Bharija SC, Singh M, Belhaj MS: Ninety-eight **fixed drug eruptions** with provocation tests. Dermatologica 1988; 177:274–279.

On challenge, 83 of the 98 fixed drug eruptions studied were caused by:

trimethoprim/sulfamethoxazole (45)
aspirin (24)
hyoscine butylbromide (8)
ibuprofen (6)

Alanko K, Stubb S, Reitamo S: **Topical provocation** of fixed drug eruption. Br J Dermatol 1987, 116:561–567.

Although per oral provocation tests are the most reliable method of discerning the cause of a fixed drug eruption, in some instances an open topical test with the drug in question will reproduce the eruption.

Apply the drug in a concentration of 10% in petrolatum over the site of the eruption and also to an area of normal skin. It may be covered or uncovered. Readings are made for 24 hours. A positive reaction is a clearly demarcated erythema appearing only in the former eruption site and lasting at least 6 hours. Alternate vehicles such as 95% ethanol or dimethyl sulfoxide may be employed to facilitate dissolving the drug or enhance penetration. These should be used if an initial provocation test with the drug in white petrolatum fails.

In this study, the following drugs produced positive topical provocation tests:

phenazone salicylate
sulfadiazine
sulfamethoxazole
trimethoprim
amobarbital
phenobarbital
carbamazepine

Doxycycline and sulfamethoxydiazine were negative in all vehicles tested.

Kanwar AJ, Bharija SC, Belhaj MS: Fixed drug eruptions **in children**: A series of 23 cases with provocation tests. Dermatologica 1986; 172:315–318.

In this remarkably comprehensive study, the offending drug was identified in each of 23 cases by challenging each child with 10 to 12 drugs. **Aspirin** proved to be the **most common cause** of fixed drug eruptions, accounting for 9 cases (39%). Other responsible drugs included hyoscine butylbromide (7 cases), erythromycin, ampicillin, phenolphthalein, and sulfamethoxazole.

The generalized **bullous form** of fixed drug eruption seen in eight children was most often **misdiagnosed as pyoderma or insect bite reaction**.

Kanwar AJ, Majid A, Singh M, Malhotra YK: An **unusual presentation** of fixed drug eruption. Dermatologica 1981; 162:378–379.

Within a few hours of taking hyoscine-N-butylbromide for abdominal pain, a 40-year-old man in Libya developed **itchy, dark-red, circular patches on the lips** and extremities. A fixed drug eruption was diagnosed and confirmed by challenge with the drug. Challenge with analgin (metamizole), an unrelated drug, also reactivated the same lesions.

Control challenges with five other drugs failed to produce any change. However, a sixth drug, tetracycline, induced totally new itchy, circular, dark-red   461

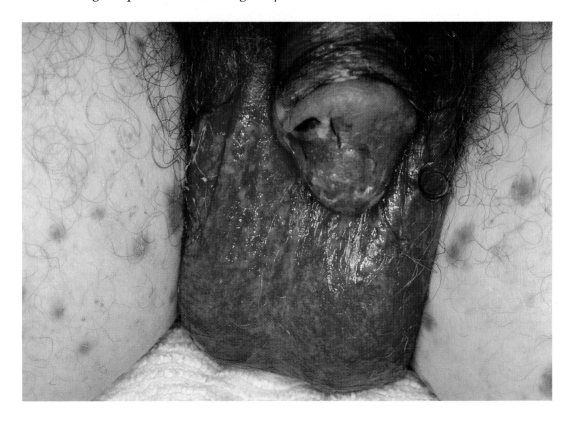

patches on the patient's back. The hyoscine-sensitive patches on the arms and legs showed no activation.

Later challenges with tetracycline and hyoscine proved the remarkable specificity of the two sets of fixed drug eruptions occurring in the same patient.

Stubb S, Reitamo S: Fixed drug eruption caused by **piroxicam**. J Am Acad Dermatol 1990; 22:1111–1112.

Application of 10% piroxicam (Feldene) in petrolatum as an open patch test to the site of a piroxicam–fixed drug eruption induced a red pruritic **reaction after only 5 hours**.

Success with topical challenge to fixed drug eruption sites is limited largely to phenazone derivatives such as Feldene.

The more perplexing the diagnostic problem, the more frequently you should see the patient.

Linear Drug Eruptions

Schwartz RA, Moore HC III, Lambert WC: **Linear localized coumarin necrosis.** Dermatologica 1984; 168:31–34.

Linear, nontender, discrete, violaceous-to-black 8-mm **papulonodules** with bright red 10-mm halos had been appearing on the forearms of a 55-year-old white man for 4 months. They formed scabs and disappeared spontaneously. He denied insect bites, catecholamine injections, or inducing the lesions himself. Biopsy showed a blood-filled vesicle overlying dermal necrosis, with no evidence of thrombosed vessels or vasculitis. Direct immunofluorescence was negative, and circulating cryoglobulins were not detected. During the next few months, two new crops appeared in linear patterns on the extremities and faded in 3 weeks without therapy.

The lesions first appeared within a few days of the start of coumarin administration for prophylaxis and treatment of pulmonary embolism. They reappeared within 3 to 10 days of a new course of coumarin and were no longer seen following cessation of the drug therapy. The diagnosis was coumarin necrosis.

Coumarin ordinarily produces a **large, solitary, tender patch of necrosis**, which begins as erythema and becomes blue-black within hours, with necrosis by the next day followed by sloughing of the affected skin and subcutaneous tissue.

The **differential diagnosis** is large:

self-inflicted lesions	disseminated intravascular coagulation
pressure necrosis	pyoderma gangrenosum
spider bites	paroxysmal nocturnal hemoglobinuria
catecholamine infusion	macroglobulinemia (Waldenström)
cryoglobulinemia	

Other reactions to coumarin (warfarin sodium) include:

ecchymoses and purpura from excessive lowering of the prothrombin time
"purple toes"
urticaria, maculopapular eruptions

The diagnosis is made in these patients by simply taking a careful history. Why were this man's lesions in a line? Ask Koebner! But a direct toxic effect of coumarin on the blood vessel wall has been suggested.

Fine J-D, Breathnach SM: Distinctive eruption characterized by linear **supravenous papules** and erythroderma following broxuridine (bromodeoxyuridine) therapy and radiotherapy. Arch Dermatol 1986; 122:199–200.

A **linear eruption** of red-to-violaceous papules precisely overlying the blood vessels of the lower aspects of both arms developed in a 56-year-old man being given concurrent radiotherapy and intravenous broxuridine for a malignant astrocytoma. An associated morbilliform eruption with plaques and papules on the trunk and scalp evolved into generalized erythroderma.

It is thought that broxuridine diffuses out from the veins into the skin where an allergic response is initiated. Notable is the fact that intravenous administration of a chemically related compound, 5-fluorouracil, produces pigmentation that marks the course of underlying arm veins, designated serpentine **supravenous fluorouracil hyperpigmentation**. Also, doxorubicin (Adriamycin) produces transient **urticaria along the vein** proximal to the injection site in up to 3% of patients receiving the drug.

Chemotherapeutic Drug Eruptions

Dufresne RG: **Skin necrosis from intravenously infused materials.** Cutis 1987; 39:197–198.

What can safely be diluted in a vein may cause skin and soft tissue necrosis as an extravasate, including hypertonic solutions, vasopressor drugs, radiologic dyes, and chemotherapeutic agents.

Some common **troublemakers** include:

dextrose 10%	norepinephrine
mannitol	dopamine
sodium bicarbonate	radiopaque dye
calcium salts	Adriamycin
potassium salts	bleomycin
nafcillin	

Bronner AK, Hood AF: Cutaneous complications of **chemotherapeutic agents.** J Am Acad Dermatol 1983; 9:645–663.

Because of their high metabolic rates, hair and mucosa are caught by chemotherapy in the same swath as the primary target of rapidly dividing tumor cells. As a result, there is **alopecia** (anagen effluvium) and **stomatitis**. The alopecia is not limited to the scalp and may be noted on the face, axilla, and pubis with long-term administration. It is, however, reversible once the therapy is stopped. The stomatitis, in turn, may become very severe because not only do the chemotherapeutic agents inhibit mucosa cell replacement but their myelosuppressive actions favor bleeding and infection.

Chemotherapy is also often associated with **darkening of the skin**. This may be generalized or localized to the nails and mucosa or to the palms and soles. The drugs, e.g., busulfan, cyclophosphamide, and bleomycin, stimulate melanocyte activity. Interestingly, when fluorouracil is given intravenously, hyperpigmented streaks may develop exactly over the arm veins used. It has the name of serpentine supravenous fluorouracil hyperpigmentation.

Dactinomycin and doxorubicin **potentiate radiation** effects so that in patients receiving radiotherapy and chemotherapy, any radiation dermatitis can be extraordinarily severe. This radiation enhancement may occur with other chemotherapeutic agents as well, and may affect other organs.

Radiation recall, classically seen with dactinomycin, represents the appearance of radiation dermatitis in a site previously treated with radiation, possibly months ago.

Similarly, these drugs **heighten the patient's sensitivity to ultraviolet light** and can reactivate an ultraviolet-induced burn. Methotrexate-treated patients may thus see an old sunburn site become erythematous and, indeed, vesicular.

The classic drug eruptions such as **urticaria**, **morbilliform eruptions**, and **erythema multiforme** also may be induced by chemotherapy, but this is uncommon.

Extravasation of most chemotherapeutic agents produces irritation phlebitis and cellulitis. **Ulcers may form** that are notoriously chronic. Any site is subject to a recall flare when the patient is given doxorubicin, even months later.

Unusual reactions include:

sclerosis of hands and feet–bleomycin
Raynaud's phenomenon–bleomycin

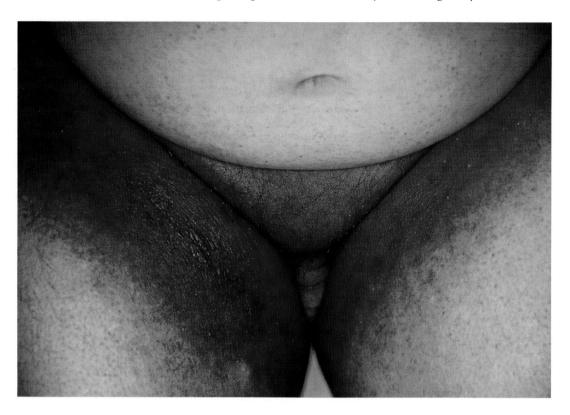

papulopustules suggesting septic emboli–dactinomycin
flushing–mithramycin

But the good news is that intravenous fluorouracil will clear your patient of
any and all actinic keratoses.

*Some diseases undergo constant change and can be recognized only
at the "right" time.*

Miscellaneous

Zijdenbos AM, Balmus KJ: **Pigmentation** secondary to **minocycline** therapy. Br J Dermatol 1984; 110:117–118.

An 83-year-old man had noticed **progressive darkening of the skin** for the past few years and generalized **pruritus** for 1 year. His face and neck showed diffuse dark-blue discoloration, especially prominent on the cheeks. Whereas the pigmentation was reticulate on the trunk and thighs, it was solid dark blue and slightly papular on the lower legs and feet. The fingernails were darkened, and the sclera showed spotty blue discoloration. Erythema was present on the hands and thighs. He had been taking **minocycline** (200 mg/day) for 9 years for chronic pulmonary disease, and minocycline-induced pigmentation was confirmed on biopsy, with brownish-black pigment and granules found within histiocytes. Special stains confirmed the presence of iron and melanin.

After discontinuation of minocycline therapy the erythema cleared. However, he died of cardiac failure, and at autopsy **the thyroid and prostate were black**, and the aorta, endocardium, and ribs showed areas of diffuse darkening.

Minocycline has now taken the place of silver in the iatrogenic darkening of the face of humans.

Penneys NS: Gold therapy: Dermatologic uses and toxicities. J Am Acad Dermatol 1979; 1:315–320.

Analysis of 37 patients showed that the most common type of eruption in patients receiving gold therapy consists of a **patchy, pruritic, erythematous, papular, eczematous dermatitis**. About 25% of gold rashes resemble **lichen**

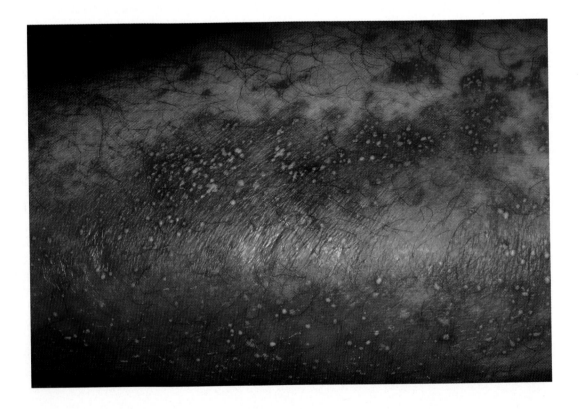

planus, clinically and histologically. Less common gold-induced eruptions include some that are pityriasis rosea–like, and erythema nodosum, erythroderma, cheilitis, and stomatitis.

After gold therapy is stopped, it takes about 10 weeks for most gold eruptions to clear (range: 10 days to 2 years). When the gold was restarted at lower doses, there appeared to be no increased risk of recurrent dermatitis, except with erythema nodosum.

Immediately after gold is injected, a vasomotor response may occur with flushing, erythema, weakness, dizziness, hypotension, and syncope. This nitritoid reaction occurs only with aqueous gold sodium thiomalate, not with aurothioglucose in oil.

Proteinuria occurring in 2 to 10% of patients with gold therapy indicates that the drug should be temporarily stopped. Gold therapy may then be restarted at lower levels after the urinary protein disappears.

Bernhard JD, Haynes HA: Non-rashes: I. The Koebner non-reaction. Cutis 1982; 29:158–164.

The total **absence of an ampicillin-induced drug eruption** from a perfect rectangle of abdominal skin was diagnosed as a nonrash. The cause proved to be radiation given at that exact site just at the time of the ampicillin administration. The **radiation portal** proved to a privileged site, incapable of developing a drug reaction.

Ultraviolet light or sunlight may have a similar protective effect, with drug rashes appearing only within the area covered by the bathing suit.

Mackowiak PA, LeMaistre CF: Drug fever: A critical appraisal of conventional concepts. An analysis of 51 episodes in two Dallas hospitals and 97 episodes reported in the English literature. Ann Intern Med 1987; 106:728–733.

Drug fever is a diagnosis of exclusion: no other cause for the fever can be ascertained and the fever resolves rapidly after discontinuation of the drug. The fever pattern gradually increases, beginning 7 to 10 days after a responsible antimicrobial was started, but much sooner for an antineoplastic drug and much later for a cardiac drug. There is little risk associated with rechallenge.

Skin rashes occurred in only 18% of cases, with urticaria in less than half of these. Eosinophilia occurred in 22% and was usually mild. Chills (53%), myalgias (25%), and headache (16%) were other major symptoms. Relative bradycardia (pulse rate <100/min) was rare. There was no association with atopy.

The most commonly implicated drugs were:

alpha-methyldopa (16)	procainamide (6)
quinidine (13)	iodide (6)
diphenylhydantoin (11)	isoniazid (5)
penicillin G (9)	bleomycin (3)
cephalothin (7)	carbamazepine (3)
methicillin (6)	

Ears

The external ear is an anatomically unique configuration of skin. As such, it becomes a favored site for certain dermatoses. It is exposed to the trauma of compression produced by sleeping on a hard pillow, boxing, or wearing a helmet. It is buffeted by the extremes of cold and sunlight. Its lobes are a site for perfuming, piercing, and pressure from earrings. Thus, we commonly see frostbite, sunburn, actinic keratoses, and nickel or perfume contact dermatitis on these special outcroppings of skin.

Besides weathering environmental exposures, the ear is an interface of skin and cartilage, so that skin damage may be accompanied by damage to the underlying cartilage. Witness chondrodermatitis nodularis chronica helicis. Primary damage to the cartilage also affects the skin, as in relapsing polychondritis, which confronts the clinician with a beefy red swollen ear. The earlobe is exempt since it possesses no cartilage.

The acral nature of the circulatory system in the external ear also accounts for some of its distinctive diseases. Discoid lupus erythematous often involves the concha as well as the fingertips, leaving discoid white atrophic scars of diagnostic significance. Likewise, the tophi of gout arise in the helix. The ear is also a natural target for the picker and scratcher. Trauma from fingernails, paper clips, or other foreign objects may induce psoriasis. The convoluted folds of the ear make cleansing difficult, and the ear canal and retroauricular folds serve as intertriginous zones with a host of ills, including seborrheic dermatitis and candidiasis. Finally, the ear is susceptible to infectious eczematoid dermatitis when there is a middle ear infection with chronic drainage into the ear canal.

Among the diagnostic memorabilia of the ear is the clinically inapparent leprosy that is unveiled by sampling the earlobe to find swarms of the lepra bacilli in smears. The blue ear of ochronosis is a physician's once-in-a-lifetime diagnostic sign, providing at once an explanation for the patient's progressive crippling arthritis.

Listen to what the ear is telling you as you travel down its canal, comparing the landscape with the color atlas of Clinical Otoscopy (Hawke M, Keene M, Albert PW, Churchill Livingstone, 1984).

It can be an exciting trip.

Hawke M, John AF: **Diseases of the Ear.** Clinical and Pathologic Aspects. Philadelphia, Lea & Febiger, 1987, 309 pp.

To increase your diagnostic skills through direct observation, pay attention to your patient's outer ear (pinna, auricle), a finely sculpted appendage that is composed of cartilage covered by skin. The surface landmarks should be learned so that descriptions of skin lesions can be anatomically accurate.

Look for:

hairy tragus Coarse hair on the male tragus is a secondary sex characteristic that occurs with aging.

hairy pinna Coarse hair over the lower portion of the helix is a Y-linked trait commonly seen in males in India but rare in North America.

Darwin's tubercle A small cartilaginous protuberance on the posterosuperior helix, which usually projects anteriorly from the concave edge, but it may project outward (posteriorly). Inherited as an autosomal dominant, it is present in 50% of the native population in England and Finland. It forms the apex of the helix in anthropoid apes.

lobule attachment This ranges from fully attached (in Orientals) to fully detached (in whites) and is an inherited racial characteristic. Attached earlobes are recessive to detached lobes.

creased lobule An oblique crease that angles diagonally back to the edge of the lobule, it appears in adults predisposed to obstructive coronary artery disease.

elongated lobule An excessively long earlobe is inherited as an autosomal dominant. It is depicted in statues of Buddha as a sign of wisdom and kindness.

preauricular pits and sinuses The pit is located just in front of the anterior crus of the helix and often discharges a cheesy substance or purulent material. Pain, redness, and swelling at points anterior to the auricle suggest an infected preauricular sinus (commonly anaerobic bacteria, such as *Bacteroides* or *Fusobacterium*).

preauricular tags These consist of one or multiple pedunculated small nubbins of soft tissue, containing skin, subcutaneous tissue, and fat.

accessory auricle A hard preauricular cartilage-containing papule, this is located just in front of the upper border of the tragus.

low-set ear Commonly seen in Down's syndrome in which the ear is usually small with a deformed helix, which meets the cranium below the Frankfort plane (a line between the outer canthus of the eye and the occipital protuberance).

Roizin H, Toren A, Berkenstadt M, Goodman RM: Congenital heart disease and external ear anomalies with hearing loss: A report of two new cases and a review of the literature. J Craniofac Genet Develop Biol 1989; 9:225–230.

Any infant born with **external ear malformations** should have a **cardiac evaluation**.

Such malformations include dysplastic ears, small low-set ears, posteriorly rotated ears, and ears crumpled forward or misplaced. Hearing loss and deafness are often associated.

Look for ear anomalies and congenital heart disease in these syndromes with skin findings:

Klippel-Feil anomaly:

low-set ears	fusion of cervical vertebrae with limited
short webbed neck	head movement
low posterior hairline	dysplastic ears with hearing loss

Fanconi pancytopenia syndrome:
    thumb/radial anomalies   eye/renal anomalies
    hyperpigmentation of skin   anemia
    café au lait spots

Noonan syndrome:
    low-set ears, posteriorly rotated   pterygium colli
    broad forehead   low posterior hairline
    ptosis

Focal dermal hypoplasia (Goltz syndrome):
    thinning ear helix/hearing loss   multiple subcutaneous fat
    atrophy/linear hyperpigmentation   herniation
    mucosal papillomas   eye/digital anomalies

LEOPARD syndrome:
    low-set ears/deafness   ptosis/epicanthal folds
    multiple lentigines   chest deformity
    triangular face   skeletal anomalies
    biparietal bossing

Howard FM: Lax ligament syndrome in children associated with blue sclera and bat ears. Br J Gen Pract 1990; 40:233–235.

Bat ears in children are prominent and stick out. They are also unfolded and remarkably soft, enabling them to be easily tweaked and bent over, like those of a rabbit.

Bat ears may occur with **blue sclera** and soft skin that bruises easily. The skin is not lax, elastic, or excessively fragile, and scars heal normally. Prominent veins may occur over the chest walls. The cheeks are usually full, and the teeth are normal.

If bat ears and blue sclera are combined with hypermobile joints, the lax ligament syndrome should be suspected. This mild collagenopathy is dominantly inherited and improves with time as more collagen cross-linkages form; it lies within the spectrum ranging from normality through joint hypermobility to the **Ehlers-Danlos syndrome**.

Joint hypermobility is present if:

    Extension of the wrist and metacarpal phalanges brings the fingers parallel to the dorsal forearm.
    Positive opposition brings the thumb to the flexor aspect of the forearm.
    The elbows or knees may be hyperextended by more than 10 degrees.
    Flexion of the trunk with the knees extended enables the palms to rest on the floor.

Other common features of the lax ligament syndrome include deep growing pains of the arms and legs, odd gait, flatfeet, lordotic posture, "toddler tummy," and epicanthic folds. Many children also have delayed milestones of motor development.

Boys with the syndrome tend to talk late and have constipation with late toilet training. They should be screened for the **fragile X syndrome**, which also features prominent ears, language delay, macro-orchidism, attention deficit, loose stretchable skin, flat feet, and hyperextensible finger joints.

The lax ligament syndrome differs from the **articular hypermobility syndrome**, which does not have any facial abnormalities.

Barker SM, Dicken CH: **Elastolysis of the earlobes.** J Am Acad Dermatol 1986; 14:145–147.

Over an 18-month period, a 15-year-old girl spontaneously developed droopy

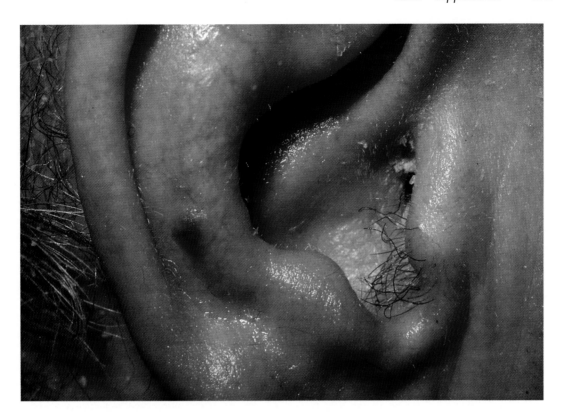

elongated earlobes with fine wrinkling. Her mother stated that her daughter's **earlobes flapped in the breeze**. Her ears had been pierced many years earlier, without any adverse reactions. She denied wearing large, heavy earrings or having easy bruisability, abnormal scars, or musculoskeletal symptoms. However, she did describe having recurrent hives for 3 to 4 years, never involving the head and neck.

Further examination revealed that the upper and lower eyelids were mildly atrophic and wrinkled, and striae were present over both breasts. She also had diffuse hypermobility of the joints, thought to be benign.

A biopsy of the earlobe revealed a marked decrease in elastic tissue throughout the dermis (elastin Giemsa stain) and a mild mononuclear cell infiltrate around blood vessels and appendages.

In a second case, a 29-year-old woman developed skin laxity first in her earlobes, with spread during 3 to 4 years to her eyelids, face, and neck. She also had suffered from generalized hives for 10 years. Skin biopsy from the neck revealed total loss of mid-dermal elastic tissue.

The diagnostic dilemma is between **blepharochalasis** (which may involve the earlobes as well as the upper and lower eyelids) and **acquired cutis laxa**. Both involve elastolysis, which causes wrinkling and drooping of the earlobes.

Hawke M, John AF: Diseases of the Ear. Clinical and Pathologic Aspects. Philadelphia, Lea & Febiger, 1987, 309 pp.

Black dermatographism is a black discoloration that develops on skin beneath jewelry when abrasive materials in powdered cosmetics remove metal particles from jewelry. It disappears with washing. It is commonly seen on the earlobe adjacent to an earring track.

van den Niewenhuijsen IJ, Calame JJ, Bruynzecl DP: **Localized argyria** caused by silver earrings. Dermatologica 1988; 177:189–191.

In a 22-year-old woman, 1-cm green-blue to **gray-blue oval macules** of the posterior earlobes had been present for more than 5 years. Only vague discoloration was seen on the front of the earlobes. She had worn silver earrings for 8 years, and 5 years previously her family physician had removed embedded earring backings from each swollen earlobe. The residual blue-gray color had remained unchanged.

Biopsy and **roentgen diffraction analysis** showed the presence of silver granules in the dermis, which accounted for the color and led to the diagnosis of localized argyria. The patient was not patch-test positive to silver nitrate (1% aqueous).

While localized argyria is very rare, it has been reported with implanted acupuncture needles, silver cones used in endodontic treatment, and silver sulfadiazine cream.

Localized argyria now joins the other daunting **hazards of pierced ears**:

staphylococcal infection   keloid
nickel dermatitis   sarcoid granuloma
cyst formation   hepatitis
bifid ear   osteomyelitis
hematoma

Acquired beauty can be hazardous to your health.

Aronsohn RS, Batsakis JG, Rice DH, Work WP: Anomalies of the first branchial cleft. Arch Otolaryngol 1976; 102:737–740.

Anomalies of the **first branchial cleft** are usually noted as a cystic abnormality near the ear shortly after birth.

Most patients give a history of recurrent or chronically infected cysts or sinus tracts, often misdiagnosed as an **abscess**. They drain in one of the following areas:

preauricular
postauricular
external auditory canal (at the bony-cartilaginous junction)
angle of mandible (anterior to sternocleidomastoid muscle)

Recurrent intermittent purulent otorrhea may be the main complaint if the sinus tract opens into the external auditory canal.

The cysts or sinuses are lined by keratinizing stratified squamous epithelium. Some of them also have adnexal skin structures and bars of hyaline cartilage.

In contrast, cysts and sinuses arising from the **second branchial cleft** are most commonly found in the carotid triangle, opening anterior to the sternocleidomastoid muscle between the hyoid bone superiorly and the suprasternal notch inferiorly. They are lined by stratified squamous epithelium that keratinizes minimally, if at all, or by mucus-secreting columnar epithelium. Abundant lymphoreticular tissue with germinal centers is found in the subepithelial tissues.

Takato T, Takeda H, Kamei M, Uchiyama K: The **question mark ear** (congenital auricular cleft): A familial case. Ann Plast Surg 1989; 22:69–73.

This congenital deformity of the auricle is characterized by a **cleft between the helix and the earlobe**. It has also been called the congenital auricular cleft. The auricle has a question mark configuration and probably results from accretion insufficiency between the fifth and sixth hillock.

In its mild form there is a notch between the helix and the earlobe, as seen in the mother in this series. Her two children (3-year-old girl, 2-year-old boy) had much more pronounced ear deformities, with complete separation of the earlobe from the upper auricle.

This deformity is apparently different from the **congenital cleft earlobe**, which results from failure of coalescence between the first and sixth hillock.

Sebben JE: The **accessory tragus**—no ordinary skin tag. J Dermatol Surg Oncol 1989; 15:304–307.

An accessory tragus is most often confused with a skin tag, located anterior to the tragus or just anterior to the crus of the helix. Less common sites include the cheek along the line of the mandible and the lateral aspect of the neck anterior to the sternocleidomastoid muscle. Occasionally, the accessory tragus is multiple or bilateral.

It is present at birth and usually presents as a protuberant fleshy papule in the preauricular area that feels soft on palpation, sometimes with a firm underlying cartilaginous component. Histologically it contains hair follicles, sebaceous glands, eccrine glands, elastic cartilage, and adipose tissue.

The tragus is the only portion of the external auricle that develops from the **first branchial arch**, which also develops into the mandible and maxilla. By contrast, the rest of the ear is derived from the second branchial arch.

The accessory tragus usually occurs as an **isolated defect**. If it is close to the mouth, however, it may be associated with other first–branchial arch abnormalities, such as cleft lip, cleft palate, and hypoplasia of the mandible. In the oculoauriculovertebral syndrome (**Goldenhar's syndrome**) accessory tragi are associated with obvious vertebral defects and epibulbar dermoid cysts.

The presence of an accessory tragus does not necessitate an extensive search for rare defects.

Wattles are a cutaneous cervical tag that represents the cervical version of the accessory tragus.

The **differential diagnosis** of an accessory tragus includes:

> epidermoid cyst
> branchial cyst and fistula (deep diffuse swelling with a small overlying pore anterior to sternocleidomastoid)
> auricular fistula (small shallow pit on helix)
> thyroglossal cyst (midline of neck near hyoid)

Mahzoon S, Azadeh B: **Elephantiasis of external ears**: A rare manifestation of **pediculosis capitis**. Acta Derm Venereol 1983; 63:363–365.

The presenting complaint of a 33-year-old woman in Iran was **erythematous, enlarged, pruritic ears**. The ears had been markedly swollen for 3 years while she had had pediculosis capitis. She gave no history of antecedent eczema, erysipelas, frost bite, or ear piercing, all known to be causes of enlarged ears. The skin over the nape and upper back was indurated and hyperpigmented.

Her scalp was heavily infested with **pediculi**, and numerous nits were present. Behind the enlarged pinnae were subcutaneous nodules, and the right cervical lymph nodes were also enlarged. Scrapings of the lobes and nasal mucosa showed no acid-fast bacilli. Biopsy of the skin showed dilated lymphatics and a chronic inflammatory cell infiltrate without granulomas. Lymph node biopsy showed only reactive changes.

A diagnosis of elephantiasis of the external ears was made, presumably the result of years of hypersensitivity reactions to the lice. Considerable reduction in the size of the ears was achieved by intralesional injection of triamcinolone acetonide (10 mg/ml).

Owens D, Humphries M: **Cauliflower ears**, opium, and Errol Flynn. Br Med J 1988; 297:1643–1644.

Cauliflower ears in elderly Chinese patients may indicate a history of **opium abuse**. Swollen misshapen auricles resulted from long periods of slumber on opium beds with hard wooden pillows.

In the past, opium was commonly taken by fume inhalation, called "chasing the dragon." Now, most addicts no longer smoke opium but use heroin by injection, smoking, or fume inhalation. The opium dens no longer exist.

Frank ST: **Aural sign of coronary artery disease.** N Engl J Med 1973; 289:327–328.

A **prominent crease in the earlobe**, which is usually bilateral, may indicate premature cardiovascular disease.

Among 20 patients who were 60 years old or younger, all but one had one or more significant risk factors for coronary artery disease (elevated cholesterol and triglyceride levels, diabetes, hypertension, recent smoker). Five of these patients already had signs of cardiovascular disease.

(This is the original paper that launched a great deal of research on earlobe creases.)

Williams RR: Myocardial infarction risk, **earlobe crease**, and sleep apnoea syndrome. Lancet 1989; 2:676–677.

A unilateral earlobe crease may indicate that the patient always sleeps on the affected ear, causing it to be folded. Such was the case in a middle-aged man with back pain, who was comfortable only if he slept on the right side.

In other studies, earlobe creases have been associated with myocardial infarction, hypertension, and obesity. Since these are all common associations with the sleep apnea syndrome, perhaps the earlobe crease develops because of the **sleeping position**.

A prevalence survey of earlobe creases in approximately 700 males and females in Utah showed that creases were generally absent before age 20 years. The incidence then gradually increased with age, creases being present in about 75% of both men and women over 60 years of age.

Shoenfeld Y, Mor R, Weinberger A, et al: **Diagonal ear lobe crease** and coronary risk factors. J Am Geriatr Soc 1980; 28:184–187.

The early appearance of an earlobe crease may indicate coronary heart disease with or without coronary risk factors.

Skin biopsies of earlobe creases revealed **significant tears in the elastic fibers**. Thickening of the prearteriole walls was also found in the earlobe biopsies from patients who also had heart disease. Possibly a diminished blood supply to the earlobe contributes to the elastic fiber tears.

In this study from Israel, earlobe creases were found in 77% of 421 patients with myocardial infarction, in contrast to 40% of 421 control patients. There was a higher incidence in Ashkenazi Jews and in patients with diabetic retinopathy or hypertension.

Wagner RF Jr, Reinfeld HB, Wagner KO, et al: **Ear canal hair** and the **earlobe crease** as **predictors for coronary-artery disease**. N Engl J Med 1984; 311:1317–1318.

Ear canal hair (one or more terminal hairs growing on the tragus, antitragus, or external acoustic meatus) is an androgen-induced trait and represents virilization of the ear.

When the presence of ear canal hair and earlobe crease is combined, there is a significant association with coronary artery disease. This combination of signs is more sensitive than the earlobe crease alone for predicting coronary artery disease.

Presumably, **androgens facilitate the development of atherosclerosis** and coronary artery disease **as well as ear canal hair**.

Papay FA, Levine HL, Schiavone WA: Facial fuzz and funny findings. **Facial hair causing otalgia** and **oropharyngeal pain**. Cleve Clin J Med 1989; 56:273–276.

Approximately 50% of all ear pain originates from other sources. Referred otalgia results from the multiple sensory innervations of the auricle, external auditory meatus, and oropharynx.

Two physicians and a lawyer experienced otalgia and oropharyngeal pain resulting from **embedding of clipped hairs in the ear or oropharynx**. Symptoms included ear pain, cough, sensation of a lump in the hypopharynx, unilateral crunching upon chewing and swallowing, and odynophagia. The cardiologist was particularly bothered by the ear pieces of the stethoscope, which presumably helped drive the hair clippings into the ear after a haircut. The surgeon, who had a full beard, probably inhaled clipped beard hairs during surgery, introducing them into his lingual tonsillar region.

Singh M, Kumar A, Paul VK: **Hairy pinna**—a pathognomonic sign in infants of diabetic mothers. Indian Pediatr 1987; 24:87–89.

Infants of diabetic mothers are usually large and plethoric and have round cherubic faces.

In five babies born in New Delhi to **diabetic mothers**, there was striking hairiness of the pinnae, with the hair 4 to 6 mm long. The dense hair growth was mostly limited to the helix of the external ears. Excessive hairiness over the forehead and back was also evident in three of the babies.

The pinnae of most normal neonates have sparsely distributed lanugo hair. In male adults, however, hairiness of the pinnae is a Y-linked trait.

The external ears of all newborn babies should be examined for excessive **hairiness**, which is a useful **clinical marker for infants of diabetic mothers**. The sign is seen in infants of either sex.

Silva JA, Leong GB, Weinstock R: A case of skin and **ear self-mutilation**. Psychosomatics 1989; 30:228–230.

Aural self-mutilation (**Van Gogh phenomenon**) is very rare. It usually occurs in psychotic patients who possibly are trying to rid themselves of persecutory voices by eliminating the organ of hearing.

Self-mutilation also serves to relieve anxiety and guilt and expiate past sins through the suffering of physical pain.

Ali AH: Borderline personality and **multiple earrings**: A possible correlation? Am J Psychiatry 1990; 147:1251.

Young women (ages 16 to 32 years old) with multiple ear piercings per earlobe may have a **borderline personality disorder**. Criteria include poor social adaptation, impulsive acting out, intense affectivity, poor interpersonal relations, and mood disorders.

Among 52 borderline personality patients in a psychiatric practice during a 6-year period, 44 had multiple earlobe piercings. The remaining patients with multiple earrings are adolescents with the diagnosis of conduct disorder. Several hundred other patients with the conduct disorder diagnosis did not have multiple earrings.

Keshavan MS: The **ear wigglers**: Tics of the ear in 10 patients. Am J Psychiatry 1988; 145:1462–1463.

Tics are sudden stereotyped and repetitive involuntary movements that often imitate coordinated acts and arise from voluntary muscles. They may involve the eye (blinking tics), nose, lips, tongue, neck (torticollis), larynx (vocal tics), breathing, and swallowing.

Ear tics are very unusual. In the patients described here, the ears moved 60 to 80 times per minute and usually also involved the scalp. One patient also had a facial tic. The tics could be voluntarily suppressed for 2 to 3 minutes in all patients, but no patient could stop the tics totally. In many cases, stress worsened the tics, and several patients had tension headaches and depression.

What is spoken of as a "clinical picture" is not just a photograph of a man sick in bed; it is an impressionistic painting of the patient surrounded by his home, his work, his relations, his friends, his joys, sorrows, hopes and fears.

FRANCIS WELD PEABODY, 1881–1927

Santucci B, Ferrari PV, Cristaudo A, et al: **Nickel dermatitis from cheap earrings.** Contact Dermatitis 1989; 21:245–248.

In Italy, wearing cheap earrings (sometimes more than one on each lobe) is common practice. This includes clip-on earrings. Among 735 schoolgirls surveyed, 92% regularly wore such earrings, and **62% reported dermatitis of their earlobes.** Relatives were similarly affected in 41%.

Nickel dermatitis is spreading very fast in Italy, presumably because of the increasing use of cheap earrings. Between 1984 and 1988 the incidence of positive patch tests to nickel increased by 27%—up to 64% of all subjects patch tested. In patients with earlobe dermatitis, 98% were patch-test positive to nickel sulfate 5% in petrolatum.

Among 300 patients who were patch-test positive to nickel, the dermatitis started on the earlobes in 70%. The mean age at onset of dermatitis was 6 years, 8 months. The dermatitis remained localized in only 5%, over the years **progressively spreading to distant sites** (hands and face) not regularly in contact with metals. Itching, erythema, and eczema were the initial symptoms. Whenever the wearing of earrings recommenced, new lesions appeared after a mean time of 5.2 hours.

Patch testing in 30 nickel-sensitive patients showed a decreasing number of positive responses with decreasing concentrations of aqueous nickel sulfate in the patches:

Concentration (%)	% Positive
5	100
2.5	78
1	53

Patch testing to the earring clasps caused eczematous reactions similar to the 5% solution in all subjects. These earrings release high quantities of nickel ions, as analyzed in artificial sweat. Plasma seems to be the most effective solution for removing available nickel from earrings. **Nickel is stored** in tissues **for hundreds of days**, which is probably significant in inducing inflammation and sensitization.

Iwatsuki K, Yamada M, Takigawa M, et al: **Benign lymphoplasia of the earlobes** induced by gold earrings: Immunohistologic study on the cellular infiltrates. J Am Acad Dermatol 1987; 16:83–88.

Three young Japanese women developed **red nodules of the earlobes** 1 to 5 months following ear piercing with 18 carat **gold earrings.** Two of them had also developed acute dermatitis of the earlobes 2 to 3 days after piercing, which resolved spontaneously within several days.

Patch tests showed extremely **strong reactions to 1% gold sodium thiomalate** at 48 hours in all three cases. Patch tests were negative to the following metals:

nickel sulfate 5%
chromium sulfate 2%
cupric sulfate 1%
potassium dichromate 0.5%
cobalt chloride 2%

Skin biopsies showed a dense lymphoid cell infiltrate with a few eosinophils and plasma cells in the dermis and subcutaneous tissue. Lymphoid follicles with germinal centers were also seen, similar to lymphocytoma cutis. The main cell types were suppressor/cytotoxic T cells and histiocytes with Leu-3a antigens (possibly Langerhans cells).

477

The lymphocytoma cutis–like nodules apparently represent an **allergic reaction to gold**. The wearing of gold earrings immediately after ear piercing permits direct contact between the earrings and dermis, with continuous solubilization of a small amount of gold into tissue fluid. Gold compound has the potential of both stimulating and inhibiting immunologic responses and can presumably modify the inflammatory reaction to induce benign lymphoplasia.

Sensitization to nickel earrings may also cause a similar reaction on the earlobe. Lymphoplasia has also been reported after **vaccinations**, repeated **hyposensitization injections**, and **tattoos**. This suggests that the main site of the immunologic reaction is in the dermis, instead of epidermal Langerhans cells.

Fisher AA: Ear piercing and sensitivity to nickel and gold. J Am Acad Dermatol 1987; 17:853.

Sensitization to nickel often occurs when ears are pierced with nickel-plated needles and when nickel-plated earrings are inserted.

Sensitization to both nickel and gold can be avoided by using an 18- to 20-gauge **stainless steel needle** for piercing and inserting **stainless steel stud earrings**. Most inexpensive gold earrings contain sufficient nickel to give a positive test with dimethylglyoxime. This test should be done on every stud earring prior to use to check for the presence of free nickel.

Stainless steel earrings should be **left in place for 3 weeks** so that the channel will be completely epithelialized. After this, any type of earring may be safely inserted.

Berth-Jones J, Norris PG, Graham-Brown RAC, Burns DA: **Juvenile spring eruption of the ears**. Clin Exp Dermatol 1989; 14:462–463.

For 3 years a 7-year-old boy had recurrent episodes of **redness**, **itching**, and **vesicles of both ears**, **beginning in spring** and persisting through the summer. The trigger was always sunlight exposure, with redness and itching appearing within the hour. In several episodes, blisters formed within a few hours. Healing required a week and left minimal scars.

The patient's father had had the same problem between the ages of 5 and 10 years. The only other family member affected was his 9-year-old brother.

Examination revealed erythematous papules, vesicles, and tense bullae, up to 1 cm in diameter in the helices and lobules of both ears. Studies failed to reveal antinuclear antibodies or any abnormal porphyrins in the blood, stool, and urine.

This **photodermatosis** of unknown etiology is mainly a boys' disease, since girls' ears tend to be hidden from the sun.

Skin biopsies in previous outbreaks of this rare dermatosis are not consistent with erythema multiforme, but the clinical course most resembles polymorphous light eruption. A combination of sunlight and cold air has been the suspected cause. Outbreaks have been reported in school children and at a summer camp.

Petrozzi JW, Warthan TL: **Malignant external otitis**. Arch Dermatol 1974; 110:258–260.

A 52-year-old man had suffered bilateral frostbite injury to his ears 30 years previously. This was followed by numerous papillomatous growths on the superior helices and external ear canals and episodes of recurrent swelling, pain, and discharge. Eventually, complete occlusion of the canals developed, and he became completely deaf. His **ears** were enlarged, **grossly deformed**, and edematous, with **purulent drainage**. Cultures revealed *Pseudomonas*, *Proteus*, *Klebsiella*, and *Staphylococcus aureus*. Surgery revealed the ear canal, middle ear, and mastoid antrum to be filled with granulation tissue, with destruction of the malleus, incus, and stapes. His blood sugar was normal, but he was found to have a squamous cell carcinoma of the lung.

Malignant otitis externa is a **severe progressive *Pseudomonas* infection** that begins in the external auditory canal, usually in elderly diabetics. The infection invades cartilage and bones, causing necrotizing osteitis that may extend to the mastoid area and temporal bone. **Deafness, meningitis, and death may follow.** Arteriosclerosis may be a predisposing factor.

Other inflammatory **disorders that may cause bony destruction** of the ear include:

> cholesteatoma with secondary infection
> acute necrotizing otitis media (mainly children; follows measles, influenza, or beta-hemolytic streptococcal pharyngitis)
> *Pneumococcus* type III otitis (indolent form of otitis media)
> external otitis due to diphtheria (exotoxins cause ulceration or gangrene)

Holmes RC, Johns AN, Wilkinson JD, et al: **Medicament contact dermatitis** in patients with chronic inflammatory ear disease. J Roy Soc Med 1982; 75:27–30.

In 40 patients with inflammatory ear disease present for more than 1 year, patch testing revealed allergic contact dermatitis to topical medications in 14 (35%).

All patients with persistent inflammatory ear disease should have **patch tests** for medicament contact dermatitis. An adequate screening battery includes neomycin, framycetin, clioquinol, gentamicin, polymyxin B, bacitracin, ethylenediamine, fragrance mix, and caine mix.

Although **ear wax solvents** rarely sensitize, they may be strong **irritants**. Ingredients include dioctyl sodium sulfosuccinate, Cerumenex, and propylene glycol.

Marks MB, Gluck JC, Lavi E, Halem-Sinclair E: An unsuspected sign of cutaneous allergy. J Am Acad Dermatol 1981; 4:519–522.

Thirty of 100 children with an atopic background of asthma or allergic rhinitis were found to have an unnoticed bilateral eczematous eruption in the superior retroauricular area. Since only 5 of 100 normal controls showed this localized eczema, the finding of **retroauricular dermatitis favors** a **diagnosis of atopy**.

Reddy AN: The stethoscope neuropathy. Ann Intern Med 1987; 106:913–914.

A physician making ward rounds noted increased warmth, burning, and, later, tingling and numbness in a bilateral symmetrical distribution on the neck and ears. While he used the stethoscope, the **paresthesia** areas suddenly felt cool and then normal. The symptoms returned a few minutes after he placed the stethoscope in its "resting position" with the metal arms around his neck. Anatomic detective work showed that the **stethoscope** was **compressing** the **great auricular nerves**.

Hawke M, John AF: Diseases of the Ear. Clinical and Pathologic Aspects. Philadelphia, Lea & Febiger, 1987, 309 pp.

Severe cold injury to the ear produces capillary vasoconstriction, and rewarming produces a bright-red color with itching and burning as the capillaries dilate. Prolonged exposure may lead to bullae. **Dystrophic calcification and heterotopic ossification of the pinna are long-term sequelae**, making the pinna stone hard. Other **causes of calcification of the pinna** include chronic trauma, sarcoid pituitary disease, and Addison's disease.

Krulder JWM, Vlasveld LT, Willemze R: **Erythema and swelling of ears** after treatment with **cytarabine** for leukemia. Eur J Cancer 1990; 26:649–650.

During a 3-year period in the Netherlands, eight patients with acute myelogenous leukemia treated with combination chemotherapy had **painful erythema and swelling of both ears**. Since the earlobes were involved, the condition was not acute perichondritis. Symptoms began during or soon after cytostatic treatment and subsided spontaneously within a week. There was no fever, and infectious causes could be ruled out.

All of the patients had been treated with **cytarabine** in combination with either daunorubicin or *m*-amsacrine. They also received allopurinol, sodium bicarbonate, and alimentary tract decontamination with neomycin, polymyxin B, amphotericin B, and nalidixic acid or pipemidic acid. Consolidation therapy with the same drugs eliminated the ear swelling except in one patient.

Cytarabine was thought to be the drug responsible for the reaction. It also causes **acral erythema with pain and dysesthesia of the palms and soles**, bulla formation, and desquamation.

Lysy J, Zimmerman J, Ackerman Z, Reifen E: Atypical **auricular pyoderma gangrenosum simulating fungal infection**. J Clin Gastroenterol 1989; 11:561–564.

A 37-year-old woman had developed **painful ulcerations of the right auricular area** 14 years before, following an episode of otitis externa. Cultures at that time yielded *Candida albicans*, and a biopsy disclosed a nonspecific dermal infiltrate. The ear eventually healed, but later she developed seronegative arthritis of the left knee, ulcerative colitis requiring a colostomy, and an ulcer on the left calf.

The **ear ulcer recurred** with a purple-red border and surrounding zone of erythema. Deep biopsies showed *Candida* spores and hyphae in the necrotic material, but systemic antifungal treatment was unsuccessful. Pyoderma gangrenosum was diagnosed, and treatment with hydrocortisone (500 mg/day IV) led to healing after 5 weeks, leaving a **cribriform scar**. Similar spreading ulcers developed on the legs at the sites of trauma and again healed with steroids (prednisone, 60 mg/day), leaving cribriform scars.

Pyoderma gangrenosum must be differentiated from deep fungal infection (blastomycosis, sporotrichosis, cryptococcosis). In this case, the presence of *C. albicans* in the ulcers represented superinfection, not an etiologic agent.

Yehia MM, Al-Habib HM, Shehab NM: **Otomycosis**: A common problem in North Iraq. J Laryngol Otol 1990; 104:387–389.

Among 219 patients thought to have otomycosis, 179 (81.7%) had positive **fungal cultures**. *Aspergillus* species constituted 92.1% of the total fungi isolated, particularly *Aspergillus niger* (70.9%). *Candida albicans* was found in 5.0% of isolates.

The dominant **bacterial isolates** found were *Staphylococcus aureus*, *Pseudomonas*, and *Proteus*, usually in mixed infections. Otomycosis is often confused with chronic otitis media and tends to be more severe in the tropics and subtropics.

The warmth, moisture, epithelial debris, and serous exudate in the external ear canal promote growth of fungi and bacteria. However, the disease is not highly infectious, as most cases of otomycosis are **unilateral**. Ear wax may aid in the heavy growth of aspergilli.

In this series, there was a higher incidence in females (65.4%), particularly housewives who while sweeping their floors are exposed to dust containing fungal spores. Young adults (16 to 30 years) were most commonly affected (48.0%).

McCreedy CA, Icken JN, Cripps DJ: **Erythematous, auricular papules**. Arch Dermatol 1990; 126:1225–1250.

A 45-year-old woman had a long history of pruritic lesions in both ears, in addition to eczematous dermatitis of the ear canals. Skin biopsies had repeatedly suggested **prurigo nodularis**. Despite treatment with intralesional steroids, multiple erythematous papules persisted. A complete blood count showed 50% eosinophils.

Another biopsy from a retroauricular papule revealed hyperkeratotic epidermis, increased vascularity in the superficial dermis with prominent endothelial cells, and clusters of lymphocytes and eosinophils in the dermis, consistent with **angiolymphoid hyperplasia with eosinophilia** (ALHE).

These red-to-violet papules, which bleed easily, may appear **like a cluster of grapes**. They have been linked to antecedent trauma or eczematous dermatitis in the involved area, mainly on the head and neck. Angiolymphoid hyperplasia is probably an inflammatory reactive process triggered by a number of external stimuli.

The clinical **differential diagnosis** includes:

> pyogenic granuloma
> Kaposi's sarcoma
> angiosarcoma
> leukemia/lymphoma cutis
> granuloma faciale

Schiavone WA, Levine HL: **Hair clippings in the external auditory canal**: Ah, there's the rub! N Engl J Med 1988; 318:54.

Clipped scalp hair may lodge in the external auditory canal and make painful contact with the tympanic membrane. This may cause intermittent noise and pain. It may be mistaken for otitis externa, which causes **otalgia** and a unilateral **crunching sound** on chewing and swallowing.

Hair dryers may blow stray hair clippings into the ear canal.

Chondrodermatitis

Goette DK: **Chondrodermatitis nodularis chronica helicis**: A perforating necrobiotic granuloma. J Am Acad Dermatol 1980; 2:148–154.

A small, painful, crusted nodule of the helix best describes chondrodermatitis nodularis chronica helicis. Removing the crust reveals, at times, a pinpoint channel that, on histologic examination, proves to be the route of transepidermal elimination of necrobiotic material (degenerated connective tissue) from the dermis.

The condition is best viewed as a **perforating actinic granuloma**. It usually occurs in older white males with actinic damage. At time, multiple lesions develop. None disappear spontaneously, and all interfere with sleep.

Dean E, Bernhard JD: **Bilateral chondrodermatitis nodularis antihelicis**. An unusual complication of cardiac pacemaker insertion. Int J Dermatol 1988; 27:122.

Within 2 months of starting to sleep on her right side following implantation of a pacemaker, a 72-year-old woman developed a painful nodule of the right antihelix. She then began to sleep on the left side, with the result that a nodule appeared on the left ear. Both were examples of **pressure–induced** chondrodermatitis nodularis helicis, as shown on biopsy.

This inflammatory disease of the ear usually appears as a nodule on the helix, just above Darwin's tubercle. Other locations include the antihelix, tragus, concha, and antitragus. Trauma leads to dermal inflammation, followed by **degeneration of the underlying cartilage due to its meager blood supply**.

Thomas JM, Swanson NA: Treatment of **perichondritis** with a quinoline derivative–norfloxacin. J Dermatol Surg Oncol 1988; 14:447–449.

A 64-year-old man developed **right ear pain**, tenderness, and swelling 7 days after undergoing Mohs' surgery for recurrent basal cell carcinoma on the concha of the right auricle. The entire auricle was edematous, erythematous, and tender, and there was yellow discharge in the surgical defect. A wound culture showed **Pseudomonas aeruginosa**, resistant to many antibiotics. Treatment with oral norfloxacin was curative.

Perichondritis of the auricle is an uncommon complication following surgical procedures and is most commonly due to *P. aeruginosa* infection. Cultures must be grown to establish antibiotic sensitivities.

Randall RE Jr, Spong FW: **Calcification of the auricular cartilage** in a patient with hypopituitarism. N Engl J Med 1963; 269:1135–1137.

Calcification of the auricular cartilage is rare. It usually follows frostbite, trauma with hematomas (cauliflower ear), or localized inflammation of the ear caused by bacteria, chondritis, or perichondritis. After frostbite, the pattern of calcification is usually confined to the upper outer rim of the helix, whereas after trauma or inflammation the calcification is spotty within the areas of deformity.

X-rays of the auricles may be obtained using dental x-ray films placed behind the folded-out pinnas.

Several metabolic disorders have been implicated in auricular calcification, with **adrenal insufficiency** being the most common. Presumably, calcification occurs as a result of some disturbance in the metabolism of mucopolysaccharide in adrenal insufficiency. **Other causes of calcification of the auricles** include:

> ochronosis
> hypercalcemia

acromegaly
hyperthyroidism
diabetes mellitus
pseudopseudohypoparathyroidism
hypopituitarism

These tend to cause bilateral symmetrical areas of calcification in several areas of the auricular cartilage. Stiffness of the pinnae may or may not be present.

A 49-year-old warehouse worker had noted for several years that his **ears** felt **unusually firm**. Although both **pinnae resisted bending**, they had normal color and shape. X-rays of the auricles disclosed symmetrical calcification and ossification in several areas of the helix, antihelix, antitragus, and borders of the concha of each pinna. He was also found to have **hypopituitarism** of several years' duration, with increasing lethargy, fatigue, cold intolerance, decreased libido, and decreased ability to tan. He shaved only every third day. The skin was thick, dry, and coarse over the distal surface of the arms and legs, with a generalized peculiar doughy feeling to the subcutaneous tissues. His forehead and face were finely wrinkled. There was scarcity of body, axillary, and pubic hair, and the hairs on the extremities were broken off and occasionally had a corkscrew appearance. Treatment with thyroid, cortisone, and testosterone dramatically improved the condition.

You can see farther if you stand on the shoulders of a good history.

Relapsing Polychondritis

Hedfors E, Hammar H, Theorell H: **Relapsing polychondritis**: Presentation of 4 cases. Dermatologica 1982; 164:47–53.

During the study of a 67-year-old Swedish man with **fever, hoarseness, episcleritis, and arthritis** of the ankle joints, it was noted that the **ears and nose were swollen, tender, and red**. Diagnostic preoccupation with the other symptoms and problems delayed for months the definitive diagnostic procedure of biopsy of the ear. Once this was done, the finding of perichondrial infiltration of neutrophils and lymphocytes led to the diagnosis of relapsing polychondritis.

The **range of presenting symptoms** may distract you from the nonspecific swelling, redness, or tenderness of the ears. But look you must, if the patient has:

eye signs of inflammation (keratitis, conjunctivitis, scleritis, uveitis)
ear problems (hearing loss, tinnitus, vertigo)
respiratory tract complaints relating to cartilage of the trachea or larynx (hoarseness, tracheal edema, tracheal collapse, which can be fatal)
polyarthritis (nonerosive, inflammatory)
nasal chondritis (swelling and redness of the nose, saddle nose deformity)

The diagnosis of relapsing polychondritis comes to those who think of the cartilage as the seat of polyorgan inflammatory disease.

Gange RW: **Relapsing polychondritis.** Report of two cases with an immunopathological review. Clin Exp Dermatol 1976; 1:261–268.

Cartilage may be injured as an **"innocent bystander"** in immune reactions, and appears to have a special affinity for immune complexes. It also has cross-reactivity with streptococcal antigens, and an increased ASO titer is found in about 20% of cases of relapsing polychondritis.

An 80-year-old man had a **swollen, tender, purple right ear**, with complete occlusion of the meatus. Four weaks earlier he had noted pain inside the ear and loss of hearing, and began having malaise and fever at night. The bridge of the nose was slightly tender, as was the right temporomandibular joint, where he had experienced pain with chewing. Laboratory findings revealed **erythrocyte sedimentation rate 118 mm/hour**, white blood count 13,800 with 93% neutrophils, hemoglobin 11.7 gm, slightly increased liver enzymes, and normal ASO titer, RA latex, and antinuclear antibodies. The ear remained enlarged and floppy without palpable cartilage following treatment with tetracosactrin depot injections.

Think of relapsing polychondritis with combinations of the following:

"cellulitis" of the pinna sparing the earlobe (which lacks cartilage)
hearing loss (collapse of ear canal or involvement of inner ear or eustachian tube)
saddle nose (cartilage loss)
breathing difficulty (laryngotracheal cartilage involved)
cardiac problems (valves involved)
arthropathy (joint cartilage involved)
eye problems (conjunctivitis, episcleritis, keratitis, iritis)

Conti JA, Colicchio AR, Howard LM: **Thymoma, myasthenia gravis**, and **relapsing polychondritis**. Ann Intern Med 1988; 109:163–164.

Erythema, swelling, tenderness, and pain of the right ear and nose occurred in a 64-year-old white man and cleared within a week without treatment. For 9 months he had also had generalized muscle weakness, most severe in the shoulders and neck and associated with ptosis and difficulty in chewing and swallowing. Four months later the **left ear became red and swollen** (exempting the cartilage-free lobule), and the **left sclera became inflamed**, with spontaneous resolution within a few weeks.

The patient was shown to have myasthenia gravis by a favorable response to edrophonium chloride (2 mg), positive serologic tests for acetylcholine receptor antibodies (22 nmol/liter—normal <0.7 nmol/liter), and positive striated muscle antibodies (titer >1:640). The erythrocyte sedimentation rate was 133 mm/hour. Muscle strength was diminished symmetrically in the neck flexors and proximal and distal upper extremities, but muscle tone and mass were normal without fasciculations. Myasthenia gravis symptoms disappeared following **thymectomy**, which revealed an epithelial **thymoma** with capsular invasion. Two months later, however, he was hospitalized with severe generalized arthralgias, episcleritis, and erythema nodosum that responded to steroid therapy.

Relapsing polychondritis was diagnosed from the history of recurrent episodes of inflammation, cartilage degeneration of the ear and nose, and episcleritis. He did not have other typical signs such as polyarthritis (nonerosive, inflammatory), polychondritis of the respiratory tract, and audiovestibular damage.

Laboratory studies in relapsing polychondritis have revealed serum antibodies directed against both cartilage matrix and type II collagen, and cell-mediated immunity against cartilage proteoglycans. Its autoimmune pathogenesis is supported through its association with myasthenia gravis, rheumatoid arthritis, systemic lupus erythematosus, Hashimoto's thyroiditis, and pernicious anemia. Patients with relapsing polychondritis should have a **complete blood count** and determination of **serum B$_{12}$**, **thyroglobulin** and **microsomal antibodies**, and **acetylcholine receptor antibodies**.

Curiosity is virtuosity in the art of diagnosis.

Growths

Lambert PR, Fechner RE, Hatcher CP: **Seborrheic keratosis of the ear canal.** Otolaryngol Head Neck Surg 1987; 96:198–201.

A 56-year-old man with drainage from the left ear for 3 months was noted to have a large papillomatous mass filling the left ear canal. Previous biopsies had been read as squamous cell carcinoma. Computed tomography showed that there was no bone erosion. The lesion was excised and proved to be seborrheic keratosis.

Seborrheic keratoses, while rare in the external ear canal, can resemble **verrucous carcinoma. Secondary bacterial infection** induces edema, inflammation, maturation of keratinocytes, and increased mitoses that may be mistaken histologically for malignancy. It is important to obtain a large biopsy specimen and carefully review it with the pathologist.

Hawke M, John AF: Diseases of the Ear. Clinical and Pathologic Aspects. Philadelphia, Lea & Febiger, 1987, 309 pp.

Neglect keratoses consist of patches of keratin debris that accumulate within the conchal bowl or behind the ears. These **pigmented, greasy, raised lesions resemble seborrheic keratoses**, but can be easily removed, revealing normal skin underneath.

Mann RJ, Peachey RDG: **Sarcoidal tissue reaction**—another **complication** of ear piercing. Clin Exp Dermatol 1983; 8:199–200.

A 14-year-old girl developed multiple soft **reddish-brown nodules** on both earlobes at the sites where, 1 month before, she had attempted (sometimes successfully) to pierce her ears herself using a gold stud. Biopsy revealed rounded granulomas with multinucleate giant cells in the dermis, with no caseation or acid-fast bacilli. Treatment with intralesional triamcinolone injections into the nodules was initially unsuccessful.

Both big girls and little girls who pierce their ears run the **risk** of:

bleeding	keloids
laceration	gold dermatitis
cleft earlobe syndrome	nickel dermatitis
postauricular pressure sores	local infection
embedded studs	septicemia
epidermal cysts	tuberculosis
sarcoidal nodules	hepatitis
scars	

Mothers, take note.

Zilinsky I, Tsur H, Trau H, Orenstein A: **Pseudolymphoma of the earlobes** due to ear piercing. J Dermatol Surg Oncol 1989; 15:666–668.

A 27-year-old white woman pierced her earlobes in 1977 and soon noted development of tumors on both earlobes. They were **thought to be keloids** and were treated repeatedly with intralesional steroids, with no improvement. By 1986 the lesions were soft, smooth, red-purple nodules 3 by 4 cm on one side and 1 by 2 cm on the other side.

Skin **biopsy** showed a dense lymphocytic infiltrate in the dermis with lymphoid follicles with typical germinal centers, characteristic of **cutaneous pseudolymphoma.**

Following complete excision of the lesions there was no recurrence at 18-month follow-up.

Nodules on the ears after ear piercing may not always be keloids!

Viani L, McCormick MS: **Duro-cutaneous fistula** caused by a congenital cholesteatoma. J Laryngol Otol 1990; 104:241–243.

A cholesteatoma is an **epidermal inclusion cyst** that forms within the middle ear and assumes the shape of the cavity in which it rests. It is assumed to be congenital if it develops behind an intact tympanic membrane in a patient without any previous history of ear infections.

In this case, a 70-year-old man had a **draining area** in the left upper aspect of the **neck, thought to be a chronically infected sebaceous cyst**. It turned out to be a cervical fistula with a sinus tract extending to the parotid gland and mastoid tip. The **mastoid sinus was opacified**, indicating chronic infection, and there was a communication with the external auditory canal. Surgery revealed **multiple sinus tracts** leading to a **congenital cholesteatoma**, which also filled the mastoid.

Carter VH, Constantine VS, Poole WL: **Elastotic nodules of the antihelix.** Arch Dermatol 1969; 100:282–285.

Elastotic nodules are discrete 4- to 6-mm semitranslucent aggregates of granular white-to-pink material with an **orange-peel–like surface** and **rolled pearly border**. They are asymptomatic, bilateral, and located on the anterior crus of the antihelix.

These nodules are apparently **induced by sun damage**. Histologically the dermal collagen is disorganized and replaced by amorphous masses of thick coalescing elastotic fibers.

Clinically the lesions may be **mistaken for basal cell carcinomas**.

Slobodkin D: **Why more keloids on back than on front of earlobe?** Lancet 1990; 335:923–924.

Earlobe keloids secondary to ear piercing were observed to occur much more commonly on the back than on the front of the earlobe in a New York City population of Puerto Ricans, Dominicans, and Afro-Americans.

The **mechanism of trauma** during ear piercing may be the differentiating factor. In the United States a mechanical punch is used to drive a sharp gold-plated hollow peg in an anterior to posterior direction through the earlobe. The peg is then held in place with a posterior fastener. Perhaps deep dermis is brought up posteriorly into contact with more superficial layers to initiate keloid formation.

Other significant factors could be preferential exposure of the anterior earlobe to sun, soap, makeup, or some other environmental factor that could be protective against keloid formation.

The only animal model available for studying keloids is the athymic mouse, which will carry transplanted human keloid cells. This model clearly implicates **abnormal fibroblasts** in the maintenance of keloid tissue.

Umeda Y, Nakajima M, Yoshioka H: **Surfer's ear** in Japan. Laryngoscope 1989; 99:639–641.

Surfer's ear refers to **exostosis of the external auditory canal**, which eventually leads to stenosis of the ear canal. It is easily visible with an otoscope.

It begins to appear approximately 5 years after the patient's onset of surfing and is more common and severe in professional surfers. It was found in 19 of 51 professionals (37%), and 5 of 43 amateurs (12%). Surfers should wear ear plugs to try to prevent the stenosis.

Stevenson TR, Zavell JF, Anderson RD: **Neurofibroma of the ear.** Ann Plast Surg 1986; 17:151–154.

A neurofibroma may cause a diffuse mass in the external ear, which fills the external canal and conchal bowl. Gradual **hearing loss** occurs, and the auricle may be displaced.

Computed tomography is helpful in evaluating the location and extent of the tumor, which may invade adjacent bone and soft tissue.

It is important to **examine the rest of the skin** for café au lait spots, axillary freckles, and other neurofibromas.

Sanchez JL: **Collagenous papules on the aural conchae**. Am J Dermatopathol 1983; 5:231–233.

Four healthy women in Puerto Rico had **smooth, firm papules**, 1 to 4 mm in size, **in the conchae** of the ears. They were asymptomatic, skin-colored, and bilateral.

Skin biopsies showed thickened papillary dermis with a small dome-shaped mass of sclerotic hyalinized collagen bundles separated by clefts. Collarettes of epidermis partially enveloped the collagenous masses, and the overlying epidermis was thinned without rete ridges. Stains were positive for collagen and negative for amyloid. Direct immunofluorescence was negative, and electron microscopy revealed collagen bundles.

There are several **papular conditions of the ear** that may be difficult to distinguish:

> colloid milia (numerous waxy papules on sun-exposed areas, basophilic aggregates in dermis)
> nodular amyloidosis (nodules or tumors elsewhere, eosinophilic homogenized masses in dermis)
> fibrous papules (solitary flesh-colored, dome-shaped papule, usually on nose, perifollicular fibrosis with angiomatous elements)
> lipoid proteinosis (papules on skin and mouth, eosinophilic hyaline material in dermis)
> erythropoietic protoporphyria (hyalinization of dermis)
> pseudocyst of auricle (solitary nodule on antihelix, band of eosinophilic homogeneous material separates the superficial and deep cartilage)
> elastotic nodules on the ears (bilateral small, pale papules and nodules on anterior surface of crus of antihelix due to actinic damage, clumped elastotic material and marked elastotic degeneration in dermis)

Hicks BC, Weber PJ, Hashimoto K, et al: Primary cutaneous **amyloidosis** of the auricular concha. J Am Acad Dermatol 1988; 18:19–25.

Small, slightly friable, **yellow, waxy or pearly papules** grouped in the concha of the ear may contain amyloid. They are not pruritic and are acquired in adulthood. One or both ears may be involved. Amyloid is found in the papillary dermis.

In the four cases presented here, there was no other sign of amyloidosis, either systemically or in the skin. Therefore, it falls into the category of primary localized cutaneous amyloidosis.

The **differential diagnosis** includes:

> elastotic nodules   colloid milium
> hyalinosis cutis et mucosae   collagenous papules of the ears

Collagenous papules of the ears appear strikingly similar, but have negative stains for amyloid (crystal violet, Congo red) and also stain like collagen (van Gieson stain).

Electron microscopy should be done to distinguish among amyloid, collagen, and colloid. Further identification can be done with immunoperoxidase staining, which in these cases appeared to be amyloid K, a keratin-type amyloid.

Schinella RA, Breda SD, Hammerschlag PE: **Otic infection due to *Pneumocystis carinii*** in an apparently healthy man with antibody to the human immunodeficiency virus. Ann Intern Med 1987; 106:399–400.

A 36-year-old Hispanic man, a former **drug addict**, had a 3- by 5-mm polyp in the left ear canal along with progressive hearing loss of the left ear. He also had widespread nontender **lymphadenopathy**, with lymph nodes 1 to 2 cm in size. Biopsy of the otic polyp showed foamy granular material characteristic of *Pneumocystis carinii*, and the organism was found with a silver stain. An **HIV test was positive**. He fit the 1985 Centers for Disease Control criteria for AIDS, having an opportunistic infection along with the HIV antibody.

Coulman CU, Greene I, Archibald WR: Cutaneous pneumocystosis. Ann Intern Med 1987; 106:396–398.

A 42-year-old man with **AIDS** had progressive hearing loss and bilateral 2- by 2-cm **polypoid lesions of the ear canals**. Later he developed dyspnea on exertion. Skin biopsy showed a perivascular mantle of amphophilic finely stippled exudate and some neutrophils infiltrating the vessel wall. A Grocott methenamine silver stain showed large numbers of *Pneumocystis carinii* cysts in the dermal exudate. The same organism was found in the sputum. Treatment with trimethoprim-sulfamethoxazole caused a marked reduction in the size of the ear masses.

Moral: Don't forget to ask for a **silver stain** in biopsies of AIDS patients.

Levine HL, Kinney SE, Bailin PL, Roberts JK: **Cancer of the periauricular region.** Dermatol Clin 1989; 7:781–795.

Approximately 5 to 10% of all skin cancers of the head and neck occur on the external ear, particularly the auricle.

The **incidence** of basal cell and squamous cell carcinoma of the ear doubles for each geographic move of 30 to 45 minutes latitude toward the equator. In addition to sun exposure, chronic irritation (such as chronic otitis externa) also predisposes to cancer of the auricle and external auditory canal. Otomycosis due to *Aspergillus*, which produces aflatoxin B1, a possible carcinogen, also predisposes to ear cancer.

Tumors on the ear tend to **recur** at a higher than expected rate because of the thinness of the skin, closeness of the perichondrium and periosteum to the surface, and the embryologic fusion planes. In general, carcinoma of the external ear spreads superficially along the plane of the perichondrium or periosteum. It also spreads from the surface deeply along the fusion planes.

Preauricular cancer spreads toward the tragus, which serves as a boundary, and then spreads deeply along the perichondrium to the parotid fissure and superficial temporal vessels. Cancers of the pretragal area may also spread up to and then along the helix. **Conchal carcinomas** spread centrifugally within the concha.

Head and neck surgeons most often see **squamous cell carcinomas** of the ear, involving the external auditory canal. In contrast, dermatologists see **basal cell carcinomas** much more often, which involve the pinna. **Melanomas** account for less than 4% of external ear cancers. Several types of cancer **metastasize** to the ear and temporal bone, particularly **from breast and kidney**.

Pain may be an early sign of ear cancer because of the rich nerve supply. Itching and bloody discharge are common. Tumor or secondary infection may obstruct the ear canal and cause conductive hearing loss. Vertigo is a late sign, occurring after invasion of the middle or inner ear. **Facial paralysis** results from involvement of the facial nerve in the mastoid and parotid gland.

Evaluation of the problem should include a thorough head and neck examination, with particular attention to the parotid and the neck. Cranial nerves VII through XII should be checked. Punch biopsies should be taken from the center and the periphery of the lesion.

Any patient with external otitis that does not respond to local treatment within 2 weeks or who develops a proliferative lesion needs a biopsy. **Computed tomography** and **magnetic resonance imaging** will also help determine the extent of a lesion, showing bony destruction and soft-tissue extension.

Lloyd KM: **Bulky, benign tumor of the external auditory canal.** Arch Dermatol 1990; 126:589–590.

A 1.5-cm smooth firm tumor with telangiectasia filled the external auditory canal of the right ear in a 76-year-old man. It had been present for over 10 years and significantly impaired his hearing.

The tumor proved to be a **cylindroma**, which did not involve the perichondrium. It was successfully removed with the carbon dioxide laser.

Murty GE, Cox NH: **Angiolymphoid hyperplasia with eosinophilia**: An uncommon tumor of the external auditory canal. Ear Nose Throat J 1990; 69:102–103, 106–107.

An 80-year-old woman had several nontender translucent **telangiectatic nodules** that bled easily in her left external auditory canal; they had been present for 6 months.

Biopsy revealed a well-circumscribed, nonencapsulated proliferation of small blood vessels in the mid-dermis with a moderate lymphohistiocytic infiltrate and scattered eosinophils. Despite a normal complete blood count, a **diagnosis of angiolymphoid hyperplasia with eosinophilia** (ALHE) was made.

Clinically and histologically, ALHE is likely to be **mistaken for angiosarcoma**. Other diagnostic considerations include pyogenic granuloma, eosinophilic granuloma, malignant lymphoma, and angiomatous lymphoid hematoma. The clinical diagnosis is rarely accurate.

Lynde CW, McLean DI, Wood WS: **Tumors of ceruminous glands**. J Am Acad Dermatol 1984; 11:841–847.

A 50-year-old man had a 9-year history of **episodic left facial paralysis** and increasing **hearing loss, diagnosed as Bell's palsy.** Examination revealed left facial asymmetry, marked facial weakness without sensory loss, and a large mass blocking the left ear canal. The mass proved to be a **ceruminous adenocarcinoma.** Following its removal and treatment with cobalt irradiation, he remained well for 9 years before metastasis occurred in the brain.

Ceruminous glands are modified apocrine sweat glands that line the external auditory meatus. Ceruminoma is a term that has been widely used for both benign and malignant neoplasms of the ear canal. Four **histologic types** are recognized: pleomorphic adenoma (mixed tumor), ceruminous adenoma, ceruminous adenocarcinoma, and adenoid cystic carcinoma.

The **symptoms** are frequently **vague** or minimal but may include progressive loss of hearing over several years, accompanied by a discharge and vague deep-seated pain. The adenoid cystic carcinoma is frequently painful, probably because of tumor invasion of nerves. The tumor usually appears as a polypoid mass in the external auditory canal or a nodule with subcutaneous induration that extends onto the preauricular skin. Although involvement of cervical lymph nodes is uncommon, **local recurrence** months to years later is common. The **differential diagnosis** includes basal cell carcinoma and squamous cell carcinoma.

Listen to your patient and look in the ear while you listen.

Shockley WW, Stucker FJ Jr: **Squamous cell carcinoma of the external ear**: A review of 75 cases. Otolaryngol Head Neck Surg 1987; 97:308–312.

Squamous cell carcinoma (SCC) on the ear is probably slightly more common than basal cell carcinoma. In this study, the most **common sites** of SCC on the ear were the helix (44%), posterior pinna (27%), and antihelix/triangular fossa (14%). All 65 patients were white, and all but two were men, with a mean age of 66 years. In the vast majority of cases, the preoperative diagnosis was nonspecific, multiple, or incorrect.

Among 40 patients with adequate follow-up, 10% had lymph node **metastasis** (cervical 5%, parotid 5%). Only 2.5% had distant metastasis. Most of the lesions were treated early and were less than 1 cm in size. The initial cure rate (after initial therapy alone) was 85%, while the ultimate cure rate was 93%.

Positive margins on histologic examination occurred in 16 lesions among the 40 patients. The recurrence rate was a surprisingly low 19%. Previous studies on basal cell carcinomas with positive margins have shown a **recurrence rate** of 33 to 35%.

Goudie RB, Soukop M, Dagg JH, Lee FD: Hypothesis: **Symmetrical cutaneous lymphoma**. Lancet 1990; 335:316–318.

Over a 6-month period a 57-year-old man developed gradual enlargement and slight **induration of both earlobes**, with local discomfort. A biopsy revealed lymphocytic lymphoma, and the lesions resolved after radiation therapy. Five years later he **developed chronic lymphocytic leukemia**.

For 3 years a 54-year-old man had swelling of the right ear, then of both ears. They were slightly painful when rubbed, particularly in cold weather. The helices and lobes of both ears had irregular nodular swellings. Biopsies showed lymphoma in the dermis. The lesions resolved after chemotherapy, leaving residual pigmentation of the ears.

Both men had **low-grade B-cell lymphomas**. The remarkable selective localization and symmetry of the skin lesions may result from preferential homing or growth of circulating tumor cells at specific anatomic sites.

Goette DK, Odom RB: **Atypical fibroxanthoma masquerading as pyogenic granuloma**. Arch Dermatol 1976; 112:1155–1157.

An 82-year-old man had a **pyogenic granuloma–like 5-mm red papule** on the **helix of his left ear**, which bled easily. It had arisen after he had incurred a scratch on the ear 5 weeks previously. Following excision, the area healed uneventfully.

The initial **histopathologic diagnosis of malignant melanoma** did not fit the clinical impression and led to further pathologic review. The tumor consisted of interlacing bundles of multinucleated pleomorphic spindle cells, with multiple mitoses and abundant eosinophilic cytoplasm. There was no junctional activity, pigmentation, or nesting tendencies. **Atypical fibroxanthoma was finally diagnosed.**

This pseudomalignancy occurs mainly on sun-damaged skin or areas of radiodermatitis on the cheeks, ears, and nose of patients over 60 years of age. The lesion is **clinically nonspecific**, being a papule, nodule, or ulcer that is usually mistaken for a basal cell or squamous cell carcinoma, pyogenic granuloma, or precancerous lesion. The prognosis is usually very good, but metastases do occur rarely.

Drago F, Parodi A, Rebora A: **Addison's disease and lupus vulgaris**: Report of a case. J Am Acad Dermatol 1988; 18:581–583.

A 54-year-old man had a 2-cm wide **red**, **violaceous plaque** of the right **earlobe**. This appeared 4 years after an initial lesion on the earlobe had shown lymphocytoma cutis on biopsy. Diascopy revealed "apple jelly" nodules, and histopathology showed tubercules and a typical tuberculous infiltrate in the dermis.

He was also suffering from dizziness, hypotension, fatigue, anorexia, weight loss (3 kg), arthralgia, myalgia, and hyperpigmentation of the whole skin, gums, and lips. **Serum ACTH and cortisol levels indicated adrenal insufficiency**, and a **solid mass** was found **on the right adrenal gland** with sonography and computed tomography. Tuberculous Addison's disease was diagnosed. Treatment with isoniazid (300 mg/day), ethambutol (600 mg/day), and rifampicin (600 mg/day) cleared the skin nodule (after 6 months) and adrenal mass (after 1 year), but the skin pigmentation and symptoms of Addison's disease persisted.

Whenever **lupus vulgaris** is found, a careful investigation should be done for **possible visceral involvement**. The finding of calcification in the adrenal gland with computed tomography is a fairly reliable marker of tuberculosis.

Glamb R, Kim R: **Pseudocyst of the auricle.** J Am Acad Dermatol 1984; 11:58–63.

An olive oil–like aspirate from a **tender swelling of the concha** of the left ear of a 31-year-old man pointed to a pseudocyst of the auricle. The viscous **yellow fluid** was easily obtained with an 18-gauge needle.

The pseudocyst recurred 3 days later, at which time a biopsy confirmed the diagnosis. The **cyst was within the cartilage** itself and apparently formed as a result of localized cartilaginous degeneration. The wearing of stereo headphones and a **motorcycle helmet** probably contributed by promoting ischemic necrosis of the cartilage.

These cysts are nontender, noninflammatory, tense swellings of the upper half of the ear. They are usually unilateral and unrelated to trauma. The intracartilaginous location is apparent on incision when one feels the gritty sensation of cutting into the cartilaginous fibrotic cyst wall. Pseudocysts that have been previously drained and then recur may yield serosanguineous fluid on aspiration.

The **differential diagnosis** focuses on:

subperichondrial hematoma (othematoma), always caused by tangential trauma to the ear and yielding blood on aspiration

seroma of the auricle, in which less viscous fluid collects outside the cartilage and the roof of the bulla is flaccid. It may be clinically identical to pseudocyst and can be distinguished only by biopsy.

relapsing polychondritis, which causes tender inflamed skin at other sites as well as the ear, and responds to steroids

cellulitis, which is highly inflammatory in contrast to pseudocyst

All of these conditions may eventuate in the scarred, deformed, collapsed auricle called **cauliflower ear**. At this end stage, the prior destructive forces can only be surmised.

Ramesh V: **Pseudocysts of the auricle.** Dermatologica 1986; 172:125–126.

A 3-cm **slowly enlarging, asymptomatic swelling** was seen over the anterior part of the upper half of the left ear in a 45-year-old man. There was mild erythema, and the swelling projected posteriorly. Aspiration yielded 4 ml of straw-colored viscous fluid, and biopsy revealed only fragmented cartilage with fibrous replacement, but no cyst wall.

Pseudocysts of the ear occur in young and middle-aged males. Possibly they are related to cauliflower ear, with **trauma** and **sun exposure** playing a role. They are localized to the upper half of the external ear, and biopsy shows intracartilaginous degeneration and fluid accumulation. The differential diagnosis includes seroma of the auricle, with exaggerated dermal edema but not cartilaginous involvement.

Hawke M, John AF: Diseases of the Ear. Clinical and Pathologic Aspects. Philadelphia, Lea & Febiger, 1987, 309 pp.

Injury to the external ear from blunt trauma may produce:

> *subperichondrial hematoma* on the lateral side of the auricle, where the skin is tightly attached to underlying perichondrium. The blood vessels between the perichondrium and auricular cartilage rupture, leading to a soft blue or **purple bulge** that distorts the normal ear contour. If the hematoma is not drained, bacterial infection and avascular necrosis of the cartilage may result, along with a cauliflower ear. If the cartilage is fractured, a hematoma may also form on the medial surface of the auricle, where the skin and subcutaneous tissue are loose and have great mobility.
>
> *traumatic seroma* with a **pale bulge** formed by subperichondrial serous or serosanguineous effusion. This persists for several days and may require aspiration.
>
> *cauliflower ear*, formed of fibrous tissue and **scar formation** that obscures the normal landmarks of the ear. Repeated blunt trauma causes devitalization of cartilage with softening and resorption.

Look for a second disease.

Edema

The accumulation of excess fluid within the skin, i.e., edema, is one of the most common signs of changed circulation. It is often barely noted, being encompassed by an overriding more exact diagnosis such as insect bite, urticaria, contact dermatitis, and postural stasis edema. In other instances it may be myxedema in which the fluid is held by the mucin deposits.

In the unexplained edema one must look for a source. Is it the edema of a failing heart or kidney? Are the serum protein levels high enough to support osmotic balance? Is it capillary leakage as in urticaria? Could it be obstruction of venous return as in venous thrombosis? Or could it be from lymphatic failure to provide its share of the circulatory return? Such failure may reflect a tumor or mass pressing on the lymphatic vessels or even congenital hypoplasia of the lymphatic vessels.

Finally, localized edema, such as that of the face, calls for examination for underlying infection such as sinusitis, deep-seated acne, a dental abscess, or even osteomyelitis.

Edema is a significant skin change. It deserves a significant etiologic diagnosis.

Hirschmann JV: **Ischemic forms of acute venous thrombosis.** Arch Dermatol 1987; 123:933–936.

Review of 73 cases:

Clinical:
Pain occurs with sudden onset in thigh, groin, or leg (usually left leg) due to compression of left iliac vein by right iliac artery.

Redness and heat overlie the thrombosed vein where it is superficial in upper inner thigh.

Edema is due to elevated venous hydrostatic pressure; skin cool, shiny, and taut; serous or hemorrhagic vesicles.

Cyanosis is due to venules engorged with trapped nonoxygenated blood.

If thrombectomy is not done by fourth to eighth day, **venous gangrene** ensues with petechiae, purpura, bullae, and finally the blackening of dead skin.

Orenstein A, Friedman B, Yaffe B, et al: **Factitious lymphedema of the hand:** A diagnostic challenge. Cutis 1987; 39:427–428.

For more than a year, attacks of **nonpitting edema** of the left arm of a 30-year-old soldier had led to repeated hospitalizations. None of the medical and vascular studies revealed any abnormality, but by close, continuous, intrahospital surveillance of the patient for 2 weeks, the cause of the lymphedema became evident: One night an **elastic bandage** was found tightly bound **around his left upper arm.**

Reed BR, Burke S, Bozeman M, et al: **Lymphedema of the lower abdominal wall** in **pregnancy.** J Am Acad Dermatol 1985; 12:930–932.

Reddish-brown elevated **ropelike tracks of induration** coursed from below the umbilicus to the pubic ramus in this 36-year-old woman who was at 40 weeks' gestation. They had been present for 6 weeks and gave a **burning sensation.** She had not noted this patterned thickening of the lower abdominal skin in any of her prior six pregnancies. Biopsy showed fibrotic dermis filled with numerous dilated lymphatics. A diagnosis was made of

lymphedema with tortuous palpable lymphatic channels due to mechanical obstruction.

Prior cases of abdominal lymphedema have been associated with massive obesity, but unlike this patient, the patients also had lymphedema of the lower extremities. When puzzling over lymphedema, one thinks of obstruction of the drainage by **postinfection fibrosis**, by **tumors**, or by **surgical damage**. But just think, here the baby did it.

Rosh MS: **Hypoproteinemic edema**: A rare complication of chronic **ulcerative colitis**. NY State J Med 1964; 64:2339–2348.

An 8-year-old girl with ulcerative colitis developed **generalized anasarca** and pallor 2 days after steroids were stopped. Eyelids and hands were puffy, 4+ pitting edema was present from the feet to the thighs, and edema was also evident on the lateral chest wall and sacral areas. The liver was palpable, and an abdominal fluid wave was present, along with dullness to percussion at the lung bases. Liver and kidney function tests were normal, and there was no proteinuria, but the total **serum protein was very low** (2.5 gm/dl) with greatly decreased albumin (1.4 gm/dl) and globulin (1.1 gm/dl). Hypoproteinemia was secondary to **increased protein loss in the gastrointestinal tract**, with increased albumin degradation and fecal excretion.

Fadell EJ, Dame RW, Wolford JL: Chronic hypoalbuminemia and **edema** associated with **intestinal lymphangiectasia**. JAMA 1965; 194:175–176.

The presence of edema with hypoproteinemia in a person without liver or kidney disease should suggest protein loss into the intestines (**protein-losing gastroenteropathy**).

A 52-year-old white woman with transient pedal edema for 30 years had gradually **increasing bouts of edema** that became more frequent and voluminous. Edema involved the pretibial areas and the abdominal and thoracic cavities, with dyspnea and abdominal distension. Serum albumin was 2.24 gm/dl, with normal complete blood count, urinary albumin, erythrocyte sedimentation rate, and remaining chemistry values. Infusions of salt-free albumin induced normal diuresis. Intravenous iodinated ^{131}I serum albumin revealed a serum half-life of 6.5 days instead of the normal 10 days, indicating **rapid loss or breakdown of albumin. Jejunal biopsy** revealed **intestinal lymphangiectasia**. Cutaneous signs included thickened ridged fingernails and clubbing of three fingers of one hand.

Mayou SC, Calderon RA, Goodfellow A, Hay RJ: Deep (subcutaneous) **dermatophyte infection** presenting with **unilateral lymphoedema**. Clin Exp Dermatol 1987; 12:385–388.

Nonpitting edema of the left leg extending to the knee developed in a 17-year-old Pakistani girl with a *Trichophyton rubrum* **infection of the feet** since the age of 3 years. The tinea pedis, which extended onto the dorsal area of the feet, had remained unaffected by long-term high-level doses of griseofulvin and ketoconazole. The infection spread to the left knee as a plaque of confluent papules and pustules, where hyphae could not be found in the scales but could be **cultured from within the biopsied dermis**. In contrast, the fungus was readily grown from scales of the feet and toenail clippings.

Within 2 weeks of the start of itraconazole therapy (100 mg/day), there was dramatic clinical improvement, and after 12 months there was complete resolution except for persistent onychomycosis of three toenails.

Kaufman RE: Trichiniasis: Clinical considerations. Ann Intern Med 1940; 13:1431–1460.

Swelling of the eyelids should suggest a search for the following:

trichinosis	acute sinusitis
acute nephritis	angioneurotic edema

Young LW: Radiologic imaging of Pott puffy tumor and other **frontal sinusitis** complications. Am J Dis Child 1986; 140:197.

Pott puffy tumor is a midforehead soft-tissue swelling resulting from acute suppurative frontal sinusitis. Aerobic and anaerobic bacteria cause **subperiosteal osteomyelitis** that extends into the forehead and scalp. Subtle neurologic signs precede epidural and subdural empyema. Serial **computed tomography** with contrast medium enhancement is the procedure of choice **for detecting empyema**.

McFadden JP, Handfield-Jones SE, Harman RRM: **Hemifacial oedema** complicating a case of **syringomyelia**. Clin Exp Dermatol 1988; 13:42–43.

A 67-year-old man with syringomyelia developed pitting edema of the right side of the face, worse on arising and most prominent around the eye. The skin was warm and erythematous, and there were decreased sweating and loss of pain and temperature sense in the area. Sinusitis and cellulitis were ruled out by absence of any clinical, symptomatic, or radiologic evidence. Neuropathic edema was diagnosed.

Syringomyelia causes asymmetric dilatation of the central canal of the cervical cord and is confirmed by myelography. This had been responsible for **paresthesias** of the right side of the face and right arm and anesthesia of the right arm for the past 3 years. The **edema** presumably **resulted from localized sympathetic dysfunction**, which favored high blood flow, vasodilatation, and arteriovenous shunting, with consequent **venous pooling**. Similar microcirculatory changes occur in the neuropathic edematous foot of the diabetic.

Truhan AP, Roenigk HH Jr: The **cutaneous mucinoses**. J Am Acad Dermatol 1986; 14:1–18.

The common denominator for an **incredibly varied set of clinical presentations** is the histologic finding of **excess mucin formation by the fibroblast**.

The cardinal diagnostic study is an **evaluation of the thyroid status**, T_3, T_4, TSH. The following **signs** demand thyroid evaluation for **hypothyroidism**:

Infant:
    periorbital puffiness
    thick lips, large protruding tongue
    skin cool, mottled, pale
    scalp hair scanty, brittle
    edema (myxedema) of external genitalia and extremities
    at 3 to 6 months, hoarseness, delayed deformed dentition

Adult:
    puffy eyelids
    lips thick, tongue large
    speech hoarse
    hands/feet swollen
    skin pale to yellow (carotenemia), cool, dry, ichthyotic, pruritic, keratotic
    hair loss, slow growth
    nails brittle, striated
    poor healing
    xanthomas

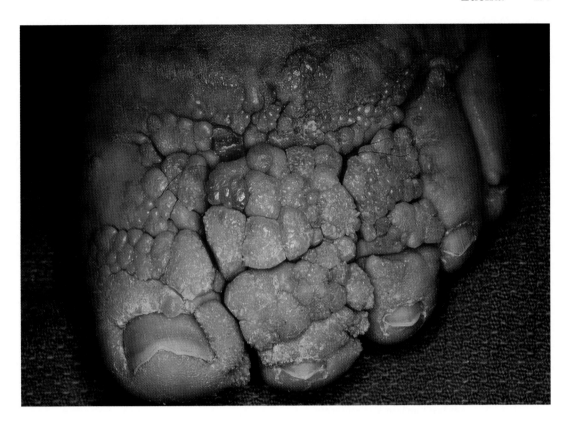

The following **signs** demand evaluation for **hyperthyroidism** (T_3, T_4, long-acting thyroid stimulator [LATS] serum level, Graves' disease, toxic multinodular goiter, excessive intake of thyroid hormone, or transient phase of subacute thyroiditis):

> pretibial myxedema—flesh-colored to yellow-brown nodules, plaques of anterior lower legs, follicles prominent (peau d'orange), possibly also associated with euthyroid or hypothyroid state
> exophthalmos
> enlarged thyroid (goiter)
> skin hot, face flushed, palms erythematous, hyperhidrosis
> onycholysis, distal nail turns upward (Plummer's nails)
> scalp hair fine, thinning
> nonspecific—pruritus, urticaria, hyperpigmentation, diffuse or patchy alopecia areata

The following **signs** demand evaluation for **paraproteinemia**:

> lichen myxedematosus:
>> generalized lichenoid papular eruption (scleromyxedema)
>> waxy papules, especially hands, elbows, face, trunk, often linear
>> skin firm, indurated, suggesting diagnosis of scleroderma
>> face—furrowed glabella
>> complaint of restricted movement—opening mouth, moving fingers
>
> papular lichen myxedematosus:
>> flesh-colored papules of trunk and extremities
>> rarely annular
>
> lichenoid plaques: resemble lichen planus
> urticarial plaques: usually evolve into other forms

Other clinically defined mucinoses:

reticular erythematous mucinosis (plaquelike mucinosis)

erythematous plaque forming reticulated pattern of upper back or chest

photosensitive: burning, itching, and flare of lesions produced by sunlight

scleredema

diffuse symmetrical hardening of skin, beginning on posterior area of neck, spreading to upper trunk, face, and upper arms; may spread for 2 weeks to 2 months

skin waxy, hard, wooden-like on palpation; may be erythematous

face expressionless

paresthesia possible

stiffness due to restriction in joint movement, e.g., jaw, elbow, chest wall

look for pleural, pericardial, peritoneal effusions, cardiac abnormalities, hepatomegaly, multiple myeloma

often preceded by streptococcal infection or other bacterial infection

usually resolved in 2 years

follicular mucinosis (alopecia mucinosa)

follicular papules, coalescing into well-defined plaques

alopecia

usually on face and neck

decreased sensory function

differential diagnosis: folliculitis, eczema, seborrheic dermatitis, neurodermatitis, mycosis fungoides (in older group)

cutaneous focal mucinosis

flesh-colored papules and nodules

solitary

any site except hands and feet

differential cyst

synovial cyst (myxoid)

smooth dome-shaped nodules over dorsal surface of interphalangeal joints of fingers, rarely face

solitary

on incision, yields viscous yellow fluid

Noppakun N, Bancheun K, Chandraprasert S: Unusual locations of **localized myxedema** in Graves' disease. Report of three cases. Arch Dermatol 1986; 122:85–88.

Firm, nonpitting, well-circumscribed flesh-colored **masses** on the shoulders of a 25-year-old Thai man proved to be **localized myxedema**. The growths, which **resembled football shoulder pads**, developed from the trauma of carrying heavy things suspended by a long stick. He had the classic signs of **Graves' disease** with an enlarged thyroid, as well as large infiltrative plaques of myxedema of the shins.

The pretibial area is the usual site of predilection for localized myxedema, but it has also been reported on the ankles, arms, hands, abdomen, face, and earlobes. The deposits of hyaluronic acid appear to favor areas of trauma. Although this myxedema **usually arises after therapy for thyrotoxicosis**, it also has been seen with hypothyroidism, thyroiditis, acute hyperthyroidism, and the euthyroid state.

In diagnosis, the coin of the realm is curiosity.

Endocrinopathy

One of the diagnostic entry points for a puzzling problem is to question an endocrine pathogenesis. Few cells escape the effects of the circulating hormones, and in significant endocrine aberrations skin disease may result.

We look to four endocrine glands as potential causes. Foremost is the pancreas. Occult diabetes may explain chronic infection, pruritus, a bullous eruption of the fingers, xanthomas, or even a red face. Similarly, a glucagonoma may explain those strange erosions.

Equally significant is the thyroid. Hypothyroidism may account for the patient's dry skin, hair loss, pruritus, or brittle nails. In turn, hyperthyroidism may explain hyperhidrosis, periorbital edema, or pruritus.

The adrenal participates in explaining the patient with Cushing's syndrome. Thus, it may account for hypertrichosis, purplish striae, poikiloderma, or acne. In the fullest development of the syndrome, the moon facies, buffalo hump, and centripetal obesity will easily ring the diagnostic bell.

Finally, the pituitary adenomas pouring out growth hormone may explain a thickened, wrinkled forehead long before the patient's change in shoe and ring size makes the diagnosis of acromegaly obvious.

The delight in "endocrine diagnosis" is in ordering the appropriate test when the symptom or sign is still subtle and the syndrome but in its infancy. Equally satisfying is the recognition of the autoimmune progesterone and estrogen dermatitides in women with cyclic flares.

Feingold KR, Elias PM: **Endocrine-skin interactions**: Cutaneous manifestations of adrenal disease, pheochromocytomas, carcinoid syndrome, sex hormone excess and deficiency, polyglandular autoimmune syndromes, multiple endocrine neoplasia syndromes, and other miscellaneous disorders. J Am Acad Dermatol 1988; 19:1–20.

Skin changes may be the initial and at times the most prominent sign of these rare endocrinopathies.

Cushing's syndrome, due to glucocorticoid excess:
    moon facies
    temporal fat pad enlargement
    fat masses, supraclavicular:
        nape
        pelvis
    smooth, thin skin
    striae—wide, purplish
    purpura, petechiae
    predisposition to tinea
    steroid acne: trunk, shoulders, arms
    hyperpigmentation, if cause is excess ACTH

Nelson's syndrome:
    hyperpigmentation due to pituitary tumor in Cushing's disease patients who had bilateral adrenalectomy

Adrenal insufficiency:
    due to melanocyte stimulation by elevated ACTH or MSH production secondary to low cortisol levels

Hyperpigmentation is rare; misinterpreted by patient as tanning, since onset is gradual.
Look for it in palmar creases, axillae, mucous membranes untouched by sunlight.
Nevi darken, new nevi become evident.
Nails develop longitudinal bands of darkening.

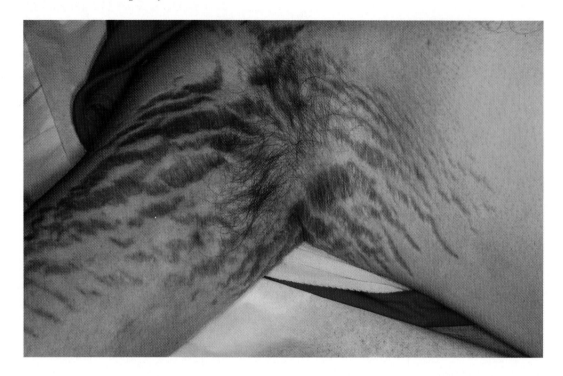

Pheochromocytoma:
  due to excess
    norepinephrine

Paroxysmal hyperhidrosis: drenching during hypertensive attacks
No flushing, pallor of anything due to vasoconstriction
Look for pheochromocytoma in mucosal neuroma syndrome (oral neuromas, large lips, flat nasal bridge)

Carcinoid syndrome:
  due to carcinoid tumor
    releasing kinins,
    prostaglandins,
    substance P, histamine,
    serotonin

Paroxysmal flushing of face, neck, upper trunk with drop in blood pressure
Periorbital edema
Attacks triggered by alcohol, eating, defecating, emotional upset, exertion
Persistent cyanotic erythema and telangiectasia; if attacks continue for years:
Think gastric carcinoids if patchy flush, sharp serpentine red borders, occurring after meals
Pellagra, hyperkeratosis, dry dark scaling on sun-exposed areas result of tryptophan being diverted to tumor to form serotonin instead of necessary niacin
Scleroderma, lower legs
Tumors due to metastases to skin

Androgen excess:
  adrenal ovarian tumors
  anabolic steroids,
    androgens, birth control
    pills

Detectable only in women;
  look for hirsutism, menses change, clitoromegaly, baldness

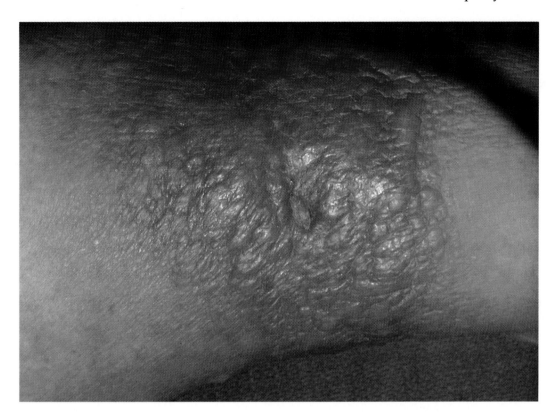

Androgen deficiency:

If prior to puberty:
  no development of facial, chest,
    abdominal hair; sebaceous and
    apocrine glands
  smooth nonoily acne-free skin
  no baldness
  tall, eunuchoid; fine wrinkling around
    eyes, lips; scrotal skin smooth;
    penis small
If after puberty:
  smooth, nonoily, acne-free skin
  hot flashes, red face, sweating attacks

Estrogen excess:
  contraceptives
  pregnancy

In men: gynecomastia
In girls: precocious puberty
In women:
  palmar erythema
  telangiectasia
  spider angiomas
  melasma
  nevi darken
  sebum production reduced with
    clearing of acne
  hirsutism
  occasionally temporary hair loss
    following and during pregnancy or
    use of contraceptive

Estrogen deficiency:	hot flashes
	atrophy of urogenital epithelium
	breasts decrease in size
Insulin resistance	Acanthosis nigricans
autoantibodies to insulin	

Huntley AC: The **cutaneous manifestations of diabetes mellitus**. J Am Acad Dermatol 1982; 7:427–455.

The following conditions should make you look for a background of diabetes mellitus:

erysipelas-like erythema
  well-demarcated erythematous areas on the lower legs of older individuals, at times purpuric or with necrotic center
gangrene
  dry form due to large vessel blockage
  wet form, inadequacy of small-vessel cutaneous circulation may lead to putrefaction
  gas gangrene due to nonclostridial organisms
absence of sweating of lower extremities, complaint of compensatory hyperhidrosis elsewhere, may develop gustatory sweating
diminished pain sensation—neuropathic ulcers (mal perforans), grossly deformed foot
Candida **infections**
  paronychia
  pruritus vulvae
  phimosis
erythrasma
  erythematous plaques on upper inner thighs
malignant otitis externa
  facial weakness, pain, persistent granulation tissue
necrobiosis lipoidica diabeticorum
  majority have diabetes
diabetic dermopathy
  skin spots, flat to red, dull-red papules due to trauma
scleredema following streptococcal infection; also may present as waxy tight skin
diabetic bullae on tips of fingers, atraumatic clear blisters
yellow skin, yellow nails
eruptive xanthomas
  crops of yellow papules with red areolae
red face
  dilatation of dermal venous plexus
hyperpigmentation
  hemochromatosis
porphyrias
lipodystrophy
acanthosis nigricans

Since 15 more skin diseases are listed as having an association with diabetes, you should look for diabetes in all your patients.

If it's an important question, ask it twice.

Epidermolysis Bullosa

With the advent of immunofluorescent and ultrastructural study of blistering diseases, physicians are left with clinical approximations until they have the pathologist's report. This is especially true for the taxonomy of inherited epidermolysis bullosa.

The essential feature of epidermolysis bullosa, whether acquired or inherited, is blister formation resulting from minor physical shearing force. The most common form is the recurrent bullous eruption of the hands and feet (Weber-Cockayne). Although nearly all of us will develop blisters with poorly fitted shoes or manual labor, these patients blister easily. The blisters result from shearing of the epidermis itself, so no scarring results. It is more evident in hot weather when the sweat increases the frictional load.

When the epidermis tears loose at the lamina lucida, the condition is designated as junctional epidermolysis bullosa, in contrast to the simplex type in which separation is within the epidermis itself. This junctional type may be so severe as to cause death in the neonatal period, since merely handling these infants denudes them.

The third type is the dystrophic type in which the epidermis and its entire basement membrane separate from the dermis. Healing occurs with scarring, and often milia are present. An unbelievable array of defects is seen in this dystrophic form. There may be loss of hair, dwarfism, and clawlike hands with the fingers lost in a mitten of epidermis. As the years pass, epitheliomas appear, both basal and squamous cell.

Electron microscopy is the only way to discern the true land of separation. Combining this with genetic history, it is possible to accurately classify the forms of this rare bullous disease.

In contrast to the inherited epidermolysis bullosa, there is an acquired form, viz., epidermolysis bullosa acquisita. In at least half of this adult-onset easy blistering dermatosis, the problem is an autoimmune one with the fault lying in the presence of antibasement membrane zone antibodies. The patients may show severe oral esophageal or ocular mucosal scarring. Thus, without immunofluorescent study, this dermatosis may be misdiagnosed as cicatricial pemphigoid. Furthermore, the widespread blisters may be viewed as bullous pemphigoid or even bullous lupus erythematosus. Even the bullous dermatosis of dialysis enters the differential.

Epidermolysis bullosa acquisita may be associated with a great variety of systemic disease. Each patient deserves review for possible lymphoma, carcinoma, and diabetes.

This amazing array of genetic and autoimmune blistering diseases testifies to the multiversity of disease that we can sense by looking at the ultrastructure and immunobiology of the skin. With new microscopes and gene mapping, there is more to come. Gone are the days when a blister was a blister and that was that.

Our future speaks to the clinician's first approximations becoming first guesses.

Fine J-D, Bauer EA, Briggaman RA, et al: Revised clinical and laboratory criteria for subtypes of inherited epidermolysis bullosa. A consensus report by the subcommittee on diagnosis and classification of the National Epidermolysis Bullosa Registry. J Am Acad Dermatol 1991; 24:119–135.

There are presently four regionally separated academic institutions in the United States that serve as centers for the federally funded national registry of epidermolysis bullosa patients.

The clinicians and other investigators involved in the registry have tried to simplify the classification of the disease. Their recommendations are presented in several tables.

503

A detailed history is vital and should include:

mapping of the family pedigree
evidence of consanguinity
age of onset
seasonal effects
fever effect on the extent of disease activity
extracutaneous disease, extent and severity (eyes, oropharynx, teeth, larynx, gastrointestinal, genitourinary, musculoskeletal, neuromuscular)

Cutaneous findings should include:

distribution: acral, inverse (flexural), generalized
morphology:
blisters (grouped)
crusted erosions
milia
scar formation (atrophic, hypertrophic)
exuberant granulation tissue (Herlitz variant)
postinflammatory pigment changes (reticulate, mottled)
scarring alopecia
nail dystrophy or absence
palmoplantar keratoderma
albopapuloid lesions
mechanical: fragility (subtle or marked)

Laboratory evaluation should include:

Transmission electron microscopy. This requires special fixatives for the skin biopsy specimens. It provides data on the level of skin cleavage and identifies three distinct groups:
simplex (epidermolytic)
junctional (lamina lucidolytic)
dystrophic (dermolytic)

It also permits direct assessment of the morphology of the anchoring filaments and fibrils.

Immunofluorescence mapping. The skin biopsy is placed into conventional immunofluorescence transport medium and shipped at room temperature. An indirect immunofluorescence technique is used to localize several basement membrane antigens (bullous pemphigoid antigen, laminin, type IV collagen) and predict the location of skin cleavage within a given skin specimen. Epidermolysis bullosa cannot be accurately diagnosed by conventional light microscopic technique in formalin-fixed specimens.

From a practical point of view, most patients can be best classified as having *one* of three major presentations (generalized, localized, inverse) of three major subsets (simplex, junctional, dystrophic). The latter two categories are subclassified as Herlitz vs non-Herlitz variants and dominant vs recessive transmitted forms, respectively.

For young infants, in whom typical phenotype features of epidermolysis bullosa may not yet be present, the term *indeterminant type* is useful as a descriptive qualifier.

Pearson RW: Clinicopathologic types of epidermolysis bullosa and their nondermatological complications. Arch Dermatol 1988; 124:718–725.

Blisters following minor skin trauma cell for a diagnosis of epidermolysis bullosa. The next diagnostic step is determining histologically the level at which the blister forms, so that it may be placed in one of three subgroups (epidermolytic, lucidolytic, dermolytic). The major subgroup is epidermolytic (EBS) with separation within the epidermal cell mass. This includes 17 types ranging from **epidermolysis bullosa simplex** to the **peeling skin syndrome**. The second, **lamina lucidolytic** (LEB) subgroup, with lysis occurring within the lamina lucida, includes six specific types. The third subgroup, **dermolytic epidermolysis bullosa** (DEB), has separation beneath the basal lamina of the epidermis and includes six types.

Confronted with 29 types of these mechanobullous diseases, one needs access to this original reference for close matching of the patients' findings with the current taxonomic nomenclature.

The range of findings is tremendous. In addition to the hallmark of blisters and erosions (with or without scars), **patients may have**:

> patterned blisters (annular, herpetiform)
> scars (milia)
> mucosal erosions (esophageal casts, corneal erosions)
> hyperkeratosis of palms and soles (diffuse or punctate)
> nail changes (loss, onycholysis, pachyonychia, dystrophy, onychogryphosis)
> hair changes (brittle, alopecia)
> teeth abnormalities (natal teeth, defective, hypoplastic pitting, anodontia)
> sweat gland abnormalities (hyperhidrosis)
> melanocyte abnormalities (hyperpigmentation and hypopigmentation, mottled, spotty)

Buchbinder LH, Lucky AW, Ballard E, et al: **Severe infantile epidermolysis bullosa simplex, Dowling-Meara type.** Arch Dermatol 1986; 122:190–198.

Long before the electron microscopists split epidermolysis bullosa into 18 types, Dowling and Meara clinically discerned a significant form of epidermolysis bullosa that now bears their names. They recognized that there was a severe version that resembled juvenile dermatitis herpetiformis and that became milder with the passage of childhood.

Five cases are presented that were diagnosed originally as recessive dystrophic epidermolysis bullosa. Each patient had an extremely severe form of the disease, with apparent subepidermal separation on biopsy. **As unexpected improvement occurred** and repeat biopsies showed intraepidermal clefting due to basal cell cytolysis, the correct and more optimistic diagnosis of the Dowling-Meara type of epidermolysis bullosa simplex was evident. Other features include milia formation, acral distribution with **herpetiform groups of blisters** in older children, intraoral lesions, and absence of scarring.

Fine J-D, Johnson L, Wright T: **Epidermolysis bullosa simplex superficialis**: A new variant of epidermolysis bullosa characterized by subcorneal skin cleavage mimicking peeling skin syndrome. Arch Dermatol 1989; 125:633–638.

Since birth, a 6-year-old boy had **fragile skin**, with any minor skin trauma leading to superficial erosions and cracking. Some lesions were linear and led to the suggestion of child abuse. Blisters were a rare finding. **Skin cleavage could be readily induced by minor rotary traction.** Finally a skin biopsy showed **cleavage between the stratum granulosum and stratum corneum**, leading to a diagnosis of epidermolysis bullosa simplex superficialis.

There are now 17 clinical variants of epidermolysis bullosa simplex. This is an additional one, unique in its high cleavage point. The others show splits within or just above the basal keratinocytes. Three variants are of major importance:

> localized (**Weber-Cockayne**): involves the hands and feet
> generalized (**Koebner**): generalized and acral lesions
> herpetiformis (**Dowling-Meara**): generalized and acral lesions

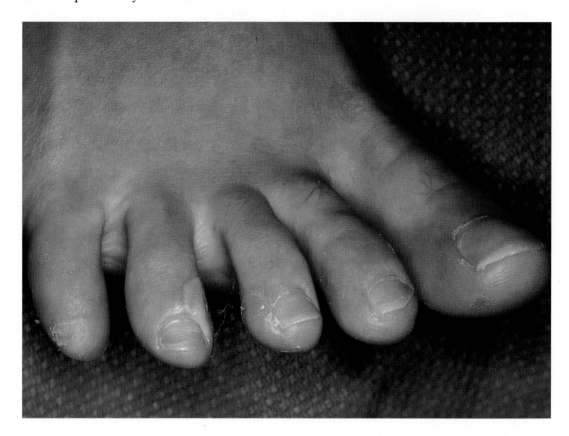

The present report includes six more patients with this superficial high-level form, which must be distinguished from the peeling skin syndrome. Although both show high-level histologic splitting of the epidermis, epidermolysis bullosa simplex superficialis is unique in presenting with blisters and not showing continual peeling.

Fischer T, Gedde-Dahl T Jr: **Epidermolysis bullosa simplex and mottled pigmentation**: A new dominant syndrome: I. Clinical and histological features. Clin Genet 1979; 15:228–238.

Mottled pigmentation with depigmented spots (2 to 5 mm) and ill-defined borders in a **mosaic pattern** was the childhood affliction of 11 members of one family. Present since birth in 10 cases, it appeared at age 1 year in one child. In spring, sunlight irritated the depigmented spots, which became red but later tanned. By adulthood the pigmentation was normal. The mottled pigmentation presumably results from **clones of keratinocytes that fail to take up melanosomes**, thus producing nonpigmented loci a few millimeters in diameter.

Each patient also experienced serous, nonscarring, mechanically induced blisters starting at birth, proven to be epidermolysis bullosa simplex. **Blister** formation usually **disappeared in adulthood**.

This pigmentary problem appears to be unique. Other considerations include:

1. **Naegeli-Franceschetti-Jadassohn syndrome** (autosomal dominant) with widespread reticular pigmentation beginning after age 2 years. Inflammation precedes the pigmentation, and bullae on the hands and feet are not induced by trauma

2. **Dyskeratosis congenita** (X-linked dominant) with similar pigment changes beginning at age 3 to 5 years. Look for skin atrophy, ridged nails, hypoplasia of dermatoglyphics, leukoplakia, blood dyscrasias, and early death due to malignant disease

3. "**Dyschromatosis universalis hereditaria**" (variable autosomal inheritance) with freckling on a depigmented background and changes in hair color

4. **Dermatopathia pigmentosa reticularis** (autosomal recessive) with similar pigment changes beginning at age 2 years along with progressive alopecia, nail dystrophy, and pigment incontinence seen on biopsy

5. **Incontinentia pigmenti** (X-linked dominant) with irregular pigment swirls on limited body areas

6. **Urticaria pigmentosa** (sporadic) with mottled pigmentation and urtication

Pearson RW, Paller AS: **Dermolytic (dystrophic) epidermolysis bullosa inversa.** Arch Dermatol 1988; 124:544–547.

This inverse form of recessive dermolytic epidermolysis bullosa is characterized by a lifelong history of **blisters and erosions of the flexural areas**: neck, axillae, submammary area, inguinal folds, and perineum.

The oral mucosa and **esophagus** are also commonly **involved**, with stenosis resulting.

Rubenstein R, Esterly NB, Fine J-D: **Childhood epidermolysis bullosa acquisita.** Detection in a 5-year-old girl. Arch Dermatol 1987; 123:772–776.

Sparse blistering of the face, trunk, and extremities as well as the mucous membranes of the eyes, mouth, vagina, and anus in a 5-year-old girl had been labeled cicatricial pemphigoid on the basis of immunofluorescence and histologic study.

However, **immunoelectron microscopy** demonstrated linear deposits of several immunoreactants in the sublamina densa region of the dermoepidermal junction, **changing the diagnosis from cicatricial pemphigoid to acquired epidermolysis bullosa.**

Clinically, cicatricial pemphigoid mimics epidermolysis bullosa acquisita, but the blister occurs within the lamina lucida and not beneath the entire basement membrane, as in epidermolysis bullosa acquisita. The distinction cannot be made in the clinic or at the light microscopy bench, but only in the transmission electron microscopy laboratory.

Traupe H, Kolde G, Hamm H, Happle R: **Ichthyosis bullosa of Siemens**: A unique type of **epidermolytic hyperkeratosis.** J Am Acad Dermatol 1986; 14:1000–1005.

Since birth, a 6-year-old girl had suffered with blisters resembling epidermolysis bullosa simplex and also **dark-gray hyperkeratosis** of the hands and feet, medial aspect of the thighs, neck, and flexural areas. Circumscribed areas of the axillae, periumbilical zone, and lower back were also involved, and the wrists, dorsal surface of the hands, elbows, knees, and ankles showed lichenification. The hands and feet were most severely involved, with blisters developing after mechanical trauma and probably related to hyperhidrosis.

Most remarkable was the **molting** of the outer skin. After "blistering," the areas became superficially denuded, with normal appearing stratum corneum evident at the bottom. There was no scarring or atrophy. The molting phenomenon was initiated by mechanical trauma, heat, and sweating. Her father, grandfather, and great-grandfather had the same disease.

On biopsy, the **blistering was seen to be intracorneal** within the ichthyotic layer, making it a **special subset of epidermolytic hyperkeratosis.** The absence of erythroderma ruled out bullous ichthyosiform erythroderma.

Erythema Multiforme

Erythema multiforme is a readily recognizable reaction pattern in the skin. With its annular and iris-shaped macules, as well as its bullous lesions of the hands and arms, it is distinctive. Involvement of the mucous membranes with erosive lesions is also characteristic of the version called Stevens-Johnson syndrome.

Some of the patients will give a history of a preceding cold sore. Indeed, it is likely that a herpes simplex viral infection accounts for half of the cases, suggesting that many examples of the primary trigger disease are occult. This viral antigen can be frequently demonstrated in the lesions by the polymerase chain reaction. Furthermore, intradermal injection of a herpes simplex antigen has reproduced the disease. The fact that so many examples of erythema multiforme are an example of a hypersensitivity reaction to the herpes virus explains the innumerable disparate causes for erythema multiforme. Each of them actually is a trigger for the appearance of herpes. Thus, fevers, foods, progesterone, sunburn, and infections have been implicated, and it is now apparent they act by initiating an attack of herpes simplex. It is well to note that erythema multiforme is a recurrent problem, even as herpes simplex. Given a patient with such recurrent erythema multiforme, diagnostic confirmation of the etiologic role of the herpes virus can be obtained by preventing or aborting an attack by immediate acyclovir therapy.

In the absence of a role for the herpes virus, look for drugs as a cause. Sulfonamides, aspirin, phenytoin, and allopurinol are a few of the many drugs known to induce erythema multiforme. Chemicals such as bromofluorine are also a possible cause. Internal malignant disease, radiotherapy, and enteric *Yersinia* infections may also be associated with erythema multiforme. In our experience, mycoplasma pulmonary infections may be as common a cause as drugs.

The primary level of diagnosis in erythema multiforme is easy. Unless herpes simplex is in evidence, the hard part is the second level of diagnosis: finding the cause.

Huff JC, Weston WL, Tonnesen MG: **Erythema multiforme**: A critical review of characteristics, **diagnostic criteria** and causes. J Am Acad Dermatol 1983; 8:763–775.

Typical primary lesion: Round erythematous macule, rapidly becoming red edematous papule, sometimes surrounded by blanching. Suggestive of diagnosis of insect bites or papular urticaria

Progression: To small plaques; may develop concentric alterations in morphology and color

Characteristic lesion: Central blister with necrotic blister roof or simple central area of epidermal necrosis. Concentric color change produces hallmark "target" or "iris" lesion.

Target lesion: Center is usually somewhat depressed, white, yellow or gray area of epidermal necrosis with darker gray to blue rim. Center may be beefy red in some individuals or dark gray in the black patient. Encircling this central area are shades of red and pink.

Progression: To coalescence, forming geographic antral erosions, crusting, polycyclic and annular figures. Central clearing in some instances. Inflammation may remit and later reactivate.

Healing: Scaling, pigmentation, no scars

Distribution: Symmetrical, dorsal surfaces of hand, extensor surfaces of extremities, centripetal spread. Mucosal lesions in 25 to 60%, erythema, edema, progressing to erosions in hours with pseudomembrane formation. May precede or follow skin lesions

Severe form: (Erythema multiforme major, or Stevens-Johnson syndrome). Morphology may be variable and atypical. At times, fine maculopapular eruption, large confluent areas of erythema, large bullae, large plaques, massive denudation of epidermis as in toxic epidermal necrolysis

Mucosal lesions are severe confluent erosions of eyes and mouth, genitalia. May extend down into pharynx and upper respiratory tract

Associated symptoms: Mild form—malaise, itching and burning of skin. Pain of mucosal erosions

Major form—also fever, myalgias, prostration

Course: New lesions in crops for 1 to 2 weeks, heal within a few weeks. Major form may take 6 weeks or longer for healing.

Complications: Major form—dehydration due to difficulty in taking fluids. Keratitis, uveitis, scarring, perforation of bulb. Permanent visual impairment in 10%. Esophagitis, pneumonia, loss of nails. Eruptive nevi appear. Sepsis, mortality

Laboratory: Nondiagnostic

Biopsy: No leukocytoclastic vasculitis; mononuclear cell infiltrate

Differential diagnosis: Discrete round lesions of erythema multiforme exclude drug eruptions, viral exanthems. Symmetry excludes fixed drug eruption. Acute episodic nature excludes chronic disease.

Precipitating factors: **Herpes simplex** (type 1 or 2) is the trigger in a majority of cases, with latent period of about 10 days (1 to 3 weeks)

Mycoplasma pneumoniae respiratory infection is significant antecedent in other patients

Sulfonamide sensitivity is the third of the major triad of causes. The latent period between onset of drug intake and skin signs is usually 7 to 14 days. In a previously sensitized patient, however, erythema multiforme may appear within hours of a single dose

Huff JC, Weston WL: Isomorphic phenomenon in erythema multiforme. Clin Exp Dermatol 1983; 8:409–413.

Expect to see erythema multiforme **lesions localizing in**:

cuts	folliculitis	bite line of buccal mucosa
scratches	traumatized nail folds	elbows, knees
surgical scars	gingivitis, focal	sunburn

In one of the 14 cases showing this isomorphic phenomenon, the erythema multiforme arose at the site of a human bite. Interestingly, Koebner, who first described the phenomenon, observed psoriatic lesions arising precisely at the site of a horse bite.

Lewis MAO, Lamey P-J, Forsyth A, Gall J: **Recurrent erythema multiforme**: A possible **role of foodstuffs**. Br Dental J 1989; 166:371–373.

Patch testing with the standard scout tray and a battery of food additives,

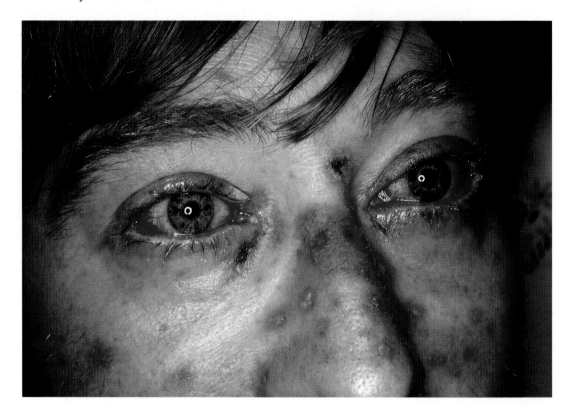

flavoring agents, and essential oils was done on seven patients with a history of recurrent acute widespread oral ulcerations. Five had associated signs of erythema multiforme. **Patch tests** were specifically positive to **benzoic acid (5%)** in all seven. By adhering to a rigid benzoate-free diet, four of the seven were able to remain free of further attacks.

Saperstein H, Rapaport M, Rietschel RL: **Topical vitamin E as a cause of erythema multiforme–like eruption.** Arch Dermatol 1984; 120:906–908.

This 31-year-old woman had a generalized eruption consisting of erythematous and edematous bullous and target lesions. She had malaise and was febrile. A diagnosis of erythema multiforme was made.

The history disclosed that for the 3 days before the eruption she had repeatedly **applied 100% pure vitamin E oil to two burn scars** on her chest. A patch test to the *d*-1 alpha-tocopherol acetate she had used was read as a 4+ positive. All materials in the patch test screening tray produced no change.

The patient had had no prior medicines, had had no herpes simplex, and was in good health. Accordingly, the erythema multiforme was viewed as reaction to the vitamin E, similar to the erythema multiforme seen in poison ivy–sensitive patients. Contactants can become and act as systemics.

Habbema L, Bruynzeel DP: **Fixed drug eruption due to naproxen.** Dermatologica 1987; 174:184–185.

Gray macules on the face of a 16-year-old girl for $1\frac{1}{2}$ years became reddish brown, elevated, and itchy before each menses and were thought to represent either progesterone autoimmune disease or erythema multiforme. Elicitation of a 2-year **history of taking naproxen** sodium the day before each menses for premenstrual pain suggested a fixed drug eruption. Challenge midperiod with 2 tablets of naproxen sodium confirmed a fixed drug eruption, with **burning, redness, and elevation of the lesions 1 hour after ingestion.** Patch tests within the lesions and scratch tests with naproxen sodium were negative.

More **common reactions to naproxen** include pruritus, photosensitivity, exanthems, and vesiculobullous eruptions. Patients must be cautioned to avoid all nonsteroidal anti-inflammatory drugs, since all of them may cross-react. Chlorambucil is also related, with cross-reactivity to be anticipated.

Milstien JB, Kuritsky JN: **Erythema multiforme and hepatitis B immunization.** Arch Dermatol 1986; 122:511–512.

Eight cases of erythema multiforme beginning 1 to 9 days after inoculation with hepatitis B vaccine have been reported to the US Food and Drug Administration (FDA). The patients were all adults (25 to 61 years), and none had mucosal involvement.

Friedman SJ, Black JL, Duffy J: **Histoplasmosis presenting as erythema multiforme** and polyarthritis. Cutis 1984; 34:396–398.

In a 55-year-old woman, an influenza-like illness in November was followed 2 weeks later by a generalized nonpruritic eruption, joint effusions, and, later, profound morning stiffness of the joints lasting 15 to 30 minutes. When seen in January she had **erythematous target lesions** over the body, typical of erythema multiforme, which was confirmed histologically.

In a wide screening search for the cause, complement-fixing antibodies to both the mycelial (1:8) and yeast (1:32) antigens of *Histoplasma capsulatum* were found. A definitive **diagnosis of histoplasmosis** was then made. The problem proved to be self-limiting, with dramatic improvement noted following prednisone therapy.

Think of histoplasmosis in both erythema multiforme and erythema nodosum, especially if polyarthritis is present.

Parodi A, Drago EF, Varaldo G, Rebora A: **Rowell's syndrome.** Report of a case. J Am Acad Dermatol 1989; 21:374–377.

A 63-year-old man had recurring **figurate lesions of the legs** of 2 months' duration. He gave a history of subacute cutaneous lupus erythematosus successfully treated with chloroquine 10 years before.

On examination, he had a large ringed lesion over the anterior right thigh. It showed necrotic sites as well as scars. There were also a typical, annular, scarring plaque of discoid lupus erythematosus on the left buttock and three erythematous, edematous, nummular plaques on the back. Finally, chilblain lesions were present on the dorsum of the fingers.

It is this **unique conjunction of subacute lupus erythematosus, discoid lupus erythematosus, and erythema multiforme–like lesions** that makes the diagnosis of Rowell's syndrome. Chilblain lesions may also be present.

The diagnosis of Rowell's syndrome was made in this patient on the basis of the clinical constellation as well as serologic evidence of anti-Ro (SS-A) antibodies in the serum. It is a diagnosis to be distinguished from the casual occurrence of erythema multiforme in any patient with lupus erythematosus.

Erythema Nodosum

Tender red nodules over the shins make the diagnosis of erythema nodosum. Rarely do they occur elsewhere, but often come in recurrent crops, each lasting for weeks. Even as erythema multiforme was a reaction pattern commonly due to herpes simplex infection or a drug, so also is erythema nodosum a reaction pattern. But here, streptococcal infection takes pride of place as the most common cause, with drugs following. In erythema multiforme the reaction was in the small superficial vessels, accounting for its superficial epidermal lesions. Here, in erythema nodosum, the hypersensitivity reaction is in the deep larger vessels, explaining its less eloquent dermal lesions.

To make an etiologic diagnosis, look for streptococcal pharyngitis, tonsillitis, erysipelas, scarlet fever, or rheumatic fever. In the absence of evidence of streptococcal infection as a source of antigen, comb the history for a drug such as sulfonamides. Contraceptives are especially suspect, and pregnancy is a known trigger. In a few instances erythema nodosum may be the sign of sarcoidosis, so that a chest plate may be helpful.

The continuing search for a causal agent centers on the colon. Acute colitis of a variety of types is well known to trigger erythema nodosum. Also, look for Crohn's disease as well as ulcerative colitis. The detailed internal medical review must continue, with emphasis on erythema nodosum being a first sign of leukemia in both its acute and chronic forms.

A variety of rare infectious diseases completes the list of causes. Thus, cat scratch disease with but a forgotten scratch may show only the regional unilateral lymphadenopathy and the erythema nodosum. Both superficial and deep fungal diseases are known causes. At times the red nodules on the shins direct one's attention simply to tinea pedis, but at other times the trail leads to coccidioidomycosis, histoplasmosis, or blastomycosis. In some patients the lesions of lymphogranuloma venereum may overshadow those of associated erythema nodosum.

Erythema nodosum is an easily recognized prototypical reaction pattern on the shins. A simple bruising of long ago has localized a blood-borne antigen to that area where bone and skin have but little fat between. We are slow to biopsy such lesions because that skin is slow to heal. But we are fast to look for infection in the throat or gut.

Hannuksela M: **Erythema nodosum.** With special reference to sarcoidosis. A clinical study of 343 Finnish adult patients. Ann Clin Res 1971; 3(suppl 7):1–64.

Look for these **causative factors**:

   sarcoidosis (33 to 47%)
   streptococcal infection (21 to 27%)
   Yersinia infection (10%)
   pregnancy (first trimester)
   oral contraceptives
   tuberculosis
   drug hypersensitivity

Erythema nodosum nodules are usually seen on the frontal surface of both legs and also frequently on the thighs and arms. After 4 to 8 weeks they disappear, leaving a livid color and scaling for a couple of weeks. Erythema nodosum migrans is a variant, with only one or a few migrating nodules of long duration. Fever and arthralgias (ankles, knees, elbows, wrists, fingers, in that order) are common accompanying symptoms.

Yersinia **infection** with erythema nodosum most frequently caused joint

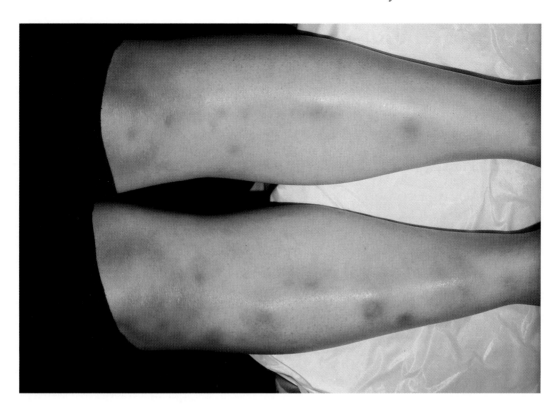

symptoms and had the shortest duration of skin lesions (3 weeks at most). Usually preceded by gastrointestinal symptoms (upper abdominal pains, diarrhea, appendicitis-like pain), it did not cause recurrent erythema nodosum.

Streptococcal infections were the most common cause of recurrent erythema nodosum.

Useful **laboratory studies**:

complete blood count
erythrocyte sedimentation rate
cryofibrinogen
serum proteins (↓ albumin, ↑ globulins)
serum protein immunoelectrophoresis (↑ IgA, IgM, and IgG)
chest x-ray
purified protein derivative skin test

The **pathogenesis** of erythema nodosum is probably immunologic. Conceivably, circulating soluble antigen–antibody immune complexes triggered by infection or drug allergy could be deposited in blood vessel walls in certain areas (locus minoris resistentiae), leading to skin lesions. Delayed hypersensitivity may be important, as most cells in erythema nodosum lesions are mononuclear. Female sex hormones and cold weather also play important roles.

Rostas A, Lowe D, Smout MS: Erythema nodosum migrans in a young woman. Arch Dermatol 1980; 116:325–326.

An **enlarging ring** of coalescing **erythematous nodules** had been present on the anterior left lower leg of this 16-year-old girl for 4 months. At the time of examination the lesion measured 15 cm in diameter, was mildly tender, and had a perfectly clear center from which the initial nodules had spread centrifugally.

A biopsy showed a perivascular infiltrate of lymphocytes and histiocytes, absence of vasculitis but the presence of **septal panniculitis**. All this was consistent with a diagnosis of erythema nodosum. The unilateral distribution, the peripherally expanding lesion, and the tenderness, however, resulted in a diagnosis of erythema nodosum migrans. It is to be histologically distinguished from subacute nodular migratory panniculitis.

In such patients, **trigger factors** center on pregnancy, streptococcal infections, or sarcoidosis. This patient had never been pregnant, had no sore throat, and took no medication or contraceptives.

Although laboratory studies for histoplasmosis, blastomycosis, and *Yersinia* infection were negative and skin tests to purified protein derivative and trichophyton were also negative, a very strong reaction to Varidase (streptokinase-streptodornase was seen at 48 hr). This suggested a streptococcal antigen entered into the pathogenesis of this eruption.

Within 5 days of treatment with 0.25 ml of saturated solution of potassium iodide three times a day, the lesions had receded. By the 21st day they were completely gone. Again, this therapeutic response favored the diagnosis of erythema nodosum.

Tami LF: **Erythema nodosum associated with *Shigella* colitis.** Arch Dermatol 1985; 121:590.

Typical erythema nodosum lesions developed on the extensor surfaces of the lower legs and forearms of this 13-year-old boy exactly 14 days after he had experienced **severe diarrhea**.

At that time, *Shigella flexneri* had been isolated on stool culture. The biopsy-proven erythema nodosum resolved within 3 weeks.

All cases of erythema nodosum need to be reviewed in terms of bowel disease as well as *Yersinia*, *Salmonella*, and *Campylobacter* gastroenteritis. It also has been reported in association with amebiasis and helminthic infection (*Ascaris lumbricoides*, *Taenia solium*).

Thus **a look at the stool and its culture** must not be neglected as one searches for bacterial antigens causing erythema nodosum.

Thomas RHM, Black MM: The wide **clinical spectrum of polyarteritis nodosa** with cutaneous involvement. Clin Exp Dermatol 1983; 8:47–59.

A few days after a streptococcal sore throat, this boy of 8 developed polyarthritis, slurred speech, muscle pain and weakness, malaise, fever, and leukocytosis. It cleared with steroid therapy, but recurrent episodes occurred over the next 3 years. At age 12 he developed **massive plaques on his hands and feet** during one of these attacks. A **biopsy suggested a diagnosis of dermatomyositis**.

Not until 2 years later, when during an attack of arthritis and myositis he developed tender red nodules of the legs, was a **definitive diagnosis** of **polyarteritis nodosa** made, on biopsy of one of the nodules.

Polyarteritis nodosa should be suspected in patients with not only nodules of the lower legs but also in patients with leg ulcers, palpable purpura, livedo reticularis, and toxic erythema. It is a multisystem vasculitic disease so that the skin is but one of the showcases. Accordingly, a skin biopsy may illuminate the nature of many of the patient's multiple complaints.

Syrjälä H, Karvonen J, Salminen A: **Skin manifestations of tularemia**: A study of 88 cases in northern Finland during 16 years (1967–1983). Acta Derm Venereol 1984; 64:513–516.

The usual sign of tularemia is an **ulcer** of the skin with lymphadenopathy, but secondary skin signs are also common:

> transitory pruritic nonspecific **papules and papulovesicles** of the arms and legs (42%), sometimes showing vasculitis on biopsy, lesions usually disappearing in 2 weeks
>
> **erythema nodosum** (22%) on the legs, numerous in some patients
>
> **erythema multiforme** (9%) usually involving the chest and upper arms, which disappeared in a few weeks
>
> A small gram-negative rod (*Francisella tularensis*) is responsible for all this. It arrives by insect bite (mosquito, horsefly, tick), handling infected animals, inhaling infected dust, or eating infected food or drinking contaminated water.

Don't forget tularemia when you see erythema nodosum or erythema multiforme! *Yersinia* infection causes similar lesions.

March LM, Webb J, Eckstein RP: **Cytophagic panniculitis.** Aust NZ J Med 1986; 16:397–401.

A 60-year-old housewife had been sick for 3 months with irregular hectic fever, sweats, malaise, weight loss, and crops of erythematous, tender, indurated, **subcutaneous nodules** on the limbs, neck, breasts, and trunk. The nodules were 1 to 4 cm in diameter. She also had generalized osteoarthritis, nontender hepatosplenomegaly, axillary lymphadenopathy, and mild proximal limb-girdle myopathy residual from an attack of polymyositis. Extensive laboratory tests were normal, except for: hemoglobin 10.7 gm/liter; white blood cell count 3.9×10^9/liter with 70% segmented neutrophils and 15% band forms, erythrocyte sedimentation rate 16 to 35 mm/hr, mildly elevated liver enzymes, and persistent isolation of herpes simplex from the throat. Lymph node biopsy showed reactive sinus histiocytosis with erythrophagocytosis.

Skin biopsy showed **florid lobular panniculitis** with histiocytes, lymphoid cells, and plasma cells. **Histiocytes showed marked phagocytosis** of nuclear debris. There was no vasculitis or granulomatous inflammation. Direct immunofluorescence and cultures of tissue were negative for bacteria, mycobacteria, and fungi. The histologic picture and persistent isolation of herpes simplex led to the diagnosis of cytophagic panniculitis versus virus-associated hemophagocytic syndrome. Erythema nodosum was excluded histologically by the absence of septal inflammation.

Cytophagocytosis is not commonly seen but does occur in:

> malignant histiocytic syndromes
> acute hemolytic anemias
> systemic lupus erythematosus
> typhoid fever
> miliary tuberculosis
> viral and bacterial infections

A compassionate listener hears more.

Erythroderma

General
Pediatric
Drug Induced
Neoplastic-Paraneoplastic
Complications

A red curtain descends over the patient with erythroderma. The entire skin is scarlet, swollen, and scaly. The patient is chilly from heat loss and excoriated from scratching. We can no longer see the players on the stage of skin; we must search the history of what was there before the curtain fell. We must go behind the curtain with our biopsy and blood studies to recognize the players. Erythroderma is a dedifferentiated dermatitis challenging you to find its cause.

Many examples are the end stage of a previously identified skin disease. Most commonly, atopic dermatitis, psoriasis, and ichthyosis present their worst scenario as erythroderma. If the history is barren of antecedent dermatitis, probe for drugs as a cause. This includes a search for contactants, from which these patients have not been able to escape. And recall that a chemical or drug known to produce contact dermatitis can produce erythroderma when introduced systemically. Unfortunately, patch tests at the time are worthless. But look for white waves of the shoreline nail as evidence of repeated drug insults causing erythroderma. Also, look for islands of normal skin in the curtain of red. This is clue for a diagnosis of pityriasis rubra pilaris, otherwise hard to make on biopsy. Secure an IgE level determination to support a diagnosis of atopic erythroderma.

In the congenital forms, search for metabolic disorders as well as consider congenital ichthyosiform erythroderma. Measure the biotin, biotinidase, as well as the urinary amino acid excretion. A streaky whorled pattern when discerned calls for peroxisomal enzyme assay in the fibroblast culture (Conradi syndrome).

Looking behind the curtain with a biopsy is invaluable. It may well reveal the players to be T cells in a lymphoma setting. It may be a generalized pemphigus foliaceous. Often the microscopic view is a disappointment, showing only the stagehands of inflammation. This calls for multiple biopsies for a better look.

If you are still bewildered, have the patient surveyed for hidden cancer or tumors. Follow any lead of ill health or dysfunction. Check the stools for occult blood. Obtain the appropriate x-rays, always including a chest plate and gastrointestinal series. In some patients, such as the elderly, a continuing series of negatives call for computed tomography and magnetic resonance imaging studies.

Look again for opportunists invading the immune-depressed or scaly terrain. Scrapings may reveal hyphae or scabies mites. Cultures may show bacterial overgrowth or the herpes simplex virus. Every visit calls for close cross-examination concerning the drug history.

When an erythrodermic patient comes in your office, it matters not whether you call it erythroderma, exfoliative dermatitis, or pityriasis rubra of Hebra. You will quickly realize you are functionally blind. There are no primary lesions, no patterns, no sites of predilection, no color plays. There is just that red curtain between you and the disease.

Thestrup-Pedersen K, Halkier-Sørenson L, Søgaard H, Zachariae H: **The red man syndrome**—exfoliative dermatitis of unknown etiology. A description and follow-up of 38 patients. J Am Acad Dermatol 1988; 18:1307–1312.

Psoriasis, **atopic dermatitis**, and **drug eruption** account for the majority of erythrodermas.

A smaller group is the consequence of contact dermatitis, seborrheic dermatitis, and internal malignant disease.

Rarest of antecedents include ichthyosis, polymorphous light eruption, parapsoriasis en plaques, pityriasis rubra pilaris, tinea, prurigo, scabies.

Beyond this, the authors identify an autonomous "red man syndrome" in 38 of their 204 erythroderma patients. It centers on a man with an idiopathic exfoliative dermatitis, keratoderma of the palms and soles, and a nonspecific histologic picture.

Note: Of these patients, 34% went on to develop mycosis fungoides (T cell lymphoma).

Boyd AS, Menter A: Erythrodermic psoriasis: Precipitating factors, course, and prognosis in 50 patients. J Am Acad Dermatol 1989; 21:985–991.

Although only about one of 40 patients with psoriasis develops erythroderma, one of every four erythrodermas is associated with psoriasis.

This study of 50 patients with **psoriatic erythroderma** revealed the following **precipitating factors**:

> systemic corticosteroids
> excessive use of topical steroids
> phototherapy
> emotional stress
> preceding illness

Cohen PR, Prystowsky JH: **Pityriasis rubra pilaris**: A review of diagnosis and treatment. J Am Acad Dermatol 1989; 20:801–807.

Clinical presentation:

> progressive erythroderma containing patches of normal skin ("islands of sparing")
> begins on head and spreads downward
> palms and soles hyperkeratotic with orange hue
> follicular papules on dorsal aspect of fingers and extensor wrists and thighs
> ectropion
> distal yellow-brown discoloration
> subungual hyperkeratosis and thickened nail plate and splinter hemorrhages

Here is a diagnosis made with more assurance by the clinician than by the pathologist.

DeSpain J, Clark DP: **Subacute cutaneous lupus erythematosus presenting as erythroderma.** J Am Acad Dermatol 1988; 19:388–392.

Generalized exfoliative erythroderma with accompanying telangiectasia had been present for 6 months in this 55-year-old woman. It had been preceded by a photosensitivity drug eruption due to trimethoprim-sulfamethoxazole taken for a urinary tract infection.

517

Antinuclear antibody testing was positive at 1:640, and Ro and La antibodies were present.

A diagnosis of subacute cutaneous lupus erythematosus was made, and combined oral prednisone and hydroxychloroquine led to complete resolution of the erythroderma in 3 months.

Ordinarily, subacute lupus erythematosus manifests itself as nonscarring plaques and annular lesions, with no systemic features. Renal and central nervous system disease are not present. This case thus represents a hitherto unknown guise for lupus.

Today it is possible to subscribe to 94 different dermatologic journals from around the world. We limit our subscriptions and scanning to the following:

Acta Dermato-Venereologica
Archives of Dermatology
British Journal of Dermatology
Clinical and Experimental Dermatology
Clinics in Dermatology
Contact Dermatitis
Cutis
Dermatologica
International Journal of Dermatology
Journal of the American Academy of Dermatology
Journal of Dermatologic Surgery and Oncology
Journal of Dermatology
Journal of Investigative Dermatology
Pediatric Dermatology
The Schoch Letter
Seminars in Dermatology
Skin and Allergy News
Yearbook of Dermatology

These "energizing eighteen" periodicals provide us with fuel for thought and new diagnostic insight every single issue. And the cost is no greater than a week at the American Academy of Dermatology Annual Meeting.

Nyhan WL: **Inborn errors of biotin metabolism.** Arch Dermatol 1987; 123:1696–1698.

A 6-week-old infant suddenly developed a **generalized erythematous scaly eruption** with marked alopecia. The appearance suggested erythroderma due to ichthyosis or seborrheic dermatitis with a monilial superinfection. By 5 months he had evidence of metabolic acidosis and ketosis, with vomiting and loss of responsiveness.

The diagnosis rested between two newly discovered inborn errors of the metabolism of biotin. This child was found to have an organic aciduria, with 3-hydroxyisovalerate the principal metabolite present, and subsequently a **molecular defect in the enzyme holocarboxylase synthetase** essential for the activation and binding of biotin, as well as the synthesis of the carboxylases whose deficiency in turn was reflected by the accumulation of the organic acids seen in the urine. The genetics were those of an autosomal recessive.

An excellent response followed therapy with biotin, 10 mg/day.

The second inborn error that could have accounted for the problem is **biotinidase deficiency**. In this deficiency, in contrast to the holocarboxylase synthetase deficiency, the skin lesions are less severe and more localized. The onset is later in infancy, some not developing the scaly dermatitis until 4 years of age. It may be associated with seizures. The biotinidase deficiency **suggests a diagnosis of acrodermatitis enteropathica**. The perioral fissuring and keratoconjunctivitis are typical. The loss of hair may be partial or complete.

These patients are at **life-threatening** risk also with episodes of acidosis and ketosis. Mental development may be delayed. They may have optic and aural deficits. The diagnosis is usually made by finding a deficiency of biotinidase activity in the serum, but there is a **spot test** for blood suitable for widespread screening. Two infants with the disease were identified in the first 81,243 infants screened. Again, this metabolic error is an autosomal recessive, with parents of the patients showing 50% normal biotinidase activity. Treatment with 10 mg/day of biotin reverses the changes, except for the auditory and optic nerve deficiencies.

These two metabolic errors account for nearly all the biotin deficiency states encountered, since biotin is in a variety of foods and the intestinal bacteria synthesize it. But, interestingly, an occasional case of hair loss and dermatitis may be seen in individuals addicted to consuming large amounts of raw eggs. It is the presence of the protein **avidin** in the raw egg that **inactivates the biotin** by binding it into an inactive form. In any event, it is well to ask the patient with thinning hair about raw egg milk shakes.

Kalter DC, Atherton DJ, Clayton PT: X-linked dominant **Conradi-Hünermann syndrome** presenting as congenital erythroderma. J Am Acad Dermatol 1989; 21:248–256.

A 5-week-old infant girl was brought to the hospital with unexplained erythroderma present since birth. The erythema was diffuse, and the thick white scaling was without patterning.

The diagnostic breakthrough came when, at 5 months, a **streaky whorled pattern of erythema** and pallor became evident. This suggested a diagnosis of Conradi-Hünermann syndrome. Confirmation came from chemical identification of the baby's **peroxisomal enzyme deficiency** as shown in fibroblast cultures from a skin biopsy.

The diagnostic trail lengthened with recognition that the mother and maternal great-grandmother had the same syndrome. It had been dismissed as "large pores and poor hair." Both also were of short stature, and both had cataracts.

Examination of the mother showed multiple patches and streaks of subtle follicular atrophoderma on the forearms and knees. Hair was sparse, coarse, and wiry on the anterior area of the scalp. She too had lowering of the peroxisomal enzyme (DHAP:AT) activity in cultured fibroblasts. Such a deficiency of enzyme activity in the peroxisomes (subcellular organelles) affects the **catabolism of long-chain fatty acids** and the oxidation of polyamines.

When one looks at erythroderma, it is like looking at a forest fire. What started it? A biopsy may give no more information than examination of a charred tree stump. In this instance, the collaboration of clinicians and chemists found that the DNA started this baby's forest fire.

Greene SL, Muller SA: **Netherton's syndrome**: Report of a case and review of the literature. J Am Acad Dermatol 1985; 13:329–337.

A 3-week-old baby boy had generalized erythematous scaling skin present since birth. A biopsy of the **erythroderma** showed chronic exfoliative dermatitis, and **Leiner's disease** was diagnosed. By age 5 years the boy had persistent erythema with accentuated periorificial involvement, resembling **acrodermatitis enteropathica**. However, he had only mild alopecia and did not have acral bullae or diarrhea. Iodoquinol (Diodoquin) therapy had no effect. Later, zinc levels were also normal. He had recurrent infections, including blepharitis, otitis externa, and chronic cellulitis of the groin and axillae. By the time he was age 13, **lamellar ichthyosis** was the diagnosis of choice, with a biopsy showing psoriasiform dermatitis and negative direct immunofluorescence.

When he was 20 years of age the erythroderma was still florid, and attention was brought to the hair. He had lost his eyelashes, and scalp hair was short, lusterless, fragile, and brittle, with spotty and diffuse loss. There was no axillary or pubic hair. **Microscopic examination** of the hair brought the answer, **revealing the trichorrhexis invaginata (bamboo hair)** of Netherton's syndrome. This telescoping of the hair shaft was confirmed under the scanning electron microscope.

Netherton's syndrome is a rare **triad of ichthyosiform dermatosis, hair shaft defects**, and **atopic dermatitis**. The ichthyosis may be ichthyosis linearis circumflexa or lamellar ichthyosis (nonbullous congenital ichthyosiform erythroderma). Diagnostic confusion arises largely because the simple examination of hair is neglected. In the 43 patients in the world's literature, all had trichorrhexis invaginata, and 14 had additional hair shaft defects (pili torti, black piedra, leukodystrophic hair, trichorrhexis nodosa, monilethrix, trichorrhexis invaginata torta).

Other common findings include mental retardation, neurologic defects, delayed growth and development, and recurrent infections (skin, respiratory, eyes, ears). The serum **IgE is usually elevated**, suggestive of the hyperimmunoglobulin IgE syndrome (15,302 IU/ml in this patient). Aminoaciduria is probably not part of the syndrome, as it is not always present and may be due to prolonged use of topical steroids.

To recognize Netherton's syndrome as it hides behind the facade of ichthyosis, atopic dermatitis, erythroderma, and acrodermatitis enteropathica, one microscopic look at the hair is worth a dozen biopsies.

Goodyear HM, Harper JI: **Leiner's disease** associated with metabolic acidosis. Clin Exp Dermatol 1989; 14:364–366.

This baby girl showed extensive **erythematous, peeling dry skin at birth**. Plasma zinc and copper levels were normal, and blood as well as skin cultures showed no bacteria. The baby failed to thrive, had persistent diarrhea, and experienced frequent infections.

At 9 months, the baby was admitted with **generalized erythroderma** and greasy crusted scaling of the face and scalp. Skin swabs grew *Pseudomonas aeruginosa* and *Staphylococcus aureus*. She was found to have a low fourth component of complement as well as a reduced neutrophil chemotaxis.

Throughout the hospital stay she showed metabolic acidosis; CO_2 content was low. Diarrhea became severe, and a rotovirus was found. The cause of the acidosis was never discerned.

A **diagnosis of Leiner's disease** was made. This is often a sign of **reduced immunologic competence**. Others have found such defects as a deficiency of C3 or C5, a yeast opsonization defect, or an immunoglobulin deficiency.

This patient's inability to combat infection led to her death a month later as a result of a *Haemophilus influenzae* respiratory tract infection.

Luy JT, Jacobs AH, Nickoloff BJ: A child with erythematous and hyperkeratotic patches. Arch Dermatol 1988; 124:1271–1274.

Sharply demarcated, scaly, **erythematous patches** and thin plaques with red borders on the face, neck, and chest had been a problem for an 8-month-old girl since she was 8 weeks old.

The patches were characteristic of **erythrokeratodermia variabilis**, an autosomal genodermatosis. The tip-off was sharply margined plaques of erythema and scaling present virtually since birth.

This genetic disorder of keratinization may range in expression from mild scaling to yellow-brown configurate plaques. Greasy fragments appear, and the border may be hyperpigmented with a striking line of erythema. The sites of predilection are the face, buttocks, and extensor surfaces of the extremities. At times, keratoderma of the palms and soles is present. The plaques may enlarge through childhood, remaining stationary after puberty.

The disease may be viewed as a **patchy localized version of congenital ichthyosiform erythroderma**.

Hebert AA, Esterly NB, Holbrook KA, Hall JC: **The CHILD syndrome**: Histologic and ultrastructural studies. Arch Dermatol 1987; 123:503–509.

A **teratogenic syndrome** for instant recognition:

1. A baby girl with a unilateral ichthyosiform and hyperkeratotic erythroderma
2. Hemiatrophy of limbs of same side
   Less obvious: cardiac, renal, pulmonary and endocrine anomalies
   Suspect cause: teratogenic insult at fourth month embryogenesis

Thus, the acronym CHILD stands for:
Congenital **H**emidysplasia, **I**chthyosiform erythroderma, **L**imb **D**efects

Dicken CH: **Peeling skin syndrome**. J Am Acad Dermatol 1985; 13:158–160.

This 7-year-old boy had a lifelong history of patches of peeling stratum corneum. At the edge of a patch, one could **easily peel back more stratum corneum**, revealing an erythematous nonoozing surface. The biopsy showed the separation to be just above the granular cell layer.

The cause of this deciduous skin is unknown, but there is no dearth of **synonyms**. It is also called:

keratolysis   skin shedding   familial continual skin peeling
peeling skin syndrome—an unusual variant of congenital ichthyosiform erythroderma

To which list we could add "**birch bark**" skin.

Drug Induced

Guin JD, Phillips D: **Erythroderma from systemic contact dermatitis**: A complication of systemic gentamicin in a patient with contact allergy to neomycin. Cutis 1989; 43:564–567.

After 15 years this 66-year-old man's exfoliative dermatitis was tracked down to a **neomycin contact dermatitis** as shown by a 3+ patch test reaction. It cleared by avoidance of the allergen and use of topical steroids.

Four years later he developed a urinary tract infection, and within 24 hours of being given **intravenous gentamicin**, he developed intense generalized pruritus. This progressed over the next 3 days to **exfoliative erythroderma**.

A diagnosis was made of systemic contact dermatitis due to gentamicin sensitivity. Once the skin had cleared, the diagnosis was confirmed by demonstrating a 3+ positive patch test reaction to gentamicin. The deoxystreptamine ring found in neomycin as well as gentamicin proved to be the common sensitizing denominator. Exposure to either of these compounds, either topically or systemically, produced an eczematous contact dermatitis type of reaction.

Such patients should **avoid** both contact and systemic therapy with the other **aminoglycosides**—kanamycin, amikacin, and tobramycin—as well. This is prudent, since cross-sensitivity may be present in as many as half the patients. The patient described proved sensitive to all five of these aminoglycosides.

Other examples of **systemic contact dermatitis** are seen in patients sensitized to ethylenediamine in topical creams, who later receive intravenous aminophylline (a theophylline compound with ethylenediamine). Mercury is another compound with this divalent potential to produce harm from within or without.

Interestingly, the distribution of systemic contact dermatitis is often initially localized to the area where the contact sensitivity was first manifested.

Carradori S, Peluso AM, Faccioli M: **Systemic contact dermatitis due to parabens.** Contact Dermatitis 1990; 22:238–239.

An injection of ampicillin containing parabens induced a generalized eczematous eruption 4 days later. The patient, a 65-year-old woman, was then shown on **patch testing** to be **sensitive to methyl and ethyl parabens**.

Sometimes a diagnosis can be made by reading labels.

Lavrijsen APM, van Dijke C, Vermeer B-J: **Diltiazem-associated exfoliative dermatitis** in a patient with psoriasis. Acta Derm Venereol 1986; 66:536–538.

Diltiazem (**Cardizem**), a new calcium antagonist, has a molecular structure **similar to chloroquine**. It joins chloroquine in its capability of rapidly inducing **exfoliative dermatitis in psoriatic patients**.

A woman born in 1913 had a history of psoriasis vulgaris. In 1981 she developed exfoliative dermatitis within 12 days of receiving chloroquine for arthritis, with rapid clearing when the chloroquine was stopped. Subsequent use of the calcium antagonist nifedipine was uneventful, but in 1984 when the nifedipine was replaced by diltiazem she developed a pruritic rash with malaise and fever within 48 hours. This rapidly progressed to exfoliative dermatitis, which cleared with 2 weeks of steroid therapy and discontinuation of the diltiazem.

A second, similar example is cited from the literature.

Zitelli BJ, Alexander J, Taylor S, et al: **Fatal hepatic necrosis due to pyrimethamine-sulfadoxine** (Fansidar). Ann Intern Med 1987; 106:393–395.

A 15-year-old white girl took four doses of pyrimethamine-sulfadoxine as **prophylaxis for chloroquine-resistant *Plasmodium falciparum*** in Ecuador. One week after the last dose she developed nausea, vomiting, sore throat, and a temperature of 40°C, followed by a macular erythematous rash over the trunk, arms, and legs. After 1 week her urine turned dark, and the rash became confluent with petechiae on the palms and soles and peeling of the skin, beginning at the nail margins. She also had edema of the hands, feet, and periorbital area, hepatosplenomegaly, icterus, generalized lymphadenopathy, nonpurulent conjunctivitis, cough, and pharyngeal edema with palatal petechiae. While initially she had 40% atypical lymphocytes on complete blood count, this fell to 15% along with 15% granulocytes and 18% eosinophils as she developed leukopenia (3100/mm^3). **She died of fulminant hepatic failure** with massive hepatic necrosis. Autopsy also showed exfoliative dermatitis and diffuse lymphadenopathy.

Extensive evaluation failed to show any cause of the illness other than the drug pyrimethamine-sulfadoxine. Available since 1982, it has caused 20 severe cutaneous reactions with six deaths. **Skin reactions** have included exfoliative dermatitis, Stevens-Johnson syndrome, and toxic epidermal necrolysis.

Schillinger BM, Berstein M, Goldberg LA, Shalita AR: **Boric acid poisoning.** J Am Acad Dermatol 1982; 7:667–673.

A suicide attempt by this 44-year-old woman involving the ingestion of half a container of **boric acid powder** (14 gm) led to **exfoliative dermatitis** within 24 hours. It began as erythema of the perioral, perineal, and buttocks area, which led to massive areas of desquamation of necrotic tissue over the entire body.

By the tenth day a patchy alopecia had developed that progressed rapidly to total alopecia.

A diagnosis of boric acid poisoning was made on the basis of history and the **classic "boiled lobster" appearance** so typical of acute poisoning with this component.

The wide availability of boric acid in antiseptics, denture adhesives, detergents, starches, foot powders, eye drops, douches, and mouthwashes calls for an awareness that **chronic exposure can lead to "idiopathic" alopecia**.

Be curious. The diagnosis may be under that next question.

Neoplastic-Paraneoplastic

Wieselthier JS, Koh HK: **Sézary syndrome**: Diagnosis, prognosis, and critical review of treatment options. J Am Acad Dermatol 1990; 22:381–401.

Sézary syndrome is a clinically **discernible variant of chronic T-cell lymphoma**. It comes in the **guise of erythroderma** so intensely pruritic and edematous as to be unusual. It comes in a patient who avoids your handshake because of his fissured painful hyperkeratotic palm. It is the hematologist who distinguishes it from the benign erythrodermas. It is the hematologist who spots the monster, hyperconvoluted, mononuclear cells circulating in the peripheral blood. First sighted by Sézary, these are now recognized as malignant helper T cells. They too are present in the skin biopsy as a dense band of atypical lymphocytes showing cerebriform nuclei and exhibiting epidermotropism that results in Pautrier's microabscesses. (It is this epidermal invasion that accounts for the **terrible itch** of this syndrome.)

Diagnosis usually rests on demonstration of at least **1000 "Sézary cells"/mm^3** of blood, although for some observers any Sézary cells in the peripheral blood cinch the diagnosis. Note that 90% of all patients with chronic T-cell lymphoma in an erythrodermic stage show such circulating Sézary cells with enrichment techniques of studying the buffy coat. The rub comes from an awareness that this Sézary cell may represent an activated T-cell state just as well as a malignant state. Thus it is seen in benign inflammatory conditions.

When evaluating **erythroderma**, it is important to recognize that the majority of cases are nonmalignant. **Only one in five is an expression of a T-cell lymphoma.** One in three represents a drug eruption. The other causes are atopic dermatitis and contact dermatitis. Furthermore, despite all studies, a significant number remain idiopathic. Yet the hunt for the preceding or precipitating causes must go on, with searches for internal malignant disease, sarcoidosis, hepatitis, lupus erythematosus, or even immunodeficiency syndrome in infants.

Grob JJ, Collet-Villette AM, Horchowski N, et al: **Ofuji papuloerythroderma.** Report of a case with T-cell lymphoma and discussion of the nature of this disease. J Am Acad Dermatol 1989; 20:927–931.

A 75-year-old woman had a pruritic dermatosis of 15 months. Although it had been diagnosed as **lichenified eczema**, it was destructive in appearance. It was an erythroderma showing the **"deck chair" sign**, i.e., all the major skin folds were completely spared. Secondly, the erythroderma was made up of coalescent flat solid papules.

Eosinophilia (3000 cells/mm^3) was present, and on biopsy the papules were made up of perivascular lymphohistiocytic infiltrates. The skin in the fold showed no infiltrate. The characteristic clinical picture made the diagnosis of Ofuji's papuloerythroderma.

Four months later the eosinophilia was even more dramatic (8200 cells/mm^3), and there was lymphadenopathy in the axillae and groin. Study of the nodes showed the presence of a T-cell lymphoma.

The intriguing question remains: Why were the folds immune?

Farthing CF, Staughton RCD, Harper JI, et al: **Papuloerythroderma—A further case with the "deck chair sign."** Dermatologica 1986; 172:65–66.

A 73-year-old man had widespread sheets of **intensely pruritic small lichenoid papules with linear patterns** on an erythematous background, which led to diagnostic frustration for 6 months at St. Johns Hospital, London. The lesions spared only the axillae and transverse abdominal folds ("deck chair

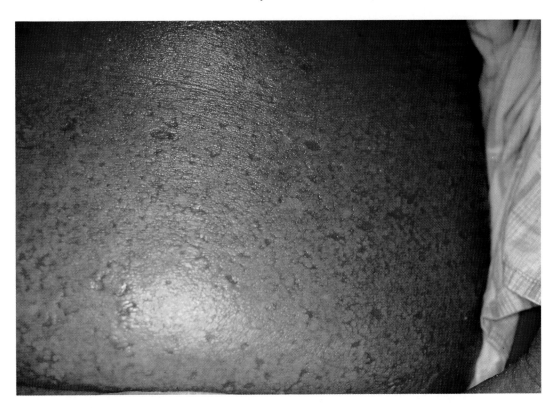

sign"), and papules appeared in linear streaks along scratch marks, although the patient did not have dermatographism. He had moderate eosinophilia (1.7×10^9/liter) and elevation of serum IgE (617 U/ml, N < 81 U/ml). Skin histology showed a dense perivascular mononuclear infiltrate in the upper dermis with increased eosinophils. Direct immunofluorescence was negative. The skin cleared with prednisone (30 mg daily), and relapse did not occur when the medication was tapered.

The final diagnosis was papuloerythroderma, first described in 1984 by Ofuji et al. It appears in older men, has associated eosinophilia, and responds to systemic but not topical steroid therapy.

Fairris GM, Kirkham N, Goodwin PG, et al: **Erythrodermic follicular mucinosis.** Clin Exp Dermatol 1987; 12:50–52.

A 36-year-old man had an **eczematous eruption on the palms and soles** that **became generalized erythroderma** over the next 2 months. Distinctive follicular papules were present on the lower legs. The erythroderma lasted 6 months and fluctuated in severity. During exacerbations he had fever and red boggy purulent plaques on the face and scalp, weeping macerated palms and soles, and purulent paronychia of all 20 digits with loss of nails and verrucous hypertrophic nail beds. Early in the course he lost all body hair and developed partial alopecia of the scalp and beard. There was generalized lymphadenopathy but no hepatosplenomegaly.

The skin showed an excellent response to prednisolone (20 mg/day) but not to methotrexate (20 mg/week) or topical steroids, which were without effect. Hair regrew in most of the areas of alopecia. Maintenance prednisolone (10 mg/day) was necessary to suppress the disease. White blood cell count was 10.4 per mm^3 with 56% neutrophils, 31% eosinophils, and a few activated T cells with atypical cytology in the peripheral smear stained with monoclonal antibodies. The bone marrow contained less than 5% lymphoid cells.

There was no sign of mycosis fungoides or other malignant disease during a 2-year follow-up.

Repeated biopsies of the trunk, limbs, and nail bed were **nondiagnostic**, but a boggy scalp plaque showed follicular mucinosis. Alcian blue staining showed free mucin in the affected hair follicles and adjacent dermis. There was also a heavy T-cell lymphocytic infiltrate in the follicles.

This erythrodermic presentation of **follicular mucinosis** is unique. It should be distinguished from the three **major clinical variants**:

1. Indurated plaques with prominent follicular openings of the head and neck, with obvious alopecia
2. Widespread follicular papules or ill-defined plaques composed of papules
3. Widespread plaques with coexisting T-cell lymphoma

Also reported are cystic forms on the face, light-induced follicular mucinoses, and generalized follicular mucinosis.

Harper TG, Latuska RF, Sperling HV: An unusual association between **erythroderma and an occult gastric carcinoma**. Am J Gastroenterol 1984; 79:921–923.

A 63-year-old black man had a **diffuse erythematous rash** that began on the face and rapidly extended over the trunk and extremities. He blamed the facial rash on a cleaning solvent, but avoidance of the solvent and taking prednisone (50 mg/day) failed to prevent erythroderma; it necessitated four hospitalizations over the next 3 months. **Skin biopsy showed eczematoid dermatitis.** Extensive studies, including a barium swallow, eventually revealed a deformed duodenal cap. At **gastroscopy** a small ulcer of the greater curvature of the stomach was seen, and biopsy revealed **adenocarcinoma**. Subtotal gastrectomy led to clearing of the rash for 6 weeks, but it then recurred, and repeat endoscopy and biopsy showed additional scattered foci of dysplasia. Following chemotherapy and radiation the rash again cleared, presumably because of elimination of tumor antigen.

Erythroderma associated with malignant disease has no distinguishing features, so that in any middle-aged or elderly patient a careful search for an occult malignant growth should be carried out. **Pulmonary carcinoma** has been the most common carcinoma associated with erythroderma, but other carcinomas have included prostatic, rectosigmoid, pancreas, liver, thyroid, stomach, tongue, cervix, and generalized carcinomas of the abdomen. Patients with idiopathic erythroderma may eventually turn out to have a diagnosable malignant disease.

van Joost TH, Vuzevski VD, Menke HE: Benign papular acantholytic non-dyskeratotic eruption: A new paraneoplastic syndrome? Br J Dermatol 1989; 121:147–148.

Multiple distinct 5- to 8-mm **papules** with a solitary distribution developed on the arms and upper trunk of a 72-year-old woman with unexplained erythroderma for 3 years. The papules were pink, smooth or scaly, and sometimes crusted. **Biopsies** showed nonspecific dermatitis in the erythroderma areas, but **suprabasilar clefts** due to acantholysis in the papules. No corps ronds were seen.

The term *benign papular acantholytic nondyskeratotic dermatosis* was coined for the diagnosis. It would seem to be a warty example of **Grover's disease**. Its significance as a possible paraneoplastic sign hinges on the fact that this patient **died of inoperable leiomyosarcoma** of the bladder 8 months after the appearance of this papular eruption.

Never stand too close to or too far from the patient.

Frost M, Parker C: **Acral hyperkeratosis with erythroderma.** Arch Dermatol 1988; 124:123–126.

A 53-year-old woman with Down's syndrome who lived in a nursing home had a 7-year history of **nonspecific dermatitis and dry skin**. Treatment with lindane lotion on two occasions had not helped, and triamcinolone lotion resulted "overnight" in the hands becoming red and swollen with heavy crusts, **followed by erythroderma**. She had extensive deeply fissured, armorlike **crusts on the hands and forearms**, with less extensive crusting on the ears, feet, and buttocks. Diffuse erythema with light scaling was present on the rest of the body. A **skin biopsy was diagnostic**.

If you thought **scabies**, you were right! The eruption cleared with overnight applications of lindane lotion 1% on days 1, 2, and 7, erythromycin (2 gm/day), and prednisone (60 mg/day).

Norwegian (crusted) scabies has been associated with:

Down's syndrome	diabetes mellitus
leprosy	Bloom's syndrome
leukemia	tabes dorsalis
lymphoma	syringomyelia
renal transplantation	Parkinson's disease
systemic lupus erythematosus	nutritional deficiencies
rheumatoid arthritis	immunosuppression (drug-induced)

It is probably due to a combination of poor hygiene, decreased cutaneous sensation, impaired cell-mediated immunity, and failure to develop hypersensitivity to the mite.

Shelley WB, Shelley ED, Burmeister V: *Staphylococcus aureus* colonization of burrows in erythrodermic Norwegian scabies. A case study of iatrogenic contagion. J Am Acad Dermatol 1988; 19:673–678.

An 85-year-old woman with a $2\frac{1}{2}$ year history of **erythroderma** suspected to be caused by drug hypersensitivity was hospitalized for emergency femoral embolectomy. Examination after surgery revealed a generalized scaling, erythematous eruption with **thick, heavy scale over the hands and feet**, but sparing the face and scalp. Excoriations were prominent.

Exfoliated scales in the bed clothes were **heavily infested with scabies mites**, and a stratum corneum biopsy of the right hand disclosed myriads of scabies mites, ova, scybala, and burrows. Scanning electron microscopy demonstrated extensive bacterial colonization of the burrows, and cultures of scybala revealed *Staphylococcus aureus*.

Within 2 days after operating on this patient the vascular **surgeon had generalized pruritus**, although he had never previously had scabies. Likewise, the anesthesiologist and chief surgical nurse developed scabies within 1 week. Over the next month the patient's daughter and seven floor nurses developed scabies. Three months later a surgical scrub nurse, who had refused treatment with Kwell because of her pregnancy, was found to have scabies, along with her husband and newborn son.

Retrospectively it was ascertained that the patient had been in **two nursing homes**, each of which then developed outbreaks of scabies in many patients, staff, and frequent visitors and family members.

The **diagnosis of erythroderma had a stultifying effect** that precluded scabies from consideration. It is important to scrape any erythroderma or palmar keratoderma, where enormous populations of mites make confirmation easy.

Deceptive forms of scabies may also masquerade as:

Darier's disease   actinic keratoses
dermatitis herpetiformis   uremic pruritus
psoriasis   urticaria
contact dermatitis

Shelley ED, Shelley WB, Schafer RL: **Generalized *Trichophyton rubrum* infection in congenital ichthyosiform erythroderma**. J Am Acad Dermatol 1989; 20:1133–1134.

This 41-year-old woman suffered from a **pustular erythroderma** for $2\frac{1}{2}$ years. Her **lifelong history of lamellar ichthyosis** blinded the physicians to a second diagnosis responsible for the erythroderma. She had a widespread **yet unrecognized *Trichophyton rubrum* superinfection of the lamellar ichthyosis**.

A biopsy had been taken, but the word-of-mouth report centered on the pathologist's confirmation of the diagnosis of lamellar ichthyosis. Only several years later when the written report was obtained was it discovered that the pathologist had also seen numerous fungal hyphae in the stratum corneum. By that time scrapings and culture had independently confirmed this second diagnosis of tinea.

Clearing was prompt once griseofulvin therapy was started.

Two lessons evolve: (1) **Trust not verbal reports.** (2) **Examine for occult fungal infections in ichthyotic patients**, especially those who have an unexplained exacerbation or erythroderma.

Verbov J: **Eczema herpeticum** in a man of 68. Dermatologica 1982; 164:410–412.

A 68-year-old man with **ichthyosis vulgaris** was hospitalized with fever, widespread exfoliative dermatitis, and multiple vesicles and erosions of the face. **Eczema herpeticum** was proven with isolation of the herpes simplex virus from vesicles. The erythroderma was later shown to be due to allergic contact dermatitis to thiuram, present in the rubber gloves he wore when caring for a disabled brother.

The **herpes simplex virus** found soil for growth in the contact dermatitis. Although atopic dermatitis is its favored haunt, **look for it also in** Darier's disease, ichthyosis, ichthyosiform erythroderma, and pemphigus foliaceous.

Diagnosis is often the art of making adequate decisions on the basis of inadequate data.

Exanthems are the red flags of systemic disease. Classically they appear in children as the skin signs of such viral diseases as measles, rubella, and bacterial infections such as scarlet fever, typhoid fever, and shigellosis. They may also reflect rickettsial disease or drug reactions.

The recognition of an exanthem rests on seeing the sudden appearance of a widespread erythematous macular, maculopapular, or papular eruption. Usually the patient is acutely ill, the rash being overshadowed by the patient's fever, chills, malaise, aching, and other focal signs, such as sore throat or diarrhea.

To step beyond a diagnosis of exanthem of unknown origin is often as hard as the step beyond the diagnosis of fever of unknown origin. Many of these rashes will be seen by pediatricians, who can make a diagnosis based on "what's going around." Without the help of epidemiology, look for the Koplik spots of **measles**. Remember, it can come in nonconforming lesions such as petechiae, purpura, and vesicles. It may elect to start on the palms and soles. It is best not to argue with the grandmother's diagnostic opinion.

Look for the strawberry tongue and raw red tonsils of **scarlet fever**. Culture for beta-hemolytic streptococci. Palpate for the occipital nodes of **rubella**, and strengthen that diagnosis by noting that the patient feels fine. Doubt the diagnosis if the rash is not gone in 3 days. Look for the "**slapped cheek**" sign of the parvovirus B19-induced erythema infectiosum with its associated reticulate rash of the arms and legs that waxes and wanes.

Delight in recognizing roseola infantum (**exanthem subitum**) in the little one who is brought in with the history of having had a high temperature for the past few days, which has now subsided. You can explain to the mother that his herpes virus type VI infection and rash will be gone within a day or two.

A special variant of the childhood exanthems is the lichenoid or papular eruption of the **Gianotti-Crosti syndrome**. This may last for weeks and is variably associated with viral hepatitis, Epstein-Barr viral tonsillitis, or enteroviral infections.

Although most of the exanthems occur in childhood, and most are due to viral infections involving the endothelial cells of the cutaneous blood vessels, exanthems may occur at any age. They may be morbilliform (measles-like) or scarlatiniform. At times they will be simply innocuous rose spots as seen in typhoid fever. Look for pharyngitis, gastroenteritis, serum sickness, a bone marrow transplant, or the generalized lymphadenopathy of the angioimmunoblastic state and the mucocutaneous lymph node syndrome of Kawasaki. Be alert to the splinter hemorrhages of the nail bed and periorbital edema signaling trichinosis. A history of eating uncooked pork, eosinophilia, and raised muscle enzyme levels plus a positive test for trichinosis antibodies secures the diagnostic knot.

A more dreaded diagnosis is that of the exanthems of rickettsial infection. Ask for a history of a tick bite, or even the possibility of such a bite. Question for rodent mite bites, lice, chiggers. These provide the entry point for the rickettsia causing such exanthems as those of Rocky Mountain spotted fever, typhus, and rickettsial pox.

Finally, ask if the patient has had the rash before. Certain drugs may produce an acute erythematous rash that is symmetrical and occurs always in the same site. 529

It is the nonpigmenting fixed drug eruption and may be seen in children as well as adults. The pseudoephedrine of various over-the-counter cold remedies is a common offender. Without the drug history, these cases are usually branded toxic erythema for the patients exhibit neither viral nor bacterial cause for their explosive exanthem.

With exanthems, there is always a race to diagnose them before they are gone. Good luck.

Childhood Exanthems

Bialecki C, Feder HM, Grant-Kels JM: The six classic childhood exanthems: A review and update. J Am Acad Dermatol 1989; 21:891–903.

One of the six childhood exanthems proved to be spurious (Dukes' disease, fourth disease), so here are the Big Five.

Measles (Rubeola)

(A rare disease since introduction of viral vaccine 40 years ago.) Koplik spots: blue-white spots on reddened base of buccal mucosa preceding rash by 2 days; may look like grains of salt sprinkled on mucosa

Exanthem:
Erythematous macules and papules first noted at hairline, behind ears, upper neck. Spreads for 3 days to cover trunk and extremities. Fades from above downward, leaving brownish stain of capillary hemorrhage.
Nonclassic form begins on palms, soles, wrists, ankles, with centripetal spread to face and trunk. Same pattern seen in Rocky Mountain spotted fever and meningococcal sepsis.
Vesicular form resembles varicella.
Petechial and purpuric lesions

Laboratory diagnosis:
Compare acute and convalescent (2 week) serum for fourfold increase in complement fixing or neutralizing and hemagglutinin inhibition antibodies. May show leukopenia.

Differential diagnosis:
Other childhood exanthems; infectious mononucleosis.

Scarlet fever

Due to toxin-producing group A beta-hemolytic streptococci. Begins as erythematous patches below ears, on chest, and in axillae. Within hours, involves face, abdomen, and extremities. Scarlet macules on erythematous background resemble sunburn with "goose pimples" and sandpaper feel.

Exanthem:
Tonsils and pharynx beefy-red with exudate. Palate shows petechiae and punctate erythema. Tongue on days 1 to 2 shows white coating with red papillae (white strawberry tongue). Days 4 to 5, coating gone, leaving red strawberry tongue
Note: Circumoral pallor. Skin folds of axilla and groin show increased intensity. Pastia's lines: transverse red streaks in skin folds due to capillary fragility persist for day or two after rash gone.
Involution begins in 1 week, desquamation a week later; may persist for 6 weeks, especially on hands and feet.

Laboratory diagnosis:
Group A beta-hemolytic streptococci found on culture of pharynx or tonsil. Blood culture positive—becomes positive in a few days if untreated.
White count elevated (12,000 to 16,000 mm^3)
95% polymorphonuclears
In second week, eosinophilia as high as 20%

Differential diagnosis:

drug eruption	mucocutaneous lymph node syndrome
erysipelas	measles
toxic shock syndrome	rubella
staphylococcic scalded skin syndrome	

531

Rubella (A rare disease since viral vaccine was introduced 30 years ago.)

Exanthem:

Discrete rose-pink macules and papules 1 to 4 mm begin on face, scalp, and neck and spread downward with fading occurring as trunk becomes involved over next 3 days.

Rapidly involutes with delicate flaky desquamation.

Mucosal change:

Petechiae or reddish spots on soft palate during prodrome or first day (Forchheimer's sign).

Laboratory diagnosis:

Hemagglutination inhibition, or complement fixation (CF) assay positive; diagnosis confirmed by fourfold or greater increase in antibody titer between serum drawn during rash and specimen 1 to 2 weeks after rash. If initial specimen drawn late, order CF antibody determination since the antibodies do not appear until after rash. Even 4 weeks after rash, enzyme-linked immunoabsorbent assay for rubella-specific IgM titer is positive.

Differential diagnosis:

Rubella distinctive in

absence of constitutional symptoms

prominent lymphadenopathy

pink-rose rash gone in 3 days

Erythema infectiosum—fifth disease—caused by B19 human parvovirus

Exanthem:

"Slapped cheek" rash—erythematous raised eruption over malar eminences, associated with circumoral pallor not seen in adults, fades in 3 to 5 days.

Reticular maculopapular eruption of extensor surface of arms and legs and on buttocks, at times palms and soles, appears concurrently or up to 5 days later.

Waxes and wanes, disappearing in 2 weeks. Flares with sunlight, bathing, exercise, or trauma.

Laboratory diagnosis:

viral particles—detect by counter-immunoelectrophoresis or DNA hybridization techniques in serum, urine, or respiratory droplets during arthralgia and fever.

Antibody titers:

IgG, IgM by radioimmunoassays or immunoabsorbent assays. IgM indicates current infection, remaining for 2 months. IgG persists for years and is evidence of immunity.

Differential diagnosis:

Recognition based on slapped cheeks and reticular pattern on trunk and extremities. Can mimic erysipelas, echovirus infection, coxsackievirus infection, and roseola infantum.

Roseola infantum (exanthem subitum)

Exanthem:

In infants under 2 years—common.

Onset: high unexplained fever for 2 to 3 days in healthy-appearing child

As fever subsides, surprise rash, maculopapular erythematous rash; each lesion surrounded by pale areola

Begins on trunk and neck; may last 2 hours only or 2 days; prodrome exanthem, erythematous macules of soft palate.

Clues:

Rash comes after rather than during fever. Child does not act sick.

Laboratory diagnosis:
    In research laboratories, detect antibodies to herpesvirus 6. Detected
    in serum 1 to 2 weeks after rash.

Roseola infantum is the baby's rash that finally explains the baby's fever.

Anon: **Rubella** and congenital rubella syndrome United States 1985–1988. Arch Dermatol 1989; 125:608–609.

During the course of a year now, only one in a million persons develops rubella. It has thus become a **vaccine-induced diagnostic rarity**.

Anon: Risks associated with human **parvovirus B19 infection**. Arch Dermatol 1989; 125:475–480.

The human parvovirus B19 is the cause not only of **erythema infectiosum** but also a variety of exanthems, including rubella-like, vesicular, and purpuric.

In the classic form of erythema infectiosum (fifth disease), the signal finding is the **slapped-cheek** appearance of the face and an associated reticulate rash on the trunk and extremities.

It is a mild childhood illness, involving a few days of malaise preceding the rash. The eruption quickly fades, but **sunlight**, **cold**, or **hot environments** or even **stress** may **recall the rash** during the following few weeks.

The B19 virus is, however, far more pathogenic as a cause not only of **arthralgias** but also **fetal defects**. It can induce chronic anemia as well as transient **aplastic crisis** in patients with sickle cell disease and other hemolytic anemias.

The most sensitive technique for detecting the virus is nucleic acid hybridization. Skin biopsies, serum, leukocytes, respiratory secretion, and urine are satisfactory sources. To test for recent infection, there is an IgM antibody assay. It becomes positive on the third day. At this time, diagnostic tests can be obtained at the Centers for Disease Control on a restricted basis.

Here is another well-defined virus the physician can have in mind when the question arises, "Is it due to a virus?"

Chorba T, Anderson LJ: **Erythema infectiosum** (fifth disease). Clin Dermatol 1989; 7:65–74.

This viral exanthem caused by the human parvovirus B19 infection is recognized thus:

    "slapped-cheek" appearance in child
    usually in epidemics in late winter, early spring
    rash spreads to trunk and extremities
    may be morbilliform confluent or circinate
    fades to give lacy appearance
    resolves in a week or so, but can be recalled by sunlight, exercise, temperature change
    easily missed in black patients

Diagnosis can be confirmed by:

    detecting B19 IgM antibodies in serum
    detecting B19 viral antigen on research level
    radioimmunoassay (RIA), enzyme-linked immunosorbent assay (ELISA)
    counterimmunoelectrophoresis

B19 DNA by hybridization
electron microscopy showing parvoviral particles

And to think, B19 wasn't even on the horizon 10 years ago.

Gillespie SM, Cartter ML, Asch S, et al: **Occupational** risk of human **parvovirus B19 infection** for school and day-care personnel during an outbreak of erythema infectiosum. JAMA 1990; 263:2061–2065.

Parvovirus B19 infection is an occupational risk for **school and day-care personnel**. Exposure to the "slapped-cheek" child can lead to adult infection, which, in the pregnant woman, can result in hydrops fetalis and **fetal death**.

Meade RH 3rd: **Exanthem subitum** (roseola infantum). Clin Dermatol 1989; 7:92–96.

Clinical diagnosis based on unique set:

> Sudden appearance of fever (temperature up to 40°C in child who is healthy, but hot)
> Fever falls in a few days, replaced by transitory red macular exanthem of trunk

News flash: **Herpesvirus type 6** has just been proven to be the cause.

Taïeb A, Plantin P, Du Pasquier P, et al: **Gianotti-Crosti syndrome:** A study of 26 cases. Br J Dermatol 1986; 115:49–59.

In **papular acrodermatitis of childhood** (Gianotti-Crosti syndrome), look for:

> a symmetrical papular, papulovesicular rash of the cheeks, limbs, and buttocks, at times showing coalescence and the Koebner phenomenon
> lymphadenopathy, particularly of cervical nodes
> acute anicteric hepatitis
> age of onset 1 to 6 years
> duration greater than 10 days and up to 16 weeks
> histology showing a nonspecific perivascular infiltrate and negative direct immunofluorescence

In the **differential diagnosis**, the distribution pattern is specific, but rule out the "four l's":

> lichen planus   lichenoid drug eruption
> lichen nitidus   Letterer-Siwe disease

Patients may have a **prodrome** of diarrhea, rhinitis, tonsillitis, fever, or pruritus. These symptoms may provide a clue toward viral etiology (tonsillitis with Epstein-Barr virus infection, diarrhea with enterovirus infection).

Associations include:

> Epstein-Barr virus infection   hepatitis B virus infection
> coxsackievirus B infection   nonhepatitis B virus infection
> cytomegalovirus infection

In general, a search should be made for preceding and concurrent viral infections (enteroviruses, adenoviruses, parainfluenza viruses, Epstein-Barr virus, and cytomegalovirus).

Spear KL, Winkelmann RK: **Gianotti-Crosti syndrome:** A review of ten cases not associated with hepatitis B. Arch Dermatol 1984; 120:891–896.

The syndrome:

> acute onset, flat-topped papules
> flesh color to erythematous, 2 to 3 mm in diameter

distribution face, limbs
lymphadenopathy
nonpruritic
self-limited, gone in 3 weeks
Association
 anicteric hepatitis
 hepatitis B antigenemia
Present study:

 Six of ten had antecedent upper respiratory infection
 Other viruses may be cause, e.g., Epstein-Barr virus
 coxsackievirus
 parainfluenza virus

Compliance diagnosis:	*When you have to agree with patient's diagnosis and don't know what it is, either.*
Coward's diagnosis:	*Naming the disease after the patient.*
Diagnosis ex juvantibus:	*Based on response to treatment.*
Provisional diagnosis:	*The first thing that comes into your mind.*
Provocative diagnosis:	*Based on response to challenge.*
Rule-out diagnosis:	*One made by other doctors.*
Sterile diagnosis:	*Suggests no therapy.*

Morbilliform–Scarlatiniform

Ruzicka T, Rosendahl C, Braun-Falco O: A probable case of **rotavirus exanthem**. Arch Dermatol 1985; 121:253–254.

A 28-year-old father developed nausea, emesis, and diarrhea the week after his two infant sons each had stool specimen–proven rotavirus **gastroenteritis**. The following week he developed a facial erythematous eruption that spread centrifugally over most of the body. Blood studies showed evidence of hepatitis, and the liver became palpable 4 cm below the costal margin. A **glovelike desquamation** of the skin of the hands and feet **followed the morbilliform eruption**.

He had taken no drugs and normal or negative serologic tests excluded recent infections with the following agents:

viral hepatitis A and B	cytomegalovirus
Yersinia enterocolitica	Epstein-Barr virus
Yersinia pseudotuberculosis	coxsackievirus B1 to B6

In contrast, a highly elevated titer of 1:256 of **rotavirus antibody** was detected in the patient's serum by the complement fixation test. This had climbed to 1:512 two weeks later when the patient's exanthem had completely subsided.

Rotavirus, the most **common cause of diarrhea** in children, must be added to the causes of exanthems. The incubation period is 1 to 3 days, and the diarrhea flushes the virus out rapidly. Thus, if the patient is not seen early, diagnosis rests on the history and complement fixation tests.

Bielory L, Yancey KB, Young NS, et al: **Cutaneous manifestations of serum sickness** in patients receiving antithymocyte globulin. J Am Acad Dermatol 1985; 13:411–417.

Serum sickness is **induced by circulating immune complexes** composed of host antibody and foreign antigen that deposit in various organs.

In 35 patients given intravenous horse antithymocyte globulin for bone marrow failure, serum sickness developed in 30. It began on day 7 as a **morbilliform eruption**, lasted 12 days, and included fever, malaise, arthralgias, myalgias, gastrointestinal complaints, and lymphadenopathy.

The morbilliform eruption began as faint pink macules in the axillae, groin, and periumbilical area. It usually became purpuric as a result of thrombocytopenia as it spread to eventually involve the entire body except the face, flanks, and scapulae. Many patients had recurrent urticarial eruptions, usually beginning during the antithymocyte globulin infusion.

In 21 patients a unique erythematous eruption developed on the sides of the fingers and toes, with a band of erythema or purpura strictly demarcating the margin between the palm and sole and the dorsal surface of the hand or foot. The linear band was the earliest sign of serum sickness, beginning on day 6. This **marginal serpiginous diagnostic sign** lasted only a day and had to be sought out but was a valuable harbinger of things to come.

Hood AF, Vogelsang GB, Black LP, et al: **Acute graft-versus-host disease.** Development following autologous and syngeneic bone marrow transplantation. Arch Dermatol 1987; 123:744–750.

Patients who receive bone marrow transplants often find their newly acquired marrow making an immunologic attack on their skin, liver, and gut. This acute reaction begins within 1 to 3 weeks after the graft and may develop even if the graft is from an identical twin. It begins as a pruritic **macular exanthem** of the palms and soles that spreads to the trunk and extremities. Small ill-defined, blanchable, erythematous macules and papules coalesce to form a diffuse confluent eruption that is either macular or contains slightly elevated plaques. The lesions may be violaceous but are not purpuric. In severe cases there is progress to vesicles, bullae, and erythroderma.

Histologically it is distinguished from a morbilliform drug eruption and viral exanthem by the presence of **vacuolization of the basal cell layer**, dyskeratosis, and superficial perivascular mononuclear cell infiltrate. In patients who have had a marrow graft but no skin lesions, there may be similar histologic evidence of cutaneous graft-versus-host disease (a subclinical form).

Since all of these patients receive an abundance of antiemetics, analgesics, and antibiotics, a drug eruption must be considered in each case, along with a viral exanthem.

The acute form of cutaneous graft-versus-host disease is distinct from the chronic form, which may develop several months later. The **chronic form** presents as a violaceous **lichenoid papular eruption**, widespread desquamation, or a **sclerodermoid eruption** with or without alopecia, diminished sweating, or sicca syndrome (dryness of the ocular and oral mucosa).

Bernstein JE, Soltani K, Lorincz AL: Cutaneous manifestations of **angioimmunoblastic lymphadenopathy**. J Am Acad Dermatol 1979; 1:227–232.

A pruritic maculopapular eruption in a patient **with generalized lymphadenopathy** points to a diagnosis of angioimmunoblastic lymphadenopathy. Histologic examination of the lymph node, not the skin, provides the answer.

A 49-year-old beautician with chronic exposure to hair dyes and bleaches and a past history of Graves' disease developed a pruritic eruption associated with fever, malaise, pharyngitis, and lymphadenopathy. It lasted 10 days and was thought to be infectious mononucleosis despite negative heterophil agglutination.

Five months later she developed an intensely pruritic erythematous maculopapular eruption on the face and neck, which then spread over much of the body. She also had generalized lymphadenopathy with somewhat tender mobile nodes up to 3 cm in size. The complete blood count showed 3800 white blood cells with 66% polymorphonuclears, 17% lymphocytes, and 9% eosinophils, and the erythrocyte sedimentation rate was 20 mm/hour.

Skin biopsies showed dermal edema and focal perivascular lymphohistiocytic infiltrates, with direct immunofluorescence negative. **Lymph node biopsy** showed proliferation of finely arborized vessels and diffuse infiltration with lymphocytes, plasma cells, and immunoblasts, characteristic of angioimmunoblastic lymphadenopathy.

Over the next year she developed gastric ulcers and an acute abdominal condition due to enlarged lymph nodes. During treatment with prednisone she developed generalized herpes zoster and died.

Miller RA, Brancato F, Holmes KK: *Corynebacterium hemolyticum* as a cause of pharyngitis and **scarlatiniform rash** in young adults. Ann Intern Med 1986; 105:867–872.

In teenagers and young adults, a **sore throat** with pharyngeal erythema and patchy white exudates, low-grade fever, nonproductive cough, and bilateral tender cervical or submandibular lymphadenopathy may be caused by *Corynebacterium hemolyticum*. A Gram stain of pharyngeal secretions shows pleomorphic gram-positive bacilli associated with polymorphonuclear leukocytes suggesting phagocytosis. Presumptive identification of *C. hemolyticum* by culture was based on the presence of hemolytic activity on 5% human blood agar and poor growth on tellurite plates, followed by biochemical tests on isolates. The organism grows poorly on sheep blood agar, commonly used for throat cultures in the United States.

In 18 of 27 patients (67%) a **scarlatiniform** (erythematous, macular, blanching) **rash** developed 1 to 4 days after onset of pharyngitis. It began on the distal surface of the extremities, involving extensor surfaces, and spread centrally over 2 to 3 days, sparing the face, palms, and soles. It was pruritic in 50%, "sandpaper-like" with fine (1 mm) papules, and was followed by mild desquamation. One patient also developed urticaria 2 days before the pharyngitis. An unidentified toxin variably present in *C. hemolyticum* strains may be responsible for the rash.

Symptoms persist and recur in patients followed without therapy. Penicillin and erythromycin are the antibiotics of choice.

Infections with *Streptococcus pyogenes* peak in the 0- to 10-year-old age group and then decrease steadily, with only 29% of isolates in the 11- to 20-year old group. In contrast, *C. hemolyticum* **affects mainly teenagers**, with 79% of isolates in this group.

By a man's fingernails, by his coat sleeves, by his boot, by his trouser knees, by the callosities of his forefinger and thumb, by his expression, by his shirt cuffs—by each of these things a man's calling is plainly revealed.

SHERLOCK HOLMES (SIR ARTHUR CONAN DOYLE)

Goscienski PJ, Haltalin KC: **Rose spots** associated with **shigellosis.** Am J Dis Child 1970; 119:152–154.

An **8-year-old white girl** had approximately **50 rose spots** on the wrists, legs, and abdomen. A few similar spots were present on the arms and legs of her sister and brother. They had been camping at a campsite with no toilet facilities or drinking water and became ill 3 days earlier with fever, vomiting, abdominal pain, lethargy, anorexia, and loose green mucoid stools. **Rectal swab cultures showed** *Shigella flexneri* **4a.** Acute and convalescent serum agglutinins were negative for typhoid O and H, paratyphoid A and B, and *Brucella* antigens. Treatment with intravenous ampicillin was curative.

Rose spots are small (1 to 4 mm), round, red, slightly raised, smooth-edged lesions that fade completely on pressure. In typhoid fever they begin to fade on the fourth or fifth day, becoming light brown or yellow with slight branny desquamation. They occasionally become pruritic or have a central vesicle followed by a crust. Skin biopsy shows dilated lymphatics and blood vessels with a mixed perivascular infiltrate and clumps of bacilli in the dermis. Cultures of rose spots in typhoid fever have yielded *Salmonella typhi.*

Rose spots have been reported in:

typhoid fever	brucellosis
psittacosis	miliary tuberculosis
leptospirosis	meningitis
trichinosis	shigellosis

Butler DF, Hough DR, Friedman SJ, et al: **Adult Kawasaki syndrome.** Arch Dermatol 1987; 123:1356–1361.

A **scarlatiniform** rash of the distal surface of the extremities appeared 5 days after a 20-year-old black woman experienced pharyngitis, fever, and arthralgia. Within a few days the rash spread to the face and trunk. On her admission 4 days later the critical skin findings were the diffuse erythematous rash and marked desquamation of the palms and soles. She had inflamed conjunctivae as well as dry, fissured lips and an erythematous pharynx. Fever persisted, and she had a **large cervical lymph node.** She gradually improved with erythromycin and aspirin therapy and was discharged from the hospital in a few weeks. Beau's lines were observed a month later.

The six cardinal findings in this patient are the centerpiece for a diagnosis of Kawasaki syndrome. Also known as **mucocutaneous lymph node syndrome,** it is a rare entity of unknown cause that usually affects children, 80% of whom are under the age of 4 years. Although the disease is self-limited, 1 in 50 affected individuals dies of later cardiac complications, particularly myocardial infarction. Only 11 patients have developed the syndrome as adults.

There is no diagnostic test for Kawasaki's syndrome, so that exclusion of other causes for the eruption lymphadenopathy and fever is necessary. The **following were excluded:**

scarlet fever: no bacteriologic or serologic evidence
viral exanthem: negative serologic tests
leptospirosis:
    negative agglutinins
    no hyperbilirubinemia
    no renal insufficiency
Stevens-Johnson syndrome: no clinical evidence
collagen vascular disease: no serologic evidence
mercury poisoning: should determine 24-hour urinary excretion level

toxic shock syndrome:
   no hypotension or shock
   no scarlatiniform rash
   no staphylococcal infection

The **association** of Kawasaki syndrome with cardiac problems ranging from transitory ECG changes to **aneurysms** and **thromboses of the coronary arteries** makes the diagnosis of this multisystem condition an important one.

Pun KK: **Rose spots and trichinosis:** Report of a case. Clin Exp Dermatol 1985; 10:587–589.

Multiple erythematous maculopapular lesions appeared on the upper abdomen of this 42-year-old police inspector. He had been sick for 10 days with myalgia and fever. **A diagnosis of typhoid fever was made**, but blood cultures and Widal tests remained negative, and chloramphenicol therapy was without effect.

Laboratory studies showing eosinophilia, elevated IgE level, and raised muscle enzymes pointed to trichinosis. However, the usual diagnostic clues of trichinosis were absent. The patient showed no periorbital edema, urticaria, petechiae, or splinter hemorrhages of the nails. Nor had he eaten undercooked pork. The **diagnosis was finally confirmed by an ELISA assay for trichinosis antibodies**. Only after this did the attending physicians elicit the history of eating semicooked boar and fox 3 weeks before the illness. A dramatic cure followed thiabendazole therapy.

Rose spots may alert you not only to typhoid fever but also to:

brucellosis   rat bite fever
shigellosis   leptospirosis
psittacosis

Burnett JW: **Rickettsioses:** A review for the dermatologist. J Am Acad Dermatol 1980; 2:359–373.

The *Rickettsiae* are **small bacteria** that can penetrate directly through host cell membranes and **replicate in the cytoplasm**. They invade humans through the vector's mouthparts, by inhalation, or conjunctival penetration of aerosolized vector feces or through broken skin or mucous membranes in contact with infected ectoparasite or vector feces. Replication occurs at the inoculation site, including endothelial cells, with subsequent hematogenous spread and widespread focal infection of blood vessels causing necrosis, thrombosis, and vascular occlusion.

Vectors:

ticks (spotted fever)   lice (typhus)
mites (rickettsialpox)   fleas (endemic typhus)
chiggers (scrub typhus)

Clinical manifestations:

erythematous macules   infarcts
vasculitis   fever
petechiae

Laboratory tests:

skin biopsy detection of organisms in dermal endothelial cells—do by
   direct staining or by direct immunofluorescence
tissue culture of frozen specimens (CDC laboratories, Atlanta, Georgia)
serologic tests (not positive for 2 to 3 weeks, too late for effective therapy

with tetracyclines)—include the Weil-Felix reaction (agglutination) and complement fixation tests

Rocky Mountain spotted fever: Latent period 2 to 14 days after tick bite. Malaise and chills as prodrome prior to severe headache, chills, fever, prostration, arthralgias, myalgias (back of legs), nausea, vomiting, photophobia and conjunctival erythema. Temperature reaches 40°C and lasts 2 weeks. On days 2 to 6, pink macules appear on wrists, ankles, palms, and soles, followed by centripedal spread to trunk. Lesions develop petechiae, then become purplish papules, and eventually desquamate.

Rickettsialpox: Transmitted by house-mouse mite. Incubation period of 10 to 24 days precedes fever. Eschar at mite bite resembles cigarette burn and is associated with regional lymphadenopathy. Intermittent temperature of 39°C appears suddenly with sweats, photophobia, myalgia, anorexia, and leukopenia. A sparse, generalized eruption of maculopapules begins evolving into firm vesicopustules with red halos. Lesions resolve in 1 week. The differential diagnosis includes chickenpox, eczema herpeticum, eczema vaccinatum, and smallpox.

Scrub typhus: Seen in the Pacific islands and Asia. Transmitted by chiggers. An eschar is apparent in initial but not recurrent infections, beginning as a papule during the 6- to 18-day incubation period. Regional adenopathy occurs with a prodrome of headache, weakness, and malaise. Within 3 days temperature of 40°C develops, along with headache, photophobia, conjunctival erythema, myalgia, and nonproductive cough. After 1 week a macular erythematous eruption appears on the trunk and extends peripherally, fading in a few days. Hepatosplenomegaly, interstitial pneumonitis, and meningoencephalitis may occur before defervescence in 10 to 21 days. The Weil-Felix test is positive in most cases, but the indirect fluorescent antibody test is the best serologic technique.

Epidemic typhus fever: Transmitted by the human body louse. Incubation period 6 to 15 days. Headache and malaise precede the acute onset of chills, myalgias (back of legs), and intense, persistent headache. Photophobia, conjunctival erythema, weakness, constipation, and a slight productive cough appear, and temperature holds at 40°C. Erythematous macules appear on days 4 to 7 of illness, beginning on the trunk and axillary folds, and spreading centrifugally. These can become purpuric and hemorrhagic, with necrosis over bony prominences. If the patient survives, recovery begins after 14 to 18 days of illness.

This disease may recur (Brill-Zinsser disease) as a result of latent rickettsiae that persist following the primary typhus infection. The Weil-Felix reaction is negative, but IgG antibodies appear rapidly.

Endemic typhus fever (*murine typhus*): Spread by rat fleas (which are not killed by the infection). The incubation period is 6 to 14 days. Symptoms are similar but milder than epidemic typhus, and skin eruption starts on days 5 to 6 of fever.

Trench fever: Transmitted by lice. Incubation period 5 to 38 days. "Saddleback" fever, headache, dizziness, photophobia, and myalgias of the back, legs, and shins. Transient erythematous macules and papules appear mainly on the trunk and fluctuate with fever. Although the disease is not fatal, convalescence may be prolonged.

Robertson HC Jr: Outbreak of **shigellosis** resembling enterovirus. South Med J 1963; 56:662–665.

In a girls' **boarding school** in South Carolina, 66 of 84 boarders, ages 14 to 17 years, became ill with fever, vomiting, and diarrhea. In the "first wave" of illness, 1 week before the severe epidemic, 12 girls were sick but recovered in 3 days without severe symptoms or skin lesions. Among the 54 students and 3 teachers sick the following week, 35 (61%) had a **fine maculopapular salmon-pink rash** on the forehead and cheeks, with spread to the upper trunk in one case and generalized spread in another. Fever, headache, diarrhea, conjunctival injection, vomiting, and meningismus were other common symptoms, which lasted 4 to 15 days. Studies on 18 hospitalized patients revealed a "saddle-back" course with initial fever and **gastrointestinal symptoms** for 2 to 3 days, improvement for 24 to 36 hours, then the return of fever accompanied by rash, headache, meningismus, and conjunctival injection, presumably due to bacteremia. **Stool cultures showed *Shigella flexneri*** in 7 of 15 patients, and the same organism was found in blood cultures of 3 of 11 patients studied. Viral studies were negative on throat washings, blood, and stools from 18 patients. Until culture results were known, an enterovirus of the Coxsackie group was suspected because of the high incidence of skin rash and central nervous system invasion. Treatment with sulfonamides was curative.

Doolittle SE: **Endemic typhus fever** in Hawaii. Ann Intern Med 1941; 14:2091–2114.

A 55-year-old man had malaise and tiredness for 5 days before developing a temperature of 103°F with delirium and muscle pains. On the seventh day an **erythematous macular rash** appeared on the lower chest and spread to the midback. The next day it involved the face, and by the tenth day the rash covered the neck, legs, forearms, and feet. The lesions were **nonpetechial** but left postinflammatory pigmentation for several days. He was hospitalized with recurring chills and diaphoresis, delirium, severe headache, cough, vomiting, and urinary frequency, which continued through the 18th day of illness. The **Weil-Felix test** was negative on days 8 and 9, **positive** 1:160 on day 10, and 1:5120 on day 17.

The typical rash appears on the fifth to seventh day of illness on the lower chest and abdomen and consists of dull red to pink 2- to 4-mm macules, which are round or oval with ill-defined margins and fade on pressure. It then spreads to the mesial surface of the arms, shoulders, and back, then to the thighs, and sometimes to the lower arms and legs, sparing the face, palms, and soles. The rash usually lasts 4 to 8 days.

Murine typhus (Brill's disease) is a rickettsial disease of rats transmitted to humans by the **rat flea**.

The Weil-Felix agglutination test becomes positive (1:160 or above) between 10 and 14 days.

Temperatures of 103° to 105°F with irregular fluctuations continues for 2 weeks. The pulse rate is slow and diaphoresis common.

In Georgia, Alabama, and Texas the disease occurs in the summer and fall.

Findlay GH: Dermatology of the **rickettsioses**. Recent Adv Dermatol 1983; 6:57–73.

The **spots** of Rocky Mountain spotted fever and the **vesicles** of rickettsialpox are due to the **actual growth of minute gram-negative bacteria**. These rickettsiae, introduced by the bites of an infected tick, flea, louse, or mite, live **within the cells of the blood vessel wall**. It is thus that they initiate the microthrombi purpura or vesicular pustules of diagnostic significance. Actually, full-thickness gangrene of the skin down to the muscle may occur. Both venous and arteriolar thrombosis have been seen. Likewise, the initial bite site may show local necrosis (tache noire) or an eschar. This entrance point may be the only skin sign of the disease.

Typhoid fever can be distinguished, since its rash is not hemorrhagic.

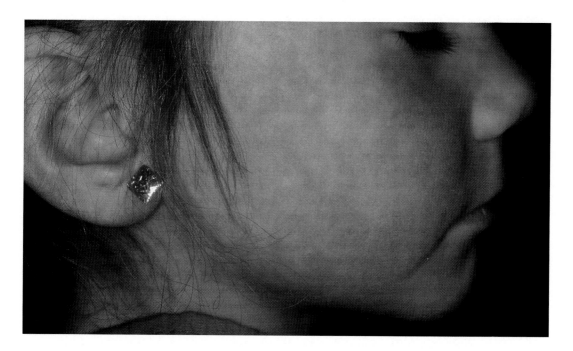

Fluorescent antibody staining of a small trephine biopsy will allow recognition of the pathogen. Do this immediately before any tetracycline therapy is initiated.

The larger the inoculum, the shorter the incubation period, and the worse the course. Thus, ticks are the most harmful, for they spend more time on the skin and introduce a longer inoculum.

Question your febrile purpuric patients for a history of travel and insect bites, and recall that the **average incubation period is 4 days.**

Crennan JM, Van Scoy RE: Eosinophilic meningitis caused by **Rocky Mountain spotted fever**. Am J Med 1986; 80:288–289.

A 25-year-old Canadian man with severe frontal headache for 5 days developed a nonpruritic diffuse **erythematous macular rash** on the distal area of the legs that spread to the arms, palms, soles, and trunk. Chills, photophobia, backache, stiff neck, myalgias, arthralgias, joint swelling, and extreme scrotal tenderness were also present. He had been **bitten by wood ticks** and mosquitos within the preceding 6 weeks.

Evaluation:

> white blood cells (11.7/mm^3 with 4% eosinophils)
> cerebrospinal fluid (60% eosinophils)
> **serum** indirect immunofluorescence **titer** for Rocky Mountain spotted fever (positive 1:256)

Other causes of eosinophilic meningitis:

> lymphocytic choriomeningitis virus
> tuberculosis
> syphilis
> pneumococcus
> coccidioidomycosis

Centers for Disease Control, Atlanta: **Rocky Mountain spotted fever**, United States, 1987. Arch Dermatol 1988; 124:1172.

Nearly 600 cases of Rocky Mountain spotted fever were reported in 1987. Of the patients in the study:

92% had fever
79% had rash
49% had rash on palms and soles
62% had a tick bite within 2 weeks
82% had onset between April and July
3% proved fatal
4 had never been outside New York City!

Ridgway HA: Adult-onset **Still's disease**. J Roy Soc Med 1982; 75:279–281.

Still's disease should be considered in any patient with a **fever**, **joint symptoms**, and a **rash** that appears particularly in the evenings.

A 54-year-old man had malaise and remittent fever that sharply increased in the latter half of the day and was associated with a **fleeting rash** of small angulated macules and maculopapules on the upper trunk and arms. Some lesions had a pale halo, and larger lesions had a central zone of pallor. Lesions appeared some hours following trauma, especially in creases and pressure lines around the waist. A more diffuse, mildly scaly rash resembling seborrheic dermatitis was present on the chest and abdomen. A skin biopsy of the exanthem revealed an upper dermal perivascular infiltrate of polymorphonuclear leukocytes and a few lymphocytes.

Other findings included an inflamed pharynx without exudate and swelling, and stiffness of the ankles, wrists, and elbows. The erythrocyte sedimentation rate was 77 mm/hr, antinuclear antibody and rheumatoid factors were negative, and the complete blood count was normal. However, three of four **blood** cultures grew a **coagulase-negative staphylococcus**. Symptoms cleared following treatment with acetylsalicylic acid, gentamicin, and cotrimoxazole but recurred 15 months later (including the rash), and blood cultures were again positive for the same organism. He soon developed a **tooth abscess** and underwent dental extraction, with no response to gentamicin. Erythromycin treatment stopped the fever and malaise, but the joint symptoms and rash persisted intermittently.

Arriving at the right diagnosis after a long journey is very satisfying to both travelers: the physician and the patient.

Shelley WB, Shelley ED: **Nonpigmenting fixed drug eruption** as a distinctive reaction pattern: Examples caused by sensitivity to pseudoephedrine hydrochloride and tetrahydrozaline. J Am Acad Dermatol 1987; 17:403–407.

Large **bright-red plaques** of the axillae, groin, face, and buttocks suddenly appeared on this 7-year-old girl. Her parents gave the history that in the past 2 years she had had two unexplained yet identical attacks with skin lesions localized to the same sites. During the first attack she had been hospitalized and studied extensively. In both instances the diagnosis of **toxic erythema** had been made, and the lesions faded within days leaving no residua.

In-depth questioning revealed that the night before the present attack, a grandparent had given the little girl an over-the-counter nighttime cold remedy, Night Time Cold Formula. A **diagnosis of nonpigmenting fixed drug eruption was made**.

Again, laboratory studies were negative, but 3 weeks later when the skin had cleared completely, a challenge partial dose of the cold remedy reproduced the eruption in the same sites 6 hours later. This remitted in 2 days, and subsequent **challenges** with the ingredients pinpointed the cause to be **pseudoephedrine**.

In contrast to the classic fixed drug eruption, the nonpigmentating form is beautifully symmetrical and quite vivid. It leaves no calling card of melanin and it leaves without a trace. You have only the patient to guide you. "It's back again in the same place." He won't say, "It's fixed." That's up to you to say.

Taylor BJ, Duffill MB: Recurrent **pseudo-scarlatina** and allergy to **pseudoephedrine** hydrochloride. Br J Dermatol 1988; 118:827–829.

Twelve attacks in 12 years victimized a 32-year-old housewife, who developed chills, fever, malaise, and erythema under the breasts and in the axillae, groin, sacrum, and popliteal fossae. The entire skin became erythematous and hypersensitive, followed by desquamation that ended on the feet 2 weeks later. Neutrophilic leukocytosis was present, but throat, vaginal, and blood cultures were negative, as were streptococcal antibody studies (ASO, AHT, ASK, anti-DNAase B).

Dénouement:

Nyal **Decongestant Cough Elixir** (Adult) New Formula had been taken hours before the last attack. **Oral challenge** with its active ingredient, pseudoephedrine (5 ml of 0.5 gm/100 ml), **produced erythema 5 hours later**. Patch testing was negative. Challenges with other ingredients, including codeine, were negative.

Goodyear HM, Laidler PW, Price EH, et al: A clinico-microbiologic study of **toxic erythemas** in children. Br J Dermatol 1990; 123 (suppl 37):18–19.

One hundred children with an acute febrile illness associated with a widespread erythematous rash of short duration were studied microbiologically.

An **infectious agent** was found responsible for the toxic erythema in 65 of the children: 47 infections proved to be associated with viruses, 13 with bacteria, and 3 with *Mycoplasma pneumoniae*; in 2 children both viral and bacterial infections were present.

The most common causal agents were the **measles virus** (producing an atypical presentation), the group A beta-hemolytic **streptococci**, and the **picornaviruses**.

545

Eyes and Eyelids

The eyelid is remarkably specialized. On one side it is covered with mucous membrane. On the other side it is covered with some of the thinnest, most permeable, and sensitive skin of the entire body surface. The immobile lower lid is skin that is loose and subject to edema. The upper lid suffers the wrinkles and folds of being constantly retracted in the interests of vision. It provides a rugose surface ideal for trapping surface antigens and irritants. In its retracted position it is truly an intertriginous site.

The eyelid margins are equally specialized and hence the site of special problems. The brush border of eyelashes may be the site of folliculitis and styes. It is here we see the marginal blepharitis of seborrheic dermatitis. The appendageal glands of Zeis and the meibomian glands give rise to apocrine or eccrine retention cysts and chalazions.

Contact dermatitis, whether irritant or allergic, is one of the most common problems seen. Cosmetics are the usual cause, but sprays or gases may be responsible. Think of nail polish as a cause of unilateral eyelid dermatitis. Note that patch tests at times fail to detect the offender, since no other area used for patch testing mimics the sensitivity of the eyelid. It is the "canary" for detecting offending contactants. The eyelid is subject to the abuse of rubbing, the sign of atopic dermatitis. It is an attempt to wipe or rub away invisible irritants causing subclinical dermatitis. It is here that tears add to the problem.

The loose corium of the eyelid favors the deposition of lipids, as in xanthelasma. But papules or nodules of all types may arise. A common example are the milia. One may find, at times, the multiple lesions of syringomas. Take time to look at the upper eyelids when the patient closes his eyes. You may see the early skin cancer he can't see with both eyes wide open.

Turning to the mucosal side of the lid, we look for the synechiae of ocular pemphigoid. There we may also see mucous gland retention cysts and always the inflammatory change of conjunctivitis, whether it be foreign body, allergic, or viral.

Color change remains the most dramatic diagnostic eyelid sign. It is here that we see the heliotrope eyelids of dermatomyositis. It is here that we see the dark shadows of fatigue (that come from writing a book like this).

Nethercott JR, Nield G, Holness DL: A review of 79 cases of **eyelid dermatitis**. J Am Acad Dermatol 1989; 21:223–230.

Most **frequent cause**: **allergic contact dermatitis** (found in 46% of cases).

Most common offending **allergens**:

    neomycin sulfate
    diazolidinyl urea
    cinnamic alcohol

Odd examples:

    contact lens solution
    eyelash curlers
    nail polish
    nickel contamination of cosmetics

Remainder of cases:

    atopic dermatitis (23%)
    irritant contact dermatitis (15%)
    other dermatoses (16%), such as seborrheic dermatitis

Moral: Don't close your eyes to patch testing.

Fisher AA: II: The management of **eyelid dermatitis** in patients with "status cosmeticus": The **cosmetic intolerance syndrome**. Cutis 1990; 46:199–201.

Intolerance of eye makeup without any apparent cause may be labeled idiopathic upper eyelid syndrome. Note is made of two women who could not tolerate mascara or eye shadow during the acute phases of chronic **sinusitis**. During that period they developed dermatitis of the eyelids upon using cosmetics that were otherwise innocuous.

Two other examples of this "**status cosmeticus**" were associated with intranasal **staphylococcal infection**. Control of the eyelid dermatitis was achieved by treatment of the nasal mucosa with Bactroban ointment. A third "promoter" for eyelid dermatitis was attacks of **herpes simplex**. In this instance, the nonspecific cosmetic sensitivity producing the eyelid dermatitis disappeared when acyclovir was prescribed.

Husz S, Korom I: **Periocular dermatitis:** A micropapular sarcoid-like granulomatous dermatitis in a woman. Dermatologica 1981; 162:424–428.

Papules and vesicles of the eyelids and outer canthi had been present for $1\frac{1}{2}$ years in a 42-year-old Hungarian technician who worked at high temperatures in a human mothers'-milk bank. Although she wore a mask, her work involved an antiseptic (potassium sulfaminochlorate) which, on contact with water, gives rise to nascent chlorine. Numerous shiny scaly faintly red papules were seen in the periorbital regions, and the eyelids were diffusely red. General studies, including x-rays of the lung and bones, were negative. A patch test to the antiseptic in high concentration proved irritating. Biopsy showed noncaseating epithelioid granuloma.

A diagnosis of a micropapular sarcoidlike **granulomatous dermatitis of Gianotti** was made. This periorbital dermatitis is considered an analogue of perioral dermatitis. It responded to long-term tetracycline therapy coupled with elimination of the chlorine-generating antiseptic from the work place.

Kaufman RE: **Trichiniasis:** Clinical considerations. Ann Intern Med 1940; 13: 1431–1460.

The most important diagnostic clue for trichinosis is edema of the eyelids or a history of **puffy eyelids**. The most characteristic ocular sign is bilateral chemosis of the bulbar conjunctiva.

Occasional skin signs:

scarlatiniform rash	strawberry tongue
rose spots	subungual splinter hemorrhages
morbilliform exanthem	erythema multiforme

Rashes **simulate**:

typhoid	
measles	German measles
scarlet fever	erythema multiforme

After an incubation period of 2 to 27 days, the trichina larvae migrate from the intestinal mucosa via the blood and lymph streams, and acute symptoms begin with **high fever** (temperature 100° to 106°F), nausea, vomiting, diarrhea, and generalized abdominal pain. Sweating and itching are common. **Myositis** causes tenderness and pain in the deltoids, biceps, gastrocnemii, and muscles around the eye. Painful breathing results if the diaphragm and intercostal muscles are involved. Edema of the masseter muscles simulates mumps. **Eye** muscle involvement causes **pain and burning**, photophobia, conjunctivitis, subconjunctival hemorrhages, paresis, and diplopia. Lymphadenopathy is not common. Clay-colored stools may occur, as well as cough, expectoration, and bronchitis with mucopurulent sputum. Reflex changes occur with loss of knee jerk and a positive Kernig's sign.

Laboratory:

leukocytosis (12,000 to 18,000 white cells) with up to 50% immature polymorphonuclears
eosinophilia (up to 80%), falls to normal after 12 months
muscle biopsy—find parasites
serum precipitin test (CDC ?)
find larvae in blood—dilute
    5 to 10 cc blood with 2% acetic acid (10 × blood volume), centrifuge and examine sediment
intradermal test

Choksi UA, Sellin RV, Hickey RC, Samaan NA: An unusual **skin rash** associated with a pancreatic **polypeptide-producing tumor of the pancreas**. Ann Intern Med 1988; 108:64–65.

A patchy, **scaly**, **erythematous**, **papular eruption** of the face, hands, trunk, and perineum developed in a 59-year-old white woman. It was pruritic and especially prominent on the eyelids. Previously, following an episode of melena, **computed tomography** (CT) had revealed a 10-cm mass in the pancreas, which proved to be a **neuroendocrine tumor** of the islet cells producing high levels of serum pancreatic polypeptide, as shown by radioimmunoassay (610 pg/ml). Surgical debulking of the tumor and chemotherapy with 5-fluorouracil and dacarbazine was associated with complete disappearance of all skin lesions as well as CT evidence of disease. The skin lesions were not those of migratory necrolytic erythema seen with glucagonoma. Significantly, fasting glucagon, insulin, gastrin, and vasoactive intestinal polypeptide levels were all normal.

One should **order** radioimmunoassays for *serum pancreatic polypeptides* in any patient with an extensive strange erythematous eruption showing non-

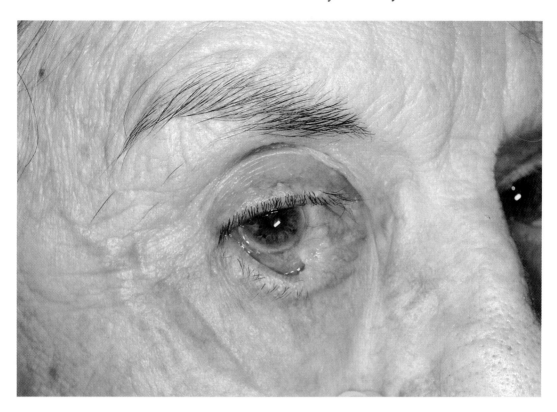

specific spongiosis and perivascular lymphocytic infiltration on biopsy. Watery diarrhea, hypokalemia, and the achlorhydria syndrome may be other signs of a neuroendocrine pancreatic tumor.

Nelson CC, Kincaid MC: **Breast carcinoma metastatic to the eyelids.** Arch Ophthalmol 1987; 105:1724–1725.

A 76-year-old woman had **left upper eyelid swelling** for 6 months, unresponsive to various ophthalmic ointments. The eyelid skin then became red and indurated, and she developed ptosis and a palpable mass just below the superior orbital rim. There were no palpable preauricular, submandibular, or cervical nodes. Excisional **biopsy** of the mass revealed large cells with granular eosinophilic cytoplasm infiltrating between muscle fibers, thought to be a benign granular cell tumor. Positive stains for mucin, cytokeratins, epithelial membrane antigen, and carcinoembryonic antigen, and negative staining for S100 protein led to a diagnosis of **adenocarcinoma**, consistent with breast as the primary site. Several years earlier she had had a mastectomy followed by radiation treatments.

Breast carcinoma is the most common tumor metastatic to the eyelid. It may cause redness, induration, ocular irritation, or a mass with surrounding redness and induration. It may also mimic a **chalazion**.

Immunohistochemical staining for S100 protein is positive in neural tumors, including the benign granular cell tumor, which was ruled out in this case.

Marsden RA, Greaves MW: Atypical **bullous dermatosis of childhood with entropion.** J Roy Soc Med 1982; 75:39–41.

A 2-year-old Syrian girl first developed an erythematous annular macular rash with lesions that extended peripherally with a serpiginous edge, followed later by crops of vesicles and bullae. At age $3\frac{1}{2}$ years, she had a widespread eruption of hemorrhagic bullae arising on urticated erythematous skin. The mildly pruritic nonscarring vesiculobullous eruption involved the eyes, mouth, face, trunk, limbs, palms, and soles, but spared the vulva. She complained of **severe eye pain**, and small **blisters** were present on the eyelids, along with bilateral cicatrizing conjunctivitis and entropion of the lower lids.

Skin biopsy showed a subepidermal blister with mild perivascular mononuclear infiltrate in the dermis (like bullous pemphigoid), but no papillary microabscesses. Direct immunofluorescence detected linear IgA and fibrin at the basement membrane zone (like chronic bullous dermatosis of childhood), while indirect immunofluorescence was negative for IgA, IgG, and C3.

Presumably she had **chronic bullous dermatosis of childhood with cicatrizing conjunctivitis** and findings similar to bullous pemphigoid. There was no evidence of dermatitis herpetiformis, although the eruption cleared with sulfapyridine.

New diagnostic tests, like new drugs, need your attention.

Wolkowicz MI: **Chalazion-like neoplasms** of the lid. Am J Ophthalmol 1962; 54:249–255.

Examination of a chalazion should include palpation of the regional lymph nodes, as **meibomian gland carcinoma** and **basal cell carcinoma** may be clinically indistinguishable from a chalazion in the early stages.

Page EH, Assaad DM: **Morpheic plaque of the lower eyelid.** Arch Dermatol 1987; 123:655–658.

An asymptomatic morpheic plaque developed on the right lower eyelid margin of this 77-year-old man. It extended down onto the skin of the eyelid, but there was loss of eyelashes in the area.

A biopsy proved it to be an invasive **sebaceous carcinoma**, requiring excision of both eyelids and radical orbital exenteration.

These carcinomas may arise from the glands of Zeis, the meibomian gland or the sebaceous glands in the caruncle, or surrounding skin. They frequently metastasize.

Beware of misdiagnosing them as a chalazion or blepharoconjunctivitis.

Sperling LC, Sakas EL: **Eccrine hidrocystomas.** J Am Acad Dermatol 1982; 7:763–770.

A 66-year-old woman had a 1-year history of multiple "bumps" under the eyes. These **bumps enlarged during hot weather** or when the patient did housework. The lesions would decrease in size over several hours with rest but never completely disappeared. Upon examination, the patient had multiple (greater than 60) pale **blue, translucent, discrete papules** on the eyelids and malar area of her face. The lesions felt soft and compressible and were not tender.

A **biopsy** determined the diagnosis of **eccrine hidrocystomas**.

Henkind P: **Sarcoidosis:** An expanding ophthalmic horizon. J Roy Soc Med 1982; 75:153–159.

Bilateral "**millet seed**" **papules** on the eyelids, including the lid margin, may be the presenting sign of sarcoid.

Falk ES: **Sarcoid-like granulomatous periocular dermatitis** treated with tetracycline. Acta Derm Venereol 1985; 65:270–272.

A 41-year-old woodwork teacher had numerous **shiny yellowish** to faint-red papules surrounded by marked erythema on the **eyelids**, paranasal area, and forehead for 6 weeks. He noted that formaldehyde fumes from sawing wall boards caused the eruption to flare. Patch tests showed a **positive reaction to formaldehyde**, but skin biopsy revealed sarcoidlike tuberculoid granulomas. Periocular dermatitis was diagnosed, and clearing occurred with oral tetracycline treatment.

The role of cosmetics, formaldehyde, or other topical allergic or toxic agents must always be considered in evaluating both perioral dermatitis and its equivalent, periorbital dermatitis.

When dermatitis comes around the eyes or the mouth, look for what else comes around these areas.

Straatsma BR: **Meibomian gland tumors.** Arch Ophthalmol 1956; 56:71–93.

These slow-growing lobulated tumors start insidiously as painless nodular **firm pink-white masses with yellow foci** on the tarsal portion of the eyelid (upper or lower). Eventually they produce hyperemia, thickening, and distortion of the eyelid. Nutrient-type vessels are prominent, and ulceration of the lid margin may occur. In malignant tumors the preauricular nodes may be enlarged.

Zina AM, Bundino S, Pippione M: **Sea-blue histiocyte syndrome** with cutaneous involvement. Case report with ultrastructural findings. Dermatologica 1987; 174:39–44.

Disfiguring exophytic, **firm nodules** on the face of a 38-year-old man began at age 14 years as eyelid infiltrations. The entire face had diffuse waxy infiltration, which was most marked on the eyelids and scalp, with the scalp corrugated as in **cutis verticis gyrata.** The hands and feet were puffy, and there was hepatosplenomegaly and nodular infiltrates in the lungs.

Skin **biopsies** showed an infiltrate of large pale macrophages loaded with yellow-brown lipid inclusions (H and E stain). The cytoplasmic granules stained blue-green with Giemsa stain, and under polarized light they were highly birefringent and showed positive yellow autofluorescence. The differential diagnosis included Niemann-Pick disease (five forms—sphingomyelin and cholesterol accumulate in tissues).

Moral: Puffy eyelids in boys is a warning sign.

Dabski K, Milgrom H, Stoll HL Jr: **Breast carcinoma metastatic to eyelids:** Case report and review of the literature. J Surg Oncol 1985; 29:233–236.

An 80-year-old woman noted multiple firm cutaneous nodules scattered on the head and neck, particularly the anterior and posterior cervical areas. Four months later she developed bilateral periorbital erythema with induration and then violaceous slightly **hyperpigmented firm plaques around both eyes. Biopsies** of an eyelid and skin nodule revealed metastatic adenocarcinoma. The primary tumor was found in the right breast.

If you haven't looked at it with the makeup off, you haven't looked at it.

Hebert AA, Jorizzo JL, Schoen I, et al: Simultaneous occurrence of idiopathic **lipemic tears** and massive seborrhea. Arch Dermatol 1985; 121:112–114.

For the past 3 months this 42-year-old man had had unexplained paroxysmal episodes of crying "**white tears**." This lacrimation lasted from 3 to 5 minutes and occurred nearly every day. There was associated massive seborrhea. The year before he had a penectomy for a squamous cell carcinoma.

The color of the tears was **due to the presence of lipids coming from** the **meibomian glands**. Analysis showed triglycerides in a concentration of 428 mg/dl.

It is postulated that concurrent hyperactivity of the meibomian and sebaceous gland accounts for the white tears and the gross accumulation of yellow sebum on the paranasal and presternal areas. The controlling factors remain unknown.

Detailed study did not bring out any evidence that this strange conjunction of fatty tears and seborrhea was a paraneoplastic process.

Carithers HA: **Oculoglandular granuloma**, eye disease of **Parinaud**. A manifestation of cat scratch disease. Am J Dis Child 1978; 132:1195–1200.

"Cat scratch disease is probably the most common cause of single node lymphadenopathy seen in children and young adults, except those caused by obvious infections of the skin or upper respiratory tract."

A child with **unilateral tender preauricular and cervical nodes**, hyperemia of one eye, and a history of exposure to young **cats** should have a careful eye examination to search for the possible inoculation site of cat scratch disease. It is usually a red polypoid granulomatous papule 0.5 to 2 cm in diameter, with an irregular border and slight surrounding erythema. It may enlarge and develop white, yellow, or gray areas of necrosis. The **inoculation site** is usually on the **palpebral conjunctiva**, but may be on the eyelid or bulbar conjunctiva. The eye is not tender, and purulent and mucoid exudate are absent.

Lymph node enlargement is usually single and unilateral unless multiple inoculation sites have occurred. Nodes vary widely in size and tenderness and regress over weeks to months. In 14 cases presented here, only one node suppurated and required drainage. All children were also afebrile.

The skin test becomes positive within 1 week after lymph node enlargement.

Lang PG, Tapert MJ: Severe ocular involvement in a patient with **epidermolysis bullosa acquisita**. J Am Acad Dermatol 1987; 16:439–443.

For 5 years this 30-year-old woman's eye problem was incorrectly diagnosed as cicatricial pemphigoid. She had initially noted tearing and burning of her eyes as well as blistering of the skin following minor trauma. A **biopsy** of the skin coupled with direct immunofluorescence studies supported the diagnosis of **cicatricial pemphigoid**. It proved recalcitrant to treatment, and the eye changes progressed from conjunctivitis to keratitis, symblepharon, and corneal opacification with loss of vision in the left eye.

A fresh review of the problem focused on the absence of:

conjunctival ulceration
cicatricial entropion
trichiasis

on the presence of:

> linear atrophic scars at sites of skin trauma
> milia

From this arose the **correct diagnosis of epidermolysis bullosa acquisita** with ocular involvement. A new biopsy of the skin under immunoelectron microscopy showed the separation was beneath the lamina densa and not just below the lamina lucida as seen in cicatricial pemphigoid. In retrospect, the severe peripheral ulcerative keratitis should have also suggested the diagnosis of epidermolysis bullosa acquisita.

Today's sophisticated **electron microscopy** provides more precision in the diagnosis of bullous diseases, although, regrettably, both cicatricial pemphigoid and epidermolysis bullosa acquisita involving the eye are largely indifferent to therapy.

Fiore PM, Jacobs IH, Goldberg DB: **Drug-induced pemphigoid**—a spectrum of diseases. Arch Ophthalmol 1987; 105:1660–1663.

Five cases of **ocular pemphigoid** are described in elderly white women with glaucoma who had been treated for more than 10 years with topical glaucoma medications. In four cases, stopping the eye drops stopped progression of the disease. No other signs of pemphigoid were present.

Implicated medications in the literature include:

> pilocarpine
> epinephrine
> timolol
> idoxuridine
> echothiophate iodide
> demecarium bromide

Ocular pemphigoid affects the mucous membranes of the eyes, causing conjunctival subepithelial inflammation (plasma cells, immunoglobulin, and complement deposits) and connective tissue invasion, with resulting conjunctival shrinkage. **Drug-induced pemphigoid** is identical clinically and pathologically with idiopathic ocular pemphigoid. Patients using long-term topical eye medications should have periodic inspection of the fornices for shortening in an effort to detect drug-induced pemphigoid in the early stages.

Synonyms include essential shrinkage of conjunctiva, chronic cicatrizing conjunctivitis, and benign mucosal pemphigoid.

For the diagnostician, the eyes are an extension of the brain. For others, they may be merely facial decorations.

van den Berg WHH, Starink THM: **Macular amyloidosis**, presenting as **periocular hyperpigmentation**. Clin Exp Dermatol 1983; 8:195–197.

An **asymptomatic pigmented eruption** had been present for 2 years in this 28-year-old man from Algeria. Examination showed a well-defined diffuse red-brown pigmented lesion **around the eyes**.

Biopsy revealed **amyloid deposits** in the dermal papillae, permitting the diagnosis of macular amyloidosis. It was not a diagnosis easily made, since routine H and E sections showed only melanin-laden macrophages and a sparse mononuclear infiltrate. It required study of frozen sections (thioflavine-T fluorescence staining) to demonstrate the amyloid. Confirmation came from electron microscopy. Interestingly, an example of what was **presumed to be nevoid hyperpigmentation** proved to be macular amyloidosis, but the **amyloid was seen only under electron microscopy**.

Rockerbie NR, Woo TY, Callen JP, Giustina T: **Cutaneous changes of dermatomyositis precede muscle weakness.** J Am Acad Dermatol 1989; 20:629–632.

The onset of cutaneous lesions in dermatomyositis may range from 4 years before to a year after the onset of muscle weakness.

Gottron's papules and the **heliotrope eyelids** call for investigation and aggressive follow-up. Don't close your eyes to this.

Spiegel J, Colton A: **AEC syndrome: Ankyloblepharon, ectodermal defects, and cleft lip and palate:** Report of two cases. J Am Acad Dermatol 1985; 12:810–815.

This dominantly inherited condition is unique for its **fusion of the eyelids** by a solid band at the medial or lateral margins. When the condition is recognized at birth, the eyelids can be surgically separated under local anesthesia.

Patients also have a diminished capacity to sweat, slow hair growth, sparse eyelids and eyebrows, dystrophic nails, and poor dental development, to say nothing of stenotic ear canals, syndactyly, and no lacrimal puncta.

The cleft palate and lip complete this sad syndrome.

Penneys NS: Skin manifestations of **AIDS**. Philadelphia, JB Lippincott Co, 1990; 164.

Marked elongation of the eyelashes may occur in HIV infection.

Richtsmeier AJ Jr, Dray P, Costas C, Martinez M: **Sarcoidosis with supraorbital swelling.** Am J Dis Child 1986; 140:189–190.

Ocular involvement approaches 100% in children under 5 years of age with sarcoid.

Prominent eyes for 3 months and bilateral supraorbital and supratemporal swelling developed in a 7-year-old black boy. He also had red eyes with watery yellowish discharge, photophobia, decreasing visual acuity, muscle soreness, and swollen knees. **Computed tomography** revealed **retroorbital masses**, and a **biopsy** of the **hyperemic conjunctiva** of the lower eyelid showed **noncaseating granulomas**.

Held JL, Schneiderman P: A review of **blepharochalasis** and other causes of the lax, wrinkled eyelid. Cutis 1990; 45:91–94.

This 55-year-old woman complained of cosmetically unappealing **lax eyelid**   555

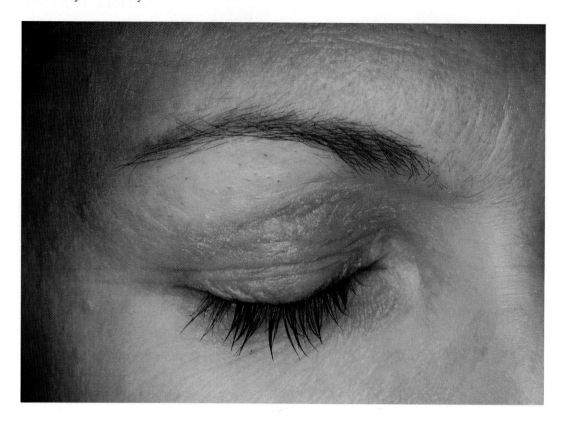

skin. A diagnosis of blepharochalasis was made, and a search for the cause undertaken. The laxity was limited to a circumscribed area of the medial upper eyelids. **Biopsy** of the baggy, wrinkled, loose skin of this site showed **elastolysis** and granuloma in the dermis. The diagnosis was revised upward to **granulomatous slack skin**. Subsequent immunologic studies showed that she had a lymphoproliferative disorder of **malignant T lymphocytes**.

Far more commonly, **blepharochalasis speaks of chronic dermatitis, cardiac failure**, or **renal disease**. Look for contact dermatitis from fingernail products. Bee stings and angioedema can be a prelude to this dropsy eyelid. Even obesity leading to eyelid eversion can result in the lax eyelid.

Cutis laxa, either hereditary or acquired following a febrile or other illness, may also explain blepharochalasis. Here, the eye sign points to increased incidence of hernias and diverticula. Inquire more into your patient's history. Similarly, osteogenesis imperfecta may be suspected when the eyelids look atrophic and translucent, even if the typical blue sclerae are absent.

Blepharochalasis in the young child may be the index sign of **congenital abnormalities**. You may find spina bifida, vertebral defects, cardiac and renal malformations or tracheomegaly. Such blepharochalasis is a constituent of two syndromes.

Ascher's syndrome:

    double lip, goiter, blepharochalasis

Meretoja's syndrome:

    familial form of systemic amyloidosis (corneal dystrophy, cranial neuropathy, polycythemia vera, ventricular hypertrophy, blepharochalasis)

Prompt diagnosis in the latter syndrome may allow for intervention to prevent vision loss. It becomes obvious that a cosmetic complaint may be of real medical significance.

Goldberg R, Seiff S, McFarland J, et al: **Floppy eyelid syndrome** and blepharochalasis. Am J Ophthalmol 1986; 102:376–381.

Recurrent episodes of painless nonpitting edema of the upper eyelids starting around puberty results in thinning, discoloration, and telangiectasia of eyelid skin and relaxation of the eyelid support structures. The **eyelids** are **lax** and easily everted. Chronic **conjunctival inflammation** (keratoconjunctivitis) may result from poor contact between the eyelid and globe.

Collin J, Gray DWR: The **eyes closed sign**. Br Med J 1987; 295:1656.

In patients with acute abdominal pain admitted to the hospital, no cause is established in approximately one third of patients. Nonspecific abdominal pain becomes an expensive diagnosis of exclusion. During palpation of the abdomen, many of these patients, particularly women, keep their eyelids tightly closed and have an embalmed beatific smile. The "eyes-closed sign" helps suggest the diagnosis of **nonspecific abdominal pain** at an early stage. Presumably these patients do not have to worry about pain that might be inflicted by the palpating hands of the surgeon, and they are not apprehensive enough to watch the examination.

Laboratory diagnoses are made by laboratories, but clinical diagnoses are made by clinicians.

Intraocular

Bardenstein DS, Katz NNK, Friendly DS, Parks MM: **Pupillary abnormalities:** Light and sight. Ann Intern Med 1987; 106:643.

Infants, toddlers, and children with abnormal pupillary reflexes (leukokoria) should be referred immediately to an ophthalmologist. This may be lifesaving in cases of **retinoblastoma**, which may present with a **white pupillary reflex** and strabismus (deviated eye or squint). **Lens opacities** in children require immediate surgery, as the human visual system continues to develop until the age of 9 or 10 years, and blockage of light interferes with normal development of the visual cortex of the brain.

Other causes of pupil abnormalities include intraocular infections, retinal detachment, inflammation, and persistent hyperplastic primary vitreous.

Norris PG, Rivers JK: Screening for **cataracts** in patients with severe **atopic eczema**. Clin Exp Dermatol 1987; 12:21–22.

Mild visual impairment in the right eye of a 21-year-old woman with lifelong atopic dermatitis became known only after direct questioning. Slit-lamp microscopy revealed a thin, dense, posterior subcapsular cataract of that eye. As a result, systemic steroid therapy was stopped and PUVA therapy avoided.

Atopic cataracts are usually subclinical, arising about 5 years after onset of atopic dermatitis. The more severe the disease, the higher the incidence of cataracts, which are present in 30% of patients with severe atopic dermatitis. They do not arise from topical steroids being used around the eye, in contrast to glaucoma, but may develop within months of starting systemic steroids. Note that 3% of subclinical cataracts progress in a few weeks to total lens opacification and visual loss.

Patients with severe atopic eczema should be screened with a **slit-lamp biomicroscope** to detect subclinical cataracts.

Toonstra J, Dandrieu MR, Ippel PF, et al: Are **Lisch nodules** an ocular marker of the neurofibromatosis gene in otherwise unaffected family members? Dermatologica 1987; 174:232–235.

The **Lisch nodule** is a raised, round, **fluffy, light-brown melanocytic hamartoma of the iris** seen in 94% of patients with neurofibromatosis over the age of 6 years. It must be viewed under **slit-lamp microscopy** to distinguish it from the flat lacy freckles of the iris seen in 30 to 40% of normal adults.

In the present report, Lisch nodules were the solitary finding in the sister and niece of a patient with neurofibromatosis, suggesting that the nodule may be a **marker for the neurofibromatosis gene.** All family members should be examined with a slit lamp in screening for neurofibromatosis, even if the case appears to be sporadic.

Jabs DA, Johns CJ: Ocular involvement in chronic **sarcoidosis**. Am J Ophthalmol 1986; 102:297–301.

Approximately 25% of patients with sarcoidosis for more than 5 years have eye problems, especially black patients. **Uveitis** is common, (19% of 183 patients), occurs early, and often resolves. Chronic uveitis with secondary glaucoma and severe visual loss occurred in 6%.

Schultz PN, Sobol WM: **Angioid streaks and pseudoxanthoma elasticum.** JAMA 1991; 265:45.

The diagnosis of pseudoxanthoma elasticum is supported by the finding of angioid streaks by direct ophthalmoscopy. Bear in mind, however, that such **angioid streaks** are associated with a host of **other systemic disorders**. Most commonly, these are Paget's disease of the bone and sickle cell disease. Less commonly one finds them in patients with Ehlers-Danlos syndrome, senile elastosis, tuberous sclerosis, Sturge-Weber syndrome, acromegaly, diabetes, and myopia itself.

What do we see with the **ophthalmoscope**? The angioid streaks are irregular, peripapillary, brown-to-red curvilinear bands that extend in a weblike manner from the optic disc. They may be confused with blood vessels, but observe that they lie below the retinal vasculature as broad shadows with tapering ends. Other notable **retinoscopy findings** are:

> yellowish mottling of pigment epithelium temporal to the macule (peau d'orange)
> punched-out depigmented peripheral lesions (salmon spots)
> drusen of optic nerve head

Statistically, over 50% of patients with angioid streaks have pseudoxanthoma elasticum, and over 85% of patients with pseudoxanthoma elasticum have angioid streaks. They are worth looking for.

The pathologist is provided with only a hundred thousandth of the skin surface that the clinician sees. Choose his peep hole carefully.

Face

The face has the most interesting skin of all. Its multifeature landscape is center stage for the adverse effects of sunlight, both the acute photosensitivity and the chronic changes of lentigines, actinic keratoses, and basal cell epithelioma. Rich in sebaceous glands, facial skin is the home of acne and seborrheic dermatitis as well as the patulous pores, comedones, and sebaceous adenomas of later years. The abundance of vessels and autonomic fibers explains the erythemas, flushing, and eventual rosacea we see in the facial area. Finally, no area is as freely endowed with elastic tissue as the face. As these fibers become frayed and clumped after years of sunlight, the tautness of youthful skin is replaced by the wrinkles and elastosis of age. Nowhere is this more evident than in the face and neck.

Although many diagnoses are easy, such as the scaly, oily, paranasal erythema of seborrheic dermatitis, or the redness of atopic cheeks in an infant, some are less evident. Here are some examples:

The unilateral scaling eruption with indistinct borders that proves to be tinea faciei. Ask about contact with cats, dogs, horses.

The faint flush that is the mask of lupus erythematosus. Secure an antinuclear antibody determination.

The basal cell epithelioma hiding in the terrain of rhinophyma.

The unilateral *Demodex* infestation producing a rosacea-like eruption. Do a scraping.

The narrow band of redness of the hairline due to psoriasis. Hold off treatment and washing for a few days to allow the diagnostic silver scale to appear.

The sclerosing basal cell epithelioma simulating an acne scar. Watch it grow or obtain a biopsy.

The actinic keratosis that looks like no more than a red spot. Employ a diagnostic therapeutic trial with 5-fluorouracil.

Granulomatous candidiasis in the perioral area simulating rosacea. Employ a therapeutic trial with ketoconazole.

A factitial ulcer that looks like an epithelioma. Obtain a biopsy.

A fixed drug eruption that appears to be a lentigo. Challenge.

A dental abscess that suggests a furuncle. Get dental x-rays.

Seborrheic dermatitis that comes as naught but a flush. Have the patient stop washing for 5 days, and diagnostic greasy scale will form.

A recurrent acneiform herpes lesion. Prevent with acyclovir.

A discoid lupus erythematosus lesion that looks like a scar. Obtain a biopsy.

Tinea versicolor that appears to be vitiligo. Scrape.

Adenoma sebaceum resembling acne. Biopsy.

Delage C, Lagace R, Huard J: **Pseudocyanotic pigmentation** of the skin induced by **amiodarone**: A light and electron microscopic study. Can Med Assoc J 1975; 112:1205–1208.

A 54-year-old white woman had a 6-month history of a **blue nose**. The gray-blue pigmentation involved the lower half of the nose and the alae nasi. Cyanosis was ruled out by the fact that it spared the perioral area and facial wrinkles and folds. Diascopy revealed violet granules in the discolored areas. Ophthalmologic examination showed small brown granular deposits on the caruncles, eyelids, and peripheral margins of the corneas.

She had previously taken the coronary vasodilator drug **amiodarone** hydrochloride for 15 months while living in Europe and had noted bluish pigmentation after 9 months of treatment (dosage 200 to 400 mg daily). The pigment was still present 17 months after discontinuation of the medication.

Skin biopsy showed histiocytes containing yellow-brown cytoplasmic granules with properties of melanin and lipofuscin.

Walton S, Keczkes K: **Trigeminal neurotrophic ulceration:** A report of four patients. Clin Exp Dermatol 1985; 10:485–490.

This 87-year-old man developed **ulceration on the left side of the nose** and upper lip 2 months after alcohol injection into the left Gasserian ganglion for treatment of longstanding trigeminal neuralgia.

On examination he had **complete anesthesia** to pain and temperature sensation in the distribution of the left trigeminal nerve. Not only did the indolent ulcer extend over the left side of the nose and upper lip, but it had also destroyed the ala nasi and adjoining nasal septum. A biopsy revealed nonspecific chronic inflammation.

The patient readily admitted to picking the area constantly to relieve the burning and pricking sensations of the area. It is this **trauma** that accounts for these nonhealing ulcers.

The same ulceration may be seen in patients who have suffered occlusion of the posterior inferior cerebellar artery with subsequent anesthesia of the nasal area. In all examples the **differential diagnosis** must include factitial dermatitis and ulcerative basal cell epithelioma.

Lober CW, Kaplan RJ, West WH: **Midline granuloma: Stewart type.** Arch Dermatol 1982; 118:52–54.

A tender, erythematous **ulceration of the tip of the nose** of a 34-year-old woman spread to involve the nasal septum. Multiple smears of a subsection biopsy showed no fungi or acid-fast organisms. Bacterial cultures showed *Staphylococcus epidermidis* and **streptococci**. A deep biopsy revealed necrotic subepithelial tissue densely infiltrated with lymphocytes, eosinophils, and polymorphonuclear cells.

Since a physical examination as well as extensive radiographic analyses and biochemical studies were otherwise normal, a diagnosis of midline granuloma of Stewart was made. **Radiation therapy** (3500 rad) provided a cure.

Without radiation therapy, one could anticipate the ulceration lasting as long as 4 years. This would be followed by painless, relentless destruction of bone, cartilage, and soft tissue with granuloma formation. The final phase would be monstrous mutilating destruction of the center face followed by death in a year due to hemorrhage, infection, or exhaustion.

At least 24 synonyms appear in the literature for these midline ulcerative lesions, but two conditions must be sharply distinguished in any differential diagnosis. These are **Wegener's granulomatosis** and **lymphoma**. In Wegener's granulomatosis the ulcerative lesions of the upper airways are not associated with nasal and facial destruction. Its hallmark is systemic disease with involvement of lungs and/or kidneys. This does not occur in midline granuloma. The granuloma in Wegener's disease is a giant cell granuloma, whereas the infiltrate in true midline granuloma is largely a pleomorphic one.

The other disease in the differential diagnosis is **malignant lymphoma** of the upper respiratory tract. It can present with features identical with midline granuloma. Only by multiple deep biopsies can distinction be made with certainty.

Champion RH: **Granulosis rubra nasi.** *In* Rook A, Wilkinson DS, Ebling FJG, et al (eds): Textbook of Dermatology, 4th ed. London, Blackwell Scientific Publications, 1986, pp 1890–1891.

This rare, heritable disease begins in childhood as **hyperhidrosis of the nose**, followed by diffuse erythema. This may extend to include the cheeks, upper lip, and chin. Sweat retention vesicles and papules are a characteristic sign. Involution usually occurs at puberty.

Stanley RJ, Olsen KD, Muller SA, Roenigk RK: Aggressive **intranasal carcinoma mimicking infection or inflammation**. Cutis 1988; 42:288–293.

Painful erythema and swelling of the nose with induration, ulceration, or draining sinuses may signal an enormous underlying intranasal carcinoma that has extended to involve nasal skin.

For 18 months a 57-year-old woman had a **tender red nose** variously diagnosed as acne rosacea, lupus erythematosus, or secondary to trauma. A skin **biopsy** confirmed **rosacea**, but therapy with tetracycline and benzoyl peroxide proved ineffective. A **deeper biopsy** of the nasal skin showed an infiltrative grade 3 squamous cell carcinoma in the lower dermis and subcutaneous layer, invading the septal cartilage. **Skull and sinus radiographs** showed partial destruction of the nasal bones, and computed tomography also showed a soft tissue mass under the bridge of the nose. Total rhinectomy with ethmoid sinus exenteration, removal of the anterior frontal sinus table, and partial left cheek excision appeared curative at 15 months follow-up.

Four additional cases of intranasal squamous cell carcinoma are described in which the presenting sign resembled cellulitis or ulcerative change.

Think of cancer of the nasal septum when:

   The nasal skin lesion progresses despite negative skin biopsies.
   Cultures and response to systemic antibiotics are repeatedly negative.
   There is nasal airway obstruction.
   The patient complains of rhinorrhea, epistaxis, epiphora, anosmia, or numbness of the nose, teeth, or palate.

Secure **rhinologic consultation**, computed tomography, and intranasal or very deep nasal biopsy. Even though it is hard to conceive of a relatively minor cutaneous disease of the nose masking such a lethal growth within the nose, this cruel diagnosis of squamous cell carcinoma must enter your thinking. Do not be misled by the slow clinical pace of this disease, the patient's history of trauma, or a patient's youthful age. Do not retreat from the diagnosis because the treatment, total rhinectomy, is so multilating and emotionally devastating to the patient. Your only chance to save your patient's life is to make the diagnosis early.

Keefe M, Wakeel RA, McBride DI: **Basal cell carcinoma mimicking rhinophyma.** Case report and literature review. Arch Dermatol 1988; 124:1077–1079.

Enlargement of the nose in an 82-year-old man was interpreted as **rhinophyma** until surgical reduction and histologic examination of the shavings revealed **basal cell carcinoma.**

Be alert: Angiosarcoma as well as basal cell carcinoma may develop insidiously in a rhinophyma. Furthermore, malignant diseases such as lymphocytic lymphoma may be misdiagnosed as rhinophyma.

Hoshaw TC, Walike JW: **Dermoid cysts of the nose.** Arch Otolaryng 1971; 93:487–491.

A **pit on the dorsal surface of the nose** with a **tuft of hair** extruding from the underlying sinus tract is typical of a congenital dermoid cyst. Sebaceous material may be present. Swelling of the cyst may cause a widened nasal bridge and root, but the cyst is usually midline, nontender, and painless. Recurrent inflammation may lead to a yellow exudate from the sinus tract.

Careful **x-ray evaluation** is mandatory prior to excision under an operating microscope.

If the classic dimple and fistula are not present, consider **other possibilities**:

Meningocele: transilluminates with bright light, drains spinal fluid if incised, becomes tense and pulsates with the Valsalva maneuver
Encephalocele: becomes tense and pulsates with jugular vein compression or the Valsalva maneuver
Nasal glioma: firm nontender mass, often slightly off to the side
Neurofibroma: superficial, attached to the skin
Sebaceous cyst: superficial, attached to the skin

Tapia A: **Rhinoscleroma:** A naso-oral dermatosis. Cutis 1987; 40:101–103.

Klebsiella rhinoscleromatis is the gram-negative diplobacillus to look for in smears and cultures in patients from Central America who have:

1. **Rhinitis** resembling a common cold that persists for months and eventually leads to epistaxis and fetid nasal discharge; thickened mucous membranes the only abnormal findings
2. Painless, reddish, waxy **infiltrates** of the nasal septum with airway obstruction
3. Laryngeal infiltrates leading to **voice changes**
4. **Tumors of the nose** with dyspnea, anosmia, massive deformity of the ala nasi and upper lip, attacks of asphyxia, and sometimes squamous cell carcinoma

A biopsy shows the bacilli in large histiocytes (Mikulicz cells) and numerous plasma cells, some of which undergo hyaline degeneration (Russell bodies).

The **differential diagnosis** centers on other forms of rhinitis and nasal polyps (which are soft and smooth). In the tumor stage, confusion can arise with lymphoma, squamous cell carcinoma, tertiary syphilis, leprosy, leishmaniasis, paracoccidioidomycosis, and rhinosporidiosis.

It is a disease with slow measured stages that must be recognized. If it is not, and the patient is denied antibiotic therapy, it is uniformly fatal.

Marsden PD: **Mucocutaneous leishmaniasis.** Br Med J 1990; 301:656–657.

In South America the appearance of a **friable granuloma** of the anterior **nasal septum** suggests a prior cutaneous infection with *Leishmania viannia braziliensis.* These granulomas eventually perforate the septum and may extend down through the floor of the nose, producing a **cobble-street appearance on the palate**. The nose and cheeks may be involved, as well as the epiglottis and larynx. Known as **espundia**, it may lead to death from suffocation due to laryngeal closure.

Diagnosis by isolating the parasite is harder in espundia than in other forms of leishmaniasis owing to problems of contamination and obtaining adequate biopsy material and the poor growth of *L. braziliensis*.

However, the typical **burnlike scar** of a previous infection adds strong support to the clinical diagnosis.

Shuttleworth D, Graham-Brown RAC, Barton RPE: Median **nasal dermoid fistula**. Clin Exp Dermatol 1985; 10:269–273.

A **small reddish pit**, exactly on the **midline of the nose**, was the presenting complaint of this 8-year-old girl. It had been present since birth and tended to swell and crust off. On examination the pit showed several small hairs, and a deep component could be palpated as a subcutaneous mass. A probe could be inserted for 1 cm. A diagnosis of median nasal dermoid fistula was made on clinical grounds.

X-rays of the nose as well as the sinuses and also **computed tomography** showed no abnormalities. Surgery under general anesthesia permitted dissection and excision of a tract, shown to be lined by keratinizing squamous epithelium with numerous hair follicles.

This rare congenital abnormality results from **sequestration of fetal ectodermal cells** during the process of nasal fusion. At times there may be a communication with the cranial cavity so that careful radiologic studies are always indicated.

If left untreated, the patient is at risk for abscess formation, osteomyelitis of the underlying bone, and even meningitis. Inadequate removal leads to recurrence, and improper removal to a saddle-nose deformity. Median nasal dermoid fistula thus is a problem in the province of the plastic surgeon.

Aram H, Mohagheghi AP: **Granulosis rubra nasi**. Cutis 1972; 10:463–464.

A 12-year-old girl had an erythematous **maculopapular eruption of the nose** that had been gradually becoming worse over the past 4 years. She had noted frequent attacks of **hyperhidrosis of the nose** as well as the face, palms, soles, and axillae. These were triggered by emotionally tense situations and lasted about 10 minutes. A biopsy showed capillary dilation and a perivascular infiltrate of inflammatory cells. This was also present around the sweat glands.

The diagnosis of granulosis rubra nasi was made. Clinically it **resembled** rosacea, lupus erythematosus, and lupus vulgaris.

Laboratory tests will put wind in your diagnostic sails but beware: too many may pull the sails down.

Williams ML, Packman S, Cowan MJ: Alopecia and **periorificial dermatitis** in biotin-responsive multiple carboxylase deficiency. J Am Acad Dermatol 1983; 9:97–103.

Laboratory demonstration of an **aminoaciduria** may explain:

hyperpigmentation, atopic dermatitis, and focal scleroderma (phenylketonuria)

erosive focal palmoplantar keratoderma (tyrosinemia—type II [Richner-Hanhart syndrome])

sparse hair, atrophic scars, telangiectasia, elastosis perforans serpiginosa (homocystinuria)

sparse hair, periorificial dermatitis (biotin deficiency)

brittle hair (citrullinemia)

brittle hair with trichorrhexis nodosa (arginosuccinic aciduria)

white hair (methionine malabsorption [Oasthouse disease])

photosensitivity (hydroxykynureninuria)

photosensitivity, alopecia, premature graying, nail streaks (Hartnup disease)

pigmentation of skin and sclerae, chromhidrosis (alkaptonuria)

skin fragility, chronic dermatitis (prolidase deficiency)

The laboratory may **also explain periorificial dermatitis**:

multiple carboxylase deficiency (serum biotin level low, lactic acidosis, organic aciduria, hypoammonuria, hypoglycemia)

chronic mucocutaneous candidiasis, acrodermatitis enteropathica (serum zinc level low)

necrolytic migratory erythema (plasma glucagon level elevated)

essential fatty acid deficiency

Brandrup F, Wantzin GL, Thomsen K: **Perioral pustular eruption** caused by *Candida albicans*. Br J Dermatol 1981; 105:327–329.

Papules, pustules, and crusts have been present for 3 weeks on the chin and perilabial area of this 22-year-old woman. She had had no prior skin disease, never been treated with steroids, nor had she been exposed to acnegenic agents. There were no signs of oral or genital candidiasis. Clinically it appeared as a severe form of **perioral dermatitis** or a mild example of **pyoderma faciale**.

Initial treatment with tetracycline for 2 weeks produced an intense flare. Nor did erythromycin provide help. A biopsy showed an intense inflammatory reaction, with patches of granulomatous change. The diagnosis was not apparent until numerous colonies of *Candida albicans* appeared on **culture of the pustules**. Bacteriologic cultures were negative.

This was a florid case of candidal infection and alerts one to the need for mycologic as well as bacteriologic culture of pustules. Noteworthy is the fact that classic perioral dermatitis may well be due to *C. albicans* at times.

Frieden IJ, Prose NS, Fletcher V, Turner ML: **Granulomatous perioral dermatitis** in children. Arch Dermatol 1989; 125:369–373.

An 8-year-old girl suddenly developed numerous small **flesh-colored papules around the nose**, mouth, and eyes. Bacterial cultures were negative as was a chest roentgenogram.

A skin biopsy showed numerous well-formed granulomas. Special stains for fungi and acid-fast bacilli were negative, and polarization did not reveal any foreign body. A diagnosis of granulomatous perioral dermatitis was made.

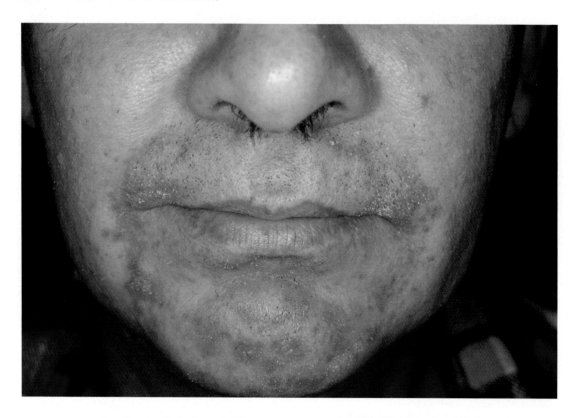

Its closest clinical resemblance was to **sarcoidosis**, but this was ruled out by absence of any findings elsewhere. Lupus miliaris disseminatus faciei and rosacea were also ruled out histologically and by the clinical absence of any rosaceal changes. Similarly, **benign cephalic histiocytosis** was eliminated from the differential diagnosis by the histologic changes. Finally, the absence of sweating and redness did not support a diagnosis of granulosis rubra nasi.

El-Saad El-Rifaie M: **Perioral dermatitis** with epithelioid cell granulomas in a woman: A possible new etiology. Acta Derm Venereol 1980; 60:359–360.

For 3 months this Arabian woman had an **itchy eruption of the face** that was resistant to topical treatment. It had begun around the mouth and within 2 weeks covered the lower face.

On examination there was a diffuse erythematous papular eruption showing scant vesicles. A diagnosis of perioral dermatitis was made and a search undertaken for one of the following **known causes** or associations:

    rosacea
    sarcoidosis
    lupus miliaris disseminatus faciei
    sarcoid granulomas
    contact allergens

A biopsy showed epithelioid cell granuloma formation consistent with the responses known to be induced by acrylic or nylon fibers. No, the culprit was not the nylon toothbrush. Rather, it was the new black synthetic **veil** she had began to wear to cover the lower half of her face. Once the veil was discarded, her perioral dermatitis essentially disappeared within 2 months.

This case is reminiscent of the little boy whose perioral dermatitis was reportedly due to bubble gum sensitivity. There is more than one way to cover your lower face!

Dameshek W, Henstell HH: The diagnosis of **polycythemia**. Ann Intern Med 1940; 13:1360–1387.

Overloading of the entire circulation with increased blood volume results in distended vessels and sensations referable to the head, cardiovascular system, gastrointestinal tract, and extremities. In most cases, emphasis is placed on only one bodily system by the patient. Symptoms may include headache, vertigo, visual disturbances, colored scotomata, and **paresthesias** or suggest vascular disturbances of the extremities with pain, warmth, and tingling of the legs resembling erythromelalgia. Patients often have a history of multiple arterial and venous thromboses and profuse hemorrhages after minor trauma.

The typical patient is plethoric with **dusky purplish-red lips**, congested conjunctival blood vessels, and **red ears**. The color is rose-red in summer but more dusky and cyanotic in winter. The hands and feet are also thick and beefy red, becoming blotchy and blue with cold exposure. The buccal mucous membranes are deep red and the tongue is large, thickly coated, and fissured. Hepatosplenomegaly and dilated retinal veins are also common.

Laboratory findings:

> bone marrow: red cell hyperplasia, megakaryocytic hyperplasia
> hematocrit: 58 to 82%
> red cell count: >6.0 million/cc
> ↑ platelets
> ↑ white blood cells (↑ polymorphonuclears)
> urinalysis: albumin

Microscopic examination of nail bed capillaries reveals increased tortuosity and distension of the capillary loops. The vessels are large, dilated, and tortuous with great distension of the venous limbs. This is analagous to the retinal veins.

Dominey A, Tschen J, Rosen T, et al: **Pityriasis folliculorum** revisited. J Am Acad Dermatol 1989; 21:81–84.

Six cases of **facial erythema with follicular plugging** were described. In each, examination of the follicular contents in mineral oil revealed numerous *Demodex folliculorum* mites. A diagnosis of **demodectic pityriasis folliculorum** was made, and five cases cleared with several weeks of treatment with 1% lindane lotion coupled with 0.01% tretinoin gel.

Ayres S Jr: *Demodex folliculorum* as a pathogen. Cutis 1986; 37:441.

It was an eruption that didn't make it into the entity class. It was simply an erythema and scaling of the cheeks of a physician's wife. It was indifferent to all the bland creams, and its host cried, "Do something!" So a **KOH preparation** was obtained, and there was the pathogen. It was *Demodex folliculorum*. Fifteen per low power field. It was an atypical rosacea, soon gone when the *Demodex* died in the sulfur fumes of Danish ointment.

Oono T, Arata J, Fukuma A, Miyoshi I: **Bloom's syndrome** with dimorphism of sister chromatid exchanges in phytohemagglutinin-stimulated lymphocytes. Arch Dermatol 1987; 123:988–989.

Mottling of the face with **depigmentation**, **pigmentation**, and **telangiectasia** was the presenting picture of this 34-year-old man.

His face had been erythematous since he was 4 months old. As the years

567

passed, some hyperkeratotic lesions resembling actinic keratosis had developed, as well as atrophic areas.

On examination there was pityriasiform scaling as well as the presenting changes. Yellowish papules were seen on the nose, lower eyelid, and outer eyebrows. His **pointed nose** and dolichocephaly gave a bird-like facies. He was short (135.5 cm) and slight in weight (29 kg). There were many small and large café au lait spots over the trunk and extremities. The high-pitched voice, the presence of diabetes mellitus, anemia, and a history of three generations of parental consanguinity made the total picture of Bloom's syndrome.

One could anticipate he will develop squamous cell carcinomas as well as possibly other neoplasms associated at times with this syndrome (lymphoma, leukemia, Wilson's tumor, meningioma).

Borkovic SP, Schwartz RA, McNutt NS: **Unilateral erythromelanosis follicularis faciei et colli.** Cutis 1984; 33:163–170.

In his early "teens," this 30-year-old man had noted a small pigmented patch on the face just anterior to the left ear. It gradually spread to involve the entire cheek, chin, and left side of the neck.

On examination these areas show a diffuse **reddish-brown discoloration** with a sharply demarcated border. On closer look one sees tiny follicular papules in crops. The reddish component is vascular and can be blanched by diascopy. The brown is epidermal pigment, accentuated by Wood's light.

On biopsy this triad of findings proved to be due to acanthosis, a lymphocytic infiltrate, dilated blood vessels, and increased pigment in the basal cell layer. Under electron microscopy the melanosomes were large and had a characteristic stippled appearance.

A diagnosis of **erythromelanosis follicularis faciei** et colli was made. Notable was its unilateral nature, its chronicity, and its progressive enlargement. Since its cause is completely unknown, all you need to know is encoded in its name. Just remember it is a mix of erythema-melanosis-follicular prominence and localizes on the face and neck.

What is this strange skin condition with red rings which expand
from the centre in widening circles?
That, says the dermatologist, is erythema annulare centrifugum.
He has spoken the words of power, and the dignity of the profession
has been upheld.

RICHARD ASHER

Fisher AA: **Perfume dermatitis** in children sensitized to balsam of Peru in topical agents. Cutis 1990; 45:21–23.

A **4-month-old infant** developed a bright-red erythematous eruption on the face whenever she came in contact with her **mother's perfume**. The significant piece of history was the fact that A & D Ointment had caused a diaper dermatitis previously.

Patch tests to the perfume, A & D Ointment, and to balsam of Peru were each positive. Since both A & D Ointment and perfume contain balsam of Peru, the common antigen was evident. Indeed, sensitivity to balsam of Peru must alert you to a fragrance allergy. Since balsam of Peru is so commonly found in baby care products, their use in the occluded diaper area may be a sensitization risk not worth taking.

Lewis JE: **Lentigo maligna presenting as an eczematous lesion.** Cutis 1987; 40:357–359.

A **chronic eczematous lesion of the right cheek** of this 65-year-old woman proved on horizontal excision (Gillette Super Blue Blade) to be lentigo maligna.

Such **lentigines** may present not only as innocuous dermatitis but also as:

> melanotic erythematous macules
> a hypopigmented patch of neurodermatitis
> nevus depigmentosus
> superficial multicentric basal cell carcinoma-like lesion
> bowenoid plaques

Obviously, atypical lentigo maligna eludes the physician reluctant to do even superficial biopsies.

No botanist is satisfied with the diagnosis of tree, nor should any physician be satisfied with the diagnosis of dermatitis.

Papules and Plaques

Alteras IA, Sandbank M, David M, Segal R: 15-year survey of **tinea faciei** in the adult. Dermatologica 1988; 177:65–69.

Tinea faciei in 100 adults **looked like**:

discoid lupus erythematosus 52
lymphocytic infiltration 15
seborrheic dermatitis 11
rosacea 8
contact dermatitis 7
polymorphous light eruption 4
granuloma faciale 3

About **70%** of these cases had been **diagnosed incorrectly**. A valuable diagnostic tip is to **look at the toenails**, since 85 of the 100 had onychomycosis due mainly to *Trichophyton rubrum*. Presumably the toenails were the source of the facial problems.

What you may miss,
Only heaven will know,
If you dismiss,
Just a peek at a toe.

Dominey A, Rosen T, Tschen J: **Papulonodular demodicidis** associated with the acquired immunodeficiency syndrome. J Am Acad Dermatol 1989; 20:197–201.

A 49-year-old man with a **pruritic eruption of the head** and neck for 2 weeks had multiple discrete erythematous papules and nodules on the posterior surface of the cheeks, jawbone, and upper neck. **AIDS** had been diagnosed 8 months before this consultation.

Skin scrapings revealed innumerable *Demodex* **mites**, and a biopsy showed the hair follicles packed with these mites. The dermis was found to have a dense lymphocytic and eosinophilic infiltrate. A diagnosis of demodecidosis was made. Application of 1% gamma benzene hexachloride lotion to the areas for each of three nights completely eradicated the pruritus, papules, and pests. Look for *Demodex folliculorum* and *D. brevis* as the **cause** of:

1. Scaly follicular eruptions with "nutmeg-grater" feel (pityriasis folliculorum)
2. Acuminate papulopustules of scalp
3. Brownish scaly hyperpigmented patches on the face
4. Edematous plaques studded with follicular pustules on the face
5. Pruritic scaly blepharitis
6. Rosacea

When you come upon a crowd of *Demodex*, you've come upon a pathogen.

Toonstra J, Wildschut A, Boer J, et al: **Jessner's lymphocytic infiltration** of the skin. A clinical study of 100 patients. Arch Dermatol 1989; 125:1525–1530.

This disease derives its name from its histology. Its clinical presentation is one of flat, **pinkish-brown**, more or less elevated lesions that usually appear on the **face**. Clearing in the center and circinate patterning are characteristic. It may last for months and then disappear without sequelae. It may recur at the same or other sites.

It is distinguished from **discoid lupus erythematosus** by absence of atrophy and follicular plugging. It mimics polymorphic light eruption, both clinically and histologically. Indeed, it may flare with sun exposure. However, negative phototests and an onset in the winter season speak in favor of Jessner's lymphocytic infiltrate.

The prognosis is good, with no threat to conversion to malignant lymphoma.

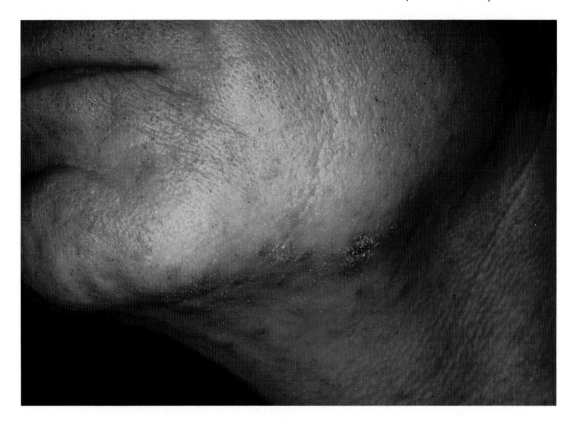

Mullen RH, Jacobs AH: **Jessner's lymphocytic infiltrate** in two girls. Arch Dermatol 1988; 124:1091–1093.

A 5-cm annular plaque composed of **coalescing erythematous papules** had been present for 6 months on a 7-year-old girl's cheek. Originally diagnosed as "**impetigo**," it temporarily resolved following a course of erythromycin. Subsequently a biopsy revealed chronic **perifolliculitis**. When a similar lesion appeared on the left upper eyelid, a second biopsy showed a dense perivascular lymphocytic infiltrate, **characteristic of Jessner's lymphocytic infiltrate**.

A second similar case is described in an 11-year-old girl with a 3-cm erythematous annular plaque on the chest and two smaller plaques on the face. The lesions waxed and waned in size and intensity, and two biopsies were required to make the diagnosis.

This benign, nonscarring, asymptomatic recurrent facial eruption has previously been reported only in adults, usually males. Jessner's benign lymphocytic infiltration should now be added to our **differential list** for facial plaques in children, which already includes:

discoid lupus erythematosus	lymphoma cutis
polymorphous light eruption	sarcoid
drug eruption	tuberculosis
lymphocytoma cutis	(and don't forget tinea faciei)

Parhizgar B, Leppard BJ: **Epithelioma adenoides cysticum.** A condition mimicking **tuberose sclerosis**. Clin Exp Dermatol 1977; 2:145–152.

A 23-year-old Iranian woman first developed **small translucent papules** on **the nasolabial folds** when she was 11 years old. Many papules showed surface telangiectasia as they gradually spread over the face, eyelids, neck, ears, and upper back. Biopsy showed tumor lobules and lacework strands of basaloid cells in the dermis, with multiple keratinous cysts. She also had periungual fibromas of both little toenails. An autosomal dominant inheritance pattern was discerned with eight relatives showing similar facial and toenail lesions. No family members had retardation or epilepsy.

The skin lesions are **clinically identical to the adenoma sebaceum** (angiofibromas) **of tuberous sclerosis** that develop early in life, seldom appear after age 9 years, and increase in size until puberty. Epithelioma adenoides cysticum lesions begin symmetrically in the nasolabial folds around puberty and then increase in size and number, with adjacent lesions sometimes becoming confluent. They may spread to the entire face, external ears, scalp, trunk, and limbs, but affect only the skin. Multiple **syringomas** and **cylindromas** may also be associated.

Moy LS, Moy RL, Matsuoka LY, et al: **Lipoid Proteinosis:** Ultrastructural and biochemical studies. J Am Acad Dermatol 1987; 16:1193–1201.

Listen for the hoarse voice.
Look at the papules of eyelids, face, cheeks, nose.
Feel the verrucous growths on shaking hands.
Examine for verrucous nodules of knees and elbows.
Find the hyalin-like material in the dermis on biopsy.

Banse-Kupin L, Morales A, Barlow M: **Torre's syndrome:** Report of two cases and review of the literature. J Am Acad Dermatol 1984; 10:803–817.

A 39-year-old woman had multiple flesh-colored, **waxy papules** of the head and trunk. Biopsy revealed these were **sebaceous adenomas.** Past history included adenocarcinoma of the uterus at age 32, and adenocarcinoma of the sigmoid colon at age 34. The conjunction of **multiple sebaceous adenomas** and **visceral carcinoma** made the diagnosis of Torre's syndrome.

Subsequent events confirmed the value of realizing that patients with multiple sebaceous adenomas are subject to visceral carcinoma. At the age of 51 years she had a second primary **adenocarcinoma of the colon.** The next year a transitional cell carcinoma of the right kidney was found and excised, and the very next year a third primary adenocarcinoma of the colon was found.

The patient's **family history** was one of **many cancers.** Her mother had cancer of the stomach and also of the colon. Three brothers had colon cancer, esophageal cancer, and renal cancer, respectively.

All of which underscores Torre's syndrome as being an autosomal dominant genetic defect.

Schwartz RA, Flieger DN, Saied NK: The **Torre syndrome with gastrointestinal polyposis.** Arch Dermatol 1980; 116:312–314.

Torre's syndrome consists of the association of numerous sebaceous adenomas, sebaceous epitheliomas, and an occasional keratoacanthoma with low-grade malignant neoplasms of the gastrointestinal tract.

The usual location of the cutaneous index sign is the face. Usually those patients present for treatment of the skin growths long after the gastrointestinal tumors have been identified and resected. Nonetheless, the presence of scores of sebaceous adenomas should alert one to the possible presence of unrecognized gastrointestinal tumors or polyposis. Since Torre's syndrome appears to be of a hereditary nature, it may be rewarding to have close relatives studied as well.

Rudolph RI: Persistent purple plaques of the face caused by gingival hyperplasia. Cutis 1981; 27:516–517.

Slowly enlarging **pruritic, purple areas** had been present on the **chin** of this

53-year-old woman for 6 months. Topical steroids had been of no help. Further history revealed that she had been edentulous for years, and that she practiced no oral hygiene. Indeed, she wore her full dentures continually day and night.

Physical examination showed several purple, firm, edematous plaques covering most of the chin. Translucent papules were seen in the center of the largest plaque. There was no lymphadenopathy. The lower gums were markedly hyperplastic, malodorous, purulent, and showed ulcerations.

The **differential of lymphocytoma cutis, sarcoidosis**, and **granuloma faciale** had to be abandoned when the biopsy of the skin showed simply marked edema with dilated lymphatics. Similarly, **malignant disease, rosacea**, and **erysipelas** were eliminated.

Because of the **purulent gingivitis**, dental sinus and actinomycosis were considered, but the critical diagnostic finding of a draining sinus was not present. The major clinical observation centered on the translucent papules. These resembled lymphangioma, but being of recent onset they were best classified as acquired lymphangiectasis.

It was presumed that the gingivitis produced a compromised lymphatic system. This view was supported by the prompt disappearance of the skin lesions within 2 months once the gingival hyperplastic tissue was excised, the dentures fitted, and oral hygiene instituted.

Schwartz BK, Demos PT, Baughman RD: **Indurated facial plaques** in a young man. Arch Dermatol 1987, 123:939–942.

Two sharply circumscribed **red plaques** had been slowly enlarging on the cheek and chin of this healthy 31-year-old man. They were asymptomatic, KOH negative, and unresponsive to oral erythromycin, as well as topical steroids.

A **biopsy** gave the answer: **follicular mucinosis**. Originally this condition was named alopecia mucinosa, because of the loss of hairs from the affected follicles. It is now realized that loss of hair is not invariably associated with the inflammatory and mucinous changes around and in the follicle.

The process usually affects the head and neck with multiple lesions, but may occur on the trunk or extremities. Although it is not pruritic, rare cases of **dysesthesia** have been reported. In the beard region the loss of hair may be striking, but reversible, since the process is nonscarring.

In children and young adults, this is a benign disease with spontaneous resolution in anywhere from 2 months to 2 years. However, in the older age group, as many as 40% are at risk of developing or having associated **lymphoma, especially mycosis fungoides**.

Ulogy-Rainey Z, James WD, Lupton GP, Rodman OG: Fibrofolliculomas, trichodiscomas, and acrochordons: The Birt-Hogg-Dubé syndrome. J Am Acad Dermatol 1987; 16:452–457.

Multiple firm facial papules are an autosomal dominant family trait that usually appears in the third or fourth decade of life. It is for the **pathologist** to sort out those that are

of hair follicle origin:

    trichofolliculomas   trichilemmomas (Cowden's)   trichoepitheliomas

of mesodermal (hair disc) origin:

    trichodiscoma   perifollicular fibroma   adenoma sebaceum of Pringle

or of mixed origin:

    fibrofolliculoma

Miscellaneous

Levit F, Casey D: **Acquired cheek dimple** caused by gingivobuccal fibrous band. Arch Dermatol 1981; 117:811–812.

The gradual appearance of a deep dimple in the left cheek of this 27-year-old woman caused concern. There was no history of trauma, dental procedures, or sinus formation.

On examination, a firm band of tissue could be felt connecting the dimple site to the gingiva above the left upper first molar. It was clearly visible on retracting the cheek. The dimple **disappeared upon excision of the band**, which proved histologically to be benign proliferation of fibrous tissue.

Reminds one of another dimple called the umbilicus.

Kuttner BJ: A productive **black facial pore**. Arch Dermatol 1989; 125:827–830.

A 4-mm facial pore that frequently extruded a black substance had been present for years on the right cheek of this 65-year-old man.

The **differential diagnosis** list included:

trichofolliculoma
pilar sheath acanthoma
dilated pore of Winer
dental sinus
scar

On **biopsy** a **trichofolliculoma** was found. This is a benign hamartoma of the hair follicle in which the key feature is a massively dilated follicle filled with keratin or hair. A bouquet of accessory hair follicles of varying degrees of maturity radiates out to the sides. By contrast, the trichoepithelioma lacks mature follicles.

Shelley WB, Burmeister V, Eisenstat BA: **A mysterious growth on facial hairs**. J Am Acad Dermatol 1986; 14:1091–1092.

Orange-pink concretions on the fine vellus hairs of the face of a 45-year-old woman appeared shortly after a Caribbean vacation. They did not wash off and had been present for 2 months.

Scanning **electron microscopy** solved the mystery. The concretions were **tight knots of synthetic fibers** attached to the villus hairs. The source was a **powder puff** purchased in the Caribbean that had become very much attached to this patient. New concretions could be readily formed by rubbing the powder puff on her face. The color came from the pigment in the face powder.

One might say she had "plica Caribbeana."

Sometimes the diagnosis is made on a global assessment. At other times it's made on a papule!

574

Factitial Dermatitis

When the patient is the pathogen, we see dermatitis artefacta. Don't expect this patient to tell you he is the "pathogen." He won't. Nor will he tell you how he produces this strange disease.

It is up to you to suspect that the patient is producing the disease when the lesions presented are **bizarre**. If they look unnatural, geometric, and angular, they may well be the work of the patient. Another clue pointing to the diagnosis of dermatitis artefacta is the failure. of the patient to describe any sequence or course to the disease. Each **lesion springs de novo** with no past. The third diagnostic lead is the affect of these patients. There is the air of nonchalance, of **la belle indifférence**. Furthermore, they, unlike their families, do not become angered when you indicate they are indeed the pathogen.

It is easy to suspect this factitial dermatitis when the pathogenic mechanism involves picking, cutting, puncturing, slashing, or burning. Far more difficult to recognize is the pathogenic injections of ink, blood, or feces. Some patients acquire the fine art of forging masterpieces of skin disease.

Such patients may or may not be consciously aware of what they do. We have surmised that some may have multiple personalities. However, others will produce disease at the time and spot you suggest. We do know that factitial lesions are induced by another group of patients who are fully aware of what they are doing, the **malingerers**. They are the ones who are in need of a disease for Worker's Compensation, for litigation, or for release from a job, a societal or parental demand, a religious order, or the armed services. They may take a drug to which they know they are sensitive. They may substitute lab specimens for analysis, or alter lab reports. Often they describe spurious symptoms. The best malingerers always outwit the trusting physician who believes there is no deceit in the doctor-patient relationship.

As to differential diagnosis, there is no limit. For almost any diagnosis you can summon, the patient may be the pathogen. The classic example is the auto-erythrocyte sensitivity syndrome. Conversely, we have misdiagnosed the bizarre pattern of vasculitis as factitial.

It is wise to take any history with a grain of salt when the lesion and the patient seem strange.

Lyell A: **Cutaneous artifactual disease.** A review, amplified by personal experience. J Am Acad Dermatol 1979; 1:391–407.

This is the negative image of medicine. The patient is there to outwit, to mislead, and to misinform you. He presents you with **synthetic disease**, a facsimile of disease—factitial, pseudodisease. He recounts a history that is unreliable, deceitful, and false. Given a disease that is not true and a history not true, what can you do?

Learn to suspect artifactual disease when the skin changes are strange *and* the patient is emotionally immature. Learn to respect it also in the individual who has much to gain or to avoid by having dermatologic disability. Witness the worker on benefits for a hand eruption and the boy saved from piano lessons by his unexplained fingertip dermatitis.

Most patients have but an elementary knowledge of how to induce skin disease. They may abrade the skin, cut it with glass, burn it with lye, inject it with feces, or simply squeeze it. Only a few have the skill of inducing drug eruptions by surreptitious dosing with a drug to which they are sensitized. Only a few know of the photodermatitis so simply induced by exposing tarred skin to sunlight. But all poison ivy–sensitive patients know of an artifactual route open to them.

Learn to suspect artifactual disease when

the lesions are bizarre, linear, or geometric, or sharply marginated

the lesions appear overnight fully developed, unlike natural disease, which involves cell recruitment

the lesions are in different stages, since the invariable course of healing demands that the patient induce fresh ones or lose its diseased status.

the patient can forecast the site and timing

no new lesions appear when patient is under total surveillance 24 hours a day

no lesions appear in an area totally guarded (metal sheet incorporated in occlusive bandage to prevent injections through the bandage and ends tightly bound to prevent entry of a wire on a long needle

the history of the early stages of the disease is kept back by the patient

the parent gives you no history of the child's problem or its course

There is little help from the laboratory or biopsy. You must be a **clinical detective** looking for clues. Hospitalize and look for a syringe in the bed, epidermis under the fingernails, and caustics or sand paper in a suitcase or purse. Observe through one-way windows. Also do multiple patch tests to the same substance under different labels while predicting one will be positive.

Given that these patients need to deceive you with their "experimental disease," what are some of the **reasonable facsimiles they can make**?

Alopecia or alopecia areata
Bullous disease
Burns
Contact dermatitis
Excoriations
Gangrene
Nail dystrophy
Nodules
Purpura
Ulcers

Remember, these patients cling to disease as vigorously as others cling to health. You will not loosen their grasp by making a diagnosis they already know. But you will enhance your grasp of how to treat them.

Lyell A: **Dermatitis artefacta** in relation to the syndrome of contrived disease. Clin Exp Dermatol 1976; 1:109–126.

Why do you miss the diagnosis of factitial disease?

You believe blindly what the patient tells you.

You think that rank, education, intelligence, devotion to duty, and an exemplary character exclude the possibility of self-inflicted lesions.

You fear missing organic disease and rare syndromes.

You feel that you are betraying the patient, the family, and the referring doctor's trust in you by making such a diagnosis.

Why do the patients do it? To gain:

Sympathy	Narcotics
Pity	Money
Attention	Escape from duties
Hospitalization	Rewards inherent in masochism

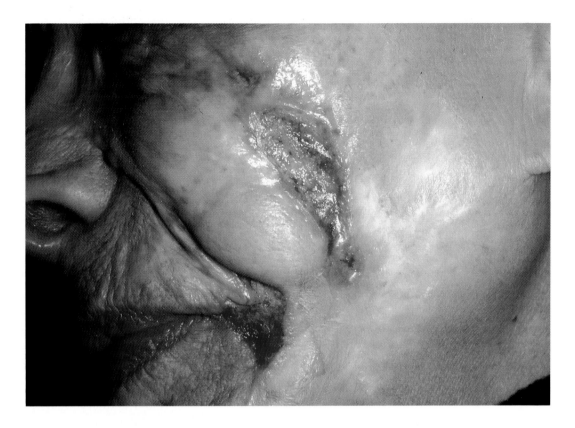

How do they do it?

Cutting	Biting
Slashing	Injecting
Slicing	Beating
Scratching	Poisoning
Burning	Puncturing

How do you recognize it?

Imagine it when confronted by the bizarre.
Think of it when you see the "unthinkable."
Consider it when lesions stop appearing under total surveillance.
Remember it if you sense that the lesions are rewarding to the patient.
Look for it in nail dystrophies.

Tucker WFG, Harrington CI, Underwood JCE: Recurrent **herpes simplex infection masquerading as dermatitis artefacta**. Arch Dermatol 1987; 123:435–436.

For 15 years this 58-year-old widow suffered **recurrent excoriated areas** on the right cheek, which evolved into ulceration and scarring. For 15 years she carried the diagnosis of **factitial dermatitis**. Not until a biopsy was made 15 years later and the herpesvirus antigen demonstrated by immunohistochemistry was the **correct diagnosis of recurrent herpes simplex** made and appropriate treatment with acyclovir started.

Egger B, Goerz G: **Artefacts** in a patient with **porphyria cutanea tarda** (PCT). Ztschr Hautkr 1990; 65:592–596.

After a year and a half of chloroquine therapy for porphyria cutanea tarda, this 56-year-old man had absolutely normal laboratory values. However, the diagnostic bullous skin changes persisted on his hands. The patient, when confronted with a diagnosis of self-induced lesions, admitted to producing the "**PCT lesions**" **by manual trauma.**

Some patients feel best when they don't feel well.

Miori L, Vignini M, Rabbiosi G: **Flagellate dermatitis after bleomycin**. A histological and immunohistochemical study. Am J Dermatopathol 1990; 12:598–602.

Within hours after the first injection of a bleomycin-containing polychemo-therapeutic mix, this patient with Hodgkin's disease experienced a **pruritic striate eruption**. Ten days later strange erythematous urticarial linear bands persisted. When the therapy was discontinued 3 weeks later, the erythema disappeared spontaneously, leaving a flagellate pattern of pigmentation. A diagnosis of **drug eruption due to bleomycin** was made. Readministration of the associated drugs (Adriamycin, vincristine, and dacarbazine) had no effect.

Gorman WF, Winograd M: Crossing the border from **Munchausen to malingering**. J Fla Med Assoc 1988; 75:147–150.

Malingering (shamming illness) is the exaggeration or **simulation of disease** to **obtain money, receive drugs, or evade responsibility**. This is not a physical or mental disorder. Look for a dramatic performance of a deceptive medical actor. Make the diagnosis cautiously using the term "probable malingering." Sometimes elements of both Munchausen syndrome and malingering are present.

Example: A 25-year-old woman claimed that while she was shopping in a store a hollow fiber glass mannequin of the upper body, natural size, became unbolted and fell from a table 30 inches high, striking her head. She stated that a previous seizure disorder had been aggravated by the head injury and later caused her to have an automobile crash, which resulted in paraplegia. She sought damages from the store. Her numerous past hospitalizations included 13 CT scans and 4 myelograms; she was taking 12 methadone tablets daily for pain. Following the car accident, which occurred while she was alone in her parked car or was parking, there was no detectable musculoskeletal or neurologic damage. However, at age 27, she appeared in a motorized wheelchair wearing an oxygen mask. The defense counsel believed that a jury would be prejudiced toward her and she was given settlement.

The *Munchausen syndrome* is a self-inflicted ("factitious") disorder in which the patient **compulsively causes medical and surgical injuries** and thereby **obtains drugs, hospitalization, and operations**. Aliases are often used. According to this article, "The signs and symptoms are limited only by the creativity, cunning, and medical experience of the patient." They include factitious fever, dermatitis, bleeding, and abscesses. Drug dependence often results from complaints of pain and demand for drugs. The patient is very familiar with medical terms and procedures and often is a health professional. Examination shows multiple surgical scars. The patient's history is dramatic, fanciful, and false but marginally plausible. Pathologic lying may include florid descriptions of unwitnessed seizures.

Example: A 36-year-old male nurse's aide with pathologic obesity and many past hospitalizations was admitted with severe left-sided chest pain, weakness of the left arm and leg, and difficulty speaking. Neurologic workup was negative and symptoms remitted. When they resumed 8 weeks later with paralysis of the left arm, a psychogenic cause was suspected. During an amytal interview, the patient moved his left arm and hand well.

Michalowski R: **Munchausen's syndrome:** A new variety of bleeding type self-inflicted **cheilorrhagia** and **cheilitis glandularis**. Dermatologica 1985; 170:94–97.

A 20-year-old woman had had 13 years of **recurrent bleeding** from the lower **lip**. She stated that she had thrombocytopenia and menorrhea lasting up to 3 weeks. The bleeding lip had required **18 hospitalizations** in 12 different hospitals, with a **recent diagnosis of cheilitis glandularis**. On admission this time a heavy crust of dried blood covered the lower lip. Removal disclosed numerous fissures, linear scars, and a score of dark red spots which discharged watery mucus on pressure. Palpation revealed nodules the size of pellets. Extensive tests, including psychiatric evaluation, revealed no hematologic or medical abnormalities. Excision (wedge-shaped glandulectomy) of the heterotopic salivary glands was followed by good healing, but the bleeding returned. It was inexplicable until another patient observed her lacerating her lip with a thread. After this revelation, she promptly fled, permitting no follow-up.

Patients with Munchausen's syndrome love to bleed. Ordinarily, they bleed from the nasopharynx, gums, ears, eyes, stomach, urinary tract, or vagina. This patient was a first: a Munchausen case who loved to munch on her lips!

Maurice PDL, Rivers JK, Jones C, Cronin E: Dermatitis artefacta with **artefact of patch tests**. Clin Exp Dermatol 1987; 12:204–206.

A **bullous eruption** of the right hand that spread up the arm to the shoulder in a 17-year-old female veterinary assistant rapidly healed under occlusive dressings. A biopsy showed a subepidermal bulla with complete necrosis of the overlying epidermis. Direct immunofluorescence of perilesional skin was negative. New bullae on the other arm and legs prompted the parents to demand patch tests for determining her "allergies." **Ten patch tests to yellow petrolatum** were applied to her back. A noninflammatory **bulla** developed 2 days later **at just one of the test sites**. The patient and her parents denied any possibility of self-inflicted disease and retreated to a homeopathic physician for further care of her factitial blisters.

Two additional experiences with other female patients are cited to alert the physician to do deceptive patch testing in the deceptive patient. The patch tests should be applied so that the patient cannot identity them, and results should be interpreted with caution.

Christie R, Bay C, Kaufman I, et al: **Lesch-Nyhan disease:** Clinical experience with 19 patients. Dev Med Child Neurol 1982; 24:293–306.

Self-mutilation by **biting the lips, fingertips, and shoulders** is a constant finding in this recessive syndrome affecting males. In this commentary the index fingers and thumbs were most often attacked, and biting broke the skin. All patients have virtually complete absence of the enzyme hypoxanthine guanine phosphoribosyltransferase, with resulting hyperuricemia and increased urinary uric acid. "**Orange sand**" in the diaper is often the earliest sign and may begin soon after birth. **Neurologic signs** begin between 3 and 5 months of age as poor motor development, spasticity, choreoathetoid involuntary movements, opisthotonos, and mental retardation.

Ishii N, Kawaguchi H, Miyakawa K, Nakajima H: Congenital **sensory neuropathy** with **anhidrosis**. Arch Dermatol 1988; 124:564–566.

An infant Japanese girl had **recurrent episodes of high fever** and hyperventilation when she was in a hot environment. Although her sweat glands were histologically normal, inability to sweat was confirmed by intradermal pharmacologic tests for autonomic nervous system functioning:

histamine 1:1000 (0.05 ml)–wheal but no axonal flare
atropine sulfate 1:10,000 (0.1 ml)–no sweating
acetylcholine chloride 1:10,000 (0.1 ml)–no sweating
epinephrine hydrochloride 1:30,000 (0.1 ml)–no sweating
neostigmine methylsulfate 1:10,000 (0.1 ml)–no sweating

An associated problem was **self-mutilation** due to her complete absence of pain sensation. She was given to biting her fingers and had bitten off much of her tongue. Before reaching 2 years of age, she died during an episode of hyperthermia.

The **differential diagnosis** included other forms of anhidrosis and inability to feel pain:

congenital ectodermal dysplasia
congenital sensory neuropathy
congenital indifference to pain
familial dysautonomia (Riley-Day syndrome)
hereditary sensory radicular neuropathy

Burket JM, Burket BA: **Factitial dermatitis resulting in paraplegia.** J Am Acad Dermatol 1987; 17:306–307.

A 56-year-old schoolteacher with a 4-year history of necrotic excoriations of the upper back eventually paralyzed herself. As shown by cultures, S. aureus from her skin produced bacteremia with organisms lodging in her vertebral bodies, causing osteomyelitis with subsequent collapse of the vertebral body of T_8, resulting in paraplegia.

The right way to take a history is to write it right away.

Flushing

The patients who come to you with the problem of flushing are not looking for a diagnosis but for the reason why. They will be asking you to find a cause other than heat, heredity, anxiety, alcohol intake, menopause, or migraine itself. These causes of vasodilatation are common knowledge and rarely lead a patient to seek a physician's aid.

You will be consulted regarding the exaggerated, unexplained episodic flush. First look to food. Is it gustatory flushing where eating itself triggered attacks? Or is there a specific food or food additive responsible? Possibly, a food diary is necessary. The patient may not realize that monosodium glutamate (Accent) used in seasoning can induce flushing. Likewise, attention should be paid to salads, hot dogs, and ham containing sodium sulfite. Hot peppers and very hot foods speak for themselves. More subtle are the flushes that result from having mushrooms and an alcoholic drink.

The explanation for cause must include a careful drug history. Metronidazole with or without alcohol may provoke flushing. Nicotinic acid as well as calcium channel blockers (e.g., nifedipine) produce flushing due to vasodilatation.

Look to the occupation. The worker in the dry atmosphere of a "sealed tight" office building may have chronic flushing due to a low-grade xerosis. Exposure to organic solvents is another occupational cause of flushing. Remember that an inappropriate degree of flushing in a worker or individual exposed to heat may be the clue that the primary cause is occult anhidrosis.

With failure to discern an exogenous cause, the search must be directed to the presence of circulating vasodilators. The simplest test is for 5-HIAA (5-hydroxyindoleacetic acid) in the urine. When found in unexplained elevated levels, 5-HIAA suggests the presence of a serotonin-secreting tumor such as the carcinoid tumor of the gut. This serotonin, acting as a vasodilator, may also act in consonance with another tumor-derived vasodilator, histamine.

Thus, measurement of a battery of vasodilators in the blood is indicated. These include serotonin, histamine, substance P, and bradykinin.

High-level serotonin directs the search to radiologic demonstration of carcinoid tumors of the gut. Elevation of the histamine levels may also suggest a carcinoid tumor or mastocytosis. Other sources of vasoactive agents may be bronchogenic carcinoma, pancreatic tumors, and vipomas.

When all the biochemical parameters remain quietly normal, you must recall that autoimmunity to estrogen or progesterone may be the cause. This can be best demonstrated by a direct intradermal or intramuscular challenge test.

Finally, the patient who has flushed and blushed all his life may come to you with the permanent flush of rosacea. It is essential in his treatment that he be made aware of all the causes of flushing.

Wilkin JK: **Flushing reactions.** *In* Rook AJ, Maibach HI (eds): Recent Advances in Dermatology, No. Six. London, Churchill Livingstone, 1983, pp 157–187.

Flushing produced by autonomic activity is associated with sweating. Vasoactive agents acting on vascular smooth muscle (without neural mediation) cause dry flushing.

I. Flushing reactions related to **alcohol**:

There is increased susceptibility in mongoloid populations. Occupational "degreaser" flush occurs in workmen drinking beer after exposure to industrial solvents such as trichloroethylene vapor, N,N-dimethylformamide, and N-butyraldoxime.

Fermented alcoholic beverages (beer, sherry) may contain tyramine or histamine, which induce flushing.

Drugs
  disulfiram (Antabuse)
  chlorpropamide (Diabinese)
  calcium carbamide (urea)
  phentolamine (Regitine)
  griseofulvin
  metronidazole (Flagyl)
  Beta-lactams with methyltetrazolethiol side chain (cephalosporin antibiotics)
    cefamandole (Mandol)
    cefoperazone (Cefobid)
    moxalactam (Moxam)
Eating mushrooms while consuming alcohol.
Carcinoid flushing–Alcohol may release a catecholamine that acts on tumor cells.

II. Flushing related to **food additives**:

Monosodium glutamate (MSG) in a large dose may cause Chinese restaurant syndrome.

Sodium nitrite in cured meats (frankfurters, bacon, salami, ham) may cause headache and flushing.

Sulfites (potassium metabisulfite) may cause wheezing and flushing.

III. Flushing associated with **eating**:

Hot beverages cause flushing through countercurrent heat exchange into blood vessels leading to the anterior hypothalamus.

Auriculotemporal flushing: unilateral flushing, heat, and sweating following parotid gland injury with misdirected regeneration of parasympathetic nerves.

Gustatory flushing: bilateral flushing, salivation, sweating, lacrimation, and nasal secretion with no history of parotid gland injury. This may be reproduced by chewing a chili pepper (Capsicum minimum) and holding it in the mouth for 5 minutes.

Dumping syndrome: Facial flushing is associated with tachycardia, sweating, dizziness, weakness, and gastrointestinal disturbances. Symptoms begin after gastric surgery and are provoked by a meal or ingestion of hot fluids or hypertonic glucose. The syndrome becomes worse with menopause.

IV. **Neurologic** flushing:

anxiety
simple blushing
brain tumors
spinal cord lesions (autonomic hyperreflexia)
orthostatic hypotension
migraine headaches
Parkinson's disease

V. Flushing due to **drugs**:

all vasodilators (e.g., nitroglycerin)
all calcium channel blockers:
  nifedipine (Procardia)

verapamil (Calan)
diltiazem (Cardizem)
nicotinic acid (not nicotinamide); flush may be blocked with aspirin or
 indomethacin
morphine
amyl nitrite and butyl nitrite (recreational drugs)
cholinergic drugs
bromocriptine (Parlodel)
thyrotropin-releasing hormone (TRH)
tamoxifen (Nolvadex)
cyproterone acetate
triamcinolone
cyclosporine A (Sandimmune)

Kasha EE, Norins AL: **Scombroid fish poisoning with facial flushing.** J Am Acad Dermatol 1988; 18:1363–1365.

A 51-year-old woman developed a sharply demarcated nonpruritic **heliotrope flush** of her face, arms, and trunk 30 minutes after having eaten broiled **mackerel**. The erythema had gone by 2 hours.

The diagnosis of scombroid (**mackerel, tuna, bonito**) fish poisoning was consistent. The patient was under no stress, had had no menopausal flushes, and had drunk no alcohol with her meal. Further checking revealed that the food had no added sodium monoglutamate or sodium nitrites. She was not taking any drug. Carcinoid flushing was ruled out since there were no additional attacks and the patient experienced no diarrhea or asthma. Also she noted no hyperhidrosis, piloerection, or hypertension, which permitted exclusion of a pheochromocytoma-associated flush.

Scombroid fish poisoning results from **bacteria** acting on improperly refrigerated fish. The histidine present is decarboxylated to form **histamine**. This can reach levels of 100 mg/100 gm of flesh. Combined with a toxin known as saurine, it can, when ingested, produce

peppery taste	diarrhea
oral burning	urticaria
flushing	headache
nausea, emesis	
cramps	

Note that cooking does not destroy the toxin and **even canned tuna** may produce such facial flushing.

Biskind MS: **Vasomotor reactions** persisting for 20 years in a male: treatment with androgens. J Clin Endocrinol Metab 1942; 2:187–188.

A 52-year-old Austrian man developed **recurrent flushes** with perspiration following bilateral inguinal herniorrhaphy and resultant testicular atrophy. Flushes occurred every half hour, lasted 2 to 3 minutes, and greatly interfered with his life. He had a feminine body contour with absent pubic and axillary hair. The testicles were not palpable. Flushing disappeared with **androgen therapy**.

Schimke RN, McKusick VA, Huang T, Pollack AD: **Homocystinuria.** Studies of 20 families with 38 affected members. JAMA 1965; 193:711–719.

Screening of patients with either ectopia lentis or presumed Marfan's syndrome revealed that about 5% have homocystinuria. Look for a **malar flush** that becomes unusually vivid in hot weather with exertion and may lead to

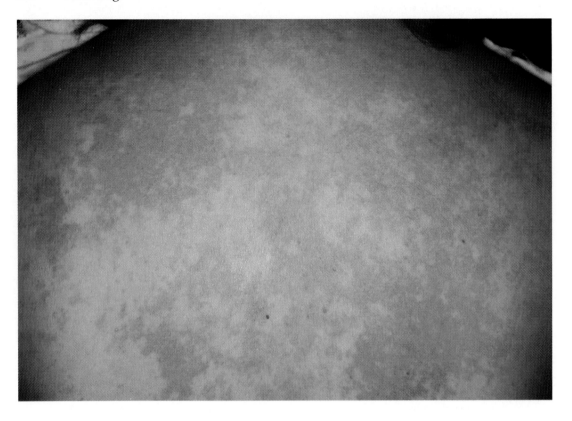

intense violaceous telangiectatic flushing of the entire face. Livedo reticularis of the trunk and extremities is frequent. Patients may die at a young age of arterial or venous thrombosis heralded by arterial bruits, loss of pulses, hypertension, and ischemia. Thrombosis of the inferior vena cava may lead to **large dilated veins** on the chest and abdomen. Recurrent thrombophlebitis in the extremities with pulmonary embolism also occurs. Seizures and localized neurologic signs reflect intracranial thromboses. Thromboses are not found in Marfan's syndrome.

The eye signs of homocystinuria and Marfan's syndrome are identical, including progressive lens displacement, myopia, retinal detachment, and glaucoma. Skeletal changes are also similar in these patients with long thin extremities, tall stature, pectus excavatum, and scoliosis. They differ, however, in that homocystinuria patients have generalized osteoporosis and a **tight feel to the joints** rather than the loose-jointedness and arachnodactyly seen in Marfan's patients. Many patients with homocystinuria are retarded, and most patients have nervousness.

Other cutaneous features of homocystinuria include light hair and skin color and sparse or coarse hair. In older patients the facial skin is coarse and wide-pored. They lack the striae distensae common in Marfan's syndrome.

Homocystinuria is autosomal recessive, in contrast to Marfan's, which is autosomal dominant. Homocystinuria and cystinuria are distinguished by high-voltage paper **electrophoresis**. Urinary stones and tissue deposits do not occur in homocystinuria, in contrast to cystinuria.

Waldhäusl W: To flush or not to flush? Comments on the chlorpropamide-alcohol flush. Diabetologia 1984; 26:12–14.

The following are the real or putative vasoactive **mediators for flushing**:

histamine	kallikrein
prostaglandins	lysyl-bradykinin
serotonin	met-enkephalin
acetaldehyde	substance P

Levine R, Taylor WB: Take tea and see. Arch Dermatol 1986; 122:856.

An extreme degree of **erythema** and slight edema enveloped the head, neck, and upper trunk of a 44-year-old man the morning after having several cups of a South Pacific **herbal tea**, Kava-Kava or kava. Despite steroid therapy, the erythema did not begin to fade for a week. The Kava-Kava tea was clearly the cause, as drinking the same tea had produced generalized erythema 3 months previously requiring hospitalization. The mechanism is not known but probably reflects an idiosyncratic toxic effect of the pyrones present in Kava-Kava, a popular drink in Samoa. To date, only lemon-yellow discoloration of the skin has been recorded as a side effect.

It would seem wise to remain a teetotaler when it comes to Kava-Kava.

Mulley GP: **Flushing.** J R Coll Physicians Lond 12:359–364, 1978.

Look for **tumors** producing catecholamines, vasoactive hormones, or other mediators, e.g., pheochromocytoma, bronchogenic carcinoma, pancreatic tumor, thyroid medullary carcinoma.

Patients with **horseshoe kidneys** experience flushing, nausea, and pain (Rovsing syndrome), which are relieved by an antiflexed position.

Flushing may signal the presence of rare tumors, such as malignant histiocytoma, neuroblastoma, ganglioneuroma, renal cell carcinoma, or basophilic granulocytic leukemia.

Diagnosis is easy; the only thing you have to know is the name of the disease.

Folliculitis

You've made the diagnosis of folliculitis. The patient has perifollicular focal erythema or pustules pierced by a terminal or vellus hair. But why?

The answer may be in the smear. You may see the commonplace gram-positive cocci of a staph infection, the unusual gram-negative bacteria of a *Pseudomonas* infection, or the pleomorphic rods of a propionibacterial infection. Or you may see the oval yeast forms of a Pityrosporum infection or the follicle mite *Demodex folliculorum.* With a silver stain you may see bacteria that are gram-stain invisible.

The answer may be in the culture. You may get a report of *Staphylococcus aureus, Pseudomonas,* or other gram-negative bacteria. If you ordered anaerobic cultures, you may receive a report of the pathogen *Propionibacterium acnes.* But naught if you forgot.

The answer may be in the biopsy. The folliculitis may be due to a retention phenomenon with follicular rupture. Or it may prove to be a necrotizing form, such as acnitis due to vasculitis. Most interestingly, it may be an eosinophilic folliculitis with swarms of eosinophils accounting for the follicular damage and inflammation. And in some biopsies of papules the diagnosis of folliculitis is the surprise.

The answer may be in the history—take one carefully. It may be the hormonally triggered folliculitis of pregnancy. It could be the folliculitis of bowel-bypass surgery. It may be due to an allergen or irritant chemical powder in the workplace that remains in the follicular pit even after washing. It may be the actinic folliculitis that comes only with sun exposure. It may be the pseudofolliculitis induced by shaving. It could be the folliculitis induced by vaseline-based topical ointments.

You made the diagnosis of folliculitis, but it was wrong. In that case you probably forgot to consider the look-alike, pustular miliaria.

Finally, do not forget that from small acorns of folliculitis great forests of inflammation may grow. These include perifolliculitis capitis abscedens et suffodiens (dissecting cellulitis of the scalp), acne keloidalis, furuncles, and carbuncles.

Blankenship ML: **Gram-negative folliculitis:** Follow-up observations in 20 patients. Arch Dermatol 1984; 120:1301–1303.

Gram-negative folliculitis:		Infection with gram-negative organisms occurring as complication of acne vulgaris.
Look for it:		Sudden flare of pustular or cystic lesions in patients resistant to treatment.
Clinical:	80%	Superficial pustules without comedones from intranasal area to chin and cheek.
	20%	Deep nodular cystic lesions.
Culture:	80%	Lactose-fermenting gram-negative rods, e.g., *Klebsiella, Escherichia, Serratia, Enterobacteriaceae.*
	20%	*Proteus* organisms in nares.
Treatment:		Responds in 2 weeks to ampicillin or trimethoprim-sulfamethoxazole.

Alomar A, Ausina V, Vernis J, de Moragas JM: *Pseudomonas* **folliculitis.** Cutis 1982; 30:405–409.

Thirty-three patients with gram-negative folliculitis due to *Pseudomonas aeruginosa* are described. All worked or had been patients in a hospital at which exposure to *Pseudomonas* in feces could have occurred. Multiple scattered **erythematous papules** were the presenting sign. These lesions were follicular in origin and some had a central pustule. The papules were recurrent and could remain, eluding diagnosis for up to 3 years. Especially significant was the finding of 9 women with lesions on the legs following **depilation**.

Cultures of the pustules was the critical diagnostic procedure and sensitivity studies essential for guidance in therapy. The best topical agent was Silvadene cream (silver sulfadiazine).

Pseudomonas folliculitis is also well known to occur in those who frequent public baths, hot tubs, and whirlpool baths. **Superhydrated skin** is especially susceptible to infections.

Lotem M, Ingber A, Filhaber A, Sandbank M: Skin infection provoked by **coagulase-negative** *Staphylococcus* resembling gram-negative folliculitis. Cutis 1988; 42:443–444.

Superficial monomorphic pustules covered the chin, cheeks, and nose of a 22-year-old electrician under long-term treatment with tetracycline for cystic acne. He had had 3 prior similar episodes of pustules covering his face and to a lesser extent his upper back and chest. They were not prevented by systemic ampicillin, tetracycline, or erythromycin. Although gram-negative folliculitis was suspected, **cultures** implicated **coagulase-negative staphylococci**. Treatment with minocycline was curative and prevented further attacks.

Presumably, tetracycline produced an imbalance of bacterial flora, permitting low-virulence coagulase-negative staphylococci to flourish as facultative anaerobes in deeper parts of the hair follicles and induce crops of follicular pustules.

Coagulase-negative staphylococci most commonly cause infections of implanted prosthetic devices. *Staphylococcus saprophyticus* types also cause acute urinary infections in women, nongonococcal urethritis in men, and occasional minor skin infections such as superficial folliculitis.

Maibach HI: **Acne necroticans** (varioliformis) versus *Propionibacterium acnes* folliculitis. J Am Acad Dermatol 1989; 21:323.

Smears of intact pustules on staining may reveal gram-positive pleomorphic rods. These are the putative *Corynebacterium acnes* (*Propionibacterium acnes*). Culture under anaerobic conditions of material taken from an intact pustule will show *P. acnes* in examples of folliculitis due to this organism.

Brozena SJ, Cohen LE, Fenske NA: **Folliculitis decalvans**—response to rifampin. Cutis 1988; 42:512–515.

A 10 × 12 cm **erythematous atrophic plaque on the scalp** with marked **alopecia** and loss of hair follicle orifices was seen in a 42-year-old woman. Around the edges of the plaque were discrete, honey-colored **pustules**. For 10 months she had experienced recurrent episodes of painful scalp infections with resultant hair loss, thought to be infected seborrheic dermatitis. However, a topical steroid solution and various systemic antibiotics, as well as oral isotretinoin (40 mg/day), had been without effect. A skin biopsy showed acute suppurative folliculitis and chronic perifolliculitis with plasma cells, and *Staphylococcus aureus* grew from the pustules. The disease progressed for the next 9 months despite a variety of treatments. Finally, rifampin (600 mg/day) for 10 weeks led to total resolution and cure.

Folliculitis decalvans is characterized by irregular, smooth cicatricial plaques with inflammatory folliculitis and pinhead-sized miliary abscesses at the periphery. It is to be **distinguished from** other forms of inflammatory scarring alopecia such as kerion, carbuncle, lupus vulgaris, morphea, atrophic lichen planus, perifolliculitis capitis abscedens et suffodiens, ulerythema, and lupus erythematosus.

Bäck O, Faergemann J, Hornqvist R: ***Pityrosporum* folliculitis:** A common disease of the young and middle aged. J Am Acad Dermatol 1985; 12:56–61.

A study of 51 patients with histologically proven and culturally confirmed *Pityrosporum* folliculitis showed the following:

Clinical picture

> small dome-shaped, follicular papules and pustules
> usually on upper back, shoulders, and chest
> sometimes on arms, legs, face, even dorsum of hands
> at times excoriated
> sought attention because of itch
> premenstrual flare of itch

Differential diagnosis—prior misdiagnoses included

> acne vulgaris
> dermographic prurigo
> chronic urticaria
> eczema
> neurotic excoriations
> superficial folliculitis pruritus
> associated disease in some cases
>> pityriasis versicolor
>> seborrheic dermatitis
>> acne vulgaris

Diagnostic tests

> Direct microscopic examination:
>> KOH show round budding yeast cells
>> Scotch tape stripping: stain with methylene blue
> Culture
>> curettement material placed on glucose-neopeptone-yeast extract medium containing olive oil. Incubated at 37°C for 3 days. *P. orbiculare* isolated in 37 of 44 patients.
> Histopathology
>> Punch biopsy shows black, round, and budding yeast cells in upper half of hair follicle.

Watch for this condition in young women complaining of itching of the upper trunk. The lack of comedones differentiates it from acne. Think of it in anyone with pruritic follicular papules.

Lim KB, Boey LP, Khatijah M: Gram's stained microscopy in the etiological diagnosis of **Malassezia (*Pityrosporon*) folliculitis.** Arch Dermatol 1988; 124:492.

In each of 30 men with *Pityrosporon* folliculitis follicular material was collected from pustular lesions using a comedo extractor and smeared on a glass slide. A Gram stain of the specimen demonstrated gram-positive yeast-like spores in clusters of 5 to 20 and unipolar conidia-bearing spores typical of *Malassezia furfur*.

Yeast folliculitis characteristically presents with erythematous follicular papules and pustules on the upper trunk and upper arms. It is common in patients with acne being treated with long-term antibiotics and may be mistaken for an extension of their acne. The diagnosis can be rapidly confirmed using the aforementioned technique.

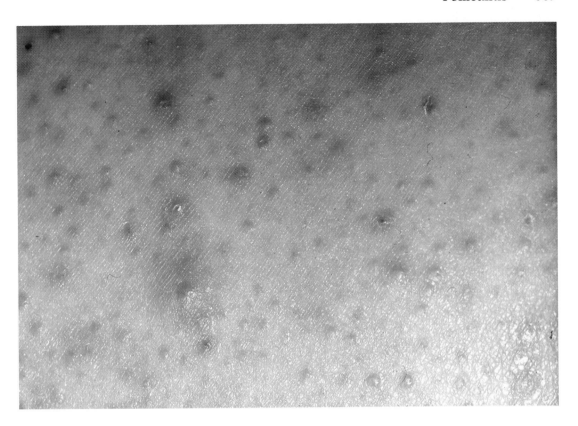

Purcell SM, Hayes TJ, Dixon SL: **Pustular folliculitis** associated with *Demodex folliculorum.* J Am Acad Dermatol 1986; 15:1159–1162.

Acute folliculitis of the right cheek of a 49-year-old man appeared to be of bacterial origin; however, dicloxacillin and erythromycin orally were without effect. The lesion was a 3-cm erythematous plaque studded with 1- to 2-mm **follicular pustules.** The possibility of tinea faciei led to a KOH scraping. This failed to reveal any hyphae but showed hundreds of elongated, transparent mites. As many as 20 mites could be seen on low power (× 40) field. Control scrapings from the left cheek showed only one mite in the entire specimen.

A diagnosis of folliculitis **due to *Demodex folliculorum*** was made. This was confirmed by complete involution of the eruption and virtual disappearance of the demodex within 12 hours of applying crotamiton (Eurax) cream twice/day.

Ofuji S: **Eosinophilic pustular folliculitis.** Dermatologica 1987; 174:53–56.

An authoritative review by the man who originally described the disease in 1970. Crops of pruritic, **follicular papulopustules** in fairly well-defined areas extend centrifugally to form annular or **polycyclic configurations**. The pustules wax and wane over long periods, leaving slight pigmentation as they subside. Lesions usually begin on the face and are present there in 85% of patients. The back and extensor surface of the arms are other common locations, and palmoplantar pustules occur in 20%. It is five times more common in males and most cases have been in Orientals. Steroids and indomethacin are effective treatments.

Laboratory studies

Bacterial cultures—no growth.
CBC—leukocytosis with eosinophilia.

Serum IgE–sometimes increased.

Histology–spongiosis, vesiculation, and an infiltrate of eosinophils, neutrophils, and mononuclear cells in the outer root sheath above the level of the sebaceous duct entry. Perivascular mononuclear cells and eosinophils surround the involved follicles.

Other conditions with eosinophilic infiltration of follicles:

AIDS
Autoimmune progesterone dermatitis of pregnancy
Eosinophilic pustular folliculitis in infancy
Erythema toxicum neonatorum
Generalized pustular toxic erythema
Pruritic folliculitis of pregnancy
Pustular eruption with eosinophilic
    abscesses

Combemale P, Courtois D, Chouvet B: **La folliculite perforante.** Ann Dermatol Venereol 1990; 117:515–520.

A disseminate papular eruption of the abdomen, flanks, and buttocks of this 20-year-old man proved on biopsy to be a **folliculitis due to perforation** of the sides of the hair follicles. There was an ensuing formation of granulomas around extruded keratin and hair debris. Pseudoepitheliomatous epithelial hyperplasia also accounted for the papules.

It is conjectured that dyskeratosis may be the cause of the perforation.

Barr DJ, Riley RJ, Greco DJ: **Bypass phrynoderma:** Vitamin A deficiency associated with bowel bypass surgery. Arch Dermatol 1984; 120:919–921.

Multiple brown-red papules and nodules with central keratotic plugs appeared on the legs and arms of this 45-year-old woman 4 years after her last intestinal bypass surgery. A biopsy showed **perforating folliculitis** and the serum vitamin A level proved to be low (5 ng/ml versus a normal of 20 to 80 ng/ml). Within a month of vitamin A therapy (50,000 U/day) not only had her skin cleared completely, but her previously unnoted night blindness had disappeared.

The vitamin A deficiency responsible for the lesions was thought to result from diminished absorption caused by the rapid intestinal transit time. The long latent period after surgery is well recognized.

Phrynoderma is an uncommon complication of bypass surgery. The usual lesions are papules, pustules, and erythema nodosum.

Strauss JS, Kligman AM: **Pseudofolliculitis** of the beard. Arch Dermatol 1956; 74:533–542.

The characteristic lesions are erythematous firm papules and pustules containing **buried hairs**, principally on the undersurface of the chin and neck. Acute impetiginization associated with coagulase-negative micrococci (normal skin residents) leads to inflammation, oozing, and crusting. Fine linear, depressed crisscrossed scars result.

This "notoriously chronic and rebellious" disease results from strongly curved hair follicles that produce **curved ingrown hairs** with inflammation. The disease is seen **only in those who shave**. Thus, shaving is another habit that may be dangerous to one's health.

Barlow RJ, Schulz EJ: **Necrotizing folliculitis** in AIDS-related complex. Br J Dermatol 1987; 116:581–584.

Pimples and painful red lumps on the back, arms, and legs were the presenting complaint of a 20-year-old homosexual man. Examination disclosed erythematous follicular papules and scaling hyperpigmented macules and papules, 3 to 6 mm in diameter. Antibodies to HTLV III were present. Biopsy of a papule showed severe necrotizing folliculitis with underlying vasculitis. No bacteria or fungi were found.

The eruption is viewed as a form of **vasculitis** that can mimic bacterial folliculitis.

Kossard S, Collins A, McCrossin I: **Necrotizing lymphocytic folliculitis:** The early lesion of acne necrotica (varioliformis). J Am Acad Dermatol 1987; 16:1007–1014.

Acne necrotica is an uncommon problem in which crops of erythematous papules undergo central necrosis and heal with varioliform scars. Usually they localize on the forehead and nose but may extend onto the anterior scalp. The midchest and interscapular area may also be involved. The course is chronic, persisting for decades.

There is a nonscarring version, **acne necrotica miliaris**, characteristically involving minute, extremely itchy follicular vesicopustules. In the scalp the only marker is minute crusted excoriations.

In the **differential**, one has to consider lupus miliaris disseminatus faciei (acnitis). Here the lesions are yellow-brown papules with central adherent crust. They do not involve the scalp, do not scar, and are usually seen on the eyelids, cheeks, or even axillae. They show a sarcoidal pattern histologically in contrast to the lymphocytic folliculitis seen in acne necrotica.

Norris PG, Hawk JLM: **Actinic folliculitis**—response to isotretinoin. Clin Exp Dermatol 1989; 14:69–71.

For the past 6 summers, this 42-year-old female had experienced intermittent attacks of a severe pruritic follicular **pustular eruption of her chin**. In addition, there were uniform erythematous 1 to 3 mm papules. The attacks occurred 6 to 24 hours after sun exposure and persisted for 3 days. She could anticipate the onset each May and a gradual development of immunity by October. However, even in winter a day with sun reflected on snow could precipitate an attack. The lesions left no scars.

The problem was not acne for there were no comedones. Furthermore, she had never had acne and had never used corticosteroids. It was not a gram-negative folliculitis; cultures showed only normal skin flora. Tetracycline orally and a sunscreen topically provided no benefit. Only the administration of isotretinoin (0.35 mg/kg/day) provided a cure.

The process most closely resembled the **Mallorca acne** (acne aestivalis) described by Hjorth, but that condition did not commonly present as a pustular eruption.

Nieboer C: **Actinic superficial folliculitis;** a new entity? Br J Dermatol 1985; 112:603–606.

Every time a 19-year-old woman **sunbathed** or used a commercial sun lamp, she developed numerous small follicular pustules the same evening on her back, upper chest, shoulders, and extensor side of the upper arms. Her face was exempt. The rash quickly evolved into a burning pustular eruption that spontaneously cleared in about 10 days of sun avoidance.

Biopsy showed intrafollicular pustules with subcorneal abscesses over the adjacent epidermis and small superficial perivascular infiltrates. Immunofluorescence was negative. It was not possible to reproduce this sterile pustular reaction by phototests or photopatch tests, although exposure to a commercial UVA sun lamp did reproduce the lesions. Accordingly, a diagnosis was made of actinic superficial folliculitis. The **differential diagnosis** included:

acne aestivalis (involves face also).
miliaria rubra pustulosa (pruritic, involves sweat glands).
transient acantholytic dermatosis (shows acantholysis).
Bockhardt's impetigo (bacteria present).
yeast folliculitis (*Pityrosporon* organisms present in large numbers).
phototoxic reaction to perfume (positive photopatch tests).

An immunocompromised patient compromises your diagnostic skill.

Genetic Disease

The fault lies not in their stars but in their genes. Very little of what is seen in practice has not been touched, altered, or actually imprinted by the patient's own DNA. Usually the influence is subtle, such as in resistance to infectious disease or actinic damage. Or it may be apparent in the history of alopecia or psoriasis as a family trait. But most dramatic of all are the morphologic manifestations of a mutant gene. Here we see congenital ichthyosiform erythroderma, epidermolysis bullosa, and neurofibromatosis. Many times we see strange rarities that send us first to our illustrated text, der Kaloustian and Kurban's "Genetic Diseases of the Skin." If no picture matches, we turn to the ninth edition of the master reference of McKusick, "Mendelian Inheritance in Man."

Once we can name the disorder, we satisfy our thirst to know of what's behind what we see by consulting Alper's splendid multiauthored 1991 volume "Genetic Disorders of the Skin." It is there that we acquire new knowledge of chromosomal abnormalities, gene mapping, gene expression, and multifactorial inheritance. It is there we read of the 100,000 transcriptionally active genes that direct our patient into health or disease. And there we find the current methods of prenatal diagnosis, which include maternal blood sampling, ultrasound, fetoscopy, and amniocentesis, as well as fetal skin and chorionic villus sampling.

Many of the genetically determined skin diseases are easily recognized as entities. Others are rare isolates reported possibly but once or twice in the literature. However, remember that every component of skin from keratin to elastin, from nerve ending to sweat gland, and from mast cell to Langerhans cell can be functionally or morphologically changed by gene edict. We can provide but a few examples to light your way inside the black box of genodermatoses.

The genetic force is powerful. Think of it when making a diagnosis.

Goldsmith LA: **Principles of genetics** as applied to dermatologic diseases. J Am Acad Dermatol 1981; 4:255–266.

Think genetics with:

disorders of pigmentation, hair, nails, keratinization, and tumors
lesion symmetry
multiple organ defects (pleiotropy)
premature aging
positive family history

Think autosomal dominant inheritance:

with the appearance of a trait in 50% of the children of an affected parent
when males and females have the trait and it appears in each generation of a pedigree

Think autosomal recessive inheritance:

with 25% of the children affected, both males and females
when parents and children of affected individuals are normal
in very rare genetic diseases where consanguinity is frequent

Think X-linked inheritance:

if only males are affected and there is no father-to-son transmission. (All daughters of affected males are carriers, and half of their sons will be affected.)

Think mutation:

if family history is negative
if there is known exposure to radiation or drugs

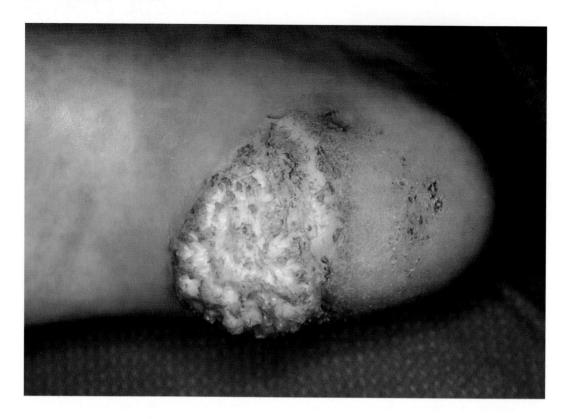

with polygenic inheritance (some traits are multifactorial, being affected by environmental influences such as diet)

if there is heterogeneity in inheritance

with increasing paternal age

when a syndrome comes in distinct molecular forms (e.g., Ehlers-Danlos syndrome)

Remember, **chance has no memory**. If the family is small in number, the chances are limited for success in genetic prediction. When your predictions fail, remember the "fudge factors" of penetrance and expressivity.

Epstein E, Jr: Workshop on linkage analysis of **hereditary skin diseases**. J Invest Dermatol 1990; 95:727–728.

Molecular diagnosis is on the way. The first step is making a linkage between inheritance of a disease and the inheritance of specific DNA markers (restriction fragment–length polymorphisms). This step is now being taken for:

atopic dermatitis	ichthyosis
Darier's disease	male pattern baldness
epidermolysis bullosa	psoriasis
Hailey-Hailey disease	

Freire-Maia N, Pinheiro M: **Ectodermal dysplasias:** A clinical and genetic study. New York, A.R. Liss, Inc., 1984, 251 pp.

The marked heterogeneity of ectodermal dysplasia is displayed here in a detailed description of 117 different types. Here is an answer to the "nosology syndrome."

Mallory SB, Paller AS: **Congenital immunodeficiency syndromes** with cutaneous manifestations. 1. J Am Acad Dermatol 1990; 23:1153–1158.

Undue **susceptibility to infection** is a sign of primary immunodeficiency. If it is cellular in nature, anticipate the full range of opportunistic viral, fungal, mycobacterial and protozoan infections. If it is an antibody deficiency, expect gram-positive bacterial infections. Disorders of phagocytosis are associated with staphylococcal, gram-negative, and fungal infections. Patients with deficiencies of early complement components may have lupus erythematosus or other autoimmune disease. Recurrent neisserial infections point to deficiencies in the alternate pathway complement components.

With any child or adult patient who has recurrent, severe, prolonged, or unusual infection, **study for the presence of one of these**:

> ataxia-telangiectasia (Louis-Bar syndrome)
> cartilage-hair hypoplasia
> Chédiak-Higashi syndrome
> chronic granulomatous disease
> hereditary angioedema
> DiGeorge anomaly
> Leiner syndrome

Burgdorf WHC: **Autosomal dominant genodermatoses** associated with cancer. Current Concepts in Skin Disorders 1987; 8:16–22.

Syndrome	Clue	Malignancy
Torre	Sebaceous neoplasia	GI, lung
Cowden	Oral papules, tricholemmomas	Breast, thyroid, GI
Multiple endocrine neoplasia 2b	Everted eyelids, facial neuromas	Thyroid, pheochromocytoma
Gardner	Cysts	Colon
Basal cell nevus	Multiple BCE, palmar pits	Central nervous system
Peutz-Jeghers	Labial macules	GI, endocrine
Carney	Myxomas, lentigines	Cardiac myxoma, endocrine, breast
Birt	Perifollicular growths	Thyroid, GI

Newton GA, Sanchez RL, Swedo J, Smith EB: **Lafora's disease:** The role of skin biopsy. Arch Dermatol 1987; 123:1667–1669.

There are a number of **invisible dermatoses** not evident to the physician or patient that are readily seen by the pathologist. A biopsy of seemingly normal skin may quickly reveal abnormal metabolic deposits similar to those in muscle, brain, and liver.

A 16-year-old girl had attacks of **generalized convulsions** for 8 months, along with progressive incoordination and weakness, and deterioration of her school performance. Extensive hospital studies were normal, but the onset of myoclonic seizures at this age suggested Lafora's disease, a progressive neurometabolic disorder transmitted by autosomal recessive inheritance. Skin biopsy confirmed the diagnosis, showing characteristic PAS-positive inclusions in eccrine sweat duct cells. These **Lafora bodies** can also be seen in apocrine glands and cutaneous nerves and are demonstrable in PAS-stained frozen sections (for rapid diagnosis).

Other invisible dermatoses with pathognomonic inclusion bodies include:

> lipofucinoses, neuronal ceroid
> glycogenosis II (Pompe's disease)
> leukodystrophies

Hagerman R, Kemper M, Hudson M: Learning disabilities and attentional problems in boys with the **fragile X syndrome**. Am J Dis Child 1985; 139:674–678.

A boy (or girl) with familial mental retardation and large, prominent ears probably has the fragile X syndrome, with a fragile locus at q 27 on the X chromosome. Examine for hyperextensible joints, enlarged testicles, and autistic behavior (hand flopping, hand biting).

Fryns JP, Haspeslagh M, de Muelenacre A, van Den Berghe H: 9_p Trisomy/18_p distal monosomy and **multiple cutaneous leiomyomata**. Another specific chromosomal site (18 pter) in dominantly inherited multiple tumors? Hum Genet 1985; 70:284–286.

A 34-year-old severely mentally retarded woman had multiple hard, reddish skin tumors 2 to 3 cm in diameter scattered over her extremities and back. They resembled keloids, with different parts coalescing into a fine linear pattern. Pressure on the tumors caused pain. Similar tumors had been present in her mentally retarded deceased sister. Skin biopsies showed **leiomyomata** arising from pilar arrector muscles. They had begun in infancy and grew slowly, with new lesions forming as others stabilized.

Multiple cutaneous leiomyomata are usually reddish-brown firm intradermal nodules less than 15 mm in diameter. They are **dominantly inherited**, as are other skin tumors of the same histologic type, including lipomas, basaliomas, glomus tumors, and neurofibromas.

Selmanowitz VJ, Stiller MJ: **Rubinstein-Taybi syndrome:** Cutaneous manifestations and colossal keloids. Arch Dermatol 1981; 117:504–506.

Look for this syndrome in the institutionalized mentally retarded. Look for broad thumbs, broad great toes, and a characteristic facies of microcephaly, retrognathia, hooked nose, deformed ears. Besides this, there is a litany of cutaneous anomalies ranging from prominent eyebrows and long eyelashes to capillary hemangiomas. Of special note are the enormous keloids that may form in the skin of these patients.

Beware of surgical procedures on these patients.

Shapiro LR, Hsu LYF, Calvin ME, Hirschhorn K: **XXXXY boy.** A 15-month-old child with normal intellectual development. Am J Dis Child 1970; 119:79–81.

A male infant of Yugoslavian extraction presented with a peculiar round "moon" facies and marked **redundancy of skin** over the posterior cervical region. Although his penis was small, the testicles were descended, and he did not evidence mental retardation. Chromosome analysis showed 49 chromosomes with XXXXY sex chromosome constitution.

Since the probability of **mental retardation** increases with the number of excess X chromosomes, this case is quite unusual and differs from previous reports of the XXXXY syndrome. Boys with this syndrome usually have mental retardation and hypogonadism with small penis and small and/or undescended testes. Clinodactyly of the 5th fingers and skeletal abnormalities of the elbows and wrists are other findings.

Sybert VP: Guide to information for families with **inherited skin disorders**. Pediatr Dermatol 1990; 7:214–217.

A complete list of support groups:

Albinism
National Organization for Albinism and Hypopigmentation (NOAH)
1500 Locust Street, Suite 1811
Philadelphia, PA 19102-4316
(215) 471-2278
(215) 471-2265

Alopecia
National Alopecia Areata Foundation
714 C Street, Suite 216
San Rafael, CA 94901
(415) 456-4644

Ataxia Telangiectasia
National Ataxia Foundation
600 Twelve Oaks Center
15500 Wayzata Boulevard
Wayzata, MN 55391
(612) 473-7666

Cockayne Syndrome
Share and Care
1294 S Street
North Valley Stream, NY 11580
(516) 825-2284

Dermatitis Herpetiformis
American Celiac Society
45 Gifford Avenue
Jersey City, NJ 07304
(201) 432-1207

Celiac Sprue Association/United States of America, Inc. (CSA/USA)
2313 Rocklyn Drive, Suite 1
Des Moines, IA 50322
(515) 270-9689

Gluten Intolerance Group of North America (GIG)
P.O. Box 23055
Seattle, WA 98102-0353
(206) 325-6980

Dysautonomia
Dysautonomia Foundation, Inc.
370 Lexington Avenue
New York, NY 10017
(212) 889-5222

Ectodermal Dysplasias
National Foundation for Ectodermal Dysplasias (NFED)
219 East Main Street
Mascoutah, IL 62258
(618) 566-2020

Eczema
Eczema Association for Science and Education
1221 Southwest Yamhill Road, Suite 303
Portland, Oregon 97205
(503) 228-4430

Ehlers-Danlos Syndrome
Ehlers-Danlos National Foundation (EDNF)
P.O. Box 1212
Southgate, MI 48195
(313) 282-0180

Epidermolysis Bullosa
Dystrophic Epidermolysis Bullosa Research Association of America, Inc.
  (DEBRA)
141 Fifth Avenue, Suite 7-S
New York, NY 10010
(212) 995-2220

Histiocytosis X
Histiocytosis X Association of America, Inc.
609 New York Road
Glassboro, NJ 08028
(609) 881-4911

Ichthyosis
Foundation for Ichthyosis and Related Skin Types, Inc. (FIRST)
3640 Grand Avenue, Suite 2
Oakland, CA 94610
(415) 763-9839

Klippel-Trenaunay Syndrome
Klippel-Trenaunay Syndrome Support Group
4610 Wooddale Avenue
Minneapolis, MN 55424
(612) 925-2596

Lupus
American Lupus Society
23751 Madison Street
Torrance, CA 90505
(213) 373-1335

Lymphedema
National Lymphatic and Venous Foundation, Inc. (NLVF)
P.O. Box 80
Cambridge, MA 02140

Neurofibromatosis
National Neurofibromatosis Foundation, Inc.
141 Fifth Avenue, Suite 7-S
New York, NY 10010
(800) 323-7983 (outside New York)
(212) 460-8980

Progeria
Progeria International Registry
New York State Institute for Basic Research
Department of Human Genetics
1050 Forest Hill Road
Staten Island, NY 10314
(718) 494-5230

Psoriasis
National Psoriasis Foundation
6443 Southwest Beaverton Highway, Suite 210
Portland, OR 97221

Scleroderma
United Scleroderma Foundation, Inc. (USF)
P.O. Box 350
Watsonville, CA 95077-0350
(408) 728-2202

Sturge-Weber Syndrome
Sturge-Weber Foundation
P.O. Box 460931
Aurora, CO 80015
(303) 693-2986

National Congenital Port Wine Stain Foundation
125 East 63rd Street
New York, NY 15021
(212) 755-3820

Trichotillomania
Obsessive-Compulsive Disorder (OCD) Foundation
P.O. Box 9573
New Haven, CT 06515
(203) 772-0565

Tuberous Sclerosis
Tuberous Sclerosis Association of America, Inc. (TSAA)
P.O. Box 1305
Middleboro, MA 02370
(617) 947-8893

Vitiligo
National Vitiligo Foundation, Inc.
Texas American Bank Building
P.O. Box 6337
Tyler, Texas 75711
(214) 534-2925

Xeroderma Pigmentosum
Xeroderma Pigmentosum Registry
UMDMJ, New Jersey Medical School
Department of Pathology, Room C-520
Medical Science Building
100 Bergen Street
Newark, NJ 07103
(201) 456-6255

For information concerning the nearest genetic center, contact the American Board of Medical Genetics, 9650 Rockville Pike, Bethesda, MD 20814, (301) 571-1825.

Dermatologic patients are invariably wrapped up in their disease.

Genital Lesions

Since contagious disease is spread by contact, the genitalia are "where it's at" when it comes to sexually transmitted disease. Any new lesion of the genitals, no matter what its size or shape, must be viewed by the diagnostician as a possible sexual contagion. It is imperative that an accurate history of incidents of sexual activity and their types be sought, since asexual transmission of venereal disease is rare. If the history indicates, a serial serologic search for **syphilis** follows. Remember that the sore precedes the serology indications and that during this serologically negative primary phase, darkfield examination for *S. pallidum* is the only satisfactory approach. Any genital ulcer must also be studied as possibly due to infection with *Hemophilus ducreyi*. This has a **soft chancre**, which contrasts with the firm hard chancre of primary syphilis. The organism is fastidious but can, at times, be cultured. An alternative is serologic complement-fixation tests.

Lymphadenopathy is common to both syphilis and chancroid, but in **lympho-granuloma venereum** (LGV) giant lymphadenopathy, i.e., buboes, is seen initially. The initial entry lesion for the *Chlamydia trachomatis* is but a transitory vesicle or erosion. Again, cultures of pus from the buboes and serologic tests are the only laboratory aids. Clinically, a crease in the buboes favors the diagnosis of LGV.

The deep beefy red ulcer of **granuloma inguinale** is a fourth venereal disease to be examined for. Here, diagnostic confirmation comes with finding the Donovan bodies in smears or biopsy. These indicate the causative organisms, *Calymmatobacterium granulomatis*.

The causes of genital lesions or erosions range from other bacteria through viruses to yeasts. Cultures are invaluable, although the gonococcus can be suspected in the presence of urethritis. Likewise, a history of a preceding group of vesicles points to the herpes simplex virus, and white pustules to *Candida albicans*.

With an accompanying vaginitis, *Candida*, *Trichomonas*, and *Gardnerella* organisms must be sought. A wet mount and culture are the favored diagnostic techniques here. A whitish discharge is typical of candidiasis, and the fishy odor of Gardnerella is diagnostically suggestive. The Gardnerella organisms adhere to the vaginal cells, producing the indistinct cell edge of the "clue" cell seen in wet mounts. In trichomoniasis, the large pear-shaped trichomonas attracts attention in the wet mount by its movement. Not only the vagina but the urethra may be infected by these.

The moist, macerated areas of the genital region favor many other infections not generally transmitted sexually. These include tinea cruris, erythrasma, furuncles, candidiasis, as well as gram-negative and gram-positive bacterial infections. Cultures are usually the fastest route to diagnosis, but clinical clues abound. These include the sharp margin of tinea, the coral red fluorescence of erythrasma, and the satellite pustules of candidiasis.

The genital skin may play host to almost any skin disease. Usually the diagnosis is obvious, as in intertrigo, warts, molluscum contagiosum, and contact dermatitis. What may not be obvious is the source of the warts or of a connubial contact dermatitis. In other examples, it is wise to mentally transpose the lesion to other, more favored sites. This allows one to more readily perceive such diagnoses as Behçet's disease, Bowen's disease, scabies, lichen sclerosus et atrophicus, as well as hidradenitis suppurativa. Lichen planus, psoriasis, and fixed drug eruptions of the glans penis may quickly come to mind when mentally viewed at their more usual sites of predilection. Down in that area you may be surprised to see alopecia areata and trichomycosis. On the scrotum you may see steroid rosacea, tinea, or annular lesions of relapsing syphilis. Don't forget to look for pediculi—they may explain an otherwise inexplicable generalized pruritus.

Felman YM, Nikitas JA: Common pitfalls in the diagnosis and treatment of **sexually transmitted diseases**. Cutis 1984; 33:28–35.

Failure

> to think of sexually transmitted disease (STD) in patients with extragenital ailments
>
> to take a sexual behavior and lifestyle history
>
> to do tests that might offend the patient
>
> to culture a sore throat for *Neisseria gonorrhoeae*
>
> to use wet mount slides for detection of *Trichomonas vaginalis*
>
> to do darkfield examination in very early syphilis when serologic tests have not yet become positive
>
> to do serologic tests for syphilis
>
> to recognize the biologic false-positive tests

Chapel TA: Primary and secondary **syphilis**. Cutis 1984; 33:47–53.

PRIMARY SYPHILIS

Any **anogenital ulcer** or ulcers should be considered syphilitic until proven otherwise. The primary lesion of syphilis, the chancre, can range in size from a few millimeters to a few centimeters. The initial change is a dull red macule that rapidly becomes a papule and erodes into an ulcer. The margins are not inflamed and the ulcer base is often clear. A few have a stippled line of hemorrhage and telangiectasia encircling the ulcer.

Classically, the ulcer **feels firm, like cartilage**. Within a week regional lymphadenopathy ensues. In some instances impaired lymphatic flow results in edema of the foreskin. If the chancre is on the anus or lower two-thirds of the vulva, there will be no recognizable lymphadenopathy, because drainage is to deep nodes only.

The common site for a chancre is the coronal sulcus of the penis. Nonetheless, remember the chancre is the crossover point for the spirochete passing from the infectious partner to your patient. Thus, a kiss may initiate a chancre on the lip. The tongue and tonsil are less likely sites. In all instances of oropharyngeal chancres, unilateral enlargement of the submental or anterior cervical **lymph nodes** is an important diagnostic lead.

Anal chancres in the homosexual are evident only if the patient's buttocks are spread. Here the chancre may be simply an indurated-appearing hemorrhage or an indurated fissure. The patients with a presenting symptom of rectal pain on defecation or mucoid- or blood-streaked stools may have a rectal chancre. This can sometimes be palpated on rectal examination. In other instances proctoscopy or even colonoscopy is required. Some lesions have been seen as far up as 20 cm. Again, indurated ulcers felt on digital examination are the most common form, but tumor-like granulomas may evolve.

Cervical chancres require speculum examination. Again, the rare intraurethral chancres require urethroscopy. Inguinal lymphadenopathy in the absence of a visible chancre may point to this need for such urethroscopy.

The most specific and immediate means of diagnosing primary syphilis is by demonstration of the pathogenic spirochete on **darkfield examination**. This requires skill and experience in expressing serous fluid from the lesion. Repeated darkfield examination may be required; in the case of oral lesions it is not recommended because of the difficulty in distinguishing *T. pallidum*   601 from the ordinary saprophytic spirochetes always present. Here, an aspirate from a regionally enlarged node is advantageous.

In the absence of darkfield examinations the diagnosis must rest on the results of the serologic tests for syphilis.

SECONDARY SYPHILIS

Subtle, faint, and overlooked are the attributes of secondary syphilis. In some of the fully apparent examples, the clinical picture is that of **pityriasis rosea**, **lichen planus**, or **psoriasis**. Usually the secondary syphilis lesions appear within 6 months of the disappearance of the chancre. Nonetheless, the chancre may still be present. Think secondary syphilis:

> papules on the palms and soles
> widespread symmetrical lesions
> > macular
> > roseolar
> > papular
> > papulosquamous
> > pustular
> generalized lymphadenopathy
> grouped annular **ring–shaped lesions**
> moist, eroded papules of labia or intertriginous areas (condylomata lata)
> sore throat that may be associated with flu symptoms, headache, meningismus, fever, hoarseness, myalgia, weight loss
> mucous patch in mucosal areas; a 1-cm papule with grayish membrane and a central erosion
> hair loss, diffuse inapparent or patchy moth-eaten; may involve eyebrows or eyelashes as well as scalp

Secondary lesions heal spontaneously and without scarring within several weeks or months. Relapses do occur, especially in cases of oral lesions.

Darkfield examination of the secondary lesion can be as rewarding as that of the chancre. Scotch tape stripping to the glistening base allows an exudate to be collected on a coverslip. Alternatively, an anesthetized papule can be crushed with a hemostat to provide serous exudate. Finally, the serologic tests provide the ultimate diagnosis. For the physician to see secondary syphilis the patient must be disrobed and must be studied in a good and varying light.

Suspicion often provides the best vision.

Falk ES, Vorland LH, Bjorvatn B: A case of **mixed chancre**. Dermatologica 1984; 168:47–49.

A 39-year-old Norwegian seaman developed two very **painful persistent ulcers** of the glans penis 6 weeks after intercourse with a prostitute in Venezuela. One ulcer localized around the urethra and the other around the frenulum. They rapidly became necrotic and were accompanied by edema of the shaft, balanitis, and inguinal lymphadenopathy.

Darkfield examination on 3 successive days showed no *Treponema pallidum*, and smears and cultures taken from the urethra were negative for *Neisseria gonorrhoeae*. However, multiple serologic tests indicated a recent syphilitic infection, and treatment with penicillin caused a marked **Herxheimer reaction**. The long incubation period also favored a diagnosis of syphilis.

Meanwhile, incontrovertible evidence of a ***Hemophilus ducreyi* infection** was obtained by the finding of multiple gram-negative bacteria in a school-of-

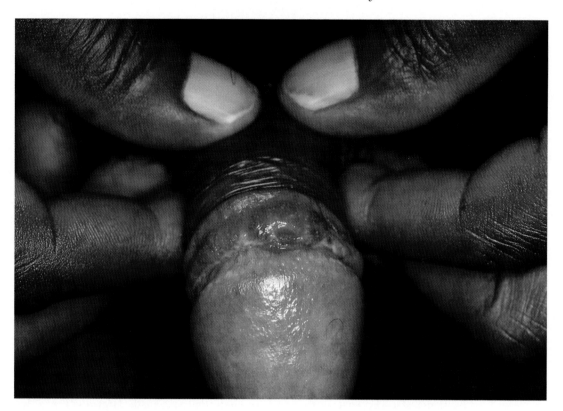

fish pattern on Gram stain preparations of the ulcers. This infection probably accounted for the severe and painful ulcerations.

A diagnosis of **mixed chancre** with both **syphilis and chancroid** was made. Concurrent treatment with benzathine penicillin (2.4 million units i.m., 2 doses one week apart) and trimethoprim-sulfamethoxazole (1 gm bid) for 3 weeks led to slow healing.

It can be assumed that this poor sailor had been hit twice in a single navel encounter. What bad luck!

Rosen T: Unusual presentations of **gonorrhea**. J Am Acad Dermatol 1982; 6:369–372.

A 22-year-old man presented with a 2-day history of an **erythematous tender nodule** with early "pointing" on the penile shaft. It resembled a furuncle, but there was no regional adenopathy, and examination of expressed purulent material revealed gram-negative intracellular diplococci. **Culture** of the pus was positive on Thayer-Martin medium. A calcium alginate swab of the urethra was negative for gonococci on both smear and culture. He admitted to casual sexual exposure 8 days prior to the onset of symptoms.

A 21-year-old woman had a 3-day history of mild dysuria and "burning bumps" in the perineal region starting one week after casual sexual contact. There was no regional adenopathy or vaginal discharge. Examination revealed pea-sized erythematous edematous papules on each side of the urethral meatus, corresponding to the ductal orifices of Skene's glands. A small bead of pus expressed from the paraurethral papules was positive for gonococci, and *N. gonorrhoeae* was also cultured from the endocervix.

The gonococcus has difficulty breaking any intact epidermal wall but thrives in traumatized skin that has been exposed to mucosal discharge. The following **types of lesions** should be incised, smeared, and cultured in search of gonorrhea:

Furunculoid lesions of the penis and scrotum

Pustules, abscesses, and erosions of the ventral penoscrotal raphe. Incomplete embryologic fusion may leave cysts, ducts, and sinuses that act as entry portals. Gland infections also occur, causing enlarged tender parafrenal papules (Tyson's glands) and deep abscess formation with rupture through perineal skin (Cowper's gland).

Abscesses of fingers

Tender labial nodules (Bartholin gland infection)

Inflamed paraurethral papules (Skene's gland infection)

Only those who look for gonorrhea of the skin will find it.

Verdich J: *Hemophilus ducreyi* **infection** resembling granuloma inguinale. Acta Derm Venereol 1984; 64:452–455.

Intercourse with a prostitute in Bangkok resulted 3 weeks later in ulcers of the frenulum and foreskin of a 21-year-old Dane. The **ulcers** were slightly tender, with varying degrees of **beefy red granulation tissue** and rolled-over borders. **Granuloma inguinale was diagnosed** since the lesions lacked the pain and lymphadenopathy characteristic of chancroid. However, biopsy failed to confirm granuloma inguinale, and there were no Donovan bodies on Giemsa stain of tissue crushed between 2 glass slides.

Syphilis was ruled out with 3 negative darkfield examinations, and herpes and lymphogranuloma venereum were ruled out by negative complement fixation tests. The **correct diagnosis of chancroid** was made after a cotton swab of the lesion was placed immediately in Stuart's transportation medium and cultured on special growth medium for *H. ducreyi*. Treatment with tetracycline and sulfamethizole/trimethoprim was curative.

Clinical diagnosis must always yield to the isolation of the causative organism.

Rosen T, Tschen JA, Ramsdell W et al: **Granuloma inguinale**. J Am Acad Dermatol 1984; 11:433–437.

An unusual epidemic of granuloma inguinale was observed in Houston, Texas, where in 8 months 19 men were found to have the disease. It was characterized by:

Painless penile ulceration

Rolled border around ulcer with friable granulation tissue base

No lymphadenopathy

Negative darkfield and VDRL

Warthin-Starry stain of biopsy showing encapsulated bacteria in histiocytes

Culture often positive for *Hemophilus ducreyi*

Excellent response to trimethoprim/sulfamethoxazole

Ackers JP, Yule A: Immunological diagnosis of **trichomoniasis**. *In* Young H, McMillan A (eds): Immunological Diagnosis of Sexually Transmitted Diseases. New York, Marcel Dekker Inc, 1988; pp 275–302.

Trichomoniasis is the most common protozoan infection in Europe and North America and is the world's most common sexually transmitted disease. In women, trichomoniasis is most commonly found in the vagina, urethra, and paraurethral glands, sparing the uterine cavity and fallopian tubes. Parasitemia does not occur. In men the urethra is the most common site, with possible penetration into the prostate. Men are usually asymptomatic, as are 25% of infected women. A purulent **frothy white vaginal discharge** is suggestive, but not diagnostic, of the disease. Vulvovaginal soreness or irritation, dysuria, urinary frequency, and dyspareunia are other common symptoms.

Wet mounts are quick and easy to perform but need to be read fairly quickly in order to see the unmistakable living motile trichomonad. However, cultures detect 20 to 30% more trichomonas infections than do wet mount examinations or fixed and stained films. Modified Diamond's medium is the most widely used culture medium worldwide, but modified Lumsden medium has the advantage of containing an indicator that changes from purple to yellow with production of lactic acid by the growing trichomonads. Penicillin does not inhibit growth and is often added to the media. Staining of smears with the fluorescent dye acridine orange is probably even more sensitive than culturing but requires a fluorescent microscope. Fluorescent antibody staining of blood will probably be the diagnostic tool of the future, but its effectiveness has been hampered so far by the failure of some infected patients to make a vigorous enough antibody response.

Jones JG, Yamauchi T, Lambert B: **Trichomonas vaginalis infestation** in sexually abused girls. Am J Dis Child 1985; 139:846–847.

Trichomoniasis is very rare in preadolescent girls and probably signals **sexual abuse**. Vaginitis with a purulent discharge is the usual presentation. Wet preps detect only 50 to 75% of cases. Other sexually transmitted diseases should be ruled out.

Kreiss JK, Coombs R, Plummer F et al: Isolation of **human immunodeficiency virus from genital ulcers** in Nairobi prostitutes. J Infect Dis 1989; 160:380–384.

Genital and anorectal ulcer disease is an important cofactor for acquisition and transmission of HIV during sexual intercourse. HIV was isolated from 4 of 36 uncontaminated ulcer cultures. Syphilis, chancroid, and anogenital or oral herpes have been associated with AIDS in other studies of homosexual men and were common here also. In this study most ulcers appeared to be **chancroid**, which was very resistant to antibiotic treatment.

Sønderbo K, Nyfors A: Skin lesions in **sadomasochism**. Dermatologica 1986; 172:196–200.

Small punched out, slowly healing ulcers of the perianal and scrotal area in a 35-year-old man proved to be caused by cigarette burns inflicted by his girl friend as part of a **sexual satisfaction ritual**.

Sadomasochists most often satisfy their lust for pain (algolagnia) by beating and whipping. Habitués of the intimate-massage clinics in Copenhagen exhibit "recreational" marks from bites, suction, binding with rope, squeezing in a pillory, pinching, cuts, and clawing, as well as the commonplace burning.

Diagnosis by recognition is easy. Diagnosis by cognition is hard.

Penis

Fisher AA: Unusual **condom dermatitis**. Cutis 1989; 44:365–366.

Condom-induced problems include:

leukoderma
  due to monobenzylether hydroquinone in rubber
contact dermatitis
  due to sensitivity to tetramethylthiuram (thiram) in condom rubber.
    Two years later oral Antabuse (tetraethyl thiuram) therapy evoked
    attack of dermatitis of penis.
  due to preservative in condom lubricant, i.e., bronopol (a formaldehyde-
    releasing compound)
consort condom dermatitis
  on thighs, abdomen, and perianal area
  may explain cheilitis and stomatitis

Revuz J, Clerici T: **Penile melanosis**. J Am Acad Dermatol 1989; 20:567–570.

Macular hyperpigmentation of the glans penis or shaft of the penis is a benign
process. On the glans the lesions are large, variegate, dark brown-black
pigmented macules of irregular outline. On the penile shaft the lesions are
round or oval sharply demarcated macules of uniform color. There may be
gradual enlargement.

Biopsy shows hyperpigmentation of the lower layers of the epidermis, but
without increase in the number of melanocytes.

Also known as **penile lentigo**, this condition is clinically and histologically
analogous to vulvovaginal melanosis and to the essential lenticular melanotic
pigmentation of the buccal mucosa and lips (Laugier-Hunziger syndrome).

The main diagnostic problem is to rule out malignant melanoma and thereby
prevent unnecessary radical surgery. **Differential diagnosis** also includes
pigmented benign neoplasms (seborrheic keratosis, melanocytic nevi) and
postinflammatory hyperpigmentation (lichen planus, fixed drug eruption).

Leicht S, Youngberg G, Diaz-Miranda C: Atypical pigmented **penile macules**. Arch
Dermatol 1988; 124:1267–1270.

Irregular patches of pigmentation on the glans penis or penile shaft always
raise the question of malignant melanoma. Although usually they are benign
penile lentigines or simple melanosis, histologic study is necessary to rule
out in situ acral lentiginous melanoma.

Three cases of dramatic variegated and retiform macular pigmentation are
presented in men ages 40, 61, and 66 years. Coloration ranged from tan to
black, and melanoma was suspected clinically in 2 of the cases. However,
each was benign despite a history of enlargement over a period of years.
Histologically, the only finding was basilar hyperpigmentation and pigmentary incontinence. There was no nuclear atypia or inflammatory dermal
reaction.

Balato N, Montesano M, Lembo G: Acquired **phlebectasia** of the glans penis. J Am
Acad Dermatol 1985; 13:824–826.

Several **blue nodules of the glans penis** that disappeared under slight pressure were the presenting complaint of a 19-year-old student. They had suddenly appeared 4 years earlier, with no antecedent injury or disease. His
only symptom was occasional tension and pain during an erection.

A diagnosis of glans penis phlebectasia was made and confirmed by phlebography. It is assumed that the lesions were hamartomas. They responded well to sclerotherapy.

Dekio S, Jidoi J: **Tinea** of the glans penis. Dermatologica 1989; 178:112–114.

An **erythematous lesion of the glans penis** was the chief complaint of this 56-year-old man. It had been present for 3 months and was a source of itching and pain.

On examination, the lesion was slightly raised, slightly scaling, and erythematous. There were no other lesions. The slight scale induced the physician to do a **KOH**. It was positive and a culture on Sabouraud's dextrose agar plate containing 50 μg/ml chloramphenicol and 500 μg/ml cycloheximide showed at 3 weeks a growth identified by later slide culture as *Trichophyton mentagrophytes*. Two weeks of topical antifungal cream cured this unusual tinea penis.

Remember, it's the early KOH test that catches the ringworm.

Kanwar AJ, Singh M, Yunus M, Belhaj MS: **Fixed eruption** to sulphasalazine. Dermatologic 1987; 174:104.

A fixed drug eruption on the penis of a 38-year-old man with ulcerative colitis proved by challenge to be due to sulfasalazine. Challenges with five other "sulfas" were negative, with the exception of sulfapyridine, a breakdown product of sulfasalazine. Attacks did not occur when prednisone (10 to 15 mg/day) was given conjointly for the colitis.

James WD: Cutaneous **group beta-streptococcal infections**. Arch Dermatol 1984; 120:85–86.

A bright red band of **superficial ulceration** had encircled the **penis** of this 20-year-old man for 1 week. It was sharply localized to the base of the foreskin, just proximal to the coronal sulcus. Fungal and bacterial cultures were obtained and treatment begun with Burow's compresses, miconazole cream, and minocycline 100 mg bid. At five days there was substantially no improvement. However, the bacterial cultures showed a heavy growth of beta-hemolytic streptococci, group B, sensitive to penicillin. All previous treatment was suspended and penicillin V potassium prescribed in a dose of 1 gm a day. The lesion promptly involuted.

Since group B streptococcus often colonizes the vaginal tract, it is assumed the patient's infection followed the minor trauma of intercourse. Ordinarily this organism causes infections in diabetics and immunocompromised hosts. However, all of this patient's extensive tests were normal including serologic tests for syphilis and scrapings for yeast and fungi.

A rosy ring around the penis can mean a pocketful of strep. Be sure to culture.

Yalisove B, Stolar EH, Williams CM: Multiple **penile papules**. Arch Dermatol 1987; 123:1393–1396.

Problem: A 4-week history of multiple asymptomatic papules of the penis in a 19-year-old man.

Exam: Multiple round to oval flesh-colored to slightly yellow soft dermal papules, 4 to 7 mm in diameter, on the dorsolateral surface of the shaft of the penis.

Diagnosis: **Syringomas**, on biopsy.

Regional **differential diagnosis** for these benign appendageal tumors of the eccrine ducts:

Face: milia, angiofibroma, trichoepithelioma

Trunk: eruptive vellus hair cysts, steatocystoma multiplex, granuloma annulare

Penis: lichen nitidus, sarcoidosis, granuloma annulare, angiofibroma, lichen planus, cysts

Usually appearing on the eyelids and upper cheeks at the time of puberty, they may evade clinical diagnosis by being in unusual sites such as the hand. Rare familial examples occur as well as a malignant variant.

Callen JP: The spectrum of **Reiter's disease.** J Am Acad Dermatol 1979; 1:75–77.

The constellation of **arthritis, urethritis,** and **conjunctivitis** is called Reiter's disease; however, each finding by itself is nondiagnostic. Likewise, the cutaneous findings in Reiter's disease taken alone are simply those of psoriasis. Most patients have the histocompatibility antigen HL-A B27.

In the urethritic arthritic, look for erythematous plaques with pustules on the palms and soles, circinate papular lesions on the glans penis, and reedy dystrophic nails. Once these are found, you have found the diagnosis.

Foucar E, Downing DT, Gerber WL: **Sclerosing lipogranuloma** of the male genitalia containing vitamin E: A comparison with classical "paraffinoma." J Am Acad Dermatol 1983; 9:103–110.

A 52-year-old man had progressive **swelling of the penile and scrotal skin** for 10 months, **diagnosed as cellulitis.** Hospitalization and intravenous antibiotics had been without effect. The scrotal and penile skin was very firm and red-brown, with discrete scattered nodules. Biopsy revealed bright yellow dermal and subcutaneous tissue filled with cystic spaces surrounded by an inflammatory infiltrate, typical of sclerosing lipogranuloma. Lipid analysis of the granuloma by thin layer chromatography showed that over half of it was tocopherol and tocopheryl acetate.

His history revealed that he had been applying **vitamin E** to the penis every day for the past 4 years to keep the skin supple. Presumably, enough vitamin E was absorbed through the permeable scrotal skin to produce a paraffinoma-like picture (which can also follow paraffin injections for cosmesis).

Kristensen JK, Scheibel J: **Sclerosing lymphangitis** of the penis: A possible Chlamydia aetiology. Acta Derm Venereol 1981; 61:455–456.

A painful **cord-like lesion of the coronal sulcus** of the penis had been noted for 2 weeks by a 20-year-old man. A urethral smear showed more than 10 polymorphonuclear leukocytes/high power field, establishing the diagnosis of urethritis. Gonococcal cultures and serologic tests for syphilis were negative, but *Chlamydia trachomatis* was isolated.

The cord lesion was recognized as a **sclerosing lymphangitis.** Similar cords may involve the dorsum of the penis. Presumably the *Chlamydia* infection was responsible, since the problem disappeared after a week of tetracycline therapy.

Brodin MB: **Balanitis circumscripta plasmacellularis.** J Am Acad Dermatol 1980; 2:33–35.

A sharply circumscribed erythematous and erosive plaque on the proximal glans penis of an 83-year-old man had been present for months and proved resistant to topical therapy. It appeared to be **erythroplasia of Queyrat**, but biopsies on two occasions showed a dense infiltrate of plasma cells, consistent with **Zoon's balanitis** (balanitis circumscripta plasmacellularis).

Circumscribed balanitis calls for STS, culture for *Candida*, history to rule out fixed drug eruption and contact dermatitis, and biopsy to rule out histoplasmosis and Queyrat's erythroplasia.

Beljaards RC, Van Dijk E, Hausman R: Is pseudoepitheliomatous, micaceous and keratotic **balanitis** synonymous with verrucous carcinoma? Br J Dermatol 1987; 117:641–646.

White laminar scales of the glans penis were associated with a verrucous keratotic tumor for 2 years in a 60-year-old man. Onset had followed circumcision. Biopsy showed no evidence of malignancy, but findings were consistent with a clinical diagnosis of **pseudoepitheliomatous micaceous and keratotic balanitis** (PMKD), first described in 1961 by Lortat-Jacob and Civatte. Excision of the tumor was followed by recurrence, and subsequent excision 4 years later showed the growth to be a **verrucous carcinoma**.

In a second patient, a 68-year-old man, there was macular erythema with telangiectasia, pale keratotic lesions, and a 1-cm erosive tumor of the glans penis. It had evolved slowly after circumcision 30 years before. Biopsy showed hyperkeratosis and acanthosis consistent with a diagnosis of PMKD. Despite excision of the tumor, there was recurrence 3 years later as a well-differentiated squamous cell carcinoma. Final treatment: partial penectomy.

Dundas SAC, Laing RW: **Titanium balanitis** with phimosis. Dermatologica 1988; 176:305–307.

A 47-year-old man had progressive **phimosis and meatal stenosis** since age 17, with a thickened foreskin adherent to the glans. Circumcision and meatotomy were performed, and histologic examination of the fibrotic foreskin ruled out balanitis xerotica obliterans. Noteworthy, however, was the presence of numerous small birefringent black granules with a moderate plasma cell infiltrate just beneath the nonkeratinizing squamous epithelium of the inside of the foreskin. Energy-dispersive analysis by x-ray (EDAX analysis) proved the granules to be titanium.

Titanium-containing creams are used in the treatment of balanitis, and such cream probably had been used by the patient many years before (he could not recall its name or composition). Presumably, after using a **titanium cream** locally he developed titanium hypersensitivity with granulomatous response, fibrosis, and phimosis.

Prior examples of **titanium sensitivity** have included reactions to joint prostheses, cardiac pacemakers, and inhaled titanium.

Helfman RJ, Poulos EG: **Reticulated porokeratosis**: A unique variant of porokeratosis. Arch Dermatol 1985; 121:1542–1543.

An erythematous rash that had a **reticulated configuration** with a slightly elevated, advancing border had troubled this 27-year-old man for 5 years. It involved the penis, scrotum, pubic area, and inguinal region. The diagnosis awaited the biopsy. Multiple well-formed coronoid lamellae in the stratum corneum and the other findings made it evident that this was porokeratosis.

As a distinctive reticulated variant it is to be **compared with** the

linear form
plaque type (Mibelli)

palmar-plantar form
disseminate form
    actinic
    nonactinic

Rosen T, Rubin H, Ellner K et al: Vesicular **Jarisch-Herxheimer reaction**. Arch Dermatol 1989; 125:77–81.

A 43-year-old black man presented with a widespread erythematous papular eruption of 2 weeks' duration. Darkfield examination of three ulcers on the penis revealed numerous spirochetes, and VDRL was positive in a titer of 1/128, confirming the diagnosis of secondary syphilis.

During the 24 hours following an intramuscular injection of 2.4 million units of penicillin G benzathine, the patient experienced chills, fever, arthralgia as well as an increased prominence of his skin lesions. In addition to this well-known **Jarisch-Herxheimer reaction**, he developed a generalized vesicular eruption. Some of the vesicles surmounted papules, and darkfield examination showed nonmotile spirochetes. A biopsy showed a subepidermal bulla. The entire eruption cleared within 2 weeks, without further treatment.

The unique feature was the appearance of vesicles, which presumably was an integral part of the Jarisch-Herxheimer reaction in this and three other similar patient reactions reported in this paper. It is important not to label the eruption a simple drug allergy but rather to recognize it as evidence of a **massive destruction of spirochetes**. Interestingly, vesicular lesions have not been previously associated with syphilis in the adult. The Jarisch-Herxheimer remains an unexplained phenomenon commonly seen within 8 hours of treatment of primary or early secondary syphilis, whether it be by penicillin, bismuth, arsenic, or mercury. In addition to the chills and fever, one sees an accentuation of or an appearance of the classic follicular, papular, papulosquamous, nodular, and pustular lesions of syphilis.

To this we must now add the appearance of vesicles.

Gaffoor PMA, George WM: **Fixed drug eruptions** occurring on the male genitals. Cutis 1990; 45:242–244.

Don't forget that a puzzling chronic, sharply circumscribed erosion of the glans penis may be due to a drug.

Salzman RS, Kraus SJ, Miller RG et al: **Chancroidal ulcers** that are not chancroid. Arch Dermatol 1984; 120:636–639.

Chancroid is a purulent, nonindurated tender ulcer with an erythematous friable base. The diagnosis can only be made by culturing ***Hemophilus ducreyi*** on a specific selective medium such as heart infusion rabbit blood–vancomycin agar.

The hazard of making a clinical diagnosis of chancroid was shown in this study of 33 darkfield-negative genital ulcers. Each was diagnosed clinically as chancroid, yet on the basis of culture only one was bacteriologically proven chancroid. Further evidence of the erroneous clinical diagnoses was the fact that the other 32 ulcers healed following therapy with a drug, sulfamethoxazole, known to be ineffective against *H. ducreyi*. In 16 of the ulcers, herpes simplex virus was isolated, suggesting that half of these 32 patients had herpetic lesions secondarily infected with pyogenic bacteria.

Clinical diagnoses of penile ulcers are obviously best made in a loud confident voice to a group of beginning students.

Czarnecki DB, O'Brien TJ, Rotstein H, Brenan J: **Leukemia cutis** mimicking primary syphilis. Acta Derm Venereol 1981; 61:368–369.

A 19-year-old man was referred for evaluation of a 5-mm **penile ulcer** that was indurated and had an erythematous halo. It had arisen without any preceding lesion and was associated with enlarged, firm, nontender lymph nodes. He gave a history of acute undifferentiated leukemia now in remission. *Treponema pallidum* could not be found on darkfield examination and serologic tests for syphilis were negative. A culture for herpes simplex virus was negative and only *Staphylococcus aureus* grew out on a swab culture. Tetracycline and penicillin therapy were without effect.

Finally, a **biopsy** revealed leukemia cutis, the only sign of relapse of leukemia. He died 4 months later of septicemia.

Hassel MA, Lesher JL: **Herpes simplex** mimicking leukemia cutis. J Am Acad Dermatol 1989; 21:367–371.

A large tender **malodorous ulcer of the glans** and distal shaft of the penis had been present for 3 weeks in a man with a 5-year history of lymphocytic leukemia. Inguinal as well as cervical adenopathy was present. Following no response to systemic tetracycline and topical gentamicin, a biopsy was taken. This showed an atypical leukemic infiltrate with a resultant histopathologic **diagnosis of leukemia cutis**. This diagnosis was consonant with the patient's history of lymphatic leukemia. Furthermore, stains for fungi, bacteria, spirochetes and Donovan bodies were all negative. Review by the dermatology service led to a Tzanck preparation of the ulcer. This showed many characteristic giant cells with viral inclusion bodies. Viral culture grew out the herpes simplex virus making the **definitive diagnosis of a herpetic ulcer** and herpetic lymphadenitis.

Two weeks of oral acyclovir therapy proved curative.

This atypical herpes infection resulted from the immunosuppressed status of this lymphatic leukemia patient.

Griffin SM, McEvilly W, Cole TP: **Pilonidal sinus** of the penis. Br J Urol 1990; 65:422–424.

A 29-year-old uncircumcised married man developed a 2 × 1.5 cm **ulcer** of the ventral corona adjacent to the glans penis. It followed a small abscess that had appeared 7 months previously. Although cultures revealed *Candida albicans* and *Staphylococcus aureus*, treatment with an antifungal agent and antibiotic agents did not help. The ulcer was indurated with a rolled border, bled on contact, and was infected. Venereal disease tests and chest x-ray were negative.

The lesion was excised under general anesthesia revealing a **sinus track** containing necrotic debris and hair. The sinus was lined by squamous epithelium and granulation tissue, typical of a **pilonidal sinus**.

Brook I: Microbiology of **infection pilonidal sinuses**. J Clin Pathol 1989; 42:1140–1142.

In 75 patients with pilonidal sinuses, aspirates of pus revealed:

anaerobic bacteria only in 58 (77%)
aerobic bacteria only in 3 (4%)
mixed aerobic and anaerobic in 14 (19%)

Among 147 anaerobes isolated, the predominant organisms were *Bacteroides* sp. and anaerobic cocci. Aerobes isolated included *Escherichia coli*, *Proteus* sp., group D streptococcus, and *Pseudomonas* sp.

This study highlights the predominance of **anaerobic bacteria** in infected pilonidal sinuses. The polymicrobial nature of the isolates probably indicates synergy among the different bacterial strains. Treatment should include antibiotics such as clindamycin, cefoxitin, metronidazole, imipenem, or the combination of a beta-lactamase inhibitor and a penicillin.

Nishigori C, Taniguchi S, Hayakawa M, Imamura S: **Penis tuberculides**: papulonecrotic tuberculides of the glans penis. Dermatologica 1986; 172:93–97.

A 4-mm erythematous **indurated ulcer of the glans penis** in a 53-year-old Japanese man was covered with whitish yellow necrotic tissue. Previous similar ulcers over a 2 year period had not responded to systemic cephalexin. Inguinal nodes were not palpable. His PPD test was positive and skin **biopsy** showed a tubercle with caseation necrosis. Chest x-ray was negative and there was no family history of tuberculosis. Therapy with isoniazid (0.5 g/day) and rifampicin (450 mg/day) gave steady improvement and complete healing with a depressed scar at 2 months.

Another man, age 61, presented with 3 indurated papules and diffuse erythema of the glans penis. An irregular-shaped sloughing ulcer was present on one of the papules. Biopsy showed widespread caseation necrosis of the lower dermis and subcutaneous tissue. His PPD was strongly positive (wheal: 17 × 15 mm; flare 20 × 18 mm).

Over 100 cases of **penis tuberculides** have been reported in Japan and several have been reported from northern Europe, but they are extremely rare in the United States. Tuberculides presumably result from hematogenous dissemination of a small embolus of tubercle bacilli in a person with a high degree of tuberculin sensitivity, with resulting rapid destruction of bacilli. A nodule arises in the deep part of the glans or around the urethral orifice and may either resolve spontaneously or ulcerate with a whitish yellow necrotic base that heals with scarring in about a month.

The **differential diagnosis** of chronic penile ulcerations include:

balanitis
Behçet's disease
chancroid
drug eruption
erythema multiforme
erythroplasia
herpes simplex
papulonecrotic tuberculide
penile cancer
syphilis

Moral: A **chronic penile ulcer** deserves a biopsy, PPD, and chest x-ray.

Chalmers RJG, Burton PA, Bennett RF et al: **Lichen sclerosus et atrophicus**: A common and distinctive cause of phimosis in boys. Arch Dermatol 1984; 120:1025–1027.

Fourteen of 100 prepubertal boys undergoing elective circumcision for disease of the foreskin were found histologically to have lichen sclerosus et atrophicus. Clinically, the majority showed gross scarring and sclerosis on the inner surface of the prepuce.

Berth-Jones J, Graham-Brown RAC, Burns DA: **Lichen sclerosus**: A review of 14 cases in young girls with emphasis on symptomatology. Br J Dermatol 1989; 121 (Suppl 34):34.

Appearing as early as the age of 2 years, lichen sclerosus may present more with symptoms than signs. These girls complain of **pain and pruritus**. The pain is associated with urination and defecation and leads to constipation, nocturia, and enuresis.

Examples are cited where the problem was mistakenly ascribed to sexual abuse or to fissures.

Tompkins KJ, James WD: **Persistent bullae** on the penis of an elderly man. Arch Dermatol 1987; 123:1392–1394.

Blisters of the penis had been this 65-year-old man's complaint for 2 years. He had several 1.0 to 1.5 cm tense noninflammatory bullae of the glans and the shaft of the penis. They were present on atrophic telangiectatic skin. Biopsy confirmed the diagnosis of **balanitis xerotica obliterans**. This condition first described in 1928 by Stühmer involves the glans, prepuce, urethral meatus, and occasionally the penile shaft. The lesions are characteristically ivory-white atrophic lesions, at times associated with pruritus and pain, as well as serous or hemorrhagic bullae. In the uncircumcised individual, phimosis frequently develops. The patient may note dysuria, as well as pain on intercourse.

Squamous cell carcinoma may rarely arise so that periodic evaluations are wise. This condition is a variant of lichen sclerosus et atrophicus and remains of equally enigmatic origin.

Cocks PS, Peel KR, Cartwright RA, Adib R: **Carcinoma** of penis and cervix. Lancet 1980; 2:855–856.

Cervical wart virus is found in approximately 1% of routine Pap smears from Quebec, Sydney, and Leeds. Warty changes range from mild dysplasia to carcinoma-in-situ. Most patients are symptom free, but there is a frequent association of penile warts in sexual contacts. A link between the **wart virus and carcinoma** of the penis and cervix seems likely, with clusters of cases occurring in spouse pairs.

The patient admires the instrument more than the instrumentalist: use the lab!

Scrotum

Fisher AA: Unique reactions of **scrotal skin** to topical agents. Cutis 1989; 44:445.

Did you ask your patient with that scrotal dermatitis

if he had used a depilatory there?
if he had used an antiperspirant there?
if he had used a deodorant there?
if he had used pHisoHex there?
if 5-fluorouracil or podophyllin had been used there or nearby?

Dr. Fisher does and he finds examples of all of the above.

The exquisite permeability of scrotal epidermis makes the scrotum very sensitive to contactants that can be used elsewhere on the skin with impunity.

Johnson WT: **Cutaneous chylous reflux**: The "weeping scrotum." Arch Dermatol 1979; 115:464–466.

For the past year this 18-year-old man had noted episodes of **weeping of a creamy fluid from his scrotum**. The attacks promptly subsided with a few days of local soaks and bed rest. Examination disclosed matting of the pubic hair with a yellow sticky material. The scrotum was thickened and leathery with numerous 2-4 mm yellow firm papules on the scrotum and adjacent medial thigh. Some of these papules were translucent.

A **biopsy** revealed dilated lymphatic channels that traversed not only the upper dermis but also the epidermis. These vessels opened to the external surface in some instances. A **diagnosis of lymphatic hyperplasia with chylous reflux** was made. It was possible to inject the lymphangiogram blue dye into the lymphatic channel of the foot and see it exude from the scrotum.

Chylous reflux may also occur in **association** with malignant disease, congenital hypoplasia of the lymphatics and filariasis. In this case, a nevoid overgrowth of the lymphatics was apparently responsible for the reflux of lymph.

Duvic M, Lowe L, Rios A et al: Superficial **phaeohyphomycosis** of the scrotum in a patient with the acquired immunodeficiency syndrome. Arch Dermatol 1987; 123:1597–1599.

Tiny brown spots appeared on the **scrotum** of a 28-year-old homosexual man with AIDS, Kaposi's sarcoma, and cytomegalovirus retinitis. Present for 3 weeks, the numerous 1- to 3-mm variably pigmented, rough, flat papules looked like dirt or small seborrheic keratoses. However, a **KOH** examination showed a mass of **mycelia**. Cultures grew out a fluffy gray-brown colony of *Bipolaris* and a velvet brown-black colony of *Curvularia*.

AIDS patients bring us a whole new world of dermatology.

Wood SM, Bloom SR: Glucagon and gastrin secretion by a **pancreatic tumor** and its metastases. J Roy Soc Med 1982; 75:42–45.

A 65-year-old man with mild diabetes, duodenal ulcer, and angina presented with an erythematous rash of the scrotum, angular stomatitis and glossitis, **arcuate erythema** with a migratory edge on the arms and trunk, and annular lesions with crusted edges in the groin. Skin biopsy showed spongiosis of the superficial layers with eosinophilic infiltration. Despite zinc therapy and initial improvement of all areas except the scrotum, over the next year the erythematous scaling rash worsened and spread with migratory margins and healed hyperpigmented centers. He also lost weight and appeared cachectic.

Laboratory evaluation showed a diabetic oral glucose tolerance curve and elevated fasting plasma gut hormone concentrations, including **glucagon**, gastrin, and pancreatic polypeptide. **A pancreatic tumor** was localized to the head of the pancreas, with metastases in the liver. Treatment with hepatic artery embolization caused clearing of the rash in 24 hours and a marked decrease in plasma gastrin and glucagon. His skin remained clear over the following months, and his diabetes and chest pain were less severe. He was believed to have a combination of the glucagonoma syndrome (necrolytic migratory erythema, mild diabetes, and severe weight loss) and the Zollinger-Ellison syndrome (hyperacidity, hypergastrinemia, and a history of duodenal ulceration).

Since hepatic metastases depend on the hepatic arterial blood supply, they become ischemically necrosed following hepatic artery embolization. Normal liver is not jeopardized, as it can survive solely on its portal blood supply.

Benson PM, Lapins NA, Odom RB: **White piedra**. Arch Dermatol 1983; 119:602–604.

Scrotal pruritus was the presenting complaint of this 22-year-old man. It had been present for 8 months, beginning about 4 months after a jungle-training exercise in Panama.

On inspection, the scrotal skin was normal but barely visible dry adherent white excrescences were noted. The hairs felt gritty. On potassium hydroxide examination the hairs showed beaded aggregates of anthrospores along the hair shaft. On culture, a mucoid growth appeared within 4 days. This was identified as the yeast-like *Trichosporon cutaneum*, the cause of white piedra. Treatment was not successful.

This **white piedra** is the analogue of black piedra, in which black concretions of *Piedraia hortae* grow on the scalp hair. Both types are well named piedra, since this is the Spanish word for "stone." Their stone-like hardness is distinctive.

T. cutaneum may involve the hair shafts of any area, although in this patient only scrotal hair was affected. It may affect horses or other animals.

Fahal AH, Hassan MA: **Fournier's gangrene** in Khartoum. Br J Urol 1988; 61:451–454.

Fournier's gangrene is a fulminant spreading infection of the scrotum in young healthy individuals. It rapidly progresses to gangrene. It may involve not only the scrotum but also the penis, perineum, and abdominal wall. Organisms reaching the subcutaneous tissue cause an **obliterative endarteritis** with the consequent gangrene. The **entry point** may be an ischiorectal or anal abscess, as well as an infected hemorrhoid. *Proteus* was the most common pathogen isolated. Others were *Pseudomonas*, *E. coli*, *Klebsiella*, and *S. aureus*, as well as a nonhemolytic *Streptococcus*.

Cultures must be taken from pus and excised tissue for both aerobic and anaerobic growth. The initial clinical presentation is **scrotal pain and swelling**, as well as a fever. Subcutaneous emphysema follows with frank gangrene and sloughing.

The mortality rate was 25%.

Slater DN, Smith GT, Mundy K: **Diabetes mellitus with ketoacidosis** presenting as Fournier's gangrene. J Roy Soc Med 1982; 75:530–532.

A 64-year-old man developed **scrotal discomfort and reddening of the genital skin** one week before becoming increasingly drowsy. Upon his admission to the hospital the scrotum was grossly swollen with early **patches of gan-**

grene, and he was dehydrated and ketotic. Blood sugar was 720 mg/100 ml, and clotting studies were abnormal. The scrotal gangrene became confluent and extended onto the penis and lower abdominal wall, and he died 6 days later. Scrotal skin biopsy showed extensive intravascular fibrin deposition, which was also present in the brain and kidney.

Although Fournier's gangrene of the scrotum has been considered to be idiopathic, Fournier in 1883 recognized that **diabetes mellitus** was a predisposing factor. Since diabetic ketoacidosis may lead to disseminated intravascular coagulation, Fournier's gangrene in a diabetic patient should suggest coagulation abnormalities.

Hashimoto T, Inamoto N, Nakamura K: Triple **extramammary Paget's disease.** Immunohistochemical studies. Dermatologica 1986; 173:174–179.

A 75-year-old man with pruritus on the legs and scrotum was found on general inspection to have an ill-defined 2-cm irregular **patch of erythema in each axilla** and a brownish erythematous plaque in the right **pubic area.** No lymph nodes were palpable. Skin **biopsies** of all lesions showed Paget's cells. Excision appeared to be curative. No internal malignancy was detected and the serum CEA remained normal. The value of examining not just the sites indicated by the patient was underscored in this report.

The serum CEA is elevated in patients with Paget's disease with widespread metastasis and is considered to be a good index for monitoring the course of the disease. Involvement of three separate body areas with Paget's disease is extremely rare, with only six previous reports in the literature.

Moy LS, Chalet M, Lowe NJ: **Scrotal squamous cell carcinoma** in a psoriatic patient treated with coal tar. J Am Acad Dermatol 1986; 14:518–519.

Psoriasis of the left half of the scrotum in a 41-year-old man cleared with topical steroid therapy, except for a residual raised **coin-shaped** 1-cm **lesion.** Skin biopsy revealed Bowen's disease.

He had been applying 5% crude coal tar (Tegrin) intermittently to his scrotal psoriasis for 17 years. With no other carcinogenic exposure, the **tar** presumably induced his scrotal squamous cell carcinoma.

Some diseases travel incognito, like your grandmother in a wig and dark glasses.

Doherty VR, Forsyth A, MacKie RM: **Pruritus vulvae**: A manifestation of contact hypersensitivity? Br J Dermatol 1990; 123(Suppl 37):26–27.

50 women with pruritus vulvae were patch tested to the standard set of contact allergens; 39 had at least one positive reaction. The most **common sensitivities** proved to be to nickel, perfume, neomycin, and local anesthetics. Avoidance of the patient's specific sensitizing allergens resulted in a lessening of symptoms in 16 of 23 patients.

McKay M: **Vulvodynia**. A multifactorial clinical problem. Arch Dermatol 1989; 125:256–262.

An unremitting burning sensation localized to the vulva is the characteristic of vulvodynia. Usually occurring in the postmenopausal years, it is labeled essential vulvodynia if no changes are seen on examination. Pruritus vulvae with its intractable itch, excoriations, and lichenification is clearly a different problem. The burning pain of glossodynia is more analogous to vulvodynia; both show a high degree of treatment resistance.

All women with vulvodynia need to be carefully examined to **rule out**

1. Vulvar dermatoses
   lichen sclerosus et atrophicus
   intraepithelial neoplasia
   contact dermatitis
   topical steroid–induced periorificial dermatitis
   lichen planus
   candidiasis
2. Cyclic vulvitis
   flare some time in menstrual period
   exhibit eruption-free days
   flare with antibiotics
3. Papillomatosis
   may be subclinical warts
   2-minute application of vinegar accentuates papillomas
4. Vulvar vestibulitis
   orifices of Skene's paraurethral and Bartholin's glands are red and painful
   minor mucosal glands may also show inflammatory change.

Rogers WB: **Shampoo urethritis**. Am J Dis Child 1985; 139:748–749.

Shampoos contain many ingredients in common with bubble bath, including essential oil fragrances. The practice of **shampooing children's hair in the bathtub** is common and should be inquired about and discontinued in children with dysuria and frequency. Shampoo used on pubic hair may cause the same problem in teenagers, as well as vulvar irritation. Urinalysis and physical examination are normal.

Guenther LC, Shum D: Localized childhood **vulvar pemphigoid**. J Am Acad Dermatol 1990; 22:762–764.

Recurrent **vulvar ulcers** had been experienced by this 4-year-old girl for the past year. They had been negative on culture and not responsive to hydrocortisone cream.

On examination, symmetrical ulcers were seen on the labia. There were no lesions elsewhere. A biopsy showed an ulcer with granulation tissue and inflammatory cell infiltrate in the dermis. The diagnosis came with **immunofluorescent studies**, which showed the lesion to be **bullous pemphigoid**.   617

Linear IgG and C_3 deposits were seen at the basement membrane. Indirect bullous pemphigoid antibody was positive at a titre of 1 to 128.

The diagnostic stumbling blocks for the clinician were the youth of the patient, the absence of lesions elsewhere, and the absence of vesicles. In solving problems like this, do not send a boy, send a "boy-opsy" for immunofluorescence.

McKee PH, Wright E, Hutt MSR: **Vulval schistosomiasis**. Clin Exp Dermatol 1983; 8:189–194.

"**Warts**" on the vulva of women coming from tropical regions, either as tourists or immigrants, may well be **schistosomiasis** and not condyloma accuminatum. The correct diagnosis comes from a **biopsy** wherein the ova are seen in a granulomatous setting. The ova can be either in microabscesses or the epidermis itself. Rarely, adult worms may be seen within the lumina of cutaneous veins.

Schistosomiasis is contracted by exposure to **snail-infested waters**. The cercariae having left the snail penetrates the patient's skin and passes to the liver, where maturation to adult wormhood occurs. The vulva is involved as the female worms pass through the vesical and uterovaginal plexus of veins.

The commonest site of cutaneous schistosomiasis is in the perianal skin: another cause of pruritus ani. It may also appear as a **pruritic lichenified eruption** around the umbilicus. Some examples appear clinically as fibromas and even **vitiligo** of the face and of the vulva has been observed.

Brook I: Aerobic and anaerobic microbiology of **Bartholin's abscess**. Surg Gynecol Obstet 1989; 169:32–34.

A review of bacterial cultures from 28 women over a 10-year period. The Bartholin's gland abscesses were surgically incised and drained at Walter Reed Army Medical Center and the Naval Medical Center, Bethesda.

Look for *Bacteroides* species (21 cases), *Escherichia coli* (6 cases), and *Neisseria gonorrhoeae* (4 cases).

Cook RL, Reid G, Pond DG: Clue cells in **bacterial vaginosis**: Immunofluorescent identification of the adherent gram-negative bacteria as *Gardnerella vaginalis*. J Infect Dis 1989; 160:490–496.

"**Clue cells**" are epithelial cells covered with adherent gram-negative bacilli, frequently observed in vaginal smears from women with bacterial vaginosis but not in clinically normal women. *Gardnerella vaginalis* is the major adherent bacterial type observed, but *Bacteroides* species and *Mobiluncus* species (anaerobic) were also detected.

Wagenberg HR, Downham TF: Chronic **edema of** the **vulva**: A condition similar to cheilitis granulomatosa. Cutis 1981; 27:526–527.

For nearly a year this 26-year-old black woman had noted marked swelling of her **vulva**. The problem began with small draining furuncles that had healed with systemic antibiotic therapy. She gave a history of engaging in **oral sex**. On examination the labia majora were extremely swollen but not tender nor was the swelling fluctuant. Peripheral pustules were present.

A biopsy culture was negative for acid-fast bacilli and fungi, but the biopsy showed diffuse edema, fibrosis, and necrotizing granulomas. The complement fixation tests for lymphogranuloma venereum were negative. A diagnosis of **chronic hypertrophic vulvitis** was considered, with the trauma of oral sex as a contributory factor. The histologic findings matched those seen in cheilitis granulomatosis.

Obstruction of the lymphatics provided the major cause of the enlarged labia in this patient. We would point to the similarity of this phenomenon to the **elephantiasis** induced by chronic streptococcal infections.

Davis J, Shapiro L, Baral J: **Vulvitis circumscripta plasmacellularis**. J Am Acad Dermatol 1983; 8:413–416.

Multiple **red-brown glistening**, **focally eroded areas** on the inner and outer aspects of the **labia minora** had been present for 3 years in this 30-year-old woman. The lesions were asymptomatic, had irregular well-defined margins, were discrete, and intermixed with scattered small white papules.

A **biopsy** gave the diagnosis: vulvitis circumscripta plasmacellularis. It is the **female analogue of Zoon's balanitis**, which is benign, circumscribed and chronic as distinguished from the premalignant erythroplasia of Queyrat. Clinically, this form of focal vulvitis is distinctive because of its brick-red lacquer-like glistening surface, its erosions, and its papules. The color comes from the abundant hemosiderin deposition. "**Zoon's**" **vulvitis** must be **distinguished by biopsy from**

Paget's disease	Fixed drug eruption
Squamous cell carcinoma in situ	Trauma
Pemphigus	Factitial lesions

Whether it's vulvitis or balanitis, it deserves a biopsy look for the plasma cells.

Haustein U-F: Localized nonscarring **bullous pemphigoid** of the vagina. Dermatologica 1988; 176:200–201.

For 2 years a 60-year-old woman suffered from **multiple erosive inflammatory lesions of the vagina**. There were no lesions elsewhere. The problem had been assumed to be candidiasis or bullous lichen planus. However, a biopsy and immunofluorescence studies proved the vaginitis to be bullous pemphigoid. Control was achieved with prednisone and azathioprine therapy.

Arul KJ, Emmerson RW: **Malacoplakia** of the skin. Clin Exp Dermatol 1977; 2:131–135.

An **indurated ulcer of the vulva** present for one year in a 75-year-old woman was heavily colonized with *E. coli* stemming from a urinary tract infection. Two punched-out ulcers on the left labium majus led into a single cavity approximately 1 cm deep. Since antibiotic therapy was without effect, the entire ulcerated lesion was excised. Microscopy revealed the diagnostic target-like Michaelis-Guttmann bodies of **malacoplakia** (Greek: *malakos*, soft; *plakos*, plaque).

Christened in 1903, it is a benign inflammatory condition probably induced by bacterial infection. The Michaelis-Guttmann bodies are inclusions in histiocytes, representing degraded bacteria encrusted with calcium phosphate. In addition to *E. coli*, pseudomonas and *Staphylococcus aureus* have been isolated from cases of cutaneous malacoplakia.

Congeni BL, Ulbrich M, Feingold M: Picture of the month: **Varicella gangrenosum**. Am J Dis Child 1985; 139:1151–1152.

A young girl with chickenpox developed erythema and swelling of the left **labia majora**, which became **blue and necrotic** within 48 hours and then ulcerated. She was thought to have varicella gangrenosum, most commonly caused by *Streptococcus pyogenes* or *Staphylococcus aureus*.

Nussbaum AR, Lebowitz RL: **Interlabial masses** in little girls: Review and imaging recommendations. AJR 1983; 141:65–71.

Colored pictures of the five most common interlabial masses seen on the vulva in young girls are featured. These can be distinguished clinically on the basis of symptoms, appearance, exact location, position of the urethral meatus, route of urine flow, and race and age.

1. *Prolapsed ectopic ureterocele*
   In white girls, this presents as a smooth round mass with variable color (pink, red, bluish purple), no evident urethral meatus, and urine exiting circumferentially around the mass. It is due to cystic dilatation of the terminal ureter in association with a stenotic orifice.

2. *Urethral prolapse*
   In black girls under 18, an edematous red-to-blue hemorrhagic mass encircles the urethral meatus, bleeds easily, and results in a central stream of urine. This prolapse of urethral mucosa through the meatus also occurs in postmenopausal women. The diagnosis can be confirmed by passing a catheter into the bladder.

3. *Paraurethral cyst*
   In neonates, this self-limited epithelial-lined cyst displaces the urethral meatus causing an eccentric urinary stream.

4. *Hydro(metro)colpos*
   A pearly gray bulging mass at the introitus with a normal urethral meatus cephalad to the mass contains mucoid material visible through the transparent hymen. Maternal estrogen stimulates secretion of uterine and cervical glands, leading to distension of the vagina and uterus. The excessive mucous secretions are trapped proximal to an imperforate hymen, transverse vaginal septum, or atretic vagina.

5. *Rhabdomyosarcoma of vagina (botryoid sarcoma)*
   A grapelike cluster of pearly gray nodules prolapses through the introitus. In infants and children under 5 years of age, this is the most common primary malignant tumor of the vagina, uterus, or bladder.

Highet AS, Warren RE, Weekes AJ: Bacteriology and antibiotic treatment of **perineal suppurative hidradenitis**. Arch Dermatol 1988; 124:1047–1051.

Streptococcus milleri was the main pathogen implicated in the pathogenesis of perineal hidradenitis suppurativa in 32 patients. Also isolated were S. *aureus*, Streptococcus, and Bacteroides.

The lesional discharge should be placed directly in Stuart's transport medium and laboratory instructed to look for S. *milleri* specifically as well as anaerobes. Appropriate sensitivity studies are to be done, although practically, erythromycin (500 mg qid) has been the most effective therapy.

Boer J, Herfst MJ, Ideler F: **Eosinophilic fasciitis**. Br J Dermatol 1982; 106:237–239.

Indurated painful areas of the back, arms, chest, and perineum had been present for 2 years in this 46-year-old woman. Examination revealed sharply margined white depigmented areas of the upper back, pubic area, and upper legs. The indurated areas were not movable over the underlying tissue.

Clinically, a diagnosis of **lichen sclerosus et atrophicus** would have been made but for the induration and pain. A **biopsy** disclosed the definitive diagnosis. With skin, fascia, muscle biopsy the skin was seen to be normal, but the fascia was thickened and had a perivascular monocellular infiltrate. The diagnosis of **eosinophilic fasciitis** was supported by the presence of a blood eosinophilia of 16%. The unusual feature in this patient was the extensive depigmentation that gave the condition a superficial resemblance to lichen sclerosus et atrophicus.

Verbov J: **Pruritus ani** and its management: A study and reappraisal. Clin Exp Dermatol 1984; 9:46–52.

In patients with pruritus ani, look carefully to see if you can make a diagnosis a notch above the one already made by the patient who told you "itch around the rectum."

Look for:

contact dermatitis	intertrigo	thread worms
seborrheic dermatitis	erythrasma	hemorrhoids
psoriasis	hyperhidrosis	diarrhea
candidiasis	lichen simplex	excessive hair
tinea	warts	

Oliet EJ, Estes SA: **Perianal comedones** associated with chronic topical fluorinated steroid use. J Am Acad Dermatol 1982; 7:405–407.

Numerous large, open comedones studded the perianal area of this 62-year-old man. The patient was totally unaware of them, having come for treatment of an erythematous scaly eruption of the groin. This proved on Wood's light to be erythrasma.

A history revealed the cause of the clustering of comedones. Because of a chronic **diarrheal-induced pruritus ani**, this patient had been applying 0.025% flurandrenolide cream 3 to 5 times daily for over 3 years. Pharmacy records suggested he had applied a grand total of about 6 pounds of this comedogenic cream. Why, no atrophy?

Guin JD: **Contact dermatitis** to perfume in paper products. J Am Acad Dermatol 1981; 4:733–734.

A 10-year-old boy had repeated episodes of **perianal itching** and a patchy erythematous **eczema of his nose** and cheeks. Patch testing revealed markedly positive vesicular reactions to cinnamic aldehyde (2% in petrolatum) and cinnamic alcohol (5% in petrolatum). With this awareness, his mother soon discovered that her son developed the facial rash whenever he used **perfumed toilet tissue** to wipe his nose. A patch test to the cardboard center roller (where the perfume is applied during manufacture), moistened with alcohol, was positive at 48 hours. Use of nonperfumed facial and toilet tissue solved the problem.

Krol AL: **Perianal streptococcal dermatitis**. Pediatr Dermatol 1990; 7:97–100.

Perianal streptococcal dermatitis comes in **3 varieties**.

Bright pink, moist erythematous tender skin extending out an inch or two from the anal orifice.
Painful fissures, dried mucoid discharge staining underclothing.
Beefy red psoriasiform eruption with yellow crusting.

Most all have associated itching and painful defecation, but there is no telltale streptococcal cellulitis. This perianal focus of streptococcal infection may trigger generalized **guttate psoriasis**, and hence all patients with guttate psoriasis deserve examination of this area and appropriate cultures.

The **differential diagnosis** includes psoriasis, seborrheic dermatitis, candidiasis, inflammatory bowel disease, pinworm infestation, and sexual abuse.

A **culture** quickly distinguishes this streptococcal dermatitis, but the physician should **alert the laboratory** to use blood agar and to isolate for group

A beta-hemolytic streptococci so that the ubiquitous *E. coli* do not obscure them. Streptococci will not grow in the selenite broth or on the MacConkey's agar commonly used to isolate stool pathogens.

Because the streptococcus loves the folds, look for it in retrovesicular dermatitis and in the flexures as well as in the perianal region.

Marks VJ, Maksimak M: **Perianal streptococcal cellulitis**. J Am Acad Dermatol 1988; 18:587–588.

A 5-year-old boy complained of perianal irritation and pruritus for 2 weeks. Moderate anal leakage and soiling and small amounts of blood were present on his underpants. He had no chills, fever, or other systemic symptoms. Examination revealed sharply demarcated **bright perianal erythema** extending 2 cm out from the anal verge onto perianal skin. There were no satellite papules or pustules and KOH examination was negative, as was a Scotch tape test for pinworms. Stool examination for ova and parasites was negative. Swab cultures from the anal canal and perianal skin were positive for group A beta-hemolytic streptococci; treatment with penicillin was curative.

Vivid perianal erythema calls for perianal swab cultures for streptococci (plated on 5% sheep blood agar) to **differentiate** perianal streptococcal cellulitis from:

>   candidiasis
>   seborrheic dermatitis
>   psoriasis
>   pinworm infection
>   inflammatory bowel disease
>   behavioral problems

Perianal tenderness, painful defecation, and fecal soiling also serve as an alert to this type of cellulitis.

Rehder PA, Eliezer ET, Lane AT: **Perianal cellulitis**. Cutaneous group A streptococcal disease. Arch Dermatol 1988; 124:702–704.

A 3-year-old boy had a 6-month history of **perianal redness** and irritation. It had not responded to soaks, topical antifungals, and topical corticosteroids. There were small perirectal fissures that yielded beta-hemolytic streptococci, group A. Interestingly, his 6-year-old brother had culture-proven streptococcal pharyngitis just before the onset of this child's perianal problem. A month of erythromycin therapy was curative, with confirmatory negative cultures.

Group A streptococcal cellulitis **may also present as** a diaper rash, chronic perianal fissures, painful defecation, fecal hoarding, or even proctocolitis. Delays in diagnosis of up to a year result from failure to culture. Often the condition is mistaken for candidiasis.

One of the five cases presented involved associated **guttate psoriasis**. Thus, perianal and pharyngeal examinations and cultures are indicated in patients with guttate psoriasis, since it may be triggered by streptococcal infection, either obvious or occult.

Friter BS, Lucky AW: The perineal eruption of **Kawasaki syndrome**. Arch Dermatol 1988; 124:1805–1810.

An **erythematous desquamating perineal rash** in a febrile child is an early diagnostic finding in Kawasaki syndrome. But also look

>   at the hands and feet for:

erythema of palms and soles
edema
desquamation of tips of digits

at the mucosa for:
conjunctival infection
dry, red lips
red pharynx and strawberry tongue

at the skin for:
polymorphous erythematous exanthem

at the neck for:
lymphadenopathy

McCuaig CC, Moroz B: Perineal eruption in **Kawasaki's syndrome**. Arch Dermatol 1987; 123:430–431.

Erythematous plaques and desquamation localized strikingly in the diaper area was the early sign of Kawasaki's disease in a pair of 2-year-olds.

The diagnosis is critical in light of the potential that this disease has for leading to coronary artery aneurysms and thromboses.

Halasz C, Silvers D, Crum CP: **Bowenoid papulosis** in 3-year-old girl. J Am Acad Dermatol 1986; 14:326–330.

Multiple **gray-brown smooth velvety papules** had been present in the **perianal area** of this 3-year-old girl for 2 months. They had been enlarging and extending into the anal canal. Bacterial cultures of the vagina, rectum, and throat showed *Neisseria gonorrhoeae* in the throat. The pharyngeal gonorrhea was treated with a single injection of procaine penicillin G (1 million units).

Biopsy of the perianal lesions showed the histologic pattern of Bowenoid papulosis (squamous cell in situ; vulvular intraepithelial neoplasia [VIN]). Until the histologic diagnosis was obtained, lichen planus, psoriasis, and condyloma acuminata had to be considered. Squamous cell carcinoma could be ruled out since it is not seen in children, other than those with xeroderma pigmentosa, albinism, dyskeratosis congenita, or epidermodysplasia verruciformis.

Bowenoid papulosis is considered to be induced by **papilloma virus**, which can be sexually transmitted. One can thus assume that this child's lesions resulted from sexual contact. The presence of the verrucally transmitted gonococcus in the throat of this child supports the view that unidentified sexual abuse may have occurred.

Over the next 8 months, the lesions regressed without therapy. Only residual depigmentation remained. Such spontaneous remission has occurred in over 20% of the patients reported and is to be compared to the high rate of spontaneous remission of common warts.

Markowitz J, Daum F, Aiges H et al: **Perianal disease** in children and adolescents with Crohn's disease. Gastroenterology 1984; 86:829–833.

Nearly 50% of 149 children with **Crohn's disease** also had **perianal disease**:

chronic deep anal fissures (anywhere in anal canal)
large, edematous skin tags (resembling external hemorrhoids)
fistulas with mucopurulent discharge (rectum to perianal, scrotal, or labial areas) but no palpable masses on digital or proctosigmoidoscopic exam.

abscesses—intensely painful masses in the subcutaneous, submucous, or ischiorectal spaces, with spontaneous drainage into the rectum or through the skin.

A careful perianal inspection is an important, but often overlooked, part of the physical examination. All anal folds should be completely separated to reveal hidden fissures. Since hemorrhoids are rare in children and adolescents, except for pregnant teenagers, Crohn's disease should be considered in any case of "**suspected hemorrhoids**."

Lookingbill DP, Spangler N, Sexton FM: Skin involvement as the presenting sign of **internal carcinoma**: A retrospective study of 7316 cancer patients. J Am Acad Dermatol 1990; 22:19–26.

Example 1

A **fluctuant purulent drainage** process in the **perianal area** was initially diagnosed as hidradenitis suppurativa. A biopsy provided the correct diagnosis. The patient had a mucinous adenocarcinoma that had spread from the rectum to the buttocks and was presenting as inflammatory abscesses.

Example 2

Erythema and edema of the malar region in this patient suggested cellulitis. Biopsy revealed the true nature of the patient's problem. It proved to be a direct extension of a cancer originating in the nasal sinus.

Example 3

A **facial ulcer** proved on biopsy to be a direct extension of an oral cavity carcinoma.

Although only 59 out of the 7316 patients studied had a skin lesion as the first sign of malignancy, it behooves one to biopsy unexplained inflammatory nodules, persistent, indurated erythema, and non-healing ulcers. Only by doing so will the skin aid in detection of otherwise unrecognized internal carcinoma.

Drusin LM, Homan WP, Dineen P: The role of surgery in **primary syphilis** of the anus. Ann Surg 1976; 184:65–67.

Rectal pain and tender lymphadenopathy were common complaints in four patients with unsuspected anal chancres. While two patients had anal fissures, one had hemorrhoids and one had a 1-cm indurated erythematous mass underlying a skin ulceration to the right of the anus. Although **chancres** are usually relatively painless, secondary infection, friction, and trauma may make them painful, especially in the anal area. Any factor that makes an anal lesion atypical for hemorrhoids, fissure, fistula, or abscess should alert suspicion for syphilis. This includes multiple anal lesions in a single patient and an **anal fissure** that occurs laterally rather than in the anterior or posterior commissures.

Kennedy CTC, Lyell A: **Perianal orf**. J Am Acad Dermatol 1984; 11:72–74.

A 7-year-old girl was referred for treatment of perianal warts of 10 days duration. On examination the **perianal skin** exhibited eroded **purplish red papules and plaques**. Close inspection disclosed a small but similar lesion on the left index finger.

Because the girl lived on a farm and had contact with orphan lambs known to have been infected with orf, this diagnosis was entertained. It was confirmed by electron microscopic examination of scrapings. Both the perianal and the finger lesions showed the diagnostic viral particles of orf. Complete resolution occurred by 2 weeks.

Horn TD, Hood AF: **Cytomegalovirus** is predictably present in perineal ulcers in immunosuppressed patients. Arch Dermatol 1990; 126:642–644.

Perineal ulcers from five consecutive immune suppressed patients proved to be infected with **cytomegalovirus**. The observations were made using commercially available monoclonal antibodies to early and late cytomegalovirus antigens. In three of the five, herpes simplex virus was also found as a resident, again using monoclonal antibodies.

The role of the cytomegalovirus is unknown. It is a herpes virus that often infects without any overt sign of its primary entry. It then persists indefinitely, residing often within the gastrointestinal tract. Thus the source of the virus may be fecal shedding. Alternatively, activities of this latent virus can lead to viremia with consequent localization of the virus in a lesion or organ. The best known pathologic results of such a virus are **retinitis** and **pneumonitis**. Cytomegalovirus remains a laboratory curiosity in the skin producing none of the specific dermatologic syndromes known, yet one may expect to find it, and at times its fellow traveller, herpes simplex, in perineal ulcers and granulation tissue.

Once cytomegalovirus is found, check the retina and lung.

Al-Najjar A, Reilly GD, Bleehen SS: **Pemphigoid vegetans**: A case report. Acta Derm Venereol 1984; 64:450–452.

A persistent **itchy eruption of both groins** in an 83-year-old man had been present for a year. Examination disclosed sharply circumscribed hypertrophic, verrucous, and vegetative lesions with no blisters. **Biopsy** revealed subepidermal cleft formation, mixed perivascular infiltrate, and intraepidermal eosinophils and lymphocytes. There was IgG deposition at the dermoepidermal junction on immunofluorescence. A diagnosis of pemphigoid vegetans was made.

Persistent vegetating eruptions have been grouped together clinically as "**dermatitis vegetans**." One of these, the distinctive **pyodermite vegetante of Hallopeau**, has chronic pustular and vegetating lesions in the groin and axillae and may point to ulcerative colitis.

Immunofluorescent studies are essential for in-depth study of any intertriginous vegetating lesion. With this tool, pyodermite vegetante of Hallopeau is recognized as a type of pemphigus. While this patient was also viewed clinically as having pemphigus vegetans, immunohistological studies revealed pemphigoid instead.

Arminski TC, McLean DW: **Proctologic problems** in children. JAMA 1965; 194:1195–1196.

An anorectal examination on a proctologic table should be part of every physical examination of children with anorectal complaints, including pain, bleeding with bowel movements, and constipation. **Examination** requires careful inspection, palpation, anoscopy and proctosigmoidoscopy with a manner that is gentle, reassuring, thorough, and resolute. Too often, pathologic abnormalities amenable to treatment are masked under a diagnosis of intestinal colic, milk allergy, and emotional problems.

Among 700 children, one third had one or more **anal fissures**. These occur in the midline and begin as an anal gland infection with resulting crypt abscess and fissure. Diarrhea often precedes the cryptitis, as forcible rectal contractions counteract the conscious holding back of liquid stool and push bacteria into the crypts and ducts of the anal glands. Once a fissure develops, **constipation** is present. A chronic anal fissure is associated with a sentinel tag (cutaneous fibroma). A fissure must be distinguished from an abrasion, which is a linear break in the anal lining. Abrasions are usually multiple and found in the lateral quadrants. They are preceded by constipation or some other cause of excessive dilatation of the anal canal and heal once the underlying cause is corrected.

Parish LC, Gschnait F (eds): **Sexually Transmitted Diseases**. A Guide for Clinicians. New York, Springer-Verlag, 1989; 388 pp.

Here is a splendid review of everything that sexual partners can give each other, besides excitement.

Parish LC, Sehgal VN, Buntin DM: Color Atlas of Sexually Transmitted Diseases. New York, Igaku-Shoin, 1991; 173 pp.

An illustrated companion piece.

When all else fails, consider one of these diagnoses:

DUO	Dermatitis of undetermined origin
Q dermatitis	Analogous to Q fever (Q indicates cause is under query)
WK syndrome	"Who knows" syndrome
Dermatitis incognita	A disease traveling incognito
Dermatitis nonrecollecta	You know the diagnosis, but can't quite remember it
_____'s disease	Insert patient's name

Geographic Disease

The question "Where have you been or where have you lived?" may be another important portal of entry into the diagnostic process. Certain diseases are endemic and contagious. Search for them and think of them when you take a travel history. There's more to geographic disease than geographic tongue.

Berger RS, Perez-Figaredo RA, Spielvogel RL: **Leishmaniasis:** The touch preparation as a rapid means of diagnosis. J Am Acad Dermatol 1987; 16:1096–1105.

With air travel reducing continents to the size of counties, here is a tropical disease, leishmaniasis, that may "fly" into your office. The cause of leishmaniasis is a **protozoon** that comes to humans by way of the bite of those extremely small **sand** flies. Carrying their gastrointestinal load of infective flagellated organisms, they can pass through ordinary window screens to bite and inoculate the tourist! Indeed, even crushing the fly on your skin puts you at risk. The sturdy organism has been known to infect also via blood transfusion, sexual intercourse, the placenta, or research laboratory accident. The incubation period correlates precisely with the number of promastigotes (flagellated organisms) that enter. Ten is the minimal infective dose. With this dose the incubation period is several months usually but can be an astounding 3 years! If millions of organisms enter, there is virtually no incubation period at all.

Of the three classic forms of the disease, cutaneous leishmaniasis due to *Leishmania tropica* is the one with the greatest spectrum of skin change. In the acute form the lesions begin as **small papules** at the exact sites of the fly bites. Thus they are usually on exposed skin. They enlarge into nodules, ulcerate and become crusted, and require 6 to 12 months for healing. The result is a scar.

Often these lesions become infected with bacteria, leading to diagnostic delay. In some instances id reactions occur as a generalized asymptomatic eruption.

There is a **chronic form** in which ulceration does not occur and the infection persists for several years. It usually occurs in elderly patients and suggests at times:

lupus vulgaris	North American blastomycosis
leprosy	deep fungal infection
syphilis	

A third form is the *recidivans* **type**, in which "new" lesions keep appearing in or near the old scars of prior disease. Examples of this may continue for decades on end. Also to be thought of is the generalized diffuse form, which simulates lepromatous leprosy. In this type the primary lesions enlarge and become disseminated in large areas of skin. They do not ulcerate and they do not involve systemic organs, but they may appear in the nasal mucosa.

Aside from these cutaneous forms of leishmaniasis there is a **mucocutaneous version** due to *L. braziliensis* and a **systemic form** (kala-azar) due to *L. donovani*. In the mucocutaneous version the primary lesion is a papule at the sand fly bite site. However, the papule then enlarges and regional lymphadenopathy as well as widespread mucocutaneous lesions ensue. Accordingly, the **differential** includes pyoderma, sporotrichosis, syphilis, yaws, chromoblastomycosis, leprosy, South American blastomycosis, rhinoscleroma, histoplasmosis, and squamous cell carcinoma. The destructive effects on skin, cartilage, and mucosa, are phenomenal.

Kala-azar, the third major form, is the systemic disease in which the reticuloendothelial cells not in the skin but throughout the body serve as host to the *L. donovani* nonflagellated organism (amastigote). Every organ may become involved; without treatment the disease kills 9 out of every 10 of its victims.

The fastest way to **diagnosis** of any form of leishmaniasis is the following:

1. Local anesthesia with epinephrine to reduce bleeding that hinders reading
2. Obtain a 6-mm punch biopsy from the edge of a lesion as far from ulcer and secondary infection as possible
3. Touch tissue to microscope slide 2 to 3 times. Do not press
4. Fix slide in methyl alcohol 3 minutes
5. Stain in Wright-Giemsa for 45 minutes (1 drop of concentrate in 1 ml distilled water)
6. Look for intracellular and extracellular organisms. They are round, 2–6 μ in length, and 1–2 μ in width with a single round nucleus

There will be a red, pointed kinetoplast from one end of parasite. Other slower diagnostic approaches are biopsy, culture, and skin tests (Montenegro).

Remember there are 12 million patients with leishmaniasis in the world today. One could walk into your office tomorrow!

Harries J: **Amoebiasis:** A review. J Roy Soc Med 1982; 75:190–197.

Amoebiasis is one of the great tropical mimics. A high index of suspicion coupled with taking a careful geographical history will help avoid diagnostic mistakes. Skin lesions include **ulcerating granulomas around the anus** or around a colostomy opening that should be scraped and examined microscopically. Only certain varieties of *Entamoeba histolytica* are pathogenic and are identified by the finding of red blood cells in the cytoplasm of the amoeba. Active trophozoites may be seen in unformed **stools** or mucus shortly after being passed, but only cysts are found in formed stools and immediate examination is unnecessary. Invasive lesions of the gut are accompanied by **serum antibodies**, detectable with an indirect fluorescent antibody test positive at a titer of 1:80 in about 70% of cases.

Amoebiasis should be suspected in any person who has visited the tropics and has had **diarrhea** for more than 2 weeks. The onset is insidious, with a windy looseness of the bowels and recurring diarrhea and constipation. Eventually, blood and mucous are found in liquid stools with an offensive odor, and abdominal tenderness occurs.

Falanga V, Kapoor W: **Cerebral cysticercosis:** Diagnostic value of subcutaneous nodules: Report of two cases. J Am Acad Dermatol 1984; 12:304–307.

One year after coming to the United States **from India**, this 24-year-old Indian man developed seizures. A CT scan of the head showed hypovascular mass that was interpreted as a falx meningioma.

In search for diagnostic help, the skin was carefully examined; two small **subcutaneous papules** were revealed, less than 5 mm in the left temporal and right postauricular area. It was serial sectioning of the **biopsy** of these that gave the diagnosis of cysticercosis. Both showed the suckers and hooks of the *Cysticercus cellulosae* scolex in the subcutaneous tissue. The neurologist could then make the definitive diagnosis of **cerebral cysticercosis**.

Cysticercosis is common in India, China, and Africa, as well as in Central and South America. It is caused by infection with the larval form of the pork tapeworm *Taenia solium*. The source is eating uncooked or partially cooked pork containing the cysts. Whereas the primary site of infestation in the pig is the muscle, in humans it is the **brain**. Usually, neurologic symptoms bring the patient to the doctor, but over half have small easily raised macules in

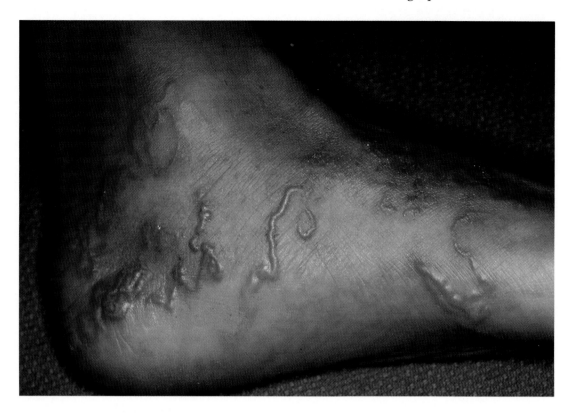

the skin that, on biopsy, reveal the disease and hence the cause of neurologic problems such as seizures.

In world travelers or in people from endemic areas:

look for subcutaneous nodules to biopsy
examine stool for eggs

In the differential diagnosis, it is well to recall that a nodule in individuals from Africa or South America may disclose onchocerciasis. Worms like to make "nodular" homes.

Milligan A, Burns DA: Ectopic **cutaneous schistosomiasis** and schistosomal ocular inflammatory disease. Br J Dermatol 1988; 119:793–798.

A group of **pruritic papules** on the left forehead of a 17-year-old Tanzanian man proved to be follicular eosinophil abscesses harboring Schistosoma ova. **Stool examination** showed the ova of *Schistosoma mansoni.* The papules had been present for only 2 weeks, appearing a month after a visit to Tanzania, highlighted by a swim in Lake Victoria. Concurrently, he had blurring of vision in his right eye, also due to the schistosomes.

Presumably, the schistosome **cercariae** penetrated his skin during the swim in Lake Victoria. After entering the circulation and spending a 3-week maturation stop in the liver, the adult flukes migrated countercurrent into the inferior mesenteric venous system to lay eggs, which normally pass directly into the feces. No one knows how the ova reached the forehead in this patient. Ectopic cutaneous localization of ova can occur in the periumbilical and genital areas and the buttocks, sometimes in a distinctively zosteriform pattern.

Always, the sign is pruritic papules. Think of schistosomiasis in anyone recently returned from an endemic area.

Lin AN, Imaeda S: A **dermatologic gazetteer.** Int J Dermatol 1990; 29:468–471.

I. PLACE VISITED	DERMATOLOGIC PROBLEM	SUSPECT
Worldwide	Erythematous pretibial lesions	Fort Bragg fever (pretibial fever) (*Leptospira autumnalis* infection) (town in North Carolina)
Worldwide	Scaling feet	Hong Kong foot (tinea pedis) (British Crown colony)
Worldwide	Erythema chronicum migrans, arthritis, neurologic changes	Lyme disease (spirochete infection) (town in Connecticut)
Worldwide	Pruritus, crusting of hands and feet	Norwegian scabies (Norway)
Germany	Hemorrhagic febrile maculopapular eruption	Marburg virus disease (German town)
Brazil	Crusted ulcers, skin, nose, mouth	Brazilian blastomycosis (South American blastomycosis) (systemic infection with Paracoccidioides brasiliensis)
South America	Pemphigus foliaceous	Brazilian pemphigus (fogo selvagem)
South America	Warts (verruga peruana) systemic illness	Oroya fever (Bartonellosis) (town in Peru)
North and South America	Hemorrhagic rash in febrile patient	Rocky Mountain spotted fever (*Rickettsia rickettsii* infection) (mountain range extending from Mexico to the Arctic)
Western America and South America	Erythema nodosum, abscesses	San Joaquin Valley fever (coccidioidomycosis) (county in California)
East Africa, New Guinea, Australia	Ulcerating nodule	Buruli ulcer (region in Uganda)
Zaire, Sudan	Hemorrhagic maculopapular eruption	Ebola virus disease (river in Zaire)
Africa, Middle East, India	Inflammatory nodules	Guinea worm infestation (*Dracuncula medinensis*) (West African country)
Africa, India, South America	Chronic draining infection of feet	Madura foot (Madurella and actinomycetes infection) (city in India)
Middle East, India, China, Africa, southern Europe	Ulcerating nodule	Baghdad boil (Oriental sore, leishmaniasis)
China, Thailand, Japan	Edema, face, and eyelids	Katayama disease (*Schistosoma japonicum* infection) (mountain in Japan)
Asia	Lymphedema and lymphadenitis	Malayan filariasis (*Brugia malaya* infection) (country in Asia)
Asia-Central America	Concentric rings of scaling	Tokelau ringworm (tinea imbricata due to infection with *T. concentricum*) (islands in Pacific Ocean)
India	*Leishmania donovani* infection with fever, lymphadenopathy, cutaneous pigmentation	Dumdum fever (town near Calcutta)
II. PLACE OF ORIGIN	PROBLEM	SUSPECT
Jews, Arabs, Armenians from Middle East	Erysipelas of legs and episodic fever	Familial Mediterranean fever
Meleda	Keratoderma of palms and soles	Mal de Meleda (Yugoslav island in Adriatic Sea)
Tangier Island	Xanthomas, large orange tonsils	Tangier disease (island in Chesapeake Bay, Virginia)

Stewart WD: **Geographic dermatology.** Int J Dermatol 1990; 29:477–478.

More dermatologic problems for the traveller.

Place Visited	Dermatologic Problem	Suspect
Western U.S. and western Canada	Fever	Colorado tick fever (Colorado) Rickettsial infection
Hawaii	Dermatitis	Pearl Harbor itch (medusa sting)
Worldwide	Chancre, rash, systemic disease	Tularemia (*F. tularensis* infection) (Tulare, California)
Africa	Intense pain, swelling of eye or face	Nairobi eye (contact with Rove beetle) (Kenya, Africa)
Africa	Painless warm, egg-size swelling	Calabar swellings (loiasis due to loa-loa filariae) (Nigeria)
Africa, Middle East, and Europe	Ulcer followed by rash (tache noire)	Marseilles fever (*Rickettsia conorii* infection, tick borne, tick typhus) (town in South Africa)
Far East, Australia	Eschar-covered ulcer with maculopapular eruption	Japanese river fever (scrub typhus, tsutsugamushi fever) Rickettsial disease caused by *R. nipponica* (major river system)

In the land of the black skin, there is much diagnostic darkness for those who come from the land of white skin.

Granuloma Annulare

A ring of papules, no matter its size or location, brings to mind the diagnosis of granuloma annulare. Still, one must step back and ask if it could be an annular syphilid, annular lichen planus, or the annular lesions of sarcoidosis. Less likely to confuse are the scaling annular lesions of tinea or the inflammatory rings of erythema annulare centrifugum.

A biopsy may be necessary to distinguish it from erythema elevatum diutinum or the annular elastolytic giant cell granuloma.

What doesn't call to mind granuloma annulare is a presentation as solitary papules or nodules as well as a solitary diffuse plaque. The giant form suggests a diagnosis of rheumatoid nodule, whereas the papules may be viewed as papular mucinosis or lipoid proteinosis.

For its disseminate form, one may be led to a clinical diagnosis of lymphoma. Micropapular and perforating lesions likewise are hard to recognize grossly. Without its ring, granuloma annulare gets lost in the crowd of granulomas.

Dabski K, Winkelmann RK: **Generalized granuloma annulare:** Clinical and laboratory findings in 100 patients. J Am Acad Dermatol 1989; 20:39–47.

Clinical forms

1. Rings of coalescing papules: center may be pigmented
2. Ring plaques with no papules: resembles erythema annulare centrifugum
3. Nonannular form: occurs in one third of cases; erythematous, macular lesions suggest drug eruption, viral infection
   symmetrical, scattered, often coalescing papules deep seated in dermis

Rarely, papules show central hyperkeratosis, resembling perforating variant.

Symptoms: itching in two thirds, burning rarely

Trigger:
   sunburn, rarely
   drug eruption, rarely

Associated diseases (20%):
   diabetes mellitus
   malignant disease

Age of onset:
   usually over 40
   more common in women

Laboratory:
   hypercholesterolemia   17%
   hypertriglyceridemia   20%
   antinuclear antibodies   56%
   elevated IgG   14%

Biopsy:
   lymphohistiocytic granuloma with varying degrees of collagen degeneration (necrobiosis), microdroplet accumulation, and mucin deposit less dramatic than localized granuloma annulare

Fulghum DD: Octopus bite resulting in **granuloma annulare.** South Med J 1986; 79:1434–1436.

A bite by an octopus landing on the dorsum of the left hand of a 53-year-old commercial fisherman produced immediate redness and swelling. Two weeks later the patient noted a red, elevated ring at the site at which the hard chitinous, parrotlike beak of the octopus mouth had punctured. A year later the clinical appearance remained unchanged and was typical of an annular **granuloma annulare**. Biopsy confirmed the clinical diagnosis.

Although the bites of the octopus introduce a toxin, the reactions are usually mild and transitory. However, some species are truly venomous, and bites produce neuralgias, visual disturbances, and even death. Previously, granuloma annulare lesions have been known to follow **insect bites**, **tuberculin** tests, **viral infections**, and a variety of **skin injuries**. This is the first example following an octopus bite.

Packer RH, Fields JP, King LE Jr: **Granuloma annulare** in herpes zoster scars. Cutis 1984; 34:177–179.

In a 66-year-old man, multiple pink papules and **irregular circinate plaques** developed in the exact sites of postherpetic scarring on the left chest. These   633

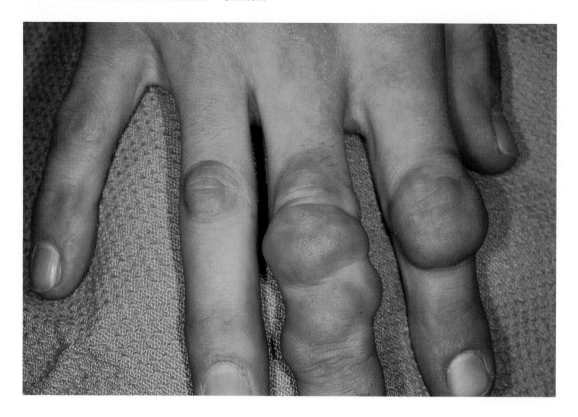

began 8 months after the onset of herpes zoster. A skin biopsy showed granuloma annulare.

Localized physical trauma, such as to the knuckles and elbows, commonly **triggers** granuloma annulare, suggesting an isomorphic response. Lesions do occur at sites of insect bites, skin tests, or warts. A good history often reveals antecedent damage to the dermis, which invites the granulomatous reparative response.

Friedman SJ, Fox BJ, Albert HL: **Granuloma annulare** arising in herpes zoster scars: Report of two cases and review of the literature. J Am Acad Dermatol 1986; 14:764–770.

Within a month of having herpes zoster of the right leg, this 72-year-old woman noted that the scars had become indurated and palpable. A diagnosis of **postherpetic granuloma annulare** was made 6 months later when a biopsy was obtained.

Other examples of granuloma annulare have been reported following varicella, verrucae, insect bites, sunlight reactions, and physical trauma.

There is no jewel in the realm of diagnosis like the jewel of knowledge.

Spencer SA, Fenske NA, Espinoza CG, et al: **Granuloma annulare**-like eruption due to chronic Epstein-Barr virus infection. Arch Dermatol 1988; 124:250–255.

Erythematous, urticarial annular lesions with yellowish borders appeared on the face of a 32-year-old nurse 1 month after she developed **infectious mononucleosis** (acute Epstein-Barr virus infection). The lesions faded with oral steroid therapy but recurred when it was discontinued. After 8 months, similar annular lesions were present on the arms, legs, and face. Repeated skin biopsies showed a lymphohistiocytic infiltrate with numerous epithelial cells. Prednisone therapy (50 mg/day) cleared the eruption and was tapered and discontinued after 6 months. She also had the fatigue, anemia, fever, and lymphadenopathy commonly seen with chronic Epstein-Barr virus infection. Intensive study did not reveal any other chronic infection, malignant disease, collagen vascular disease, or immunodeficiency disorder.

Other **clinical impressions** that were ruled out included:

annular elastolytic giant cell granuloma
drug eruption
granuloma annulare
lichen planus
lupus erythematosus (systemic discoid subacute cutaneous)
necrobiosis lipoidica
sarcoidosis
syphilis
tinea corporis
xanthomatosis

This granuloma annulare–like eruption may be a cutaneous marker for chronic Epstein-Barr virus syndrome.

Jain HC, Fisher BK: **Annular syphilid** mimicking granuloma annulare. Int J Dermatol 1988; 27:340–341.

Several dermatologists **misdiagnosed** a 26-year-old black man's erythematous annular lesions as **granuloma annulare**. Present for 3 months, these annular lesions were found on the trunk, thighs, and face, but not the palms. There was associated lymphadenopathy. Scrapings were negative for fungi, and a **biopsy** was interpreted as compatible with **pityriasis lichenoides chronica**.

The correct diagnosis became apparent when a VDRL test was reactive to 1:128 and the confirmatory **FTA test was strongly positive** to 4 +. The lesions disappeared in the month following benzathine penicillin therapy (2.4 million units IM, twice in 2 weeks).

Annular lesions also **suggest**:

erythema multiforme	sarcoid
seborrheic dermatitis	tuberculosis
lichen planus	leprosy
gyrate erythema	gumma

Triana AF, Matis WL, Peterman AR: **Annular plaque** on the shoulder. Arch Dermatol 1987, 123:1709–1712.

An annular plaque composed of discrete and confluent scaly, erythematous **brown papules** had been present on the right shoulder of a 62-year-old woman for more than 8 months. She had a history of having been treated for "bad blood" in 1943. A rapid plasma reagin (RPR) titer of 1:4096 and rapid disappearance of the lesions following penicillin (2.4 million units IM

635

once a week for 3 weeks) confirmed the clinical diagnosis of **tertiary syphilis, nodular type**. The differential diagnosis included psoriasis and cutaneous tuberculosis.

The annular lesions of tertiary syphilis stand in marked contrast to its other presentation—the **gumma**, a deep mass that becomes necrotic, leaving a nonspecific punched-out ulcer.

Amato DA, Silverstein J, Zitelli J: The prodrome of **bullous pemphigoid.** Int J Dermatol 1988; 27:560–563.

Intensely **pruritic annular erythematous plaques** on the dorsal surface of the hands, forearms, and neck of a 70-year-old woman had persisted without a diagnosis for 10 months. Vesicles or bullae had never been exhibited, and biopsy showed mild subacute dermatitis with eosinophils scattered through the dermis. Months later another biopsy showed subepidermal clefts and deposits of C_3 at the dermal-epidermal interface. A diagnosis of **prodromal bullous pemphigoid** was made. A month later vesicles appeared, and both direct and indirect immunofluorescent studies were positive for IgG and C_3 binding at the dermal-epidermal junction. Finally, multiple tense bullae appeared.

Think of prodromal bullous pemphigoid whenever you have a patient in this age group complaining of severe burning and itching. It may last for years before the diagnostic blisters and pathology become evident.

Brodell RT, Miller CW, Eisen AZ: Cutaneous lesions of **lymphomatoid granulomatosis.** Arch Dermatol 1986; 122:303–306.

A 33-year-old man gave a history of widespread, progressively **expanding annular lesions**. Originally they had appeared as pea-sized erythematous nodules of the right forearm, which then enlarged with flat erythematous centers and spread to the chest and back. Some lesions showed hypoesthesia, others hyperesthesia. Numerous hospital studies were noncontributory except for the skin biopsy findings: lymphohistiocytic infiltrate with atypical cells consistent with lymphomatoid granulomatosis. Chest x-ray revealed several poorly defined dense areas, which at **open-lung biopsy** were yellow, hard pea-sized nodules showing lymphomatoid granulomatosis histologically. All cultures for bacteria, fungi, and atypical mycobacteria were negative. Treatment with cyclophosphamide and prednisone controlled the skin lesions.

Important points:

1. Skin lesions may precede pulmonary changes by months to years. This patient had no pulmonary symptoms during the 4-year-course of the disease.
2. Suspect lymphomatoid granulomatosis if the nodules or plaques are painful or if the nodules on the lower legs ulcerate.
3. Thirty-three per cent of patients have peripheral neuropathy, with perineural infiltration in the skin causing hyperesthesia and hypoesthesia.
4. No laboratory tests are available to confirm the diagnosis other than tissue biopsies, which show a characteristic polymorphous angiocentric and angiodestructive granulomatous vasculitis with atypical and occasionally bizarre cells.
5. Anergy is present in 50 to 60% of patients.

The **differential diagnosis** includes:

sarcoidosis
mycosis fungoides
figurate erythema
subacute cutaneous lupus erythematosus

Prendiville J, Griffiths WAD, Russell Jones R: **O'Brien's actinic granuloma.** Br J Dermatol 1985; 113:353–358.

A 56-year-old woman noted raised **polycyclic and annular lesions** on the anterior area of the neck and upper chest, beginning with papules that enlarged, cleared in the center, and formed various sized rings up to 4 cm in diameter. The lesions were persistent, asymptomatic, and limited to sun-damaged poikilodermatous skin. Biopsy revealed small necrobiotic foci surrounded by a granulomatous epithelioid infiltrate. It lacked the tidy palisaded arrangement of granuloma annulare, the extensive necrobiotic change of necrobiosis lipoidica, and the pure epithelioid cell infiltrate of sarcoid. Elastotic material was seen outside, but not within, the annulus, and phagocytosis of elastic material by histiocytic cells was present. A diagnosis of **O'Brien's actinic granuloma** was made. Although intralesional steroid treatment was successful, new lesions continued to appear in the sun-damaged elastotic skin of the neck.

Actinic granuloma is a distinct entity. It occurs only in areas of elastosis, unlike granuloma annulare. It should not be confused with granuloma multiforme seen in nonexposed as well as exposed skin sites in black women in Central Africa. It must also be distinguished from elastosis perforans serpiginosa and pseudoxanthoma elasticum.

Actinic granuloma is the skin's way of ringing off and disposing of old, worn-out elastic tissue.

Billings JK, Milgraum SS, Gupta AK, et al: **Lipoatrophic panniculitis:** A possible autoimmune inflammatory disease of fat. Arch Dermatol 1987; 123:1662–1666.

A 6-year-old girl had insulin-dependent diabetes, Hashimoto's thyroiditis, and **tender erythematous nodules** on the legs, which slowly expanded annularly and left central hyperpigmentation and atrophy. Large atrophic hyperpigmented annular plaques with erythematous indurated borders were present. Superficial blood vessels were easily visualized, as there was total loss of palpable fat. Skin biopsy revealed lobular panniculitis with lymphocytes and mononuclear phagocytes, an inflammatory response not normally seen in either partial or total lipodystrophy.

In the **differential diagnosis** were the lipoatrophies of insulin injection, lupus profundus, and factitial panniculitis.

Similar inflammatory panniculitis was seen in two other children:

A 3-year-old boy had firm nontender erythematous nodules on the sole that flared following tonsillectomy. He later developed seronegative juvenile rheumatoid arthritis.

A 9-year-old boy had erythematous indurated nodules on the thighs and ankles that flared after streptococcal pharyngitis and temporarily subsided after tonsillectomy. He later developed insulin-resistant diabetes and hypertriglyceridemia. An initial punch biopsy of a nodule was interpreted as "scleroderma."

Could inflammatory lobular panniculitis with lipoatrophy be triggered by underlying streptococcal infection?

The pathologist is the diagnostician's best friend.

Granulomatous Disease

Sarcoidosis
Foreign Body Reactions
Syphilis, Tuberculosis, Leprosy
Miscellaneous

When you are in a diagnostic corner, it is wise to ask, "Could this be a granuloma?" Admittedly, *granuloma* is not a clinical term. It is the pathologist's lesion, i.e., one made up of "granules" of histiocytes and other inflammatory cells. But the question does awaken you to consider that those papules, or that plaque, could be sarcoidosis or a foreign body reaction. Or could it be the systemic infection of syphilis, tuberculosis, or leprosy? Might it be a deep fungal infection? Should we think of sporotrichosis or ask about actinomycosis or blastomycosis? Dare we consider coccidioidomycosis, cryptococcosis, or chromoblastomycosis? Has histoplasmosis a place in our diagnosis? Is iododerma possible, or might it be lymphomatoid granulomatosis?

Those quiet lumps and bumps in the skin before us will not answer. But the pathologist will.

Kerdel FA, Moschella SL: **Sarcoidosis:** An updated review. J Am Acad Dermatol 1984; 11:1–19.

Think of sarcoidosis:

Chronic violaceous nodules or plaques on nose, cheeks, ears

Papules, plaques, nodules on face, extremities, buttocks, shoulders; if telangiectasia prominent on these

Maculopapular eruption, symmetrical on face, dorsum hands, feet, nuchal area

Enlarging scar or scar of venipuncture site

Ichthyosis, lower extremities

Erythroderma

Hypopigmentation

Subcutaneous mass

Discoid lupus erythematosus–like

Scarring alopecia

Psoriasiform lesions

Mutilating lesions

Ulcerative lesions

Lichenoid papules of face suggestive of hamartoma

When you think sarcoidosis, think biopsy. It's the only way to know.

Spiteri MA, Matthey F, Gordon T, et al: **Lupus pernio:** A clinico-radiological study of 35 cases. Br J Dermatol 1985; 112:315–322.

Lupus pernio (purple lupus) refers to **chronic violaceous skin lesions** with a predilection for the nose, cheeks, ears, and fingers. It may vary from a few small buttonlike nodules under the tip of the nose to exuberant plaques covering the nose and spreading across both cheeks. Similar plaques or nodules are seen on the eyelids and pinnae. As a distinct subset of sarcoidosis, lupus pernio often occurs in association with lymphadenopathy, and sarcoidosis of the upper respiratory tract, kidney, and lacrimal gland. In this study of 818 patients with sarcoidosis, 251 (31%) had erythema nodosum, 35 had lupus pernio, and 147 had other skin lesions.

Serum **angiotensin-converting enzyme** (SACE), produced by metabolically active sarcoid granulomas, was a useful test for monitoring therapy in lupus pernio patients. SACE levels were elevated in 12 of 16 patients not taking steroids, but in only one of 15 patients receiving steroid treatment.

Gupta AK, Haberman HF, From GLA, Lipa M: **Sarcoidosis** with extensive cutaneous ulceration: Unusual clinical presentation. Dermatologica 1987; 174:135–139.

A 70-year-old white woman with insulin–resistant diabetes mellitus developed **erythematous infiltrated papules and plaques** on the knees, cheeks, arms down to the fingertips, and legs down to the toes. Marked yellow-orange discoloration with mild atrophy and scattered **ulceration** was present within the asymmetrical plaques on the legs. Skin biopsy showed a granulomatous reaction consistent with sarcoid. The ulcers healed dramatically with prednisone given for hypercalcemia.

Laboratory findings:

hypercalcemia
elevated angiotensin-converting enzyme

639

decreased serum parathyroid hormone
diffuse hypergammaglobulinemia
elevated 1,25-dihydroxyvitamin D
chest x-ray normal

Raman VV: **Sarcoidosis** of the skin and larynx. Arch Otolaryngol 1971; 93:324–326.

Hoarseness in a patient with sarcoid deserves full evaluation by an ear, nose, and throat specialist. A 44-year-old woman with raised bluish plaques (6 to 8 cm in diameter) on her face and arm for 11 years finally developed hoarseness. Nodular granulomatous lesions were found on the vocal cords, aryepiglottic folds, and epiglottis. Sarcoidosis was confirmed microscopically.

Kennedy C: **Sarcoidosis** presenting in tattoos. Clin Exp Dermatol 1976; 1:395–399.

Itchy, raised, faintly brown, translucent, scaly **patches and plaques** appearing in **11-year-old tattoos** proved on biopsy to be the only cutaneous manifestation of systemic **sarcoidosis**. Lesions involved all colors (red, blue, green, black, nonpigmented) in the tattoos, which were located on the forearms.

Tattoos may also be the **localizing point** for:

Darier's disease
discoid lupus erythematosus
keloids
lichen planus
malignancy
photosensitivity
psoriasis
syphilis

Blobstein SH, Weiss HD, Myskowski PL: **Sarcoidal granulomas** in tattoos. Cutis 1985; 36:423–424.

A 40-year-old man with chest pain, dyspnea, and previous renal calculi had noted **discomfort and induration in two tattoos**, corresponding with the onset of pulmonary symptoms. Both tattoos were red and blue but had been placed at different times on opposite arms. Only the red areas of one and the blue areas of the other were scaly and indurated, showing sarcoid on biopsy.

Moral: Biopsy the reactive tattoo!

The diagnostician's crystal ball is his eyeball.

Morgan RJ: A case of **silica granuloma**. Cutis 1986; 38:95.

During dynamiting in Colorado, a 24-year-old man had multiple fragments of radioactive uranium-silica ore and mammoth bones blown into his skin. Healing was uneventful, but 3 years later pearly, bluish-red, telangiectatic nodules began appearing in many of the scars. Some lesions became thick, **lichenified, scaly plaques**. He then became feverish and short of breath and developed lymphadenopathy. The **differential diagnosis** included sarcoidosis, hypertrophic lichen planus, epithelioma, and metastatic malignant disease.

Skin **biopsy** showed sarcoidlike **foreign body granulomas**, presumably due to silica. Foreign body granulomas were reproduced with subcutaneous implants of silica and ore from the mine. This man's experience shows that "internal" radiation therapy was of little value for these granulomas; clearing occurred with systemic steroids.

Lupton P, Kao GF, Johnson FB, et al: Cutaneous **mercury granuloma:** A clinicopathologic study and review of the literature. J Am Acad Dermatol 1985; 12:296–303.

Recurrent nodular lesions of the upper arm and lower extremities were associated with malaise and fever in this 28-year-old man. The following **differential** was considered:

sarcoidosis	lymphomatoid granulomatosis
nodular vasculitis	deep fungal infections
panniculitis	acute febrile neutrophilic dermatosis

The original pathologist's report on biopsy was nodular and diffuse dermatitis. **Reexamination** showed foreign body granulomas surrounding dark spherical globules, which were suggestive of metallic mercury. Indeed, on **energy dispersive x-ray analysis**, the foreign body did prove to be metallic **mercury**. A final diagnosis of granuloma due to mercury was made. It was assumed the patient was injecting mercury into his skin at these sites, although he strongly denied this.

Such mercury granulomas can result either from accidents, e.g., a broken thermometer, or from **self-injection**, e.g., as in Philippine natives who inject mercury to protect against bullets. Although the acute response seen in weeks to months is inflammation and necrosis, months to years later the typical foreign body granuloma may appear. **Serum and urine levels of mercury** may be high, attesting to systemic absorption and mercury poisoning with or without acute symptoms.

The absorbed mercury may produce **acrodynia**. Even more serious is embolization of the mercury. Look for evidence of this in the **chest plate**. Renal failure and death can ensue. Experience with this patient underscores the value of a second histologic opinion in puzzling problems.

Macaulay JC: Occupational **high-pressure injection injury.** Br J Dermatol 1986; 115:379–381.

A 33-year-old farmer was referred because of presumed **cellulitis of the penis and scrotum**. The history disclosed that for 10 days he had concealed being hit by a **high-pressure stream of lubricating oil** while at work. The penis was yellowish, cool, grossly enlarged, distorted, and subject to constant painful erections. A small pit on the underside of the penis revealed the entrance site for the oil. Biopsies revealed lipid granulomatosis. Although systemic steroids were helpful, the problem required extensive plastic surgical excision of the thick yellow indurated oil-laden tissue.

In all **high-pressure injection injuries**, the injury site is pinhole size, since the lubricant nipple opening is only 1 to 2 mm. The pressures are so enormous (5000 to 10,000 kg at 3 to 5 cm) that the oil penetrates gloves as well 641

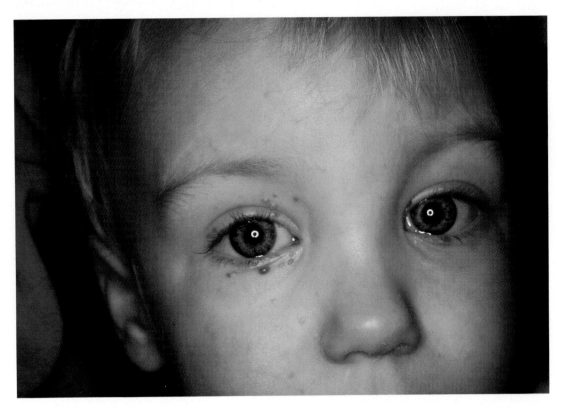

as clothing. There is a latent anesthetic period followed by gradual onset of swelling, pain, and ischemic problems. The injected materials (turpentine, chock oil, lubricating greases) continue to spread in the subcutaneous tissue. X-ray (if the grease contains lead) or xeroradiology (for nonopaque grease) will delineate the affected tissues. Rapid decompression, complete cleansing, and plastic surgery are recommended.

This type of injury has also been **factitial** in individuals seeking to avoid army service.

For a fresh look at your patient, pretend you are a consultant called in.

Perry HO, Lofgren RK: Secondary and tertiary **syphilis** presenting as sarcoidal reactions of the skin. Cutis 1984; 34:253–258.

Brownish-red gyrate and arcuate granulomatous lesions with central atrophy and depigmentation were scattered over the left upper arm and anterior area of the neck of a 68-year-old woman. The lesions had been present for 40 years! A **histologic diagnosis of sarcoidosis** was made, and search was made for the cause. This came quickly when serologic tests for syphilis were consistently positive. The diagnosis was **revised to tertiary syphilis**, and complete clearing occurred after four weekly injections of benzathine penicillin (2.4 million units) intramuscularly. Forty years of undiagnosed skin disease was diagnosed and cured in 4 weeks!

A 36-year-old man developed a lump in the neck, followed by lymphadenopathy in the inguinal areas and right axilla. Node biopsies showed inflammatory reactions. A few months later he developed a faint erythematous papular eruption of the arms and legs, histologically diagnosed as sarcoidosis. He recalled patchy hair loss 6 months previously but denied genital lesions or urethral discharge. The **riddle of the "sarcoidosis"** was solved by finding a 4+ positive FTA-ABS test. A history of no sexual contacts other than with his venereal disease–free wife was then amplified to include an extramarital contact 1 year previously. A diagnosis of secondary syphilis was made, and he was treated with penicillin.

It is well to think of syphilis when the pathologist is thinking sarcoid.

Matsuda-John SS, McElgunn PSJ, Ellis CN: **Nodular late syphilis.** J Am Acad Dermatol 1983; 9:269–272.

A group of **violaceous, pruritic nodules** had been present on the back of this 52-year-old man for 10 months. He had a history of penicillin-treated secondary syphilis 12 years before.

A biopsy showing a large number of plasma cells, and a VDRL test positive at a titer of 1:128 confirmed the clinical **diagnosis of syphilis**. Therapy with benzathine penicillin G (2.4 million units IM once a week × 3) resulted in complete resolution of the nodules within 3 months. There was a relapse $1\frac{1}{2}$ years later with new nodules appearing; 12 million units of penicillin G given intravenously every day for 10 days again cleared the skin.

Obviously, some spirochetes won't play by the rules.

Graham WR, Duvic M: **Nodular secondary syphilis.** Arch Dermatol 1982; 118:205–206.

Asymptomatic **erythematous nodules and plaques** of the genitalia, arms, and hands of this 57-year-old man had been present for the past 4 months. He had no other complaints, and the **differential diagnosis** centered on lymphoma, sarcoidosis, and deep fungal infection.

Skin biopsy revealed multiple granulomas with an inflammatory cell infiltrate. No organisms were seen on special stains. The VDRL test titer was 1:128 with a reactive FTA-ABS test. A diagnosis of **secondary syphilis** was made, and the patient finally admitted to prior sexual contact with a prostitute.

Although syphilis is still with us, it sits in the back row of diagnoses.

Ghigliotti G, Ciaccio M: A young woman with **nodules** on her face and trunk. Arch Dermatol 1989; 125:551–556.

Violaceous red nodules had been growing for the past 2 months on the abdomen, arms, and face of this 27-year-old woman. They were firm and   643 asymptomatic. In the nasolabial fold the lesions had a vegetating appearance. A biopsy showed a dense perivascular infiltrate of lymphocytes, epithelioid cells, and plasma cells.

In the clinical differential, the following were considered:

sarcoidosis	tuberculosis
granulomatous rosacea	tertiary nodular syphilis
granuloma annulare	mycosis fungoides

The diagnosis of **tertiary syphilis** carried the field when, in addition to numerous plasma cells found on biopsy, the serologic tests for syphilis were all positive (VDRL positive at 1:80, *Treponema pallidum* agglutination 1:5120, and a positive FTA-ABS result). Penicillin therapy gave prompt improvement, and by 3 months the skin lesions were entirely gone.

Even though skin lesions of late syphilis are rare today, the diagnosis of the tubercular gummatous lesions of tertiary syphilis should enter the differential diagnosis of every chronic inflammatory or destructive lesion of the skin.

These tubercular lesions are small firm nodules with a brownish-red, copper, or violaceous hue. Scaling may or may not be present. They tend to grow in over circles or bands, although this clue was absent in this patient. Had the lesions remained untreated they would have progressed to the **nodulo-ulcerative form**. Spontaneous healing would have left areas of superficial atrophic scarring as well as pigmentation of the borders. At this stage, clinical awareness of the correct diagnosis would have been heightened. The gummatous form begins in the subcutaneous tissue and becomes necrotic with an ulcer showing clean-cut edges and a torpid base.

The age of syphilis has passed, but the age of awareness of it must linger.

Katz RA, Matis WL, Hood AF: Multiple **facial nodules** in a young woman. Arch Dermatol 1987; 123:1708–1712.

Soft **crusted granulomatous nodules** scattered over the face of a 34-year-old woman had been present for 4 months. It began with what was thought to be impetigo. A VDRL titer of 1:512 and rapid disappearance of the lesions following treatment with penicillin (2.4 million units IM once a week for 3 weeks) confirmed the clinical diagnosis of **secondary syphilis**. The wide range of skin changes in secondary syphilis places nodular-papular lesions among the rarities. Interestingly, the patient's initial lesions were probably a pustular syphiloderm that mimics impetigo.

Commonly, the secondaries are **multiple, rose-pink macules** of the trunk. The appearance of dark red (raw-ham color), round, discrete indurated papules or nodules on the palms, soles, genitals, face, and trunk makes the diagnosis highly probable. A special variant is the **split papule**, the lesion that pulls apart in the nasolabial folds and the angles of the mouth. Another variant is the dull red, large, round, sessile warty lesions of the anogenital and intertriginous sites. Large plaques may regress, may be widespread, may encircle other plaques (corymbose lesions), or may cause loss of hair (moth-eaten alopecia of the scalp). At times, the syphilitic papules may scale and form indurated plaques that appear to be psoriasis or lichen planus.

In the **mouth**, one may expect to see round grayish patches that may ulcerate. Such lesions can extend down into the larynx and vocal cords, producing a husky voice change. Look for the **leukoderma colli syphiliticum** (collar of Venus) where the inflammatory response is manifested only by the loss of pigment. Rarely the lesions are **pustular** and may present as miliary pustular syphilis located in the hair follicles, flat pustular syphiloderm with superficial flat pustules, and deep pustules that ulcerate.

Brown FS, Anderson RH, Burnett JW: **Cutaneous tuberculosis.** J Am Acad Dermatol 1982; 6:101–106.

CLINICAL CLASSIFICATION	APPEARANCE	SITE
Primary inoculation tuberculosis (chancre)	Papule, painless ulcers with regional lymphadenopathy	Face, hands
Lupus vulgaris	Red papules forming plaques of apple jelly nodules	Face
Tuberculosis verrucosa cutis (prosector's warts)	Verrucous plaques with inflammatory border	Hands, fingers
Tuberculosis cutis colliquativea	Bluish-red papules, swelling overlying tuberculous lymph node or bone, breaking down to form undermined ulcer	Neck
Tuberculosis cutis orificialis	Yellow-brown papules rapidly becoming painful shallow ulcer	Mucocutaneous orifices
Tuberculosis cutis miliaris disseminata	Papules, pustules, vesicles becoming necrotic, tiny ulcers	Widespread

Duhra P, Grattan CEH, Ryatt KS: **Lupus vulgaris** with numerous tubercle bacilli. Clin Exp Dermatol 1988; 13:31–33.

A brownish-red plaque with **apple jelly nodules** appeared on the right jaw of a 45-year-old man, and within 3 months it covered the whole right mandible. Although there was no history of foreign travel or exposure to active tuberculosis, a few weeks before the lesion appeared he had cut himself while shaving around an old excision scar. **Lupus vulgaris** was diagnosed, and the biopsy showed epithelioid granulomas with acid-fast bacilli in every section (Ziehl-Nielsen stain). After 4 months of treatment with daily isoniazid (30 mg) and rifampicin (600 mg), no acid-fast bacilli were seen on repeat biopsy.

This is the most comon form of cutaneous tuberculosis and is almost always on the head and neck. It does not heal spontaneously (as does pulmonary tuberculosis) but rather enlarges by peripheral extension. If untreated, it may be complicated by contractures, lymphedema, and basal cell and squamous cell carcinomas.

Stevens CS, VanderPloeg DE: **Lupus vulgaris:** A case that escaped diagnosis for 28 years. Cutis 1981; 27:510–517.

An extensive, irregular, **annular, hyperpigmented patch** with a nodular border was noted on the buttocks of a 65-year-old Mexican man. The history was remarkable. He had been seen by a dermatologist 28 years ago because of "ringworm," which began on the right buttock. The lesion was KOH negative, and although the eruption spread to the thighs and to the other buttock he was lost to follow-up. Although he had periodic physicals for years, he covered the lesions with his hands during rectal examinations until they were eventually discovered when they grew too large to cover.

Continued treatment with antifungals and steroid preparations gave no help. At this time a biopsy from the border disclosed epithelioid tubercles with caseation necrosis. A **chest film** showed infiltrates consistent with a diagnosis of miliary tuberculosis. **Sputum cultures** grew out *Mycobacterium tuberculosis* at 6 weeks. A **diagnosis of lupus vulgaris** with disseminate tuberculosis was made. The lesions completely resolved after 4 months of isoniazid-rifampin therapy.

Modlin RL, Rea TN: **Leprosy:** New insight into an ancient disease. J Am Acad Dermatol 1987; 17:1–13.

Think tuberculoid leprosy

plaques–asymmetrical, anesthetic, sharply marginated
nerve trunk palsies
no bacteria on biopsy

Think lepromatous leprosy

nodules–numerous, poorly defined, with symmetrical widespread distribution
acral anesthesia that is symmetrical
swarms of bacteria on biopsy

Mann RJ, Harman RRM: Cutaneous anaesthesia in **necrobiosis lipoidica.** Br J Dermatol 1984; 110:323–325.

A 38-year-old English woman who had spent many years working in Thailand had a smooth, dry, **hypopigmented plaque** on the shin, confirmed on **biopsy** as **tuberculoid leprosy.** Repeated tests showed anesthesia of the area to light touch, heat, cold, and pinprick. When a second histologic opinion failed to support the diagnosis of leprosy, a **second biopsy** was done, which showed **necrobiosis lipoidica.** No evidence of diabetes or leprosy was found, and the patient was delighted at the changed diagnosis.

The concept that an anesthetic lesion is a leprosy lesion was destroyed by the authors' finding that 11 of 12 patients with typical necrobiosis lipoidica showed partial or complete **anesthesia** of affected skin. Five of these patients had had prior ulceration, and five were nondiabetic. The anesthesia probably results from neural entrapment within the necrobiotic process.

Sensory changes in cutaneous granulomas are usually neglected unless leprosy is suspected. Sensory tests should include the use of cotton wool, tubes of hot and cold water, and pinprick.

A diagnosis makes a dandy stick for beating the therapeutic bushes.

Jambrosic J, From L, Assaad DA, et al: **Lymphomatoid granulomatosis.** J Am Acad Dermatol 1987; 17:621–631.

A 38-year-old Jamaican man developed **violaceous plaques on the face, upper trunk,** and upper extremities. The lesions were indurated and had been present for 1 month. A biopsy was interpreted as a nondiagnostic lymphohistiocytic infiltrate. He was hospitalized because of a 30-pound weight loss, and **nodular infiltrates** were found on **chest x-ray.** On open lung biopsy these proved to represent lymphomatoid granulomatosis. Review of the original skin biopsy led to a **revised diagnosis of lymphomatoid granulomatosis.**

This condition first described in 1972 has been recorded in more than 180 published cases. It has a **high mortality rate** because of progressive interference with pulmonary function. The skin changes may be the first problem for which the patient seeks attention, although granulomas occur in the central nervous system and kidney as well. The skin lesions may occur before the pulmonary changes, but recall that they are not diagnostic. The violaceous appearance suggests lymphoma or leukemia cutis. One can also think of granuloma annulare, sarcoidosis, and leprosy. However, it is the biopsy that counts, and only then, as you have seen, when it is read by a skilled dermatopathologist.

Akagi M, Taniguchi S, Ozaki M, et al: Necrobiosis-lipoidica–like skin manifestation in lymphomatoid granulomatosis (Liebow). Dermatologica 1987; 174:84–92.

Three **indurated erythematous lesions** on the right **shin** of a 50-year-old man were initially viewed on **biopsy** as **necrobiosis lipoidica diabeticorum.** Lesions were erythematous indurated plaques that gradually enlarged and ulcerated with localized gangrene. Chest x-ray revealed an irregular pulmonary mass in the left upper lobe, proven on **open lung biopsy** to be **lymphomatoid granulomatosis.** Later, a nasal mass showed the same angiocentric and angiodestructive granulomatosis and lymphohistiocytic infiltrate. Review of the initial and subsequent skin biopsies confirmed that skin changes were part of the lymphomatoid granulomatosis. Direct immunofluorescence showed heavy deposition of IgG, IgM, IgA, and C3 in dermal and subcutaneous blood vessel walls.

Lymphomatoid granulomatosis, first described in 1972 by Liebow, is now considered to be a **lymphoma of T-lymphocyte origin.** It affects the lung most commonly; however, it additionally involves skin in 50% of patients. The **skin may be the first organ afflicted,** usually as subcutaneous or dermal nodules but also as erythema, ulcers, and maculopapular lesions.

Alessi E, Crosti C, Sala F: Unusual case of **granulomatous dermohypodermatitis** with giant cells and elastophagocytosis. Dermatologica 1986; 172:218–221.

A 4-cm firm, **reddish, asymptomatic plaque** developed slowly on the back of a 27-year-old Italian man over 1 year. It was sharply demarcated, bound down to the underlying structures, had a surface like an orange peel, and continued to grow. It was totally excised 1 year later. Histologic sections revealed thinned dermis resulting from a histiocytic granulomatous band of infiltrate replacing the deep dermis. Many epithelioid cells and multinucleated giant cells were seen in the subcutis.

The **differential diagnosis** centered on sarcoid vs the progressive, atrophying, chronic granulomatous dermohypodermatitis described in 1973 (Convit, J et al: Progressive, atrophying, chronic granulomatous dermohypodermatitis: autoimmune disease? Arch Dermatol 1973; 107:271–274.) and also labeled **granulomatous slack skin** (Ackerman). Convit's patient had widespread   647 multiple papules that formed plaques that progressively transformed into acquired cutis laxa because of elastolysis.

Eventually, **Hodgkin's disease** was diagnosed in the lymph nodes at postmortem study.

Sutphen JL, Cooper PH, Mackel SE, Nelson DL: Metastatic cutaneous **Crohn's disease.** Gastroenterology 1984; 86:941–944.

A 38-year-old woman with quiescent Crohn's disease developed a tender erythematous indurated 8- by 10-cm **plaque on the left calf**. It contained several punched-out ulcers up to 2 cm in diameter, which drained straw-colored fluid. Skin biopsy showed granulomatous dermatitis and panniculitis, with multinuclear giant cells concentrated at the dermal-subcutaneous interface, but no vasculitis or necrosis. Stains for microorganisms were negative, as was a tuberculin test. Chest x-ray disclosed a small calcified granuloma but no hilar lymphadenopathy.

Differential diagnosis:

metastatic Crohn's disease	mycobacterial infection
erythema induratum	deep fungal infection
sarcoid	

A 16-year-old boy with Crohn's disease had persistent painful **perianal fistulas** and progressively enlarging erythematous nodular serpiginous plaques on the left forearm and left lower leg. The surfaces were shiny and irregularly alopecic but lacked crust or scale. The margins were indurated, with scattered small pustules. Skin biopsy showed granulomatous inflammation and discrete granulomas.

Differential diagnosis:

deep fungal infection	erythema induratum
Majocchi's granuloma	cutaneous Crohn's disease
lichen sclerosus et atrophicus	

Other **skin lesions associated with Crohn's disease**:

indolent undermined granulomatous ulcers (perianal, peristomal, perifistular)
pyoderma gangrenosum
erythema nodosum
cutaneous polyarteritis nodosa—painful hemorrhagic nodules and ulcers in areas of livedo reticularis

Taieb A, Dufillot D, Pellegrin-Carloz B, et al: **Postgranulomatous anetoderma** associated with Takayasu's arteritis in a child. Arch Dermatol 1987; 123:796–800.

A 9-year-old boy with **idiopathic hypertension** had small keratotic or lichenoid brownish papules on the upper trunk. They appeared in crops of a dozen or more lesions, which progressed to whitish atrophic lenticular scars within a few weeks to months. Present since infancy, some showed herniation, as in **anetoderma.**

Clinically it was suggestive of:

Darier's disease	disseminated granuloma annulare
lichen planus	sarcoidosis
lichen nitidus	

However, a biopsy exhibited noncaseating tuberculoid granulomas with focal loss of elastic tissue.

After $3\frac{1}{2}$ years of study of the hypertension, angiographic studies revealed the underlying problem to be **Takayasu's arteritis**. The aorta showed an irregular alternating pattern of stenosis irregularity and ectasia. This usually reflects granulomatous change in the vessel wall. This rare disease of unknown cause (2.6 cases/million/year) has **hypertension** as its signal finding. Cutaneous signs are nonspecific, but in a patient with hypertension the following could alert one to the diagnosis, which is so often made after long delay:

> pyoderma gangrenosum
> papulonecrotic tuberculoid-like eruptions
> erythema induration
> erythema nodosum
> papular erythematous lesions of fingers and hands
> Raynaud's phenomenon
> lupus-like rash of face
> scaly erythema of the face

When you don't know what to do next, measure the blood pressure and look in the eyes for vascular change. That is what Takayasu did in 1908 when he first sighted this entity.

Brunken RC, Lichon-Chao N, van den Broek H: Immunologic abnormalities in **botryomycosis:** A case report with review of the literature. J Am Acad Dermatol 1983; 9:428–434.

A large, **pebbly surfaced**, **well-defined raised lesion** had been present in the left submandibular area of this 47-year-old man for many months. There were no sinus openings or drainage, but the odor was foul.

The biopsy showed marked hyperplasia of the epidermis, and dense accumulations of polymorphonuclear cells. **Gram stain** revealed both gram-positive and gram-negative bacteria, some clumped into **granules**. The culture of minced skin specimens grew out *Staphylococcus epidermis* and *Escherichia coli*, both sensitive to penicillin. A **diagnosis of botryomycosis** was made, and intravenous penicillin therapy was begun. Progress was moderate, even after 6 weeks, so the remaining verrucous lesion was excised.

Botryomycosis was first described as grapelike (botryoid) clusters of nodules seen in the lungs of horses and was erroneously ascribed to be fungous infection (mycosis). Today it is recognized as a unique clinical entity in the skin of man as well as horses. Visceral forms are seen as well. The **causative organisms** are a variety of bacteria, including S. *aureus, Proteus, Pseudomonas, E. coli,* and alpha-hemolytic streptococci. Why the bacteria form granules simulating fungal granules is not known, but may reflect a symbiotic accommodation.

Whittaker SJ, Smith NP, Russell Jones R: **Solitary morphoea profunda.** Br J Dermatol 1989; 120:431–440.

Solitary morphea profunda is a condition that may cause considerable difficulty in diagnosis. It presents as an ill-defined, indurated, **deeply tethered plaque** on the upper trunk. Yellowish-brown pigmentation, a nodular or peau d'orange surface, and a peripheral rim of telangiectasis round out the typical presentation. There is no atrophy. It may begin as an erythematous plaque, which fades into a pale sclerotic area. The persistence is as remarkable as its lack of progression or involvement elsewhere.

Clinically, morphea profunda **mimics** cutaneous lymphoma, sarcoidosis, dermatofibrosarcoma protuberans. The histologic diagnosis is evasive. One 72-year-old woman had a nodular crescentic interscapular plaque under observation for 17 years with the following sequence of histologic diagnoses:

first biopsy: consider lymphoma, tertiary syphilis, morphea
second biopsy (edge of lesion): consider sarcoidosis, necrobiotic granuloma
last biopsy (year later): atypical morphea

Holden CA, Winkelmann RK, Wilson Jones E: **Necrobiotic xanthogranuloma:** A report of four cases. Br J Dermatol 1986; 114:241–250.

Yellow indurated plaques around the eyes was the singular clinical diagnostic sign in each of four women, ages 55 to 85 years. The plaques were well demarcated, and in some instances showed black to brown or purplish hemorrhagic centers. Ulceration and scarring occurred in some plaques with residual atrophy and telangiectasia. In all cases, similar plaques were seen elsewhere on the face and trunk. Lymphadenopathy was usually not present, but splenomegaly was present in two patients.

The singular diagnostic **laboratory finding** was **paraproteinemia,** but no patient developed myeloma based on bone marrow examination and skeletal survey. Leukopenia, anemia, and an elevated erythrocyte sedimentation rate were common. Histologically the necrobiosis and granulomatous infiltrate could lead to an erroneous diagnosis of atypical necrobiosis lipoidica, granuloma annulare, or sarcoidosis.

Boudoulas O, Siegle RJ, Grimwood RE: **Iododerma** occurring after orally administered iopanoic acid. Arch Dermatol 1987; 123:387–388.

Multiple **vesiculopustular**, **vegetating nodular lesions** with ulceration appeared on the face, trunk, and extremities of a 45-year-old man 2 days after taking Telepaque tablets orally for cholecystography. He had taken six of these iodide contrast tablets twice within a week. A skin biopsy showed acanthosis with ulceration and a polymorphonuclear cell infiltrate in the dermis.

A **diagnosis of acute iododerma** was made after ruling out:

blastomycosis   anthrax
syphilis   lymphoma
tuberculosis   metastatic tumors
mycosis fungoides   pemphigus vegetans
glanders

Soria C, Allegue F, España A, et al: **Vegetating iododerma** with underlying systemic diseases: Report of three cases. J Am Acad Dermatol 1990; 22:418–422.

For 3 weeks a 76-year-old man had experienced rapidly enlarging red verrucous **vegetating masses** on the neck, chest, back, and groin. The history gave the tip to the diagnosis. He had been taking **potassium iodide** (260 mg tid) daily for 8 months because of chronic obstructive pulmonary disease. The clinical diagnosis was confirmed by a skin biopsy, as well as complete clearing of the eruption within 5 days of stopping the iodide. Furthermore, challenge with potassium iodide induced a papulopustular eruption of the face 5 days later. On further study, he proved to have hypercalcemia, an elevated IgA level on serum protein electrophoresis, and 60% plasma cells in a bone marrow aspirate, confirming **multiple myeloma**.

Two other patients with iododerma and underlying disease (polyarteritis nodosa, monoclonal gammopathy) are presented with the observation that polyarteritis and paraproteinemia may predispose patients to the development of iododerma.

Be careful in history taking. A single dose of iodide contrast dye can produce a fever and a variety of lesions ranging from acneiform to nodular and ulcerative lesions.

Welch KJ, Burke WA, Park HK: **Pyoderma vegetans:** Association with diffuse T cell lymphoma (large cell type). J Am Acad Dermatol 1989; 20:691–693.

A 29-year-old black man had **generalized exfoliation** and multiple firm annular and nodular plaques with oozing eroded centers. They had a blastomycosis-like appearance, but cultures grew *Staphylococcus aureus, Streptococcus* species (*beta-hemolytic* group A), and *Proteus mirabilis*. A skin **biopsy** confirmed the diagnosis of pyoderma vegetans.

Five months later he developed a tumor of the scalp shown on biopsy to be a **T-cell lymphoma**. Presumably the original vegetating tissue reaction to bacteria was due to a lymphoma-compromised immune system.

In any patient with pyoderma vegetans, look for:

ulcerative colitis
alcoholism
malnutrition
halogen ingestion
cellular immunodeficiency

Don't's for diagnosticians:

1. *Don't be too clever.*
2. *Don't diagnose rarities.*
3. *Don't be in a hurry.*
4. *Don't be faddish.*
5. *Don't mistake a label for a diagnosis.*
6. *Don't diagnose two diseases simultaneously in the same patient.*
7. *Don't be too cock-sure.*
8. *Don't be biased.*
9. *Don't hesitate to revise your diagnosis from time to time in a chronic case.*

SIR ROBERT HUTCHINSON

Hair Shaft Disorders

Individuals seek a diagnosis or explanation for hair that won't grow, hair that breaks off, and hair that can't be combed. Much of your answer comes from an examination of the hair shaft itself.

Any infant with sparse, lusterless, or broken-off hair should have a hair mount (Permount and coverslip) to search for the signs of genetic defects that may signal impending neurologic and mental defects. These are **trichorrhexis nodosa**, **pili torti**, **trichothiodystrophy**, and **trichorrhexis invaginata**. All deserve urinary or blood amino acid screening for metabolic defects. The hair shaft itself should be analyzed for the low cystine or sulfur content trichothiodystrophy. Any one of these four fragile-hair syndromes may herald mental deficiency, which may be prevented by proper measures.

Patients with hair that won't comb deserve determination of serum copper levels to rule out Menke's syndrome and biotin and biotinidase levels to rule out the uncombable hair syndrome.

Finally, patients with hair that won't grow need to be checked by hair mount for trichorrhexis nodosa of the proximal hair shaft and for the presence of monilethrix and pseudomonilethrix. Awareness of their presence can do much to instruct and to reassure the patient on the importance of gentle grooming for those genetic defects that are unique in being limited to the hair alone.

Failure to examine a hair mount and to do specific blood and urine studies can leave you and your patient with a diagnosis only of "funny hair." Both of you deserve more.

Price ML, Griffiths WAD: Normal body hair—a review. Clin Exp Dermatol 1985; 10:87–97.

Human **hair follicles** tend to be **grouped** in threes, occasionally fives, with one hair larger than the others. Both sexes have the same total number of hair follicles, approximately 5 million. There are about 1 million follicles on the scalp, including 100,000 terminal hairs. In men, 90% of the hairs on the chest, trunk, shoulders, legs, and arms are terminal hairs, in contrast to 35% in women.

Approximately 85% of hairs are in **anagen**, with 15% in **telogen**. Terminal scalp hairs have a very short resting period. The duration of anagen is genetically determined and is a racial characteristic. Hair grows faster and longer in summer than in winter, and beard hair grows faster in the tropics.

The growth of **sexual hair** (beard, axillary, pubic) is dependent on androgens. Pubic hair starts to grow about 2 years before axillary and facial hair. Estrogens also play a role; in ovarian agenesis administration of estrogen leads to full development of pubic and axillary hair. In women, the level of sex hormone–binding globulin (SHBG) is important, lower levels being associated with increased metabolically available testosterone and hirsutism.

Diffuse alopecia is a common feature of hypothyroidism, with a reduction in mean hair diameter. Increased terminal body hair growth occurs in acromegaly. Body hair coarsens and becomes sparse and dry in hypoparathyroidism.

Carcinoembryonic antigen (CEA) may influence the type of hair produced by hair follicles. Its increase in certain carcinomas may stimulate **lanugo hair growth**, leading to hypertrichosis lanuginosa acquisita.

Samlaska CP, James WD, Sperling LC: **Scalp whorls**. J Am Acad Dermatol 1989; 21:553–556.

When the fetus is 3 months old, **hair follicles** have evolved to the point at which their **slope** is subject to the **mechanical shearing forces of an expanding cranium**. The hair alignment may thus pattern into whorls at the epicenters of this expansion. Such scalp whorls and associated cowlicks can be seen at any location, but especially along the frontal hair line. Likewise, single, double, and even triple scalp whorls may be normal. Furthermore, such whorls are not limited to the scalp, but may be seen at any body site.

However, abnormal scalp whorls such as those with midline confluence may point to the presence of a variety of congenital malformations (e.g., microcephaly) or dysmorphic syndromes (e.g., Down's).

Trichoglyphics tell us of the swirling skin of embryogenesis.

Price VH: Structural anomalies of the hair shaft. *In* Orfanos C, Happle R (eds): Hair and Hair Diseases. New York, Springer-Verlag, 1990, pp 363–422.

Structural hair malformations are easily diagnosed by a **hair mount**:

- Place four short, selected segments of hair on microscopic slide, side by side, and cover with coverslip.
- Place 3 drops of balsam or synthetic mounting medium at edge of coverslip and promote capillary action with gentle alcohol lamp heat. Do not use water or KOH.
- View hair with microscope, realizing that hair is often oval with the result that if the hair is twisted, your two-dimensional view of the three-

653

dimensional hair will make you think the diameter is variable and mislead you into a diagnosis of monilethrix.

Here is what you see and here is what it means:

1. **Microscopic changes**. Possibly the most common change to be seen is the **Pohl-Pinkus mark**, which is a constriction of the hair shaft due to severe illness. It is the analogue of Beau's line in the nail plate. Unusual formations that may be seen include multiple hair shafts arising from a single follicle (**pili multigemini**) and pili bifurcati. The pili multigemini represent a bundle of two or more hairs, each with its own inner root sheath, but all surrounded by a common outer root sheath. **Pili bifurcati** are a variant in which a single hair shaft divides into two and then re-forms back to a single shaft. It is not a split hair, since each of the two rami has its own cuticle. Another

Usually observed incidentally in examining a patient for some other reason, **pili annulati** consist simply of a condition in which the hair is studded with beadlike bright spots. It is due to discrete focal air cavities within the shaft and hence is analogous to leukonychia. Under the microscope, transmitted light displays these spots as black, since the air absorbs the light. The hairs are otherwise normal, and the patient can be reassured that her pili annulati are an adornment no brunette can possess. Black hair, like the black hole, allows for no reflectance.

A **pseudoform exists** in which the alternating bright and dark rings are due to the optical effects of having hair that is elliptic in cross-section and partially twisted in an oscillating fashion. Examination shows the bands of brightness only if the light strikes at right angles to the long axis of the hair. The fiber must be optimally rotated on a trial basis to see the phenomenon. Transmitted light reveals no air pockets as in the true form, but it does reveal the deception in fiber diameter as a result of the twist of elliptic fiber. Again, it is seen only in blond hair.

2. **Combability**. The classic example of this is **uncombable hair**. Here, blond hair has a frizzy, stand-away, uncombable appearance easily recognizable at a glance. Many of the hair shafts have a triangular grooved shape with a resultant resemblance in appearance to spun glass. This spun-glass problem does not reveal its diagnosis on a simple mount. It is not twisted hair, but polarized light examination does disclose abnormal alignment in the hair shaft. Histologic examination and also scanning electron microscopy give the answer that the hair abnormality results from an asynchrony in internal root sheath formation in the follicle and the hair shaft. The shaft morphology gives the condition its formal name, pili trianguli et canaliculi, more easily remembered as uncombable hair. One can anticipate spontaneous disappearance of these hair changes during adolescence.

Two other conditions account for hair that is difficult to manage. One is **wooly hair**; in this condition, the child, at birth or shortly after, develops *tight curly hair* that is difficult to brush. By adulthood, the wooly nature of the patient's hair growth may disappear. It may represent a dominant or a recessive gene. In the recessive form, the hair never grows to more than an inch or so in length. This is due to the shortened anagen phase. A *nevoid form of wooly hair* has also been described in which one or more patches of fine curly hair may appear on the scalp. It is often associated with a linear nevus elsewhere.

An eye examination is suggested in all cases of wooly hair disease, since abnormalities of the eye may occur concomitantly.

Finally, tight curly hair may appear not at birth, but in adult life. This has been called **acquired progressive kinking** of the hair. It is usually localized. No associated changes have been recorded.

3.   **Fragility**. By far and away the most common cause of hair breakage is **trichorrhexis nodosa**. It is easily recognized on the hair mount as a hair fracture, resembling two brushes pushed into each other. It may be of congenital or acquired origin. In the case of trichorrhexis nodosa in infants and children, there may be an inborn error of urea synthesis. Mental retardation occurs by the age of 2 years. The syndrome is due to a deficiency of arginosuccinate lyase. The hair is dry, brittle, matted, and stubby, but at birth may have been normal.

It is essential to make the diagnosis as early as possible to institute proper dietary therapy (high arginine, low protein) to prevent brain damage from the accumulation of arginine succinic acid. Once the trichorrhexis is seen, an amino acid screening study of blood or urine readily detects this serious metabolic disorder.

Acquired forms of trichorrhexis nodosa may be proximal or distal or circumscribed. The proximal form is seen in black patients exclusively. The hair breaks off a few centimeters from the scalp. It appears to be a result of a barber, but actually occurs spontaneously by breakage. The patient complains that the hair won't grow. It can occur at any age. The usual cause is thermal or chemical hair straightening, the use of metal combs, or tight fitting head covering. But, in others, no cause is evident. Usually the entire scalp is not affected. A hair mount quickly provides the diagnosis.

Distal trichorrhexis nodosa is a result of cumulative cuticular damage. White specks seen along the shaft are the diagnostic clue. They are not dandruff, but rather the fractures of trichorrhexis. It occurs distally because only the older hair has sustained enough damage to essentially destroy the cuticle. A hair mount reveals the diagnosis, and scanning electron microscopy shows the worn-out or damaged cuticle. Once the cuticle barrier is gone, the detergent shampoos dissolve the cement substance of the cortex and the hair buckles. This results in a skimpy ragged appearance. The affected hairs are long, lusterless, and oddly faded.

A rare hair shaft defect is **pili torti**. Here the shaft is flattened and twisted on its own axis. Reflected light produces a striking spangled look. More importantly, the hairs are brittle, fragile, broken, and short. It often occurs with other ectodermal defects such as keratosis pilaris and dental and nail abnormalities, as well as hearing defects.

Pili torti is diagnosable under a hair mount as closely grouped twists of a flattened hair. However, it is the most misdiagnosed hair defect. It is confused with monilethrix because oval forms, where twisted, resemble fibers with diameter variations. Another source of error is the fact that pubic and axillary hairs are normally twisted. Scalp hairs and weakened hairs may show up as occasional examples of this as well.

The congenital form of pili torti usually appears in infancy, in blond females, and all patients deserve auditory tests for sensorineural hearing loss. In the late-onset form, appearing after puberty, the hair is usually black, and areas of alopecia occur.

Pili torti is an index finding in patients with **Menkes' kinky hair disease**. Here the twisted hair results from an X-linked recessive disorder of copper metabolism. Markedly decreased levels of copper are present in serum, brain, and liver, with resultant decreases in essential copper-dependent enzymes, such as tyrosinase. Paradoxically, the copper level is pathologically high in skin and other organs.

The hair resembles steel wool, and the appearance in the infant is basically a failure to thrive, seizures, and deficient visual development. But the bedside diagnosis is made from the sparse, depigmented, lusterless hair that feels like **steel wool** and stands on end. The skin has a doughy consistency and may hang in loose folds, as in cutis laxa. A hair mount confirms the diagnosis, and serum copper and copper oxidase levels sight the cause.

Noteworthy is the fact that scarred areas, as in cicatricial alopecia, may beget the hairs of pili torti. Thus, the hairs from scleroderma, pseudopelade, and lupus erythematosus may show multiple twists of flattened hairs.

The third major hair defect of critical importance in medicine is **trichothio-dystrophy**, i.e., sulfur-deficient brittle hair. It is a rare congenital disorder of hair in which the scalp hair, eyebrows, and eyelashes are all brittle, broken, short, uneven, and sparse. The hair has an irregular, slightly undulating contour with fractures, both as a diminutive trichorrhexis nodosa and as a clean transverse break (trichoschisis). The shaft is notably flattened and can even fold on itself. Under polarizing light, birefringence is seen as alternating bright and dark domains when cross-polarizers are used. Under scanning electron microscopy, the cuticle scale pattern is reduced. The key diagnostic finding is **cystine content** less than half of normal. Measure total sulfur content of hair or do an amino acid analysis of the hair.

Patients with sulfur-deficient hair syndrome may exhibit mental deficiency as well. Often this is masked by a smiling talkative nature. Additional clinical clues are facial appearance of a receding chin and protruding ears, short stature, defective nails, ichthyosis, and neurologic disorders. Nonetheless, the hair defect may be the only finding, yet all patients should be checked for their response to ultraviolet light. Some have impaired DNA repair with or without **photosensitivity**, which may eventuate in skin cancer.

Another hair defect readily recognized on a hair mount is the bamboo hair of **trichorrhexis invaginata**. It is also known as **Netherton's syndrome**, since he first described this ball-and-socket deformity of the hair. It is important to look for it in all patients with an ichthyosiform eruption. Usually it is a distinctive feature of ichthyosis linearis circumflexa, although it may appear as a congenital ichthyosiform erythroderma.

It is basically an autosomal recessive disease, appearing as redness and scaling of the body and face in the first few days of life. Subsequently, migratory serpiginous erythematous scaling lesions appear with characteristic **double-edge scale**. All of this is on an atopic background. The hair is dry, lusterless, and so fragile it never grows to normal length. This is due to the abnormal invagination so readily recognized on a hair mount. Aminoaciduria is present at times, so that checking for this is also advisable.

The fifth and final type of fragile hair syndrome is covered in the next entry, i.e., in the discussions of monilethrix.

Don't file your nails while taking a history. You need them to dig with!

Whiting DA: Structural abnormalities of the **hair shaft**. J Am Acad Dermatol 1987; 16:1–25.

GLOSSARY

Fractures

trichoschisis: clean transverse fracture seen in brittle hair, associated with low sulfur content (trichothiodystrophy)

trichoclasis: "greenstick" type of fracture with cuticle intact and serving as a splint

trichorrhexis nodosa: brush fracture with bead at site of splayed hair fibrils, usually due to trauma

trichorrhexis invaginata: bamboo hair in which nodule is ball-and-socket juncture, seen in ichthyosis

tapered fracture: pencil-point fracture caused by inhibition of hair synthesis associated with alopecia areata, cytostatic drugs

trichoptilosis: "split ends," like frayed ends of a rope, caused by trauma

Hair shaft structure

pili trianguli et canaliculi: uncombable hair

pili bifurcata: shaft divides into two, then reunites

pili multigemini: tufts of flat individual hairs coming from one follicle in which there are multiple papillae

trichostasis spinulosa: tufts of multiple hairs from one follicle and one papillae, due to retention of hairs

pili annulati: attractive, alternating bright and dark rings due to patterned deposition of air between cortical fibers

pseudo-pili annulati: same; not air pockets but periodic flattening of shaft accounts for banding

monilethrix: elliptic nodes about 1 mm apart with intervening tapered nonmedullated constrictions

pseudomonilethrix: transient change considered artifact from inadvertent mechanical pressure

tapered new anagen hairs: tapered hypopigmented tips of normal uncut hair

tapered hairs: tapering due to inhibition of cell division, e.g., alopecia areata

Pohl-Pinkus mark: constriction of hair analogous to Beau's lines in nails

bayonet hairs: spindle-shaped expansion just proximal to tapered tip; seen in cytostatic drug response, ichthyosis, etc.

trichomalacia: hair root deformed, twisted as result of plucking

Hair shaft topology

pili torti: twists 180 degrees on own axis, giving beaded appearance

corkscrew hair: coiling like corkscrew

wooly hair: tightly coiled hair

whisker hair: popular term for short, dark, curly hairs around ears of young men

trichonodosis: knotted hair possibly due to friction

circle hairs: unusual coil of hair growing in stratum corneum

Bentley-Phillips B: **Monilethrix** and pseudo-monilethrix. *In* Orfanos C, Happle R (eds): Hair and Hair Diseases. New York, Springer-Verlag, 1990, pp 422–441.

Although the lanugo hair is normal at birth, this is soon replaced by dry, brittle, lusterless hair in cases of **monilethrix**. The hairs break easily, leaving a stubble of less than 1 inch in length. Under the microscope, the hairs are

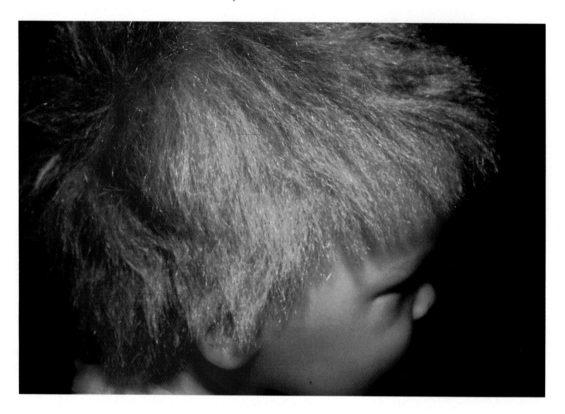

distinctive, showing regular nodes and internodes about 1 mm apart. It is this appearance of a string of beads that gave the condition its name, i.e., *monile* (Lat) "necklace" and *thrix* (Gr) "hair."

Monilethrix can involve hairs anywhere on the body and may explain localized **patches of alopecia** on the scalp. The unbroken hairs are never long. Palpation of the scalp allows a sensing of the gritty feel of an associated follicular hyperkeratosis. Keratosis pilaris of the scalp and elsewhere is commonly present.

Monilethrix is rare and is inherited as a **dominant trait**. It is important to note that unlike the other genetic hair defects, it appears in normal healthy individuals. No metabolic abnormality has been discovered to explain the regular periodic thinning of the hair shaft. It is at these thinned internodes that the hair breaks, leaving brushlike ends.

Far more common is **pseudomonilethrix**. It too exhibits nodes, but they are illusions of thickening. Under scanning electron microscopy, they can be observed to be indentations in the shaft, the sides thus protruding beyond the normal diameter of the shaft. These indentation nodes occur at irregular intervals, unlike the exquisite regularity of the monilethrix beading. Furthermore, the internodes are the thickness of a normal hair shaft, whereas in monilethrix the internodes represent a thinning of the shaft. The pseudomonilethrix hairs are fragile and lead to varying degrees of alopecia. Again, both pseudomonilethrix and monilethrix are dominant gene disturbances.

It is important to do hair mounts on all patients complaining of poor-quality, thin hair, or alopecia. Only in this way can pseudomonilethrix be recognized and the patient made aware of the weak spots along the hairs. Good growth can follow gentle grooming.

Levit F, Scott MJ Jr: **Circle hairs**. J Am Acad Dermatol 1983; 8:423–425.

Black circular lesions on the back of this 68-year-old man proved on scraping to be superficial coils of ingrown hairs.

The condition is an asymptomatic curiosity of no known cause or with no clinical correlates. It has been previously described as spiral hairs.

Van Neste D, Houbion Y: Office diagnosis of **changes in hair cuticular cell patterns**. Arch Dermatol 1986; 122:750–752.

A hair shaft cast can be easily made in the office by placing a hair in a small drop of **cyanoacrylate glue** on a glass slide. After polymerization occurs (about 30 sec), the hair is gently removed and discarded. The cyanoacrylate replica remaining on the slide is then examined using light microscopy. Although this technique provides less detail than scanning electron microscopy, it is more convenient, cheaper, and faster than SEM.

The cuticular scale pattern is significantly modified by environmental factors such as bleaching or permanent waving. Hair mismanagement with various noncompatible hair care products may result in irreversible damage to the hair shaft.

Fabbri P, DiFonzo EM, Palleschi GM, Pacini P: **Hair casts**. Int J Dermatol 1988; 27:319–321.

Months of nightly combings and frequent pediculicide shampoos failed to cure an 8-year-old girl of presumed pediculosis capitis. Her mother kept seeing many small grayish refringent formations, which resembled nits, on scalp hairs. These "nits" were actually **hair casts**, which, unlike the eggs of the head louse, were fragile and could be slid along the hair shaft, which they completely encircled like cylinders.

These "**pseudonits**" or keratin hair casts represent periodic exfoliation of the root sheath. Both Huxley's sheath and Henle's layer can be seen in the 3-mm-long casts. Hundreds of casts may be present, with multiple casts on a single hair. They are apparently shed whenever the adherence of the root sheath is greater to the hair shaft than to the follicle wall.

Mothers, schoolteachers, and nurses need to know of the innocuous hair cast that hatches nothing except anxiety.

Scott MJ Jr, Roenigk HH Jr: **Hair casts**: Classification, staining characteristics, and differential diagnosis. J Am Acad Dermatol 1983; 8:27–32.

A variety of materials may encircle the hair shaft, at times suggesting the presence of nits. Most of these **hair casts** are bands of extruded external root sheath. They can easily be distinguished from nits, since any traction slides them along the hair, in contrast to the nits, which are firmly cemented in place.

Rarely the internal root sheath is extruded, and this sheath can be distinguished from the external sheath by its selective red staining by DACA (Cytosol Labs Inc., Boston, MA) 1% in 0.5 N HCl, 30-second immersion on glass slide. The **stain is for citrulline**, which is absent in the external sheath as well as in parafollicular keratin debris, which may be extruded also on the hair. These casts are especially common in psoriasis and seborrhea.

Artifactual hair casts can result from aerosol hair spray, paints, protein shampoo, or occupational exposure to any adherent particulate matter. The last has occurred with denture-manufacturing technicians. Other sources of diagnostic concern are trichomycosis axillaris and piedra.

Kalter DC, Tschen JA, Cernoch PL, et al: Genital **white piedra**: Epidemiology, microbiology, and therapy. J Am Acad Dermatol 1986; 14:982–993.

Soft, white, red, brown, or greenish, **fine concretions** adherent to the hair make the diagnosis of this yeastlike fungous infection with *Trichosporon beigelii*. These sleeve-like concretions, whether discrete or confluent, are more easily stripped off than the black concretions of black piedra, caused by *Piedraia hortai*. The hairs may break, since the cuticle is invaded. Any terminal hair is vulnerable, whether scalp, eyelash, moustache, or perigenital. Indeed, even the nails may be infected. Its significance extends to the development of systemic infection in immunocompromised hosts.

Clinically, **white piedra** cannot be distinguished from the bacterial sleeve of trichomycosis. KOH examination does permit distinction, and the trichosporon is easily cultured on Sabouraud's dextrose agar plates, incubated at 30°C for 7 days. The colony is waxy and cream colored.

The **differential diagnosis** includes not only trichorrhexis nodosa but also black piedra, hair casts, nits, and developmental hair anomalies.

Although usually asymptomatic, white piedra of the perigenital hairs can be the cause of treatment-resistant **intertrigo**. Sometimes looking at the hairs can be more instructive than looking at the skin.

If you'd like a cram course in diagnosis, read all those journals crammed in your office.

Césarini JP: **Hair melanin** and hair color. *In* Orfanos CE, Happle R (eds): Hair and Hair Diseases. New York, Springer-Verlag, 1990, pp 165–197.

The natural coloring of hair is due to the presence of black, brown, and red particles of the biopolymer **melanin**. This melanin is found between the keratin fibrils of the cortex and to a lesser degree in the medulla. There is essentially none in the cuticle. All of it is formed in melanosomes in the melanocytes of the hair matrix where it is transferred to the adjacent keratinocytes.

The melanosomes here are much larger and in greater number than in the epidermis itself. Furthermore, there is one melanocyte for every five keratinocytes. By contrast, the epidermis has only one melanocyte for every 25 keratinocytes. The preponderance of melanocytes and large melanosomes permits adequate coloring of the hair.

Melanin in the hair comes in two forms: **eumelanin**, which accounts for dark-brown or black hair, and **phaeomelanin**, which accounts for red hair. Varying mixtures of these two melanins are found in reddish-brown hairs. Blond hairs are thin and show essentially no medulla or pigment. White hair has no melanin in the cortex and very little in the medulla. Red hairs contain essentially only red melanin. This is a form of phaeomelanin that some label erythromelanin.

Axillary and genital hairs often have a reddish tint. The beard, in turn, is lighter in color than the scalp hair. During puberty, hair color often darkens, but the gray of aging begins to appear in the 30s.

Cline DJ: **Changes in hair color**. Dermatol Clin 6:295–303, 1988.

Many examples of hair color change are missed or dismissed by the physician because they remain in the normal range of hair coloring. Many examples are hidden by today's custom of bleaching and coloring. Many serve no diagnostic function, as in the case of genetic disease in which blond hair is common.

However, the following deserve attention:

> Periods of severe malnutrition may be manifested by lighter hair. When this is episodic, the reappearance of bands of normal marker hair results in the "flag sign."
> Vitamin B_6 supplement will darken the light hair of patients with homocystinuria.
> Premature graying is associated with the vitamin B_{12} deficiency of pernicious anemia and is reversible with B_{12} supplement.
> White hair may be seen in celiac disease. Following a gluten-free diet, the anagen hairs darken at the roots.
> Essential fatty acid deficiency associated with intravenous hyperalimentation will induce depigmentation of hair.
> Chloroquine may cause hypopigmentation of scalp hair.
> Excessive copper in shower water or swimming pools may turn hair green.

Hori Y, Seiji M: **Hypomelanotic hair disorders**. *In* Orfanos C, Happle R (eds): Hair and Hair Diseases: New York: Springer-Verlag; 1990:443–466.

The presence of a white forelock on the scalp alerts one to **piebaldism** or to the **Waardenburg-Klein syndrome**. In piebaldism, the localized areas of congenital loss of pigment in the skin may be confused with vitiligo. The distinctive features of piebaldism are that it is inherited as an autosomal dominant trait and that islands of normal and hyperpigmented skin appear within the white skin sites.

In Waardenburg-Klein syndrome, heterochromia of the irides, fused eyebrows, and **deafness** are associated findings. Interestingly, the white forelock in these patients may repigment in later life.

Patches of white hair (poliosis) may alert one to the **Vogt-Koyanagi-Harada** syndrome. These, with accompanying patchy alopecia and vitiligo, are the permanent markers for a prior episode of an acute infection, possibly viral. A lesser degree of pigment loss involving all of the scalp hairs occurs in several other conditions. It is subtle, but a brown-haired child's parents with black hair alerts one to the possibility of **phenylketonuria** as a cause of the pigment dilution. Here the high levels of phenylalanine inhibit the tyrosinase so critical in the formation of melanin. A PKU urine test is indicated to demonstrate this autosomal recessive disorder.

A second condition to consider in children with surprisingly blond or silver-gray hair is the **Chédiak-Higashi syndrome**. They also exhibit translucent irides and pale retinas, accounting for their photophobia and nystagmus. A blood smear will show the diagnostic large granules in the leukocytes and on electron microscopy of the large nonmelanized melanosomes and will be seen in the melanocytes.

Finally, the cardinal loss of hair color is that seen in **albinism** (oculocutaneous). Classically the hair is white, the skin pink, and the child photophobic, exhibiting severe nystagmus. The hair bulbs form no pigment on in vitro incubation in tyrosine or L-dopa solution. A remarkable variant is the type 1B albinism in which the child by age 1 year develops yellow or yellow-red hair and a moderate ability to tan. This represents an ability to form the yellow-red phaeomelanin. Simple incubation of the hair bulbs in tyrosine and cysteine solution demonstrates this by the appearance of yellow or yellow-red pigment. Note that the brown and black melanin, called eumelanin, does not form.

In type II albinism the child also develops small amounts of pigment in the hair and skin as he grows. Pigmented nevi may appear, and irides become brown. In this type, the hair-bulb incubation test with L-dopa is positive. A further rarity is the type IV albinism (**Hermansky-Pudlak syndrome**). In this, the unique feature is an associated hemorrhagic diathesis. Other examples of albinism may exhibit a variety of defects, including oligophrenia (**Cross syndrome**).

Sato S, Jitsukawa K, Sato H, et al: Segmented **heterochromia** in black scalp hair associated with iron-deficiency anemia: Canities segmentata sideropaenia. Arch Dermatol 1989; 125:531–535.

A 15-year-old Japanese girl was referred because of a **dusty appearance** of her scalp hair. This had been present for 2 years. Since early childhood her scalp hair had been dark brown rather than the black that is characteristic of her race.

Examination showed discrete alternating light and dark bands along the hair shafts. The light bands varied from 2 to 50 mm in length. Laboratory studies were normal except for low levels of hemoglobin and serum iron (4 μmol/liter vs the normal of 14 to 18 μmol/liter). The serum zinc and copper levels were normal, as were numerous other tests.

After the diagnosis of iron deficiency anemia was made, ferrous sulfate (525 mg/day) therapy was started, and the serum iron climbed to normal. The newly synthesized hair shafts could be seen emerging black by the end of the second month. After more than a year of iron supplementation, no hypopigmented bands could be seen.

This newly described role of iron in melanogenesis led to designating the heterochromic hair as **canities segmentata sideropenica**. It is a diagnosis right out of a cantata.

Juhlin L, Ortonne JP: Red **scalp hair** turning dark-brown at 50 years of age. Acta Derm Venereol 1986; 66:71–73.

Nicknamed "Carrot" for his lifelong red hair, a 57-year-old man noted that for the past 4 years his scalp hair had turned dark brown, while his axillary and pubic hair remained red. He worked in vineyards with products that could have contained arsenic, and the explanation is advanced that arsenic exposure was responsible for the hair color change. Arsenic levels in the blood, nails, scalp hairs, and pubic hair were above normal, although arsenic levels in the axillary and pubic hair were ten times lower than that in the scalp hair. **Arsenic** binds easily to thiol groups and probably caused conversion of phaeomelanogenesis to eumelanogenesis.

Kellen RI, Schrank B, Burde RM: **Yellow forelock**—A new neuro-ophthalmological sign. Br J Ophthalmol 1990; 74:509–510.

When this 63-year-old gray-haired man complained of 2 months of progressive painless loss of vision in both eyes, his ophthalmologists noted that he had a **yellow forelock**. This proved to be the cutaneous sign for a diagnosis of optic neuropathy due to tobacco abuse. He had been pipe smoking well over a half pound of tobacco a week for more than 15 years.

The yellow of the hair was a tobacco smoke stain. The nicotine content of the forelock proved to be 21.7 ng/mg, whereas the occipital hair nicotine content was 2.2 ng/mg.

Smoke can not only get in your eyes, it can also get in your hair.

It's easy to diagnose a reaction pattern. It's hard to discern the cause.

Broken Hair

Itin PH, Pittelkow MR: **Trichothiodystrophy**: Review of sulfur-deficient brittle hair syndromes and association with the ectodermal dysplasias. J Am Acad Dermatol 1990; 22:705–717.

Presentation; short, sparse, brittle, unruly hair at scalp, eyebrows, eyelids. Hair easily broken, feels dry

Associated findings: nail dysplasia, ichthyosis, photosensitivity, mental and growth retardation

Diagnostic clues:

microscopy:
clean, transverse fractures (trichoschisis)
twisting
trichorrhexis nodosa
polarization microscopy: alternating light and dark bands (tiger-tail pattern)
scanning electron microscopy: cuticle damaged or absent, longitudinal grooves
chemical analysis: at least 50% decrease in cystine/cysteine sulfur of hair

Suspect in:

short-statured Amish patient (Amish brittle-hair syndrome)
mental retardation (Sabinas syndrome)
ichthyosis (Tay syndrome)
chronic neutropenia
photosensitivity
congenital abnormalities of ectodermal and neuroectodermal nature

Etiology: autosomal recessive defect

For want of sulfur, cuticle was lost. For want of cuticle, hair was lost.

Lucky PA, Kirsch N, Lucky AW, Carter DM: **Low-sulfur hair syndrome** associated with UVB photosensitivity and testicular failure. J Am Acad Dermatol 1984; 11:340–346.

Hair loss and erythema were the presenting complaints of this 15-year-old boy. He stated that he had persistent redness and pruritus of the skin, especially on the face and upper chest. The symptoms were worse in the summer. His hair had always been short, lusterless, and brittle, never longer than an inch because of spontaneous breakage. Biopsies had been consistently read as congenital ichthyosiform erythroderma.

Phototesting with UVB showed marked persistent erythema and edema to 0.5 joule. The erythema remained for more than 6 weeks. Examination of the hair showed trichoschisis (clear transverse fractures of hair shaft), as well as variations in the diameters of the hair shaft. Under polarization microscopy, there were alternating light and dark bands where the axis of the hair was aligned with the direction of one of the polarizing filters. X-ray analysis revealed a moderately low sulfur content of scalp hair (2.8% vs normal of 4.6 to 5.2%). Sun screens gave relief of symptoms, and the hair grew longer when the pruritus lessened and the breakage from scratching was eliminated.

Diagnosis of **low-sulfur hair syndrome** was made. Sulfur-deficient, brittle, fragile hair is the index marker for this syndrome. It is also known as:

trichothiodystrophy
BIDS syndrome (brittle hair, intellectual impairment)
trichoschisis with alternating birefringence and low-sulfur hair

The low sulfur content reflects a low concentration of cystine and thus can be detected on **amino acid analysis** of the hair shaft. The syndrome fits best into the ectodermal dysplasias, since these patients show:

mental and growth retardation	ichthyosiform skin changes
hypoplastic nails	ocular dysplasias
dental caries	testicular deficiency

Patel HP, Unis ME: **Pili torti** in association with citrullinemia. J Am Acad Dermatol 1985; 12:203–206.

For 3 weeks a 2½-year-old girl had been **losing scalp hair** on combing. Examination revealed that 90% of the scalp hairs were broken, leaving stubble less than 1 mm long. A patch of frontal hair remained, but these hairs were easily broken, and showed 180-degree twisting of a flattened hair shaft under the microscope. Pili torti was diagnosed.

This correlated with the fact that she had **citrullinemia** (argininosuccinate synthetase deficiency), profoundly delayed development, cerebral palsy, microcephaly, and recurrent infections. Because of the enzyme deficit, the urea cycle was disturbed, leading to a deficiency of the end product, arginine (9 μmol/liter, normal 15 to 115), and an accumulation of citrulline (5,149 μmol/liter, normal 10 to 34) and ammonia (162 μmol/liter, normal 11–35).

Arginine is essential in protein synthesis and probably affects hair growth. In another arginine deficiency state, argininosuccinicaciduria due to lack of arginosuccinate lyase, fragile hair, trichorrhexis nodosa, and pili torti may occur. Pili torti is the hair follicle expression of ectodermal dysplasia and may be part of a syndrome of corneal opacities, dental abnormalities, keratosis pilaris, and dystrophic nails. Pili torti also occurs in four other conditions, which should be searched for:

1. Menkes' syndrome (progressive psychomotor retardation, convulsions, low serum levels of copper and ceruloplasmin, failure to thrive, arterial degeneration, temperature instability, scorbutic bone changes, sex-linked recessive)
2. Björnstad's syndrome (sensorineural deafness, autosomal recessive)
3. Crandall's syndrome (deafness, hypogonadism, sex-linked recessive)
4. Hidrotic ectodermal dysplasia (characteristic facies, dental defects, autosomal dominant)

Fragile hair calls for a look under the microscope, and pili torti calls for a laboratory look at the amino acid, copper, and ceruloplasmin levels.

Hart DB: **Menkes' syndrome**: An updated review. J Am Acad Dermatol 1983; 9:145–152.

Depigmented, twisted, or broken hairs in a little boy call for determination of the serum copper level. If it is low, he fits into the Menkes' syndrome characterized by **kinky or steely hair**. The pili torti, monilethrix, trichorrhexis nodosa, or trichopoliodystrophy seen under the microscope are diagnostic markers of a disease usually fatal by the age of 5 years because of cerebral degeneration, cerebellar atrophy, seizures, growth failure, and respiratory infection. All patients look alike, with pale skin, a pudgy face, horizontal tangled eyebrows, and a "cupid's bow upper lip." Seborrheic dermatitis of the scalp is also common.

This X-linked recessive disorder does not affect girls. All patients have **low serum copper** and low serum ceruloplasmin levels because of poor absorption of copper from the intestine. Moreover, copper is stored in large amounts in certain tissues such as the kidney, with resultant deficiency in other tissues, including blood.

Looking at the hair and documenting a copper deficit may explain myoclonic seizures, which commonly are the presenting problem of these young boys. Regrettably, copper supplementation is without therapeutic benefit in this congenital copper storage disease.

Brown VM, Crounse RG, Abele DC: An **unusual new hair shaft abnormality**, "bubble hair." J Am Acad Dermatol 1986; 15:1113–1117.

For the past 4 months this 16-year-old girl had noted a strange area of hair loss on the right side of her scalp. The hair in that site had lost its soft curly nature, becoming straight and stiff. As it broke off, it left a "singed" appearance to the short hairs remaining.

Exhaustive biochemical analysis of both the patient and the hair revealed no clues other than the finding of **bubbles** along the hair shaft, both on light and electron microscopy. Strangely, these bubbles could be mechanically induced by localized pressure, e.g., compression of a glass slide over hairs that crossed each other.

Elimination of the use of electric rollers and hot blow drying led to improvement, so that by 10 months the area of hair was back to normal. (We suspect the area exhibiting this bubble hair was actually singed by the patient inadvertently or advertently.)

A single ray from the spectrum of a disease may light the path to diagnosis.

Mortimer PS: **Unruly hair**. Br J Dermatol 1985; 113:467–473.

Unruly scalp hair has many adjectives: crinkly, wooly, kinky, crimped, frizzy, steely, spun glass. It may be congenital or acquired, with or without hair shaft abnormality.

Extreme **unruliness of scalp hair** in babies (hair that stands up over the top of the head from the posterior parietal whorl toward the frontal hairline) may correlate with brain growth deficiency and is common in microcephaly, de Lange syndrome, and Down's syndrome. It also occurs in 2% of normal infants.

Wooly hair is curly hair that does not group into locks or lie down, with a curl diameter of approximately 5 mm. Hair-shaft microscopy is normal except for excess weathering. Wooly hair is noted soon after birth and is impossible to brush or comb. Diffuse or generalized scalp involvement is either an autosomal dominant (hereditary wooly hair) or recessive trait (familial wooly hair). A localized form (wooly hair nevus) may be associated with ipsilateral epidermal nevi.

Uncombable hair (cheveux incoiffables, spun-glass hair, pili triangulati et canaliculi) is disheveled with a tendency to stand on end as if controlled by electrostatic forces. It is noted in infancy when the hair starts to grow (age 3 to 9 months) and is blond or straw-colored with a characteristic sheen and spangled appearance. It does not break off (in contrast to pili torti) and improves with age. Scanning electron microscopy reveals triangular cross-sectional shape and a longitudinal canal extending along the hair shaft. Light microscopy may also reveal a dark homogeneous band along one edge of the hair shaft.

Pili torti is a structural defect in which the hair shaft is twisted 180 degrees on its axis at a few or many points along its length, with resulting fragility, breakage, and alopecia. The spangled hairs of various lengths stand on end and appear disheveled, particularly over the vertex. Present at birth, it improves with age.

Pili torti is associated with several syndromes:

> hypohidrotic ectodermal dysplasia
> Menkes' syndrome
> Björnstad's syndrome
> Bazex syndrome
> Crandall's syndrome
> pseudomonilethrix
> acquired focal scarring alopecia

Acquired progressive kinking of the hair (whisker hair) is a prelude to androgenic alopecia. It has no pathognomonic features under the microscope, but resembles pubic or whisker hair interspersed with normal hairs in the frontoparietal regions and vertex of the scalp. The kinky hair is dry, coarse, wiry, darker than normal, and impossible to comb. It must be distinguished from the reversible kinking of hair of the entire scalp seen in patients receiving etretinate.

Shelley WB, Shelley ED: **Uncombable hair syndrome**: Observations on response to biotin and occurrence in siblings with ectodermal dysplasia. J Am Acad Dermatol 1985; 13:97–102.

Clinical:

> blond, straw-colored hair that will not lie flat on combing
> onset in infancy, persists into teenage years if untreated

Diagnosis:

    hair shaft triangular with canal-like indentation in shaft
    seen on horizontal section biopsy, or cross-section of hair samples, or on
       scanning electron microscopy

Ravella A, Pujol RM, Noguera X, de Moragas JM: Localized **pili canaliculi** and trianguli. J Am Acad Dermatol 1987; 17:377–380.

A 3-year-old boy had two patches of uncombable hair on the scalp. Each grew unruly strawlike light-brown straight hairs. Elsewhere the scalp hair was normal, pliable, brown hair. Electron microscopy confirmed the diagnosis by demonstration of the canaliform grooves as well as trihedron-shaped abnormal hairs.

In previous accounts of the uncombable hair syndrome, all of the scalp hairs had been affected.

Rebora A, Guarrera M: **Acquired progressive kinking** of the hair. J Am Acad Dermatol 1985; 12:933–936.

This boy's hair began to curl when he was 15 years old. Within 2 years, the entire scalp was covered with curly hair. Examination revealed that the hair was wooly, lusterless, and darker than the rest. Under the microscope many hairs showed a sharp reduction in diameter. Some showed ill-defined spindle-shaped swelling and beading of the shaft, and others were twisted in their own axis. Pili canaliculi were seen as well on scanning electron microscopy.

A diagnosis of acquired kinking of the hair was made. This condition does not appear until late in the teens and is to be distinguished from:

    hereditary wooly hair
    familial wooly hair
    sporadic wooly hair
    wooly hair nevus

These appear early in life and disappear with aging.

Also in the differential is acquired wooly hair seen in adults as a result of trauma, such as radiation.

Mortimer PS, Gummer C, English J, Dawber RPR: **Acquired progressive kinking** of hair. Report of six cases and review of literature. Arch Dermatol 1985; 121:1031–1033.

In this 19-year-old man, the frontal, temporal and vertex regions of the scalp began to show thinning of the hair. The new hair was wiry, kinky, and resembled the hairs of the pubic area. Under the microscope the hairs were darker and tortuous with curls and half twists. Biopsy showed no abnormalities.

A diagnosis of acquired progressive kinking of the hair was made. It was possible to rule out wooly hair nevus since this is present since birth and manifests itself as a sharply circumscribed area of lighter colored, tightly curled hair.

Menkes' kinky hair due to copper deficiency is easily distinguished by its pili torti appearance. Similarly, uncombable hair and true pili torti again arise in childhood and show structural changes in the hair shaft. Acquired progressive kinky hair is an unusual prodrome of androgenetic hair loss. It would appear to be the product of follicles fighting senescence. Once the kinky hair falls out, end-stage baldness appears.

Marshall J, Parker C: **Felted hair untangled**. J Am Acad Dermatol 1989; 20:688–690.

A 40-year-old woman noted extensive tangling of her hair immediately after routine shampooing. Her hair was long, not having been cut since she was 16. During the shampoo, the hair had been piled on the top of her head and vigorously scrubbed.

On examination, there was a solid mass of matted hair on the scalp. A diagnosis of felted hair was made. Other terms used to describe this problem are **plica neuropathica**, felting of the hair, bird's-nest hair.

The patient elected to manually tease the hair apart rather than cut away her treasure of 24 years. It took 150 hours of knitting-needle labor on the part of her and her family over the next $2\frac{1}{2}$ months to unsnarl this mess.

Dawber RPR, Calnan CD: **Bird's nest** hair. Matting of scalp hair due to shampooing. Clin Exp Dermatol 1976; 1:155–158.

While using a new 2% cetrimide cationic detergent shampoo, three women were shocked to find their hair suddenly matted into a tangle over the entire occipital parietal areas. The mats defied all attempts at disentangling and had to be cut away.

Scanning electron microscopy revealed fluid "welds" where hair fibers were in contact. This viscous fluid welding probably contributed to the matting, as did the physical phenomenon of **felting** in which imbricated scales on the hair surfaces became interlocked through frictional forces. The matting could be reproduced within 30 seconds in normal plucked hair from six women by wetting the hair, adding the 2% cetrimide shampoo, and rubbing the hairs together. The hair could not be disentangled, even under the dissecting microscope.

Doctor: "Well, Bob, it looks like a paper cut, but just to be sure, let's do lots of tests."

THE NEW YORKER, *Cartoon, February 5, 1990*

Hand Eruptions

The skin of the hand is an anatomic mosaic. As such, it presents a remarkable number of diagnostic challenges for such a small area. It has interdigital and paronychial folds with their predilection to maceration and consequent bacterial and yeast infection. It has on the one side the thick mitotically active palmar skin sensitive to circulating antigens and toxins. On the other side is the thin epidermis preyed on by solvents, detergents, and contact allergens.

The palm is, moreover, so richly supplied in sweat glands that it is a unique site of hyperhidrosis as well as the corollary of the sweat-retention phenomena. It is this trapped sweat that converts a banal eczema into a vesicular or even bullous dyshidrosiform eruption. By contrast, the backs of the hands are without sebaceous glands, favoring the asteatotic eczema of dish-pan hands. Its thin epidermis favors contact dermatitis in contrast to the palm covered with keratin armor plate.

The circulation of the hand is a remarkable terminal bed of blood flow under sympathetic control. It is here that we see the Raynaud's phenomenon, the painful reflex sympathetic algodystrophy, and the glomus tumors. Even richer than the blood supply is the palmar nerve supply serving a sensory prowess and the symptoms of acrodynia.

All of the keratinization defects of congenital origin are greatly magnified in the palmar skin. It is here that we see the hereditable keratodermas, as well as the pits of the basal cell nevus syndrome. It is here that we see the fissured sharply circumscribed patches of psoriasis. The palms may not only trap sweat but also the neutrophils of the psoriatic epidermal invasion: Witness pustular psoriasis. At times, the palm may caricature in keratin the papules of lichen planus or play host to fungi as in piedra.

It is in the hand that we feel the early hardness of scleroderma, and it is here that we see the calcium deposits and the ultimate ulceration and gangrene of acrosclerosis. It is the hand that shows the atrophy of aging and the atrophic constriction band of ainhum. It is here that subjacent joints push up the ganglion on the back of the hand as well as the synovial cysts of the fingers.

A striking element of the mosaic of the skin of the hand is the fingernail. Its diagnostic implications range from the ridging of aging to the dystrophy of fungal infections. These are reviewed in the section "NAILS."

Unique as the hand is in its anatomic mosaicism, it is even more remarkable in its degree of exposure to "the slings and arrows" of the hostile environment of the work place, the sports world, and even the hobby center. It is the hand that dips into the cutting oils at work, the poison ivy patch on the golf course, and the mycobacterial-infested aquarium. Not even the gloved hand of the dentist may be safe from the vinyl and acrylic resins it contacts. Indeed, the glove itself may be the cause of the hand dermatitis. It is the hand that suffers the dermatitis as a result of the irritants used simply to clean it.

It is the hands that are constantly traumatized physically, as well. Such trauma accounts for the writer's middle-finger callus, the fingertip psoriasis of the violinist, and the purpura of the aged. It accounts for the frayed nail of the nail biter, the knuckle callus of the bulimic patient, and the bizarre skin lesions of factitial origin.

As if contactants and direct physical trauma were not enough, the skin of the hands is bombarded with ultraviolet rays that regularly and inevitably induce photoaged hands. These are the hands that exhibit lentigines, actinic keratoses, and squamous cell carcinomas. In the photosensitive porphyria cutanea tarda patient, erosions on the dorsae of the hands may be the only telltale marks of prior blisters.

Diagnostically, one's major effort must be directed toward distinguishing the various forms of hand eczema. Contact dermatitis is surely the most common. But is it an irritant dermatitis from chemicals, from washing, or simply from wet work? Exactly how does the patient cleanse his hands? Does he use steel wool, turpentine, or a scrub brush? How does he shampoo his hair? Shampoos are the most overlooked cause of hand dermatitis because they cause no scalp problem. Is it of allergic origin? Recall that patchy areas of dermatitis may still be due to allergens coming in contact with the entire hand. Nickel sensitivity is a classic example.

Is the hand dermatitis really an atopic dermatitis? Here, flares may come not only from external contactants, but they may be due to inhalants or foods from within. Secure an IgE determination. An elevated level favors an atopic type of dermatitis and a very prolonged course. Could the hand eruption be an id reaction due to tinea pedis? Examine the feet. If the eruption is on only one hand, you may have an example of the one-hand–two-feet tinea syndrome.

Watch for premenstrual flares so characteristic of the autoimmune progesterone sensitivity. Have the patient keep a food diary to correlate unusual foods with flares. We have seen coffee, pork, tomatoes, eggs, and corn, among other foods, cause hand eczema. It is serious business, since an allergen undetected can be responsible for years of hand eczema.

Could the eczema have an underlying psoriasis that has become eczematized? Is the eczema the result of sensitization to bacteria, as in acrodermatitis perstans? Could it be eczematized scabies? Is there secondary bacterial infection? Is there primary tinea? Do a scraping. Is it an allergic contact dermatitis? Do patch tests.

You won't get a handle on hand eruptions unless you keep asking questions. And if you don't look for something, you won't see it.

Color Change

Gonzalez JR, Botet MV: **Acromelanosis**. A Case report. J Am Acad Dermatol 1980; 2:128–131.

Jet-black pigmentation of the dorsal phalanges of all fingers of the right hand of this 2-year-old boy proved to be due to benign proliferation of melanocytes in the epidermis. It is viewed as the epidermal version of a blue nevus. The solid black of this acromelanosis is to be distinguished from the reticulate and freckling hyperpigmentation seen in the reticulate acropigmentation of Kitamura and the acropigmentation of Dohi.

As the child ages, there is the distinct possibility of progression to other sites, leading then to a diagnosis of acromelanosis progressiva.

Crotty CP, Dicken CH: Blue fingertips associated with **myxedema**. Arch Dermatol 1981; 117:158–159.

A **mat of telangiectases**, of red-blue hue, symmetrically covered the ventral aspect of each fingertip of a 42-year-old woman. It persisted for over a year and had not abated following bilateral carpal tunnel surgery for paresthesias of the hands. Slow verbal responses, thinning scalp hair, cold intolerance, and a puffy face suggested hypothyroidism, confirmed by a low total serum thyroxine level of 0.7 μg/dl (normal 5.0 to 13.5 μg/dl), low free thyroxine value of 0.1 ng/dl (normal 0.8 to 3.3 ng/dl), and a high thyroid-stimulating hormone level of 282 μU/ml (normal 0 to 15 μU/ml). The skin was generally dry and thick, and there was mild cracking of the fingertips.

A **diagnosis of primary myxedema** was made, and 2 months after she started taking levothyroxine sodium (0.15 mg/day), the bluish discoloration and telangiectases of the fingertips had completely disappeared. There was no recurrence during the subsequent 2-year course of thyroid replacement.

The telangiectases apparently resulted from vascular occlusion due to **mucin** deposited around small cutaneous vessels. Doppler ultrasound studies initially showed reduced pulse volumes in the proximal phalanges, with significant improvement 3 months after the starting of thyroid treatment.

Broussard RK, Baethge BA: Peripheral gangrene in **polyarteritis nodosa**. Cutis 1990; 46:53–55.

This 28-year-old woman was seen in the emergency room because of **pain and discoloration of the fingertips** that had been present for several weeks. Actually, 3 months earlier she had noted paresthesias and stiffness of the fingers. Her family physician had made a diagnosis of Buerger's disease. The history was remarkable in that she was addicted to cigarettes and to intravenous methamphetamine.

On physical examination there was **gangrene** of the tips of the right second and third fingers. Tests for HIV virus (ELISA assay), antinuclear antibody, and cryoglobulin gave negative results. Echocardiography failed to reveal any endocarditis, vegetations, or intracardiac thrombus. However, mesenteric and renal vessel arteriography showed irregular arteriolar narrowing of the renal vessels as well as microaneurysms at vessel branch points. These findings permitted a diagnosis of **periarteritis nodosa**.

The history and the laboratory studies ruled out these **causes of gangrene**: emboli, Raynaud's syndrome, overwhelming infection, systemic lupus erythematosus, crutch pressure arteritis, cold injury (cold agglutinins, cryoglobulinemia, cryofibrinogenemia), arteriosclerosis obliterans, and thromboangiitis obliterans.

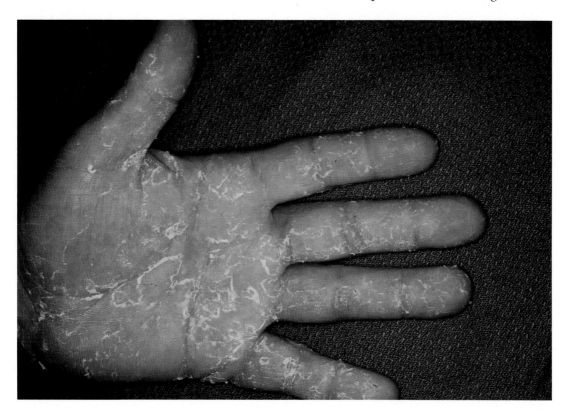

Cohen SR, Bilinski DL, McNutt NS: **Vibration syndrome**: Cutaneous and systemic manifestations in a jackhammer operator. Arch Dermatol 1985; 121:1544–1547.

Hand discomfort and swelling had been the lot of this 57-year-old jackhammer operator. It had begun as episodic hand pallor, **numbness, and tingling** within the first 6 months of employment. Each attack terminated with cyanosis and hyperemic and transient hand edema. As the years went on the attacks worsened and increased in frequency. Despite promotion 4 years later to bridge inspector, and the end of working with pneumatic tools, the hand problem has remained, elicited now by trivial exposure to cold. The hand swelling was no longer transient but continuous. He was found to have hearing loss and to be under psychiatric care for depression.

A skin biopsy showed striking dilatation of the blood vessels as well as mucinous deposits and the dermis thickened by the presence of numerous small collagen fibrils. The diagnosis was **vibration syndrome** or a variant of Raynaud's syndrome due to long-term exposure to vibratory equipment. It is also referred to as dead-hand syndrome or white-finger disease.

The condition went unrecognized for 11 years, indicating the need for greater awareness of the danger of vibration tools damaging the blood vessels, nerves, muscles, and joints of the hands that use them. There is loss of muscle strength and hand coordination. The incessant sound produces hearing loss, tinnitus, and mental depression. Half of these operators, whether they were using pneumatic drills or chain saws, noted headaches, forgetfulness, irritability, and sleep disturbances, as well as a depressed mood. Others had neck and elbow pain, shoulder stiffness, and lumbago.

Look for this in miners, road builders, aircraft workers, and tree surgeons. If it is found early, a job change can reverse the syndrome. If found late, the changes are irreversible, as in this patient.

Vesicles, Bullae

Shelley WB, Shelley ED: Chronic **hand eczema** strategies. Cutis 1982; 29:569–585.

Approach the patient with hand eczema as a problem in medical sleuthing. Be relentless in learning **every single manual contactant** the patient has in a single sample workday. Extend it to a sample weekend day. Force the patient to track each hour. Do not neglect the occasional contactants. They may trigger dermatitis that persists for days in their absence.

Find out if the patient is an atopic or not. Atopic patients regularly develop persistent hand eruptions when exposed to irritants that produce only transitory dermatitis in the nonatopic. The signs of the atopic state include not only a history of infantile eczema or asthma, but dry skin, itching after bathing, sensitivity to wool, an elevated IgE level, and also a family history of atopy. These **atopics** are the ones in whom the net for causes must be expanded to include foods, drugs, and inhalants.

Look at the feet for **fungal infection**. The hand eczema may be an id or even primary tinea. Look for sinusitis, cholecystitis, or urinary tract infection as a trigger for bacterial id eruptions of the hands. Look for streptococcal pharyngitis to explain keratolysis exfoliativa.

Examine the patient's skin in toto in **good light** for evidence of a diagnostic sign elsewhere, such as contact dermatitis at sites of nickel underclothing clasps. Look for a contactant patterning that may explain the origin, for example, fingertip dermatitis at the site of holding color-printed newspaper.

Test by patch testing, oral challenges, scrapings, and cultures.

Sander-Jensen K, Thomsen K: -Id reaction associated with chronic *Trichophyton rubrum* infection: Flare-up induced by cimetidine. Dermatologica 1987; 174:103–104.

Over a 2-year period, cimetidine (1 gm/day) was given for duodenal ulcer on three separate occasions to a 62-year-old man with chronic *Trichophyton rubrum* infection of the feet and toenails, each time precipitating a pruritic vesicular eruption of the palms, fingers, feet, and forearms. Symptoms began within 3 days of starting cimetidine in the second two episodes.

Cimetidine treatment augments the delayed-hypersensitivity skin test reaction to trichophyton antigen and presumably stimulated the cell-mediated response to trichophyton infection, with resulting id reactions.

Marks, JG: **Allergic contact dermatitis** to *Alstroemeria*. Arch Dermatol 1988; 124:914–916.

The chronic fingertip dermatitis of two florists was tracked to their work. However, wearing vinyl gloves gave no protection; this fact eliminated nearly all of the allergens to which they were exposed. Plant allergens that were patch tested included:

    tuliposide A (0.1% petrolatum)
    marguerite (1% petrolatum)
    laurel (bay leaf) (2% petrolatum)
    alantolactone (0.1% petrolatum)
    chrysanthemum (1%)
    primin (0.01%)

The mystery was solved when both were shown to have **positive patch tests** to the petal and stem (not the leaf) of the recently popularized Peruvian lily *Alstroemeria* (named after Klas Alstroemer, who brought seeds back from Peru in 1754). The responsible antigen produced positive patch tests even through a vinyl barrier. The principal allergen is tuliposide A, which also causes "**tulip finger**" in those who work with tulips.

Florists and dermatologists must watch out for the Peruvian lily, as well as the tulip, when vinyl gloves provide no protection at work.

Fisher AA: **Burns** of the hands due to ethylene oxide used to sterilize gloves. Cutis 1988; 42:267–268.

Gloves, shoes, gowns, masks, and drapes sterilized with ethylene oxide, but not sufficiently aerated, can cause irritant contact dermatitis in hospital workers and patients. Lesions sometimes resemble localized Lyell's disease or bullous impetigo.

Chapel J, Chapel TA: **Disuse contractures** in a patient with tinea manuum and irritant contact dermatitis. Cutis 1985; 36:55.

This 58-year-old woman gave a history of having **deep fissures** of the palmar creases of the left hand for the past 4 months. Movement of the hand had become so painful that the patient kept the hand in a flexed position. After 2 months she could no longer extend the fingers. The flexion contracture of the left third, fourth, and fifth fingers had resulted in a 50% loss of normal range of motion. Deep tendon reflexes, muscle strength, and sensation to pinprick and cotton were normal, indicating absence of nerve damage.

KOH examination of scabs from the palm and from the soles showed hyphae, which on culture proved to be *Trichophyton rubrum*. The history revealed her to be a compulsive housewife, washing, scrubbing, and polishing barehandedly.

The diagnosis was tinea pedis, tinea manuum, an irritant contact dermatitis, and disuse contracture of the flexor tendons of the last three fingers of the left hand.

Any chronic fissured hand dermatitis can lead to **contracture deformities** that are not readily reversible.

Miura T, Matsuda M, Yanbe H, Sugiyama S: Two cases of **autoimmune progesterone dermatitis**. Immunohistochemical and serological studies. Acta Derm Venereol 1989; 69:308–310.

This 25-year-old woman had insisted that for the past year she had had a widespread pruritic **erythematous rash** that appeared about 1 week before her menses and persisted until the period began. The eruption was ill-defined but included vesicles of the hands and lower legs. The periods were regular, and she had never taken contraceptives. She did have a history of atopic dermatitis, and blood studies showed eosinophilia and a high serum level of IgE. Progesterone and estrogen levels were normal.

The diagnosis of autoimmune progesterone dermatitis was made by demonstrating a positive intradermal **skin test** to aqueous progesterone suspensions (0.1 mg/ml). Within 20 minutes, a 12- by 12-mm wheal formed. Next, an IgG in her serum was shown to bind to rat corpus luteum. Finally, the indirect basophil test for progesterone was positive.

Progesterone sensitivity manifests itself in many other ways: Eczema, urticaria, erythema multiforme, and papulopustular, vesicular, and bullous lesions. The skin test to progesterone should be done, watching for both immediate and delayed responses.

In our practice, the hard part of making this diagnosis is in developing the patient's awareness of the premenstrual flare. Many patients fail to note the temporal relationship on their own, since the eruption never seems to really go away.

Veien NK, Hattel T, Justesen O, Nørholm A: **Dermatosis** in coffee drinkers. Cutis 1987; 40:421–422.

Five patients with recurrent **vesicular hand eczema** and a history of drinking more than 10 cups of coffee a day noted resolution of the hand eczema on stopping the coffee drinking.

Resumption of the excessive coffee intake resulted in reappearance of the hand eczema.

Milgraum SS, Friedman DJ, Ellis CN, Waldinger TP: **Pemphigus vulgaris** masquerading as dyshidrotic eczema. Cutis 1985; 35:445–446.

This 80-year-old woman had blisters on the soles. On examination she showed symmetrical vesiculobullous and pustular lesions of the plantar surfaces of the feet. The skin and mucous membranes were otherwise clear.

Ten days later the palms showed similar lesions. Scrapings and culture gave no evidence of fungi. A diagnosis of **dyshidrotic eczema** was made. Not until biopsy of a new lesion on the side of the foot was the diagnosis made. The specimen showed the typical immunofluorescent pattern of **pemphigus vulgaris**. A pemphigus antibody titer of 1:160 confirmed the diagnosis.

Within a week of the making of the diagnosis, the clinical picture enlarged. Flaccid bullae and erosions now appeared on the arms and abdomen, making the clinical diagnosis much less difficult than when the presenting problem was strictly vesicles of the palms and soles.

Rongioletti F, Parodi A, Rebora A: **Dyshidrosiform pemphigoid**. Report of an additional case. Dermatologica 1985; 170:84–85.

For 1 year a 72-year-old woman had had a pruritic vesicular eruption of the hands, diagnosed as **pompholyx**. Topical steroids were beneficial, but when tense bullae began to appear on the soles, along with a few red macules on the back, she sought a second opinion. Biopsies of the palms and back revealed **localized pemphigoid**, with heavy deposits of IgG and C_3 at the dermoepidermal junction on direct immunofluorescence.

Without biopsy and immunofluorescent studies, many examples of dyshidrosis may be dys-diagnosed!

Dawber R, Baran R: Painful **dorsolateral fissure** of the fingertip—an extension of the lateral nail groove. Clin Exp Dermatol 1984; 9:419–420.

A minor yet painful and disabling fissure of the thumb or index finger commonly occurs in atopic, psoriatic, or hyperkeratotic hands. It is strikingly uniform in its location, precisely as a trough extending out from the lateral nail groove. Adult atopics with irritant contact dermatitis commonly develop this problem in winter.

Perhaps an accidental pull on the lateral nail fold initiates this "anatomic" split.

Gawkrodger DJ, Cook SW, Fell GS, Hunter JAA: **Nickel dermatitis**: The reaction to oral nickel challenge. Br J Dermatol 1986; 115:33–38.

Nickel sulfate heptahydrate given orally in a dose ten times that found in a normal daily diet induced **pompholyx** in six nickel-sensitive subjects who had a history of pompholyx and a contact reaction to jewelry. In three subjects there was a flare of the patch test site as well as mild toxic erythema, and four subjects had itching of the palms without an eruption. The dose required to induce pompholyx was 5.6 mg of elemental nickel, given as $NiSO_4 \cdot 7H_2O$. Lower doses (0.4 mg, 2.5 mg) were without effect.

The estimated average daily intake of nickel is 300 to 600 µg, with foods high in nickel including whole wheat, rye, oats, cocoa, tea, gelatin, baking powder, kippered herrings, soya, red kidney beans, and peas. Stainless steel cooking utensils can increase the nickel content of acidic foods, and canned food may have more nickel than the fresh equivalent. The absorption and metabolism of nickel vary considerably between individuals. It is not known how the systemically induced nickel reaction is mediated.

Burrows D, Creswell S, Merrett JD: Nickel, hands and hip **prostheses**. Br J Dermatol 1981; 105:437–444.

Despite the fact that stainless steel and vitallium (chrome-cobalt) hip prostheses contain 12% and 2.5% nickel, respectively, these replacements do not sensitize patients to nickel. Nor does the presence of nickel allergy lead to rejection of a hip replacement.

Despite the fact that large amounts of nickel given orally as a challenge may aggravate nickel dermatitis, the amount of nickel in an ordinary diet plays no role in the **hand dermatitis** of nickel-sensitive patients.

Shelley ED, Shelley WB, Burmeister V: **Naproxen-induced pseudoporphyria** presenting a diganostic dilemma. Cutis 1987; 40:314–316.

A 72-year-old farmer's nonspecific **erosions** of the dorsa of the hands elicited interest because he claimed they were preceded by bullae.

The problem appeared to be routine **porphyria cutanea tarda**, and the biopsy findings were consistent with this. However, porphyria screening was negative. Epidermolysis bullosa acquisita was considered, but he had no lesions at sites of trauma outside the light-exposed areas. Nor were milia seen. The problem had been present for years but was becoming worse. A look at his drug intake revealed no less than 10 different ones taken every day. Cautious elimination of four of the less critical drugs resulted in complete clearing. The specific offending agent, **naproxen**, was identified when the patient's arthritis led him to resume taking it. Within a week, a large bulla appeared on the dorsum of the right hand.

Naproxen was discontinued, and there has been no recurrence of bullae during the following year, despite his continuing to take six of his original ten drugs.

Shelley WB, Shelley ED: **Blisters** of the fingertips: A variant of bullous dermatitis of hemodialysis. J Am Acad Dermatol 1989; 21:1049–1051.

For 3 months this 49-year-old man had had a sequence of recurring **blisters** of the fingertips. They appeared morphologically to be the blisters of burns of the pads of the fingertips. However, the only history of trauma elicited was that of manual digging of potatoes.

An initial diagnosis of **blistering dactylitis** was made but abandoned when antibiotics were without effect. A normal porphyrin screen ruled out porphyria cutanea tarda, and absence of diabetes eliminated the possibility of the burnlike bullae seen in diabetics. Elimination of furosemide therapy had no effect, and the absence of lesions elsewhere, as well as absence of milia formation, did not favor the diagnosis of acquired epidermolysis bullosa.

The critical determinant proved to be hemodialysis. For the past 8 months the patient had been undergoing hemodialysis because of renal failure. A diagnosis of **bullous dermatitis of hemodialysis** was made, and this was supported by the histologic findings. The unique feature was the presence of the blisters on the volar finger pads. It thus differs from the classic porphyria cutanea tarda–like lesions seen on the dorsa of the hands in patients undergoing long-term hemodialysis.

Feuerman EJ, Ingber A, David M, Weissman-Katzenelson V: **Lichen ruber planus** beginning as a dyshidrosiform eruption. Cutis 1982; 30:401–404.

Numerous **blisters** on the palms and soles of this 39-year-old woman had been present for 2 months. Some of the lesions were pustular, and cultures revealed *Escherichia coli*. Fungi were not found on KOH examination or on culture. A diagnosis of **dyshidrosis** with secondary infection was made.

Not until 3 months later did the full clinical picture evolve. Small, shiny purple papules then appeared on the flexor aspects of the extremities as well as firm vesicles of the palms. Biopsy of the forearm lesions showed a picture typical of **lichen planus**. A palmar vesicle showed similar changes.

The final diagnosis was lichen planus, presenting initially as dyshidrosis.

O'Reilly K, Snape J, Moore MR: **Porphyria cutanea tarda** resulting from primary hepatocellular carcinoma. Clin Exp Dermatol 1988; 13:44–48.

A 90-year-old woman experienced **bullae**, erosions, and crusts on the scalp, face, and dorsal aspect of the hands for 1 month, **attributed to frequent falls**. Hyperpigmentation and facial hypertrichosis were present, but she was taking no medications and did not drink alcohol. Liver function tests were abnormal, and a total urinary porphyrin level was 586 mmol/liter (normal 3 to 44). An ultrasound scan of the liver showed a large mass in the right lobe. Porphyria cutanea tarda in association with a hepatic lesion was diagnosed. After she died from bronchopneumonia, an autopsy revealed **malignant hepatoma**. The tumor was 11 by 10 by 10 cm, and the hepatoma cells fluoresced red, with a porphyrin level of 18.3 nmol/gm wet weight (normal 0 to 3.0). The majority of porphyrins found in the liver and the hepatoma on high-pressure liquid chromatography (HPLC) were protoporphyrins and coproporphyrins.

This patient's lesions, at first thought to be trivial abrasions, were really a **paraneoplastic phenomenon**. Reading the backs of the hands, rather than the palms, told the future.

Snyder MH, Snyder WH: Traumatic **thrombosis** of deep palmar vein. JAMA 1938; 111:2007–2008.

A 67-year-old blacksmith experienced sudden immediate **pain in the palm** of the left hand while holding an anvil on which he was pounding. A mass appeared at the injury site soon after, and he experienced pain whenever he used that hand. On examination 1 month later a firm, movable mass 1 by 2.5 cm could be palpated at the base of the hypothenar space. It did not move with flexion and extension of the fingers. There were no cutaneous lesions, but there was a slight decrease in sensation in the palmar aspect of the fourth and fifth fingers. A diagnosis was made of a "**ganglion**" with post-traumatic tenosynovitis.

At surgery, the mass proved to be a **thrombosed, dilated vein** under the palmar fascia. It extended from the fourth digital vein upward within the deep ulnar vein to the wrist. Excision was followed by pain-free full use of the hand and return to work in 3 weeks.

Grange JM, Noble WC, Yates MD, Collins CH: **Inoculation mycobacterioses**. Clin Exp Dermatol 1988; 13:211–220.

For want of a diagnosis, fingers have been amputated unnecessarily in cases of infection with *Mycobacterium gordonae* as well as *M. marinum*. One young woman was saved from amputation of a leg by the chance visit of an African physician who recognized that the problem was a postinjection abscess due to *M. fortuitum*.

*Think of **inoculation tuberculosis***

  in those doing autopsies (The great French physician Laennec realized his own fatal tuberculosis had begun as a "prosector's wart" on his left index finger acquired when he sawed through the vertebra of a tuberculous cadaver.)
  in those handling needles, instruments around patients with tuberculosis
  in those in laboratories where a broken test tube containing a culture of *M. tuberculosis* may be the instrument of inoculation
  in those performing mouth-to-mouth resuscitation, a source of subsequent nasolabial-inoculation tuberculosis
  in immunologic experiments involving tubercle bacilli
  in butchers and milkmaids around bovine tuberculosis
  in patients receiving injections given by a nurse with open pulmonary tuberculosis
  in cases of self-inoculation of tubercle bacilli to produce a factitial eruption or even to commit suicide
  in instances of reuse of an inadequately sterilized needle previously used to aspirate a tuberculous abscess
  in a circumcision performed by a rabbi with open pulmonary tuberculosis
  in ear piercing or tattooing in the crude form as performed in prisons
  in legs, buttocks, genitalia of children playing and sitting on pavements contaminated with tuberculosus sputum

*Think of **bacille Calmette-Guérin (BCG)***

  Intentionally induced BCG vaccination heals spontaneously in several weeks.
  in needle-stick accidents involving medical personnel

*Think of **leprosy***

  in those with tattoos
  in those with dog bites (latent period 3 to 5 years)

in abrasions

in insect bites

in those in direct contact with armadillos, a potential animal carrier of the disease

Think of *other mycobacteria*

in postinjection abscesses, especially following injections with poor technique, poor hygienic conditions, contaminated multidose vials

in swimming pool or aquarium abrasions

in cat scratches

in animal kicks

in auto, bicycle, motorcycle accidents

in nail, splinter, or wire injuries

in thorn pricks

in scorpion stings

in gunshot wounds

in surgical implants

in augmentation mammoplasty

in stripping of varicose veins, due to contaminated antiseptic used to prepare skin

Make the diagnosis

bacteriologic culture of biopsy material

biopsy material from wall of abscess far better than pus for culture

culture at 30° and 37°C

Remember these mycobacteria do not like warmth. The two most common, *M. chelonei* and *M. fortuitum*, were initially isolated from a turtle and a frog, respectively. And they love only our cool skin.

If you don't ask about a lot of things, you won't know about a lot of things you see.

Coulson IH, Marsden RA, Cook MG: Purpuric **palmar lichen nitidus**—an unusual though distinctive eruption. Clin Exp Dermatol 1988; 13:347–349.

A reddish-brown hyperkeratotic umbilicated papular eruption on the palms and lateral fingers of a 50-year-old roofer for 8 years had been dismissed as dermatitis. When the monomorphic 2-mm papules failed to respond to topical steroids, a biopsy revealed the lesions to be lichen nitidus.

While only a handful of these cases have been reported, have you missed one for want of a biopsy?

Huntley AC: **Finger pebbles**: A common finding in diabetes mellitus. J Am Acad Dermatol 1986; 14:612–617.

A pebbly appearance to the knuckles and distal finger skin may be seen in 75% of patients with diabetes mellitus. It reflects a thickening of the skin that occurs in this population. Such thickening also accounts for the finding of decreased wrinkling of these patients following immersion in water.

The change is subtle and suggests the term "finger sand" to us more than finger pebbles.

Abdul Razack EM, Premalatha S, Raghuveera Rao N, Zahra A: **Acanthosis palmaris** in a patient with bullous pemphigoid. J Am Acad Dermatol 1987; 16:217–219.

"**Tripe palms**" is a distinctive form of acanthosis of the palms in which the ridges are exaggerated and the furrow accordingly deep. This gives the palm the appearance of the rugose surface of bovine foregut mucosa known as tripe. It may at times herald malignancy, although here it was the strange accompaniment of bullous pemphigoid.

Cross DF, Ellis JG: Occurrence of the Janeway lesion in **mycotic aneurysm**. Arch Intern Med 1966; 118:588–591.

Two patients with *Pseudomonas* infections of the brachial arterial wall following angiography developed multiple nontender **hemorrhagic macules** on the finger pads downstream from the infection. One patient had several splinter hemorrhages on the same hand, while the other patient also had a 1-cm erythematous tender nodule on one finger pad. Neither patient had endocarditis. Excellent color photographs are presented.

Rapaport MJ: **Pellagra** in a patient with anorexia nervosa. Arch Dermatol 1985; 121:255–257.

A mild **pruritic eruption** of the dorsa of the hands and the extensor surface of the forearms proved to be pellagra. It had come on after Maytime sun exposure in a 20-year-old girl who was under care for anorexia nervosa.

The photosensitivity was mild, there were never any blisters, and the biopsy was rather nonspecific. Light tests for minimal erythema dose (MED) were within normal limits. However, it was possible to show on 24-hour urine tests that she suffered from a niacin deficiency. Excretion of 1-methyl-5 carboxyl-amide-2-pyridone was 2.8 mg/24 hours (normal 6 to 51 mg) and N-1 methyl nicotinamide was 0.5 mg/24 hours (normal 1.6 to 14.8 mg).

Oral niacin (100 mg tid) cleared the eruption in 21 days. The diagnostic skill here was in relating the erythema, dermatitis edema, and scaling of the backs of the hands to sunlight exposure. It is important to recognize that one third of patients with a deficiency of niacin or its precursor, tryptophan, suffer only **photosensitivity**. They do not have the diarrhea and dementia so long taught in the textbooks as an essential part of the 3-D triad of pellagra.

Nor is pellagra seen only in the poor undernourished. Your next patient with pellagrous photosensitivity may be the patient who has a diet of alcohol, the one who eats nothing and tells you his diet is normal, the patient with malabsorption, the patient taking isoniazid, or the one with an unrecognized carcinoid syndrome.

If the diagnostic sun is to shine in your office, you must think of pellagrous photosensitivity to explain some of those banal mild dermatitides of the exposed areas, in the rich and poor alike.

Harper KE, Spielvogel RL: **Nevus comedonicus** of the palm and wrist. J Am Acad Dermatol 1985; 12:185–188.

This 18-year-old white man had had **blackheads** on the right palm and forearm since he was 6 years of age. They had begun as tiny dark wartlike papules on the palms. Only recently had they appeared on the wrists. Expression of the blackhead left a pit that would rapidly refill.

Examination revealed numerous slightly raised, well-circumscribed, firm, flat-topped papules on the right palm and wrist. The papules were arranged in a linear pattern, and the larger ones were filled with a central yellowish hyperkeratotic plug.

A diagnosis of nevus comedonicus was made. The **differential diagnosis** includes:

punctate porokeratosis of mibelli
palmar keratosis
keratosis punctate (in flexural creases)
arsenical keratoses

Nevus comedonicus remains most likely a vestigial variant of linear epidermal nevus.

Russell G: **Bulimia nervosa**: An ominous variant of anorexia nervosa. Psychol Med 1979; 9:429–448.

Oval **reddish-brown calluses** and scars over the second, third, and fifth metacarpophalangeal joints of the right hand are shown in a 17-year-old girl with bulimia for 3 years. She told her mother they resulted from boils, but they were really caused by the upper incisors rubbing against her skin.

Patients with **bulimia** have an irresistible urge to overeat but a morbid fear of becoming fat and therefore resort to self-induced vomiting. In contrast to patients with anorexia nervosa, they tend to be heavier, more likely to be sexually active, and have regular menses. Depression may be severe with a high risk of suicide.

Williams JF, Friedman IM, Steiner H: Hand lesions characteristic of **bulimia**. Am J Dis Child 1986; 140:28–29.

Abrasions, calluses, or scars on the dorsal aspects of the metacarpophalangeal joints on one or both hands in an adolescent girl may be an early sign of bulimia. **Self-induced emesis** is most often accomplished by inserting two fingers into the mouth to stimulate the gag reflex, thereby abrading the skin against the maxillary incisors.

The estimated incidence of bulimia in the United States is 10% for women 15 to 30 years old, compared with a rate of 1% for anorexia nervosa in the same population.

Joseph AB, Herr B: Finger calluses in **bulimia**. Am J Psychiatry 1985; 142:5.

A 22-year-old woman college student had depression and significant callus formation on the dorsal aspect of each index finger over the metacarpophalangeal joint. She admitted to inducing emesis with the tip of either index finger over an 8-year-period, and the calluses formed where her teeth came in contact with her fingers.

Yoneda K, Kanoh T, Nomura S, et al: **Elastolytic cutaneous lesions** in myeloma-associated amyloidosis. Arch Dermatol 1990; 126:657–660.

Night sweats and fatigue led to a general physical examination of this 62-

year-old man. The singular feature observed was the soft, loose, **redundant skin around the fingertips**. After pressure indentation, the skin returned to normal very slowly. He was unable to grasp a pen because it cut into his fingertips. Similar loose skin was seen on the soles, but not elsewhere. The tongue was normal in size, but petechiae were noted on the palms. The only other finding was a papable liver.

A biopsy revealed a decrease and fragmentation of elastic tissue (Verhoeff-van Gieson) as well as **amyloid deposits** (Congo red, cotton-dye stains). General laboratory studies were negative except for an elevated serum calcium level. A bone marrow aspirate showed numerous immature plasma cells, and urinary immunoelectrophoresis revealed large amounts of Bence Jones protein. Osteolytic areas were also seen on a skeletal survey. A diagnosis of **myeloma-associated amyloidosis** was made.

The cutaneous finding of loose skin is unusual, but the long-lasting depression after pressure called for an explanation. It proved to be localized **cutis laxa** due to the destructive effects of amyloid on the elastic tissue. Such cutis laxa may also be seen in neutrophilic dermatosis, but this patient showed no neutrophil infiltrate.

Amyloidosis is the great mimic. Its repertoire is not limited to "**pinch purpura**." It may also come to your office in the guise of glassy or waxy papules, nodules, and plaques. Or it may enter as a bullous eruption, scleroderma, or even as mundane hair loss. Recognition calls for biopsy and stain.

Good JM, Neill SM, Rowland Payne CME, Staughton RCD: **Keratoderma** of myxoedema. Clin Exp Dermatol 1988; 13:339–341.

A 67-year-old man had dry, **thickened**, **painful palms**, thought to be chronic endogenous eczema. Topical steroids and keratolytics were unsuccessful. Because of the pain, superficial radiotherapy was employed, but it provided only a 6-week remission.

Finally the development of severe morning headaches and ataxia led to hospitalization, where routine blood studies revealed profound **hypothyroidism**: free thyroxine 6.6 pmol/l (normal 9 to 24); thyroid-stimulating hormone 24.3 μmol/liter (normal 0.3 to 3.5); and the presence of thyroid autoantibodies. Within 3 days of starting thyroxine therapy (0.1 mg/day) the headache and ataxia resolved, and within a week the palms had improved. Within a month he no longer had any keratoderma or pain, and the remission persisted.

Puzzling patients with keratoderma (or even without keratoderma) deserve a **health profile**!

Aratari E, Regesta G, Rebora A: **Carpal tunnel syndrome** appearing with prominent skin symptoms. Arch Dermatol 1984; 120:517–519.

Erythematous lesions of the left hand of this 68-year-old woman had defied diagnosis and therapy for 7 years. The left first, second, and third fingers showed a reddish chilblain-like discoloration as well as small areas of necrosis. The second finger was anhidrotic and lacking in hair. There was no pain or itching, but there were recurrent shocklike sensations. The radial side of the left wrist was deformed, the result of a wrist fracture many years before.

Many studies finally revealed markedly reduced sensory conduction velocity of the left median nerve. A diagnosis of **carpal tunnel syndrome** was made, and hand surgery was followed by disappearance of all the skin changes.

Carpal tunnel syndrome is a compressive neuropathy of the median nerve due to ligamentous entrapment. It usually is the result of a wrist fracture, trauma, or dislocation. This case eluded diagnosis for 7 years because the classic signs of **numbness and tingling** were absent, as well as the later signs of motor nerve impairment such as inability of the thumb to touch the fingers. The signs related more to autonomic fiber compression. In every disease there is a forme fruste.

Feingold, M: Picture of the month: Syndromes associated with **thumb abnormalities**. Am J Dis Child 1985; 139:529–530.

Rubinstein-Taybi syndrome: The terminal phalanges of the toes and thumbs are broad and angulated.

Holt-Oram syndrome: A triphalangeal thumb resembles a finger in the same plane. There may also be aplasia or hypoplasia of the thumb.

Marfan's syndrome: The hand is large with arachnodactyly. When the fist is closed with the thumb inside, the thumb extends beyond the ulnar border.

An admiring and inquiring patient can pump a lot of diagnostic energy into a doctor.

Hands and Feet

The hands are bare and subject to a thousand environmental insults never suffered by the reclusive feet hidden within shoes. Yet the hands and feet are homologous. As a result, hand eruptions often bespeak a foot eruption and vice versa. This is especially true of genetic defects or of any eruption in which the pathogens are circulating and become lodged in the circulation of the hand and foot. Examples include the hereditary diseases such as keratodermas. Other examples are the hormonally induced changes seen in acromegaly and acrokeratosis. The hands and feet will also be the site of localization as seen in Raynaud's phenomenon and in hyperhidrosis. Another example of the tandem hand and foot eruption is erythema multiforme due to herpes simplex viremia. Nail changes are commonly shared, as well as the scabietic mite.

Make no mistake: if the patient complains of a hand eruption, look at the feet. And if the patient complains of a foot eruption, examine the hands. When both are involved, think first of an internal cause.

Lines and Signs

Bernhard JD, Rhodes AR, Melski JW: **Wallace's line** in serum sickness and Kawasaki disease. Br J Dermatol 1986; 115:640.

Cutaneous changes delineated sharply at the margin between the dorsal and plantar skin of the foot (**Wallace's line**) or dorsal and palmar skin of the hand may reflect the presence of immune complexes, as well as the anatomy of the lymphatic and vascular systems. These factors may help explain how rashes localize.

In **serum sickness** a serpiginous, erythematous, purpuric eruption may occur in these areas of the hands and feet. Similar findings occur in Kawasaki disease, with scalloped erythema on the hands and feet.

Rowland Payne CME, Branfoot AC: **Wallace's line**. Br J Dermatol 1986; 114:513–514.

Wallace's line is the sharp transition line between the ventral and dorsal surfaces of the hands and feet. Certain dermatoses, such as lichen planus and pompholyx, are delineated sharply at these lines on the medial and lateral borders of the hands and feet. Stasis ulceration never occurs distal to Wallace's line. Sweat glands, dermatoglyphics, hair, and sometimes pigmentation all alter sharply at this line.

Distal to Wallace's line the **lymphatics** are plentiful, and drainage is rapid and efficient, whereas the lymphatic drainage of the dorsal surface is poorer, resulting in delayed clearance of unwanted material such as ecchymoses, interstitial fluid, and antigens. Therefore, Wallace's line may reflect lymphatic drainage more than any other anatomic factor.

It is respected by surface markings, pigmentation, appendages, lymphatics, function, anatomy, and diseases.

Cardullo AC, Silvers DN, Grossman ME: **Janeway lesions** and **Osler's nodes**. A review of histopathologic findings. J Am Acad Dermatol 1990; 22:1088–1090.

The **Janeway lesion** is a hemorrhagic lesion on the palms or soles that is associated with bacterial endocarditis. Histologically one finds a neutrophilic abscess in the dermis with bacteria present. This results from **septic emboli** coming from the heart.

The **Osler node** is the other sign of endocarditis. Clinically it is a painful erythematous nodule with a pale center. Appearing suddenly, usually on the fingertips, it fades away without ulceration. Histologically it is a sterile **embolus** producing a microabscess in the glomus body.

The asymptomatic hemorrhagic macule belongs to Janeway and the tender papule belongs to Osler.

Kerr A Jr, Tan JS: Biopsies of the Janeway lesions of **infective endocarditis**. J Cutaneous Pathol 1979; 6:124–129.

In three men with infective endocarditis caused by *Staphylococcus aureus*, small (2 to 5 mm) **reddish**, **nontender macules** developed on the palms, fingertips, and soles. In two patients, prior to therapy the organism was cultured from these skin lesions, and skin biopsies showed epidermal and dermal microabscesses. In the third patient the lesions developed during antibiotic therapy, and skin biopsy showed lack of inflammation and no vasculitis.

Presumably the **Janeway lesion** results from a bacterial, embolic, suppurative, process in acute infection, without involvement of immune complexes leading to vasculitis (in contrast to Osler's nodes).

Breathnach SM, Wells GC: **Acanthosis palmaris**: Tripe palms. A distinctive pattern of palmar keratoderma frequently associated with internal malignancy. Clin Exp Dermatol 1980; 5:181–189.

A search for visual analogies led this 70-year-old man to describe his palms as looking like tripe. In other words, they had the appearance of the rugose convoluted surface of the **cow's foregut**, sold as tripe in the butcher shop. The change had been progressive for the past 8 months. His appetite had been fading for 6 months, and there had been associated diarrhea for the last 4 months. The palms showed a distinctive ridged, patterned thickening that accentuated the normal skin markings. It was not unlike the appearance induced by prolonged soaking of the palm in water.

Study of the patient revealed he had **bronchogenic carcinoma** with metastasis. The "**tripe palm**" is viewed as a restricted version of acanthosis nigricans. As such, it may herald internal malignant disease.

Nordstrom KM, McGinley KJ, Cappiello L, et al: **Pitted keratolysis**. The role of *Micrococcus sedentarius*. Arch Dermatol 1987; 123:1320–1325.

Superficial **crateriform pits** in the stratum corneum of the soles is the typical presentation of pitted keratolysis. The usual sites are those of the weight-bearing surfaces of the feet. On the palms it occurs rarely and then as collarettes rather than pits. The pits are 1 to 7 mm in diameter, but may coalesce into large irregular areas of eroded stratum corneum. It is, in general, asymptomatic, but at times is accompanied by plaques of reddened thickening and distinct tenderness. Nearly always the condition is associated with **hyperhidrosis**, occlusive shoes, and/or moist conditions. Malodor due to thiolsulfides and thioesters is also present.

The pathogenesis centers on digestion of the stratum corneum and elaboration of odor by bacteria that grow in abundance in the wet stratum corneum. The offending organism was found to be *Micrococcus sedentarius* in eight consecutive patients in this study. This bacterium is well named for its sedentary job of nibbling at feet.

Gillum RL, Hussain Qadri SM, Al-Ahdal MN, et al: **Pitted keratolysis**: A manifestation of human dermatophilosis. Dermatologica 1988; 177:305–308.

Pitted defects in the soles of a 44-year-old physician proved to be due to the bacterium *Dermatophilus congolensis*, which had simply attached to the thick stratum corneum of the soles. It was seen on KOH examination as motile coccoid organisms and branched septate filaments around the keratin fragments. The coccoid forms were gram-positive and appeared as rough gray colonies on anaerobic blood agar plates.

This organism produces crusting exudative dermatitis with thick crusts and alopecia in cattle, horses, deer, and sheep, as well as many wild animals. In sheep it also causes "strawberry footrot" and "lumpy wool" (known in higher circles as dermatophilosis), while in cattle it causes "mycotic dermatitis." In man this organism can produce **furuncles** in those handling infected deer.

Previously the only other pathogen isolated from pitted keratolysis was a species of *Corynebacterium*.

Zaias N: Pitted and ringed **keratolysis**: A review and update. J Am Acad Dermatol 1982; 7:787–791.

This entity represents focal loss of stratum corneum due to keratolysis by colonies of saprophytic corynebacterium growing on the moist thick skin of the palms or soles.

The **pits** or rings may vary from 1 mm in size to confluent lesions covering the entire sole. When present in the interdigital spaces, they may simulate the lesions of candidiasis (erosio interdigitalis blastomycetica). Clinically the lesions are dramatically accentuated by soaking the palm or sole for 15 minutes in tap water. By this maneuver, the inapparent becomes apparent as a result of differential swelling of the uninvolved and involved stratum corneum. A culture (anaerobic at 35 to 37°C) on 5% brain-heart infusion produces a profuse spidery growth of **diphtheroid organisms**.

"Microbial"-eaten soles are more often a curiosity of inspection than an object of referral.

In making a dermatologic diagnosis, look for the distinctive face of the disease, not its featureless arms, legs, and trunk.

Stack KM, Churchwell MA, Skinner RB: **Xanthoderma**: Case report and differential diagnosis. Cutis 1988; 41:100–102.

A lifelong history of **yellow-orange palms** and soles in a 29-year-old man from Liberia was found to be due to high **dietary** intake of red palm oil containing yellow beta-carotene. Excess carotene is deposited in the skin, with a predilection for fat and stratum corneum (particularly thick on the palms and soles). The serum carotene level was 229 μg/dl (normal 50 to 200) after he had been away from the palm oil for 3 months in the United States.

Xanthoderma refers to yellow-orange discoloration of the skin. If jaundice is ruled out (normal bilirubin, no bilirubin in urine, nonicteric sclerae and mucous membranes), **hypercarotenemia** (aurantiasis, carotenosis cutis) is likely. A deeper red-orange color of the palms, soles, and palate indicates **lycopenemia** (an isomer of carotene).

In a patient with yellow-orange discoloration of the skin, look for:

> yellow sclerae (binding of bilirubin and quinacrine to elastic tissue)
> discoloration of palms and soles (hypercarotenemia, lycopenemia, riboflavinemia)
> elevated levels of serum lipids, which bind the lipophilic carotenes (diabetes mellitus, hypothyroidism, nephrotic syndrome)
> drug or chemical ingestion or exposure (quinacrine, fluorescein, saffron, santonin, dinitrophenol, tetryl and picric acids, acriflavine)
> diet high in intake of:
>> carotenoids (vegetable oils, carrots, oranges, squash, spinach, green vegetables, butter, eggs)
>> lycopenes (tomatoes, rosehips, bittersweet berries)
>> riboflavin (vitamins)
> multiple myeloma (elevated IgG level possibly binding riboflavin, causing yellow hair and skin)
> an inborn error of beta-carotene metabolism to vitamin K (no lipidemia, no overingestion of carotene)

Ryan TJ: **Vibration**: Good or bad? Clin Exp Dermatol 1981; 6:179–189.

The "**dead finger**" Maurice Raynaud described in 1862 was an intermittent, segmental whitening due to a sudden decrease in blood supply, induced by cooling. Today the sign intermittent pallor of the fingers calls for consideration of the following known causes:

Vasospasm

> cold, fear, anxiety, vasoconstrictors: nicotine, ergot, beta-adrenergic blockers
> carpal tunnel syndrome   shoulder girdle compression
> thoracic outlet syndrome   syringomyelia

Connective tissue disease

> scleroderma   rheumatoid arthritis
> vasculitis   dermatomyositis
> systemic lupus erythematosus

Occlusive disease

> vinyl chloride exposure   thromboangiitis obliterans
> arteriosclerosis

Blood

cold agglutinins	macroglobulinemia
cryoglobulins	emboli
cryofibrinogen	platelet aggregation
hyperviscosity	

Vibration

tools, pneumatic	typing	piano playing

Raynaud would be impressed at the many directions in which his finger now points.

Mufson I: Intermittent limping—**intermittent claudication**; their differential diagnosis. Ann Intern Med 1941; 14:2240–2245.

If the superficial circulation is patent, skin color depends on an adequate arterial blood supply. To test for this, elevate the leg and flex the foot several times to render the skin colorless. Then lower the leg to a dependent position and watch for prompt return of the pink color. A definite delay in color return shows an insufficient **arterial blood supply**. However, delay may also occur if the skin is cool or the patient is very anxious with a strong vasoconstrictive reflex.

Sparrow GP: A **connective tissue disorder** similar to vinyl chloride disease in a patient exposed to perchlorethylene. Clin Exp Dermatol 1977; 2:17–22.

A 19-year-old white man had constant coldness of the hands and feet for 3 months and **Raynaud's phenomenon** occurring not only on the hands and feet, but also on the knees, elbows, and even the tongue. The affected areas would not become red upon rewarming. The cause of this and associated severe muscle weakness and pain in his arms, shoulders, and legs was traced to exposure to the solvent, **perchlorethylene**, used in the dry cleaning shop in which he had worked for 4 years.

Although his fingers become swollen and he could not grip tightly, he did not show the acral osteolytic lesions often seen in workers exposed to vinyl chloride. A skin biopsy showed mild edema of blood vessel walls with sparse perivascular round cell infiltrate, but no sign of scleroderma, which ruled out mixed connective tissue disease. He also had mild hepatic dysfunction, impotence, and a high titer of ANA (1:10,240) in a speckled pattern.

The skin of the hands was diffusely swollen and thickened, and multiple nail-fold hemorrhages were prominent.

Ross JB, Cohen AD, Ghose T: **Goodpasture's syndrome** associated with skin involvement. Arch Dermatol 1985; 121:1442–1444.

Areas of **erythema** suddenly appeared on the **instep** of this 48-year-old man who was hospitalized for the treatment of a longstanding hemoptysis and hematuria. The major change on skin biopsy was seen as a perivasculitis and in the immunofluorescent demonstration of linear deposits of IgM and C3 along the basement membrane.

Renal biopsy indicated necrotizing glomerulonephritis with the same antibody deposits around the walls of the glomerular capillaries. The serum anti-GBM (glomerular basement membrane) antibody titer was high, and it is this same antibody that participated in the pulmonary alveolar damage and hemoptysis he experienced.

The progressive life-threatening pulmonary hemorrhage and severe necrotizing glomerulonephritis made the diagnosis of **Goodpasture's syndrome**. It is like the red macules of his instep were but a previously undescribed cutaneous sector of this autoimmune syndrome.

Davies GE, Triplett DA: Corticosteroid-associated **blue-toe syndrome**: Role of anti-phospholipid antibodies. Ann Intern Med 1990; 113:893–895.

This 71-year-old man experienced pain in the left toes and the left sole within a few days of being given prednisone (60 mg/day) for asymptomatic thrombocytopenia. Examination on the 13th day showed **patchy purple macules**, most vivid on the tip of the great toe. Simply stopping the prednisone led to rapid lessening of the pain in 2 days and return to normal skin color in 3 weeks.

The **differential diagnosis for a unilateral blue toe** in the presence of palpable pulses includes microembolism of fibrin-platelet debris or cholesterol crystals from a proximal atherosclerotic lesion. In this patient the laboratory finding of high levels of antiphospholipid antibodies (lupus anticoagulant) suggested that the pain and blue toe were due to the formation of **capillary thrombi**.

Harms M, Feldman R, Saurat J-H: Papular-purpuric **"gloves and socks"** syndrome. J Am Acad Dermatol 1990; 23:850–854.

A 16-year-old boy experienced progressive pruritic **reddening and swelling of his hands** and feet 10 days after being treated with oral chymotrypsin for a sprained left ankle. This was associated with a mild fever. On examination the hands and feet showed symmetrical edema and erythema that was sharply marginated on the wrist and ankle. These borders presented confluent erythematous and flat papules. On the backs of the hands and feet there were purpuric macules. Poorly demarcated patches of erythema were seen on the knees and elbows, as well as the face. The axillary and inguinal lymph nodes were tender and enlarged. By the fifth day, petechiae developed, as well as buccal erosions. Clearing of the skin lesions was gradual.

This is one of five patients with an identical clinical picture. Although each had a preceding history of drug intake, drug eruption was considered unlikely in the absence of prior reports and the fact that each had taken a totally different class of drugs. Nonetheless, attention is directed to the destructive **acral erythema** observed in patients taking doxorubicin and cytarabine chemotherapy for myelogenous leukemia.

Further diagnoses considered and rejected included the serpiginous erythematous and purpuric eruptions on the hands and feet along the palmoplantar border (Wallace's line) seen in serum sickness. Erythema multiforme was ruled out by the absence of target lesions. Viral infection, such as Coxsackie type A or even hand, foot, and mouth disease, was considered, but there were no vesicles, and unlike the asymptomatic lesions of these infections, all five patients experienced marked pruritus. Moreover, serologic tests, including those for measles and viral cultures, were negative.

The eruption was distinguished from Gianotti-Crosti (papular acrodermatitis) syndrome, which extends up the limbs and onto the trunk. There was no history of tick bites or travel to endemic regions to indicate a diagnosis of rickettsiosis such as Rocky Mountain spotted fever, nor were the palms and soles involved. Finally, Kawasaki disease was eliminated by the absence of conjunctival injection, hypertrophied lingual papillae, enlarged cervical lymph nodes, and laboratory data changes.

When a patient comes to you wearing **red gloves and socks**, think of this new syndrome, which affects mainly young people in the springtime.

Frankel DH, Larson RA, Lorincz AL: **Acral lividosis**—a sign of myeloproliferative diseases. Hyperleukocytosis syndrome in chronic myelogenous leukemia. Arch Dermatol 1987; 123:921–924.

Bluish-purple discoloration of the distal phalanges of the hands and feet as well as the distal part of the penis in a 44-year-old man with chronic myelogenous leukemia was the result of **ischemia** due to occlusion of the small cutaneous blood vessels by **myeloblasts** that are so large, so nondeformable, and so numerous (more than 50,000/mm^2) as to produce a microvasculature shutdown. This affects not only the skin, but many other organs with signs most evident in the cardiopulmonary system (dyspnea, chest pain) and central nervous system (syncope, ataxia, lowered mentation). This forms the leukocytosis syndrome in which leukostasis is the critical result.

Look for polycythemia vera and essential thrombocythemia as the two other chronic myeloproliferative diseases causing acral lividity. In these, hyperviscosity of the blood and thrombosis are the cause.

What is archaic in clinical medicine today is the idea that the complex natural phenomena occurring in diseased people can be adequately classified by a taxonomy devoted only to disease.

ALVAN R. FEINSTEIN

Ritter MM, Richter WO, Schwandt P: **Acromegaly** and colon cancer. Ann Intern Med 1987; 106:636–637.

A 61-year-old woman was found to have two malignant adenomatous colonic polyps. She had been well until 17 years earlier, when she noted a change in facial appearance and also that her **wedding ring** and old gloves, shoes, and hats had become too tight. Acromegaly and a pituitary tumor had been diagnosed 5 years later, when she also had macroglossia, carpal tunnel syndrome, a deep voice, and oligomenorrhea. The acromegaly did not recur following hypophysectomy.

Patients with acromegaly are thought to be at increased risk for colon cancer and should have regular colonoscopy.

Goette DK: **Thyroid acropachy**. Arch Dermatol 1980; 116:205–206.

During the past 8 years this 48-year-old man had watched his **shoe size** enlarge from a 10 to a 12. In the same period his wedding ring had to be enlarged twice. Not only were the hands and feet enlarging, but there was concomitant enlargement of the supraorbital ridges, nose, and tongue. Two hospitalizations had failed to support the clinical diagnosis of acromegaly.

The diagnostic mystery was solved 6 years later when a diagnosis of hyperthyroidism and **thyroid acropachy** was made. The remarkable feature here was the fact that the acral enlargement preceded the clinical hyperthyroidism. Often associated exophthalmos tips off the clinician to the diagnosis of thyroid acropachy. Thyroid acropachy is recognized by its manifestations of digital clubbing. The x-rays will show actual new bone formation occurring in the diaphyses. One looks for it in the phalanges as well as in the distal long bones. Rare, such acropachy occurs in only 1% of patients with Graves' disease.

A **differential** diagnostic list for acral enlargement includes:

acromegaly
pachydermoperiostosis
pulmonary osteoarthropathy
osteoperiostitis

None of these, however, shows the distinctive new bone formation seen in acropachy.

Big hands and feet may mean a big thyroid problem.

Wiedemann H-R, Burgio GR, Aldenhoff P, et al: The **Proteus syndrome**. Partial gigantism of the hands and/or feet, nevi, hemihypertrophy, subcutaneous tumors, macrocephaly or other skull anomalies and possible accelerated growth and visceral affections. Eur J Pediatr 1983; 140:5–12.

Although the title says it all, the pictures of four boys show an amazing array of asymmetrical gigantic fingers and toes, cutis verticis gyrata–like changes on the soles, linear epidermal nevi, and hemihypertrophy. The subcutaneous tumors were histologic combinations of lipomas, lymphangiomas, and hemangiomas.

Diagnosis sometimes calls for distinguishing a small crow from a large blackbird.

Dermatitis, Blisters

Mackie RM, Husain SL: **Juvenile plantar dermatosis**: A new entity? Clin Exp Dermatol 1976; 1:253–260.

Glazed fissured skin and burning or itching of the weight-bearing areas of the feet in 102 children proved to be unique. Erythema, scaling, and fissuring of the ball of the foot and undersurface of the toes was a constant feature, with the heels and insteps less commonly involved. The toenails and dorsal area of the feet were spared. Study proved that it was not contact dermatitis, psoriasis, fungal infection, or atopic dermatitis. The problem is chronic, painful, and at times disabling. It is a childhood disease with onset at the time of entrance into primary school (age 5 years).

Frictional forces associated with games, as well as the wearing of nylon socks, may play a role. Response is best to wearing cotton socks and applying a weak corticosteroid preparation. Exacerbations and remissions often occur for several years before the problem involutes.

Weismann K, Hjorth N: **Microbial eczema** of the feet. Br J Dermatol 1982; 107:333–337.

Eczema of the medial interdigital spaces and dorsal medial toes is often due to **bacterial sensitization**. It presents as a well-defined scaly erythema without pustules, crusts, or fissures. In all 27 patients studied, *Staphylococcus aureus* and/or hemolytic streptococci were isolated. In contrast, scrapings for fungi were uniformly negative (microscopic examination and culture). The patient will commonly give the history that antifungal therapy has been ineffective. The pathogenic role of bacterial colonization accounts for the excellent results obtained with topical and systemic antibiotics. However, relapses are common in this bacterial sensitivity state, which may persist for 1 to 10 years.

This **microbial eczema** must be **distinguished from**:

tinea pedis (affects lateral toe webs and adjacent plantar areas rather than medial toe webs and dorsal areas)
gram-negative bacterial infection (do a culture)
bacterial infection (produces a pattern of erysipelas, impetigo, or folliculitis)
juvenile plantar dermatosis (young age, negative culture)
shoe dermatitis (spares the interdigital spaces, isolated patch on dorsal surface of foot)
hyperhidrotic maceration (affects bases of toes, backs of feet, and ankles)

Although intradermal and patch tests to *S. aureus* antigens elicit a delayed eczematous reaction in patients with microbial eczema, they are of little diagnostic use, since they are commonly positive in controls.

Wenger JD, Spika JS, Smithwick RW, et al: Outbreak of ***Mycobacterium chelonae*** **infection** associated with use of jet injectors. JAMA 1990; 264:373–376.

Soon after being treated by a podiatrist, six patients developed pain, redness, and swelling near the site of **local anesthetic injections**. Cultures taken by incision showed the problem to be a *Mycobacterium chelonae* infection.

Investigation then disclosed that the **jet injector** used had been sterilized in a disinfectant diluted with distilled water. Cultures showed the distilled water to be the source of the mycobacterium, stored as it was in a reusable nonsterilized container. Notable was the observation that patients treated later in the day were at less risk, the disinfectant having had time to kill the pathogens introduced during the morning dilution routine.

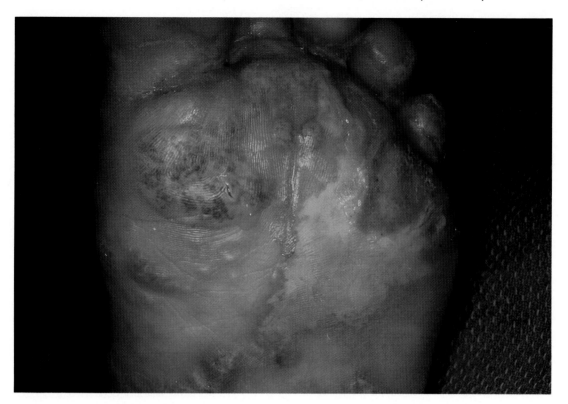

The patient reported here is unique in having a series of seven eccrine poromas appear in an area of radiodermatitis on his right calf over a period of 14 years. This sequence began 34 years after x-ray was given for osteomyelitis.

Pentland AP, Anderson TF: **Plantar fibromatosis** responds to intralesional steroids. J Am Acad Dermatol 1985; 12:212–214.

Slowly enlarging **nodules on the soles** of this 52-year-old woman had been present for 26 years. They were painful and gave the sensation of walking on marbles. A biopsy showed the sclerotic spindle cell proliferation of plantar fibromatosis. After five monthly intralesional injections of triamcinolone acetonide (40 mg/ml), the lesions became soft and smaller. Four months later the patient took up jogging.

Plantar fibromatosis is a characteristic benign entity in which large and small nodules grow out from the plantar aponeurosis. The patient may exhibit other fibroproliferative processes. These include:

Dupuytren's contracture, an analogue on the palm
Peyronie's disease (fibrous cavernitis of the penis)
knuckle pads

With these patients, look for epilepsy, since long-term **phenytoin** or anticonvulsant therapy favors fibromatosis.

Ashinoff R, Werth VP, Franks AG Jr: Resistant **discoid lupus erythematosus** of palms and soles: Successful treatment with azathioprine. J Am Acad Dermatol 1988; 19:961–965.

This 39-year-old black woman had a 7-year history of painful, brightly erythematous, **atrophic lesions of the soles**. They had begun as painful plaques of the great toes. At the time of examination she could not walk or put on shoes. The pink patches of the instep showed erosions and a hyperpigmented scaly border, giving a discoid pattern. There were no lesions elsewhere. She had been given a variety of ineffective treatments, including topical, systemic, and intralesional steroids, the latter producing bullae on the soles. She also had received dapsone and antimalarials.

A biopsy showed sparse changes, but the immunofluorescent studies showed deposition of IgA, IgG, and fibrin along the basement zone, consistent with discoid lupus erythematosus. Several months of oral azathioprine therapy (50 mg/day) resulted in improvement to the point of walking normally.

Discoid lupus erythematosus rarely attacks the palms or soles, but when it does it is most disabling. It also adds the risk of squamous cell cancer in this site.

Kelly JW, Dowling JP: **Pernio**: A possible association with chronic myelomonocytic leukemia. Arch Dermatol 1985; 121:1048–1052.

Raised **violaceous plaques** had been appearing on the extremities of this 63-year-old man during each of the last three winters. They receded in the summer. The lesions on the shins, fingers, and toes were erythematous nodules that developed central purpuric areas, then resolved over a period of weeks, leaving a depressed hemosiderin-pigmented site. A biopsy showed lymphocytic vasculitis.

The summer remissions and the prevention of new lesions by the avoidance of cold made firm the clinical diagnosis of **pernio**. Interestingly, pernio affects all the chilly acral areas, including the nose and ears. Usually occurring in young and middle-aged women, it has no known medical correlates.

In the present example, study revealed a marked increase of 12 to 55% in the number of monocytes in a white count ranging from 3400 to 6000/mm. The monocytosis proved on further study to result from the myelomonocytic leukemia. Four other examples of pernio in the older individual were shown to be associated with **monocytic leukemia**.

Pernio in the elderly calls for more than an admonition to bundle up and keep warm.

McGinnis MR: **Chromoblastomycosis** and phaeohyphomycosis: New concepts, diagnosis and mycology. J Am Acad Dermatol 1983; 8:1–16.

Chromoblastomycosis begins as small, pink, **scaly papules**, usually on the foot, following trauma and usually in a farmer in the tropics. The papules grow to nodules and expand to form **purplish irregular plaques**, eventually becoming large papillomatous growths. Satellite lesions arise, often from scratching.

Chronicity is the rule, some lesions remaining for 20 years, to the point of fibrosis and ensuing elephantiasis. The lesions become ulcerated, infected, and malodorous. **Tumors** may become enormous, resembling the head of a cauliflower.

The **differential diagnosis** includes:

verrucae	tertiary syphilis
blastomycosis	mossy foot
leprosy	tropical lymphangitis
leishmaniasis	

The distinctive diagnostic feature is the presence of **sclerotic bodies**. Look for them in scrapings, crusts, pus, or biopsy material of verrucous lesions. Clearing is done with KOH and special attention paid to black dots when seen on the surface of the epidermis. The sclerotic bodies are chestnut-brown muriform structures (10 um) alone or in clumps. Muriform refers to the presence of septa within the cells of the sclerotic bodies.

Culture the crusts, exudate, pus, or tissue specimen on Sabouraud glucose agar with and without cycloheximide and chloramphenicol. Not until a month at 25 to 30°C can the culture be considered negative. The most common fungus to be isolated is *Fonsecaea pedrosoi*, which grows in the soil, wood, and vegetable debris through which these patients walk. The colony will be olive to black in color and the organism can be identified by conidial analysis, there being at least a half-dozen fungal pathogens.

In contrast to chromoblastomycosis, **phaeohyphomycosis** is an opportunistic fungal infection in which a solitary subcutaneous nodule develops, often at the site of a **puncture wound**.

The **differential** includes:

ganglion	epidermal inclusion cyst
Baker's cyst (synovial cyst of popliteal space)	foreign body granuloma

The nodule in time may become an **abscess** from which gray, viscid, purulent material can be aspirated. A KOH examination will reveal the brownish (phaeo) hyphae and some brown yeastlike cells. There are no sclerotic bodies. Culture permits precision in identification of the common pathogen *Exophiala jeanselmei*.

Cats, fish, frogs, and toads join humans in allowing this fungus to get under their skin.

Noel SB, Greer DL, Abadie SM, et al: Primary **cutaneous phaeohyphomycosis**. Report of three cases. J Am Acad Dermatol 1988; 18:1023–1030.

A **violaceous erythematous plaque** with central ulceration persisted for months on the side of the right foot of this immunocompromised 66-year-old woman. Systemic antibiotic therapy was not helpful.

The diagnosis rested on **biopsy and culture**, for this was a deep dermatomycosis. Inoculation had probably occurred as a result of contact with vegetation or soil where the facultative pathogen lives. The biopsy showed pigmented (Greek *phaeo* "dusky gray") septate hyphae and yeastlike cells. A black dematiacious mold grew out on each culture but eluded precise identification, since spores never formed in the culture.

Macules, papules, subcutaneous nodules, plaques, or chronic ulcers must always be looked upon with suspicion when they develop in patients receiving chemotherapy. A good full-thickness biopsy and tissue culture are the only way to convert your position from "I don't know" to "I do know."

Brown MD, Headington JT: Solitary **plaque** on the foot. Arch Dermatol 1990; 126:815–817.

For 2 years this 47-year-old man had watched a crusted, indurated, violaceous **plaque** slowly enlarge on the dorsum of his right foot. Although at times it drained small amounts of pus, it was not tender and did not interfere with his daily activities. Early studies, including a **biopsy** that revealed only nonspecific inflammation, had led to the conclusion that this was a deep fungal infection. However, no organism had been cultured, and systemic potassium iodide as well as ketoconazole therapy had been without effect.

At the time of this examination the lesion was rather sharply circumscribed and measured 3.5 cm by 2.5 cm. An x-ray of the foot showed no bone involvement.

A wide excision biopsy was taken for histologic study, as well as bacterial, fungal, and mycobacterial cultures. Potassium hydroxide and acid-fast bacilli stains were negative as were all subsequent fungal and mycobacterial cultures. However, bacterial cultures isolated two strains of staphylococci. The biopsy itself was diagnostic, showing a central area of suppuration within which were basophilic grape-like granules. They were PAS positive and showed an amorphous eosinophilic coating. The granules had centers of bacteria. The patient thus had **botryomycosis** (actinophytosis).

"Botryomycosis" is a term from Greek *botrys*, which indicates the grape-like appearance, and mycosis, the originally suspected fungal cause, but it is now a misnomer. It is now known to be an **unusual response to bacteria**, usually *Staphylococcus aureus*, as in this instance. However, *Pseudomonas*, *Proteus vulgaris*, *E. coli*, *Streptococcus*, and gram-negative *Coccobacillus*, and even *Propionibacterium acnes* have been incriminated. How these bacteria induce this fungus-like granule formation is unknown. They are indifferent to antibiotics. It took laser therapy to cure this patient.

Hay RJ: A thorn in the flesh—a study of the pathogenesis of **subcutaneous infections**. Clin Exp Dermatol 1989; 14:408–415.

Painless subcutaneous swellings, which in time form numerous sinus tracts to the surface, are the hallmark of **mycetomas**. Often the bone is involved as well. It is a chronic disease of the tropics, often hailed as **Madura foot**, reflecting the geographic source of many cases in India.

The mycetomas are true infections caused by filamentous bacteria (actinomycetes) or fungi. The unique feature is the formation of grossly visible aggregates of the pathogen. These are the well-known "**grains**." The organisms that are present in the soil or vegetation are implanted deep in the skin by a puncture wound as from a thorn. They prove remarkably resistant to host defenses and to therapy by virtue of both an extremely thick cell wall and of a cement substance that forms a rather impenetrable matrix.

Culture of the grains permits classification of the mycetomas into either the true mycetomas caused by fungi or the actinomycetomas due to actinomycetes, i.e., filamentous bacteria. The predominant organism varies with the geographic site. Thus the black fungal grains of *Madurella mycetomatis* are most common in the Sudan, and the small actinomycete grains of *Nocardia brasiliensis* are predominant in Mexico. Over a dozen such pathogenic fungi and filamentous bacteria have been specifically incriminated as causative.

The mycetomas are a class of subcutaneous infections in which the pathogen hides, not behind, but within a cement wall.

Hay RJ, MacKenzie DWR: **Mycetoma** (Madura foot) in the United Kingdom: A survey of forty-four cases. Clin Exp Dermatol 1983; 8:553–562.

Multiple sinuses and swelling of the right hand of this 34-year-old Turkish businessman had been present for 6 years. There was no tenderness. The diagnosis of mycetoma was made on finding fungal grains within the biopsy specimen and by culturing *Streptomyces somaliensis*. A year of clotrimoxazole therapy resulted in a cure.

The **diagnostic grains** in the exudate are often large enough to be seen with the naked eye. There are multiple fungi or actinomycetes that can be the cause of this exquisitely chronic subcutaneous infection usually seen in the tropics. They enter from the soil or vegetation at the site of an injury. Thorns are especially suspect as agents of inoculation. Not only skin but local bone infection may occur, so that x-rays are indicated.

Particularly confusing are the simple painless swellings with no sinus tracts. Remember, it is a **disease of the tropics**. All but one of the 44 patients recorded here were from the tropics, with nearly half from the West Indies. And the diagnostic shoe really fits if the patient is from Madura.

Friedman SJ, Herman PS, Pittelkow MR, Su WPD: **Punctate porokeratotic kerato-derma**. Arch Dermatol 1988; 124:1678–1682.

Tiny horny spines have been appearing on the palms and soles of this 72-year-old man. Although asymptomatic, they resembled music box spines and made his handshake most unwelcome. There was no history of arsenic intake. These keratotic plugs proved resistant to all local treatments tried in the past 13 years.

Under microscopy, the spine proved to be a compact column of parakeratotic stratum corneum as seen in porokeratosis. Electron microscopy allowed distinction from porokeratosis of Mibelli and disseminated superficial actinic porokeratosis.

Kalter DC, Stone MS, Kettler A, et al: **Keratosis punctata** of the palmar creases: Extremely uncommon? J Am Acad Dermatol 1986; 14:510–511.

Hyperkeratotic pits of the flexion creases of the palm were seen in one out of three black patients in Texas. So the answer to the question in the title of this article is no.

Weiss RM, Rasmussen JE: **Keratosis punctate** of the palmar creases. Arch Dermatol 1980; 116:669–671.

Punctate keratosis limited to the creases of the palms is seen only in black skin. It affects as many as 3% of black patients, but only rarely, and then only because of tenderness is it called to the attention of the physician.

Cox NH, Finlay AY: **Crossed-leg callosities**. Acta Derm Venereol 1985; 65:559–561.

The repetitive minor trauma of sitting cross-legged produced thick **callosities** on the dorsal surface of the feet in three women (ages 28, 30, 35 years) with long-term psoriasis. The lesions were not psoriasiform, but rather hyperkeratotic or lichenified. Apparently, trauma does not induce psoriasis when the patient is in a non-Koebner sensitization phase. Hyperextensible ankle joints with bony prominence at the callosity site may be predisposing factors. Poor-fitting footwear was not a factor.

These callosities are similar to the "**prayer nodules**" seen on the forehead and lateral malleolus of Muslims.

Pratt AG: **Hyperkeratosis of heel** caused by foreign body (hair). Arch Dermatol 1956; 74:469–470.

A 47-year-old white woman had a very **painful callus** on the right heel. This resulted from partial paralysis of the right leg with heel dragging following spinal anesthesia 6 years previously. The 0.3-cm thick yellowish-white callus covered the entire plantar surface of the heel and included a 2-cm long zone of deeply embedded black dots on the medial edge. The entire foot was cool and perspiring, but had ample arterial pulses. Aseptic necrosis was suspected, but a KOH examination of the dark areas revealed short thick fragments of **beard hair** (which fell on the bathroom floor when her husband shaved). Removal of the soft, degenerated horny material with embedded hairs cured her pain.

Sybert VP, Dale BA, Holbrook KA: **Palmar-plantar keratoderma**. A clinical, ultrastructural, and biochemical study. J Am Acad Dermatol 1988; 18:75–86.

The hereditary palmar-plantar keratodermas are distinguished on the basis of:

703

inheritance pattern
sites of involvement
associated abnormalities

This report describes a family (nine members, three generations) with a new autosomal dominant condition similar to mal de Meleda and Greither's disease. The 34-year-old male proband had lifelong erythema and scaling of the palms, soles, gluteal cleft, and groin, with eventual spread to the elbows, knees, dorsal surface of the hands and feet, posterior area of the forearms, and anterior aspect of the legs. Severe **hyperkeratosis** led to digit deformities and spontaneous amputations. He was greatly helped by isotretinoin (Accutane 80 mg/day).

Other **autosomal dominant keratodermas** include:

1. Unna-Thost disease: involves palms, soles, and occasionally knees
2. Howel-Evans' syndrome: associated with esophageal carcinoma
3. Greither's disease, "transgrediens form": involves extensor surfaces of hands and feet
4. Vohwinkel's disease: starfish-shaped keratoses associated with fibrous bands and autoamputation
5. Epidermolytic hyperkeratosis: recognized on biopsy

Mal de Meleda keratoderma differs from the above in being autosomal recessive and was first recognized on the Dalmation island of Meleda in the Adriatic Sea.

Hamm H, Happle R, Butterfass T, Traupe H: **Epidermolytic palmoplantar keratoderma of Vörner**: Is it the most frequent type of hereditary palmoplantar keratoderma? Dermatologica 1988; 177:138–145.

Twenty-six patients with hereditary palmoplantar keratoderma fell into the following categories:

epidermolytic (Vörner)	12
progressive (Greither)	4
mal de Meleda	3
Papillon-Lefèvre syndrome	2
striate (Siemens)	2
acrokeratoelastoidosis	2
Richner-Hanhart syndrome	1
	26

Correct classification of these keratodermas is impossible without a biopsy.

The most common form is Vörner's epidermolytic hyperkeratosis:

autosomal dominant inheritance
onset in first year of life
strictly limited to palms and soles (nontransgradiens)
diffuse or punctate (localizing at points of trauma)
erythematous border
superficial blister formation from trauma
biopsy: perinuclear vacuolization of keratinocytes and thick stratum granulosum

The other most common form of palmoplantar keratoderma is the Unna-Thost-Greither type:

autosomal dominant inheritance
onset later in childhood
diffuse or punctate
may involve dorsal area of hands and feet, elbows, and knees (transgradiens)
biopsy: no vacuolization of keratinocytes (nonepidermolytic)

Kanitakis J, Tsoitis G, Kanitakis C: Hereditary **epidermolytic palmplantar kerato-derma** (Vörner type). J Am Acad Dermatol 1987; 17:414–422.

Since the age of 2 months, this 20-year-old man has suffered diffuse, thick, yellowish keratosis of the palms and soles. He is one of 21 persons in the last six consecutive generations to have this keratoderma.

Histologically, the keratosis proved to be typical localized epidermolytic hyperkeratosis of the Vörner type separable from the other dominantly trans-mitted Thost-Unna type. There are forms associated with destructive change (Vohwinkel mutilans type) as well as with deafness. Two other types carry the eponymic baggage of Greither type and Howel-Evans' syndrome. Re-cessively transmitted keratodermas include the Meleda type as well as that seen in the Papillon-Lefèvre syndrome.

Circumscribed keratodermas include:

> punctate forms (Brauer-Buscke-Fisher)
> striate forms (Brunauer-Fuhs)
> porokeratosis of Mantoux
> pachyonychia congenita (Jadassohn-Lewandowsky)
> hereditary painful callosities
> tyrosinosis keratoderma (Richner-Hanhart)

A history and a biopsy will carry you a long way down this nosologic trail.

Balato N, Cusano F, Lembo G, Santoianni P: **Tyrosinemia type II** in two cases previ-ously reported as Richner-Hanhart syndrome. Dermatologica 1986; 173:66–74.

All patients with linear or punctate **palmoplantar keratoses** and/or pseudo-herpetic **keratitis** should be screened for tyrosine and its metabolites to rule out oculocutaneous tyrosinemia (type II, Oregon type). Plasma and urinary tyrosine levels should be checked. Elevated levels result from a deficiency in the liver enzyme, tyrosine-aminotransferase.

Immediate early reduction of tyrosine and phenylalanine in the **diet** prevents mental retardation and produces dramatic improvement within days or weeks in the keratoses and keratitis, which resolve without scarring. The seasonal improvements noted by some could reflect dietary changes.

A literature survey of 56 patients with tyrosinemia type II (Richner-Hanhart syndrome) revealed the following clinical features:

1. Skin: Keratoses of the palms and soles: bilateral, asymmetrical, ver-rucous, localized, striate, painful, onset in infancy to teenage years. Bullae, eczema on the palms and soles, and leukokeratoses in the mouth were also occasionally seen.
2. Eye: Dendritic keratitis with persistent dendritic herpetiform ulcers leading to conjunctival plaques and corneal opacities. Cataracts, pho-tophobia, redness, pain, and tearing may also occur.
3. Mental retardation: Slight to severe, it is preventable with diet.

Hunziker N: Richner-Hanhart syndrome and tyrosinemia type II. Dermatologica 1980; 160:180–189.

Since the age of 14, a 40-year-old man had painful fissured **hyperkeratotic lesions on the fingertips** and toes and also sharply circumscribed hyperker-atotic plaques on the palms and soles. His brother had identical thickenings of the palms and soles, attributed to his work as a bricklayer.

The diagnosis was never made until **tyrosine levels** were obtained from the blood and urine. The finding of tyrosinemia (1160 μmol/liter, normal 33 to 82) and tyrosinuria (3918 μmol/24 hr, normal <1) made it evident that the skin changes were part of the Richner-Hanhart syndrome (tyrosinemia type II).

This **autosomal recessive disease** often presents with keratitis, keratoderma, and mental retardation. It is an inborn error in the metabolism of tyrosine and phenylalanine, due to a deficiency of hepatic tyrosine aminotransferase. Large amounts of tyrosine accumulate, with crystals even in the tissue.

Once the condition was diagnostically recognized, this man (who had neither keratitis nor mental retardation) went on a low phenylalanine/tyrosine **diet**. Within 3 weeks the hands and soles were much improved.

Bergman R, Friedman-Birnbaum R: **Papillon-Lefèvre syndrome**: A study of the long-term clinical course of recurrent pyogenic infections and the effects of etretinate treatment. Br J Dermatol 1988; 119:731–736.

Recurrent pyogenic infections were a major problem in six members of a family with the Papillon-Lefèvre syndrome (**hyperkeratosis** of the palms and soles, keratotic plaques of the elbows and knees, and **periodontosis** leading to early loss of deciduous and permanent teeth). The infections had been especially severe in infancy and early childhood, with involvement of both skin and internal organs. One person died of an abdominal abscess, and another had a hepatic abscess that ruptured into the lung. In adolescence the infections were confined to the skin, with *Staphylococcus aureus* in all cultures.

Etretinate therapy markedly improved the keratoderma and induced complete remission of the pyoderma on both normal and abnormal skin.

Nielsen PG: **Psoriasis** and hereditary palmoplantar keratoderma complicated with a dermatophyte infection: Case report. Dermatologica 1984; 168:293–295.

A 29-year-old woman with **psoriasis** of the elbows, knees, and legs developed scaly patches and thick fissured hyperkeratotic plaques on the soles. These were believed to be psoriasis until it was learned that the patient's mother had hereditary palmoplantar **keratoderma** (Unna-Thost). A biopsy confirmed the keratoderma but also revealed numerous hyphae that vividly stained with PAS in the thickened stratum corneum of the sole. A fungal culture grew *Epidermophyton floccosum*.

By study, rather than by simply looking, this clinician found three diagnoses where others had seen but one.

Nazzaro V, Blanchet-Bardon C: **Progressive symmetric erythrokeratodermia**. Histological and ultrastructural study of patient before and after treatment with etretinate. Arch Dermatol 1986; 122:434–440.

A 24-year-old white man had erythematous **hyperkeratotic plaques** on the backs of the hands and feet with sharp cutoffs at the wrists and ankles. He first developed erythematous keratoderma of the palms and soles 2 months after birth. Other lesions then appeared during the next few years, gradually involving the knees, elbows, and gluteal cleft with sharply demarcated symmetrical erythematous hyperkeratotic plaques. There had been gradual extension up to the age of 12, but no change thereafter. No one else in the family was affected, suggesting a new mutation.

The **erythrokeratodermias** are a heterogeneous group of inherited disorders with discrete sharply marginated lesions of hyperkeratosis and erythema. Progressive symmetrical erythrokeratodermia is very rare (25 cases reported) and involves the extremities and buttocks, with 50% having palmoplantar keratoderma. It is clearly related to **erythrokeratodermia variabilis**. Both are lifelong disorders of cornification that appear in infancy and are transmitted in an autosomal dominant fashion. In the variabilis form, however, lesions continuously change their morphology, color, and localization over hours to days and appear on the extremities, buttocks, abdomen, face, and thorax. These patients may show physical retardation, neuropathy, and deafness. The **differential diagnosis** must include pityriasis rubra pilaris and psoriasis vulgaris.

Deschamps P, Leroy D, Pedailles S, Mandard JC: **Keratoderma climactericum (Haxthausen's disease)**: Clinical signs, laboratory findings and etretinate treatment in 10 patients. Dermatologica 1986; 172:258–262.

Keratoses limited to the palms and soles occasionally appear in **postmenopausal women** (age of onset 47 to 69 years). They begin at pressure points of the sole with erythema and thick hyperkeratosis, which commonly fissures, making walking painful. They may advance to the margins of one or both soles. Later involvement of the palms is localized to the proximal medial palm. Biopsies show lichenified eczema with evidence of mechanical irritation. The condition is idiopathic, although the majority of patients are overweight. Patients had no history of prior disease or hormone therapy.

Differential diagnosis:

arsenical poisoning	Reiter's disease
eczema (atopic, allergic, irritant)	secondary syphilis
pityriasis rubra pilaris	tinea pedis
psoriasis	

Blanchet-Bardon C, Nazzaro V, Chevrant-Breton J, et al: **Hereditary epidermolytic palmoplantar keratoderma** associated with breast and ovarian cancer in a large kindred. Br J Dermatol 1987; 117:363–370.

Yellowish, smooth hyperkeratosis uniformly covering the entire palms and soles was the **genetic marker for malignant disease** in eight women who developed either breast or ovarian adenocarcinoma (or both). Appearing during the first weeks of life, the keratoderma remained unchanged and asymptomatic except for moderate hyperhidrosis and bromhidrosis. It was demarcated from normal skin by a distinct band of erythema. No other skin lesions were present. Histologically the thick yellow plaques proved to be **epidermolytic keratoderma**. Among 61 family members in four generations studied, 25 had palmoplantar keratoderma.

Acquired palmoplantar keratoderma has frequently been associated with late-onset cancer of the bronchus, breast, esophagus, stomach, colon, or skin. It also may accompany paraneoplastic skin syndromes (acanthosis nigricans, Bazex's syndrome, paraneoplastic acrokeratosis), which reflect carcinomas of the upper respiratory and digestive tracts.

Inherited palmoplantar keratoderma is only infrequently found with internal malignant disease. The first association noted was esophageal carcinoma in 18 of 48 patients with autosomal dominant keratoderma of the palms and soles (Howel-Evans syndrome). Recently, punctate palmoplantar keratoderma was associated with adenocarcinoma of the colon. None of these patients had epidermolytic keratoderma, so that this report is unique in having the first example of internal malignant disease associated with an autosomal dominant inheritance of epidermolytic hyperkeratosis.

Duvic M, Reisman M, Finley V, et al: **Glucan-induced keratoderma** in acquired immunodeficiency syndrome. Arch Dermatol 1987; 123:751–756.

In an attempt to reverse the failing immune system in AIDS, an immunostimulant, glucan, was given intravenously twice weekly to 20 patients. Within 2 weeks, six homosexual men developed **keratoderma of the palms and soles**. It began as persistent pruritus and moccasin-like erythema and salmon-pink or yellow hyperkeratosis of the soles and palms; within a few weeks it progressed to thickening, scaling, and painful fissuring. Over the dorsal surfaces of several proximal interphalangeal and metacarpal joints were discrete, symmetrical, pink scaly papules and plaques. In some, the keratoderma was limited to the sites of greatest pressure. Only the soles were involved in two patients. The **glucan infusions** were stopped after 8 weeks, and within 2 weeks the lesions virtually cleared.

The **glucan keratoderma** most closely resembled psoriasis, pityriasis rubra pilaris, or Papillon-Lefèvre syndrome (without the dental manifestations). Tinea, lichen planus, and contact dermatitis seemed unlikely, as did the genetic disorders of Unna-Thost, mal de Meleda, and Richner-Hanhart. Also considered were the keratodermas seen after castration, menopause, arsenic poisoning, esophageal or bronchial carcinoma, and mycosis fungoides.

Glucan is a β-1,3 polyglucose oligosaccharide derived from the inner cell wall of the **yeast**, *Saccharomyces cerevisiae*. Its presence in the cell wall of other yeasts, fungi, and certain bacteria adds speculative delight to thinking about keratodermas and infection.

Protonotarios N, Tsatsopoulou A, Scampardonis G: **Right ventricular cardiomyopathy** and sudden death in young people. N Engl J Med 1988; 319:175.

Diffuse palmoplantar keratosis, as well as hair and nail dysplasia, was associated with arrhythmogenic right ventricular dysplasia in 18 patients from eight families from the Greek island of Naxos.

Thus the **hyperkeratosis of the palms and soles** should direct the clinician's attention to the possibility of **arrhythmia** and cardiac problems of a potentially lethal nature. Echocardiography may aid in evaluation of the cardiomyopathy. These problems are thought to be transmitted as an autosomal dominant trait with incomplete penetrance, so that genetic counseling is appropriate.

Atherton DJ, Sutton C, Jones BM: Mutilating **palmoplantar keratoderma** with periorificial keratotic plaques (Olmsted's syndrome). Br J Dermatol 1990; 122:245–252.

At age 16 months this boy developed **keratoderma of the soles**. Seven months later it had extended to the palms. Initially it was only focal, but in the months that followed it spread over the entire palm and sole with maceration and pitting. The pain was so severe as to limit function. Shaving down the keratin with a razor blade afforded the only relief. His mother also suffered palmoplantar keratoderma.

On examination of the patient at age 3 years, the palms and soles and undersurface of fingers and toes showed diffuse, thick, yellow keratoderma. The borders were erythematous, hyperpigmented, and tender, with the keratoderma splitting into thick sheets. The nails were all thickened and transversely ridged. The finger joints showed **flexion contractures** with deep and painful fissures of the joint creases. Pus drained from a defect in the epidermis over the center of the left palm. Elsewhere the only change noted was a brownish-yellow crusted plaque of the lower lip. Biopsy showed massive thickening of the horny layer with retained nuclei.

The perioral eruption progressed, becoming hyperkeratotic and more extensive. It spared the vermilion but later arose around the nares.

A diagnosis of **Olmsted's syndrome** was made. This is a mutilating keratoderma in which the oral, nasal, and anal orifices may be involved. The mutilation comes from the autoamputation of a digit by a constricting band of keratin. This was also described by Vohwinkel, and the condition carries his eponym as well.

Trauma may be an initiating factor. One may expect this child to develop further areas of hyperkeratosis. Development is generally retarded in these children, since the profound and painful keratoderma interferes not only with their ability and willingness to walk and to gain manual skills, but with their social and scholastic development.

It is apparent that **biopsy** should be done of all linear epidermal nevi to see if they represent linear epidermal hyperkeratosis. Only in this way can the individual be apprised of the small but definite possibility that an offspring might have the universal form, i.e., congenital bullous ichthyosiform erythroderma.

Widespread **linear epidermal hyperkeratosis** can be distinguished from the generalized form by noting the normal skin areas, the linear patterning, and the absence of transverse verrucous streaking in the axillary folds in the more localized linear form. It is also possible to differentiate widespread linear epidermolytic hyperkeratosis from **ichthyosis hystrix** (Curth-Macklin). Electron microscopy shows ichthyosis hystrix to have concentric perinuclear shells of aggregated tonofilaments, but none of the distinctive clumping of linear epidermolytic hyperkeratosis.

Finally, although this family did not exhibit it, there is a third type of **epidermolytic hyperkeratosis**, i.e., the palmoplantar form. Known as Vörners keratoderma, it is the most common inherited diffuse palmoplantar condition. Again, it is of autosomal dominant inheritance, but it is not linked to date with the generalized form. It has the same clinical presentation as **Thost-Unna** disease.

Although these are the major presentations of what the pathologist with his electron microscopy can link together, "spots" of epidermolytic hyperkeratosis may be seen in epidermolytic acanthoma or in a variety of acquired solitary skin lesions.

Let the electron microscope serve as a telescope to see farther into your patient's skin problem.

Mikhail GR, Babel D: ***Trichophyton rubrum* infection** and keratoderma palmaris et plantaris. Arch Dermatol 1981; 117:753–754.

In the past few years this 42-year-old man had noted worsening of a **genokeratoderma** of his palms and soles. He had had diffuse, yellow thickening of these sites since birth. However, in the last 3 years painful fissures had developed. The skin had become thicker, more indurated, and tender. Scaling was present, which extended between the toes, but the nails remained unaffected.

Multiple potassium hydroxide preparations of scrapings from both the palms and soles revealed branched segmented hyaline hyphae in all specimens. *Trichophyton rubrum* grew in the culture.

A diagnosis was made of keratoderma palmaris et plantaris with superimposed tinea infection. Griseofulvin (500 mg bid, 2 weeks/month) was initiated with resultant prompt improvement. The scabs disappeared, and the skin became softer and less thick. Relapses occurred whenever the griseofulvin was withheld for 8 weeks. At this time, he has been taking griseofulvin for more than 6 years.

Griffiths WAD: **Pityriasis rubra pilaris.** Clin Exp Dermatol 1980; 5:105–112.

Pityriasis rubra pilaris is an erythematous scaling disorder characterized by follicular plugging, perifollicular erythema tending to be confluent, and hyperkeratosis of the palms and soles, as well as fine powdery scaling of face and scalp.

Think of it in **erythrodermas** and look for small islands of unaffected skin, as well as an orange-yellow hue best sensed on the palms. Ectropion is common. The nails show subungual hyperkeratosis, longitudinal ridging, but not the onycholysis and salmon patches of psoriasis. Circumscribed versions may be seen on the knees and elbows as sharply demarcated erythematous plaques with follicular hyperkeratosis. The **differential diagnosis** of pityriasis rubra pilaris centers on:

> psoriasis
> follicular eczema
> follicular ichthyosis
> lichen planopilaris
> keratosis pilaris
> drug eruption

However, rarities may **mimic** pityriasis rubra pilaris to a degree. These include:

> parakeratosis variegata
> symmetrical progressive erythrokeratodermia
> generalized eruptive keratoacanthomas
> familial dyskeratotic comedones
> infundibulofolliculitis

Histologically the follicular papule affords little information. Go for an erythematous site.

Areas of dermal scarring such as a prior herpes zoster remain unaffected by pityriasis rubra pilaris. **Subclinical scarring** thus may account for the small diagnostic islands observed in a sea of erythema.

Richard M,Giroux J-M: **Acrokeratosis paraneoplastica (Bazex' syndrome).** J Am Acad Dermatol 1987; 16:178–183.

A 55-year-old man noted **redness** of the ears and thickening of the palms and soles. This was followed by redness of the nose, lips, cheeks, and chin, eventually involving the elbows and knees.

At the time of examination the erythema in these areas had a violaceous hue, and scaling was present.

A diagnosis of **Bazex syndrome** was made, but bronchoscopy, gastroscopy, and otorhinolaryngologic examination revealed no tumor. Six months later the patient was completely studied again with negative findings on bronchoscopy, esophagogastroscopy, and otorhinolaryngologic studies. However, swallow-function radiography revealed compression of the esophagus by a mass that on exploration proved to be an enlarged lymph node with metastatic **squamous cell carcinoma**.

The unique findings of Bazex syndrome call for exhaustive serial tests for carcinoma of the respiratory and upper digestive system. Recall that:

> The skin changes can antedate any other evidence of a neoplasm by as much as a year.
> The skin changes disappear when the tumor is treated and recur with relapse of the neoplasia.
> Bullae may appear on the dorsae of the hands and feet and ears, suggesting porphyria cutanea tarda.

Bazex syndrome ranks with acanthosis nigricans, erythema gyratum repens, and migratory necrolytic erythema as the **mask of neoplasia**. Once seen, the tumor must be unmasked.

Herpes Simplex/Zoster

The diagnosis of herpes simplex can be easy; but is it always easy? No, it is not easy when it comes as multiple **deep**, **chronic ulcers** in the patient with leukemia or AIDS. These may persist for months, and you will need a culture or the response to Zovirax (acyclovir) to tear you away from a diagnosis of ecthyma.

Nor is it easy when herpes simplex comes as a **paronychial lesion**. You will have to remember to suspect it in nurses, dental hygienists, and others who put their fingers in other people's mouths, a natural lair for the herpes simplex virus. It is not easy to diagnose when it appears as a **vesicular eruption of the toes** or sole looking exactly like vesicular tinea pedis.

It is not an easy diagnosis when it comes in a **zosteriform** patterning or with pain. Short of culture, your clue is its return to the same site, something herpes zoster never does.

It is not an easy diagnosis when it comes as widespread multiple lesions. It may come as **folliculitis** of the beard, seeded by the patient's razor. There is also the form we see in wrestlers, i.e., herpes gladiatorum, in which friction lesions from the mat grant multiple portals of entry.

Nor is it easy to remember to diagnose herpetic **superinfection in atopic dermatitis**. It may produce only an inexplicable flare with herpetic erosions that you see as excoriations. Even mild eczema herpeticum in the patient with Darier's disease may elicit only the diagnosis of secondary bacterial infection.

No, it's not easy to recognize herpes simplex as a **sore on the tongue**, or in its expression as severe **primary gingivostomatitis**. It is not easy to sense herpes simplex as the cause of **facial palsy**. Herpes simplex of the mucosa is especially hard to recognize. It may cause **unilateral conjunctivitis**, which, if untreated, can lead to blindness. Indeed, herpes simplex is the most common cause of blindness due to disease. Herpes may appear on the penis and look like a **chancre** or chancroid. It may be within the urethra and pose as nonspecific **urethritis**. It's hard to remember that herpes lesions may swarm around the anus in the homosexual. But hardest of all is thinking of herpes as the cause of what appears to be streptococcal **pharyngitis**. Nor is the diagnosis easy in cases of herpetic vulvitis and vaginitis.

No, the diagnosis is not easy in the newborn who doesn't develop the vesicles until a few weeks after birth.

Nor is it easy to even find the primary causal herpes simplex lesion in the midst of an attack of bullous **erythema multiforme** or Stevens-Johnson syndrome.

No, the diagnosis of herpes simplex is not always easy. Conversely, some diagnoses are missed because the lesions are erroneously considered to be herpes simplex. These include impetigo contagiosa, since herpes is so often impetiginized. Local contact dermatitis in the site of recurrent herpes simplex may easily be dismissed as another herpes lesion. And other viral infections producing vesicles, such as those of *Coxsackie* infection and cowpox, may be dismissed as herpes simplex for want of a culture or the immunofluorescent slide test now widely available.

To turn to **herpes zoster**: Here is a disease so unusual in patterning distribution and symptoms that it can be diagnosed over the phone. "Doctor, I have been having this neuralgia and now I have a rash on that side" clinches the diagnosis. But before the vesicles come, the pain may lead to a clinical impression that the patient has angina, a duodenal ulcer, a kidney stone, appendicitis, or glaucoma, 711 depending on the nerve trunk involved. We recall vividly having seen the telltale vesicles appear in the fresh scar of a craniotomy and also of an appendectomy.

And remember, if the patient says, "Doctor, this is the second time I have had the shingles," the diagnosis is not recurrent herpes zoster but rather recurrent zosteriform herpes simplex. Distinguishing these two entities is about the only challenge in differential diagnosis. Zosteriform herpes simplex may be painful and is unilateral, but it does not scar, leaves no significant postherpetic neuralgia, and most importantly will recur at the same site.

It is important to note that the neuropathy of herpes zoster can spill over into the **motor nerves**. Accordingly, we may see bladder and anal sphincter tone lost in sacral zoster, loss of muscle strength of the abdominal muscles (with T-10 to L-1 involvement), which leads to unilateral abdominal protrusion. The unilateral facial paralysis is a well-known sign of involvement of the facial and auditory nerves in **Ramsay Hunt syndrome**.

Young individuals experience little pain, and immunocompromised or AIDS patients may develop gangrenous and hemorrhagic lesions with deep ulcers. When there is any diagnostic doubt a viral culture or electron microscopy is indicated. The triggers for that attack of zoster are not known, and extensive medical examinations are no longer considered indicated. Still, the immune status is key, and patients who develop zoster before the declining immunity of aging has occurred might wisely be checked for HIV infection.

Verbov J: **Eczema herpeticum** in a man of 68. Dermatologica 1982; 164:410–412.

A 68-year-old man with ichthyosis vulgaris was hospitalized with fever, widespread **exfoliative dermatitis**, and multiple vesicles and erosions of the face. Eczema herpeticum was proven with **isolation of the herpes simplex virus** from vesicles. The erythroderma was later shown to be due to an allergic contact dermatitis to thiuram, present in rubber gloves he wore when caring for a disabled brother.

The herpes simplex virus found soil for growth in the contact dermatitis. Although atopic dermatitis is its favored haunt, **look for it also in** Darier's disease, ichthyosis, ichthyosiform erythroderma, and pemphigus foliaceus.

Smith MD, Scott GM, Rom S, Patou G: **Herpes simplex virus** and facial palsy. J Infection 1987; 15:259–261.

An 8-year-old boy developed **ulcers** of the lower lip, gums, tongue, and hard palate. There were erosions on the tonsils and uvula as well as cervical lymphadenopathy and fever.

By the 10th day he developed an obvious lower motor neuron **facial paralysis**. Before that, slight facial asymmetry had been attributed to his severe mouth pain. The paralysis persisted for a week, gradually resolving over the following month.

The diagnosis of primary **herpetic gingivostomatitis** was proven by isolation of HSV type 1 in a mouth swab taken on the fifth day of illness. The cytopathic effect on human embryo lung fibroblasts was neutralized by polyclonal HSV antibody. It was then shown to be HSV type 1 by indirect immunofluorescence with type–specific monoclonal antibody. Coxsackie and zoster-varicella virus infections were eliminated by serial serologic studies.

This example speaks strongly for the immediate treatment of acute facial (Bell's) palsy with Zovirax, whether a cold sore be evident or not.

Purcell SM, Dixon SL: **Allergic contact dermatitis** to dyclonine hydrochloride simulating extensive herpes simplex labialis. J Am Acad Dermatol 1985; 12:231–234.

Application of 1% dyclonine gel for the treatment of **presumed herpes simplex** of the upper lip of this 24-year-old woman provided no relief and was followed by progressive extension of the blistering. Examination revealed edema and erythema of both lips with golden-yellow crusts. Moist erythematous plaques studded with tiny 0.5-mm vesicles extended across the vermilion borders of both lips.

Swabs for bacterial and viral cultures were taken, but no pathogens were found. **Contact dermatitis** to the dyclonine gel was suspected. Discontinuance of the gel followed by the use of wet compresses and erythromycin ointment led to rapid healing in 48 hours. A patch test to dyclonine gel was 2+ positive at 48 hours. Dyclonine is an anesthetic and under the trade name Resolve has been marketed for the treatment of herpes simplex.

Here is an unusual example of a case in which the patient and sometimes the physician can't distinguish the treatment from the disease.

Scott MJ Jr, Scott MJ: Primary cutaneous *Neisseria gonorrhoeae* infections. Arch Dermatol 1982; 118:351–352.

A 26-year-old man had a group of **tender pustules** of the medial aspect of the **right middle finger**. Present for 2 days, they appeared to be herpes simplex.

713

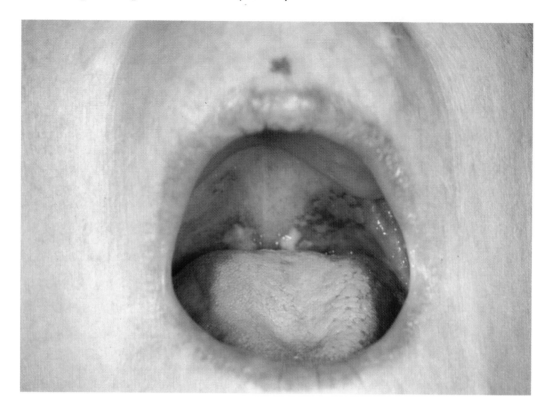

But it was the history that prepared one for the finding of numerous gram-negative diplococci on a stained smear. Five days before the lesions appeared, the patient had foregone intercourse with his female friend because she suspected she had gonorrhea. Instead, he had engaged in **vaginal massage** using only the same right middle finger.

Conclusive proof of primary **gonorrheal infection** of the skin was secured by culturing *Neisseria gonorrhoeae* from the pustules and from the urethral discharge of his female contact. The latter had no history of herpes progenitalis. This diagnosis can be missed in culture studies of pustular lesions, since *N. gonorrhoeae* requires enriched media, and a high CO_2–low O_2 environment at 34 to 36°C.

In this patient, penetration of the gonococcus was favored by the fact that prior to his intimacy episode, he had been using a silicone rubber bathtub caulk, which had resisted removal by soap, detergent, water, and chloride bleach. Only by vigorous rubbing and peeling was the silicone peeled off, no doubt along with stratum corneum. If only he had left the rubber on!

Casemore DP, Emslie ES, Whyler DK, et al: **Cowpox** in a child acquired from a cat. Clin Exp Dermatol 1987; 12:286–287.

A blister on the lower lip of a 10-year-old girl rapidly evolved into a large indurated swelling surmounted by a **hard black crust**. There were deeply fixed indurated nodes in the submental and right superior cervical areas. When she was seen 3 weeks later the diagnoses considered were orf, actinomycosis, herpes simplex, and anthrax.

A **biopsy** revealed poxvirus particles on electron microscopy. Tissue culture inoculation produced the cytopathic effects of cowpox, and confirmation of cowpox was made by inoculation onto chorioallantoic membranes of fertile hens' eggs. The serum was strongly positive for antibody to orthopoxvirus.

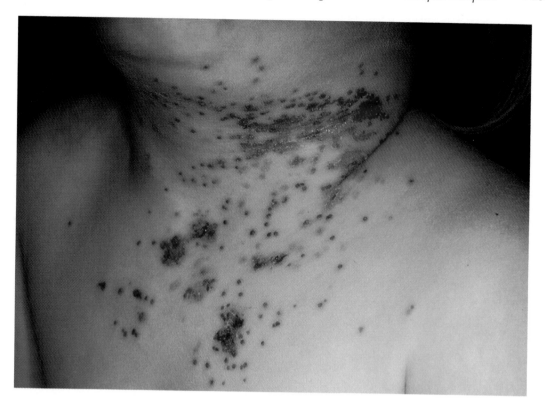

Since she had had no contact with cows, pigs, sheep, or dogs, the source of infection remained hidden until the mother observed that her daughter had acquired a **new kitten** with a lesion on its face, which then resolved. The circle of investigation was closed when serum from the kitten showed a high antibody titer to *Orthopoxvirus*. Control studies on the serum of two other cats, including the mother of the kitten, were negative.

Feline cowpox probably will be increasingly recognized once serologic testing is routinely employed.

Goldstein GD, Bhatia P, Kalivas J: **Herpetiform protothecosis**. Int J Dermatol 1986; 25:54–55.

For 2 months this 61-year-old woman had had **painful grouped vesicles** on the presternal area. No serologic or cultural support could be obtained to support a diagnosis of pemphigus, pemphigoid, or herpes simplex.

The biopsy provided the diagnosis, for in the epidermis and in the inflammatory infiltrate in the dermis were seen numerous **algae**. These organisms were thick walled, 3 to 5 μm in diameter, and stained intensely with periodic acid–Schiff stain. A distinct morula (spokes in a wheel) pattern identified the invader to be *Prototheca*, which is a genus of algae that lack chlorophyll.

Thus, plants as well as molds can grow in the skin. Not only is their presence evidenced by vesicles, but also by papules, pustules, plaques, ulcers, and deep nodules.

These plants don't grow very big, so you'll need the microscope to see them.

Curiosity is the catalyst of diagnosis.

Herpes Zoster

Solomon AR, Rasmussen JE, Weiss JS: A comparison of the Tzanck smear and viral isolation in **varicella** and **herpes zoster**. Arch Dermatol 1986; 122:282–285.

To prepare a **Tzanck smear**:

1. Scrape the base of the vesicle vigorously with the edge of a scalpel blade. Touch the blade to a glass slide several times. Air dry.
2. Stain for 15 seconds with an aqueous solution of 1% toluidine blue O. Rinse with tap water. Air dry.
3. Apply a coverglass over permanent mounting media (Permount).

To recognize a positive smear: Find multinucleated giant cells with nuclei having faceted or molded contours and ground-glass chromatin. You will not see intranuclear viral inclusions with the monochromatic stain.

In this study, all 11 patients with varicella had positive Tzanck smears, whereas only 7 had positive viral cultures. In addition, 12 of 15 patients with herpes zoster had positive Tzanck smears, but only 9 had positive cultures.

Conclusion: The Tzanck smear is a useful and cost-effective test for confirming the clinical diagnosis of varicella and herpes zoster.

Lambert WC, Okorodudu AO, Schwartz RA: **Cutaneous nasociliary neuralgia**. Acta Derm Venereol 1985; 65:257–258.

In a 42-year-old man, severe **constant pain of the left eye** and periocular area for 12 hours suggested incipient herpes zoster. At 18 hours a typical acneiform papule in the left nasolabial fold, which had arisen at the onset of the pain, spontaneously ruptured, with instant clearing of symptoms. The ophthalmodynia disappeared, leaving no sequelae.

This acute unilateral neuralgia (**Charlin's syndrome**) was caused by irritation of the nasociliary branch of the ophthalmic division of the trigeminal nerve, which innervates both the skin and eye. Conceivably, this cutaneous-neurologic mechanism may also be responsible for headaches, particularly if facial skin lesions are manipulated and chronically irritated by the patient.

Referred pain in the face may be very complex because of the variable courses of cutaneous sensory nerves in the nose, eyes, eyelids, and sinuses.

Janier M, Hillion B, Baccard M, et al: Chronic **varicella zoster infection** in acquired immunodeficiency syndrome. J Am Acad Dermatol 1988; 18:584–585.

A 27-year-old man with AIDS had ten **vesiculopustular lesions** on the trunk, neck, legs, and thighs for 2 months. Each lesion had central evolution toward necrosis and ulceration. Chronic herpes simplex infection was suspected, and a skin biopsy showed vacuolated keratinocytes full of eosinophilic inclusions. However, cultures of specimens showed **varicella zoster virus**. Over the following 12 months new necrotic pustules appeared, some leading to extensive ulcerations. The virus appeared to be resistant to acyclovir.

Muller SA, Winkelmann RK: Cutaneous nerve changes in **zoster**. J Invest Dermatol 1969; 52:71–77.

In 23 patients with active or recently healed lesions of herpes zoster, the presence or absence of a histamine flare correlated with the severity of nerve damage and the severity and duration of herpetic neuralgia.

Intradermal injections of histamine phosphate (0.1 to 0.2 cc of 1:100,000) solution were made in a paired comparison manner into normal-appearing skin of the affected dermatome and into a symmetrical site in the paired unaffected dermatome on the opposite side. The size of the axon flare was

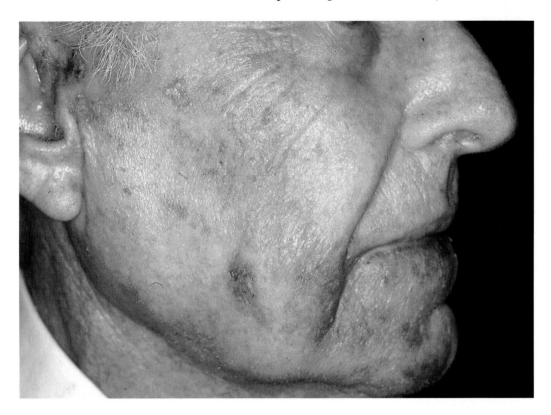

measured in 2 diameters, and a significant change was considered present only if the axon flare was nearly absent in the affected dermatome. The skin of the trunk was the best site for eliciting axon flares.

The **histamine flare** is an indication of functional integrity of the sensory afferent nerves in a dermatome. Patients with absence of flares had longer and more severe pain and also had severe loss of nerve fibers, as seen in skin biopsies that were frozen and stained with acetylcholinesterase.

Imagination and insight are as necessary as observation in the diagnosis of factitial disease.

PHILIP C. ANDERSON

Hirsutism and Hypertrichosis

The woman who consults you about unwanted hair usually comes because she has **polycystic ovaries**. Her abnormal ovaries are secreting an excess of androgen hormones with the result that she is growing an excess of hair in the areas of skin, such as the face and chest, that are reserved for male hair growth. She has hirsutism, a diagnosis limited to women.

It is unlikely that she comes because her hair growth is a family trait. It is also unlikely that she comes because of underlying acromegaly or Cushing's disease. But if the hair growth is of recent and sudden onset, an **adrenal or ovarian tumor** must be ruled out. This is done by finding a normal or only slightly elevated level of plasma total testosterone. Tumors causing hirsutism invariably are associated with high androgen levels in the plasma. It is unlikely that she comes because of androgen intake or use of a high-progesterone contraceptive, but a careful history of **drug intake** is necessary.

If the unwanted hair is generalized in distribution, it is not of androgen origin. In these instances, both men and women come under study. They have hypertrichosis. It may reflect **porphyria**, as well as use of drugs such as minoxidil or cyclosporine. Often, this hypertrichosis, especially in the male, is subtle and not a complaint. You must look for it and cross-examine.

Far more dramatic, but a rarity of rarities, is **hypertrichosis lanuginosa**. Here the patient becomes covered with a coat of fine vellus hair. When acquired, it demands immediate total study for internal malignant disease. When congenital, consider drug intake by the mother (hydantoin, alcohol, minoxidil) or an autosomal dominant genetic problem.

Localized hypertrichosis may be congenital as well, e.g., in the ponytail of spinal diastrophism or in the nevoid form. If the localized hypertrichosis is acquired, it may be a cosmetic oddity. Examples include idiopathic forms such as hairy elbows or the examples due to repeated trauma (biting of the wrists seen in the mentally retarded), occlusion under a cast, topical steroids, pretibial myxedema, POEMS syndrome, and linear scleroderma.

Always a hair follicle that is active when it should be at rest deserves an explanation. And this is especially true when the follicle signals to us that it is being spurred by a circulating androgen.

Rittmaster RS, Loriaux DL: **Hirsutism**. Ann Intern Med 1987; 106:95–107.

The clinical spectrum of **excess body hair** in women ranges from mild hirsutism with normal menses to generalized hirsutism with irregular menses and signs of virilization. Mild clitoral enlargement is common. Total testosterone levels are often normal, whereas the unbound (free) testosterone is usually increased. Most women note the onset of hirsutism around puberty, with slow progression over many years. Rapid weight gain and menstrual irregularity may coincide with hair growth. The family history is often positive for hirsutism. Combined ovarian and adrenal factors are probably responsible.

The primary task in evaluating hirsutism is to exclude serious underlying **disease**. Alarming historical points include:

> onset of hirsutism *not* around puberty
> rapid progression of hair growth
> virilization signs and symptoms (balding, deepening voice, increased libido)

In **idiopathic hirsutism** the skin metabolism of androgens is increased and may be an important factor. In the skin 5α-reductase converts testosterone into dihydrotestosterone, the androgen that regulates hair growth. Men with 5α-reductase deficiency develop sparse secondary sexual hair. Androgens promote the conversion of vellus hairs to terminal hairs in responsive hair follicles located on the pubis, axillae, back, face, chest, and abdomen. The amount and distribution of excess hair are important. Terminal hair on the face, lower abdomen, and around the areolae is normal, whereas that on the upper back, shoulders, sternum, and upper abdomen suggests a more marked androgenic effect.

Look for:

> clitoral enlargement (> 100 mm^2)
> ovarian and adrenal masses
> acanthosis nigricans (suggests insulin resistance, especially in a thin woman)
> Cushing's syndrome (central obesity, increased dorsocervical and supraclavicular fat, hypertension, facial plethora, acne, thin skin, striae, proximal muscle weakness)
> drugs (especially in athletic women reluctant to admit taking anabolic steroids)

HIRSUTISM AND OBESITY

Many hirsute women are obese, especially those with polycystic ovarian syndrome. Weight loss may reverse the hyperandrogenism and menstrual disturbance. Obesity is associated with hyperinsulinemia and insulin resistance, and human granulosa cells secrete more androgens in the presence of insulin. Adipose tissue can also convert preandrogens into testosterone, possibly contributing to increased testosterone production in obese women. In obesity the biologic effects of increased testosterone may also be amplified by reduced plasma concentrations of sex hormone–binding globulin. This globulin binds testosterone in a biologically inactive form, so that when it is decreased there is an increased percentage of active free unbound testosterone.

DRUG-INDUCED HIRSUTISM

Androgens, anabolic steroids, and birth control pills may stimulate hirsutism. Drug-induced hirsutism, other than that caused by these androgens, consists of increased vellus hair (rather than terminal hair), which appears anywhere on the body and is not restricted to androgen-dependent areas.

Causative drugs:

minoxidil   glucocorticoids
diazoxide   cyclosporine
phenytoin

ANDROGEN-MEDIATED CAUSES OF HIRSUTISM

ovarian:

polycystic ovarian syndrome   insulin resistance   tumors

adrenal:

Cushing's syndrome (ACTH dependent)
tumors
congenital adrenal hyperplasia

combined: ovarian and adrenal

idiopathic (mostly ovarian)
polycystic ovarian syndrome secondary to adrenal hyperplasia

exogenous medications

LABORATORY EVALUATION OF HIRSUTISM

A.   Hirsutism + regular menses:

serum testosterone (> 200 ng/dl suggests virilizing tumor or severe
   insulin resistance)
plasma 17-hydroxyprogesterone (> 350 ng/dl suggests congenital adrenal hyperplasia with 21-hydroxylase deficiency and should be followed by an ACTH stimulation test)

B.   Hirsutism + irregular menses:

serum prolactin (to exclude a prolactin-secreting tumor)
serum testosterone
plasma 17-hydroxyprogesterone

C.   Optional tests:

dehydroepiandrosterone (DHEA) sulfate (extreme increase suggests
   ovarian or adrenal cancer)
gonadotropin (if ovarian failure is suspected)
urinary free cortisol (if Cushing's disease is suspected)
overnight dexamethasone suppression test if urinary cortisol is increased
   (Cushing's disease)
serum insulin and insulin response to glucose load (insulin resistance)

D.   If a virilizing tumor is suspected, computed tomography of the adrenal
   glands and ultrasonography of the ovaries should be done.

Kvedar JC, Gibon M, Krusinski PA: **Hirsutism**: Evaluation and Treatment. J Am Acad
   Dermatol 1985; 12:215–225.

This is a disease of the female hair follicle in which the diagnosis is made
by the patient but the cause is made evident by the physician. It is a disease
of excessive growth of terminal hair in women. It grows and grows in follicles
that lie dormant until awakened by the **male hormone**. And where are these
androgen-responsive follicles? They are present at the sites of masculinity—
the mustache, the goatee, and the hairy chest, lower abdomen, anterior
thighs, and preauricular area. Thus hirsutism is to be sharply distinguished
from **hypertrichosis**, in which there is an increase in hair growth anywhere
on the body. It is usually of nonendocrine origin.

Hirsutism can be an early sign of **virilism**. Be alert to other evidence of
virilism in these patients: acne, temporal balding, breasts becoming smaller
and muscles bigger, a deep voice, and clitoromegaly.

And where do the male hormones come from in the woman with hirsutism or virilism? They come from the **ovary** and the **adrenal**, and they come from nonendocrine organs such as the liver and skin, which can synthesize them. Although in the usual hirsute woman the excessive hair growth is a racial characteristic, all these patients deserve a search for elevated circulating androgen levels. Once found, the search is on for the source.

The **polycystic ovary** is a prime suspect. Similarly, ovarian hyperthecosis may account for androgen excess. More ominous are the androgen-producing tumors of the ovary, arrhenoblastoma, hilus cell tumor, luteoma.

The second major source is the adrenal in which congenital **adrenal hyperplasia** or idiopathic adrenal overproduction of androgens may be responsible. Again tumors must be considered, i.e., adrenal adenoma, adrenal carcinoma. And since the master gland, the pituitary, oversees all, Cushing's disease may be implicated, as well as acromegaly.

Knowing these sources, what are the tests of value? One of the better "tests" is simply asking about the menses. If there are major disturbances in the cycle, referral to an endocrinologist is advisable. Likewise, simple inspection for cushingoid changes or for acromegaly may lead directly to the endocrinologist. But from the laboratory standpoint order determination of:

1. Testoterone
   if less than 2 ng/ml proceed to treatment
   if over 2 ng/ml, it suggests a gonadal neoplasm and need for referral
2. Dehydroepiandrosterone sulfate (DHEA)
   if less than 9000 ng/ml, proceed to treatment
   if over 9000 ng/ml, it suggests an adrenal neoplasm and need for referral

Ehrmann DA, Rosenfield RL: **Hirsutism**—beyond the steroidogenic block. N Engl J Med 1990; 323:909–911.

Clinical assessment involves first distinguishing abnormal hair growth that is androgen dependent (hirsutism) from that which is androgen independent (hypertrichosis). Because small amounts of male pattern (androgen-dependent) hair growth is normal in women, hirsutism is defined as being present when a woman has a score of 8 or more on the **Ferriman and Gallwey scale**. This score is based on each of the nine androgen-sensitive areas being rated from 0 (none) to 4 (frankly virile).

Since the problem of hirsutism reflects elevated androgen levels, evaluation is done biochemically. The best single measure of hyperandrogenism is the **plasma *free* testosterone** level since total levels in hirsute women may be deceptively lowered by a low level of the testosterone-binding globulin. But recall that androgen secretion is episodic, so a single determination can be very misleading if normal. An initial goal is to identify women who have an androgen-secreting tumor. This is done by demonstrating elevated plasma levels of *total* testosterone (> 200 ng/dl) and of dehydroepiandrosterone (DHEA) sulfate (> 800 μg/dl). The exact source is next sought by looking for an **ovarian or adrenal mass** (ultrasonography, computed tomography, magnetic resonance imaging).

With tumors eliminated as a cause, the search focuses on whether the source of the testosterone is an **ovary** that is polycystic or an **adrenal** gland that is deficient in the enzymes needed for the biosynthesis of cortisol. The 5-day dexamethasone (2 mg/day) suppression test makes this distinction, since it selectively suppresses adrenal testosterone production but not that from the ovary. Accordingly, when by the fifth day the testosterone levels show no change, the evidence points to a diagnosis of polycystic ovarian syndrome. Conversely, in those women in whom the testosterone source is the adrenal, the plasma free testosterone level will be back to normal by the fifth day of dexamethasone administration.

In turn, an **ACTH test** will permit recognition of late-onset congenital adrenal hyperplasia as a precise cause of the elevated androgen production and hence hirsutism. In this condition, enzyme deficiencies prevent the synthesis of cortisol. As a result, the biosynthetic precursors are diverted into the production of excessive 17-ketosteroids (including testosterone). It is a mild form of the classic congenital adrenal hyperplasia. An ACTH test is positive when the androstanedione is increased or the plasma 17-hydroxyprogesterone goes to levels above 44 mmol/liter.

In the absence of excess androgen produced by tumors, polycystic ovaries, or enzyme-deficient adrenals, a diagnosis of **idiopathic hirsutism** remains. The need for a precise diagnosis is underscored by the need for proper therapy. Thus, the tumors call for surgery, the polycystic ovaries call for suppression of serum gonadotropins by contraceptives, the adrenal hyperplasia calls for corticosteroids, and the idiopathic hirsutism calls for spironolactone or flutamide to inhibit androgen binding.

Vasiloff J, Chideckel EW, Boyd CB, Foshag LJ: Testosterone-secreting **adrenal adenoma** containing crystalloids characteristic of Leydig cells. Am J Med 1985; 79:772–776.

A 49-year-old woman had plethora, facial telangiectases, intermittent facial flushing, **hirsutism**, and temporal baldness. Other symptoms included asthenia, weight loss, diarrhea, heat intolerance, tremulousness, and palpitations. Past history revealed hypertension, polycystic kidneys, and an old myocardial infarction.

Increased serum testosterone (520 to 1408 ng/dl) with normal urine and 17-ketosteroids suggested a virilizing ovarian tumor, but computed tomography showed focal enlargement of the right adrenal gland. At surgery she was found to have atrophic (postmenopausal) ovaries and an **adrenal** cortical **adenoma** with Leydig cells.

Rose BI, LeMaire WJ, Jeffers LJ: **Macromastia** in a woman treated with penicillamine and oral contraceptives. A case report. J Reprod Med 1990; 35:43–45.

This 25-year-old woman with Wilson's disease began to develop dark facial hair 10 months after starting **penicillamine** therapy (1500 mg/day). She continued the treatment and 6 months later showed **marked hair growth** on the face, but not elsewhere. There was no clitoromegaly or other signs of virilization or galactorrhea. Hormonal assays were normal.

An attempt to treat the hirsutism with Ortho-Novum 7/7/7 resulted only in greatly enlarged breasts. When the contraceptive and penicillamine were both stopped, the facial hypertrichosis abated. This complication of penicillamine had not been previously reported.

Conway GS, Jacobs HS: **Hirsutism**: Treatable and usually caused by the polycystic ovary syndrome. Br Med J 1990; 301:619–620.

Polycystic ovary is clearly the source of excess androgen in most hirsute women. In fact, 92% of women with hirsutism now can be shown on **ultrasonography** to have the morphology of the polycystic ovary.

The induction of excessive synthesis of ovarian androgens may occur through stimulation by luteinizing hormone, ACTH, overactivity of the cytochrome P-450 c 17α-enzyme complex, or insulin. Since most hirsute women are more **obese** than nonhirsute women and, in turn, show **hyperinsulinemia**, reduction in weight with its concomitant lowering of insulin can be of therapeutic benefit.

Reed OM, Mellette JR Jr, Fitzpatrick JE: Familial **cervical hypertrichosis** with underlying kyphoscoliosis. J Am Acad Dermatol 1989; 20:1069–1072.

Congenital spinal hypertrichosis calls for orthopedic and radiologic review, since it is a marker for the following defects:

spina bifida
meningocele
diastematomyelia
scoliosis

kyphosis
chest deformities
foot deformities

Any congenital localized hypertrichosis must be distinguished from:

congenital nevus
nevoid circumscribed hypertrichosis
Becker's nevus
familial hypertrichosis of palms and soles
congenital spinal hypertrichosis
linear epidermal nevus

In contrast, one sees *acquired* localized hypertrichosis following:

local trauma
chronic inflammation
cutaneous hyperemia

peripheral neuropathy
pretibial myxedema
topical medications

Look for it also in:

scars
vaccination sites
friction sites
thrombophlebitis

stasis dermatitis
lichenification
x-rays, ultraviolet light treatment

Cox NH, McClure JP, Hardie RA: **Naevoid hypertrichosis**—report of a patient with multiple lesions. Clin Exp Dermatol 1989; 14:62–64.

Scattered discrete areas of **excessive hair growth** have been present since birth in this 6-year-old girl. The sites, which included both scapulae, the upper arms, the buttocks, and upper lip, showed ginger-colored terminal hairs in abundance. The underlying skin was normal in appearance and the child in good health. There was no visible alteration on rubbing the affected skin.

Spinal radiographs showed no spinal dysraphism known to be associated with hypertrichosis. A biopsy showed increased numbers of normal hair follicles, making the diagnosis nevoid hypertrichosis.

Three other conditions had to be considered in the differential diagnosis:

1. Congenital smooth muscle hamartoma:

    may show associated hyperpigmentation in half of the cases
    may show a pseudo-Darier sign, consisting of transient elevation of the affected skin, piloerection, or even vermicular squirming as a result of stimulating the nevoid smooth muscle by rubbing

2. Congenital hairy nevi:

    clinically pigmented

3. Becker's nevus

    presents at early age
    pigmentation precedes hypertrichosis

Only by biopsy can the definitive diagnosis be made.

We recently saw an 85-year-old woman who had had a lifelong history of a congenital hairy nevus of the left leg. At the time we saw her, only the nevoid hypertrichosis remained, the melanocytic nevus having faded away many years before. The life cycle of the nevoid follicular organ proved to be longer than that of the nevoid melanocytes.

Rudolph RI: **Hairy elbows**. Cutis 1985; 36:69.

Long blond-brown curly terminal hairs on the lateral aspect of the elbows had been present and unchanged for the past 3 years in this 5-year-old girl. The elbow hairs measured up to 3.5 cm in length, but hypertrichosis was noted nowhere else on the skin or in the family history.

Complete studies revealed no associated findings. A diagnosis of **hypertrichosis cubiti** was made. Other examples found in the literature were equally benign and idiopathic.

Jackson CE, Callies QC, Krull EA, Mehregan A: **Hairy cutaneous malformations** of palms and soles. Arch Dermatol 1975; 111:1146–1149.

Scant, localized, bilaterally symmetrical areas of hair growth were noted on the palms and soles of four individuals representing four consecutive generations of a Canadian family. Hair follicles were found on biopsy.

The pattern of inheritance was autosomal dominant.

Wysocki GP, Daley TD: **Hypertrichosis** in patients receiving cyclosporine therapy. Clin Exp Dermatol 1987; 12:191–196.

A study of 56 diabetics receiving long-term **cyclosporine** therapy indicated that 94.6% developed unequivocal **hypertrichosis**. The phenomenon was evident within 3 months of starting the drug and generally peaked at about 6 months. It was more common and more severe in the younger age group. It occurs in both males and females in nonandrogen–stimulated skin sites such as the glabella, nose, ear lobes, and upper spine. It is **reversible**, the hair being lost within 6 months of stopping the cyclosporine.

The major **side effects of cyclosporine** are hepatotoxicity, nephrotoxicity, and lymphoma. Minor side effects also include mild anemia, transient tremors, acral paresthesias, gingival hyperplasia, and gastrointestinal reactions.

Rousseau C, Willocx D, Bourlond A, et al: **Hypertrichosis** induced by diazoxide in idiopathic hypoglycemia of infancy. Dermatologica 1989; 179:221.

A large number of terminal as well as vellus hairs began to grow on the forehead, cheeks, back, and extensor aspect of the limbs of this 2-month-old infant girl. The history revealed the cause. Over a month ago, **diazoxide** therapy had been started for the treatment of severe hypoglycemia discovered at birth.

Later, an 85% pancreatectomy permitted withdrawal of the diazoxide. Following this, the **hypertrichosis** faded slowly. By 6 months the skin was essentially normal.

Minoxidil and **diphenylhydantoin** are fully capable of producing the same disturbing facial hypertrichosis. All of these iatrogenic examples must be distinguished from congenital and hereditary syndromes (**Cornelia de Lange**).

Soyuer U, Aktas E, Ozesmi M: Postphlebitic localized **hypertrichosis**. Arch Dermatol 1988; 124:30.

Thrombophlebitis of the legs was followed by a **linear band of hair growth**

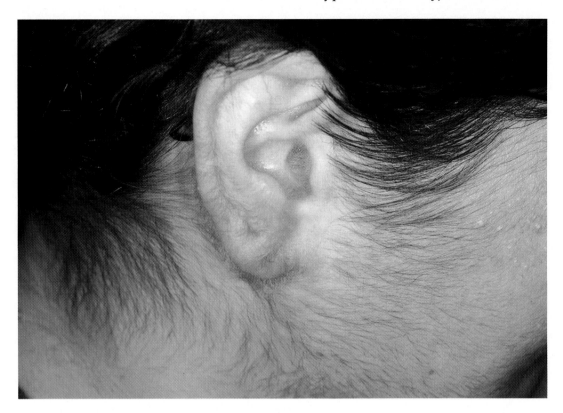

and hyperpigmentation over the inflamed indurated **veins** in a 42-year-old woman with congestive heart failure and tricuspid valve insufficiency secondary to chronic obstructive pulmonary disease.

Hair growth over superficial varicose veins is very rare. More common manifestations of the postphlebitic syndrome are edema, increased pigmentation, dermatitis, and indurated cellulitis. Localized sweating may also be seen.

Casanova JM, Puig T, Rubio M: **Hypertrichosis** of the eyelashes in acquired immunodeficiency syndrome. Arch Dermatol 1987; 123:1599–1600.

Prominent very **long eyelashes** may occur in patients with AIDS. This is a unique form of hypertrichosis and as yet is unexplained. The following known causes of acquired hypertrichosis were ruled out:

drugs: phenytoin, diazoxide, minoxidil, streptomycin, steroids, benoxaprofen, penicillamine, psoralen, cyclosporine

porphyria

malnutrition: anorexia nervosa

dermatomyositis

hypothyroidism: pretibial myxedema

pregnancy

cerebral disturbance

acrodynia

Jester HG: **Lymphedema-distichiasis**. A rare hereditary syndrome. Hum Genet 1977; 39:113–116.

Since early childhood, this 18-year-old man had noted **double-row eyelashes** (distichiasis). In the last 2 years he had developed edema of both legs. On examination he was found to have uvula bifida, palatoschisis, and hyperextensible fingers. His father had similar findings, and a diagnosis of the lymphedema-distichiasis syndrome was made.

These patients may also have ectropion, pterygium colli, extradural spinal cysts, and vertebral fusion. The lymphedema was due to an inadequate perforating vein system.

Price ML, Hall-Smith SP: **Hypertrichosis lanuginosa acquisita**. Clin Exp Dermatol 1985; 10:255–257.

For 2 months a 63-year-old woman had noted a sore tongue and long fine hairs on the face, arms, and trunk. Two years previously she had undergone sigmoidectomy for carcinoma of the colon, with no evidence of recurrence on colonoscopy. **Hypertrichosis lanuginosa acquisita** was diagnosed, and a search was made for an underlying malignant disease. The carcinoembryonic antigen level was 118 μg (normal less than 10 μg), and multiple metastases were seen on liver scan.

Carcinoembryonic antigen is a glycoprotein found in normal fetal colon and gastrointestinal, lung, and breast tumors. It may be a trophic substance that causes adult hair follicles to revert to producing fetal hair. Most patients with hypertrichosis lanuginosa acquisita have **underlying carcinomas** (22/24 cases reported), and 25% also have glossitis.

The appearance of a fetal hair fuzz in an adult demands the same intensive search for internal cancer as does a case of dermatomyositis.

Jemec GBE: **Hypertrichosis lanuginosa acquisita**. Arch Dermatol 1986; 122:805–808.

A 48-year-old woman had a 2-month history of increased facial and eyebrow hair, which began 1 month after starting chemotherapy (chlorambucil and prednisolone) for non-Hodgkin's **lymphoma**. A fine layer of silky, white, soft, downy hair approximately 1 cm long covered her face. She had no signs of virilization or seborrhea (in contrast to hirsutism), but had simultaneously developed 10 to 15 seborrheic keratoses on the dorsal aspect of the hands. She also had burning pain on the tip of the tongue, which appeared normal.

Malignant down points to internal malignant disease or lymphoma, especially in the lung or colon, but also in the breast, gallbladder, ovary, uterus, and pancreas.

Before assuming that the hypertrichosis is a paraneoplastic sign, however, check for drugs that stimulate hair growth, including corticosteroids, spironolactone, dilantin, penicillamine, or streptomycin. (Don't forget minoxidil.)

Additional "**cancer alert**" **signs** in these patients include:

glossitis—tender red tongue
cherry-red spots on the tongue
disturbed ability to taste or salty taste
pigmentation of oral mucosa

Watch out that your laboratory reach does not exceed your diagnostic grasp.

Histiocytosis

Histiocytosis X comes wearing the mask of **seborrheic dermatitis**. Its crusted exudative lesions of the scalp and trunk will fool you into a misdiagnosis of seborrheic dermatitis. Or it may come as the bronzed pigmentation of Addison's disease. There may be the hemorrhages of a petechial or purpuric eruption. Unexplained nodules, ulcers in the groin, or diaper dermatitis may be your only clue to this systemic disease that affects bones, lungs, and many other organs. Indeed, it may never surface to the skin.

Your definitive diagnosis comes from the pathologist who finds the dermal Langerhans' cell to be the root of this evil. Electron microscopy will find the racquet-shaped Birbeck's granules and place the disease in the right court.

Although histiocytosis X is the generic diagnosis, a few specific brands are observable. The most serious is **Letterer-Siwe disease**, an aggressive variant with a poor prognosis. **Hand-Schüller-Christian** type shows not only the skin lesions but also exophthalmos, diabetes insipidus, and cysts of the bones. It may occur in adults as well as children. In the third subset, the **eosinophilic** type, granulomas are present with strange keratotic ulcerative tumors whose diagnosis remains a secret until they are seen by a pathologist.

At this masquerade ball there may be the rarest of all, malignant histiocytosis. Your pathologist, again, is the one to unmask it. It's all very chilling to the clinical diagnostician, but imagine how the pathologist feels when he finds the Langerhans' cell came to the party under an assumed name, Monsieur Histiocyte.

Gianotti F, Caputo R: **Histiocytic syndromes**: A review. J Am Acad Dermatol 1985; 13:383–404.

Proliferation of the monocyte-macrophage lineage of cells produces a wide spectrum of clinical findings with a variety of names:

Histiocytosis X

Letterer-Siwe disease
Hand-Schüller-Christian disease
eosinophilic granuloma

Non-X histiocytosis

self-healing reticulohistiocytosis
benign cephalic histiocytosis
juvenile xanthogranuloma
sinus histiocytosis with massive lymphadenopathy
generalized eruptive histiocytoma
papular xanthoma
xanthoma disseminatum
multicentric reticulohistiocytosis
progressive nodular histiocytosis

A. Histiocytosis X.

1. Acute disseminated (Letterer-Siwe disease). This occurs in infants (sometimes congenital) or adults and is usually fatal. Crops of small translucent rose-yellow papules occur on the trunk and scalp. They may scale and crust or become pustular or purpuric. When confluent on the scalp the eruption looks like seborrheic dermatitis. Mucosal ulcerations occur, but lymphadenopathy is rarely prominent. Look for pulmonary involvement, hepatosplenomegaly, and painful osteolytic lesions.

2. Chronic progressive (Hand-Schüller-Christian disease). This begins in early childhood but has fewer (although similar) skin lesions than

727

Letterer-Siwe disease. The course is chronic and fatal in half of the cases. Look for exophthalmos, osteolytic lesions of the skull, and diabetes insipidus.

3. Localized benign (eosinophilic granuloma). This begins in early adulthood, usually with an osteolytic lesion leading to a spontaneous fracture. Otitis media is common, and noduloulcerative skin lesions occur around orifices and on mucous membranes.

    If the skin lesions resemble seborrheic dermatitis, also think about:

candidiasis	miliaria
Darier's disease	lichen nitidus

    If the skin lesions are nodular, consider:

urticaria pigmentosa	benign cephalic histiocytosis
eruptive histiocytoma	granuloma faciale
papular xanthoma	self-healing reticulohistiocytosis

B. Non-X histiocytosis.

1. Self-healing reticulohistiocytosis. Multiple red-brown nodules are present at birth or neonatally. They grow in the first few weeks, become crusted, and peel off, leaving white atrophic scars. Remission occurs within 3 months, and there is no recurrence and no systemic disease. Urticaria pigmentosa and juvenile xanthogranuloma are in the differential diagnosis.

2. Benign cephalic histiocytosis. Erythematous yellow papulonodular lesions occur on the scalp, upper face, ears, neck, shoulders, and arms of children. After a few years the lesions involute, leaving round atrophic pigmented macular scars. The differential diagnosis includes:

histiocytosis X	urticaria pigmentosa
sarcoidosis	papular xanthoma
juvenile xanthogranuloma	

3. Juvenile xanthogranuloma. Usually occurring in infants and children, it may appear as:

    Small nodular form. Numerous red-brown 2- to 5-mm papules quickly turn into small yellow nodules on the upper part of the body. They are frequently associated with café au lait spots of neurofibromatosis.

    Large nodular form. One or a few round 1- to 2-cm translucent red nodules with telangiectasia occur on the skin or mucous membranes. These flatten and disappear in 3 to 6 years.

    The differential diagnosis includes:

urticaria pigmentosa	self-healing reticulohistiocytosis
benign cephalic histiocytosis	benign juvenile melanoma
eruptive xanthomas	

4. Sinus histiocytosis with massive lymphadenopathy. In this self-limited disease of children, painless cervical lymphadenopathy is associated with fever, leukocytosis (neutrophilia), elevated ESR, and hypergammaglobulinemia. Other nodes may also be involved. Skin lesions occur in 10% of cases and consist of red-brown or yellow-brown papules or nodules. The lesions resemble dermatofibromas, but are distinguished histologically.

5. Generalized eruptive histiocytoma. These self-healing dark-red or

bluish 3- to 10-mm papules in adults are numerous (up to 1000) and occur in successive crops. They are symmetrical on the face, trunk, and proximal area of the limbs. Lesions disappear after a few years.

6. Papular xanthoma. In this normolipidemic condition 2- to 15-mm round yellowish papulonodular lesions occur in a generalized distribution on skin and mucous membranes. They do not form confluent plaques or become red or brown, in contrast to xanthoma disseminatum. They are self-healing in a few years.

7. Xanthoma disseminatum (Montgomery syndrome). This is associated with diabetes insipidus and a normal lipid profile. Hundreds of red-brown papules become yellowish, symmetrically involving the trunk, face, proximal area of the extremities, and flexural folds. The eyelids, conjunctivae, lips, pharynx, and larynx are infiltrated with red or yellow plaques. The skin lesions and diabetes insipidus disappear after several years.

8. Multicentric reticulohistiocytosis. Occurring in adults over 40 years of age, translucent yellow-rose or yellow-brown papulonodular lesions up to 2 cm occur symmetrically on the face, fingers, hands, juxta-articular regions, and oral and nasal mucosa. There is associated severe destructive polyarthritis. It is not self-limiting. Nodular leprosy and progressive nodular histiocytosis must be ruled out.

9. Progressive nodular histiocytosis. Widespread symmetrical papules and nodules tend to merge on the face, leading to leonine facies as in leprosy. The patient remains in good health and there is no arthritis or involvement of mucous membranes. New lesions continue to develop.

Gianotti F, Caputo R, Ermacora E, Gianni E: Benign **cephalic histiocytosis**. Arch Dermatol 1986; 122:1038–1043.

The diagnosis of histiocytosis X is frightening, forecasting involvement of mucous membranes, liver, lungs and bones, with little hope of cure. The histiocytosis X cells are S100- and OKT6-positive and show Langerhans' granules on electron microscopy.

Fortunately, in children, a **benign self-healing histiocytosis** can be sorted out, with 13 cases described herein. All initially involved the face, with slightly raised, round, or oval pink and brownish-yellow papules. Later, lesions appeared elsewhere. All appeared in the first 3 years of life and regressed or disappeared months to years later. None showed systemic involvement, and all spared the mucous membranes. Significantly, the histiocytic infiltrate contained no lipids and was S100- and OKT6-negative. All were examples of benign cephalic histiocytosis, which must be distinguished from other benign self-healing conditions:

1. Generalized eruptive histiocytoma: (localized on trunk and extremities).
2. Juvenile xanthogranuloma (disseminated, easily recognized histologically by the foam cells, lipid droplets, and giant cells).
3. Urticaria pigmentosa (look for the diagnostic Darier's sign).

Goodfellow A, Cream JJ, Seed WA: **Histiocytosis X** with unusual facial and axillary ulceration responding to topical nitrogen mustard. J R Soc Med 1982; 75:279–281.

A 31-year-old white man had a **pinkish-brown papular rash on the cheeks** and forehead intermixed with pustules, discrete crusted papules, and crateriform ulcerations. Many yellow crusted papules were present on the scalp, with a few on the ears and chest. In each axilla he had 1-cm exudative ulcers with thick raised smooth margins. He also had bilateral sensorineural deafness, polyuria, polydipsia, and exertional dyspnea. Two fingernails were dystrophic, with clippings showing *Candida tropicalis*. Past history revealed mouth ulcerations, alcoholism, and an eosinophilic granuloma of the left mandible treated with radiotherapy and partial maxillectomy.

Skin biopsies from facial lesions and an axillary ulcer showed histiocytes in the upper dermis extending into the epidermis and a dense lymphocytic infiltrate beneath the histiocytes. Electron microscopy revealed Langerhans' cell granules in the histiocytes, characteristic of histiocytosis X. Diabetes insipidus was confirmed, along with pulmonary disease characteristic of **Hand-Schüller-Christian disease**.

Treatment with prednisone had no effect on the skin lesions, but they cleared with topical nitrogen mustard.

Oral ulceration may be an early manifestation of chronic disseminated histiocytosis X. Ulcers may also occur on the vulva, vagina, perineal, and perianal areas. Axillary ulcerations are rare and may be confused with hidradenitis suppurativa.

Moayed MJ, Kanitakis J, Nabai H, Mauduit G: **Regressing atypical histiocytosis** (of Flynn). Report of a new case. Dermatologica 1987; 174:253–257.

A massive 10-cm ulcerated vegetating tumor of the left temple of 3 months' duration in a 24-year-old female farmer from Iran was associated with marked eyelid swelling. Cultures showed *Pseudomonas aeruginosa* and were negative for tuberculosis, deep mycosis, and leishmaniasis. Although the tumor had histologic features of malignancy (dense infiltrate of large atypical cells with ill-defined cytoplasm, large nuclei, abundant mitoses), it disappeared spontaneously within 6 months. She had had a similar "**self-destruct" tumor** of the left elbow 6 months prior.

Disparities between histologic prognosis and clinical course have also been reported under the titles of:

lymphomatoid papulosis
persistent insect bite reaction
giant pseudomalignant granuloma
cutaneous histiosarcoma
histiomonocytoid reticulosis

All such lesions require a guarded long-term prognosis.

The frequency of making a given diagnosis depends not only on the frequency of the disease but also on the frequency with which it comes to mind.

Hyperhidrosis

Hyperhidrosis does not summon the question, "What is it?" but rather the question, "Why is it?" Normally the sweat glands provide sweat for evaporative cooling as in a hot environment or in the presence of a fever. In such instances, hyperhidrosis is a physiologic response under hypothalamic control and mediated by cholinergic fibers of the sympathetic nerves.

However, in the absence of thermal or febrile stress, generalized hyperhidrosis suggests an **autonomic discharge**. Shock, hypoglycemia, anxiety, hyperpituitarism, and drugs are examples of triggering factors. Brain injury, a stroke, or even the smell of perfume may also initiate such generalized hyperhidrosis. Close attention to the context of attacks is essential as shown in the example of sugar-induced attacks seen in a patient with fructose intolerance.

Much more common is the localized hyperhidrosis associated with ingestion of **foods**. This gustatory sweating may occur most commonly on the face, but we have seen it localized on the knees—and in this instance, amazingly, in both a husband and his wife.

Any localized hyperhidrosis suggests **peripheral neuropathy** or the encroachment of a tumor, a cervical disc, or arthritic spur on the sympathetic chain. Patchy hyperhidrosis can be seen in diabetics in whom it reflects a compensatory hyperhidrosis resulting from extensive diabetic neuropathic anhidrosis. Indeed, extensive sympathectomies can result in a very disturbing compensatory hyperhidrosis whenever the patient is in a hot environment.

The usual presentation of hyperhidrosis is in the palms, soles, and axillae. These areas exhibit sweating in response to emotional rather than thermal stimuli. The presence of localized hyperhidrosis in such areas is indicative of a genetic trait in which there is marked hypersensitivity of these glands to acetylcholine.

Finally, it is important to note that hyperhidrosis will be completely inapparent in a hot, dry, windy environment in which the sweat evaporates before being seen. Likewise, hyperhidrosis of the axilla may require the challenge of mental arithmetic to be seen. And the thick keratin of the palms and soles soaks up the sweat so no droplets are seen. Only the white, wet, macerated skin is your diagnostic marker.

Sato K, Kang WH, Saga K, Sato KT: Biology of sweat glands and their disorders: II. **Disorders of sweat gland function**. J Am Acad Dermatol 1989; 20:713–726.

Hyperhidrosis of palms and soles:

increased sympathetic response through T2-3 ganglia.
occurs in:
nail-patella syndrome
keratosis palmaris et plantaris
Raynaud's disease
erythromelalgia
atrioventricular fistula
cold injury
rheumatoid arthritis

Hyperhidrosis of axillae: increased sympathetic discharge, T4 ganglion.

Localized hyperhidrosis due to previous spinal cord injury (profuse sweating months to years later):

may be triggered by orthostatic hypotension associated with cervical cord transection
may be due to post-traumatic syringomyelia. In paraplegics requires surgical drainage

may result from autonomic dysreflexia associated with spinal cord lesions at or above T6.

may be triggered by skin irritation, pain, visceral inflammation of bowel or bladder distension

may have clinical triad:
episodic profuse sweating, hand, neck and upper extremity
flushing, nasal congestion
throbbing headache

Hyperhidrosis associated with peripheral neuropathies

familial dysautonomia:
no axon reflex after histamine intradermally
absence of fungiform papillae of tongue
reduced pain sensation
Ashkenazic Jewish ancestry

congenital autonomic dysfunction:
universal pain loss, accidental self-mutilation

cold-induced hyperhidrosis:
neck and thorax
muscle weakness

Hyperhidrosis associated with brain lesions:

malformations or episodic decrease in hypothalamic temperature set point results in hypothermia
cerebrovascular accident
brain injury
examples triggered by smell of perfume

Localized hyperhidrosis:

unilateral circumscribed idiopathic hyperhidrosis
usually on face or arm
triggered by heat, mental stimulation, or foods
lacrimal sweats in supraorbital area

Unilateral hyperhidrosis associated with intrathoracic neoplasm:

paroxysmal
due to encroachment of tumor on sympathetic trunk or ganglion
may result from cervical rib, osteoma

Generalized hyperhidrosis with illness:

diabetes mellitus
congestive heart disease
thyrotoxicosis
hyperpituitarism

anxiety
menopause
pheochromocytoma
drugs: antidepressants

Localized hyperhidrosis associated with skin disease:

blue rubber bleb nevus
glomus tumor
POEMS syndrome
Gopalan's syndrome (burning feet)

causalgia
pachydermoperiostosis
painful ulcers

Hyperhidrosis of gustatory sweating:

preauricular and infra-auricular area
can reflect invasion of cervical sympathetic by tumor (Pancoast's syndrome)
sympathectomy
diabetes mellitus
herpes zoster

parotitis
Frey's syndrome: follows parotid gland surgery after 1 month to 5 years

Hyperhidrosis at night:

tuberculosis	pheochromocytoma
endocarditis	carcinoid syndrome
lymphomas	drug withdrawal
hyperthyroidism	infectious disease
diabetes mellitus	acromegaly
insulinoma	Prinzmetal angina
vasculitis	

Grice K, Verbov J: **Sweat glands** and their disorders. Rec Adv Dermatol 1977; 4:155–198.

Expect hyperhidrosis:

infection
familial dysautonomia (Riley-Day syndrome)
hypoglycemia, shock, pheochromocytoma
hirsutism
tetanus
gustatory: look for diabetes, sympathetic nerve trauma
auriculotemporal syndrome (Frey's syndrome; after parotid surgery)
Parkinson's disease
spinal cord lesions
peripheral nerve lesions: causalgia
menopause
hyperthyroidism
hyperpituitarism

Stewart PA: **Adrenal phaeochromocytoma** in familial neurofibromatosis with initial control of hypertension by labetalol. J Roy Soc Med 1982; 75:276–278.

A 45-year-old woman with neurofibromatosis and a family history of cancer in three siblings had experienced **episodes of profuse sweating** for many years. Her blood pressure fluctuated from 150/80 to 220/120. Repeated 24-hour urinary catecholamine assays were elevated, and a 5-cm diameter pheochromocytoma was located on the upper pole of the right kidney. Following surgery, she became normotensive and remained free of episodes of sweating.

Normal values of urinary catecholamines do not exclude a pheochromocytoma because a short paroxysm of catecholamine secretion during a 24-hour urine collection may be insufficient to raise the total value above normal because of the dilutional effect of the urine. The catecholamine levels may be falsely increased or decreased by certain drugs and foods, as well as smoking and stress.

Coulson IH, Marsden RA: Ross' syndrome. Br J Dermatol 1985; 113 (suppl 29):96–97.

A 45-year-old man noted severe **hyperhidrosis** in **patchy small islands** over his left buttock, sacral area, and above the umbilicus. This had become progressively severe for 8 years. The palms were dry and scaly, and he had noted inability to sweat in many areas. Examination using 2% edicol ponceau powder in starch revealed scattered areas of hyperhidrosis. Elsewhere he was anhidrotic, with no sweat elicited by acetylcholine, heat, or exercise. The **pupils** were small and of unequal size with sluggish light and accommodation reflexes, and **deep tendon reflexes** were absent. Biopsy revealed normal eccrine sweat glands in both the anhidrotic and hyperhidrotic areas.

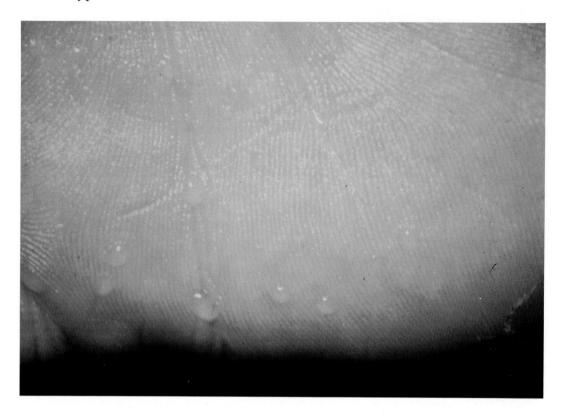

He showed no evidence of diabetes or syphilis, and cardiovascular autonomic function tests were normal.

A diagnosis of Ross' syndrome was made on the basis of sweat pattern, pupillary findings, and absence of tendon reflexes.

McCoy BP: Apical **pulmonary adenocarcinoma** with contralateral hyperhidrosis. Arch Dermatol 1981; 117:659–661.

The dermatologic complaint of this 58-year-old man was an erythematous, pruritic, **papulovesicular eruption** of the entire right side of the trunk. Of acute onset, it also involved the right arm and right side of the face. His general medical problem was one of weight loss, anorexia, asthenia, fever, and dyspnea on exertion for the past 6 months.

Although the patient had not recognized it, he had **hyperhidrosis** of the same half of the body. In the hospital the eruption subsided with compresses and cloxacillin therapy, but the unilateral hyperhidrosis continued.

Studies revealed the presence of metastatic **adenocarcinoma** of the upper part of the upper lobe of the left lung. It was felt that the hyperhidrosis resulted from the tumor encroaching on or compromising the sympathetic nerves on the contralateral side.

We assume that the presenting eruption was miliaria rubra induced by the persistent hyperhidrosis.

Eedy DJ, Corbett JR: Olfactory hyperhidrosis responding to amitriptyline. Clin Exp Dermatol 1987; 12:298–299.

In the past 5 years, this 42-year-old woman has noted **profuse sweating** on both cheeks whenever she comes in contact with **perfume**, perfumed items, or individuals wearing perfume. Nothing else triggered this response other than stress, such as induced by mental arithmetic. She had no palmar or axillary hyperhidrosis. The facial hyperhidrosis of diabetes was ruled out as well as any neurologic lesion.

A challenge with perfume produced beads of sweat on the malar areas within a few minutes. It continued for 30 minutes after the olfactory stimulus was removed. There was no associated flushing or any symptoms. A single daily dose of **amitriptyline** (25 mg) has completely blocked this hyperhidrosis for the past 3 years.

Cunliffe WJ, Johnson CE: **Gustatory hyperhidrosis**: A complication of thyroidectomy. Br J Dermatol 1967; 79:519–526.

For the past 28 years, this 57-year-old woman has experienced profuse **sweating** of the right side of the face, scalp, neck, and upper back **on eating** most types of foods. It began 6 months after a thyroidectomy and has been the source of anxiety and depression. Significantly, there was hypohidrosis on the right side in response to thermal stimulation.

Analysis indicated that the most likely explanation was that there had been **surgical damage** to the cervical sympathetic trunk and that subsequently cholinergic fibers had sprouted from the vagus into the sympathetic trunk.

Other reports in the literature have discerned a **variety of causes** of gustatory hyperhidrosis. These include lesions of the cervical sympathetic trunk induced by sympathectomy, carcinoma of the lung, and osteoma of the spine. It has also occurred in association with diseases of the central nervous system, such as encephalitis and syringobulbia. However, most examples remain idiopathic in nature.

Cox TM: An independent diagnosis: A treatable **metabolic disorder** is diagnosed by molecular analysis of human genes. Br Med J 1990; 300:1512–1514.

This 30-year-old man with a 10-year history of unexplained episodes of **hyperhidrosis**, followed by convulsions and loss of consciousness, made his own diagnosis by reading the newspaper. He recognized his problem to be identical to the newspaper description of patients with hereditary **fructose intolerance**.

His physicians were then able to confirm the diagnosis by doing genomic analysis on a simple saline mouth rinse. With the polymerase chain reaction, the buccal epithelial cell sample provided sufficient DNA to show that there was a **deficit of aldolase B_1**, the enzyme responsible for normal fructose metabolism. A challenge with fructose reproduced the symptoms and revealed a dramatic triggering drop in the blood glucose level.

Hereditary fructose intolerance is a rare autosomal recessive disorder in which ingestion of fructose, sucrose, or related sugars induces abdominal pain, vomiting, and hypoglycemia. The affected infants quickly acquire an aversion to sweet-tasting foods, as well as fruits and vegetables. Should these children be forced to eat the "forbidden fruit and sweet," their growth is retarded, and progressive renal and hepatic disease can lead to death.

Until the patient described became fully informed, he had had 10 years of grand mal seizures, had his driver's license withdrawn, and had to change jobs as well as live in constant fear.

Listen to patients who bring in **newspaper clippings**. Maybe what they say is not hogwash but calls for a mouthwash in your diagnostic work-up. And don't forget to get that blood glucose level during the course of the episode of hyperhidrosis.

Pfeifer MP, Hardison JE: **Profuse diaphoresis** relieved by coronary angioplasty. Am J Med 1989; 86:338–339.

Simply walking 100 feet would trigger a **drenching sweat** for this 65-year-old man. As a result, he was obliged to change his underclothes upon any degree of exertion, even in the cold. The attacks had been occurring for over a year and were unrelated to any feeling of exertion, dyspnea, or chest pain. They abated upon rest and never occurred when the patient was at rest. The patient's health was good, aside from hypertension.

General physical examination and an electrocardiogram were normal. However, an exercise test reproduced the attack of hyperhidrosis, again with angina. Attacks could be alleviated by the administration of sublingual nitroglycerin. At this point, coronary angiography showed 90% stenosis of the left anterior descending artery. Following angioplasty the patient was able to walk for miles without sweat.

Hyperhidrosis as a phenomenon of **myocardial ischemia** usually occurs in association with the pain of angina. Here it was the solitary sign. Presumably it arose as a cardiac-induced reflex increasing autonomic discharge.

Hu C-H, Michel B, Farber EM: Transient **acantholytic dermatosis** (Grover's disease): A skin disorder related to heat and sweating. Arch Dermatol 1985; 121:1439–1441.

Nine days after open reduction of a right femur fracture, an 86-year-old man developed multiple pruritic, flesh-colored to slightly **erythematous papules** on the back.

The biopsy demonstration of acantholysis above the basal cell layer confirmed the diagnosis of Grover's disease or transient acantholytic dermatosis.

It is postulated that prolonged bed confinement induced an occlusive environment, sweating, and **sweat retention** due to poral closure. The trapped sweat and/or local heat favored the acantholytic cleavage seen in the lesions.

Most patients with transient acantholytic dermatosis relate this eruption to heat and excessive sweating.

What does the patient think the cause is?

Hyperpigmentation

You've looked at the patient's dark spots. Now comes the history to confirm or to conjure a diagnosis. First, could the problem be genetic? Has he had it since early childhood? Do other members of his family have it? Could it be multiple lentigines? Are the lesions localized on the lips, face, fingers, and toes (Peutz-Jeghers syndrome), suggesting the presence of gastrointestinal polyposis? Should you look for other parts of the syndrome called LEOPARD? Is there hypertelorism, deafness, cryptorchidism, or short stature? Are the pigmented spots those of the nevi or freckling that speak of myxomas of the heart or of the neurofibromas of the NAME and LAMB syndromes?

Is the pattern of pigmentation reticulated as in dyskeratosis congenita? Here the clue leads to looking for the ectropion, cataracts, lacrimal duct obstruction, and dental dystrophies of the Zinsser-Cole-Engman syndrome. Is the pattern whorled and streaked and in a girl, thus leading to a diagnosis of incontinentia pigmenti? If so, look for the confirming findings of missing or conical teeth, a history of vesicles in rows, as well as verrucous lesions.

Is the pigment a café au lait spot? Is it in the axillae? Do you see the "coffee" spot that awakens you to a diagnosis of neurofibromatosis with its endocrine, skeletal, and central nervous system ramifications? Does it explain the patient's seizures, delayed development, and future malignant disease?

Is it a large brown patch with jagged coast-of-Maine border? Should you look for the rarefactions of the long bones, hyperostotic lesions of the skull, and the precocious puberty of Albright's syndrome (polyostotic fibrosis dysplasia)?

Could the pigment signal underlying mastocytoma (urticaria pigmentosa)?

Continue to pursue the history. If the pigment is of recent origin, can the patient relate it to prior inflammation? Has he had radiation therapy or chemotherapy, such as bleomycin? Could it be due to a drug being taken, such as minocin, amiodarone, Dilantin, or quinidine? Could it be of hormonal origin such as an oral contraceptive or an estrogen? Is it a sign of Addison's disease or malignant melanoma? Is it a metal deposition, as in argyria or chrysiasis? In the genital area could it be Bowen's disease? Ask the patient if he is taking cathaxanthin, the "sun tan pill," if the color is salmon pink. For yellow palms, the question is how much carotene or carrot juice is being taken.

Turn the questioning to contactants. Is it work related? Does the patient handle dyes or organic compounds? Has the patient had long-term usage of hydroquinone? Ironically, this bleaching agent turns to hyperpigment by inducing focal ochronosis.

Ask and keep on asking while you think and maybe read some more.

General

Fulk CS: Primary disorders of **hyperpigmentation**. J Am Acad Dermatol 1984; 10:1–16.

Skipping over the hyperpigmentation of the nevoid lesions, the hamarto-matous growths, and recognizable skin lesions, we come to the following examples of hyperpigmentation, many of which are congenital or familial:

1. *Patchy hyperpigmentation*

   acromelanosis: Dorsal distal digits show brown to black hyperpigmen-tation in infancy, which generally fades in early childhood.

   acromelanosis progressiva: Initially before the age of 1 year, the dorsa of the fingers are hyperpigmented. It progresses to involve the ex-tremities, perineum, and areas of the head and neck by the age of 5 years. The border is sharp, and the color may be as black as India ink.

   congenital diffuse pigmentation (Wende-Bauckus): This is hyperpig-mentation that begins on the scalp and face and extends over the whole body during early childhood. By the age of 5 years the hy-perpigmentation faded leaving pinpoint white spots over the clavicle and in general areas.

   familial progressive hyperpigmentation: Very dark irregular patches began to appear in childhood involving not only the skin, but also the oral mucosa and conjunctiva.

   universal acquired melanosis (carbon baby): When this baby was 2 weeks old his skin and oral mucosa turned completely black in a short time. Only a few areas on the palms and soles maintained their regular color.

2. *Punctate and reticulate hyperpigmentation*

   reticulate acropigmentation of Kitamura: Distal, reticulate, slightly atrophic, polygonal, hyperpigmented macules appear in childhood and extend proximally. Look for pits and breaks in the epidermal ridge patterns on the palms. The pigmentation begins in childhood and gradually extends.

   acropigmentation symmetrica of Dohi: Acral, punctate, and reticulate hyperpigmentation appears in childhood. The distinctive features are coalescence into stellate patches and interspersed leukoderma of the face, trunk, flexor extremities, and palms. Pigmentation con-tinues to progress until adulthood, at which time it remains stable.

   reticulated pigmented anomaly of the flexures (Dowling-Degos dis-ease, dark dot disease): reticulated macular hyperpigmentation of antecubital fossae and inframammary areas, especially; usual onset is in adolescence. Look for pitting at angles of mouth.

   Franceschetti-Jadassohn-Naegeli syndrome: punctate hyperpigmen-tation of neck, waist, and axilla from early childhood. Look for as-sociated palmar-plantar hyperkeratosis, hypohidrosis, yellow teeth, lost finger-pad ridges.

   Dermatopathia pigmentosa reticularis: reticulate hyperpigmentation of trunk and extremities beginning in infancy. Look for anonychia, alopecia, atrophy of hands, feet, elbows, and knees.

   Cantu's syndrome: tiny brown macules becoming confluent to form patches on face, dorsal surfaces of forearms and feet. Onset in ado-lescence. Look for hyperkeratotic palms and soles.

   Ectodermal dysplasia: generalized pigmentation with superimposed raindrop hypopigmented macules. Look for hypoplastic digitalized thumbs, alopecia, endocrinopathy.

738

3. *Dyschromatosis:* hyperpigmentation in multiple shades. Distinguished from poikiloderma where telangiectasia and atrophy are also present.

> dyschromatosis universalis: progressive dyschromia of trunk and extremities with onset in early childhood.

> dyschromatosis symmetrica: dyschromia in sun-exposed areas or in seborrheic distribution, usually macules of varying color coalesce to make a reticulum over normal colored skin.

> Berlin's syndrome: mottled dyschromia of extremities with focal poikiloderma on elbows and telangiectasia of lips. Look for plantar hyperkeratosis, thick lips, thin intelligence, and absence of teeth and lanugo hair.

> Da Costa's syndrome: scattered bullae before the age of 3 years followed by reticulate dyschromia of cheeks and extremities. Look for alopecia, mental or physical retardation.

> acromelanosis albopunctata (Siemens): diffuse hyperpigmentation with small white maculae of dorsa of hands and of palms, axillae, groin, and antecubital areas. Look for short, thick, silky hair, platyonychia, and strabismus.

4. *Unclassified Primary Disorders of Pigmentation*

> periorbital melanosis, familial: darkening of lower eyelid during adolescence followed by similar darkening of the upper eyelid, to be distinguished from secondary type due to atopy

> pigmentary demarcation lines: best perceived in pigmented races.
> > Type A: along upper extremities
> > B: on legs
> > C: on chest
> > D: posteromedian
> > E: oblique hypopigmented macules of chest
> > May be atavistic remnant where dorsal skin is more pigmented than ventral, providing better protection from sun.

Oh, what a tangled DNA brings on this tangle of pigmentation.

James WD, Carter JM, Rodman OG: **Pigmentary demarcation lines**: A population survey. J Am Acad Dermatol 1987; 16:584–590.

Avoid eponyms. Pigmentary lines of demarcation are classified as Type:

> A: lateral aspect of upper anterior arms, across pectoral area
> B: posteromedial portion, lower limbs
> C: vertical hypopigmented line in sternal area
> D: posteromedial area of spine
> E: midthird of clavicle to periareolar skin

Types A and B are present in over 50% of black females. Type C is most common in black males.

Fitzgerald PH, Donald RA, Kirk RL: A true **hermaphrodite** dispermic chimera with 46, XX and 46, XY karyotypes. Clin Genet 1979; 15:89–96.

When a 16-year-old boy was seen for acne, examination of the trunk revealed an astounding **checkerboard patterning of segmental pigmentation**, with wide rectangular pigmented bands alternating with nonpigmented bands. These geometrically precise color bands met at the midline on each side, giving a checkerboard appearance. Skin biopsy showed absence of melanocytes in the nonpigmented skin.

The patient was a true **hermaphrodite**, with a functioning left testis, rudimentary uterus, and right fallopian tube and ovary. Both XX and XY cells were present. The patient's checkerboard skin spoke of dual inheritance, apparently from fertilization of the ovum by two separate sperm.

Happle R: **Lyonization** and the **lines of Blaschko**. Hum Genet 1985; 70:200–206.

In contrast to dermatomes, which are the cutaneous representation of spinal ganglia, the lines described by Blaschko in 1801 have remained a mysterious develomental patterning of the skin. They show a classic **V shape** on the back over the spine, and an **S shape** on the lateral and anterior trunk. Whorls are often present on the abdomen, and perpendicular lines appear on the limbs. On the scalp the pattern is a spiral, converging on the center of the crown. The dorsal **V** configuration may result from asynchrony in the transverse and longitudinal embryonic growth. The ventral **S** may reflect the curved form of the embryo. In various heterozygous X-linked skin disorders the lines of Blaschko visualize for us the clonal proliferation of two different populations of cells during early embryogenesis.

The concept of the two-cell population stems from Lyon's (1961) observations on mice with variegated coat patterns (mottled, brindled, tortoise shell, tabby), which are heterozygous for X-linked genes. These genes can give rise to clearly discernible linear patterns, similar to chimeric mice. Lyon hypothesized that this was the result of **X inactivation**, which created two functionally different populations of cells.

Human **X-linked gene defects** with patterns corresponding to the lines of Blaschko include:

1. **Incontinentia pigmenti** (X-linked dominant) with pigmented **V** shapes on the back and **S** shapes and whorls on the abdomen.
2. **Focal dermal hypoplasia** (X-linked dominant) with **V** and **S** patterning of linear pigmentation, widespread dermal hypoplasia with herniated fat, and severe bone defects.
3. **Chondrodysplasia punctata** (X-linked dominant) with ichthyosis, atrophoderma, and sometimes pigmentation in a linear dorsal **V** shape and abdominal **S**-shape pattern. These lines were the first signal that this disease was X linked. Punctate calcifications of the epiphyses, asymmetrical shortening of the long bones, and asymmetrical lenticular opacities are other findings.
4. **Hypohidrotic ectodermal dysplasia** (X linked) with bands of hypohidrosis that swirl in perfect alignment with the lines of Blaschko, demonstrable on the back using a starch-iodine test for sweating.
5. **Menkes' syndrome** (X-linked recessive) with linear hypopigmented **S**-shaped patterns on the abdomen, showing sharp midline separation in heterozygous girls. The pigmentary disturbance may reflect the role of copper in tyrosinase activity. This neurodegenerative disorder, which is due to a defect in copper ion transport, also includes kinked and twisted hair, mental retardation, skeletal deformities, and hypothermia.

Moral: When you see a **V** pattern on the back or an **S** shape on the abdomen, think of X-linked genetic disease. The lines of Blaschko separate the girls from the boys, as few males survive these serious X-linked diseases.

Fuller RL, Geis S: The significance of skin color of a newborn infant. Am J Dis Child 1985; 139:672–673.

Racism in western culture focuses on skin pigmentation. Minority (black) and interracial parents worry greatly about a newborn's skin color. Distress over darker or lighter newborn skin may raise questions of paternity and

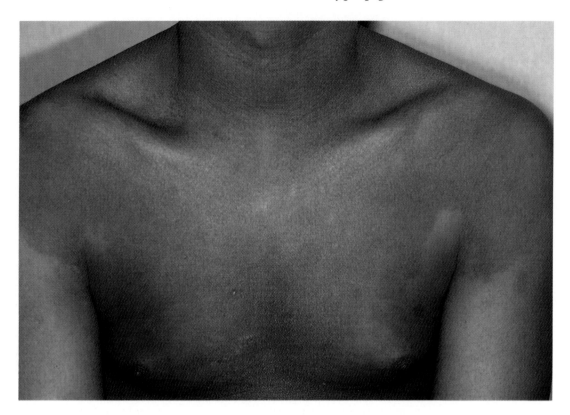

cause rejection, abuse, or neglect. These worries are seldom discussed with physicians.

Variations in skin tones are described as mocha, mahogany, ebony, cinnamon, pecan, walnut, and so on. Skin color darkening or "coming in" in light-skinned newborns occurs over 4 to 6 weeks. The "real" color appears first around the ears and nails.

Your retina picks up 50,000 discrete bits of information at a glance. Use them.

Nevoid

Person JR, Longcope C: **Becker's nevus**: An androgen-mediated hyperplasia with increased androgen receptors. J Am Acad Dermatol 1984; 10:235–237.

This 16-year-old boy was noted incidentally to have a collection of irregular **hyperpigmented macules** with a local increase in **terminal hairs** on the right pectoral area. A diagnosis of Becker's nevus was made.

The known **increase in sebaceous gland activity**, the aberrant terminal hairs, and dermal thickening suggest that androgen stimulation may be responsible. To study this, a biopsy was taken of both the nevus and normal skin from the opposite side of the chest. Measurement of androgen cytosol–receptor levels revealed the nevus to have a level of 634 fm/mg protein and the contralateral control skin to have a level below 2.

This finding supports the view that a local segmental increase in androgen sensitivity is responsible for appearance of this nevus at or after puberty when androgen levels climb.

Rustin MHA, Bunker CB, Gilkes JJH, et al: **Polyostotic fibrous dysplasia** associated with extensive linear epidermal naevi. Clin Exp Dermatol 1989; 14:371–375.

Albright's syndrome will come to you as a café au lait spot. It is indistinguishable from the café au lait spots of neurofibromatosis, although melanotic macules that are larger, fewer in number, unilateral, or segmental favor the presence of Albright's syndrome. But most of all, a jagged, serrated margin (coast of Maine) to the large café au lait spot asks for further investigation into the possibility of the two major indices of Albright's syndrome.

The one is an **endocrine survey**, classically spurred on by a history of precocious puberty. One may find endocrine adenomas, acromegaly, or a host of endocrinopathies. The other is the search for **bone changes** either gross or radiographic. Deformities of bowing, swelling of the bone, or fracture suggest the essential presence of polyostotic fibrous dysplasia. Under the x-ray, the scene may be one of cysts, sclerosis, or a thickened cortex. The femur is a favored locus.

So when we see a café au lait spot that looks not like a splash of coffee but like coffee spilled on the skin, we search for Albright's child.

Moss C, Ince P: Anhidrotic and achromians lesions in **incontinentia pigmenti**. Br J Dermatol 1987; 116:839–849.

In a 22-year-old woman streaks of alopecia on the scalp and bizarre Chinese figurate hypopigmented streaks on the backs of the legs were of mysterious origin. Present since the age of 2 years, the streaks on the scalp represented cicatricial alopecia. The **hypopigmented streaks** on the backs of the legs showed atrophy, loss of hair, and loss of the ability to sweat. She also had hard, tender, warty periungual tumors of three fingers and two thumbs, with the adjacent nail being dystrophic. These disappeared spontaneously over an 8-month period.

By history, there had been no prior skin disease, but screening of the pediatrician's neonatal records solved the mystery. There had been papules, vesicles, and plaques in a linear distribution that indicated that this patient's problem of 20 years was the burned-out scarring phase of **incontinentia pigmenti**.

Study of ten other women with incontinentia pigmenti confirmed the view that hypopigmented and/or alopecic streaks are a feature of incontinentia pigmenti. This should prove to be of diagnostic usefulness in women who know of no skin disease prior to the appearance of their streaks.

The streaky loss of sweat glands may be so extensive as to be responsible for heat intolerance, as observed in one of their patients.

O'Brien JE, Feingold M: **Incontinentia pigmenti**: A longitudinal study. Am J Dis Child 1985; 139:711–712.

Long-term follow-up of 15 patients (14 females) with **incontinentia pigmenti** revealed great variability in skin lesions, with occasional persistence of bullous lesions to age 6 and verrucous lesions to age 11. Vesiculobullous lesions were the first sign in most children.

Skin lesions:

hyperpigmented	15
at birth	2
verrucous	9
bullous	13
partial alopecia	9
pegged or widespread teeth	12

Development was normal in 12, but 2 patients had neonatal seizures and developmental delay.

Avrahami E, Harel S, Jurgenson U, Cohn DF: Computed tomographic demonstration of brain changes in **incontinentia pigmenti**. Am J Dis Child 1985; 139:372–374.

Diffuse brain atrophy was found by computed tomography in two girls (ages 2 and 11 years) with incontinentia pigmenti and central nervous system symptoms.

Tanigaki T, Endo H: A case of **epidermodysplasia verruciformis** (Lewandowsky-Lutz, 1922) with skin cancer: Histopathology of malignant cutaneous changes. Dermatologica 1984; 169:97–101.

A 34-year-old Japanese man had dark-brown plaques and **red plaques** intermixed with **flat wartlike lesions** on the chest wall and shoulders. A clinical diagnosis of **pityriasis versicolor** and **actinic keratoses** was made. However, he had first developed verrucous lesions on the forehead, chest, back, and extremities at age 7 years, and when he was in his 20s, invasive squamous cell carcinoma and multiple actinic keratoses and lesions of Bowen's disease had appeared. Eventually, recurrent **squamous cell carcinoma** near the left eye necessitated removal of the eyeball.

Epidermodysplasia verruciformis commonly presents as a pityriasis versicolor-like eruption with disseminate flat warts. Watch out for malignant change.

Gross G, Ellinger K, Roussaki A, et al: Epidermodysplasia verruciformis in a patient with Hodgkin's disease: Characterization of a new papillomavirus type and interferon treatment. J Invest Dermatol 91:43–48, 1988.

Tinea versicolor-like lesions (reddish, slightly scaling plaques) of the neck, face, scalp, and pubic region in a 42-year-old man with Hodgkin's disease proved on biopsy to be **epidermodysplasia verruciformis**. The lesions were limited to previously irradiated and ultraviolet light–exposed areas. A new human papillomavirus (**HPV 46**) was found in the lesions.

Allegue F, España A, Fernandez-Garcia JM, Ledo A: Segmental **neurofibromatosis** with contralateral lentiginosis. Clin Exp Dermatol 1989; 14:448–450.

Partial unilateral lentiginosis has been suspected as a forme fruste of neurofibromatosis (NF). The complete linkage is provided in this 37-year-old woman who had **multiple hyperpigmented macules** on the left side of the trunk since infancy. On biopsy, they proved to be lentigo simplex, making the diagnosis of partial unilateral lentiginosis.

By the time she was age 22 years, soft pigmented papules appeared in a dermatomal distribution on the right breast. Two large café au lait spots were also seen on the left side of the abdomen. Biopsy of the papules revealed them to be **neurofibromas**. This favored viewing her problem as a conjunction of lentigines and NF. Each respected its half of the body, but both may be presumed to have a common genetic background.

Interestingly, no one else in the family, including the grandparents, had any ephelides, lentigines, café au lait spots, or other stigmata of NF.

The urge to classify now leads to **eight types of NF**:

NF1:   Von Recklinghausen's classic of multiple café au lait spots, Lisch nodules of the iris, multiple neurofibromas
NFII: Acoustic form with bilateral acoustic neurofibromas as well
NFIII: Mixed expression of NF1 and NF2
NFIV: Variant form with variable family history
NFV: Café au lait spots or neurofibromas in unilateral segment
NFVI: Only café au lait spots
NFVII: Onset after age of 30 years
NFVIII: None of above.

Precision diagnosis may be possible in the near future now that NF is known to represent a gene on chromosome 17 and NFII on chromosome 22.

Sparrow GP, Samman PD, Wells RS: Hyperpigmentation and hypohidrosis (the **Naegeli-Franceschetti-Jadassohn syndrome**): Report of a family and review of the literature. Clin Exp Dermatol 1976; 1:127–140.

Early in life (2 to 6 years), seven individuals from one family developed:

symmetrical, freckled hyperpigmentation (neck, upper trunk, axillae, groin, antecubital and popliteal fossae) with ill-defined margins and ephelid-like areas. Possibly postinflammatory.
heat intolerance (functional hypohidrosis) with flushing and discomfort in hot weather and inability to work outdoors
hand and foot changes, with combinations of:
dry palms
punctate hyperkeratosis (palms, soles)
onycholysis (toenails, fingernails)
subungual hyperkeratosis (fingers, toes)
fingerprints with loss of ridging (acquired hypoplastic dermatoglyphics) on the palms and soles, possibly secondary to hypohidrosis
blisters on the soles
patchy atrophy of the cheeks
yellow spots on the teeth (from defective enamel and multiple caries)

The **differential diagnosis** of hyperpigmentation, hypohidrosis, and onychodystrophy includes:

1.   Dyskeratosis congenita

Similarities:

pigmentation (widespread, sheeted or reticulated)	fingerprint hypoplasia
hyperkeratosis (palmar, plantar)	atrophic changes
	bullae on feet

Differences:
normal heat tolerance
normal sweating (except hyperhidrosis of palms, soles)

leukoplakia (early death from squamous cell carcinoma of tongue, esophagus, rectum, cervix)
gingivitis
sparse hair
tearing (closed lacrimal puncta)
anemia (Fanconi type) with splenomegaly
X-linked recessive transmission

2. Pachyonychia congenita

Similarities:

pigmentation (rare)	neonatal onset
autosomal dominant transmission	hyperkeratosis (palmar, plantar)

Differences:

normal sweating	anomalies of teeth, hair, eyes (rare)
thick nails	follicular hyperkeratosis
leukoplakia	normal fingerprints

3. Anhidrotic ectodermal defect

Similarities:

heat intolerance	fingerprint hypoplasia
hypohidrosis	dental anomalies

Differences:

normal pigmentation	alopecia
X-linked recessive	normal nails

4. Incontinentia pigmenti

Similarities:

bullae on feet	hyperpigmentation	dental anomalies

Differences:

onset 0 to 2 months	no hyperkeratosis
alopecia	erythematous phase
normal nails	normal fingerprints
X-linked dominant (lethal in males)	eye anomalies

Rebora A, Crovato F: The spectrum of **Dowling-Degos disease**. Br J Dermatol 1984; 110:627–630.

The basic diagnostic triad of Dowling-Degos disease consists of reticulate pigmented macules, hyperkeratotic follicular lesions with or without pitted scars, and facial erythema. This autosomal genodermatosis, with variable expression, appears in the literature as:

Dowling-Degos disease (reticulate dark macules in flexural areas, medial aspect of the thighs, neck, wrists, scrotum, face, scalp; comedo-like hyperkeratotic follicular lesions; pitted acneiform scars on face)

Haber's syndrome (flushed face with telangiectases, hyperkeratotic follicular papules, pitted scars.)

Kitamura's acropigmentatio reticularis (reticulate, slightly depressed pigmentation on extensor surfaces of hands and feet; milia-sized keratotic papules on palms and fingers)

Pigmentatio reticularis faciei et colli with cystomatosis (brown-black reticulate macules on face, neck; multiple epithelial cysts on chest, back)

Familial multiple follicular hamartoma (miliary, whitish, cystic nodules on cheeks, eyelids, chest; larger cysts on forehead, labia majora, perineum, perianal area)

Perhaps Dowling-Degos disease should be thought of as the "United States" of reticulate, pigmented macules.

Rhodes AR, Silverman RA, Harrist TJ, Perez-Atayde AR: Mucocutaneous lentigines, cardiomucocutaneous myxomas, and multiple blue nevi: The **"LAMB" syndrome**. J Am Acad Dermatol 1984; 10:72–82.

During infancy and early childhood, small **brown spots** had appeared on the face of this girl. They were also present on the lips, but caused no concern. At age 9, discrete black macules first appeared on the vulva.

Sudden onset of congestive heart failure when she was 10 led to the discovery of a right atrial mass, partially occluding the tricuspid valve. Resection of this friable gelatinous tumor immediately corrected the cardiac failure. Over time, she developed opalescent papules and nodules on various sites, including the tongue and the vulva.

When she was seen at age 13, biopsies of the brown macules revealed lentigines; the black papules were blue nevi. The cardiac tumor was an **atrial myxoma**, and the opalescent papules and **dermal nodules** were **also myxomas**.

The acronym LAMB was used to describe this constellation of *l*entigines, *a*trial myxomas, *m*ucocutaneous myxomas, *b*lue nevi. An alternate acronym is NAME (*n*evi, *a*trial myxoma, *m*yxoid neurofibromas, *e*phelides). Individuals with multiple melanocytes and myxomatous tumors of the skin and mucosa deserve complete cardiac study for atrial myxomas.

A LAMB by any other NAME calls for biopsy of insignificant papules or nodules in a search for the cutaneous or mucosal myxoma pointing to curable heart disease. The lentigines will alert you.

Iijima S, Naito Y, Naito S, Uyeno K: **Reticulate hyperpigmentation** distributed in a zosteriform fashion: A new clinical type of hyperpigmentation. Br J Dermatol 1987; 117:503–510.

There have now been four cases of this **reticulate pigmentation** in children reported from Japan. Widespread hyperpigmentation in a linear and **zosteriform pattern** appeared in a $1\frac{1}{2}$-month-old baby, with no previous history of inflammatory lesions. It was asymptomatic, sparing the face, palms, and soles. No pigment incontinence was seen on histology. After age $1\frac{1}{2}$ years the spots started to fade. Eosinophilia was present with a 13% increase (absolute count 1.2×10^9/liter). The family history was negative for incontinentia pigmenti.

Review of the literature leaves a **differential** of:

progressive cribriform and zosteriform hyperpigmentation (adolescence, lower torso, single zosteriform area)

progressive zosteriform macular pigmented lesions (lower torso, mild itching at first)

nevoid macular amyloidosis (lower abdomen and legs, linear or arcuate confluent macules, biopsy showing amyloid)

reticular acral pigmentation (acropigmentatio reticularis) (acral, may be reticulate, lesions depressed, biopsy showing epidermal atrophy)

familial pigmentary anomaly (positive family history, chin, neck, freckle-like, reticulate lesions)

familial progressive hyperpigmentation (positive family history, present at birth, zosteriform reticulate whorls and streaks, buccal mucosa and conjunctival hyperpigmentation).

incontinentia pigmenti (Bloch-Sulzberger syndrome, neonatal females, generalized, zosteriform whorls or streaks, preceded by erythema and bullae, later hyperkeratosis)

incontinentia pigmenti achromians (Ito). (neonatal, generalized, zosteriform whorls and streaks of hypopigmentation in reverse pattern to incontinentia pigmenti)

Granstein RD, Sober AJ: Drug- and heavy metal–induced **hyperpigmentation**. J Am Acad Dermatol 1981; 5:1–18.

A few examples:

blue-black: antimalarials, tetracyclines
slate gray: mercury, silver
blue gray: bismuth, gold, amiodarone
bronze: arsenic, ACTH
brown-black: busulfan, bleomycin, doxorubicin, 5-fluorouracil

yellow: beta-carotene
red: clofazimine
violet: phenothiazines

Heavy metals produce increased pigmentation because of deposition of metal particles in the dermis and increased epidermal melanin production.

Gingival hyperpigmentation is seen with mercury, silver, bismuth, and lead exposure.

Arsenic causes diffuse bronze pigmentation with "raindrop" areas of sparing or depigmentation, most prominent on the trunk.

Mercury causes slate-gray pigmentation, which is increased in the skin folds and most pronounced on the eyelids, nasolabial folds, and folds of the neck.

Silver causes slate-gray pigmentation most prominent in sun-exposed areas with relative sparing of skin folds. The sclerae, nails, and mucous membranes become hyperpigmented.

Bismuth causes a distinctive blue-black line at the gingival margin and may cause generalized blue-gray pigmentation resembling argyria, including the conjunctivae and oral mucosa.

Gold causes argyria-like blue-gray pigmentation (chrysiasis) limited to sun-exposed areas and very pronounced about the eyes.

Lead causes a "lead hue," which is a mixture of pallor and lividity of the skin. It also produces a lead line at the gingival margin.

Iron salts may cause dark-brown discoloration at sites of application to broken skin.

Many systemic drugs produce diffuse or localized pigmentation:

antimalarials:
phenothiazines:
tetracyclines:

blue-black
violet to deep-purple–gray metallic
blue to gray-black
yellow-brown conjunctivae
  (methacycline)

busulfan (Myleran):
bleomycin:
doxorubicin (Adriamycin):
5-fluorouracil:

brown
brown streaks
black-brown
brown

Dark pigmentation or bands of pigment of the nail beds may occur with several chemotherapeutic agents: cyclophosphamide, melphalan, bleomycin, doxorubicin, daunorubicin.

Gross DJ, Dellinger RP: **Red/orange person syndrome**. Cutis 1988; 42:175–177.

An 18-year-old Hispanic woman brought into the emergency room at 5:30 AM gave a history of having awakened at 3:30 AM with generalized pruritus, to find that her **skin, tears, and urine had turned orange overnight**. She also had headache, lethargy, and nausea.

The cause: 40 **rifampicin** capsules (300 mg) she had taken at 12:30 AM to commit suicide.

The course: normal color skin by the second day, although the bilirubin peaked at 2.8 that day. The urine and body secretions remained bright orange for a much longer period.

In the emergency room, other color changes in the urine or blood may point to ingested poisons or drugs. The urine ferric chloride test turns purple with salicylates and brown with phenothiazines. Wood's light illumination of urine reveals fluorescence due to antifreeze poisoning. In the blood, a chocolate-brown color occurs with methemoglobinemia.

Rogers SCF, McCabe MMM: **Skin pigmentation** due to minocycline therapy for acne vulgaris. Br J Dermatol 1984; 111 (suppl 26):59–60.

Blue-black pigmentation, resembling tattooing from coal dust, appeared in facial acne scars of a 22-year-old woman. Initially the pigmentation was thought to be due to deposition of aluminum silicate from a face mask. However, biopsy showed perivascular macrophages filled with gray pigment suggestive of sulfur on electron-probe analysis.

She had been taking minocycline (100 mg bid) for 5 months, known to produce pigmentation at sites of inflammation. **Minocycline-induced** pigmentation was confirmed by the fact that it completely disappeared 9 months after the minocycline was stopped.

Mahler R, Sissons W, Watters K: Pigmentation induced by quinidine therapy. Arch Dermatol 1986; 122:1062–1064.

Slowly progressive **bluish-gray** discoloration of the shins, hard palate, tip of the nose, ears, and forearms puzzled an 83-year-old man and his physician. He also had horizontal blue-gray striations on the fingernails and toenails that did not advance over several months. He was not taking minocycline, chlorpromazine, or chloroquine. Biopsy showed an unidentifiable pigment in perivascular dermal histiocytes. For 9 years, however, he had been taking quinidine sulfate (600 mg qid). Since **quinidine** is structurally related to chloroquine, a well-known cause of similar pigmentation, the quinidine was discontinued. Within months the skin reverted to normal color.

Guillet G, Guillet M-H, de Meaux H, et al: Cutaneous pigmented stripes and bleomycin treatment. Arch Dermatol 1986; 122:381–382.

The **factitial-like streaks of pigmentation** seen in bleomycin-treated patients actually represent the exact sites of **scratching** or rubbing.

It was seen in 10 of 15 patients treated with polychemotherapy that included **bleomycin** sulfate (160 mg). Although the patients denied pruritus, the linear stripes of pigment could be reproduced in the hospital with gentle skin rubbing in all patients. Possibly a dermographic mechanism with local vasodilatation caused excessive accumulation of bleomycin and subsequent increased melanin production.

Merenich JA, Hannon RN, Gentry RH, Harrison SM: Azidothymidine-induced **hyperpigmentation** mimicking primary adrenal insufficiency. Am J Med 1989; 86:469–470.

A 32-year-old black woman with human immunodeficiency virus, recurrent mucocutaneous fungal infections, and a profoundly depressed CD_4 lymphocyte count was given azidothymidine (AZT, 200 mg every 4 hours).

Six months later a **bluish discoloration of the nail lunulae** was noted. Several months later the palmar creases became hyperpigmented, and punctate dots of pigment were seen on the face, trunk, extremities, and on the soft palate, gingiva, lips, and tongue. It was erroneously assumed that the pigmentation was evidence of an adrenal insufficiency state, but corticosteroid therapy was stopped when the ACTH level was found to be normal.

Within 2 months of stopping the AZT therapy, all of the skin and oral lesions decreased in size, number, and intensity. A diagnosis of **AZT-induced hyperpigmentation** was made.

The blue lunulae of AZT therapy may also be mistaken for cyanosis. But it is the mucosal and palmar crease hyperpigmentation that can lead to a misdiagnosis of adrenal insufficiency.

Shelley WB, Shelley ED, Burmeister V: **Argyria**: The intradermal "photograph," a manifestation of passive photosensitivity. J Am Acad Dermatol 1987; 16:211–217.

The treatment of varicose veins with a silver nitrate sclerosant 41 years ago accounted for the dark **blue-black pigmentation** of this elderly man's legs, face, and neck. All sun-exposed areas were pigmented, since the photoreduction of the silver compounds leads to a tattoo of elemental **silver**.

Electron-probe microanalysis allowed distinction of the metallic pigmentation of skin from that of gold, bismuth, or mercury.

Larsen FS, Boye H, Hage E: **Chrysiasis**: Electron microscopic studies and x-ray microanalysis. Clin Exp Dermatol 1984; 9:174–180.

A permanent **bluish discoloration** of the face and hands in a 71-year-old woman became evident after 4 years of intravenous **aurothiosulfate** (100 mg/week). The color was most obvious in light-exposed areas, especially the forehead and periorbital regions, and became more prominent in cold weather. Cyanosis, chrysiasis, and argyria were the main diagnostic considerations. Skin biopsy revealed coarse brown to blue deposits in the perivascular histiocytes.

X-ray microanalysis of a skin biopsy showed deposits of **gold** in macrophages, leading to a diagnosis of chrysiasis. The concentration of gold in the skin, determined by neutron activation analysis, was 75 parts/million.

Chrysiasis occurs in all aurothiosulfate-treated patients receiving a total dose of more than 150 mg/kg of body weight, but not in those receiving less than 50 mg/kg.

Green P, Eviatar JM, Sirota P, Avidor I: Secondary hemochromatosis due to prolonged iron ingestion. Isr J Med Sci 1989; 25:199–201.

A 45-year-old man with chronic paranoid schizophrenia had diffuse, dark-yellowish **pigmentation** of the skin. The liver and spleen were palpable just below the costal margin. For over 15 years he had taken up to 1000 mg of iron (ferrum fumarate tablets) daily. Blood studies showed hemoglobin 15.0 gm/dl, serum iron 280 µg/dl, total iron-binding capacity 428 µ/dl, transferrin saturation 66%, and serum ferritin 3,125 ng/ml (normal range 20 to 150).

The liver was shown to be slightly enlarged on isotope scan, and a liver biopsy showed evidence of fibrosis with excessive stainable iron in hepatocytes and Kupffer cells, compatible with hemochromatosis.

Since he had no evidence of familial idiopathic hemochromatosis, alcoholism, or hemolytic anemia, it was assumed that the **hemochromatosis** was secondary to longstanding massive **iron ingestion**. Similar cases are very rare.

Teitelbaum DT, Kier LC: **Arsine poisoning**—report of five cases in the petroleum industry and a discussion of the indications for exchange transfusion and hemodialysis. Arch Environ Health 1969; 19:133–143.

Arsine gas (AsH_3) was produced by interaction between zinc-galvanized pipe and hydrochloric acid (HCl) containing sodium meta-arsenite ($NaAsO_2$). Of five men exposed one died within 30 minutes following tingling of the hands and feet, vomiting, and chest pain; three had minor exposure without major symptoms; and one had massive hemolysis and renal failure.

This last patient was a peculiar **mottled gray-green color** and initially noted tingling of the hands and feet and violent nausea and vomiting. He then became extremely flushed and had headache and severe abdominal pain. Serum and urine were a deep burgundy-red, and urine had 4+ albumin and a few red blood cells. The following day the skin was a coppery hue with patches of gray-green cyanosis over the trunk and extremities. The sclerae were red, suggesting massive subconjunctival hemorrhage. Hands and feet were icy cold, he was anuric, and had profuse vomiting and green diarrhea. He appeared moribund, but recovered after immediate exchange transfusion and hemodialysis. The copper hue disappeared after 3 days.

Arsine gas binds to red blood cells and causes massive hemolysis in a non-dialyzable form, leading to renal failure. This patient's blood arsenic level was 220 µg/liter 24 hours after exposure and 20 µg/liter after exchange transfusion and dialysis. Five days after the accident the arsenic level was 60 µg/liter in the nails and 960 µg/liter in the hair.

1st level diagnosis—name the disease
2nd level diagnosis—name the associations
3rd level diagnosis—name the cause

Ackerman Z, Michaeli J, Gorodetsky R: Skin discoloration in **chronic idiopathic thrombocytopenic purpura**: Detection of local iron deposition by x-ray spectrometry. Dermatologica 1986; 172:222–224.

Diagnostic x-ray spectrometry, a method employing soft x-ray fluorescence analysis, can be used for noninvasive determination of trace elements in skin. It was employed here to assay iron and zinc in black-brown pigmentation of the lower legs, revealing a striking increase in iron content. The ankles showed an iron level of 550 µg/gm, with only 9 µg/gm in the noninvolved arm. Zinc levels were normal in all sites tested.

The patient was a 46-year-old woman with idiopathic thrombocytopenic purpura for 32 years, who over 1 year developed deep **brown-black discoloration** of the legs. The pigmentation was most apparent on the knees, calves, ankles, and dorsal aspect of the feet. This type of pigment is commonly associated with **iron overload**, which presumably accumulated because of recurrent purpura of the legs.

Marks VJ, Briggaman RA, Wheeler CE Jr: Hyperpigmentation in megaloblastic anemia. J Am Acad Dermatol 1985; 12:914–917.

For 2 years this 65-year-old woman had watched her **entire skin gradually darken**. There was associated fatigue, shortness of breath, loss of taste and smell, tingling of the fingers and toes, and, ironically, lightening of hair color.

Serum B_{12} proved to be less than 50 pg/ml (normal 180 to 900 pg/ml) and hemoglobin was 11.3 gm/dl. Values for serum folate, iron, iron-binding capacity, ferritin, cortisol, adrenocorticotropic hormone, and routine chemistry were normal. A diagnosis of **pernicious anemia** was made.

Cyanocobalamin (B_{12}) 1 mg intramuscularly a month after a loading dose of 1 mg/week for the first month produced notable pigment lightening within 3 months. She no longer saw the streaks of dark in the nail beds. By 9 months, skin color was back to normal.

B_{12} deficiency is a definite cause of hyperpigmentation even as folate deficiency is. Both are reversible.

In all instances of **generalized acquired hyperpigmentation**, think of:

Autoimmune disease:	systemic sclerosis
Endocrinologic disease:	myxedema, Graves' disease, Addison's disease
Nutritional causes:	malnutrition, starvation
Liver disease:	cirrhosis, hemochromatosis, Wilson's disease
Metabolic disorder:	porphyria
Chemicals:	arsenic, busulfan

Morlock CG: **Hemochromatosis**: Report of a case in which tuberculous peritonitis was a complication. Ann Intern Med 1940; 13:2341–2346.

A 54-year-old electrical engineer with abdominal pain, enlarged liver, and ascites had a striking dusky, cyanotic, **grayish-brown color of the face** that began 8 years earlier. The skin was dry, and definite brown metallic pigmentation was noted on the hands, forearms, and legs, and to a lesser extent on the rest of the body. The palmar creases were sharply defined by the pigment. No pigment was present in the mouth, but the mouth and tongue were smooth and cherry-red. Slight scleral icterus was present. Ascitic fluid contained a high concentration of protein. At autopsy the liver was dark bronze.

Hyperpigmentation in **hemochromatosis** is due to two pigments, hemosiderin (iron containing) and hemofuscin (related to melanin, no iron). In this patient, hemosiderin was found in most organs, including the skin, in which it was localized in the sweat glands.

Felty AR: **Chronic arthritis** in the adult, associated with splenomegaly and leucopenia. A report of five cases of an unusual clinical syndrome. Johns Hopkins Hosp Bull 1924; 35:16–23.

All five **Felty's syndrome** patients had **yellowish-brown pigmentation** of the skin, confined to exposed surfaces in four, but also over the abdomen, axillae, and flexor surface of arms in one patient.

Toone EC Jr: Cerebral manifestations of **bacterial endocarditis**. Ann Intern Med 1941; 14:1551–1574.

Café au lait coloring associated with clubbed fingers, splenomegaly, and conjunctival petechiae suggests acute bacterial endocarditis, with emboli to the brain and resulting meningoencephalitis. Cardiac signs may be absent.

Stuckey BG, Mastaglia FL, Reed WD, Pullan PT: **Glucocorticoid insufficiency**, achalasia, alacrima with autonomic and motor neuropathy. Ann Intern Med 1987; 106:62–64.

A 21-year-old white woman with alacrima (no tears) since infancy had hyperpigmentation of the nipples, abdominal scar, and extensor surface of forearms, with no vitiligo. Fungiform papillae were present on the tongue. The pupils were fixed and dilated, and symmetrical distal muscle wasting was marked in the limbs, along with mild global weakness.

Past history revealed that the hyperpigmentation was present at age 6 years, along with hypoglycemia, low plasma cortisol level, and lack of response to cosyntropin. At age 12 years she was found to have achalasia, with vomiting of undigested food, nocturnal cough, and recurrent chest infections.

She appeared to have a previously described syndrome of glucocorticoid deficiency, achalasia, and alacrima, together with widespread autonomic neuropathy and progressive loss of adrenal function.

David M, Shanon A, Hazaz B, Sandbank M: Diffuse, progressive **hyperpigmentation**: An unusual skin manifestation of mycosis fungoides. J Am Acad Dermatol 1987; 16:257–260.

For the past year this 80-year-old man had been troubled with very pruritic patches of **hyperpigmentation**. They were appearing progressively on the face, axillae, chest, abdomen, and groin. The borders were ill defined, and virtually the whole back was hyperpigmented. There were no other signs of disease.

A **skin biopsy** disclosed the cause: **mycosis fungoides**. The patient refused treatment and died 6 months later during staphylococcal sepsis.

In its early phases, mycosis fungoides may simulate seborrheic dermatitis, psoriasis, or eczema. Indeed, atypical bullous hyperkeratotic or verrucous forms may occur. Although hypopigmentation may occur, this is the first example of hyperpigmentation being the initial and solitary sign of mycosis fungoides. Significantly, such hyperpigmentation is recognized as a nonspecific sign of leukemia and cancer, as well as Hodgkin's lymphoma.

Sexton M, Snyder CR: Generalized **melanosis** in occult primary melanoma. J Am Acad Dermatol 1989; 20:261–266.

The patient was a 34-year-old white woman who reported a 2-month history of progressive **slate-gray pigmentation**. She had lost 10 to 12 pounds because of associated nausea and vomiting.

Examination showed pigmentation most noticeable over hands and face, accentuated over acne scars, and present in sclerae as well as oral mucosa. Biopsy showed no hyperpigmentation in the epidermis and no melanoma cells, but did show free melanin in the dermis. Darkening was rapidly progressive, and hospitalization studies were indicated.

Computed tomography of the abdomen revealed ascites, and on paracentesis, 2 liters of dark-brown fluid were removed. A subsequent scan disclosed a mass behind the uterus. On laparotomy the peritoneum and bowel were melanotic and the ovaries deep black, as well as enlarged to several times normal. The ovaries were removed and found to be diffusely replaced by **metastatic melanoma**. The patient survived for 6 months, but the primary site of the melanoma was never found.

Occult melanoma must enter the diagnosis of any case of unexplained darkening of the skin, whether it be gun metal in color, slate-gray, slate blue, or blue-black.

Nelson BR, Ramsey ML, Bruce S, et al: **Asymptomatic progressive hyperpigmentation** in a 16-year-old girl. Arch Dermatol 1988; 124:769–772.

This girl had an asymptomatic **hyperpigmented macular eruption** of the entire body for 4 years. The bluish-gray macules began on the arms and gradually enlarged and coalesced, often with transitory erythematous raised borders that faded in a few days. They spared the scalp, palms, soles, and mucous membranes.

This is an example of **erythema dyschromicum perstans** (erythema perstans group). It has eluded all attempts to find its cause, except that there have been reports associating it with whipworm infection and ammonium nitrate ingestion.

The **differential diagnosis** includes:

fixed drug eruption	argyria
figurate erythemas	Addison's disease
urticaria pigmentosa	hemochromatosis
lichen planus	pinta (carate)
pediculosis (maculae ceruleae)	

Hisler BM, Savoy LB: **Acanthosis nigricans** of the forehead and fingers associated with hyperinsulinemia. Arch Dermatol 1987; 123:1441–1442.

Asymptomatic **darkening of the forehead** and neck for 7 years led a 64-year-old obese man to medical attention. The lesions were hyperpigmented velvety plaques of the forehead, elbows, dorsal interphalangeal joints, axillae, and posterior area of the neck. **Acanthosis nigricans** was confirmed by biopsy. He also had palmar and plantar hyperkeratosis.

Despite a normal blood sugar level, he had a greatly elevated fasting serum insulin level of 89 μU/ml (normal 7 to 25 μU/mL). There were no antibodies to insulin, indicating tissue resistance to insulin. Since insulin binds to and activates receptors for growth-promoting factor (thereby favoring cell growth), the **high insulin levels** were felt to account for the acanthosis nigricans.

Al Rustom K, Gérard J, Piérard GE: **Extrapituitary neuroendocrine melanoderma**: Unique association of extensive melanoderma with macromelanosomes and extrapituitary secretion of a high molecular weight neuropeptide related to pro-opiomelanocortin. Dermatologica 1986; 173:157–162.

For 10 years a 47-year-old woman had noted progressive **darkening** of the skin, first involving sun-exposed areas and later extending over the entire body. Examination showed **addisonian-like pigmentation**, particularly marked in the palmar and plantar creases, but unevenly distributed on the trunk. It was mottled in the darker areas with confluence of multiple hypopigmented and hyperpigmented macules 2 to 4 mm in diameter. The oral mucosa was studded with many gray-brown spots. Skin biopsy showed that the melanin content of the keratinocytes and dermal macrophages was increased, with many macromelanosomes observed. Focal necrosis of solitary epidermal cells was also present.

Laboratory study disclosed a **high ACTH level** of 800 pg/ml (normal 10 to 100 pg/ml) due to the presence of a cross-related melanocyte-stimulating neuropeptide, possibly an aggregate of pro-opiomelanocortin (a precursor molecule of ACTH). By intravenous catheter sampling, it was possible to selectively localize the source of this neuropeptide to the lower cerebral stem, showing that it was of ectopic and not pituitary origin. However, computed tomography and other procedures failed to disclose any tumor.

Goldblatt J, Beighton P: Cutaneous manifestations of **Gaucher disease**. Br J Dermatol 1984; 111:331–334.

In 50 South African patients with type 1 non-neuropathic adult Gaucher disease, the singular skin finding was **yellow-bronze hyperpigmentation** with easy tanning. Another nonspecific finding of "diagnostic-alert" value was brown macules, which had a flitting course.

These patients, most often of Ashkenazi Jewish ancestry, have a disorder of glycosphingolipid metabolism due to an autosomal recessive **deficiency** of the lysosomal hydrolase, **acid-beta-glucosidase**. This favors **increased melanocyte activity**. Other observers have recorded streaky chloasma-like patches of nonspecific distribution, black scars following hemorrhagic furunculosis on the extremities, and symmetrical hyperpigmentation of the lower legs with sharp cutoffs just below the ankle and knee. Rarely these patients also show a malar flush.

Secondary skin changes include purpura, ecchymoses, pallor, jaundice, and spider angiomas resulting from liver and bone marrow infiltration. Splenomegaly, dyshemopoiesis, and bone cysts may also be found. The course is chronic and not life threatening.

Noppakun N, Swasdikul D: Reversible **hyperpigmentation** of skin and nails with white hair due to vitamin B_{12} deficiency. Arch Dermatol 1986; 122:896–899.

For 1 year a 43-year-old Oriental man in Bangkok suffered from weakness, weight loss, and progressive **hyperpigmentation** of the skin, which began as multiple spots on the dorsal area of the hands and feet, on the palms and soles, soon spreading to the nose and face. He was anemic (hemoglobin 7.1 gm/dl), but folic acid therapy was without effect. By the time of hospitalization, his entire skin was very dark. The fingernails and toenails appeared bluish-black with transverse and longitudinal pigmented streaks. In contrast, his **hair was totally white** and his tongue was beefy red and tender, with darkening of the mucosa. He also had paresthesias of the tips of his fingers and toes, and weakness of the proximal arm and leg muscles. The medical history provided no clues, as his diet was normal, the family history was noncontributory, and he denied illness, alcoholism, or drug abuse.

The answer came with hematologic study that showed **pernicious anemia**. Within 24 hours of cyanocobalamin therapy (100 mg IM) he felt much better, and with continued **vitamin B$_{12}$** therapy for a month the tongue and hemoglobin were normal. In the second month of treatment the hyperpigmentation decreased. After 3 months skin color was normal, and after 6 months 90% of the scalp hair was black. He continues to receive cyanocobalamin (100 mg IM) monthly.

Leibowitz MR, Weiss R, Smith EH: **Pityriasis rotunda**: A cutaneous sign of malignant disease in two patients. Arch Dermatol 1983; 119:607–609.

A 60-year-old South African black man in the hospital for evaluation of hepatosplenomegaly was noted to have eight strikingly **round patches of scaling** on the chest, abdomen, and back. They measured 3 to 10 cm in diameter and were noninflammatory.

No fungi could be found on microscopic examination or culture. A biopsy showed mild hyperkeratosis, absence of granular cell layer, and absence of acanthosis. This permitted a diagnosis of **pityriasis rotunda**. Further investigation showed the patient had a leukocyte count of 137,000/mm^3 and the hematologic pattern of chronic myeloid leukemia.

The skin changes of pityriasis rotunda always suggest a diagnosis of **tinea corporis**, tinea versicolor, or erythrasma. The biopsy is consistent with the pattern of ichthyosis, and indeed pityriasis rotunda may be a subset of ichthyosis.

The pathogenesis is **mysterious**, but a small percentage of these patients do have malignant disease. Also noteworthy is the fact that this circle of scaling does not occur in Americans or American blacks. It has appeared only in South African, West Indian black, or Japanese skin.

History-taking, the most clinically sophisticated procedure of medicine, is an extraordinary investigative technique: in few other forms of scientific research does the observed talk.

ALVAN FEINSTEIN

Contactants

Coffman K, Boyce WT, Hansen RC: **Phytophotodermatitis** simulating child abuse. Am J Dis Child 1985; 139:239–240.

Bizarre linear, digitate, and loop-shaped patterns of uniform deep-brown **hyperpigmentation** on the chest, back, and arms occurred in two children. Both had been exposed to lime juice and sunlight.

A 4-year-old girl developed these "bruises" 3 days after returning from Mexico and had lesions on the back in a handprint configuration, although trauma was denied. She had been exposed to lime juice at a beach party. A 14-month-old boy had also been touched during a party by adults with lime juice on their hands from preparing margaritas. Within a few days he developed handprint lesions.

Plants causing **phytophotodermatitis** include fig, lime, lemon, parsley, and celery.

Serrano G, Pujol C, Cuadra J et al.: Riehl's melanosis: **Pigmented contact dermatitis** caused by fragrances. J Am Acad Dermatol 1989; 21:1057–1060.

For 5 years this patient had been unsuccessfully treating a **patchy pigmentation** of the cheeks and forehead with **2% hydroquinone creams** and sun protection. On examination she had patchy, brown macules surrounded by ill-defined erythema. The presumed melasma was not associated with birth control pills, and she experienced no flare during pregnancy.

A focused history elicited an onset just 2 months after starting the use of a compact face powder. The diagnosis centered on pigmented contact dermatitis when laboratory tests for antinuclear and anti-DNA antibodies as well as urinary porphyrins were normal. Immunofluorescent studies of the biopsy also ruled out hyperpigmented lupus erythematosus.

Standard patch testing with the scout tray as well as the cosmetic face powder gave no evidence of the cause. To indict the face powder, and it still remained the prime suspect, it was necessary to apply it to the antecubital fossa twice a day for 2 weeks. Within 4 days a pruritic erythematous reaction developed, followed by light hyperpigmentation. The precise offending allergen was identified by patch testing with a 2% fragrance mix (hydroxycitronellal, geraniol, and lemon oil). Photosensitivity was ruled out by showing that irradiation of the patch test sites was without effect.

A diagnosis of **Riehl's melanosis due to perfume sensitivity** was made. Within 2 months of stopping the face powder (and the hydroquinone!) there was considerable improvement. By 6 months the skin color was completely normal.

Other examples of Riehl's melanosis in the literature have been due to dyes (orange II, brilliant lake red) in cosmetics.

Mallory SB, Miller OF III, Tyler WB: *Toxicodendron radicans* dermatitis with black lacquer deposit on the skin. J Am Acad Dermatol 1982; 6:363–368.

Twenty-four hours after playing football in the woods, this 17-year-old boy noted asymptomatic black lesions scattered over the trunk and forearms. Examination disclosed **black macular changes** overlying erythema and vesiculation.

The diagnosis was poison ivy dermatitis and a **black lacquer deposit** of undiluted sap from the poison ivy vine. It is well known that the poison ivy sap dries and blackens, but few patients have such gross exposure to the sap. The patient's clinical findings were completely reproduced by placing a drop of sap directly on the skin. Indeed, the same black lacquer deposits were noted on the plastic bag used to transport the plants to the doctor's office.

People who know more see more.

Lawrence N, Bligard CA, Reed R, Perret WJ: **Exogenous ochronosis** in the United States. J Am Acad Dermatol 1988; 18:1207–1211.

Patchy or speckled **hyperpigmentation** of the face in a black woman should make you wonder if she is using any one of a dozen over-the-counter bleach creams containing **hydroquinone**. A biopsy will show a finely granular achromatic pigment in the dermis. This deposit results from the inhibition of homogentisic acid oxidase by the hydroquinone, permitting accumulation of homogentisic acid, which then polymerizes to form the insoluble pigment.

The analogy with alkaptonuria is fascinating. The alkaptonuric patient's urine and skin are darkened, since these patients lack the enzyme homogentisic acid oxidase. In the bleach cream user, the same enzyme is locally inactivated by the bleach, with the same resultant accumulation of **homogentisic acid** and subsequent polymerization to a pigment.

Be alert to other chemicals on the skin that can produce this **paradoxical**, pigmenting ochronosis. These include such homogentisic acid oxidase inhibitors as phenol and benzene derivatives. Finally, the oral antimalarials have also been incriminated as inducing ochronosis.

Connor T, Braunstein B: **Hyperpigmentation** following the use of bleaching creams. Arch Dermatol 1987; 123:105–108.

Progressive darkening of the face for the past month brought this 72-year-old black woman to the clinic. Physical examination revealed confluent hyperpigmented blue-black macules and patches on the forehead, malar, and temporal regions. The sclerae, conjunctivae, ears, and oral mucosa were normal.

The change was symptomless. There had been no history of laxative ingestion or chemical exposure, nor was there a family history of skin disorders. However, the patient had been using a hydroquinone bleaching cream on her face since childhood.

A 2-mm biopsy showed many yellow and brown pigment granules in the dermis with the staining properties of ochronotic pigment. A diagnosis of **localized exogenous ochronosis** was made. It is to be sharply distinguished from endogenous ochronosis, since only the local skin area is affected. It is a paradoxical effect of hydroquinone in which the "lightener" becomes the "darkener."

The condition involutes once the hydroquinone usage is stopped.

Cullison D, Abele DC, O'Quinn JL: Localized **exogenous ochronosis**. Report of a case and review of literature. J Am Acad Dermatol 1983; 8:882–889.

This 50-year-old black woman had used a **2% hydroquinone bleaching cream** twice a day for 6 months to brighten her complexion. To her dismay, the **skin darkened**, so she tripled her efforts, applying the cream six times a day for the next 2 years.

When seen, her face showed a sooty blue-black hyperpigmentation. It was relatively uniform, but with some accentuation of the malar eminences and skin creases. The eyelids and ears were not involved.

On biopsy, a yellow-brown pigment was seen in swollen broken collagen bundles. A diagnosis of ochronosis was made, and negative urinary studies for homogentisic acid proved it to be **localized ochronosis**.

The continual application of hydroquinone had resulted in the formation of the **brown pigment**, **homogentisic acid**, a hydroquinone metabolite of tyrosine. Its presence in the collagen produced the blue-black color as a result of the Tyndall effect, as is seen in the blue nevus. By discontinuing the bleaching cream and using a 2.5% hydrocortisone cream, the patient's color returned to normal within $1\frac{1}{2}$ years.

Such exogenous ochronosis can be produced by other chemicals, namely, phenol, puric acid, and mercury. When used in treating ulcers for long periods, they induced local blackening similar to that produced by hydroquinone. The **differential diagnosis** for all of these must include the pigmentation seen with drugs such as the antimalarials, phenothiazines, minocycline, and amiodarone.

When asked for a diagnosis, the student replied, "It might be a fracture, sir, or it might be only sprained." To which Treves responded, "The patient is not interested to know that it might be measles, or it might be a toothache. The patient wants to know what is the matter, and it is your business to tell it to him or he will go to a quack who will inform him at once."

Sir Frederick Treves

Rycroft RJG, Calnan CD, Allenby CF: **Dermatopathia pigmentosa reticularis**. Clin Exp Dermatol 1977; 2:39–44.

Generalized **reticulate hyperpigmentation** was present in a 16-year-old girl. It began at age 2 as fine brown macules of the axillae, groin, and toe webs and spread over the trunk and limbs over the next 3 years. At age 5, hypopigmentation was noted between the dark macules, with sun exposure being unpleasant because of burning and the skin becoming leathery. At age 13 the pigment darkened on the abdomen, lower back, and breasts, and the nipples became completely black. Skin biopsy showed numerous clumps of melanin-laden macrophages in the dermis, whereas the epidermal melanin content was normal. There was no atrophy, scaling, erythema, or telangiectasia (apart from the cheeks, a family characteristic). The dermatoglyphic pattern was lost over all fingertips. Mucous membranes were normal, but the toenails were soft and atrophic with longitudinal ridging and lamellar splitting. Scalp hair was lost, especially over the vertex. Other abnormalities included partial syndactyly of the toes and slight curving of the little finger.

The **differential diagnosis** of finely reticulate hyperpigmentation includes:

1. Dyskeratosis congenita: Develops after age 5, X-linked recessive, leukoplakia, blood dyscrasia in childhood
2. Naegeli-Franceschetti-Jadassohn syndrome: Pigmentation beginning at age 2 and fading in adolescence; no alopecia
3. Familial pigmentation (Moon-Adams): Progressive pigmentation up to 6 cm in diameter in three females in one family; mucous membrane hyperpigmentation; no alopecia
4. Familial pigmentation (Becker): Pigmentation in three sisters that progressed in one after hysterectomy; no nail dystrophy or alopecia

Kalter DC: Acquired **intertriginous pigmentation**. Arch Dermatol 1985; 121:401–404.

For 5 years this 28-year-old woman has noted mild progression of multiple **oval brown macules** in the axillae, antecubital fossa, groin, and neck. Some showed a lace-like configuration of pigment, others a mild degree of hyperkeratosis, while a few were wrinkled and shiny.

The clinical **differential diagnosis** included:

acanthosis nigricans	xeroderma pigmentosum
Gougerot-Carteaud syndrome	Darier's disease
Crowe's sign of neurofibromatosis	Haber's syndrome
lentiginosis profusa	Kitamura's acropigmentation reticulosis

It proved to be none of the above, but rather "**dark-dot**" **disease of Dowling-Degos disease**. This familial nevoid anomaly shows a distinctive dappled and reticulate pattern of melanin. Small, pigmented, hyperkeratotic, follicular, and comedo-like lesions dot the neck and axillary margin. It is another rare disease to be spotted.

Brown WG: **Reticulate pigmented anomaly** of the flexures. Case reports and genetic investigation. Arch Dermatol 1982; 118:490–493.

A 35-year-old moderately retarded woman had noticed increasing pigmentation in the flexural areas for 6 years. Examination revealed symmetrical, reticulated, **brownish macules** of the neck, axillae, antecubital, intergluteal, inguinal, and popliteal areas.

Four uncles and an aunt exhibited the same delayed onset of reticulate pigmentation of the flexural areas, suggesting that the problem was an autosomal **genodermatosis**.

The pigmentation differs from that of acanthosis nigricans in that affected sites do not have a confluent, uniform, velvety appearance. The lesions do   759 not show the localization of confluent and reticulate papillomatosis (Gougerot-Carteaud) in the sternal and interscapular areas. Nor are the lesions colonized by *Pityrosporum orbiculare*. Characteristic lesions in reticulate pigmented anomaly of the flexures are brown to black hyperpigmented macules in flexural areas, which are discrete at the periphery and confluent in the center.

Hamilton D, Tavafoghi V, Shafer JC, Hambrick GW: Confluent and reticulated **papillomatosis of Gougerot and Carteaud**. J Am Acad Dermatol 1980; 2:401–410.

An intermammary localization of reticulated reddish or **brown papules** with a trace of atrophy is the classic presentation, detailed in four patients. The slightly cornified surface of the lesions soon becomes verrucous. The papules, which become confluent, do not show a true scale but rather a mealy deposit on their surface.

The **differential diagnosis** includes acanthosis nigricans (favors intertriginous areas), pseudoacanthosis nigricans (obese persons), and tinea versicolor (KOH positive).

Sau P, Lupton GP: **Reticulated truncal pigmentation**. Arch Dermatol 1988; 124:1272–1275.

An 8-month history of **dark-brown keratotic patches** on the trunk and axillae of this 14-year-old black boy led to the **diagnosis of tinea versicolor**. Failure to show fungal elements on scrapings, as well as failure to respond to selenium sulfide lotion, led to restudy.

The unique feature of the eruption was the reticulated appearance of the areas in which the verrucous keratotic lesions were not confluent. The primary lesion was a brown flat-topped papule without a true scale. Scraping produced only a mealy deposit. It was these features that led to the correct diagnosis of confluent and reticulated papillomatosis of **Gougerot and Carteaud**. Histologically the characteristic hyperkeratosis, papillomatosis, and acanthosis were all present.

Always to be considered in the **differential diagnosis** is Darier's disease and acanthosis nigricans. Darier's disease can easily be recognized histologically. Benign acanthosis nigricans does not present with a reticulated pattern, and pseudoacanthosis nigricans has the diagnostic clue of obesity.

Connor JM, Teague RH: **Dyskeratosis congenita**: Report of a large kindred. Br J Dermatol 1981; 105:321–325.

This 25-year-old man exhibited widespread **reticulate hyperpigmentation** as well as pigmented striae along the axillary folds and back. It began when he was 10 years old and had gradually increased. Also noted were patchy areas of skin pallor and atrophy.

The nails had been markedly dystrophic since he was 10. Although there were no leukoplakic patches on the buccal mucosa, they were seen on examination of the conjunctival sac. Bilateral epiphora and palmar hyperhidrosis completed the constellation of findings. The **family history** indicated X-linked recessive inheritance as well as association with a malignant potential. One cousin with the same skin findings died of Hodgkin's disease at age 25. Another relative with the pigmentary and nail changes died of adenocarcinoma of the pancreas at age 29.

A diagnosis of **dyskeratosis congenita** was made on the basis of the patient's presentation. No abnormalities were found in extensive studies of the health or immunologic status. This is an important diagnosis to make so that the patient can have close continuing surveillance for malignant disease in its early treatable stage.

The family history is your walking stick to a diagnosis in a young man with reticulate hyperpigmentation and poor nails.

Duncan WC, Tschen JA, Knox JM: **Terra firma–forme dermatosis**. Arch Dermatol 1987; 123:567–569.

A 12-year-old girl was brought in for evaluation of a **dirty neck**. Neither the mother nor the child could wash the skin clean of brownish hyperpigmentation that encircled the neck.

The clinical **differential diagnosis** list included tinea versicolor, Gougerot-Carteaud, acanthosis nigricans, epidermolytic hyperkeratosis, and idiopathic deciduous skin.

The answer came when an alcohol sponge was rubbed over the area in preparing for biopsy. The neck was immediately transformed to clean, pink skin. It is viewed as a benign cosmetic maturation defect in the keratinocyte, leading to **abnormal retention of a pigmented stratum corneum**.

Hashimoto K, Ito K, Kumakiri M, Headington J: Nylon brush **macular amyloidosis**. Arch Dermatol 1987; 123:633–637.

Poikilodermatous, reticulated, **mottled hyperpigmentation** developed on the back of a 53-year-old woman. Biopsy showed the presence of amyloid K in the papillary dermis. This **amyloid** is a modified keratin that had formed as a result of the damage inflicted on the epidermis by the patient's 10-year habit of using a nylon brush for back massage.

Considerable improvement in the discoloration was noted 4 months after the patient stopped using the nylon brush.

Miyachi Y, Yoshioka A, Horio T, et al: **Prurigo pigmentosa**: A possible mechanism of action of sulfonamides. Dermatologica 1986; 172:82–88.

A 31-year-old Japanese woman had a 4-year history of occasional attacks of itchy red papules on the back, which spread over the back with subsequent reticular pigmentation. The itching became intractable, with no help from oral antihistamines or topical steroids. Examination showed clusters of miliary-sized red papules and brownish plaques with scales or crusts and irregularly shaped **reticular hyperpigmented** areas on the back. Skin biopsy showed spongiosis, exocytosis, and liquefaction degeneration. A diagnosis of **prurigo pigmentosa** was made, and the eruption cleared rapidly with sulfamethoxazole (2.0 gm/day), with lightening of the pigmentation.

Prurigo pigmentosa occurs mainly in **adult women**, with sudden onset in the spring or summer. The pruritic red papules coalesce into a reticular pattern on the trunk and subside, leaving mottled, marble-like reticular pigmentation. The nonspecific histologic appearance is often lichenoid with incontinence of pigment. Dapsone or sulfamethoxazole may produce dramatic improvement. More than 100 cases have been reported since its first description in Japan in 1971.

The **differential diagnosis** includes:

lichen pigmentosa: pigmentation of the trunk following pruritus, but is not reticular and begins slowly—a variant of lichen planus
prurigo melanotica: itchy papules with pigmentation on the back associated with hepatic disease
pigmented contact dermatitis: contact allergy to the optical whitener, Tinopal (CH3566), causing red papules and reticular pigmentation, particularly in elderly women
dermatitis herpetiformis

Cox NH: **Prurigo pigmentosa**. Br J Dermatol 1987; 117:121–124.

A 21-year-old Chinese student developed a pruritic rash of his trunk and upper arms 3 years previously while living in Hong Kong. It resulted in a striking pattern of gross **reticulate pigmentation**, suggestive of **erythema ab igne**. Erythematous scaling papules were present in some areas of the upper trunk, neck, and shoulders, with secondary eczematization and excoriations. The papules were strictly confined to the hyperpigmented areas. Symptoms were most marked after sun exposure and exertion. Skin biopsy showed a nonspecific lichenoid reaction with dyskeratotic keratinocytes throughout the epidermis. Direct immunofluorescence was negative. A diagnosis of **prurigo pigmentosa** was made.

In prurigo pigmentosa the initial lesions are pruritic red papules that coalesce, form urticarial plaques, or become eczematized. The lesions resolve in a few days, leaving nonpruritic reticulate or mottled hyperpigmentation, particularly on the upper back, nape, and upper chest. Treatment with dapsone is quite effective. It is of unknown origin but may reflect a tendency of Oriental skin to develop **postinflammatory hyperpigmentation**.

Shimizu H, Yamasaki Y, Harada T, Nishikawa T: **Prurigo pigmentosa**: Case report with an electron microscopic observation. J Am Acad Dermatol 1985; 12:165–169.

The entire back of this 18-year-old man showed diffuse, gross, **reticular pigmentation**. Superimposed were numerous red papules with some excoriations. On the front of the chest there was a similar change forming a confluent V-shaped plaque. The eruption had been present for 2 years.

Extensive studies revealed no cause, but dapsone therapy was remarkably successful. Immunofluorescence studies ruled out dermatitis herpetiformis. It is best thought of as a lichenoid tissue reaction such as pigmented contact dermatitis, lichen pigmentosa, or erythema dyschromicum perstans.

Kumakiri M, Takashima I, Iju M, et al: **Eruptive vellus hair cysts**—a facial variant. J Am Acad Dermatol 1982; 7:461–467.

A 29-year-old man complained of **pigmentation of the forehead**. On examination, some 50 barely noticeable slate-colored macules were seen on the forehead. Each macule was 1 to 3 mm in size.

On **biopsy**, round **keratinous cysts** were found in the mid-dermis. Each contained vellus hair shafts and laminated keratinous material. A diagnosis of eruptive hair cysts was made with note of the unusual site.

These slate-colored to brownish lesions more evident to the patient than to the physician are to be distinguished from the white milia or the black comedones.

If you can't make a diagnosis looking at it, try thinking about it.

Hypopigmentation

Possibly the most significant area of hypopigmentation you will see is the one hardest to see. This is the ash leaf–shaped macule in the infant. The mother may not point it out to you. You may need the Wood's light to sight it in blond skin; but once seen, it is the augury of bad things to come. These ash leaf macules—and there may be more than one—are the early warning signs of tuberous sclerosis. They precede the other index signs of central nervous system disease. Thus, shagreen patches of collagen plaques, periungal fibromas, alopecia, and adenoma sebaceum appear much later. It is these faint areas of hypopigmentation that alert the physician to possible hydrocephalus, seizures, and renal malformation. They are tiny holes in the curtain of melanin that let us see into the future.

If the ash leaf macule is the most significant example of hypopigmentation to the diagnostician, it is **vitiligo** that is the most significant to the patient. Here the insidious progressive symmetrical patchy lack of color is a cosmetic threat. And the threat is directly proportional to the darkness of the normal skin and the size and location of the pigment loss. This may vary from a small patch at the site of an injury or a distinguished premature graying of the hair to great round pigmentless spots over the entire body. You won't find a cause, but it may be an autoimmune rejection of the melanocyte, since other autoimmune states such as thyroid disease and diabetes mellitus may be present. It is this immune rejection state that accounts for the white halos of Sutton's nevi as well as the ominous and widespread "vitiligo" developing in some patients with malignant melanoma. At times you may uncover a familial but unpredictable trail.

Be sure your patient has true idiopathic vitiligo. Some examples of tinea versicolor in the well-washed will fool you if you fail to do a KOH examination. Another deception occurs with sarcoidosis, in which pigment loss may be the only sign aside from the histologic finding of granulomas beneath. At a glance, nevus anemicus also deceives, but slapping the area quickly reveals that its whiteness is due to lack of blood, not lack of melanin.

Be sure to cross-examine. Could the patient have had a prior inflammatory change such as a thermal burn, a sunburn, or a chemical burn? Most importantly, be sure the patient has had no exposure to phenolic disinfectants or depigmenting chemicals such as hydroquinone. One other consideration is the possibility of a fixed depigmenting drug eruption.

Patients with vitiligo usually are healthy but deserve to be checked for thyroid antibodies, pernicious anemia, and eye changes. The eye is a central feature in the Vogt-Koyanagi syndrome. Here the melanocyte destruction in the eye, the meninges, and the ear accounts for the finding of an attack of uveitis, meningitis, and dysacusis. It is remarkable that but a few white eyelashes may permit the diagnostician to recognize this syndrome.

Vitiligo is acquired. When the same blotchy pigment loss is congenital, the diagnosis is **piebaldism.** In this condition, the index sign is the white forelock of hair seen at birth or early in infancy. Later, piebaldism is distinguished from vitiligo by the fact that hyperpigmented macules may be present as well as hyperpigmented borders or areas of intermediate coloring. The hereditary nature of piebaldism is evident in the family name Whitlock, and some members inherit only the white forelock.

All patients with congenital depigmentation or with piebaldism need to be checked for the congenital deafness of Waardenburg's syndrome, in which loss of pigment may be associated. At least three forms are described. Look to the family history. 763

A few children with congenital "vitiligo," i.e., leukoderma, may have other associated neurologic defects, including mental retardation.

Most dramatic of all is *albinism,* in which the children are born without the capacity to form any of our protective melanin. It is the absence of melanin in the eye that accounts for their poor vision. Their constant nystagmus is as though the eyes are in continual movement to escape the sun's damaging rays. Albinism comes in nine "flavors" or types, each characterized by tyrosinase or other eyzymatic aberrations.

Type I is the most common (tyrosinase negative), and only one of these types (type VI) is recognized by the clinician. In this example the patients bruise easily, may experience gingival bleeding, menorrhagia, and postsurgical bleeding. This is due to a platelet storage pool deficiency. They also accumulate and deposit ceroid, which can lead to colitis and lung fibrosis. This is known as the Hermansky-Pudlak syndrome. Still, skin cancer remains the greatest threat to all albinos, since their skin has an SPF of zero.

Trivial examples of depigmentation occur. These include pityriasis alba and guttate hypomelanosis, but some are not trivial. Be sure the local patch of depigmentation you are looking at is not the lead sign of leprosy or syphilis. Check for hypesthesia and check the serologic test for syphilis.

Sharquie KE: **Vitiligo.** Clin Exp Dermatol 1984; 9:117–126.

Clinical characteristics:

variously sized patches of depigmentation of skin that enlarge and coalesce
white lesions with borders hyperpigmented or erythematous
asymptomatic, often first evident as focal failure to tan in summer
usual onset before age of 20 years.

Sites:

face	umbilicus
backs of hands	genitalia
axillae	elbows, knees
groin	areas of trauma (isomorphic phenomenon)

Types:

complete vitiligo
segmental vitiligo: dermatomal or trigeminal distribution
ocular
halo nevus
gray hair

Associations:

diabetes mellitus	lichen sclerosus et atrophicus
hyperthyroidism or hypothyroidism	myasthenia gravis
hypoparathyroidism	melanoma
alopecia areata	autoimmune hemolytic anemia
pernicious anemia	Addison's disease
scleroderma	

Differential:

chemical vitiligo: phenolic compounds

Johnson DB Jr, Ceilley RI: Basal cell carcinoma with **annular leukoderma** mimicking
leukoderma acquisitum centrifugum. Arch Dermatol 1980; 116:352–353.

A halo of depigmentation may develop not only around a nevus but also
around a:

malignant melanoma	psoriasis
neurofibroma	lichen planus
blue nevus	sarcoidosis
angioma	basal cell carcinoma
fibroma	

Look closely—that halo nevus may really be a halo pigmented basal cell
carcinoma.

Bolognia JL, Pawelek JM: Biology of **hypopigmentation.** J Am Acad Dermatol 1988;
19:217–255.

The clinical patterns of lack of melanin include:

VITILIGO

Circumscribed macules and patches of amelanosis best seen under Wood's
light (long wavelength ultraviolet, 340 to 400 nm)

Variants:

inflammatory vitiligo: erythematous halo

trichrome vitiligo: border intermediate level of color
rimmed vitiligo: border hyperpigmented
generalized vitiligo: total loss over entire skin
type A: common form—patches
type B: segmental dermatomal distribution

Localization:

flexor, wrist
extensor, extremity
intertriginous
periorificial

oral mucosa
Koebner sites of trauma
retina choroid: discrete areas

Associations:

Vogt-Kayanagi-Harada syndrome
    (uveitis, tinnitus, hearing loss, dysacusis, poliosis, alopecia)
Alezzandrini's syndrome (retinitis, facial vitiligo, poliosis)
sympathetic ophthalmia
autoimmune disorders (usually thyroid)

HALO NEVI (Sutton's nevus, leukoderma acquisitum centrifugum)

Rim of depigmentation around nevus that may lighten in color and disappear

Associations:

melanoma
vitiligo
Vogt-Kayanagi-Harada syndrome

halos of hypopigmentation also seen around:

histiocytoma
basal cell carcinomas
neurofibromas

seborrheic keratoses
flat warts

CHEMICAL LEUKODERMA

due to cytotoxicity of catechols, phenols
specifically: rubber gloves, rubber products; germicides; hydroquinone,
    photographic developer
indistinguishable from vitiligo on simple inspection

OCULOCUTANEOUS ALBINISM

decrease or absence of melanin in eyes, skin, hair
unlike vitiligo, melanocytes present
ten forms described, including:
   Hermansky-Pudlak syndrome
   ceroid deposits in leukocytes
   Chédiak-Higashi syndrome
   giant lysosomal granules
   Cross syndrome
     blindness
     usually autosomal recessive
     exhibit: dilution in skin and hair color, photophobia, nystagmus, de-
      creased visual acuity

PHENYLKETONURIA

blond hair, fair skin, blue eyes
dermatitis
rarely scleroderma

mental retardation
seizures

PIEBALDISM (PARTIAL ALBINISM)

autosomal dominant

    localization:
        white forelock   ventral trunk
        scalp beneath forelock   midregion: upper, lower extremities
        forehead
    contrast with vitiligo
        present at birth
        normal or hyperpigmented islands within symmetrical areas of
            hypomelanosis
        possibly darken with UVL

WAARDENBURG'S SYNDROME

congenital hearing loss   piebaldism
eyebrow hypertrichosis   heterochromia of iris
white forelock

TUBEROUS SCLEROSIS

ash leaf spot of leukoderma (partial loss of pigments)
    present at birth as index sign (use Wood's light to see)
dull-white macules, may be numerous
can be oval polygonal, lance-ovate;
    can be confetti-like, dermatomal
often spares mustache area
very common in children
usually face and neck

INFLAMMATORY DISORDERS

Hypomelanosis seen occasionally with:

    alopecia mucinosa   sarcoidosis
    pityriasis lichenoides chronica   T-cell lymphoma

Postinflammatory hypopigmentation:

    atopic dermatitis   guttate parapsoriases
    psoriasis   lichen striatus
    dermatitis   pityriasis lichenoides chronica
    discoid lupus erythematosus

INFECTIOUS DISEASE

Hypopigmentation seen in:

    tinea versicolor   yaws
    secondary syphilis   leprosy
    late pinta   onchocerciasis: looks like leopard skin

Additional later signs:

    poliosis: fibromas: gingival, ungual
    connective tissue nevi (shagreen patch)   soft fibromas of neck, axilla
    café au lait spots   fibrous plaques of forehead

Differential diagnosis:

    nevus depigmentosus (less melanin in keratinocyte, histologic distinction)
    nevus anemicus (can't see in Wood's light)
    vitiligo (occurs on face)

NEVUS DEPIGMENTOSUS

present at birth   may be isolated (circular, or rectangular):
hypomelanotic   dermatomal
                        systematized (whorls or streaks)
                        predominantly unilateral

Differential diagnosis:

hypomelanosis of Ito (neurocutaneous findings)
segmental vitiligo

nevus anemicus
ash leaf spot

HYPOMELANOSIS OF ITO (incontinentia pigmenti achromicans)

Mimics pattern of marble cake; sworls, streaks, patches of hypopigmentation:

streaks running along lines of Blaschko
is negative image of late-stage incontinentia pigmenti
can be unilateral or bilateral
usually on trunk
appears at birth or in first year of life
may repigment later
may show alopecia, transverse ridging of nails, dental abnormalities, strabismus, hypertelorism

IDIOPATHIC GUTTATE HYPOMELANOSIS

off-white macules (2 to 8 mm)
  no scale or atrophy
may be circular or angulated

acquired, usually in old age
usually on extensor arms and legs
does not repigment

Differential:

confetti-like lesions of tuberous sclerosis
tinea versicolor
postinflammatory hypopigmentation
lichen sclerosus et atrophicus
vitiligo

PITYRIASIS ALBA

Scaly hypopigmented patches with indistinct borders or raised erythematous border

Falabella R, Escabar C, Giraldo N, et al: On the pathogenesis of **idiopathic hypomelanosis.** J Am Acad Dermatol 1987; 16:35–44.

Idiopathic guttate hypomelanosis is a common finding in women. It manifests itself as small (2 to 5 mm) hypopigmented and achromic macules with irregular borders. Some of the lesions may be punctate, others as large as 1.5 cm. The cause remains unknown.

Wilson PD, Lavker RM, Kligman AM: On the nature of **idiopathic guttate hypomelanosis.** Acta Derm Venereol 1982; 62:301–306.

Idiopathic guttate hypomelanosis consists of multiple sharply defined, partly to completely depigmented angular macules between 2 and 8 mm in diameter, most commonly found on the legs.

Extensive studies of 20 cases revealed that the focal lack of color was indicative of a reduction not only in number but also in size and activity of the melanocytes in these areas.

The cause of this melanocyte shrinkage and disappearance remains a mystery, but there is concurrent focal keratinocyte shrinkage and reduction. We do know that these "drops" of hypomelanosis are not minivitiligo, age changes, actinic dermatoses, postinflammatory changes, or scars.

Thus, we know what these dots of white are, and what they are not, but not what they are from.

Oppenheimer EY, Rosman NP, Dooling EC: The late appearance of **hypopigmented maculae in tuberous sclerosis**. Am J Dis Child 1985; 139:408–409.

Infants and children with seizures and/or mental retardation of unknown cause deserve repeated **Wood's light examinations**. In four children with seizures, hypopigmented macules appeared at age 5.5 months, 9 months, 18 months, and 6.5 years, respectively.

Hypopigmented macules appear eventually in 80% of patients with tuberous sclerosis and vary from 1 to more than 100. They resemble a thumbprint or ash leaf (rounded at one end, tapered at the other) or have irregular borders. They may occur along cleavage lines or dermatomes. The lesions are **pale-white**, in contrast to the chalk-white lesions of vitiligo.

Buzas JW, Sina B, Burnett JW: **Hypomelanosis of Ito**. Report of a case and review of the literature. J Am Acad Dermatol 1981; 4:195–204.

A whirlpool of **hypopigmented streaks** appeared on the back of a 4-month-old boy. The streaks were asymmetrical, sharply defined, and pointed and also involved the abdomen and right thigh. Biopsy showed normal melanocytes, but decreased melanin, consistent with Ito's hypomelanosis. When he was age 17 months, the hypopigmented areas became slightly darker.

Because the streaks and whirls resemble a negative image of the dark patterns of incontinentia pigmenti, Ito coined the label, *Incontinentia pigmenti achromians*. Sometimes the two conditions coexist (as a black and white version). The hypopigmentation may be unilateral or bilateral, involve any site, and appear at birth, infancy, or early childhood, with no preceding visible inflammatory change. There may also be dysplastic teeth and hair changes ranging from alopecia to hirsutism.

A majority of patients show **other organ abnormalities**. Neurologic problems include seizure disorders, retarded development, hearing loss, and poor gait. Eye defects are numerous, ranging from strabismus to opaque cornea. Limb hypertrophy and multiple musculoskeletal abnormalities also occur. Always the prognosis remains guarded.

Ito's hypomelanosis must be distinguished from **nevus depigmentosus**, a more localized pigmentary abnormality that is permanent, present at birth, and involves the trunk and proximal surface of the extremities with circular or rectangular hypopigmented macules or whorls.

Ito's hypomelanosis suggests that the embryonal batter of melanocytes was insufficiently stirred.

Takematsu H, Sato S, Igarashi M, Seiji M: **Incontinentia pigmenti achromians** (Ito). Arch Dermatol 1983; 119:391–395.

This 12-year-old girl had developed **bizarre bands of hypopigmentation** of the trunk and extremities at the age of 1 month. There was no preceding inflammatory change, and the many hypopigmented areas had grown more pronounced as she aged.

She had had **seizures** throughout childhood, requiring anticonvulsant therapy. Growth and mental development had been retarded. Biopsy showed a weakly positive dopa stain in the hypopigmented areas.

This is an example of Ito's nevus, which is the hypopigmented analogue of incontinentia pigmenti. Both have distinctive whorled or linear patterns of pigmentary change. And both show other congenital anomalies of the CNS, as well as ocular, dental, and musculoskeletal anomalies.

769

The **CNS anomalies** center on motor and mental retardation and seizure disorders, but ataxia and deafness have been recorded. Other patients have shown hypertelorism, deformed auricles, and dwarfism. Sweating may be reduced in areas of hyperpigmentation.

It indeed is a congenital neurocutaneous disease in which the swirls and eddies of depigmentation give evidence of a tempestuous embryonic past.

Rozycki DL, Ruben RJ, Rapin I, Spiro AJ: **Autosomal recessive deafness** associated with short stature, vitiligo, muscle wasting and achalasia. Arch Otolaryng 1971; 93:194–197.

Vitiligo of the neck and trunk was seen in two siblings under 5 feet tall (20-year-old male, 19-year-old female) from a consanguineous marriage. They also had profound muscle atrophy of the hands, feet, and legs; congenital deafness due to sensorineural hearing loss; and difficulty swallowing, with frequent vomiting.

Cole GW, Barr RJ: **Hypomelanosis** associated with a colonic abnormality. A possible result of **defective development of the neural crest**. Am J Dermatopathol 1987; 9(1):45–50.

A newborn black infant boy had **loss of normal dark coloration** except for a few isolated areas on the trunk. His hair was uniformly black. A biopsy of hypopigmented skin showed infrequent brown melanin pigment granules in the basal layer, with only a small number of melanosomes seen on electron microscopy.

After passing bright red blood at the age of 5 days, he was found to have massive dilatation of the distal colon, thought to be **aganglionic megacolon**. He also had idiopathic hypertrophic subaortic stenosis, premature closure of the cranial sutures, and generalized encephalopathy, and died at 5 months of age.

Differential diagnosis:

> piebaldism and vitiligo: complete absence of melanocytes
> albinism: normal number of melanocytes, but maturation arrest of melanosome development
> nevus depigmentosus: melanosomes poorly developed and aggregated

Mukamel M, Weitz R, Metzker A, Varsano I: **Spastic paraparesis, mental retardation, and cutaneous pigmentation disorder**. Am J Dis Child 1985; 139:1090–1092.

Six children in one Arab family with high consanguinity in Israel had gray hair at birth, multiple **café au lait spots** and freckles, and numerous hypopigmented macules. Two children died at 3 to 4 months of age, while the others developed severe muscle wasting, progressive spastic paraparesis, skeletal deformities, mental retardation, and microcephaly. Inheritance is probably autosomal recessive.

Leal I, Merino F, Soto H, et al: **Chédiak-Higashi syndrome** in a Venezuelan black child. J Am Acad Dermatol 1985; 13:337–342.

A baby born to consanguineous parents had **marked depigmentation** of the skin and ash-gray hair. A sister with similar hypopigmentation, recurrent infections, and ecchymoses had died at an early age. At 2 weeks of age, he had pyoderma of the scalp, which cleared with antibiotics. Skin color gradually returned to normal over several months, and physical and psychomotor development was normal.

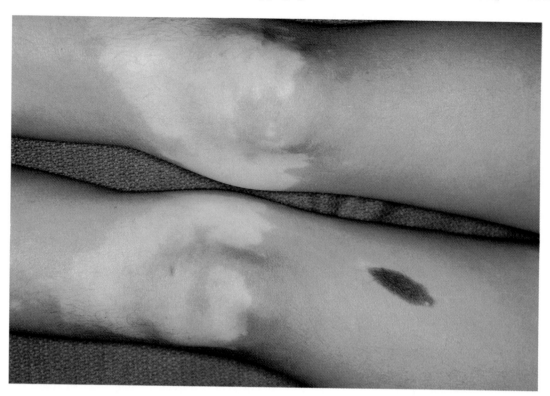

White cells exhibited large azurophilic granules in the cytoplasm of lymphocytes and polymorphonuclear neutrophils, typical of **Chédiak-Higashi syndrome**. Neutrophil function revealed marked impairment of digestive ability against *Candida albicans*.

Chédiak-Higashi syndrome is the likely diagnosis in any baby born with **albinism and ash-gray hair**. Patients may also show photophobia and nystagmus and are prone to repeated bacterial infections of the skin, ears, and upper respiratory tract. It is a rare recessive syndrome.

Wood C, Graham D, Willsen J, Strefling A: **Albinism and amelanotic melanoma**: Occurrence in a child with positive test results for tyrosinase. Arch Dermatol 1982; 118:283–284.

A **nodule** of 9 months' duration just below the lateral part of the left knee in this 14-year-old albino boy had been dismissed as a **keloid** requiring no treatment.

As it continued to enlarge, anxiety returned, and a second opinion was sought. A punch biopsy showed it to be an atypical spindle cell nevus. It was decided to excise the entire lesion, and microscopic examination of this gave the tertiary and definitive diagnosis of **malignant amelanotic melanoma**.

Although the tumor was not tested for tyrosinase, an anagen hair bulb incubated for 24 hours in levodopa (1 mg/ml, 0.1 M phosphate buffer, pH 6.8) became black, indicating the presence of tyrosinase.

There is a grave need for sun protection, sunscreens, and biopsy of innocent looking bumps in albinos.

Rare diseases sneak into your office in twos or threes.

Differential Diagnosis

Mathias CGT, Maibach HI, Conant MA: **Perioral leukoderma simulating vitiligo** from use of a toothpaste containing cinnamic aldehyde. Arch Dermatol 1980; 116:1172–1173.

For 6 months this 25-year-old woman had had slowly enlarging **leukoderma around the mouth**. The leukoderma was sharply marginated by a thin border of hyperpigmentation. No scaling or dermatitis was present. A diagnosis of vitiligo was made. However, patch tests revealed a 2+ positive 48-hour reaction to **cinnamic aldehyde**, with complete loss of pigment at the test site several months later. Inasmuch as cinnamic aldehyde was a component of the toothpaste she was using, she was asked to switch to one free of this sensitizer. By 6 months the perioral area had almost completely repigmented.

It was thus obvious that she had occult **contact dermatitis to the toothpaste**, manifested only by the loss of pigment. She did not have vitiligo. Significantly, patch testing with the original toothpaste gave no reaction at 48 hours or loss of pigment at 3 months. The perioral loss of color came from months of repeated contact of the moist lips with the toothpaste foam. This cannot be reproduced by a single 48-hour exposure.

Many examples of vitiligo may be due to long-term exposure to contactants that produce little or no eczematous change following the standard 48-hour test exposure. There is real need for a standardized **vitiligo patch test** that specifies the diluent and concentration of the contactant, the duration of patch test exposure, and the time of reading for depigmentation with a Wood's light. It is not possible to detect the effect of a chemical on the melanocyte synthesis of melanin until the overlying reservoir of preformed melanin is shed by the epidermis. This mandates a **reading at 4 to 6 weeks**, no sooner.

Fisher AA: Highlights of the AAD post-graduate course. **Recent developments in contact dermatitis and occupational dermatology** sponsored by the AAD with the North American Contact Dermatitis Group, San Diego, May 21–28, 1988. Part I. Cutis 1988; 42:93–95.

Occupational **contact leukoderma can mimic vitiligo**. Always ask if there is a clustering of cases of leukoderma in the plant or if there is a known depigmenting agent in the environment. Be wary of making the diagnosis of vitiligo if your patient has had exposure to known depigmenting chemicals. A biopsy, even with electron microscopy, will not distinguish vitiligo from chemically induced leukoderma.

To assess the depigmenting potential of a chemical, use black guinea pigs or do a cautious patch test on the buttock. Avoid testing black skin if possible.

Depigmenting chemicals:

Hydroquinone or its ethers:
monobenzylether
monomethylether (p-methoxyphenol, p-hydroxyanisole)
monoethylether (p-ethoxyphenol)
p-*tert*-butylphenol
p-*tert*-butylcatechol
p-isopropylcatechol
p-methylcatechol
p-octylphenol
p-nonylphenol
p-phenylphenol
p-*tert*-amylphenol
p-cresol

mercaptoamines: N-12 mercaptoethylodimethylamine, β-mercapto-ethylamine, hydrochloride (MEA), physostigmine (eserine), disopropyl, fluorophosphate, thiotepa (N, N′, N″-triethylene thiophosphoramide)

Dupré A, Ortonne J-P, Viraben R, Arfeux F: **Chloroquine-induced hypopigmentation** of hair and freckles. Association with congenital renal failure. Arch Dermatol 1985; 121:1164–1166.

Thirty days after starting **chloroquine sulfate** (100 mg/day) as malaria prophylaxis this 15-year-old girl noted her freckles and dark red hair were becoming lighter. The chloroquine was discontinued $2\frac{1}{2}$ months later.

Examination disclosed a 2-cm zone of **hypopigmentation** at the base of each scalp hair. The eyelashes, eyebrows, axillary and pubic hair were similarly affected. But why? Further history disclosed that since early childhood she had suffered from renal failure (nephronophthisis). It is likely that this patient had abnormally high levels of chloroquine because of failure of renal tubular excretion and that this may have interfered with melanin synthesis. Interestingly, when the chloroquine was stopped, the freckles redarkened and the band of hypopigmented hair grew out.

Chloroquine can cause the same phenomenon in individuals with normal renal function. It affects light brown or red hair, but not dark brown. Appearing 2 to 5 months after starting, it is dose related and reversible.

Sanchez JL, Vasquez M, Sanchez NP: **Vitiligo-like macules in systemic scleroderma.** Arch Dermatol 1983; 119:129–133.

In systemic scleroderma a **salt-and-pepper** patterning of **depigmentation** is common. It mimics vitiligo that is undergoing repigmentation, in that the pigment present is dotted and follicular in origin.

Frithz A, Lagerholm B, Kaaman T: **Leukoderma syphiliticum**: Ultrastructural observations on melanocyte function. Acta Derm Venereol 1982; 62:521–525.

The appearance of multiple large macules of **hypopigmentation on the penis** of this 24-year-old homosexual proved to be the herald sign of **secondary syphilis**.

On examination, he had enlarged inguinal and axillary lymph nodes as well as positive serologic tests for syphilis. Biopsy showed loss of melanin, but little else. No spirochetes were seen in the Warthin-Starry stained specimens. On electron microscopy the melanocytes were seen to be reduced in number with small incompletely melanized melanosomes. A clinical diagnosis of **leukoderma syphiliticum** was made.

Treatment with penicillin reversed the Wassermann test but not the TPI or the leukoderma. It is typical for these treponemal leukodermas to remain permanently.

Hall RS, Floro JF, King LE Jr: Hypopigmented lesions in **sarcoidosis**. J Am Acad Dermatol 1984; 11:1163–1164.

This 32-year-old black man complained of unexplained **white spots** and an itchy scaly rash of both legs of 2 months' duration. He was known to have had sarcoidosis for a number of years, which involved the lungs, lymph nodes, and eyes.

Examination showed numerous nonindurated hypopigmented macules on both arms and an ichthyosiform rash with faint hypopigmented macules on both legs. Biopsy examination showed no underlying sarcoidal granulomas, but did show a reduction to absence of granular cell layer consistent with the pattern seen in ichthyosis.

The skin lesions gradually became more prominent, and 3 years later papules developed in the middle of, eccentric to, and outside the hypopigmented macules in a miliary or disseminate pattern. Biopsy of the firm hypopigmented macules or papules now clearly showed an **underlying sarcoidal granuloma** pattern. Again the impalpable macules showed no evidence of sarcoidosis. Sarcoidosis usually produces papules, plaques, and nodules, sometimes erythema nodosum, and, on such an occasion as this patient, acquired ichthyosis and hypomelanotic spots. A biopsy of the *firm* light spots should be done if you wish to confirm or to discern sarcoidosis.

The black skin hides erythema from us, but in turn it allows us to see variations in melanocyte activity never perceived in white skin. The invisible in the whites thus becomes the visible in the blacks.

Zackheim HS, Epstein EH Jr, Grekin DA, McNutt NS: **Mycosis fungoides** presenting as areas of **hypopigmentation**: A report of three cases. J Am Acad Dermatol 1982; 6:340–345.

A 22-year-old black woman gave the history of having **white spots** for the past 5 years. Numerous slightly scaly hypopigmented patches up to 10 cm in diameter were present on the face, extremities, and buttocks. There was no erythema, scarring, loss of sensation, or central clearing. KOH examination for fungi was negative. On repeated biopsies a diagnosis of **patch-stage mycosis fungoides** was made.

The lesson here is that white spots in black skin deserve a biopsy.

Misch KJ, Marsden RA: **Hypopigmented mycosis fungoides**. Br J Dermatol 1985; 113 (suppl 29):94–95.

For 7 years a 19-year-old West Indian woman had noted gradual development of mildly itchy, pale patches on the left arm and right buttock. They were oval, hypopigmented, sharply bordered macules with a trace of atrophy but normal sensation. General medical studies were normal. Skin biopsy revealed mycosis fungoides.

Kossard S, Commens C: **Hypopigmented malignant melanoma** simulating vitiligo. J Am Acad Dermatol 1990; 22:840–842.

For 10 years this 66-year-old woman had noted a slowly enlarging yet asymptomatic area of **hypopigmentation** on the right calf. The entire area measured 6 cm. For the past 2 years there had been slow patterned repigmentation of the center. Biopsy of the central area showed the process to be **superficial spreading melanoma**, Clark level II.

The patient was viewed as having an amelanotic melanoma that, after 8 years, developed a pigmented clone of tumor cells. Amelanotic melanomas may not only present as "vitiligo," but also as Bowen's disease or persistent dermatitis or even nevus pigmentosus. But, recall that perilesional vitiligo can occur as a halo around not only a nevus, but also a malignant melanoma. Finally, loss of pigment may reflect **regression of a melanoma**.

The only way to spot "vitiligo maligna" is by biopsy.

If things don't add up, try dividing the problem up.

Ichthyosis

In ichthyosis the scale tells all. In ichthyosis vulgaris it is white and branny, whereas in X-linked ichthyosis it is dark and large. In epidermiolytic hyperkeratosis, it is row on row and rough, while in lamellar ichthyosis it is armor plate attached like a button.

As for the rarities, run for the book. They range from the CHILD syndrome (congenital *h*emidysplasia with *i*chthyosiform erythroderma and *l*imb *d*efects) to Rud's syndrome, in which the brain, the gonads, and stature are "rudimentary." We like to think of Conradi's disease as ichthyosis written in curlicue Cs—chondrodystrophia calcificans congenita beginning as a collodion baby with cartilages that show characteristic calcified stippling on x-ray. Note that in this disease the whirl and swirl pattern of ichthyosis clears in infancy leaving a pattern of pigmentation to fool you into thinking it is incontinentia pigmenti.

Making the diagnosis of the KID syndrome calls for a kid who can't hear you. Erythrokeratoderma variabilis has a keratoderma as variable as the weather, whereas if you don't spot the retinitis pigmentosa you are blind to Refsum's disease. If all this leaves you paralyzed, that is the sign of Sjögren-Larsson syndrome.

It is exciting to know that the laboratory can diagnose **X-linked ichthyosis** by lipoprotein electrophoresis. The steroid sulfatase lacking in these patients results in elevated cholesterol sulfate levels in the keratin which, in turn, makes low-density lipoproteins migrate faster than normal. The pathologist can diagnose **Sjögren-Larrson syndrome** by a formazan frozen section stain. In these patients the defect is a fatty acid metabolic defect, i.e., low fatty alcohol (hexanol) dehydrogenase.

Finally, don't just be satisfied with the diagnosis of ichthyosis. In adults, look behind it for a cause. It can be triggered by a malignancy or malnutrition. It can come as a manifestation of sarcoidosis, leprosy, or lupus erythematosus. Do a biopsy. Take a drug history. Nicotinic acid in high dose can produce ichthyosis. Other cholesterol control drugs may also be responsible.

Last, but not least, do a KOH. You may find that your patient with ichthyosis has a second diagnosis, tinea corporis.

General

Traupe H: The **ichthyoses**: A Guide to Clinical Diagnosis, Genetic Counseling, and Therapy. New York, Springer-Verlag, 1989, 253 pp.

This is a reference masterpiece. Here, one finds precise directions for distinguishing more than 20 types of ichthyosis. Could your patient have:

Dorfman's syndrome (neutral lipid storage disease with ichthyotic erythroderma)
Hystrix-like *ichthyosis* with *deafness* (HID syndrome)
Keratitis, ichthyosis-like hyperkeratosis and *deafness* (KID syndrome)
Ichythyosis follicularis, atrichia, and *photophobia* (IFAP syndrome)
Peeling-skin syndrome, type A, type B
Congenital ichthyosis and keratoderma
Hereditaria mutilans of Vohwinkel
Congenital migratory ichthyosis with neurologic and ophthalmologic abnormalities

Despite the genetic heterogeneity of ichthyosis, with this book at your side you will welcome the nosologic challenge of your next patient with scaling skin.

Gianotti F: **Inherited ichthyosiform dermatoses** in infants with children. *In* Marks R, Dykes PJ (eds): The Ichthyoses. New York, SP Medical and Scientific Books, 1978, pp 137–148.

Differential diagnosis

1. Ichthyosis vulgaris
   Trunk and extensor limbs, not flexural
   Fine white branny scales
   Granular layer absent
   Autosomal dominant

2. X-linked ichthyosis
   Large dark scales on neck, trunk, lower limbs
   Involves flexural areas
   Worsens with age

3. Epidermolytic hyperkeratosis (congenital ichthyosiform erythroderma)
   Large flaccid bullae at birth, later skin thick
   Gray brown furrowed hyperkeratosis of flexures

4. Lamellar ichthyosis
   Large thin scales, thick palms, soles
   Persistent erythema

5. Collodion baby
   Baby enveloped in collodion-like membrane
   May evolve into X-linked or lamellar form

6. Harlequin fetus
   Most severe form fatal
   Thick fissured keratin plaques

Very rare forms with associations:

1. Sjögren-Larsson syndrome
   Spastic paralysis, mental retardation

2. Rud's syndrome
   Oligophrenia, epilepsy

3. Conradi's syndrome
   Short limbs, whorl pattern ichthyosis

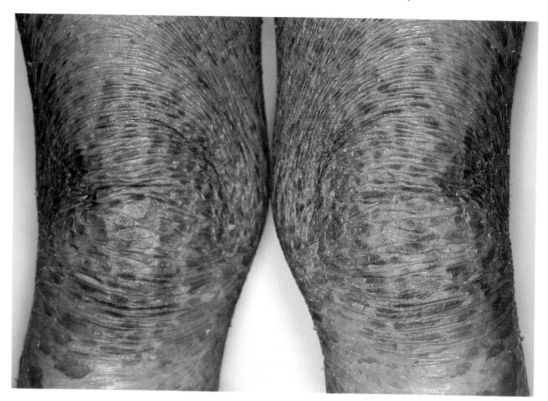

4. Tay's syndrome
    Pili torti, progeria
    Mental retardation

5. Erythrokeratoderma variabilis of Mendes da Costa
    Hyperkeratosis
    Areas of erythroderma show change in size and location day to day

6. Ichthyosis linearis circumflexa of COMEL
    Migratory serpiginous lesions of scaling and erythema
    Double-edged scale at borders

7. Refsum's disease
    Late in childhood
    Retinitis pigmentosa
    Phytanic acid in serum

The older the clinician, the fewer the laboratory tests ordered.

Types

Unamuno P, Martin C, Fernandez E: **X-linked ichthyosis** and cryptorchidism. Dermatologica 1986; 172:326–327.

In your patient with X-linked ichthyosis look for:

Mental retardation
Hypogenitalism

Cryptorchidism
Hypertrophic pyloric stenosis

In the women carriers be alert to:

Abortions
Stillbirths
High perinatal mortality

Goldsmith LA: Look at the **genes**, see what's in the jeans. Arch Dermatol 1990; 126:585–586.

It is prudent to have male patients with **X-linked ichthyosis** remove their jeans so their testes can be examined. Incompletely descended testes in these patients can be a prelude to **testicular carcinoma**.

These are the patients who have complete deletion of the **steroid sulfatase** gene, residing as it does on the short arm (p arm) of the X chromosome near the terminal (ter) portion of that chromosome related to a cytogenetically determined band 22.3. Thus, this enzyme, so critical in keratinization, has a home address or zip code of X p 22.3-pter. Now that we know the address, we can see if anyone is at home.

Høyer H, Lykkesfeldt G, Ibsen HH, Brandrup F: **Ichthyosis** of steroid sulphatase deficiency. Clinical study of 76 cases. Dermatologica 1986; 172:184–190.

Steroid sulfatase (STS) deficiency is the biochemical basis for recessive X-linked ichthyosis that occurs in males. These patients cannot metabolize cholesterol sulfate, which accumulates in keratinocytes and interferes with keratinization. The gene is on the short arm of the X chromosome and surprisingly is only partially inactivated in the female, resulting in women having a higher steroid sulfatase enzyme level than men. The assay for STS enzyme is usually done on peripheral leukocytes, with both the patient and the female carrier having lowered levels. If the enzyme level is normal, the patient has autosomal dominant ichthyosis vulgaris, which may be indistinguishable clinically from recessive X-linked ichthyosis with STS deficiency. In addition to ichthyosis, these patients often have **cryptorchidism** with subsequent testicular cancer.

Characteristic scales: polygonal and brown with narrow lighter zones between them. The scales are largest on the extensor aspects of the lower legs and forearms and smallest on the trunk. A honeycomb pattern of scale appears on the scalp, with the hair being normal. The flexures, palms, soles, and nails are spared. Sun exposure and sea bathing are beneficial.

Characteristic course:

Infancy. Universal peeling usually begins at 1 to 3 weeks of age, leaving polygonal dark scales on the lower legs. All 76 patients had developed lesions by age 1 year.

Childhood. The scalp develops large yellow, crusty scales and the forehead, neck, and preauricular areas have a "dirty" look. These gradually clear, leaving the trunk and extremities as the major sites.

Adulthood. Polygonal brownish scales persist on the trunk and extremities, with greatest intensity on the distal trunk and extensor aspects of the extremities, giving the appearance of ichthyosis nigricans.

Judge MR, Lake BD, Smith VV, et al: Depletion of alcohol (hexanol) dehydrogenase activity in the epidermis and jejunal mucosa in **Sjögren-Larsson syndrome**. J Invest Dermatol 1990; 95:632–634.

Sjögren-Larsson syndrome is an inherited disorder comprising ichthyosis, spastic diplegia or tetraplegia, and mental retardation. The initial presentation may be as a collodion baby. Glistening dots on the macula are considered pathognomonic.

It is now possible by **staining for fatty alcohol dehydrogenase** in frozen skin sections to make a definitive diagnosis of this syndrome. In these patients, staining reveals the critical absence of the enzyme formazan, which is essential in keratinization.

McGrae JD: **Keratitis, ichthyosis, and deafness (KID) syndrome**. Int J Dermatol 1990; 29:89–93.

A composite of the skin changes in 39 cases:

Red, dry, thickened, leathery skin at birth.
Plaques of verrucous, ichthyotic doughy rugal or elephant skin develop on face and extremities during first year.
Plaques are sharply marginated and map-like in contour.
Furrows may appear on chin and transverse ripples on knees.
Follicular keratoses are seen on face and extremities.

Palms have pebbly excrescences, and keratoderma here suggests heavily grained leather. Stippling may be so patulous as to give moth-eaten appearance.

Hair is sparse, fine, and sometimes absent on scalp; may simulate pseudopelade. Eyebrow and eyelash alopecia are in evidence.

Nails show dystrophy or are absent.

There is predisposition to infections, e.g., otitis externa and media.

Hearing loss may be total and is of neurosensory nature. Eye problems center on vascularizing keratitis.

Nazzaro V, Ermacora E, Santucci B, Caputo R: **Epidermolytic hyperkeratosis**: Generalized form in children from parents with systematized linear form. Br J Dermatol 1990; 122:417–422.

This 12-year-old girl was born with generalized erythema and focal superficial erosions of the skin. During the first weeks of life, her skin became scaly and as the years passed it became progressively thickened.

Physical examination disclosed a **generalized hyperkeratosis** with erythema and areas of blisters. The major skin folds exhibited thick verrucous scales with transverse striations. On biopsy there was compact hyperkeratosis with clumps of tonofilaments as well as cytolysis in the suprabasal keratinocytes. These histologic findings of epidermolytic hyperkeratosis confirmed the clinical diagnosis of bullous congenital ichthyosiform erythroderma.

Significantly, the patient's mother had hyperkeratotic skin changes as well. These were bilateral but asymmetric linear and reticulate configurations that followed the lines of Blaschko. The primary lesions were 2- to 4-mm brown hyperkeratotic papules. Again, on both light and electron microscopic studies the changes of epidermolytic hyperkeratosis were found. A diagnosis of **linear epidermolytic hyperkeratosis** was made.

Thus both the daughter and the mother suffered the same **tonofilament system disorder**. The daughter's universal skin defect is inherited usually as an autosomal dominant trait and can be diagnosed prenatally as early in fetal life as 18 weeks. It is a disease of generalized erythema, bullae, and verrucous hyperkeratosis. In its localized form, as seen in this mother, it is not transmitted; however, the possibility of the generalized form appearing in an offspring is a real one.

Wolf R, Zaritzky A, Pollak S: Value of looking at leukocytes in every case of **ichthyosis**. Dermatologica 1988; 177:237–240.

The simple demonstration of **fat droplets within the granulocytes** on a blood smear permitted precise typing of a 3-year-old boy's congenital ichthyosiform erythroderma. He had the **Chanarin-Dorfman syndrome**, an autosomal recessive neutral lipid storage disorder. Born as a collodion baby, his skin fissured and peeled within the first week and eventually he was left with dry erythematous plaques on the flexor areas of his body. Skin biopsy showed slight hyperkeratosis and acanthosis, mild monocytic inflammation in the dermis, and clear intracellular lipid droplets in the basal layer and around skin appendages. A peripheral blood smear stained by the May-Grünwald-Giemsa method revealed round vacuoles in 25% of the neutrophils, which otherwise appeared normal. This is the best way to make the diagnosis, since automated blood counts never sense the abnormality.

One piece of the skin biopsy specimen was frozen in liquid nitrogen, sectioned on a cryostat, and stained with oil red O, revealing lipid droplets in pilosebaceous epithelium and faint staining also of the basal cell layer. Most patients with this disease also have prominent fat droplets in the basal and granular cell layers.

This novel error of lipid metabolism presents as ichthyosis, leukocyte vacuoles, and involvement of other organs. Deafness, cataracts, myopathy, fatty liver, and central nervous system disorders may occur in these patients. It is a defect in intracellular triglyceride pathways, distinct from **acid lipase deficiency** (**Wolman's disease**) or from carnitine deficiency. In the skin, look for generalized scaling, mild erythroderma, and ectropion.

If the baby scales, don't forget to do a blood smear.

Unamuno P, Pierola JM, Fernandez E, et al: **Harlequin foetus** in four siblings. Br J Dermatol 1987; 116:569–572.

Two stillborn and two premature infants born of one mother had the grotesque features of harlequin fetus. Their cutaneous surface was covered with an enormous horny shell (armor-like) of keratin which showed deep fissures separating large polygonal plates. The limbs remained in rigid semiflexion. The nose and ears were entirely hidden, whereas the eyes and mouth were accentuated by severe ectropion and eclabium. The one premature infant died shortly after delivery; the other lived 4 days.

Since first described in 1750, the condition of harlequin fetus has remained a shockingly identifiable **lethal form of ichthyosis**. It is thought to be the most severe form of either congenital ichthyosiform erythroderma or X-linked ichthyosis, although it might be an entirely different form of ichthyosis. It is of genetic origin, with an autosomal recessive pattern of inheritance. The mother and father in this instance had to trace back eight generations to find the marriage link between their two families.

Mevorah B, Frenk E, Saurat JH, Siegenthaler G: **Peeling skin syndrome**: A clinical, ultrastructural and biochemical study. Br J Dermatol 1987; 116:117–125.

Also known as skin shedding (keratolysis exfoliative congenita) or deciduous skin, the peeling skin syndrome has been reported in 22 individuals.

A 28-year-old woman suffered from a variably pruritic ichthyosiform dermatosis all her life. Her skin had been diffusely red at birth and soon became generally encrusted. The erythema faded except on her face, and much of her skin became covered with erythematous scaling migratory patches on a dirty-gray thickened surface. Remarkably, large sheets of **stratum corneum could be peeled away** from the underlying erythematous epidermis. Skin biopsy showed psoriasiform features with separation of the stratum corneum just above the granular layer.

In this condition detachment of the stratum corneum occurs spontaneously in a **cyclical pattern**, evident as migratory peeling patches. Inflammation appears to initiate the process. The defect is reduced adherence of an abnormally thick stratum corneum to the stratum granulosum. It does not respond to isotretinoin or etretinate.

Levy SB, Goldsmith LA: The **peeling skin syndrome**. J Am Acad Dermatol 1982; 7:606–613.

The dry scaly skin of this 24-year-old woman suffering from dwarfism was unique. By simply grasping the edge of a scale, one could peel off a large sheet of skin revealing an underlying erythematous epidermis. She had had generalized dry pruritic skin since birth; the condition had been diagnosed simply as **ichthyosis**. Although she never had blisters, the peeling phenomenon had always been present, leaving erythematous patches with annular and serpiginous borders.

On study, the sheets that peeled off proved to be full-thickness stratum corneum; a diagnosis of peeling skin syndrome was made.

It is distinguished from **ichthyosis linearis circumflexa**, which also shows migratory polycyclic lesions, but with no peeling. Furthermore, in ichthyosis linearis circumflexa, one sees a double-edged scale at the edge of the lesion, and much of the skin is entirely normal.

Idiopathic is one of the most dangerous words in medicine because it fosters intellectual surrender before the diagnosis battle even starts.

Jeffrey D. Bernhard

Causes

Williams ML, Feingold KR, Grubauer G, Elias PM: **Ichthyosis** induced by cholesterol-lowering drugs. Arch Dermatol 1987; 123:1535–1538.

Dry scaly skin was first noted years ago as a response in patients who took **high-dose nicotinic** acid. Since then a variety of experimental drugs that inhibit the later steps in cholesterol metabolism have also proven to be "ichthyogenic." In addition to ichthyosis, they have induced loss of hair pigment, loss of the hair itself, and palmoplantar keratoderma. Significantly and unexpectedly, the new cholesterol-lowering agent lovastatin (Mevacor) does not have these effects.

New drugs that induce similar changes include butyrophenone, an antipsychotic drug linked to palmoplantar keratoderma, and dixyrazine, a major tranquilizer, which may produce the triad of white hair, alopecia, and dry skin.

Ruze P: **Kava-induced dermopathy**: A niacin deficiency? Lancet 1990; 335:1442–1445.

Heavy consumption of the popular South Pacific beverage kava (or kava-kava) induces a reversible **ichthyosiform eruption**. Clinically, the scale seen is a fine polygonal one. This scaling is widespread but the flexural areas are exempt. The palms and soles become thickened, and changes on the naso-labial folds resemble seborrheic dermatitis. The findings are slow to develop and slow to improve when the kava intake is stopped.

Although the problem has been viewed by some observers as pellagra, there are no other findings of pellagra and administration of nicotinamide has no benefit.

DiBisceglie AM, Hodkinson HJ, Berkowitz I, Kew MC: **Pityriasis rotunda**. A cutaneous marker of hepatocellular carcinoma in South African blacks. Arch Dermatol 1986; 122:802–804.

Multiple large, **scaly hyperpigmented circular lesions** of the back and buttocks should arouse suspicion of hepatocellular carcinoma. The disclike lesions are flat and scaly with a crazy-paving pattern and have sharply demarcated edges without inflammation. Diameters range from 1 cm to over 30 cm, and some lesions coalesce into arcuate patterns. Skin biopsy shows hyperkeratosis and atrophy of the granular layer, similar to ichthyosis.

Pityriasis rotunda may be regarded as a localized form of acquired ichthyosis. In this report, all 10 patients who had it also had **hepatocellular carcinoma**.

Banse-Kupin L, Pelachyk JM: **Ichthyosiform sarcoidosis**. Report of two cases and a review of the literature. J Am Acad Dermatol 1987; 17:616–620.

A 36-year-old black woman was being treated for a pruritic scaling eruption of the legs. It had been present for 3 weeks with a presumptive diagnosis of **venous stasis dermatitis**.

Not until a **biopsy** was taken was the correct diagnosis made. Although the epidermal changes were those of ichthyosis, noncaseating granulomas were lying beneath, permitting the diagnosis of **cutaneous sarcoidosis**. Ichthyosiform sarcoidosis is a rare yet specific form of sarcoidosis. It presents as large thick adherent polygonal scales of the lower extremities. Once the condition is diagnosed, a search is made for systemic sarcoidosis, but the ichthyosis may precede any other sign of sarcoidosis by as much as 2 years.

The **differential diagnosis** includes acquired ichthyosis. This may be due to malignancy, e.g., Hodgkins, reactions to medications, e.g., nicotinic acid, or diseases, e.g., hypothyroidism.

Immunosuppression

This is the age of immunosuppression. Patients come to you with the acquired immunodeficiency syndrome (AIDS), as well as with the iatrogenically suppressed immunity necessary in chemotherapy, and with organ transplants or bone marrow grafts. These are the immunosuppressed patients of the 1990's. They present the same problem of severe and strange skin infections we have seen for years in the primary hereditary immunodeficiency syndromes of childhood.

We may expect to see bacterial, fungal, and candidal infections in children born without B lymphocytes and, hence, without gammaglobulins. This is the X-linked agammaglobulinemia of Bruton. Cell immunity is intact. By the age of 6 months, pyogenic and viral infections become commonplace.

Specific classes of immunoglobulin may be deficient or absent in other patients. A deficiency of IgM particularly leads to severe infections. Paradoxically, the hypergammaglobulinemia E syndrome also is associated with furuncles, carbuncles, and abscesses. More serious is the predicament of children born without T cells. This leads to severe combined immunodeficiency disease, with its devastating triad of oral candidiasis, diarrhea, and pneumonia, in which death comes before the age of 2. Any abnormality of the thymus also interferes with development of normal immune defenses against infection. Again, anticipate that patients with either ataxia, telangiectasia, or Wiskott-Aldrich syndrome will suffer infections.

Today the AIDS virus creates the greatest diagnostic challenge. It amplifies disease in the skin by infecting the T_4 lymphocytes, among other cells, thereby weakening the patient's immunity. Not only does it favor "disease gigantism," it also allows saprophytes to become pathogens. Not only may the patient have myriads of large molluscum lesions, but he may also have an ulcer that is the result of an *Alternaria* infection.

Any severe version of disease in a younger person is a signal to think of AIDS. Conversely, any patient with AIDS calls for in-depth diagnostic studies for obscure, rare pathogens. The AIDS patient with skin lesions may well need a biopsy and full spectrum cultures of even innocuous-appearing lesions. The presence of the AIDS virus demands your diagnostic imagination and your best laboratory support. When any disease of the skin comes in amplified form, it is time for an HIV test. AIDS has now entered the inner circle of differential diagnosis.

General

Rapini RP: Practical evaluation of **skin lesions** in immunosuppressed patients. Cutis 1988; 42:125–128.

In the immunocompromised patient with AIDS, malignancy, or organ transplant, things may not be what you think. Nothing is certain without a skin biopsy and appropriate cultures of skin lesions.

Beware of banal-appearing lesions that may represent unusual infections, malignancy, or reaction patterns (drug eruption, erythema, vasculitis). For instance:

PRESENTATION	CLINICAL DIAGNOSIS	HISTOLOGIC DIAGNOSIS AND CULTURE
Purpuric papules	Vasculitis	Biopsy: vasculitis
	Leukemia	Culture: *Candida* sepsis
Small ulcer	Ulcer	Cryptococcosis
Large perirectal ulcer	Chronic ulcer	Biopsy: Herpesvirus infection
Exudative dermatitis, scrotum	Intertrigo	Tzanck smear: Herpesvirus infection
Red macule	Erythema	Kaposi's sarcoma
Nodule	Panniculitis	Biopsy: neutrophilic panniculitis
		Culture: *Staphylococcus aureus* sepsis
Grouped pink nodules	Lymphoma	Biopsy: Chronic Herpesvirus infection

In these patients:

1. Culture all skin biopsies, especially if vasculitis or panniculitis seems likely.
2. Ask for special stains on all biopsy specimens.
3. Remember that **false-negative serologic tests** for various infections will occur due to immune suppression, concealing syphilis, Epstein-Barr virus, cytomegalovirus, human immunodeficiency virus, and hepatitis B virus.
4. In obtaining a biopsy for culture, use as little lidocaine (0.5%) as possible (preferably without preservatives), to minimize its antibacterial properties. Rush the specimen to the laboratory, where it should be ground or minced before plating.
5. Always consider the possibility of drug eruption, even if eosinophils are not present in the biopsy.

Radentz WH: Opportunistic **fungal infections** in immunocompromised hosts. J Am Acad Dermatol 1989; 20:989–1003.

The most common causes of fungal infection in immunocompromised hosts are *Candida* and *Aspergillus* species. However, many fungi once viewed as insignificant contaminants have become powerful pathogens in the skin of these relatively defenseless patients.

Examples shown include:

An erythematous nodule in a heart transplant patient, representing localized phaeohyphomycosis.
Erythematous macules and papules in leukemia patient due to candidiasis.
Purpuric plaque with central ulceration in patient with disseminated zygomycosis.
Indurated red nodule due to *Trichophyton rubrum*.

The range of reactions is astounding:

I. Yeasts

Candida

Discrete, firm, raised red nodules in disseminate candidiasis. Biopsy makes diagnosis; aspiration biopsy culture gives species in 66%.

Other skin changes seen are erythematous macules, purpura, pustules, papules, central necrosis.

Cryptococcus (from soil, pigeon excreta)

Disseminate cryptococcosis may produce cellulitis, ulcers, molluscum contagiosum–like lesions, herpes-like lesions, panniculitis, vasculitis, acneiform lesions, abscesses, vegetating plaques.

II. Zygomycoses

Rhizopus–most common pathogen. As a primary infection of skin, look for vesiculopustules, gangrene, and ulcers.

Dematiaceous fungi

Phaeohyphomycosis produces cysts, ulcers, verrucous plaques, nodules, seborrheic keratosis–like lesions.

III. Hyaline Hyphae

Aspergillus fumigatus most common pathogen. If disseminate aspergillosis, expect maculopapular lesions, granulomas, subcutaneous abscesses. Simulates drug or viral infection.

Dermatophytes

Widespread scaling

Abscesses

Sinus tracts

Dimorphic fungi

Histoplasmosis

Erythematous rash

Cellulitis

Indurated plaques

Erythema nodosum–like lesions

Culture very slow growth

Need biopsy identification

Coccidioidomycosis

Papulopustules, nodules

Granulomas, abscesses, ulcers

Sinus tracts

Biopsy for diagnosis

Sporotrichosis

Painless fluctuant swellings with ulceration

Papules

Nodules

Periorbital swelling

Weitzman I: **Saprophytic molds** as agents of cutaneous and subcutaneous infection in the immunocompromised host. Arch Dermatol 1986; 122:1161–1168.

In the past molds used to grow mainly on inanimate objects, but in today's world of immunosuppressive therapy you can expect to see some of these unusual saprophytic fungi growing in your patients as **opportunistic pathogens**. *Candida*, *Aspergillus*, and *Cryptococcus neoformans* are the most common "carpetbaggers," but a score of others (with names known only to the mycologist) can colonize and invade, causing similar clinical manifestations. Be on the lookout for these in the leukemic child, the transplant patient,

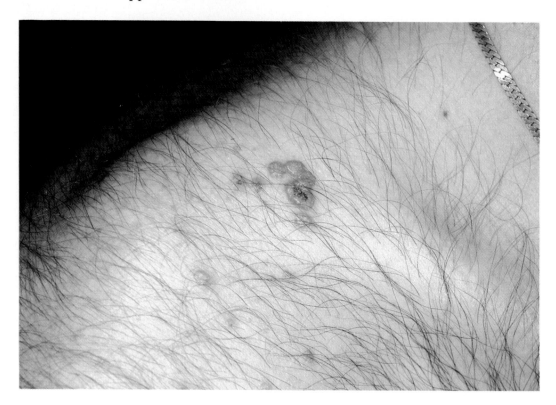

and the person with neutropenia. Touch preparations, KOH examination of a blister roof, and frozen sections all hasten a diagnosis otherwise made only slowly by biopsy and culture.

Cutaneous aspergillosis may present at an IV site as:

cellulitis   granulomas
abscesses   ulcers
toxic erythema   necrotic plaques
maculopapular eruption   eschars
hemorrhagic bullae

Mucormycosis, caused by such strangers as *Apophysomyces, Saksenaea,* and *Mucor* itself, is a special threat to the diabetic patient, with blood vessel wall invasion, thrombosis, and infarction leading to enlarging ulcers with black eschars and gangrene. Cheesy yellow necrosis of the skin, fascia, and muscle was also caused by *Saksenaea vasiformis* infection at a catheter site.

Other molds that may prove responsible for cellulitis, nodules, or black ulcers in your immunocompromised patients include:

Fusarium   *Exophiala*
Penicillium   *Wangiella*
Paecilomyces   *Bipolaris*
Alternaria

When you are faced with these "new" pathogens from the soil, air, and water about us, the mycologist may become your best diagnostic friend!

Watch out—some patients give deliberately misleading histories.

Straka BF, Whitaker DL, Morrison SH, et al: **Cutaneous manifestations** of the acquired immunodeficiency syndrome in children. J Am Acad Dermatol 1988; 18:1089–1102.

Suspect AIDS with

HIV-infected mother
atypical or severe forms of infections
persistent candidiasis
serious staphylococcal infections
extensive herpes simplex or herpetic gingivostomatitis
molluscum contagiosum of face
extremely long eyelashes

Do not suspect AIDS in

disease appearing in first 3 months of life

Penneys NS, Hicks B: **Unusual cutaneous lesions** associated with acquired immunodeficiency syndrome. J Am Acad Dermatol 1985; 13:845–852.

Patients with AIDS present the diagnostician the challenge of common diseases in uncommon disguises and uncommon diseases in common disguises. Be prepared to do KOH examinations, Tzanck preparations, viral cultures, and biopsies or be wrong.

Vivid photographic examples are given of

PRESENTATION	CONFIRMED DIAGNOSIS
Erythema multiforme lesions	Tinea faciale
Flat-topped papules on neck	Tinea corporis
Dyshidrosis palms	Herpes simplex infection
Leg ulcers	Herpesvirus infection
Discoloration, ill-defined papules	*Mycobacterium avium–intracellulare* granuloma
"Molluscum contagiosum" lesions	*Cryptococcus neoformans* infections
Keratotic papules, palms	Histoplasmosis
Papule on thigh	Amebiasis cutis
Palpable purpura lower legs, feet	Cytomegalovirus infection
Rusty oval plaques of upper trunk	Kaposi's sarcoma
Verrucous hyperpigmented lesions of legs	Pellagra

Rau RC, Baird IM: Crusted **scabies** in a patient with acquired immunodeficiency syndrome. J Am Acad Dermatol 1986; 15:1058–1059.

A 22-year-old man with AIDS presented with an extensive nonpruritic **papular hyperkeratotic eruption** that was most prominent around the waist, in the axillary folds, and on the posterior neck. The lesions strikingly resembled **Darier's disease**. A scraping of a papule from the side revealed over 20 adult and well-formed young mites, egg fragments, and fecal pellets in great abundance. He died $2\frac{1}{2}$ weeks later.

Seven months previously he had had more typical scabies and was treated with 1% lindane lotion over a 3-month period. As his clinical condition worsened he developed crusted (**Norwegian**) **scabies**, although typical scabies burrows remained on the wrists.

Watch out for scabies that look like Darier's disease!

Rufli T: **Syphilis** and HIV infection. Dermatologica 1989; 179:113–117.

Since syphilis and HIV infection use the same sexual route of transmission,   787 every patient with a positive syphilis serology should be tested for HIV antibodies and every HIV-positive patient must be tested for syphilis.

The clinical presentation of syphilis in HIV-infected individuals may take the form of **syphilis maligna**: ulcers covered with scabs and thick crusts (**rupia syphilitica**) which develop from papular, vesicular, and pustular lesions. This is a necrotizing reaction pattern and there is an associated headache, high fever, arthralgia, bone pain. It may present as a widespread **ecthyma syphiliticum** mimicking ecthyma of bacterial origin or as **variola syphilitica**, suggesting the vanished disease of smallpox.

It may also come as a perianal ulcer, alopecia or psoriasiform plaques, even keratoderma blennorrhagicum. To add to the **diagnostic challenge**, these lesions, unlike the chancre, are darkfield negative. Furthermore, the palms and soles are often lesion free, leaving the clinician without a favorite diagnostic indication. But in all of these patients the serologic tests for syphilis are fully reactive.

Not only are the cutaneous signs of syphilis highly magnified in the HIV infected, but also the chance of **neurosyphilis** is greatly increased. Cerebrospinal fluid tests for syphilis are needed in all HIV infected individuals who have a reactive blood serology. This is true whether or not there are neurologic symptoms.

Fivenson DP, Weltman RE, Gibson SH: Giant **molluscum contagiosum** presenting as basal cell carcinoma in an acquired immunodeficiency syndrome patient. J Am Acad Dermatol 1988; 19:912–914.

For 6 months, this 51-year-old man had watched a growth on his right cheek as it slowly enlarged. On examination, the lesion was a 1.2 cm pearly, smooth-surfaced, **dome-shaped nodule** surrounded by numerous fine telangiectatic vessels.

The attending staff all agreed that the growth was a **basal cell epithelioma**; because the man was an HIV-positive homosexual, radiotherapy was elected as the treatment of choice. To everyone's surprise, a biopsy showed the lesion to be a **giant molluscum contagiosum**. One session of cryotherapy resulted in a cure.

Coldiron BM, Bergstresser PR: Prevalence and clinical spectrum of skin disease in patients infected with **human immunodeficiency virus**. Arch Dermatol 1989; 125:357–361.

It's simple to diagnose the florid examples of the common diseases routinely seen in AIDS patients, e.g., seborrheic dermatitis, candidiasis, dermatophytosis, and xerosis.

What is hard to remember is that

  a seemingly innocuous crusted papule may be the cutaneous sign of immunoblastic **lymphoma**
  a large inflammatory plaque studded with erosions and tufts of white granulation tissue may be a **herpes simplex** infection
  a deep ulcer may be due to *Mycobacterium avium* infection
  conjunctivitis may really be **Kaposi's sarcoma**

Prose NS: **HIV infection** in children. J Am Acad Dermatol 1990; 22:1223–1231.

No single indication is pathognomic of HIV infection in children. It is the failure to respond to therapy, the persistence of illness, the recurrence, and the severity that tend to suggest HIV infection.

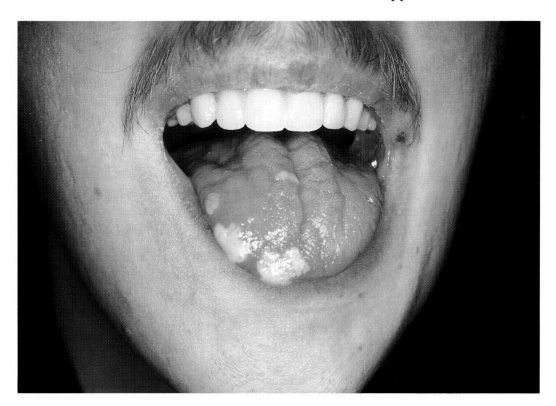

Think of HIV infection in a child with:

    onychomycosis and paronychia
    ecthyma
    disseminate molluscum contagiosum
    extensive flat warts or condyloma accuminatum
    vasculitis

Then think of HIV testing.

With AZT (zidovudine) available and other drugs in the offing, here's a diagnosis worth making.

Gibson IH, Barnett JH, Conant MA et al: Disseminated ecthymatous **herpes varicella-zoster virus infection** in patients with acquired immunodeficiency syndrome. J Am Acad Dermatol 1989; 20:637–642.

Ecthyma in AIDS patients may be due to varicella-zoster virus as shown on viral culture and by excellent response to acyclovir therapy.

Winchester R, Bernstein DH, Fischer HD et al: The co-occurrence of **Reiter's syndrome** and acquired immunodeficiency. Ann Intern Med 1987; 106:19–26.

All patients with Reiter's syndrome should have HIV testing.

Among 13 patients diagnosed with both conditions in one New York City hospital, diarrhea was the most common illness triggering the severe reactive arthritis. Possibly, a novel bowel pathogen responsible for inducing **Reiter's syndrome** could be present at higher frequency among these patients.

Another patient with spondyloarthropathy simultaneously developed extensive psoriasis and signs of AIDS: A 37-year-old woman, a former IV drug abuser who had had progressive symmetrical inflammatory polyarthritis for 10 years, had experienced weight loss, lymphadenopathy, fatigue, and oral candidiasis for 2 years. Pancytopenia developed, followed immediately by widespread **hyperkeratotic fissured psoriasis**. Skin biopsy revealed extensive lymphocyte infiltration. She then developed septic arthritis and herpes zoster and was found to have HIV antibodies, hypergammaglobulinemia, and an elevated sedimentation rate.

Picon L, Vaillant L, Duong T, et al: Cutaneous **cryptococcosis** resembling molluscum contagiosum: A first manifestation of AIDS. Acta Derm Venereol 1989; 69:365–367.

Round papular and **nodular lesions** had appeared on the face and later spread to the trunk and extremities of this 30-year-old homosexual man. Some were umbilicated, suggesting a diagnosis of **molluscum contagiosum**. However, the patient's homosexual status prompted further study. He proved to be HIV seropositive.

A biopsy showed encapsulated yeast structures (4 to 7 μm) with a mucin capsule. Culture identified them as *Cryptococcus neoformans*.

The patient developed a fever, weight loss, generalized lymph node enlargement, and depletion of the T helper cell population; he died a few months later of disseminate cryptococcosis.

Rico MJ, Penneys NS: Cutaneous cryptococcosis resembling molluscum contagiosum in a patient with AIDS. Arch Dermatol 1985; 121:901–902.

Numerous 2- to 4-cm dome-shaped, firm ivory-white **papules** were scattered over the face and neck of a 29-year-old Haitian man. They appeared to be **molluscum contagiosum**, but when a fresh tissue crush preparation failed to reveal intracytoplasmic inclusions, a biopsy was done. This showed numerous basophilic organisms in the papillary dermis, which proved to be *Cryptococcus neoformans* on culture. (The organism grows readily on Sabouraud's agar at 20°C and 37°C.)

Histoplasma duboisii is another fungus that can appear in the skin in the guise of molluscum contagiosum.

A rapid presumptive diagnosis of cutaneous cryptococcosis can be made by examining an India ink or Wright's stain preparation of a smear, which reveals the encapsulated organisms 8 to 20 μm in size.

Several special stains of biopsies will also reveal the organisms in various colors:

red	PAS and mucicarmine
blue	colloidal iron
brown	silver methenamine
green	alcian green

Patterson JW, Kitces EN, Neafie RC: Cutaneous **botryomycosis** in a patient with acquired immunodeficiency syndrome. J Am Acad Dermatol 1987; 16:238–242.

What appeared to be a commonplace **prurigo nodularis** proved on biopsy to be **botryomycosis** with gram-positive cocci clumped into granules in abscesses in the papillary dermis. The patient was a 25-year-old homosexual man who had had pruritic papules and nodules over his chest, back, and upper arms for 3 weeks.

Granules are a characteristic finding in botryomycosis. It is these granules that suggest a diagnosis of actinomycosis or mycetoma, yet botryomycosis is a bacterial infection in which a wide variety of gram-positive or gram-negative organisms may be isolated and cultured.

The lesions are indolent and unresponsive to antibacterial therapy and may need to be excised.

Yebra M, Segovia J, Manzano L et al: Disseminated-to-skin kala-azar and the acquired immunodeficiency syndrome. Ann Intern Med 1988; 108:490–491.

A 37-year-old Spanish homosexual man with leukopenia and oroesophageal candidiasis had two **purplish macules** on his face. Skin biopsy revealed typical Kaposi's sarcoma together with an intense parasitization by *Leishmania* amastigotes, which were also present in normal-appearing skin. Although serologic tests for leishmaniasis were negative, a bone marrow biopsy also showed heavy infiltration by **Leishmania organisms**. He died 5 months later after developing fever and diarrhea.

Asymptomatic visceral leishmaniasis with cutaneous dissemination is likely to become common in AIDS patients in countries where kala-azar is not uncommon (e.g., Spain, Italy, France). Atypical dissemination and lack of symptoms probably result from deeply impaired immunity.

Sometimes you can make the diagnosis by the way the patient looks . . . at you!

Chemotherapy

Cogolludo EF, Antunez PA, Martinez AA, et al: **Neutrophilic eccrine hidradenitis**: a report of two additional cases. Clin Exp Dermatol 1989; 14:341–346.

Look for **neutrophilic eccrine hidradenitis** in patients with underlying malignant disease, usually on chemotherapy. May be ushered in with fever.

Clinical

erythematous papules and plaques, at times tender, often on upper limbs, trunk.

Diagnosis made histologically

neutrophil infiltrate around eccrine sweat gland coils.

This relative of Sweet's syndrome is frequently a fellow traveler with myelogenous leukemia.

Grossman ME, Silvers DN, Walther RR: Cutaneous manifestations of **disseminated candidiasis**. J Am Acad Dermatol 1980; 2:111–116.

A 52-year-old woman on **chemotherapy** for acute myelogenous leukemia had thrush and purpuric erythematous papules with pale centers, pustules, and petechiae on her abdomen and knee. Although both an aspiration smear and a culture of a skin lesion were negative, a biopsy stained with methenamine silver showed clusters of pseudohyphae and spores in an inflamed dermis. Blood cultures later showed the offending yeast to be *Candida tropicalis*. Despite treatment with amphotericin B and 5-fluorocytosine she died 3 weeks later.

Disseminated candidiasis speaks of yeast invasion in every organ and early death.

Veglia KS, Marks VJ: *Fusarium* as a pathogen. A case report of **Fusarium sepsis** and review of the literature. J Am Acad Dermatol 1987; 16:260–263.

A 44-year-old woman with acute lymphocytic leukemia developed a dozen or so indurated **purpuric papules and nodules** on the trunk and extremities. Some had necrotic centers; a clinical diagnosis of **septic emboli** was made.

Biopsy revealed branching hyphae in the dermis, and repeat punch biopsy for culture allowed identification of *Fusarium moniliforme*.

This is a normal cutaneous contaminant that grows on plain Sabouraud's agar. Here in the immunocompromised patient it was growing as a pathogen, and it proved lethal.

Magid ML, Prendiville JS, Esterly NB: **Violaceous nodules** on the arm of a child with acute lymphocytic leukemia. Arch Dermatol 1988; 124:122–125.

Any new lesion in an immunocompromised patient calls for immediate biopsy as well as bacterial and fungal cultures.

A 4-year-old boy undergoing chemotherapy for acute lymphocytic leukemia developed a 4-cm tender **violaceous, poorly demarcated nodule** on the left forearm with 2 crusted areas within the nodule, but no discharge. Several centimeters away there was a 0.5-cm nodule. The lesions were located at the site of previous contact with an arm board. A punch biopsy revealed fungal hyphae within the dermis; these were septate and branching at an acute angle. No spores were seen. **Fungal culture** of the tissue grew *Aspergillus flavus*.

Since 1970 there have been a score of patients (mostly children) with acute lymphocytic leukemia who developed similar lesions at the sites of intravenous cannulas or arm board friction. Lesions begin as erythematous papules, especially on the palm and progress to violaceous edematous indurated plaques or hemorrhagic bullae with black eschars over ulcers. They represent primary cutaneous aspergillosis due to infection with *Aspergillus flavus*.

The **diagnosis** is made by (1) seeing the hyphae in the dermis on biopsy (PAS staining helps but is not essential) and (2) culture on Sabouraud's dextrose agar producing a velvety yellow-green or brown colony with characteristic conidiophores. For speed, use frozen sections of an ulcer scraping or a KOH exam of a bulla roof and fluid. Blood cultures are negative.

Differential diagnosis:

> Staphylococcal cellulitis
> Group A beta-hemolytic streptococcal cellulitis
> Vasculitis
> Ecthyma gangrenosum
> Pyoderma gangrenosum
> Mucormycosis
> Cryptococcosis
> Hepatitis B infection

Aspergillus is second only to *Candida* as a cause of mycotic infection in patients who are immunocompromised.

Junkins JM, Beveridge RA, Friedman KJ: An unusual **fungal infection** in an immunocompromised oncology patient. Arch Dermatol 1988; 124:1421–1424.

Tender maculopapular lesions showing central necrosis were suddenly noted on both knees of a 69-year-old man who had been receiving chemotherapy for a glioblastoma multiforme.

The biopsy showed granulomatous inflammation, abscess, and thick-walled septate mycelia of the common soil and airborne fungus **Alternaria**. Amphotericin therapy was successful. This opportunistic fungus constantly awaits a site of trauma for entrance into an immunocompromised or debilitated patient. Once in the skin it can induce a focal eruption of ulcerative plaques and papules of the hands, knees, face, and forearms, persisting for as long as 25 years. Yet it does not induce systemic infection.

With more chemotherapy being given, we can expect to see more **cutaneous alternariosis**.

Horn TD, Redd JV, Karp JE et al: **Cutaneous eruptions** of lymphocyte recovery. Arch Dermatol 1989; 125:1512–1517.

Macular and papular eruptions in patients receiving bone marrow suppressive chemotherapy may appear 1 to 3 weeks after the start of chemotherapy. The onset of these rashes in 10 patients studied prospectively was not related to a drug sensitivity or to a blood transfusion. It proved to be specifically associated with the **reappearance of lymphocytes** in the blood following their chemotherapeutic-induced disappearance. The rash spontaneously faded days after the recovery of immunologically competent cells.

Whether these cells showed a transient graft versus host type of reaction or whether their presence permitted a viral or a drug reaction to be expressed is not known. In any event, the **lymphocyte recovery eruption** should be considered whenever immunologically competent cells return after an absence. Interestingly, the rash of measles appears on the 14th day of the infection at a time when the lymphocytes are escaping from their initial viral immunosuppression.

Organic Transplants

Itin P, Rufli T, Rüdlinger R, et al: **Oral hairy leukoplakia** in a HIV-negative renal transplant patient: A marker for immunosuppression? Dermatologica 1988; 177:126–128.

Patchy white, **hairy lesions** developed on the left side of the **tongue** in a 58-year-old renal transplant patient. A clinical diagnosis of oral hairy leukoplakia was confirmed by biopsy and a positive Southern blot analysis for the presence of Epstein-Barr virus. The patient had taken cyclosporine, steroids, and azathioprine for 2 years but was not HIV-1 or HIV-2 positive.

Until this report, **oral hairy leukoplakia** was considered a specific sign for HIV infection. Now it appears that nonspecific or drug-induced immunosuppression can cause the same change.

Abel EA: Cutaneous manifestations of immunosuppression in **organ transplant** recipients. J Am Acad Dermatol 1989; 21:167–179.

Don't forget:

1. Cyclosporine causes hypertrichosis, gingival hyperplasia, and xerosis as well as renal damage.
2. The most common cause of death in organ transplant recipients is infection.
3. Culture and biopsy of skin lesions in these immunocompromised patients may reveal the cause of infection.
4. Expect to see molluscum contagiosum, warts, herpes as well as such rarities as *Pneumocystis carinii* and cytomegalovirus infections.
5. Recognize that B cell lymphomas and genital and perianal carcinoma as well as Kaposi's sarcoma may develop in these patients after 4 or 5 years of immunosuppression.
6. Immunosuppression favors conversion of dysplastic nevi to malignant melanoma.
7. Sebaceous adenomas, porokeratosis, and pyoderma gangrenosum are favored by immunosuppressed skin.

Sindhuphak W, MacDonald E, Head E, Hudson RD: *Exophiala jeanselmei* infection in a postrenal transplant patient. J Am Acad Dermatol 1985; 13:877–881.

A **boggy verrucous plaque** with an occasional pustule developed on the anterior thigh of this 35-year-old man. It had been present for a month and a half, was asymptomatic, and was enlarging. A similar lesion had recently appeared on the patient's abdomen. The patient had had a renal transplant and was azathioprine and prednisone immunosuppressed. He worked in a seafood plant where he carried wooden boxes balanced on his right thigh and pressing against his abdomen.

A touch preparation of the biopsy, examined in KOH, gave instant evidence of a **fungal infection**. Numerous brown hyphae and swollen cells filled the field. Culture of the biopsy material grew out *Exophiala jeanselmei*. Histologically the biopsy showed light brown spherical bodies within giant cells, as well as budding yeast forms and hyphae in the granulomatous infiltrate.

The diagnosis of **phaeohyphomycosis** was made, although the lesions had the clinical and histologic picture of chromoblastomycosis. Surgical excision was curative.

All immunosuppressed patients are candidates for strange opportunistic infections. Only by suspicion can you think of them and only by your KOH and culture takes can you identify them.

Basuk PJ, Scher RK: **Onychomycosis** in graft vs host disease. Cutis 1987; 40:237–241.

Half the individuals who have a bone marrow graft find that the graft becomes a pathogen. Within weeks they experience generalized pruritus and then an erythematous macular eruption spreading from the trunk to the palms and soles.

The graft may produce further immunologic damage in the chronic graft versus host disease. This includes

Papulosquamous lesions	Bullae, ulcers
Sclerosis, atrophy	Dry mouth, stomatitis
Poikiloderma	White plaques of mucosa
Photosensitivity, lupus erythematosus	Loss of teeth
Reticulate hyperpigmentation, vitiligo	

In the patient discussed, leukonychia trichophytica appearing several months after a bone marrow transplant was the first cutaneous sign of his graft vs host disease. This was followed by reticulated hyperpigmentation and a lichenoid eruption of the face.

Any cutaneous sign can be a critical determinant in the recognition and management of graft vs host disease.

Leyva WH, Santa Cruz DJ: **Cutaneous toxoplasmosis**. J Am Acad Dermatol 1986; 14:600–605.

Multiple purpuric nodules of the scalp, forearm, groin, and back appeared 3 weeks after this 53-year-old man had received a bone marrow transplant in the treatment of his myelogenous leukemia. On biopsy the keratinocytes contained 3 μm oval organisms that on electron microscopy were typical of the protozoan *Toxoplasma gondii*.

Toxoplasmosis is a diagnosis rarely made other than serologically. The condition may present not only as purpuric nodules but also in a spectrum including purpura, papulopustules, and lichenoid vegetating and erythema multiforme–like lesions.

The source of this man's infection was unknown, but the possibilities included reactivation of previous latent infection or transmission through the graft or nosocomial sources.

Goldberg NS, Ahmed T, Robinson B et al: Staphylococcal **scalded skin syndrome** mimicking acute graft-vs-host disease in a bone marrow transplant recipient. Arch Dermatol 1989; 125:85–87.

A 33-year-old man with an 11-month history of chronic myelogenous leukemia had a bone marrow transplant after conditioning with total body irradiation and cyclophosphamide.

The appearance of a **generalized erythematous rash** on the 14th day was interpreted as a graft vs host reaction as was a second attack on day 73. These were suppressed by progressively higher doses of systemic steroids.

On day 90 the patient developed a **necrolytic eruption** of the chest and elbow. This was viewed as a toxic epidermal necrolysis, associated with a grade 4 cutaneous GVHD. Despite a daily dose of 6 gm of methylprednisolone sodium succinate, the rash progressed with large sheets of epidermis separating from most of the skin surface. The underlying skin was erythematous and moist. Honey-colored crusts were noted around the nose and mouth. A skin biopsy showed an intraepidermal split at the granular layer. A diagnosis of **staphylococcal scalded skin syndrome** was made. Confirma-

795

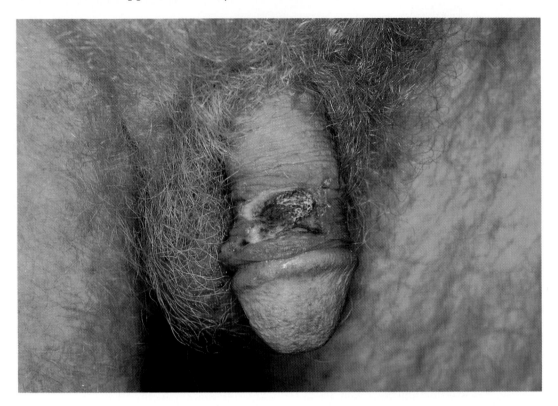

tion came from multiple cultures of blood, crusts, and sputum showing *S. aureus*. There was consequently a good therapeutic response to nafcillin.

Staphylococcal scalded skin syndrome occurs mostly in children under the age of 5 years. Its appearance in this man presumably reflected his suppressed immune status following large steroid dosage. The portal of entry for the staphylococci was presumably a central venous catheter.

A frozen section histologic examination permits rapid distinction from toxic epidermal necrolysis where the split is below the epidermis. Rapid diagnosis is necessary because of the urgent need for immediate appropriate antibiotic therapy.

Too much data can create a traffic jam on the highways of your mind.

Keratoses and Hyperkeratoses

Rough skin calls for an explanation. Although often the roughness is due to obvious scales or to the inapparent scaling of xerosis or atopic dermatitis, focal lesions deserve more specific diagnoses. These are the keratoses and are to be distinguished from the keratodermas, in which the epidermis is uniformly thickened.

The most common examples of focal roughness all arise in the orifice or pit of the hair follicle. The classic form is the mundane **keratosis pilaris** of the upper arms and thighs. It is mimicked by follicular ichthyosis, which is widespread and is best distinguished on biopsy by the fact that it involves the entire follicle. Inflammatory forms of keratosis pilaris usually occur on the face and can be labeled keratosis pilaris rubra. Of the more serious diseases, we may see the rough skin of **pityriasis rubra pilaris** and **keratosis follicularis**; each primary lesion is centered in the hair follicle.

The spiked lesions of lichen spinulosus, as well as follicular lichen planus and the alopecic lesions of lichen planopilaris, attract attention. Rarely, as in Kyrle's disease (hyperkeratosis in cutem penetrans), the keratoses grow into the skin. On occasion, the sudden appearance of spiked keratoses late in life may be a sign of internal cancer. In this way it resembles acquired ichthyosis in being a paraneoplastic change. In contrast, follicular keratoses present since childhood make one ask "Is this change just the tip of a congenital syndrome iceberg such as the KID syndrome?"

Turning from the keratosis of the hair follicle to the form arising from the sweat pore, diagnosis is based on an entirely different finding. Here we see the faint threadlike keratotic border of a central atrophic area. Initially the lesion is a keratotic plug in the sweat pore, but this is no longer the diagnostic feature when the patient sees you. At that time the only trace of the primary lesion remains in the name, which is **porokeratosis**. This may occur in children as but a single lesion or multiple lesions in linear, random, or zosteriform distribution. In older individuals it is the result of sun damage, e.g., disseminate superficial actinic porokeratosis. Immunosuppression also favors the appearance of porokeratosis.

Nonappendageal keratoses appears as papules on the extremities as in stucco keratoses as well as Flegel's disease (hyperkeratosis lenticularis perstans). Keratoses of the palms and soles suggest a congenital origin or the result of exposure to arsenicals.

On the face and back, greasy keratotic papules of all shades growing in later life generate the diagnostic thought of seborrheic keratoses. In black skin the genetic form of this condition is called dermatosis papulosa nigra. These lesions are slow growing and benign in contrast to the rapid flowering of a keratoacanthoma or cutaneous horn.

The **actinic keratosis** is the example of focal rough skin that always deserves our attention. Its scales and redness brought on by sun exposure through the years are the prelude to skin cancer. It must not only be recognized but also treated.

Keratosis Pilaris

Watt TL, Kaiser JS: **Erythromelanosis follicularis faciei et colli**: a case report. J Am Acad Dermatol 1981; 5:533–535.

A 15-year-old boy had a symmetrical blotchy, irregularly marginated but well-defined **pink-brown macular eruption of the temples and cheeks**, with extension onto the neck near the ears. Close examination revealed fine lighter-colored follicular papules with slight scaling and patchy loss of vellus hairs in the beard. A KOH examination was negative for fungi but showed trichostasis of epilated hairs. Biopsy showed capillary dilatation and mild perivascular lymphocytic cuffing in perifollicular areas. During the following year the erythema decreased to red-brown with marginal spread, but pigmentation increased. Whisker growth also appeared within areas of patchy hair loss. Notable keratosis pilaris was present on the upper arms.

The **differential diagnosis** includes:

chloasma
poikiloderma of Civatte
erythema péribuccale pigmentaire of Brocq
ulerythema ophryogenes (keratosis pilaris atrophicans faciei)
folliculitis ulerythematosa reticulata (atrophoderma vermiculare)

This polysyllabic entity, erythromelanosis follicularis faciei et colli, which occurs in adolescent males, differs from keratosis pilaris rouge (red cheek syndrome) only by its extension down onto the neck and by the presence of some pigmentation.

Both have:

blotchy erythema
telangiectasia
fine follicular papules of cheeks
generally dry skin
keratosis pilaris of arms
the same histologic findings

Whittaker SJ, Griffiths WAD: **Erythromelanosis follicularis faciei et colli**. Clin Exp Dermatol 1987; 12:33–35.

Increasing pigmentation over the left cheek was the presenting complaint of a 15-year-old Greek boy. Examination revealed a bilateral well-demarcated, reddish brown eruption of the preauricular region, with numerous pinhead-sized follicular papules that gave it a granular texture on palpation. The erythema blanched on diascopy, bringing the brown pigmentation into prominence. Increased growth of beard hair was seen within the areas. No scarring or atrophy was present. Mild keratosis pilaris was noted on the upper arms. Skin biopsy revealed acanthosis, spongiosis around the openings of pilosebaceous follicles, and an upper dermal perivascular mononuclear cell infiltrate.

A diagnosis of **erythromelanosis follicularis faciei et colli** was made, based on the triad of erythema with telangiectasia, fine follicular papules, and hyperpigmentation. First described in 1960 in Japanese males, it begins in the second decade and is associated with keratosis pilaris. It can affect the neck, eyebrows, and cheeks as well as its typical preauricular site. Photosensitivity is not a component.

Closely related conditions have been called keratose pilaire rouge (Brocq keratosis pilaris with marked erythema) and lichen pilaris faciei. If atrophy or scarring is present, the term *ulerythema ophryogenes* has been used ("ul" referring to scarring and "ophryogenes" to eyebrow involvement). Other synonyms include keratosis pilaris atrophicans faciei, atrophoderma vermiculata, and folliculitis ulerythematosa reticulata.

Hazell M, Marks R: **Follicular ichthyosis**. Br J Dermatol 1984; 111:101–109.

Four unrelated patients with generalized follicular hyperkeratosis since early childhood had a unique form of **follicular ichthyosis**, with lesions more prominent on the head and neck. Three of the four patients also had acanthosis nigricans–like changes in the axillae, and two had comedo-like lesions on the dorsal fingers and cheeks. Two patients had abnormal dental occlusion with similar facies. One patient had white hyperkeratotic patches on the buccal mucosa.

The lesions were distinguished from keratosis pilaris on **biopsy**. In follicular ichthyosis the hyperkeratosis in the follicle is compact stratum corneum that not only expands the orifice but extends deeply into the follicle. In contrast, in keratosis pilaris the hyperkeratosis is a loose basketweave type of stratum corneum that does not distend the follicle nor extend below the infundibulum. **Scanning electron microscopy** revealed a compact horn plugging the follicles and displacing abnormal hairs in follicular ichthyosis but only a small amount of horny material around a normal hair in keratosis pilaris.

The **differential diagnosis** for dermatoses with a follicular distribution is lengthy:

Keratosis pilaris	Vitamin B$_2$ deficiency
Keratosis follicularis (Darier)	Vitamin C deficiency
Follicular ichthyosis	Pityriasis rubra pilaris
Follicular psoriasis	Lichen spinulosus
Kyrle's disease	Lichen planopilaris
Phrynoderma (vitamin A deficiency)	Folliculitis decalvans

Burnett JW, Schwartz MF, Berberian BJ: **Ulerythema ophryogenes** with multiple congenital anomalies. J Am Acad Dermatol 1988; 18:437–440.

Multiple brownish-red papules of the forehead and absent eyebrows were the presenting signs of ulerythema ophryogenes in a 7-month-old black baby boy. The classic findings of pitted depressed scars and atrophy were not present. He also had patchy scalp alopecia, sparse eyelashes, hyperkeratotic palms, and extensive keratosis pilaris–like hyperkeratotic hyperpigmented papules on the extensor arms and legs. **Skin biopsies** from the eyebrow area and thigh showed acanthosis, follicular plugging, and perifollicular infiltration with mild fibrosis. Other **developmental defects** included dysmorphic face (hypertelorism, flat nasal bridge, bulbous nasal tip), ptosis, undescended testes, and mental retardation. A CT scan showed cerebellar degeneration.

Except for the facies this child's condition resembled **Noonan's syndrome**, sometimes associated with ulerythema ophryogenes. The cardiofaciocutaneous syndrome with patchy hyperkeratosis and generalized ichthyosis was also considered. Ichthyosis follicularis (a follicular papular dermatitis) with inflammatory spinous follicular hyperkeratotic papules on the dorsal fingers, knees, and extensor aspects of the legs was another possibility.

It is well to look beyond the eyebrows for congenital defects in youngsters with inflammatory keratotic papules.

The only thing predictable about disease is its unpredictability.

Porokeratosis

Shumack SP, Commens CA: Disseminated superficial **actinic porokeratosis**: A clinical study. J Am Acad Dermatol 1989; 20:1015–1022.

A raised, **sharply marginated**, **keratotic border** is the essential clinical feature of this autosomal dominant condition. The initial lesion is a small follicular cone-shaped papule topped with keratotic plug. The papule enlarges centrifugally, leaving an atrophic central area and raised thin keratotic rim. The border is ovoid, petalloid, or circular. It comes in six clinical variants.

Disseminated superficial actinic porokeratosis
   Small anhidrotic keratotic rimmed lesions in sun-exposed areas of legs, arms, face spared, worse in summer. Onset often in 3rd or 4th decade of life.

Porokeratosis of Mibelli
   Single or few discrete rimmed lesions. Onset in infancy or childhood. Can be in mucous membranes.

Porokeratosis palmaris et plantaris disseminata
   Lesions on palms and soles.
   Many lesions elsewhere later.
   Punctata version may occur.
   Plantar corn may simulate (porokeratosis plantaris discreta).

Linear porokeratosis
   Linear or zosteriform arrangement.

Reticulated porokeratosis
   Salmon-pink plaques with reticulated surface.

Malignant disseminated porokeratosis
   Basal cell–squamous cell carcinomas appear rarely.

Any diagnostic doubt concerning porokeratosis is erased by the distinctive coronoid lamella seen on biopsy.

Tatnall FM, Sarkany I: **Porokeratosis of Mibelli** in an immunosuppressed patient. J Roy Soc Med 1987; 80:180–181.

After a year of therapy with azathioprine (50 mg/day) for presumed active hepatitis and alcoholic cirrhosis, a 63-year-old man developed two lesions of **porokeratosis** (red, scaly plaques with raised borders) on his right upper arm. It was thought that azathioprine-induced immunosuppression was responsible for his lesions by allowing clones of mutant epidermal cells to proliferate.

Other examples are given of the induction, exacerbation, and spread of porokeratosis following drug-induced immunosuppression.

Schwarz T, Seiser A, Gschnait F: Disseminated superficial "**actinic**" **porokeratosis**. J Am Acad Dermatol 1984; 11:724–730.

A review of 110 cases.

Clinical:

   Annular minimally hyperkeratotic brownish-red plugs 1 to 20 mm.
   Border is hyperkeratotic, slightly elevated.
   Center minimally atrophic or depressed.
   May be pigmented, erythematous, or even depigmented.
   Rarely circinate, ulcerate.
   Number: a few to a few hundred.
   Distribution symmetrical, usually on legs.
   Pruritus in half of the cases.

Origin:

> Genodermatosis; 70% have positive family history.
> Women primarily affected.
> Average age of onset 43.
> Role of sunlight debated.

Bencini PL, Crosti C, Sala F: **Porokeratosis**: Immunosuppression and exposure to sunlight. Br J Dermatol 1987; 116:113–116.

Three renal transplant patients immunosuppressed with methylprednisolone and azathioprine, and one patient with chronic active hepatitis receiving prednisone alone, developed **disseminated superficial actinic porokeratosis** (DSAP). The lesions were lenticular or rounded crateriform brown spots surrounded by a whitish hyperkeratotic ring, located on the arms and legs. Noteworthy is the **trigger role of sunlight**, which is immunosuppressive in its own right. It may interact with viral infection or immunosuppression produced by drugs to produce the lesions. DSAP lesions have also been associated with PUVA therapy.

Venencie PY, Verola O, Puissant A: **Porokeratosis** in primary biliary cirrhosis during plasmapheresis. J Am Acad Dermatol 1986; 15:709–710.

Two superficial cornified lesions on the right knee of a 41-year-old woman with primary biliary cirrhosis were identifiable as porokeratosis, both clinically and histologically.

It is suggested that her diminished immunologic status was responsible. Similar examples have been observed in immunodepressed patients, e.g., following renal transplantation.

Kossard S, Finley AG, Poyzer K, Kocsard E: **Eruptive infundibulomas**: A distinctive presentation of the tumor of **follicular infundibulum**. J Am Acad Dermatol 1989; 21:361–366.

Hundreds of hyperpigmented irregular lesions 2 to 15 mm in diameter appeared on the upper chest and shoulders of this 23-year-old man. The distinctive feature was the angulated shape of complex **bizarre patterning**. The lesions were dry and rough to palpation and presented in actinically damaged skin.

The **diagnoses** entertained were actinic porokeratosis, discoid lupus erythematosus, pityriasis versicolor, and acne scars.

The **biopsy** revealed the lesions to be **infundibulomas**, i.e., tumors of the follicular infundibulum.

The asymptomatic subtle presentation of these tumors excites little interest on the part of the physician and patient until their sheer numbers attract attention.

If you can't make a diagnosis, it may be too early in the course of the disease.

Seborrheic Keratosis

Westrom DR, Berger TG: The sign of **Leser-Trélat** in a young man. Arch Dermatol 1986; 122:1356–1357.

Radiotherapy of a pineal body tumor (germinoma?) in a 22-year-old man was followed 1 month later by an efflorescence of multiple seborrheic keratoses over his back.

Such an explosive appearance of seborrheic keratoses, known as the **sign of Leser-Trélat**, occurs before, during, or after the appearance of an underlying cancer. Such cancers usually include adenocarcinoma of the gastrointestinal tract, squamous cell carcinoma of the lung, lymphomas, and leukemias.

The impressive feature of this example is the youth of the patient. Ordinarily, doubt arises as to the significance of this sign in the older age group, since in these patients malignancies and seborrheic keratoses are common enough to coexist by chance.

Grimes PE, Arora S, Minus HR, Kenney JA Jr: **Dermatosis papulosa nigra**. Cutis 1983; 32:385–386.

Round or filiform smooth surface, papular lesions of the face, neck, and upper trunk are the hallmark of **dermatosis papulosa nigra**. As many as four out of five black patients may exhibit this entity. It is much more common in women but less likely to be seen in fair complexioned blacks. It is not seen in children, but the lesions show an arithmetic progression as the patients age.

The clinical differential diagnosis includes:

nevi
verrucae
adenoma sebaceum
acrochordon
seborrheic keratosis

And it is the latter diagnosis that is most likely on your biopsy. By their numbers and their race you will know them.

Subrt P, Jorizzo JL, Apisarnthanarax P et al: Spreading pigmented **actinic keratosis**. J Am Acad Dermatol 1983; 8:63–67.

A 47-year-old Australian woman of Irish ancestry presented with a light-**brown macule of the right cheek**. It measured 3 × 4 cm and was an oval smooth patch with regular borders. The patient questioned the possibility of its being a malignant melanoma since it had shown a steady enlargement during its 4 years of existence. Her skin, exposed to the rigors of a Texas sun, showed senile lentigines, actinic keratoses, and actinic elastosis.

Although the lesion in question was given a clinical diagnosis of seborrheic keratosis, histologically it fit into a class of spreading pigmented actinic keratosis.

Here, the clinical diagnosis must yield to the histologic one. At times, it is clinically impossible to make a definitive distinction between:

senile lentigo
lentigo maligna
lentigo maligna melanoma
melanocytic nevus
seborrheic keratosis
spreading pigmented actinic keratosis

It is at these times your pathologist must guide you to the correct diagnosis.

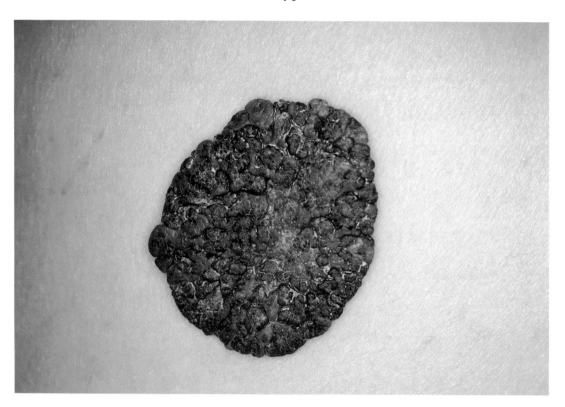

Steiner A, Konrad K, Pehamberger H, Wolff K: **Verrucous malignant melanoma**. Arch Dermatol 1988; 124:1534–1537.

Slowly growing verrucous tumors, clinically diagnosed as seborrheic keratoses in each of five patients, proved on curettage removal to be **malignant melanomas**.

Since clinical distinction is not easily made, it is imperative:

1. To remove all atypical seborrheic keratoses.
2. To interrupt curettage and do a total full-thickness surgical excision of any lesion that proves tough and fleshy, i.e., one that does not have the friable consistency of a keratosis.

Learn to order diagnostic, not agnostic, laboratory tests.

Hyperkeratoses

Garcia-Bravo B, Rodriguez-Pichardo A, Camacho F: Uraemic **follicular hyperkeratosis**. Clin Exp Dermatol 1985; 10:448–454.

A patient in **chronic renal failure** may come to your office complaining of:

keratotic follicular papules
dry, itchy, hyperkeratotic, hyperpigmented skin
bullous dermatosis mimicking porphyria cutanea tarda
calcifications in the skin
"half and half" nails
uremic frost

A bad kidney leads to bad skin.

Friedman SJ: **Lichen spinulosus**. J Am Acad Dermatol 1990; 22:261–264.

Clinical:
Follicular keratotic papules grouped into large symmetric patches.
Often on elbows, knees, extensor arms, abdomen, and buttocks.
Look for flat to conical projections (1- to 3-mm diameter) with hair-like, horny spines.
Nutmeg grater–or thorny feel. Removal of spine leaves tiny orifice in papule.
Onset at age 16 years ± 10, appearing in crops or all at once.
Differential diagnosis:
Keratosis pilaris–common, diffuse, develops slowly; entire lesion is removed with plug.
Follicular hyperkeratosis
Pityriasis rubra pilaris
Darier's disease
Associations:
Fungal infection id
Drug eruption
Seborrheic dermatitis
Hodgkin's disease
Syphilis

Rodriguez-Pichardo A, Garcia-Bravo B, Sanchez-Pedreno P, Camacho-Martinez F: **Progressive symmetric erythrokeratodermia**. J Am Acad Dermatol 1988; 19:129–130.

Circumscribed plaques of persistent or fluctuating erythema and hyperkeratosis is the central feature of this autosomal dominant disease. It begins at an early age and involutes at puberty. The usual presentation is **warty, hyperkeratotic lesions** on the elbows, knees, hands and feet.

Two of the five cases reported have involved tinea infection superimposed. In both, *Trichophyton rubrum* was isolated from the groin and knee.

Look for it in children with "**toilet seat**" **red scaly plaques** of the buttocks.

Laur WE, Posey RE, Waller JD: **Lichen planus–like keratosis**. A clinicohistopathologic correlation. J Am Acad Dermatol 1981; 4:329–336.

This single discrete velvety pinkish-orange to rusty-violaceous **lichenoid keratosis** is slightly raised with a sloping periphery, 3 to 10 mm in size, pruritic or painful, and develops rapidly. It is usually located on the face, forearm, or hand of older women and is frequently preceded by a lentigo, which may still be present.

The **differential diagnosis** includes:

actinic keratosis	lichen planus
Bowen's disease	melanoma
flat wart	seborrheic keratosis
intradermal nevus	

Flannigan SA, Tucker SB, Rapini RP: Recurrent **hyperkeratotic papules** following superficial trauma. Arch Dermatol 1985; 121:1554–1558.

A thick keratotic papule appeared at almost any site of trauma to the skin of this 30-year-old-man. This had been true since childhood; the lesions could appear anywhere—the face, arms, and hands being the most common sites. The **hyperkeratotic papules** enlarged for a month or so and then the hyperkeratotic plug fell out, permitting healing with mild atrophy and hypo- or hyperpigmentation.

A biopsy gave away the diagnosis of **reactive perforating collagenosis**. In this condition, the trauma transforms normal collagen into a foreign material which is subsequently removed by transepithelial elimination. The trauma can vary from acne to insect bites. It is hereditary in a will-o'-the-wisp fashion. If it begins in adulthood, look for diabetes or neural disease as associations of record.

The **differential diagnosis** centers on the perforating diseases:

perforating folliculitis, involves hair follicle
elastosis perforans serpiginosa
  increased elastic tissue around and in material extruded
hyperkeratosis follicularis et parafollicularis in cutem
  penetrans (Kyrle's disease)
  greater epidermal proliferation and greater inflammatory infiltrate

One should also note that a hyperkeratotic plug can prove to be a flushing out of:

granuloma annulare	osteoma
pseudo xanthoma elasticum	chondrodermatitis
injected steroid or foreign material	nodularis helicis
calcinosis	

A perforated epidermis can be a grand portal of escape for many things, but don't let the diagnosis escape you.

Aloi FG, Molinero A, Pippione M: Parakeratotic horns in a patient with **Crohn's disease**. Clin Exp Dermatol 1989; 14:79–81.

A 38-year-old woman was concerned over multiple **filiform horny projections** of the trunk and arms. They had been present for 2 years and were increasing in number. On examination the lesions were white-yellow in color and cylindrical (1–5 mm in height but less than 1 mm wide); they did not arise from hair follicles and were easily removed by a curette. The patient had had Crohn's disease for over 6 years controlled by sulfasalazine, prednisone, and metronidazole.

A biopsy showed tall columns of parakeratotic cells without any dyskeratosis or dermal changes. There was no association with underlying appendages.

The following **diagnoses for spine-like lesions** were considered and discarded:

Follicular hyperkeratosis
  orthokeratotic cells associated with sebaceous gland

Filiform verrucae
  usually on face
  acanthosis prominent
Punctate parakeratosis
  localized to palms and soles
  may be linear
  dyshidrotic or vacuolar cells in addition to parakeratotic columns
Multiple minute digitate hyperkeratosis (disseminate spiked hyperkeratosis)
  orthohyperkeratosis
Kyrle's disease
  horny plugs
  dyskeratotic cells
  epidermal penetration
Postirradiation digitate keratosis
  actinic or x-ray exposure

The diagnosis of parakeratotic horns remains the correct one. It probably bears no relationship to Crohn's disease, since exacerbations produced no known change in the horns.

Happle R, Steijlen PM, Kolde G: **Naevus corniculatus**: A new acantholytic disorder. Br J Dermatol 1990; 122:107–112.

This 33-year-old man had had an epidermal nevus of the trunk since birth. It was arranged in streaks, involved the whole body, and followed the lines of Blaschko. The individual lesions were **hornlike processes** of variable size. They could be removed without pain, leaving a pit in the keratin base.

Biopsies showed not only the keratotic excrescence but also blister formation within the epidermis. The clefting caused by the acantholytic keratinocytes produced the histologic picture of a dilapidated brick wall.

The nevus was viewed as a new entity and was named **nevus corniculatus**. Its horn formation stands in contrast to the Darier type of lesions observed in acantholytic dyskeratotic epidermal nevus. Nor is it to be confused with relapsing linear acantholytic dermatosis, in which the lesions are both inflammatory and transitory.

The horny processes are the clinical hallmark of this disorder. Most likely it originates as a somatic mutation early in embryogenesis. The time at which this event occurs determines whether the involvement is widespread or localized.

Bessems PJMJ, Jagtman BA, van de Staak WJBM et al: Progressive, persistent, hyperkeratotic lesions in **incontinentia pigmenti**. Arch Dermatol 1988; 124:29–30.

A 24-year-old woman had scattered erythematous, **hyperkeratotic** verrucous and atrophic **lesions** present for 4 years on her left leg in the whorled pigmented residua of incontinentia pigmenti. Removal of hyperkeratotic crusts disclosed erosions. Her fingernails also showed subungual hyperkeratosis and dystrophy.

Past history revealed that soon after birth her trunk and extremities were covered with linearly arranged erythematous vesiculobullous lesions. These were followed by hyperkeratotic lesions, which left reticular hyperpigmentation. At age 2 she had persistent eosinophilia (54%), scarring alopecia of the scalp, tooth dystrophy and hypodontia, atrophy of the left leg, cerebral cortical atrophy, and spina bifida occulta. At age 11 she had another attack of bullae and verrucous lesions, also localized to the pigmented areas of the left leg.

Persistent hyperkeratotic lesions in areas of hyperpigmentation, as well as subungual hyperkeratosis, should arouse suspicion of **incontinentia pigmenti**.

Grob JJ, Breton A, Bonafe JL et al: **Keratitis, ichthyosis, and deafness (KID) syndrome**. Vertical transmission and death from multiple squamous cell carcinomas. Arch Dermatol 1987; 123:777–782.

A father and daughter are presented with this rare syndrome. The father died at age 37 of metastatic squamous cell carcinoma.

The catchy acronym is misleading, since these patients do not have an ichthyosis with scaling but rather a hyperkeratosis with keratoderma, follicular keratosis, and perioral wrinkling. The condition falls into the class of congenital erythrodermas with overtones of congenital ectodermal defect.

To make the diagnosis look for:

> A history of erythematous dry skin since infancy.
> Reticulated hyperkeratosis of the cheeks and nose (diagnostic facies).
> Erythrokeratotic plaques of the elbows and knees.
> Small grayish, dry, warty growths over the entire body.
> Reddish-orange keratoderma "transgrediens" of the palms and soles with a surface like heavy-grain leather. Such stipple-and-dot grainy conformations make dermatoglyphics undecipherable.
> Acanthosis nigricans–like nipples
> Other ectodermal defects
> > hypohidrosis overall, but hyperhidrosis on palms and soles
> > buccal leukoplakia
> > dental anomalies
> > alopecia–sparse or absent hair on all parts of the body, including eyelashes and eyebrows
> > unmanageable hair
> metabolic disturbances
> > low blood zinc levels
> > vitamin A deficiency
> > glycogen accumulation in tissues
> > susceptibility to infection
> > > bacterial
> > > mycotic
> > > scabietic (such a wonderful stratum corneum for long-term housing).

You still don't have a diagnosis of KID syndrome until you confirm dual sensory impairment of vision and hearing dating back to infancy. The deafness is neurosensory, while loss of vision and photophobia result from bilateral keratitis with vascularization and opacification of the cornea.

What might confuse you?

> Refsum's disease (ichthyosis, retinitis pigmentosa, neurosensory deafness).
> Rud's syndrome (ichthyosiform erythroderma "*rud*imentary" physical and mental characteristics, dwarfism, hypogonadism, mental deficiency).
> Thick skin diseases without dual sensory loss:
> > pachyonychia congenita
> > erythrokeratodermia variabilis
> > erythrokeratoderma, symmetrical progressive
> > follicular hyperkeratosis
> > ichthyosis follicularis

Moral: Check the **eyesight** and **hearing** of any infant or child with rough skin if you want to find that kid who has KID syndrome!

History taking requires fine tuning . . . some patients give you a history so filled with static that you can't hear the message.

Cunningham SR, Walsh M, Matthews R, et al: Kyrle's disease. J Am Acad Dermatol 1987; 16:117–123.

Hyperkeratotic plugs—big, little, and small—are the centerpiece of Kyrle's disease. They make their entrance on the lower legs and posterior thigh but may arise anywhere except the palms, soles, and mucous membranes. Some of the keratotic plugs are large and verrucous; others are no more than a scale with a promise. When they are removed there is an underlying shallow crater, usually not at the site of a hair follicle. The biopsy is rather unexciting, showing mainly a mass of orthokeratin with a touch of parakeratosis and basophilic debris. The plug does not often penetrate into the papillary dermis, and only a slight inflammatory cell response is seen in the underlying dermis.

It is a disease of genetic origin but with marker significance for systemic disease. It is a chronic disease that over a decade can result in keratotic plugs sprouting out on the arms and trunk.

Look to the pathologist in ruling out

perforating folliculitis
Flegel's disease (hyperkeratosis lenticularis perstans)
reactive perforating collagenosis
elastosis perforans serpiginosa

Pearson LH, Graham Smith J Jr, Chalker DK: **Hyperkeratosis lenticularis perstans** (Flegel's disease). Case report and literature review. J Am Acad Dermatol 1987; 16:190–195.

Small hyperkeratotic papules of the dorsa of the feet and lower legs of adults is the presenting sign of this rare genodermatosis. It is a chronic process that may eventually involve arms, palms, soles, and even oral mucosa.

It is distinguished from

Kyrle's disease–variable size
Stucco keratosis–gray-white keratosis
Porokeratoses of Mibelli–occurs in childhood, few lesions
Disseminated superficial actinic porokeratosis–border distinctive

Price ML, Wilson Jones E, MacDonald DM: A clinicopathological study of **Flegel's disease** (hyperkeratosis lenticularis perstans). Br J Dermatol 1987; 116:681–691.

Scaly papules (1 to 5 mm) on the lower legs, upper arms, and pinnae of the ears appearing in adulthood are the characteristic findings of Flegel's disease. This focal hyperkeratosis, not seen until adulthood, is of autosomal dominant transmission in some instances and appears to be a disorder of keratin proliferation.

It is to be **distinguished** clinically from other focal hyperkeratotic disorders such as stucco keratoses and actinic porokeratosis. Biopsy reveals discrete foci of hyperkeratosis with some parakeratosis over an attenuated and partially spongiotic epidermis. The lesion might be primarily inflammatory, as the earliest histologic changes consist of inflammation in the papillary dermis with edema extending as spongiosis into the lower epidermis.

Balus L, Donati P, Amantea A, Breathnach AS: Multiple minute **digitate hyperkeratoses**. J Am Acad Dermatol 1988; 18:431–436.

A 48-year-old woman had **hundreds of dark keratotic lesions** roughening the skin of her back, shoulders, chest, arms, and thighs. Some papules were tiny and spiked, while others were 2- to 3-mm flat-topped or dome-shaped. It was a dominant family trait. The skin felt like sandpaper, but the lesions were asymptomatic and not follicular.

The **differential diagnosis** included:

keratosis pilaris
porokeratosis
follicular lichen planus
pityriasis rubra pilaris
Kyrle's disease (hyperkeratosis in cutem penetrans)
Flegel's disease (hyperkeratosis lenticularis perstans)

The skin eruption of Flegel's disease is similar to the present case but involves predominantly acral keratotic papules and differs histologically, having a bandlike lymphocytic infiltrate. In one reported case, similar spiked papules were associated with a carcinoma of the larynx. These improved after surgical treatment of the tumor.

Other names of this condition are disseminated spiked hyperkeratosis, hyperkératose piliforme disséminée familiale, and minute aggregate keratosis.

Taxonomy would be easy if skin diseases bred true as birds and beetles do.

Palms

Larsson P-A, Lidén S: Prevalence of **skin diseases among adolescents** 12 to 16 years of age. Acta Derm Venereol 1980; 60:415–423.

Circumscribed, erythematous, hyperkeratotic thickenings over the proximal interphalangeal joints may make you think they are **knuckle pads**. However, on looking at the palm and seeing the thickened yellowish surface, it becomes evident that they are a part of the **Unna-Thost hereditary palmar-plantar hyperkeratosis**.

In problematic cases, the keratoderma is made more evident by immersion of the hands in water for 10 minutes.

Stasko T, Vander Ploeg DE, DeVillez RL: **Hyperkeratotic mycosis fungoides** restricted to the palms. J Am Acad Dermatol 1982; 7:792–796.

Hyperkeratotic pits and plaques had been present for 6 months on the palmar side of the fingers of this 45-year-old man. Although the initial impression was hand eczema, this was not supported by analysis of his occupation, hobbies, and history. Furthermore, patch tests were negative. Keratolytics and high-potency topical steroids used for months proved ineffective.

Biopsies on two occasions, as well as electron microscopy, showed the pattern of mycosis fungoides. Application of nitrogen mustard (10 mg in 50 ml water) twice daily for $2\frac{1}{2}$ months resulted in complete clearing.

Although mycosis fungoides may appear localized to the hands, this is the first report of this lymphoma strictly limited to the palms.

A biopsy was the way they caught the nature of the thing.

Rapini RP, Hebert AA, Drucker CR: Acquired perforating dermatosis: Evidence of combined transepidermal elimination of both collagen and elastic fibers. Arch Dermatol 1989; 125:1074–1078.

In any patient with adult-onset acquired perforating dermatosis, look for underlying diabetes mellitus and/or renal disease.

The cutaneous presentation is a **hyperkeratotic papule** that histologically proves to be a transepidermal elimination of degenerated material, including both collagen and elastin. The generic diagnosis is acquired perforating dermatosis. However, four categories have and will continue to be recognized:

> perforating folliculitis–follicular location
> elastosis perforans serpiginosa–annular, favors the neck
> reactive perforating collagenosis–Koebner phenomenon
> Kyrle's disease–epithelial hyperplasia

Nielsen PG: The prevalence of **dermatophyte infection** in hereditary palmoplantar keratoderma. Acta Derm Venereol 1983; 63:439–441.

The first appearance of hereditary palmoplantar keratoderma ranged from birth to age 13. It manifested itself as a diffuse homogeneous hyperkeratosis with distinct demarcation from normal skin. In a few patients, the border shows hyperkeratotic papules. Pad-like keratoses of the knuckles are also often present. Some patients noted intermittent scaling and a few showed fissuring. Immersion in water produced a spongy appearance in all.

Ironically, nearly everyone had hyperhidrosis that had persisted well into adulthood. As the sweating waned, the hyperkeratotic skin remained rough and dry.

Study of 60 patients with this hereditary keratoderma revealed that 40% had proven **dermatophyte infections**. Obviously, the keratoderma provides a favorable home for fungi.

Schwartz BK, Clendenning WE: A cutaneous sign of **bulimia**. J Am Acad Dermatol 1985; 12:725–726.

Callus-like crusted papules and nodules over the knuckles of the hands proved to be the index diagnostic sign of previously unrecognized bulimia in a 20-year-old atopic woman.

The lesions reflected the fact that after every meal for the past several years, she had induced vomiting by putting either hand deep into her mouth. During this emetic maneuver the knuckles were repeatedly traumatized by the teeth.

By their knuckles, ye shall know them.

Perret C: **Schöpf syndrome**. Br J Dermatol 1988; 120:131–132.

A 4-H Club genodermatosis:
Hidrocystomas of eyelids.
Hyperkeratoses of palms and soles.
Hypoplastic teeth.
Hypotrichosis.

It is associated with cancer proneness (and residency gamesmanship). In this case, a 75-year-old man with the syndrome also had an interdigital tumor on one hand, diagnosed as a squamous cell carcinoma.

The more diagnoses you can think of, the more likely you'll think of the right one.

Legs

Look to the legs for the diagnoses of **circulatory incompetence and failure**. It is here that dependent edema is seen. It is here that diabetic dermopathy and necrobiosis lipoidica diabeticorum herald small vessel damage. And it is here that we see stasis dermatitis and ulceration, as well as islands of dermatitis overlying incompetent perforator veins.

The legs are the home of antigen antibody complex deposition in the slow-moving capillary stream. It is here we see pigmented purpuric eruptions such as Schamberg's disease and the purpura annularis telangiectoides of Majocchi.

And it is in the skin of the legs that we see the effects of physical trauma inflicted on a dermis hammered on the subjacent tibia. Here we see erythema nodosum, nodular vasculitis, and the picture of panniculitis.

The compromised slowed circulation of the legs, our price for an erect posture, sets the stage for thrombophlebitis, with its tender inflamed nodules. And it is here we see the infarcts of atrophie blanche and atrophie noir.

When you look at the legs you are looking for diagnoses centered on the frailties of cutaneous circulation.

Angeloni VL, Salasche SJ, Ortic R: Nail, skin, and scleral **pigmentation** induced by minocycline. Cutis 1987; 40:229–233.

A 47-year-old white man was referred for evaluation of a color change of his lower legs that had been considered to be due to **stasis dermatitis**. Discoloration of his toenails was thought to be bruises. He denied any ingestion of heavy metals, antimalarials, or phenothiazines. However, he had been taking minocycline (200 to 300 mg/day) for 8 years for treatment of an acneiform eruption.

When the patient was seen by the authors, his entire skin had a muddy discoloration, accentuated in the sun-exposed areas. Numerous gray macules were seen on the lower legs. The nail beds of the great toes showed a blue-gray color. Likewise, the anterior sclerae were bluish.

A biopsy showed numerous pigment granules and pigment-laden macrophages in the dermis. Perls' stain for iron was mildly positive.

The patient's discoloration is another example of the cutaneous pigmentation produced by high-dose long-term **minocycline** therapy. Not only is the skin involved but also the teeth may be discolored, the bones greenish, and the thyroid black, with black galactorrhea.

The major **differential** includes:

argyria
chloroquin (antimalarial) pigmentation
chlorpromazine (phenothiazine) pigmentation
and with the blue nail plate, don't forget Wilson's disease.

Fishman HC: Pigmented purpuric **lichenoid dermatitis** of Gougerot-Blum. Cutis 1982; 29:260–264.

Dull red split pea–sized papules, in ill-defined groups, were the presenting complaint of this 45-year-old male alcoholic. The lesions, which included macules, were present on the legs, thighs, waist, and forearms. They had been present for 7 months and showed improvement when his drinking abated.

A diagnosis of the **pigmented purpuric lichenoid dermatitis of Gougerot-Blum** was confirmed by the biopsy findings of extravasated red cells and a perivascular infiltrate.

The erythematous papules and scaling distinguished this condition from the closely related **Schamberg's disease** (progressive pigmentary dermatosis), in which the rust-colored pigmentation is so prominent. It is also distinguished from **Majocchi's purpura annularis telangiectodes**, in which telangiectasia is the dominant finding.

Barnhill RL, Braverman IM: Progression of pigmented **purpura-like eruptions** to mycosis fungoides: Report of three cases. J Am Acad of Dermatol 1988; 19:25–31.

Widespread erythematous patches had been present on this 33-year-old man's skin for 7 years. They had a golden-brown pigmentation and clinically suggested **Schamberg's disease** or lichen aureus. Biopsy showed a pattern consistent with a pigmented purpuric eruption. Three years later, with new lesions appearing, a biopsy showed **mycosis fungoides**, patch stage.

Two other patients with chronic purpuric lesions, one of whom was thought to have **lichen aureus**, showed progression of a pigmented purpuric eruption to histologically recognizable mycosis fungoides over a period of 6 and 12 years, respectively. Persistent widespread pigmented purpuric eruptions must be included in the spectrum of premalignant disease.

813

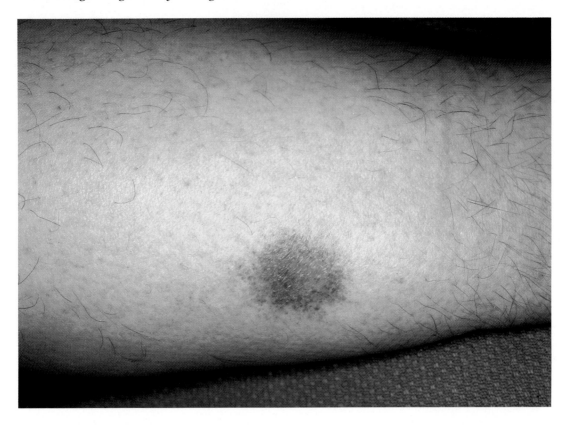

Bergman W: **Lichen aureus** with underlying arteriovenous shunt. Br J Dermatol 1989; 121:800–801.

A progressively enlarging purple patch on the right medial malleolus of this 10-year-old girl proved on biopsy to be **lichen aureus**. It had been present for 4 years.

The presence of an underlying small-caliber arteriovenous shunt was demonstrated by **Doppler** ultrasound studies. The purple patch exhibited a venous vessel sound accompanied by a soft heartbeat sound.

Shelley WB, Swaminathan R, Shelley ED: **Lichen aureus**: A hemosiderin tattoo associated with perforator vein incompetence. J Am Acad Dermatol 1984; 11:260–264.

A 61-year-old man presented with a 6-cm circular plaque of dermatitis with petechiae on the medial aspect of his right lower leg. It had appeared suddenly and was localized over an incompetent posterior tibial perforating vein.

Within weeks the lesions took on a burnt orange or golden hue. A diagnosis of **lichen aureus** was made. This rare entity, first named lichen purpuricus, can present with a variety of "aureus" shades: burnt orange, yellow, gold, golden brown, or even purple. It appears usually on the leg, but may be seen elsewhere. Usually a solitary plaque with varying degree of lichenification, it shows a distinctive histologic picture of extravasated red cells and the inevitable hemosiderin end product appearing in the macrophages. It is this **hemosiderin** that accounts for the golden diagnostic clue tattooed into each lesion.

If the lesion looks strange, and the patient does also, think factitial.

Owens CWI, Al-Khader AA, Jackson MJ, Prichard BNC: A severe "stasis eczema," associated with **low plasma zinc**, treated successfully with oral zinc. Br J Dermatol 1981; 105:461–464.

This 82-year-old woman had had 3 months of an extremely itchy confluent erythematous and excoriated rash with lichenification of both lower legs. The backs of the hands, the forearms, and thighs showed a similar yet less severe picture.

The problem had been confidently diagnosed as **stasis dermatitis** with autosensitization dermatitis of the hands. She had given no evidence of alcohol abuse, renal disease, diabetes, malabsorption, rheumatoid arthritis, collagen disease, or excess phytate (legumes, grains) ingestion. General medical studies and chemical profiles were normal.

Because dry skin (eczema craquelé) as well as warty or psoriasiform changes on the extremities can result from a zinc deficiency, a plasma zinc level was secured. It proved to be low (6.7 μmol/liter vs normal 11.4 to 18.4 μmol/liter). A diagnosis of **zinc deficiency dermatitis** was made and confirmed by a disappearance of the itching within 1 week of zinc supplementation (220 mg $ZnSO_4 \cdot 7 \, H_2O$/day). Within a month the so-called stasis dermatitis was gone and the zinc level was up to high normal. Noteworthy was the improvement in her gait and strength.

Further proof of the correctness of the diagnosis came when the zinc supplement was stopped 2 months later. Within 6 weeks, the pruritus was back, and by 10 weeks the rash of the legs and hands had returned. Again, with resumption of oral zinc, the skin returned to normal.

The cause of the zinc deficiency was never determined but it may have been due to an inadequate diet taken by a listless, sick old lady.

Butler DF, Berger TG, Rodman OG: **Leukemia cutis** mimicking stasis dermatitis. Cutis 1985; 35:47–48.

A 23-year-old man with chronic lymphatic leukemia presented with a 3-day history of an enlarging painful red area on the medial aspect of his left lower leg. The lesion was a large, warm, tender, **purpuric edematous patch**. Numerous petechiae were present on the extremities.

Even as the biopsy was being read as a specific **leukemia cutis**, the blood studies showing a white blood cell count of 148,000/mm^3 were interpreted as a blast crisis of this young man's chronic lymphatic leukemia.

Look for the unusual in the medical background of a young patient with a "stasis dermatitis." In history taking, ask for details: it is the details that can surprise and instruct you. Examples **from our practice**:

consumption of 2 gallons of milk a day. ("Milk makes muscle" and cystic acne)
consumption of 40 cups of coffee a day (florid rosacea)
consumption of 20 cola drinks a day (rosacea)
a diet consisting of candy bars (led to hospitalization for cystic acne)
daily application of deodorant to scrotum (the cause of scrotal dermatitis)
consumption of 3 to 6 packs of beer a day (associated with failure of penile ulcer to heal)
eyedrops (cause of erythroderma)
acne cyst that "migrated" across the cheek (dirofilarial infection)
antidandruff shampoo (scalp hair loss)
intake of large doses of OTC vitamin A (cause of hair loss and pseudotumor cerebri)

8 years of daily oral steroids based on a single prescription given 8 years earlier (Cushing facies, striae, hypertension, diabetes, osteoporosis, peptic ulcer)

Wyre HW: Cutaneous manifestations of **Noonan's syndrome**. Arch Dermatol 1978; 114:929–930.

Lymphedema and stasis dermatitis of the lower legs had been present in this 37-year-old man for nearly 20 years. In casting about for an explanation of this **early onset of stasis dermatitis**, it was noted that defects suggested a genetic origin. His right testicle had never descended. He had had surgical intervention for atrophic maxillae and for an inguinal hernia. He exhibited neck webbing, hypertelorism, and prominent ears. Finally, his short stature, curly hair, and numerous nevi all pointed to a diagnosis of Noonan's syndrome, a multisystem disorder of wide spectrum.

Noonan's syndrome lives in a foggy family of eponymic siblings. Out of a commonality of congenital defects, one tries to discern a singular finding that permits an appropriate eponym. This is the scrotum that overrides the penis in Aarskog-Scott syndrome, the pulmonary valve dysplasia in the cardiofaciocutaneous syndrome, the lentigines in the LEOPARD syndrome, and the occurrence in girls of ovarian agenesis in Turner's syndrome, as well as the short neck in the Klippel-Feil variant.

Learn to recognize these family members so you can call them by their first names.

Taking a good history requires not only a patient but also a patient doctor.

Lebel M, Lassonde M: **Erythema induratum of Bazin**. J Am Acad Dermatol 1986; 14:738–742.

Multiple brownish-red **nodules**, punched out ulcers as well as atrophic scars had been present for over 3 months **on the calves** and shins of this 41-year-old woman. They had been indifferent to treatment with systemic tetracycline, penicillin, and dicloxacillin as well as topical antibiotics.

Work-up for connective tissue disease, blood levels for iodides and bromides, as well as health profiles and chest roentgenogram were all negative. Cultures for acid-fast bacilli from sputum and skin were negative. However, *S. aureus* and *E. coli* were cultured from the ulcers. The skin biopsy showed a granulomatous and necrotic reaction in the fat. A PPD test (5 units) gave a 3-cm area of induration at 48 hours.

The cardinal finding of microbiologically and radiologically confirmed pulmonary tuberculosis 13 years ago led to the diagnosis of **erythema induratum of Bazin**. Isoniazid (300 mg/day) therapy resulted in significant improvement in 6 weeks and complete resolution in 1 year, with only atrophic hyperpigmented scar remaining.

Erythema induratum is a rare disease:

> usually seen in women
> presents as persistent recurrent nodules
> site of predilection is posterior lower leg, lower third of calf
> ulcerates in cold weather
> ulcers are irregular and shallow with bluish, tense borders
> may show spontaneous healing in months
> significant number of patients have history of tuberculosis
> pathogenesis–severe vasculitis

Rademaker M, Lowe DG, Munro DD: **Erythema induratum** (Bazin's disease). J Am Acad Dermatol 1989; 21:740–745.

Presentation
> Violaceous indurated nodules 1 to 2 cm in diameter that were painful, occasionally ulcerative, and could heal without scarring.

Occurs in middle-aged women.

Location: legs, also arms, thighs, feet, buttocks.

Course: evolve for several weeks, heal in several months, appear in crops over many years.

Most common misdiagnosis: recurrent thrombophlebitis.

Best diagnostic test: tuberculin-purified protein derivative (PPD) strongly positive at 1/10,000. Use 1 Unit (10 U may produce deep ulcer at skin test site. Be certain injection is in dermis and not in fat.

Good response to antituberculosis therapy.

Too much lab data can add to diagnostic doubt.

Atrophie Blanche

Shornick JK, Nicholes BK, Bergstresser PR, Gilliam JN: **Idiopathic atrophie blanche**. J Am Acad Dermatol 1983; 8:792–798.

Primary lesions:

Recurrent painful purpuric macules and papules that undergo superficial necrosis and ulceration.

Diagnostic secondary changes:

Porcelain white atrophic scars with peripheral telangiectasia and hyperpigmentation.

Location:

Lower extremities, rarely forearms.

Biopsy:

Vascular occlusion by fibrin. No necrotizing vasculitis.

Differential diagnosis:

Secondary atrophie blanche due to:
stasis dermatitis
dysproteinemia
cryoglobulins
macroglobulins
connective tissue disease
lupus erythematosus
rheumatoid arthritis
diabetes mellitus
arteriosclerosis
hypertension

Synonyms:
Segment hyalinizing vasculitis.
Livedo reticularis with summer ulceration.

Sadick NS, Allen SL: **Atrophie blanche** in chronic myelogenous leukemia. Cutis 1988; 42:206–209.

A 69-year-old woman with chronic myelogenous leukemia developed left calf pain with marked edema and a reticular erythematous eruption with vasculitic papules over the left lateral malleolus. This was followed by ulceration, **eschar formation**, and foci of atrophic porcelain white scarring. Direct immunofluorescent studies showed IgM, C3, and fibrin deposits in blood vessel walls. She then developed burning of both feet and similar lesions on the right ankle. No gammopathy was found on serum protein electrophoresis. Treatment with prednisone (60 mg/day) and control of her leukemia with busulfan cleared the atrophie blanche lesions.

Fatigue is the cataract of the diagnostic eye.

Miller JA, Machin SJ, Dowd PM: **Cutaneous gangrene** with hyperparathyroidism. Clin Exp Dermatol 1988; 13:204–206.

Extremely painful **necrotic bruises** appeared on the lower legs and thighs of a 70-year-old woman hospitalized for renal failure. Indeed, dressing changes were so painful as to require nitrous oxide anesthesia. Skin biopsy of a tender indurated area showed a thrombosed vessel in the subcutaneous fat but no inflammation, vasculitis, or calcification in blood vessel walls.

Her serum calcium was elevated at 3.25 mmol/liter (normal 2.2 to 2.6); and the **infarcts** were thought to be due to **hyperparathyroidism**. Removal of a right upper parathyroid adenoma led to significant pain reduction in a few days, and after 3 months the ulcers had completely healed.

Coagulation studies revealed an increase in the von Willebrand factor (compared with factor VIII activity), which is synthesized, stored, and released into the circulation by vascular endothelial cells. Its elevation occurs when there is endothelial damage. The cause of the vascular damage is unclear in patients with renal impairment and elevated parathormone levels. In this patient other factors that promote thrombosis and infarction were normal (protein C, plasminogen, lupus anticoagulant screen, and antithrombin III).

Itin P, Stalder H, Vischer W: Symmetrical **peripheral gangrene** in disseminated tuberculosis. Dermatologica 1986; 173:189–195.

In a 66-year-old alcoholic bricklayer with hereditary hemorrhagic telangiectasia, the sudden appearance of purplish discoloration followed by **necrosis of the toes** led to amputations of the forefeet. The veins were normal, but every acral arterial vessel was occluded by thrombi, which may have been microembolic *M. tuberculosis* from disseminate miliary tuberculosis with bacteremia.

Symmetrical peripheral gangrene is an ischemic necrosis which simultaneously affects the distal parts of two or more extremities without obstruction of the greater arteries. The most common cause is gram-positive sepsis (*Staphylococcus aureus*, *Streptococcus pyogenes*, pneumococci), although gram-negative sepsis (meningococci, *Hemophilus influenzae*, enteric organisms) has also been reported.

Other causes for this rare symmetrical **peripheral gangrene** occurring in the presence of good pulses include:

   I. Hypotension: Shock, cardiac failure, use of betablockers

   II. Vasoconstriction: Shock, frostbite, Raynaud's phenomenon, vasoactive agents (dopamine, ergotamine, vasopressin, chloroquine)

   III. Endothelial damage: Sepsis (bacterial, treponemal, rickettsial, viral), bleomycin, arsenic ("black foot disease"), carbon monoxide poisoning, vasculitis, collagen disease, Kaposi's sarcoma, arterial calcification (uremia, oxalosis)

   IV. Vascular obliteration:
      a. Thromboembolic occlusion: Disseminated intravascular coagulation, emboli (cholesterol, septic), thrombocythemia, sickle cell anemia, heparin-induced thrombosis, malaria, polycythemia vera
      b. Hyperviscosity states: Cryoglobulinemia, paraproteinemia, hypernatremic dehydration
      c. Venous thrombosis

Kirk CR, Dorgan JC, Hart CA: **Gas gangrene**: A cautionary tale. Br Med J 1988; 296:1236–1237.

A 6-year-old boy suffered a deep **laceration** of his right knee after a fall,   819 through which the joint capsule was visible. A radiograph revealed air within the joint. Deep soiling was present upon wound exploration, but following extensive cleansing and hematoma evacuation the skin was sutured and the leg was placed in a split cylinder of plaster of Paris. Due to a previous rash and facial swelling from amoxicillin, he was given erythromycin prophylactically. Three days later he developed a fever, WBC 32,000, and swelling of the right leg. Pus was found when the wound was re-explored, from which ***Clostridium perfringens*** and *Citrobacter freundii* were cultured and sensitivities determined. Despite treatment with intravenous cefuroxime, trimethoprim, and metronidazole, and hyperbaric oxygen, the edema progressed to the other leg, abdominal wall, and lower chest, and his condition deteriorated over 3 days. He had convulsions and required ventilation and cardiovascular support. The skin of the right thigh and lower abdomen became mottled, erythematous, and indurated with blisters over the thigh and dorsum of the foot. A test dose of Augmentin (amoxicillin trihydrate and clavulanic acid) was given without adverse effects; it was then started in high dose. After 24 hours he was weaned from the respirator and by 10 days after starting the medication the edema had resolved. The wound healed by secondary intention, but a split skin graft was required to repair the full-thickness skin loss over the thigh where blistering had occurred.

Gas gangrene is usually associated with wartime injuries. It is now rare since soiled or penetrating wounds are managed with debridement, prophylactic antibiotics, and delayed primary closure. In this case, immediate closure of the wound predisposed to the gas gangrene.

Penicillin is the drug of choice as it can penetrate edematous avascular tissue as well as septic joints. Even with a history of possible penicillin allergy, it should be given in a test dose, taking necessary precautions.

Center your reading on the patient. In my experience, it makes reading more meaningful and enhances retention.

Robert G. Petersdorf

Graham-Brown RAC, Sarkany I: **Chronic leg ulcers** with hyperlipidaemia. J Roy Soc Med 1982; 75:478–479.

In two brothers, ulcers of the feet and legs began at the age of 16 years, resulting in areas of **atrophie blanche** with small, painful, indolent, hard to heal ulcers on the feet and scarring and pigmentary changes on the lower legs. Both men, ages 27 and 33, had type IV hyperlipidemia, with elevated triglyceride levels. Control of the **hyperlipidemia** with clofibrate and diet resulted in healing of the ulcers, which promptly reappeared when therapy was stopped.

Both brothers also had increased whole-blood viscosity, possibly due to altered red blood cell deformability.

Skin biopsy adjacent to an ulcer showed numerous capillaries with focal endothelial proliferation and thickening of the wall due to PAS-positive materials consistent with atrophie blanche.

Verdegem TD, Sharma OP: **Cutaneous ulcers** in sarcoidosis. Arch Dermatol 1987; 123:1531–1534.

Four cases of **ulcers** on the anterior surface of the lower legs in black women (ages 27 to 51 years) are presented. **Biopsies** revealed noncaseating granulomas, and all of the women had chest x-rays showing hilar adenopathy. Successful treatment consisted of combinations of prednisone and chloroquine/hydroxychloroquine.

Ulcers with necrotic bases and serosanguineous purulent exudate, although a rare sign of **sarcoidosis**, have been reported in more than 30 patients. Usually located on the anterior surface of the lower legs (a site of trauma), they have also been seen on the face, arms, trunk, abdomen, and perineum. Infectious causes of granulomatous ulcers must be ruled out by cultures of biopsy specimens. Work-up should also include skin tests for tuberculosis, histoplasmosis, and coccidioidomycosis, and sputum smears and cultures.

Caro I, Calnan CD: **Hereditary sensory neuropathy**. Report of a case. Clin Exp Dermatol 1976; 1:91–92.

A 66-year-old man had suffered **recurrent ulceration of the feet** for 35 years, necessitating amputation of six toes. The family history revealed a father with syringomyelia, a paternal grandfather whose leg was amputated because of ulcers, and a son and daughter with ulcers of the feet and diminished sensations of the lower legs and the feet. The patient reported infrequent paroxysms of stabbing pain in the feet and lower legs and dermatitis around the ulcers. Examination revealed two deep ulcers on the left sole and right ankle and superficial sensory loss of pain below the knees. The peripheral nerves were not thickened.

A diagnosis of **hereditary sensory** (**radicular**) **neuropathy** was made. This autosomal dominant disease reflects dorsal root ganglia degeneration and peripheral nerve degeneration and fibrosis. The first sign is often a painless trophic ulcer on a pressure-bearing area of the foot, beginning in the second to third decade. Loss of sensation to pain and temperature is found in the lower legs and the feet. Sympathetic function and tendon reflexes are depressed or absent in involved areas, but motor function is normal. Progressive nerve deafness may develop, along with lancinating pain in the legs similar to tabes dorsalis. Spontaneous amputation of digits, osteolysis, and shortening of the phalanges and metatarsal bones are also characteristic.

Other **sensory neuropathies** considered:

syringomyelia
leprosy
familial sensory neuropathy with anhidrosis
familial amyloidosis
familial dysautonomia
congenital sensory neuropathy
congenital indifference to pain with total body analgesia

Leoni A, Cetta G, Tenni R et al: **Prolidase deficiency** in two siblings with chronic leg ulcerations. Clinical, biochemical and morphological aspects. Arch Dermatol 1987; 123:493–499.

Ragged-edged ulcers of the lower third of the legs, 3 to 4 mm deep, with vertical margins and a necrotic base were the presenting complaint of a 37-year-old woman. The surrounding skin was atrophic, scarred, nonhairy, and inflamed. The ulcers had appeared when she was 12 years old and had persisted despite 16 skin grafts.

After a frustrating series of negative tests for autoantibodies, complement abnormalities, cryoglobulinemia, lupus erythematosus cells, Doppler evaluation of circulatory disturbance, as well as chromosomal analysis, the problem was identified as a hereditary disease by measuring (1) immunodipeptides in a 24-hour urine sample after 3 days of a nonprotein diet; (2) prolidase activity of the erythrocytes. The immunodipeptides level was high, and prolidase was only 2% of normal.

The disease is characterized by a **lack of prolidase** (proline dipeptidase), **which splits dipeptides** containing hydroxyproline or C-terminal proline. The absence of this splitting results in accumulation of dipeptides containing an amino acid at the C-terminus, thereby inhibiting the normal recycling of proline for the synthesis of collagen.

Her ulcers and those of her sister can be viewed as the result of trauma to skin that has **faulty collagen synthesis**.

Think of prolidase deficiency in children with chronic ulcers of the lower legs and in adults who have ulcers since childhood, and think of it in a mentally retarded child who has strange inexplicable purpuric, papular, erythematous eruptions, and think of it with **telangiectasia and photosensitivity**. It is rare, but its major manifestation is common, i.e., leg ulcers that won't heal. If you can't think of it, your amino acid analyzer can't either.

Lewis JE: **Cutaneous epitheliomas** on the lower extremities. Cutis 1981; 27:499–502.

A large **chronic ulcer** had been present on the calf of this 70-year-old white woman for 9 years. Her personal physician who had been treating it for 4 years diagnosed the problem as "ulceration from weak blood vessels."

On biopsy the ulcer proved to be not a stasis ulcer but an **ulcerated basal cell carcinoma**. From the history came the major contributory factor in the pathogenesis of this leg ulcer: The patient had spent a lifetime working in the cotton fields of the south.

Twenty-two such patients with epitheliomas of the legs are recorded from one county in Arkansas. All were women whose dress allowed exposure to the sun, unlike the men, who wore trousers.

Chronic leg ulcers in elderly white women who live and work in sunny climes should arouse a suspicion of epithelioma.

Kardaun SH, Kruis-De Vries MH, Oosterhuis JW et al: **Epithelioid sarcoma**. Br J Dermatol 1988; 118:843–844.

A pretibial ulcer, 3 by 3.5 cm, with central deep necrosis and smooth, slightly elevated, undermined margins on the right lower leg of a 23-year-old man eluded diagnosis for 6 months. Two punch biopsies had been nondiagnostic. Only by histologic study of the completely excised ulcer was the diagnosis of **epithelioid sarcoma** finally made. The tumor cells were in strings and showed eosinophilic cytoplasm, atypical nuclei, and atypical mitoses. They were intermixed with granulation tissue and a dense polymorphous infiltrate beneath an acanthotic epidermis. Eight months later an enlarged inguinal lymph node appeared, filled with metastatic tumor cells.

It is recommended that ulcers of unknown nature be subjected not to punch biopsies but rather to **wedge excisions**. Prolonged follow-up of epithelioid sarcoma is always indicated, since there are recurrences in 77% and metastases in 45% of cases, as long as 19 years later. First described by Enzinger in 1970, it is very rare and occurs mostly in young men on the distal portions of the arms and legs.

Shelley WB: An idiopathic leg ulcer as the presenting sign of **lymphoma**. Cutis 1981; 28:43–44.

This 53-year-old woman developed a series of evanescent tender nodular masses on the legs; however, one over the right medial malleolus became ulcerated and persisted. A biopsy showed a nonspecific inflammatory change, and the ulcer was viewed as venous in origin.

Within months a large fungating lobulated mass developed in the ulcer. The **differential diagnosis** included lymphoma, amelanotic melanoma, bromoderma, squamous cell carcinoma, blastomycosis, and tertiary syphilis. Histologic examination proved the tumor to be a **malignant histiocytic lymphoma**.

Sometimes you have to wait for a disease to grow up before a diagnosis can be made.

Castellani A: A pleomorphic slime organism associated with **ulcerative dermatosis** of the leg. Lancet 1964; 2:72–73.

In two cases of nonpainful, nontender chronic leg ulcers with gummalike lesions and open sores, slime-producing organisms were isolated. They had features of both Myxobacteriales (slime bacteria) and Myxomycetes (slime molds), organisms that grow on damp decayed wood and vegetable material. The term *myxo-ulcus cruris* is used.

Many physicians lack not the ability but the time to solve difficult diagnostic problems.

Lichen Planus

Ordinarily, lichen planus is as easily recognizable as an old friend. He greets you with an itch and wears iridescent purple patches in all the old familiar places on wrist and ankle. See those lacy gray curtains? And if that is not enough, a drop of oil reveals his signature in white.

But sometimes lichen planus does not come as a diagnostician's friend; he may come in disguise. He may present only thick hypertrophic plaques on the shins that suggest lichen simplex chronicus. He may come dressed in bullae and lead you to think you are seeing pemphigoid. He may come presenting only ulcers of the palms or widespread annular plaques. He may show you naught but atrophic spots or nails mysteriously deformed or lost. He may even come as a sunlight reactor or as one without some hair. For these encounters your pathologist may be needed to see behind the mask to spot your old friend. Then with experience you will learn to recognize your friend by his masks. You will come to know him sans itch, sans papule, and sans Wickham's striae.

But always remember that your friend can be impersonated by a drug reaction.

Banse-Kupin L, Morales A, Kleinsmith D'A: Perforating **lichen nitidus**. J Am Acad Dermatol 1983; 9:452–456.

This 22-year-old black man had numerous discrete dome-shaped papules of the trunk and thighs for the past month. Flat-topped violaceous papules and plaques were also seen on his wrists and forearm. A biopsy of the latter gave a diagnosis of **lichen planus**. In contrast, the biopsy of dome-shaped papules showed **lichen nitidus** with a heavy mononuclear and histiocytic infiltrate permeating and breaking through the epidermis.

Although confluent, vesicular, hemorrhagic, as well as palmar and plantar variants of lichen nitidus have been described, this is only the second case of perforating lichen nitidus recorded. The coexistence of lichen planus and lichen nitidus is also noteworthy. Both show the Koebner phenomenon and may be versions of one disease. However, lichen planus heals with hyperpigmentation, whereas lichen nitidus does not.

Lichen planus comes in a great many forms:

bullous	hypertrophic	guttate
ulcerative	atrophic	giant
actinic	linear	planopilaris

The finding of lichen nitidus showing a perforating form adds to the list of diseases in which an altered dermis is being eliminated through the overlying epidermis. One also sees this phenomenon in:

> elastosis perforans serpiginosa
> perforating folliculitis
> perforating granuloma annulare
> Kyrle's disease
> reactive perforating collagenosis
> chondrodermatitis nodularis helicis

As patients often say, "What's bad has got to come out."

Matta M, Kibbi A-G, Khattar J et al: **Lichen planopilaris**: A clinicopathologic study. J Am Acad Dermatol 1990; 22:594–598.

There are 3 types of lichen planopilaris.

> Follicular lichen planus–individual keratotic papules
> Plaque type–erythematous to violaceous plaque in which follicular prominence is seen.
> Cicatricial alopecia type–spinous or acuminate follicular papules of scalp with concomitant or subsequent scarring alopecia.

Let the pathologist help you rule out discoid lupus erythematosus, and pseudopelade of Brocq.

Salman SM, Kibbi A-G, Zaynoun S: **Actinic lichen planus**. A clinicopathologic study of 16 patients. J Am Acad Dermatol 1989; 20:226–231.

Clinical presentation of this variant of lichen planus:

> Appears in spring and summer on exposed areas (face, dorsal hands, forearms).
> Annular pigmented plaques have light brown to slate blue center.
> Violaceous papules
> Reticulated brown patches
> Asymptomatic

Differential diagnosis:

Melasma
Drug-induced photosensitivity
Pityriasis alba

Synonyms

Lichen planus tropicus
Actinic lichenoid eruption
Lichenoid melanodermatitis

Salman SM, Khallouf R, Zaynoun S: **Actinic lichen planus** mimicking melasma. A clinical and histopathologic study of three cases. J Am Acad Dermatol 1988; 18:275–278.

Two patients were **misdiagnosed as having melasma** until skin biopsies demonstrated actinic lichen planus. The major clinical clue is a slate blue component in contrast to the true brown of melasma. It is not pruritic and occurs during the spring and summer on exposed areas. The presence of periorbital involvement and extrafacial lesions favors the diagnosis of actinic lichen planus over melasma.

Differential diagnosis

Drug eruption from:
    phenytoin
    oral contraceptives
    isoniazid
    chlorothiazide
    tolbutamide
Topical photosensitivity
    perfumes
    tars
    hormones

Prost C, Tesserand F, Laroche L et al: **Lichen planus pemphigoides**: An immunoelectron microscopic study. Br J Dermatol 1985: 113:31–36.

A 26-year-old woman had 5 months of a generalized intensely pruritic eruption, followed by an acute vesiculobullous eruption. Innumerable **violaceous papules** with a glossy surface and a tendency to coalesce were intermixed **with vesicles** and large bullae. The buccal mucosa exhibited a network of white streaks and patches, as well as bullae. A diagnosis of lichen planus pemphigoides was made.

Biopsy of a lichenoid papule revealed typical lichen planus, while the blisters showed subepidermal bulla formation with linear deposits of IgG and C3 along the basement membrane of perilesional skin. Immunoelectron microscopy of a blister revealed cleavage within the lamina lucida, with the floor being lamina densa with deposits of IgG and C3, as in bullous pemphigoid. However, the absence of IgG and C3 from the roof of the bulla differed from bullous pemphigoid.

This patient provides the option of making the diagnosis of two coexisting diseases (lichen planus and bullous pemphigoid) or a single diagnosis of lichen planus pemphigoides. Take your choice.

Mora RG, Nesbitt LT Jr, Brantley JB: **Lichen planus pemphigoides**: Clinical and immunofluorescent findings in four cases. J Am Acad Dermatol 1983; 8:331–336.

An 18-year-old black man gave a history of widespread pruritic eruption of a month's duration and blisters on his lower legs for the past 2 weeks.

Examination showed **violaceous hyperpigmented macules** and papules of the chest, arms, and legs. In addition, there were tense **bullae** on the arms and legs.

The papules were typical of lichen planus, both clinically and histologically. Immunofluorescent studies of a bullous lesion showed the C3 pattern of deposition at the dermoepidermal junction diagnostic of bullous pemphigoid. The basement membrane zone antibodies were also shown to be present in the serum and blister fluid.

The diagnosis of lichen planus pemphigoides was made and the lesions healed completely with steroid therapy over the next few months. The **immunofluorescent** studies permit its distinction from bullous lichen planus.

Laskaris GC, Papavasiliou SS, Bovopoulou OD, Nicolis GD: **Lichen planus pigmentosus** of the oral mucosa: A rare clinical variety. Dermatologica 1981; 162:61–63.

A month after his wife died, a 54-year-old Greek man developed roughness in his mouth with extensive pigmented reticular lesions interspersed with whitish patches on the entire buccal mucosa. They were palpably rough. Biopsy confirmed the clinical diagnosis of **lichen planus pigmentosus** of the mouth. He gave no history of recent infection, exposure to drugs, toxic fumes, or heavy metals. He had no allergies, was not a smoker, and followed a normal diet.

Since lichen planus can leave a diagnostic trail of pigment in the skin, this would appear to be an analogous phenomenon in the mucosa.

Todd P, Garioch J, Lamey PJ et al: Patch testing in **lichenoid reactions of the mouth** and oral lichen planus. Br J Dermatol 1990; 123(Suppl 37):26.

Improvement in **oral lichen planus** was achieved:

  in 4 patients who were cinnamaldehyde/benzoic acid patch test positive, by dietary restrictions or change

  in 2 patients who were rubber mix patch test positive, by replacing rubber pillows

  in 1 patient who was formaldehyde patch test positive, by change in toothpaste.

The golden diagnostic coin has two sides: What is it and why is it?

Differential Diagnosis

Bauer F: **Quinacrine hydrochloride drug eruption** (tropical lichenoid dermatitis). Its early and late sequelae and its malignant potential: A review. J Am Acad Dermatol 1981; 4:239–248.

The antimalarial drug Atabrine (quinacrine), taken by thousands of servicemen in World War II, produced a bizarre **lichen planus–like eruption** in as many as 1 out of every 500. The eruption was polymorphous, with combinations of lichenoid, eczematoid, hypertrophic, and atrophic lesions. Some areas were slate blue to purple, others were depigmented, and some were atrophic, mimicking disseminated lupus erythematosus. Sweat gland damage produced **anhidrotic tropical asthenia**. There was widespread hair loss as well as ulceration of the mucosal tissue. Nearly 10% of patients went on to develop an exfoliative dermatitis.

In the years that followed, some of these patients noted:

permanent inability to sweat
recurring lichenoid lesions and ulceration of the mucosa
development of peculiar, well-defined red plaques of the palms
warty keratodermas of the palms, eventuating in squamous cell carcinomas
permanent depigmentation

Apparently, quinacrine is deposited in the spiral portion of sweat ducts, where it remains several years and can cause destruction of the sweat gland apparatus. Rupture of the sweat ducts may deposit quinacrine in the skin, reactivating lichen planus.

Some drug eruptions never go away, even though the drug exposure goes away.

Penneys NS: **Gold therapy**: Dermatologic uses and toxicities. J Am Acad Dermatol 1979; 1:315–320.

Analysis of 37 patients showed that the most common type of eruption in patients receiving gold therapy consists of a **patchy pruritic**, **erythematous**, **papular eczematous dermatitis**. About 25% of gold rashes resemble lichen planus clinically and histologically. Less common **gold-induced eruptions** include pityriasis rosea–like, erythema nodosum, erythroderma, cheilitis, and stomatitis.

After gold therapy is stopped, it takes about 10 weeks for most gold eruptions to clear (range: 10 days to 2 years). When the gold was restarted at lower doses, there appeared to be no increased risk of recurrent dermatitis, except with erythema nodosum.

Immediately after gold is injected, a vasomotor response may occur with flushing, erythema, weakness, dizziness, hypotension, and syncope. This nitritoid reaction occurs only with aqueous gold sodium thiomalate, not with aurothioglucose in oil.

Proteinuria occurs in 2 to 10% of patients with gold therapy and indicates that the drug should be temporarily stopped. Gold therapy may then be restarted at lower levels after the urinary protein disappears.

Lidén C: **Occupational dermatoses** from photographic chemicals. With special reference to contact allergy and lichenoid reactions from colour developing agents. Acta Derm Venereol Suppl 1988; 141:1–37.

The art of photography was introduced in 1831 with mercury poisoning an occupational problem at first. However, for the past 30 years it has been the **lichenoid dermatitis** and **contact dermatitis** due to color film developers that has excited interest. These agents are derivatives of paraphenylenediamine

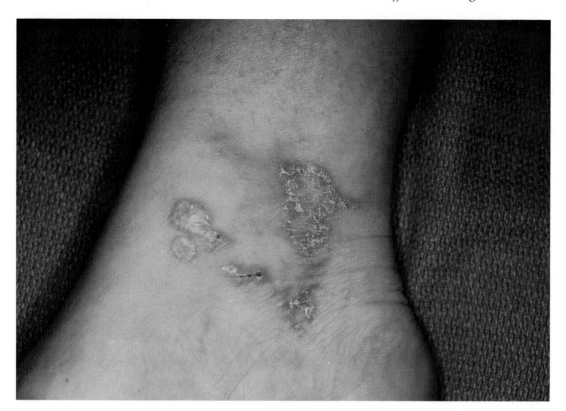

(a "color developer" for hair) which also induces lichenoid and contact dermatitis. Another compound used is hydroquinone, a color developer for black and white film. It does not "develop" color in the skin but rather produces loss of color, a contact vitiligo. Numerous other hazardous chemicals are used, and especially to be noted as contact allergens are persulfate bleach accelerator (PBA-1), potassium dichromate, formaldehyde, ethylenediamine and metol.

This study involved 114 of the 5,000 people employed in Sweden in film laboratories. It was found that the **color developer** agents frequently induce a lichen planus–like eruption, which differs from true lichen planus in that it occurs only at the contact sites, involutes promptly on avoidance of exposure, and does not cause oral lesions. It is similar to lichenoid reactions caused by black stockings or contact with paraphenylenediamine-dyed objects. It cannot be reproduced by patch testing.

Vasily DB, Bhatia SG: **Lichen striatus.** Cutis 1981; 28:442–446.

Papules in dusky **violaceous plaques** spread up the fourth finger, over the dorsum of the hand, and up the volar forearm and dorsal upper arm of this 21-year-old girl. The fourth fingernail was dystrophic. The lesions were intensely pruritic and had evolved in a 2-month period; some areas appeared to have a herpetiform vesiculation. Skip areas were present.

The skin biopsy showed intraepidermal vesiculation and a nonspecific lymphohistiocytic perivascular infiltrate. A diagnosis of **lichen striatus** was made. This disease presents a variable picture of lichenoid, diamond-shaped punctate scaling, and verrucous papules. In dark skin, loss of pigment in a linear band is common.

Before a diagnosis of lichen striatus is made the other linear dermatoses must be ruled out. These include:

linear lichen simplex chronicus   linear lichen planus
linear porokeratosis   linear epidermal nevus
linear psoriasis

Here again, the pathologist gives you the greatest help.

Quiroz-Kendall E, Wilson FA, King LE: **Acute variegate porphyria** following a Scarsdale gourmet diet. J Am Acad Dermatol 1983; 8:46–49.

This 34-year-old woman developed a pruritic **macular rash in the light-exposed areas.** The lesions on the dorsum of the hands became encrusted and formed dark scars. The first dermatologist to see her made a diagnosis of **lichen planus.**

The sun sensitivity persisted and the patient became aware of its association with colicky abdominal pain and drug intake (alcohol, barbiturates, estrogens, and sulfonamides). More probing into her history revealed that the abdominal pain had led to a cholecystectomy years ago that had not produced relief. Furthermore, her urinary porphobilinogen had been elevated at that time. She had also found out that her niece had "porphyria."

It was now apparent that this patient had **variegate porphyria.** Her plasma fluoresced with an emission wavelength maximum of 626 nm and the total porphyria level in the plasma was 2 μg/dl (normal, below 0.69 μg/dl).

At this time the patient went on a Scarsdale diet, losing 8 pounds in 3 weeks. Nausea, vomiting, abdominal pain, and occipital headaches followed with an additional 5-pound weight loss and eventual coma. Hospitalization and intravenous hematin therapy became necessary.

This patient's variegate porphyria induced a **sun sensitivity** that led to understanding her abdominal pain. She had a hereditary enzyme deficiency (protoporphyrinogen oxidase) that led to inability to synthesize heme and a consequent set of gastrointestinal and neuropsychiatric symptoms. Not only drugs but the mere act of fasting strains the heme synthesis system by stimulating a competitive hemoprotein, cytochrome p-450. The other inherited heme-deficient porphyrias are acute intermittent porphyria and hereditary coproporphyria, each requiring the same therapy.

Ask about episodes of unexplained abdominal pain in the patient with sun sensitivity. Ask about episodes of fasting and screen for drug intake as well as for porphyrins. The authors list 33 drugs that can precipitate these porphyric attacks.

Nabai H, Mehregan AH: **Keratosis lichenoides chronica**. J Am Acad Dermatol 1980; 2:217–220.

A 37-year-old Iranian woman suffered for 21 years with erythematous scaling plaques of the face and purplish lichenoid and papulonodular lesions and plaques of the buttocks and extremities. Many nodules on the legs were distributed in a linear fashion. Ophthalmologic examination revealed bilateral trichiasis and destruction of the eyelid margins with scarring. She also had bilateral central corneal scarring and peripheral vascularization.

Skin biopsies revealed chronic lichenified dermatitis, lichen planus–like epidermal changes, telangiectasia, and a heavy dermal infiltrate of lymphocytes, histiocytes, and plasma cells. This suggested a diagnosis of **keratosis lichenoides chronica,** which is probably a subset of lichen planus. Her VDRL was nonreactive and fungal cultures were negative. Intradermal skin tests and leukocyte migration tests indicated immunologic depression.

Keratosis lichenoides chronica features a distinctive erythematous scaling eruption with **telangiectasia of the face**, resembling seborrheic dermatitis or rosacea. Lesions on the arms, legs, and buttocks are purplish papulo-nodules and plaques, often with linear configuration.

The clinical **spectrum of lichen planus** now includes several new entities:

actinic (tropical) lichen planus: brown to purple circular plaques on light-exposed areas of the face and arms. Affects children and young adults in middle eastern countries.

discoid lupus erythematosus–like lichen planus: plaque-like facial lesions and lichen planus-like lesions of the extremities.

bullous lichen planus: resembles bullous pemphigoid.

Lang PG Jr: **Keratosis lichenoides chronica**. Successful treatment with psoralen–ultraviolet-A therapy. Arch Dermatol 1981; 117:105–108.

A retiform pattern of hyperkeratotic lichenoid papules on the arms and legs was the cardinal sign in this 24-year-old patient. Confluent plaques of such papules were also seen on the thighs and buttocks. There were mucosal aphthae present, and a nonspecific whitish coating of the tongue. All this had been present since infancy. Initial diagnostic considerations were given to lichen planus, as well as a variegate form of parapsoriasis and Darier's disease.

Biopsies revealed a bandlike infiltrate of mononuclear cells as well as acanthosis and atrophy of the epidermis. When detailed medical studies were noncontributory, a diagnosis of keratosis lichenoides chronica was made.

It is possible that this diagnosis has a number of aliases. It may be reported as having been sighted as:

lichen ruber moniliformis
lichen verrucosus et reticularis
porokeratosis striata lichenoides
keratose lichenoide striae

But they are all "oids" in the lichen family.

Ryatt KS, Greenwood R, Cotterill JA: **Keratosis lichenoides chronica**. Br J Dermatol 1982; 106:223–225.

A reticulate, linear eruption of violaceous papules and nodules has been present for 3 years on the dorsal surface of the hands and feet of this 16-year-old boy. In addition, there was a scaly erythematous eruption of the forehead, cheeks, and perioral region.

A biopsy was unremarkable except for acanthosis. The diagnosis of keratosis lichenoides chronica was made on the typical clinical presentation of linear and **reticulate patterns of keratotic or lichenoid violaceous papules** in a patient with a seborrheic-like dermatitis of the face.

Personally, we still call this disease by the name that Kaposi gave it, viz., **lichen ruber moniliformis**. However, you will find it wandering through the dermatologic woods and answering to the call of porakeratosis striata lichenoides, and keratose lichénoide striée, or keratosis lichenoides chronica. We think of it as lichen planus, with a lacy pattern in the skin analogous to what is seen in the oral mucosa.

Remember, violets are blue and lichen planus is too.

To diagnose without a history is to sail without a chart.

Linear Lesions

The linearity of a lesion can spark the synaptic flash point for a diagnosis. We all think of poison ivy or a plant dermatitis when we see the streak of contact. Linear streaks of pigmentation bespeak a perfume dermatitis. We think of dermographism when we see the mark of the scratch, and a bizarre array of linear cuts suggests factitial dermatitis. Flagellate bands of dermatitis make one ask if bleomycin is responsible.

Likewise, the Koebner phenomenon may expose itself as a linear lesion. Here the disease such as psoriasis, lichen planus, or warts is expressed in an easily recognizable state. Thus, the challenge is not in the primary diagnosis but rather in what triggered this Koebner phenomenon. It may represent a tight wristwatch band or a shoulder strap.

A line of nodules directs one's diagnostic thoughts to sporotrichosis. It is the line determined by lymphatic spread of organisms from a distal portal of entry. Such a sporotrichoid pattern is seen in other infectious diseases such as coccidioidomycosis. When the trail of disease involves the blood vessels, a continuous linear band may be the diagnostic tip of an underlying thrombophlebitis. A specific example is the linear cord of Mondor's disease seen, for instance, on the chest. In turn, a linear band of disease determined by the nerves is herpes zoster.

Often the linear configuration provides the glance diagnosis of a linear epidermal nerves, a lichen striatus, or an inflammatory linear verrucous epidermal nevus (ILVEN). Other times the diagnosis of nevus or a disease such as morphea is self-evident. It is the linearity that summons the question of why. In some instances, such as incontinentia pigmenti, the lesions are in the lines of Blaschko. These are the lines that reflect the mosaicism of the skin of some patients. The alphabetic swirls of V-, U-, or S-shaped lesions always suggest a genetic factor of "twin skins." The patient has inherited two distinct cutaneous cell lines that remain seemingly identical until struck by disease. Only one of the twin skins is afflicted with a resultant mosaic pattern following the lines of Blaschko. It is a line the lesion cannot cross.

Jackson R: The **lines of Blaschko**: A review and reconsideration: Observations of the cause of certain unusual linear conditions of the skin. Br J Dermatol 1976; 95:349–360.

By precisely outlining on a doll the exact localization of 83 examples of nevoid linear skin diseases and of 63 examples of acquired linear skin diseases, Blaschko developed in 1901 a series of lines that still bear his name. They may represent bands of skin with genetically distinct origins producing a banded mosaicism.

The **lines of Blaschko** correspond to the patterning of a variety of **linear nevi** as well as the linear patterning of such common acquired diseases as psoriasis, scleroderma, and lichen planus. The **V shape over the upper spine**, the **S shape of the abdomen**, and the inverted **U shape from the breast area** onto the upper arm, as well as the perpendicular lines down the lower extremities are unique to the Blaschko lines. They cannot be explained by the boundaries of the areas of distribution of the main cutaneous nerves, known as Voight's lines. Neither can they be explained by the lines of cleavage (Langer's lines). Nor do they follow the course of blood vessels or lymphatics.

Significantly, the lines of Blaschko delimit for you the discrepant morphologic findings, not only for the epidermis and its appendages but also for the dermis, the fat, and all their constituents. Thus, one may see bands of hyperpigmentation, hyperhidrosis, pruritus, or eczema respecting the territorial claims of Blaschko.

Katz M, Weinrauch L: Differentiating **vesicular linear lichen planus** and lichen striatus. Cutis 1987; 40:151–153.

A 62-year-old woman had a 5-month history of an asymptomatic interrupted linear eruption on the posterior left thigh. Small lichenoid pink papules and vesicles in groups began in the left popliteal fossa and extended linearly up the posterior thigh. White lacy streaks and plaques also developed on the left margin of the tongue. Skin biopsy showed vesicular lichen planus.

If the patient has a linear eruption, think along these lines:

lichen striatus	lichen nitidus
linear psoriasis	contact dermatitis
lichen planus	verruca vulgaris linearis
nevus	incontinentia pigmenti
porokeratosis	lichen simplex chronicus linearis
Darier's disease	

Geffner RE, Goslen JB, Santa Cruz DJ: Linear and **dermatomal trichoepitheliomas**. J Am Acad Dermatol 1986; 14:927–930.

A 10-year-old black girl showed multiple discrete flesh-colored papules of the face and left shoulder in a dermatomal pattern. She also had a linear band of these papules on the posterior portion of her left lower leg.

They had been present since age 4; on biopsy they were shown to be **trichoepitheliomas**. The appearance of such papules in a linear band always calls for biopsy since the following adnexal tumors can show a linear distribution:

basal cell nevus syndrome	eccrine poroma
comedonal nevus	syringomas
eccrine nevus	trichoepitheliomas
eccrine spiradenomas	

Bouwes Bavinck JN, Van de Kamp JJP: **Organoid naevus phakomatosis**: Schimmelpenning-Feuerstein-Mims syndrome. Br J Dermatol 1985; 113:491–492.

A 19-year-old woman had linear and V-shaped orange-brown verrucous plaques on the left side of her back, left axilla, and left chin since birth. Her left eye was abnormal with a coloboma of the upper eyelid, microcornea, and a cloudy cornea with ingrowth of blood vessels. She also had four atrophic bald spots on the left side of the scalp. Starting at age 2 years she had several spontaneous fractures of long bones due to nonossifying fibromas (visible as multiloculate cystic spots on x-ray).

A diagnosis of organoid naevus plakomatosis was made. This special type of epidermal nevus syndrome (**Schimmelpenning-Feuerstein-Mims syndrome**) consists of a unilateral linear epidermal or sebaceous nevus associated with ipsilateral dysplasia of the eye. Other findings may include spotty alopecia, mental retardation, epilepsy, neural deafness, and skeletal deformities.

Aloi FG, Pippione M: **Porokeratotic eccrine ostial and dermal duct nevus**. Arch Dermatol 1986; 122:892–895.

When a 6-year-old girl with numerous bands of yellowish-brown comedolike keratotic papules was first seen, her mother would not allow a biopsy. The asymptomatic 1 to 2 mm papules, present since birth, ran down her arms from the axillae to the finger tips and also involved her feet. Some papules were surmounted by filiform excrescences, while others on the palms appeared as filiform warts or comedones.

For 16 years the clinicians could only play a cutaneous version of "What's my line?" Was it any of the following linear nevoid dermatoses?

Linear verrucous epidermal nevus? (unlikely, since the nevus had comedones)

Inflammatory linear verrucous epidermal nevus (ILVEN)? (unlikely, since the nevus was not inflammatory)

Nevus comedonicus? (possible)

Linear and punctate porokeratosis? (unlikely, since the nevus had no annular atrophic lesions)

Porokeratotic eccrine duct and hair follicle nevus? (possible)

Finally, the answer came when the patient reappeared at age 22 and gave permission for multiple biopsies, which revealed coronoid lamellae associated with hyperplastic and dilated eccrine sweat ducts. Sweat tests revealed anhidrosis in the affected areas. Accordingly, the 16-year wait was climaxed by a diagnosis of **porokeratotic eccrine ostial and dermal duct nevus**. And now the wait is for a treatment.

Herbst VP, Kauh YC, Luscombe HA: **Connective tissue nevus** masquerading as a localized linear epidermal nevus. J Am Acad Dermatol 1987; 16:264–266.

A zosteriform pattern of shiny smooth, soft, grouped, hyperpigmented papules had been present on the left forearm of this 22-year-old woman since infancy. A clinical diagnosis of a localized **linear epidermal nevus** was made but not confirmed on biopsy.

The patient proved to have a connective tissue nevus.

Pucevich MV, Latour DL, Bale GF, King LE Jr: Self-healing **juvenile cutaneous mucinosis**. J Am Acad Dermatol 1984; 11:327–332.

Linear and grouped papules formed plaques over the sternum and sacrum as well as the left submandibular region in this 15-year-old black male. Nodules were present on the dorsa of the fingers as well as the forehead. There was an associated arthralgia.

Mucinous material oozed out when a biopsy of the sternal lesions was done. Stains of the biopsy specimen showed the presence of hyaluronic acid and a diagnosis of papular mucinosis was made.

Five months later the skin lesions had spontaneously resolved and remained so for the following 2 years. This benign course led to a final diagnosis of self-healing **juvenile cutaneous mucinosis**.

The differential diagnosis of cutaneous nodules occurring in a patient with arthralgias and arthritis is complex and calls for a consideration of:

juvenile rheumatoid arthritis	Farber's disease
systemic lupus erythematosus	amyloidosis
rheumatic fever	deep fungal infection
multicentric reticulohistiocytosis	hepatitis B infection

Finding mucin deposition provides essential diagnostic help.

Burket JM, Zelickson AS, Padilla RS: **Linear focal elastosis** (elastotic striae). J Am Acad Dermatol 1989; 20:633–636.

Yellow-orange palpable linear lesions were seen extending out from the vertebral column in three elderly men.

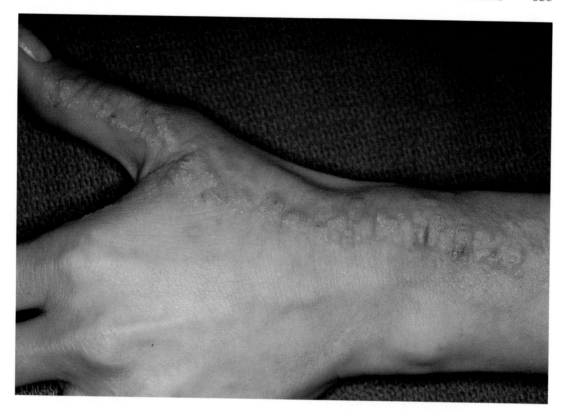

Biopsy showed dermal elastosis making the diagnosis of **linear focal elastosis**. Noteworthy is the fact that sunlight played no role in its pathogenesis.

Vincent F, Prokopetz R, Miller RAW: **Plasma cell panniculitis**: A unique clinical and pathologic presentation of linear scleroderma. J Am Acad Dermatol 1989; 21:357–360.

A 64-year-old woman presented with a tender red linear eruption of her left arm. Present for the past 11 months, it was made up of large indurated **dusky-red plaques** of the medioventral aspect of the forearm, extending over the dorsum of the wrist and involving the fourth and fifth digits. The upper arm showed a reticular pattern of violaceous patches.

Biopsy revealed an intense plasma cell infiltrate extending throughout the dermis and into the fat, and a diagnosis of a plasma cell panniculitis was made.

During the subsequent 3 years, the lesions evolved into a firm sclerotic band characteristic of **linear scleroderma**.

Lindae ML, Hu C-H, Nickoloff BJ: **Pruritic erythematous linear plaques** on the neck and back. Arch Dermatol 1987; 123:395–398.

Large, brightly erythematous **pruritic linear plaques** and patches adorned the patient's neck and lower back. Of acute onset, they were associated with the chemotherapy she was receiving for lymphoma.

A diagnosis of "**flagellate**" **erythema secondary to bleomycin** therapy was made. The linear bands may well represent a Koebner-like scratch marking. When bleomycin was eliminated from her schedule, the eruption completely faded over the next 6 weeks.

Bleomycin has a track record of inducing not only these streaks but also hyperpigmentation of hands, elbows, and knees in 30% of those receiving it. Hyperkeratotic plaques of the elbows and knees may also appear. Even sclerosis and gangrene have been reported.

O'Doherty CJ, Savin JA: **Dermatologic dyspnea**. Int J Dermatol 1986; 25:58–59.

It was not auscultation but rather a look at the skin that revealed why this 54-year-old woman had **shortness of breath**. There on her left shoulder, left neck, and left upper chest were scattered brown macules. The brown macules were the residua of C4 herpes zoster that had been treated 3 weeks earlier by her family physician.

Recalling the mnemonic "C3, 4, and 5 keep the diaphragm alive," it was evident that the zoster had induced a persistent diaphragmatic paralysis.

Recall that motor as well as sensory nerves may be damaged in an attack of shingles.

Jaworsky C, Bergfeld WF: **Metastatic transitional cell carcinoma** mimicking zoster sine herpete. Arch Dermatol 1986; 122:1357–1358.

Two weeks of severe left-sided back pain accompanied by localized erythema of the left flank in a 61-year-old man led to a provisional diagnosis of **herpes zoster**. The area of erythema and hyperesthesia was a dermatomic band from the 3rd through 10th thoracic segments. The absence of vesicles favored a more specific diagnosis of zoster sine herpete. Two important facts were brought out in the history. The patient had had a previous episode of herpes zoster involving the right shoulder. Secondly, he had had a cystectomy 4 years ago for a transitional carcinoma of the bladder.

CT scan of the chest revealed a soft tissue density of the left posterior chest wall, and on thoracotomy metastatic transitional cell carcinoma was found touching the 9th rib. It was deemed likely the tumor had invaded the dorsal root ganglia, accounting for the dermatomal erythema and pain.

This patient's problem could be clearly distinguished from carcinoma erysipeloides and zosteriform inflammatory metastatic carcinoma in that there was no palpable border nor was the area warm to touch. One other possibility considered was the zosteriform metastasis of a prostatic carcinoma, in which there is perineural lymphatic spread.

So often metastatic disease produces such nonspecific changes that diagnosis is delayed.

Heng MCY, Feinberg M, Haberfelde G: **Erythematous cutaneous nodules** caused by adulterated cocaine. J Am Acad Dermatol 1989; 21:570–572.

Multiple **nodules** trailing **along a vein** suggests an intravenous use of cocaine with granulomatous reactions to the material that missed the "main line." Biopsy can show birefringent needlelike crystals of talc, which is poorly degradable.

Remember that when the addict injects cocaine, he may be injecting numerous fellow-travelers such as sucrose, lactose, dextrose, and starch as well as procaine, lidocaine, quinine, and caffeine.

Marsch WCh, Haas N, Stüttgen G: **Mondor's phlebitis**—a lymphovascular process. Light and electron microscopic indications. Dermatologica 1986; 172:133–138.

A subcutaneous **cord-like lesion** of sudden onset on the abdominal wall of a

45-year-old woman proved on histologic study to be a thrombotic process within a lymph channel. The authors believe that Mondor's disease is not thrombophlebitis but rather thrombolymphangitis. The cords are too narrow for venous structures and do not follow the distribution of subcutaneous veins. A similar lymphothrombotic process occurs on the penis (sclerosing lymphangitis, lymphangiofibrosis thrombotica occlusiva).

Nusbacher J: **Migratory venous thrombosis** and cancer. NY State J Med 1964; 64:2166–2173.

Migratory (multiple) **thrombophlebitis**, particularly involving the arms, may be the earliest sign of an occult carcinoma of the pancreas, lung, or stomach. Histologic examination of thrombosed veins for tumor cells is urged. Pulmonary emboli occurred in 50% of the 80 cases reviewed.

Samlaska CP, James WD, Simel DL: **Superficial migratory thrombophlebitis** and factor XII deficiency. J Am Acad Dermatol 1990; 22:939–943.

For 3 years this 29-year-old man had suffered from **intermittent painful nodules** and swelling of the ankle. Punch biopsy specimens were repeatedly nondiagnostic and venograms normal. On examination, a unique feature was the linear arrangement of both the erythematous nodules and the postinflammatory hyperpigmentation. A deep wedge-shaped biopsy revealed the presence of **polyarteritis nodosa**. The process remained completely refractory to a wide variety of treatments.

Finally, $2\frac{1}{2}$ years later, again, there was no deep venous thrombosis on venogram. A second deep excisional biopsy of one of the cords now palpable showed the presence of a thrombosed vein, consistent with the diagnosis of a superficial thrombophlebitis. **Reassessment** of the former biopsy showed the "polyarteritis nodosa" to actually be a **thrombosed vein**.

The hunt was on for the causes of his long-term **hypercoagulable state**. It was heightened by the history that when the patient was 10 years old he had been hospitalized for intravenous heparin therapy of a venous thrombosis of the right thigh. He now proved to have a very low factor XII (17% normal) (a specific plasma protein, the Hageman factor). This is an autosomal recessive defect in which a hypercoagulable state occurs. The mechanism is obscure, but the original patient, John Hageman, died of a thrombosis. The sophistication of modern testing for the nature of a coagulation problem is highlighted by the fact that over 30 specific blood factors and functions were assayed in the study of this man. Incidentally, his protein C and protein S levels were normal, as were factors VIII, IX, XI, and factor XII inhibitor.

The fact that this patient did not respond to steroids reduced the diagnostic possibility of polyarteritis nodosa. **Other conditions** one had to think of as possibilities were cocaine abuse, pseudothrombophlebitis of AIDS, sarcoidal granulomas, and Buerger's disease. Sometimes, a second opinion and a second biopsy are necessary in making the correct diagnosis. Do not forget to make the biopsy big and deep. A simple "punch" is not enough. You need a "knock-out" biopsy.

Once superficial thrombophlebitis is identified, **one looks behind the diagnosis for** Hodgkin's disease, multiple myeloma, secondary syphilis, rickettsial infection, Behçet's syndrome, and Trousseau's syndrome. None of these was present in this patient.

Samlaska CP, James WD: Superficial thrombophlebitis. I. Primary **hypercoagulable states**. J Am Acad Dermatol 1990; 22:975–989.

Superficial thrombophlebitis may be the presenting sign of a genetically determined tendency to intravascular clotting. Suspect such a primary hypercoagulable state when there is:

1. Family history of thrombosis.
2. Recurrent thrombosis without an apparent precipitating factor.
3. Thrombosis occurring before age 30.
4. Thrombosis occurring at a site other than the leg.
5. Resistance to antithrombotic therapy.

When such a primary hypercoagulable state is suspected, look for:

antithrombin III and heparin cofactor II deficiencies
protein C and protein S deficiencies
plasminogen activator defects (inability to lyse the fibrin clot)
dysfibrinogenemia
factor XII (Hageman trait) deficiency (partial thromboplastin time prolonged)

Be cautious in assessing values. They may be a coincidental abnormality, or artefact associated with blood drawing techniques or anticoagulant used, or may be wrong because of inexperience of the laboratory. What the patient with a hypercoagulable state needs is a good hematologist.

Harpster EF, Mauro T, Barr RJ: **Linear granuloma annulare**. J Am Acad Dermatol 1989; 21:1138–1141.

A **linear band** of coalescing firm subcutaneous papules had been present for 1 month on the right lateral chest of this 62-year-old man.

A diagnosis of Mondor's disease (superficial thrombophlebitis of the thoracoepigastric veins) was made; however, the biopsy showed it to be linear granuloma annulare.

Might we call it "granuloma lineare"?

Brownstein MH, Silverstein L, Lefing W: Lichenoid epidermal nevus: "linear lichen planus." J Am Acad Dermatol 1989; 20:913–915.

Some cases previously reported as linear lichen planus are actually epidermal nevi with a lichenoid tissue reaction.

Some cases previously reported as linear psoriasis are actually cases of inflammatory linear verrucous epidermal nevi (ILVEN) with psoriasiform features.

A working diagnosis simply means you have more work to do.

Lipomas

A soft, freely movable symptomless subcutaneous mass makes for an easy diagnosis of lipoma. Yet there are atypical forms. Some of these are distinctive because of **pain** (angiolipomas and also Dercum's disease). Others are puzzling because of their tremendous size (Launois-Bensaude lipomatosis). Some show a mixed picture with progression and, at times, a striking yellow verrucous surface (Zurhelle's nevus lipomatosis). But the ones posing the greatest diagnostic challenge are those located below the fascia. On the scalp, lipomas beneath the galea may be so firm as to suggest the diagnosis of an osteoma or a dermoid tumor. On the forehead they may extend deep into the frontalis muscle. In the sacral area lipomas may be the sign of **spinal dysraphism**. X-ray studies are advisable. Beware of thinking of lipomas of the neck as simple encapsulated masses of fat. They may also extend beneath other fascia deep into the muscles.

Clinically, the differential diagnosis of lipomas centers on distinguishing them from keratinous cysts. It extends to insulin lipohypertrophy occurring at the sites of insulin injections. It also extends to cysts of fat necrosis, herniation of fat lobules, and panniculitis. Large lipomas may actually prove to be **liposarcomas**.

In looking at any lipoma, always consider trauma as an initiating factor.

Zitelli JA: **Subgaleal lipoma**. Arch Dermatol 1989; 125:384–385.

> A firm, fixed nodule on the forehead may be a lipoma located below the galea and thus require incision through this fascia for exposure and removal. A lipoma in such an unusual location summons a clinical **differential** that includes sarcoma, dermoid tumors, and osteomas.
>
> Other **heterotopic lipomas** include intramuscular lipomas, lipomas of tendon sheaths, and intraneural lipomas as well as those beneath fascia other than the galea. Lipomas may also be diffuse and infiltrating (lipomatosis, e.g., of the neck and pelvis). Such extensive forms can suggest the presence of liposarcoma.
>
> As clinicians, we are usually "tongue-tied" to the diagnosis of lipoma, but the pathologist can extend our vocabulary. He verbalizes such **variants** as angiolipoma, spindle cell lipoma, pleomorphic lipoma, benign lipoblastoma, and angiomyolipoma. Next time you cut away the fat, think of that!

Ruzicka T, Vieluf D, Landthaler M, Braun-Falco O: Benign symmetric **lipomatosis Launois-Bensaude**. J Am Acad Dermatol 1987; 17:663–674.

> **Massive symmetric overgrowth** of the subcutaneous tissue of the neck and shoulder girdle gives these patients a pseudomuscular appearance. With a median onset at age 45, the change is progressive for a year or two. As many as a thousand confluent lipomas may appear. Its stable phase is often accepted by these patients as a part of their build. Rarely, dyspnea may be present as a result of compression of the airway. The overlying skin becomes tense and livid in color and exhibits telangiectasia.
>
> Alcohol abuse is the most common associated finding, although malignancy occurs in a few.
>
> In the **differential diagnosis** consider:
>
> > lipomatosis dolorosa (Dercum's)
> > neurolipomatosis
> > multiple lipomas due to intracranial lesions (Froehlich syndrome)
> > hereditary lipomas
> > von Recklinghausen's disease

buffalo neck of Cushing's disease
muscular dystrophy with pseudoathletic appearance
lymphoid tumors
cervical cysts

But always, the perfect symmetry of the lesions and histologic finding of normal fat makes the diagnosis an easy one.

Findlay GH, Duvenage M: Acquired symmetrical **lipomatosis of the hands**—a distal form of the Madelung-Launois-Bensaude syndrome. Clin Exp Dermatol 1989; 14:58–59.

For 6 months this 55-year-old Bantu male had noted a **progressive bilateral swelling** of the distal half of the palm and the proximal phalanges. The swellings were painless but interfered with finger movement. The patient was both a diabetic and a chronic alcoholic.

Radiographs showed the soft tissue swelling, but no bony change. On incision fat globules poured out of the skin. The biopsy showed a nonlobulated mass of mature normal-appearing adipocytes extending from the subcutis to the lower dermis.

A diagnosis was made of acquired symmetrical lipomatosis of the hands. This is an inverse distribution of the "**fat neck**" described by Madelung and the lipomatosis described by Launois and Bensaude. The site of predilection is the neck and it may extend into the mediastinum. Other areas such as the face are exempt. It occurs usually in alcoholic, white males of middle age.

This lipomatosis differs from the common lipoma by being symmetrical and by not being encapsulated.

Dotz W, Prioleau PG: **Nevus lipomatosus cutaneus superficialis**. A light and electron microscopic study. Arch Dermatol 1984; 120:376–379.

Multiple large, soft, nontender nodules had been appearing on the right side of the abdomen of this 68-year-old man for the past 25 years. Biopsy showed the growths to be made up of extensions of mature fat into the collagen bundles of the dermis. A diagnosis of **Hoffman and Zurhelle's nevus lipomatosus was made**.

Ordinarily, this nevus appears far earlier in life and usually appears on the **buttocks and sacral areas**. There are no associated abnormalities or disease associated with nevus lipomatosis. The nodules, which rarely cross the midline, may be domed, sessile, or pedunculated. They may be **yellow** in color reflecting their nature. Although the surface is usually smooth, it may be wrinkled, verrucoid, or even have a peau d'orange appearance. Follicular accentuation and comedone formation have been recorded.

Usually the lesions, although variable in size, all appear at one time and remain unchanged. It is the one that continues to enlarge that provokes anxiety.

Schiazza L, Occella C, Bleidl D, Rampini E: **Insulin lipohypertrophy**. J Am Acad Dermatol 1990; 22:148–149.

Soft masses of the thighs and arms of this 10-year-old boy began to appear after he started to use human highly purified **insulin** in the treatment of his diabetes. When injection sites were continuously changed, the masses began to regress.

A diagnosis of insulin lipohypertrophy was made. In explanation of this benign enlargement of the fat cells, note is made of insulin as a growth hormone.

Hurt MA, Santa Cruz DJ: **Nodular-cystic fat necrosis**: A reevaluation of the so-called mobile encapsulated lipoma. J Am Acad Dermatol 1989; 21:493–498.

Clinical: Movable nodules in subcutis; usual site is elbow or hip; women frequently affected, often with a history of trauma.

Origin: Infarct of fat lobule; encapsulation of ghost fat cells.

Comparable:

Battered buttock syndrome
Traumatic herniation of buccal fat pad
Traumatic fat necrosis of face
Posttraumatic lipomas.

Differential diagnosis:

Lipoma–normal adipocytes
Angiolipoma–painful
Pancreatic fat necrosis:
    pancreatitis or pancreatic carcinoma present
    membranous fat necrosis–diffuse, not encapsulated
Alpha-antitrypsin deficiency panniculitis–enzyme assay.

Each patient is an anecdote, and the more you know about him or her, the better the anecdote.

Livedo Reticularis

The blue network we see in livedo reticularis is **patterned cyanosis**. It signals a slowdown in blood flow, but not to the degree that turns the skin uniformly blue. Here, in livedo, we are seeing a marginal loss of oxygenated blood. The pattern reflects the anatomy of the cutaneous vasculature. The annular blue bands are the surface markings of the marginal vascularization that exists between the arborescent or inverted conical modules of blood supply coming up into the skin.

When blood flow slows, these bands are the peripheral regions first to show the blue of deoxygenated blood. Accordingly, livedo has many causes. We see it when the skin is chilled and blood flow slowed.

We see it more commonly in the legs in which stasis slows the flow. We see it in patients in whom blood flow is impeded by emboli or by the thickened blood vessel walls of arteriosclerosis. Indeed, livedo may herald a stroke, as in Sneddon's syndrome. It occurs when blood itself is thickened by cryoglobulinemia with a consequent sluggish flow. Livedo in infants may result from vascular **malformations** with a consequent slow blood flow. Look for other genetic malformations in such children.

Perhaps the commonest cause of persistent acquired livedo reticularis is **vasculitis**. This may be a manifestation of lupus erythematosus, of a viral infection, or even of a drug eruption. Always it speaks of the presence of blood so slow in transit that pausing in the skin it depletes its oxygen, becoming the blue blood of reduced hemoglobin.

It is well to remember that localized patchy livedo may occur. This indicates a focal lesion impairing blood flow. The sequence is not always a simple color change. The skin may ulcerate and atrophy for want of oxygen.

Interestingly, the blue bands of poorly oxygenated skin may serve as **loci minoris resistentiae**. As a result, think of livedo in the background to explain the localization of such annular eruptions as lichen planus, psoriasis, or drug eruptions. Livedo favors Koebner reactions. Perhaps the best example is erythema ab igne wherein the thermal burn is limited precisely to the livedo network. Its bands are precisely the sites of poor heat transfer or dissipation.

The mottling of livedo reticularis can be recognized at a glance. What takes time is finding out exactly why the flow is slow. The most recent example we have seen was the prodrome for tryptophan-induced scleroderma.

Page EH, Shear NH: **Temperature-dependent skin disorders**. J Am Acad Dermatol 1988; 18:1003–1019.

Livedo reticularis is a mottled bluish (livid) discoloration of the skin occurring in a netlike pattern. It is persistent, ranging in color from reddish blue in warm and dark blue in cold. Its persistence distinguishes it from cutis marmorata, a common transient pattern induced by cold. The blue color pattern outlines the less well-oxygenated venous outflow, permitting contrast from the fully oxygenated skin of each central arterial cone.

Interference with either the arterial inflow or the venous outflow accentuates the cyanotic reticular pattern. Thus we see it as a sign of arteriolar disease, hyperviscosity of blood, or obstruction of venous outflow. In severe forms, ulceration may develop.

In **patchy livedo reticularis** look for systemic lupus erythematosus, periarteritis nodosa, or cryoglobulinemia. A sudden onset can result from emboli, cryoglobulinemia, heart failure or paralysis.

As always, drugs can be responsible, especially quinine, quinidine, amantadine.

Piscascia DD, Esterly NB: **Cutis marmorata telangiectatica congenita**: Report of 22 cases. J Am Acad Dermatol 1989; 20:1098–1104.

Cutis marmorata telangiectatica congenita presents at birth as a reticulated blue-violet patterning of the blood vessels in the skin. It may be generalized or it may be localized as a segmental process sharply demarcated at the midline. The areas of skin within the marbled markings may be normal or erythematous, at times showing telangiectases and venous lakes. With time, involution may or may not occur.

Atrophy and ulceration with scarring are common complications. Furthermore, other congenital defects may be present. These include hypo- or hyperplasia of a limb, mental retardation, nevus flammeus, and glaucoma.

The **differential diagnosis** centers on:

Diffuse phlebectasia (Bockenheimer's syndrome)
    Onset in childhood
    Multiple large painful venous ectasias

Klippel-Trenaunay-Weber syndrome
    Port wine stain   Venous varicosities   Hypertrophy of limb

Port wine stain with reticulate pattern

Physiologic cutis marmorata

    Homocystinuria

    Down's syndrome shows physiologic cutis marmorata

    deLange syndrome shows physiologic cutis marmorata

    Neonatal lupus erythematosus–livedo pattern, but serology distinguishes

Giudice SM, Nydorf ED: **Cutis marmorata telangiectatica congenita** with multiple congenital anomalies. Arch Dermatol 1986; 122:1060–1061.

At birth a baby girl showed a **reddish-purple marbled pattern** over the entire right leg and right hemipelvis. Within this area of livedo reticularis there were multiple linear telangiectases up to 2 cm in length. Further examination disclosed multiple congenital anomalies, including an imperforate anus, rectovaginal and urethrovaginal fistulas, absence of urethral meatus and clitoris, spina bifida with overlying lipoma in the sacral region, and bilateral syndactyly of toes 2 and 3.

Cutis marmorata telangiectatica congenita usually heralds **congenital anomalies**, both hypo- and hyperplastic in nature. The range of findings is astonishing:

aplasia cutis	short stature
dystrophic teeth	scoliosis
cleft palate	scaphoid scapulae
high-arched palate	acral cyanosis
capillary hemangiomas	glaucoma, congenital
asymmetry of the skull	patent ductus arteriosus
micrognathia	atrophy or enlargement of a limb
triangular face	mental retardation

It may be referred to as Van Lohuizen's syndrome by those with a congenital aversion to Latin or Greek.

van Eijk CLA, De Wit RFE: **Phlebectasia congenita** (Bockenheimer's syndrome). Br J Dermatol 1987; 116:602–603.

A congenital lesion of **patterned veins** was slowly progressing over the right upper chest and right arm of a 3-year-old boy. This was viewed as a hamartomatous malformation of the superficial venous system. It was possible by noninvasive tests (arterial Doppler examination) to rule out a diagnosis of arteriovenous fistulas. There were also no cardinal findings of a Klippel-Trenaunay-Weber syndrome.

Such phlebectasia may be associated with dysplasia in the deep venous system. In some instances, rapid growth may be associated with ulceration, bleeding, thrombosis, or even abnormal development of the affected limb.

Bruce S, Wolf JE Jr: Quinidine-induced photosensitive **livedo reticularis-like eruption**. J Am Acad Dermatol 1985; 12:332–336.

Purplish bruiselike spots suddenly appeared on the lower legs of this 39-year-old man while he was camping. Within 2 days they had spread to the trunk and upper arms. The legs were swollen and tender to the point of interfering with walking.

On physical examination, a **purpuric eruption in a reticular pattern** was present in the sun-exposed areas of his swollen legs with a sharp cutoff at the ankles and mid thighs. The lesions were nonpalpable purpura with dark red borders and gray-blue areas suggesting ischemia. The overall pattern was that of livedo reticularis. Similar changes but to a lesser degree were present on the chest and upper arm. The face, posterior legs and back were exempt.

Biopsy revealed simple purpura, with an absence of inflammatory change and vasculitis. The major diagnostic clue was in the history. The patient had been taking quinidine sulfate 800 mgm qid as an antiarrhythmic and he had been in the sun 7 hours a day while camping. A diagnosis of **photosensitive quinidine drug eruption** was made. Quinidine was discontinued, the purpura faded, and at one week the gray areas began to desquamate.

In the **differential** drug-induced lupus was considered because of the photosensitivity and the fact he had a positive ANA titer. Against this diagnosis was a negative immunofluorescent study of the biopsy and the fact his ANA titer was quite low 1:160 (normal in their lab 1:80). Also it should be noted that the purpura distinguishes this eruption from true livedo reticularis, in which purpura is absent. Livedo reticularis eruptions caused by sunlight have been reported previously in patients taking quinidine. They reflect a specific damage to the blood vessels rather than the diffuse photodermatitis induced by quinidine sensitivity.

Quinidine not only produces photosensitivity reactions but also a host of other skin problems:

Pruritus	Flushing
Fixed drug eruptions	Urticaria
Lichen planus–like eruptions	Exfoliative dermatitis
Purpura, thrombocytopenia	Contact dermatitis
Morbilliform eruptions	

It is clear that while it helps the heart, quinidine may produce a lot of arrhythmia in the skin.

Weigand DA, Burgdorf WHC, Tarpay MM: Vasculitis in **cytomegalovirus infection**. Arch Dermatol 1980; 116:1174–1176.

Erythematous papules and plaques had been present for 2 days on the thighs and legs of this 7-year-old girl. Some had an element of purpura. Some of the lesions were in an annular configuration, others in a livedo pattern. She had a low-grade fever and arthralgia of the left knee and ankle.

The initial CBC showed a monocyte count of 11% with 20% atypical lymphocytes. A biopsy revealed a lymphocytic small vessel vasculitis. By the

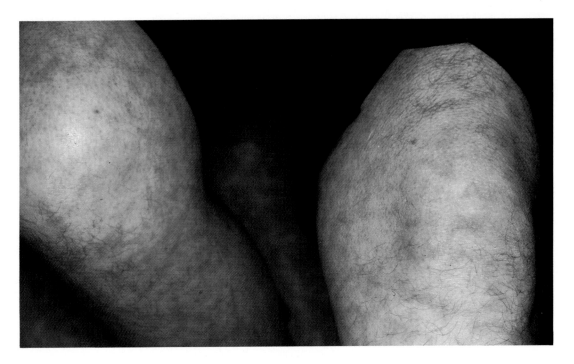

6th day splenomegaly and lymphadenopathy was detected. A provisional diagnosis of **atypical Rocky Mountain spotted fever** was made. However, complement-fixing titers to cytomegalovirus antigen were present in a concentration of 1:1024. As the rash faded over the following weeks, these titers dropped to 1:256 (3 weeks) and 1:128 (3 months).

A diagnosis of **cytomegalovirus mononucleosis** was made. It is rare but similar to the infectious mononucleosis associated with the Epstein-Barr virus. Usually it is seen in children under the age of 18 months, presenting as a maculopapular, vesicular, or petechial rash. Even the blueberry muffin lesions of dermal erythropoiesis may be seen. In many others, there is no accompanying rash.

Look to the monocytes and lymphocytes to help you think of CMV infection.

Weinstein C, Miller MH, Axtens R et al: **Livedo reticularis** associated with increased titers of anticardiolipin antibodies in systemic lupus erythematosus. Arch Dermatol 1987; 123:596–600.

The persistent **reticulated pattern** of livedo reticularis is caused by stagnation of blood in dilated superficial capillaries and venules. Thus, the purple or cyanotic network represents areas of skin with marginal blood flow and inadequate oxygenation. Such a patterned cyanosis stems from interference with blood flow in the very deep vessels. It can reflect transient spasm of the deep arterioles or it may result from intravascular clotting. Thus, it is seen in thrombotic disorders such as thrombotic thrombocytopenic purpura and atheromatous vascular disease, as well as connective tissue disease such a systemic lupus erythematosus. The association of severe livedo reticularis with cerebrovascular thrombosis is known as **Sneddon's syndrome**.

The clinician must recognize that livedo reticularis in systemic lupus erythematosus can be a cutaneous marker for vasculitis, renal disease, or central nervous system disease.

In moderate to severe examples of livedo reticularis, the patients often show an increase in anticardiolipin antibody. Unlike the lupus anticoagulant, this immunoglobulin favors coagulation, and its presence suggests that the livedo in systemic lupus erythematosus is due to thrombosis occurring in the underlying vessels.

Determination of this **anticardiolipin procoagulant antibody** has become valuable in the finer analysis of not only livedo reticularis but also of necrotizing processes such as atrophie blanche, Degos' disease, and ischemias. It also sheds light on the false-positive VDRL reactions in lupus patients, since the VDRL antibodies are also directed against cardiolipin.

Lubach D, Schwabe C, Weissenborn K et al: **Livedo racemosa generalisata**: An evaluation of 34 cases. J Am Acad Dermatol 1990; 22:633–639.

Nineteen of 34 patients with generalized **livedo racemosa** experienced one or more **cerebral infarctions**, and in six epilepsy was present. This association of livedo and cerebrovascular disease is known as Sneddon's syndrome. One should look also for cardiac abnormalities, vascular changes in the ocular fundus, and Raynaud's phenomenon.

Diagnosis is the mother of therapy.

Deffer TA, Berger TG, Gelinas-Sorell D: **Sneddon's syndrome**. J Am Acad Dermatol 1987; 16:1084–1087.

This 38-year-old mildly hypertensive obese woman had nonfluent speech, acalculia, agraphia, finger agnosia, and a right homonymous hemianopia. The diagnosis of **Sneddon's syndrome** could be made, since she not only had cerebrovascular disease but also an extensive nonulcerating **livedo reticularis**. It had gradually extended up from the lower extremities to cover the trunk.

A biopsy from a white area of the affected skin showed a thick-walled thrombotic vessel. Note that repeated biopsies from the red areas showed no abnormalities. The **vascular occlusion** occurs not only in the skin but also in the brain, as Sneddon was the first to observe. In the skin the lacy pattern results from stasis of blood in the superficial venous drainage system. In the brain, where collateral circulation is less, the occlusive ischemia may result in transient or permanent damage to vital tissue. Thus Sneddon's patient suffered hemiplegia and aphasia. The outcome is variable, ranging from complete recovery to ultimate death.

This is a rare association of the central nervous system and the skin. Such livedo reticularis (livedo racemosa), i.e., persistent netlike mottled red to blue discoloration of the skin, has also been **associated** with

emboli	neoplasms	vasculitis
pancreatitis	infection	drug sensitivity
hematologic disorders	metabolic disorders	

Nonetheless, over half of the examples remain idiopathic.

Kalter DC, Rudolph A, McGavran M: **Livedo reticularis** due to multiple cholesterol emboli. J Am Acad Dermatol 1985; 13:235–242.

Painful purpuric lesions of the right sole and several of the toes was the chief complaint of this 26-year-old man for the past month. A red-blue mottling covered the right lateral malleolus. Detailed blood studies and roentgenograms were all negative but a biopsy showed fibrin clots with **cholesterol** clefts in the small vessels in the lower dermis.

Angiography of the right iliac artery showed a large thrombus that was responsible for the distal microembolism, purpura, and livedo reticularis. Extirpation of the right iliac artery and a Goretex graft returned the skin to normal.

Falanga V, Fine MJ, Kapoor WN: The cutaneous manifestations of **cholesterol crystal embolization**. Arch Dermatol 1986; 122:1194–1198.

Microemboli of cholesterol crystals measuring 100 to 200 μ can lodge in the small arterioles of the skin and produce signs of vascular occlusion.

The most common sign is **livedo reticularis**; however, cyanosis, purple mottling of the toes, and macular purpuric lesions may also result. In severe forms ulcers and gangrene may occur.

The diagnosis comes only to those who biopsy and look for cholesterol clefts in a thrombus-filled vessel.

Spiers EM, Sanders DY, Omura EF: Clinical and histologic features of **primary oxalosis**. J Am Acad Dermatol 1990; 22:952–956.

A mottled, **bluish reticular change** on the legs of this 45-year-old woman was recognized as livedo reticularis. The background was believed to be a hypercoagulable state or a systemic vasculitis. The patient, however, proved to be in acute kidney failure. Development of a complete heart block led to a right ventricular biopsy that showed birefringent crystalline material in the arteries and capillaries.

A **Johnny-come-lately biopsy** of the skin then showed these same crystals in radial array. They were **calcium oxalate**—the evidence of her primary oxalosis, which accounted for her renal and cardiac problems. The primary oxaluria leads to recurrent urinary tract infections, calcium oxalate stones, and ultimately renal failure. Similarly, the oxalate crystals form in the cardiac conduction system and produce arrhythmias, failure, and even complete heart block. In the vessels these crystals produce the vasospasm and small vessel thrombosis behind livedo reticularis, Raynaud's phenomenon, and gangrene. The skin may also be the diagnostic lead-in because of whitish calcium deposits on the face or fingers.

Note that routine urinalysis is not usually helpful.

Brownstein MH: **Invisible** dermatoses versus non rashes. J Am Acad Dermatol 1983; 9:599–600.

Dermatoses invisible to the clinician:

Symptoms
pruritus of systemic disease
prodrome period of herpes zoster

Imagined changes
delusional states

Subclinical disease
clinically normal skin showing amyloidosis or hemochromatosis on biopsy

Disease not present at time of visit
urticaria

Areas of sparing
normal skin under wristwatch band in a light-related dermatosis

To this we would add:

All dermatoses in areas unexamined, e.g., scalp, mouth, groin, feet.

Lupus Erythematosus

To know lupus is to know medicine. Few diseases involve more organs or have a greater diversity of lesions. Nor is this surprising, for in lupus the body is involved in self-destruction. It has turned on itself with all the weaponry of autoimmunity and the forces of the complement system. Autoantibodies attack nuclear proteins of both the DNA and RNA types wherever they appear. Injury must first release them, and for this reason, the skin battered by ultraviolet light, chemicals, and physical trauma is a primary site for this disease. They form immune complexes that may clog the vessels of any organ. Likewise, antiphospholipid antibodies disrupt the clotting system and may account for anything from heart attacks to psychoses. And we see all of the drama of such internal disease played out on the stage of the skin.

Lupus is a disease that has an enormous range from the cosmetic to the fatal. Fortunately, its mild form is common, its lethal form rare. We see it in a chronic form, a subacute form, and an acute form. The chronic form known as discoid lupus erythematosus appears classically as dull red macules with scales seemingly "tacked" onto the skin. Removal shows an undersurface covering with horny prongs. Healing occurs initially with permanent residual scarred atrophic white patches. The pigmentation is spotty, and diagnostic telangiectasia is seen. The clinical changes may appear to be those of actinic keratosis; at other times, seborrheic dermatitis, lichen planus, or simple hyperkeratosis. On the scalp there is hair loss in scarred plaques, and in the ears a depigmented scaly spot may be the best clinical sign. Lesions on the lips and tongue are often erosive.

Although the **discoid form** is typically on the face, it may be widespread. Look to the paronychial areas to see the telangiectasia and dermatitis suggestive of lupus. The array of skin changes is daunting to the diagnostician who thinks only in terms of discoid lesions. You may see hyperkeratotic forms that look like warts, keratoacanthoma, or hypertrophic lichen planus. Only a biopsy will tell.

You may see subcutaneous masses that are termed lupus profundus. These are the areas of panniculitis that may make you think of sarcoid. You will see photosensitivity reactions identical to those produced by drugs. The patient's palms may show erosions and ulcers as the only sign. Repeated experience with the many faces of lupus proves it is wisest to let the pathologist take you by the hand and lead you to the diagnosis. In older days the consultant's cry was, "Is it syphilis?" Today comes the cry, "Is it lupus?"

The second major class is **subacute cutaneous lupus erythematosus**. In this form, commonly seen in women, there is no scarring. Rather, one sees large circinate polycyclic lesions suggestive of erythema annulare centrifugum. The primary change is scaly papules on the trunk and arms. Lesions may be present on the scalp and palate as well. Drug eruptions will fool you here. Indeed, drugs such as procainamide may induce lupus, and others such as thiazides may cause it to flare.

The third form, acute cutaneous lupus erythematosus, comes as the famed butterfly rash or simple blotchy erythema and edema of the face. It may last for a day or a month, leaving without trace. More extreme is the appearance of vesicles or bullae.

Through all of this the question arises, does this patient have systemic lupus? Are organs other than the skin significantly affected? The first question is, "Is the patient sick?" Are there signs or symptoms of arthritis, anemia, fatigue, fever, cystitis, weakness, gastrointestinal upsets? The list is endless and a hypochondriac's delight.

It is time to look for **laboratory help** in making a diagnosis of systemic lupus erythematosus. These are the key starting points:

1. Urinalysis for albuminuria, red cells, and casts
2. Blood count for hemolytic anemia, leukopenia, lymphopenia, and thrombocytopenia
3. Sedimentation rate elevation
4. ANA. If ANA is negative, systemic lupus erythematosus (SLE) is excluded unless the patient has marked photosensitivity. In this case, lupus will be revealed by a positive anti-Ro antibody test. *Note:* old people may develop a positive ANA, but a titer over 1:64 calls for further study at any age.
5. Anti-nDNA and anti-Sm antibody tests are positive in SLE patients.
6. Complement C3, C4 will be low.
7. Biopsy for positive immunofluorescent lupus band test. (Granular deposits of immunoglobulins and complement along dermoepidermal junction occur in normal skin only in SLE.)

If your patient passes all seven tests, she does not have laboratory-confirmed SLE; but if she continues to have vague complaints with or without skin lesions, repeat the tests from time to time. If you believe it may be drug induced, order an antihistone antibody test, positive at times in this type of lupus. But remember, none of the autoantibody tests is consistently positive in any patient with lupus. You still have to be a clinician in making the diagnosis after all the evidence is in.

General

Tuffanelli DL: **Lupus erythematosus**. J Am Acad Dermatol 1981; 4:127–142.

Cutaneous lupus erythematosus (LE) occurs predominantly in women and flares with sunlight, ultraviolet light, use of oral contraceptives, pregnancy, and administration of certain drugs.

Chronic discoid LE is benign, with skin lesions showing persistent erythema, telangiectasia, follicular plugging, atrophy, scarring, depigmentation, and hyperpigmentation. Alopecia (scarring and nonscarring) may occur, along with scarring on the palms, soles, conjunctivae, and mouth.

Persistent facial erythema suggestive of LE mimics seborrheic dermatitis, rosacea, poststeroid erythema, polymorphic light eruption, lymphocytic infiltrate of Jessner, actinic reticuloid, and tinea faciale.

Subacute cutaneous LE refers to widespread nonscarring skin lesions that may be annular or papulosquamous.

Systemic LE (as seen in skin) includes a wide spectrum of lesions:

> butterfly blush
> photosensitivity
> alopecia (nonscarring, scarring)
> acute erythema
> erythematous maculopapules
> discoid lesions (chronic)
> mucous membranes: gingivitis, hemorrhage, erosions, ulceration (Be sure
>   to check the hard palate.)
> urticaria
> erythema multiforme
> livedo reticularis
> Raynaud's phenomenon
> necrotic ulcers (palms, soles, legs)
> digital gangrene
> erythromelalgia (red discoloration, elevated skin temperature, and burn-
>   ing after heat exposure)

LE due to drugs (isoniazid, hydralazine, procainamide)

LE panniculitis. Firm, well-defined nodules (up to 5 cm), often with normal overlying skin, leave deep depressions on resolution. They commonly affect the face, back, upper arms, and buttocks and may appear with trauma. They are clinically similar to:

> morphea profundus
> Weber-Christian disease
> pancreatic disease
> traumatic panniculitis

Neonatal LE occurs in infants of LE mothers and causes discoid LE lesions with prominent telangiectasia around the eyes. Leukopenia, thrombocytopenia, and congenital heart block may also occur.

Laboratory studies—obtain at initial visit:

> CBC
> ESR
> urinalysis
> ANA
> anti-DNA
> chemistry profile
> C3
> CH_{50}
> skin biopsy (H & E and immunofluorescence)

If SLE is suspected, also obtain determinations of:

> anti-extractable nuclear antigens (ENA)
> anti-RNP (mixed connective tissue disease)
> anti-Sm (Raynaud's phenomenon, more benign SLE)
> immune complexes (C1q, Raji cell assay)
> cryoglobulins
> immunoglobulins (quantitative)
> rheumatoid factor
> Coombs' test
> renal function
> VDRL test

The clinical differential diagnosis of lupus is a yard wide and a mile long.

Callen JP: Systemic lupus erythematosus in patients with **chronic cutaneous (discoid) lupus erythematosus**: Clinical and laboratory findings in seventeen patients. J Am Acad Dermatol 1985; 12:278–288.

Lupus erythematosus is not a fixed static clinical entity, as evidenced by its progression from a localized skin disease to widespread discoid lupus erythematosus with systemic disease in two patients.

Thus it is necessary to continually reevaluate discoid lupus erythematosus in these patients so that therapy can be altered appropriately.

As your discoid lupus patient begins to move across the lupus erythematosus spectrum, look for:

> extending discoid lesions
> Raynaud's phenomenon
> necrotic pits of fingertips
> periungual telangiectasia
> arthritis
> pericarditis, pleuritis

And check:

> CBC (anemia/leukopenia?)
> urine (proteinuria? hematuria?)
> ANA (antibodies to nuclear or cytoplasmic components)
> renal function (creatinine clearance?)

Tan EM, Cohen AS, Fries JF et al: The 1982 revised criteria for the classification of **systemic lupus erythematosus**. Arthritis Rheum 1982; 25:1271–1277.

The presence of four or more of these criteria serially or simultaneously satisfies the requirements for a clinical diagnosis of systemic lupus erythematosus.

1. Malar erythema
2. Discoid LE
3. Photosensitivity
4. Oral ulcers
5. Arthritis (nonerosive)
6. Serositis (pericarditis, pleurisy)
7. Nephropathy (albuminuria, cellular casts)
8. CNS disorder (seizures, psychoses)
9. Hematologic disorders (anemia, leukopenia, lymphopenia)
10. Anti-nDNA, anti-Sm antibodies, false-positive STS
11. Positive ANA

Complications

Keith WD, Kelly AP, Sumrall AJ, Chhabra A: **Squamous cell carcinoma** arising in lesions of discoid lupus erythematosus in black persons. Arch Dermatol 1980; 116:315–317.

A small **area of irritation** on the upper lip developed in an old, inactive, hypopigmented atrophic lupus lesion in a 46-year-old black man with an 18-year history of discoid lupus erythematosus. Within a week, the area developed into a shallow ulcer. His physician, thinking it was a reactivation of the lupus, prescribed prednisone, but within a month a large fungating mass grew in the site.

Biopsy proved the lesion to be **squamous cell epithelioma**. This report emphasizes the need for black patients to use a sunscreen preparation on all areas lacking their normal protective cover of pigment.

Farber JN, Koh HK: **Malignant fibrous histiocytoma** arising from discoid lupus erythematosus. Arch Dermatol 1988; 124:114–116.

Watch for squamous cell carcinomas and malignant fibrous histiocytomas arising in the scarred lesions of discoid lupus erythematosus.

A 63-year-old Hispanic man with discoid lupus erythematosus had a 2-cm ulcerated **verrucous plaque** on the dorsal aspect of the nose, within a scarred atrophic hypopigmented plaque of DLE. Biopsy of the plaque revealed a dense pleomorphic spindle cell infiltrate with a high mitotic rate throughout the dermis. Immunoperoxidase stains were negative for cytokeratin and epithelial membrane antigens.

The overall pathologic picture was consistent with malignant fibrous histiocytoma, a type of soft tissue **sarcoma**. It presents as a firm asymptomatic flesh-colored tumor, with occasional ulceration and adherence to the underlying soft tissue or bone. It usually arises in deep musculature. Chronic severe inflammation may be a predisposing factor. The prognosis is poor because of aggressive local recurrence and metastasis.

Rongioletti F, Rebora A: **Papular and nodular mucinosis** associated with systemic lupus erythematosus. Br J Dermatol 1986; 115:631–636.

A 24-year-old woman had a "**lumpy back**," best appreciated with tangential lighting. She had numerous indolent 5- to 15-mm skin-colored papules and nodules of the chest, back, and arms, some showing a reddish central depression. Histologically the lesions were gross deposits of mucin. One year earlier she had developed a rash after sunbathing that waned spontaneously but recurred the following summer after sunbathing. She also complained of low-grade fever, fatigue, diffuse hair loss, and arthralgia in the fingers. Laboratory tests revealed ESR 41 mm/hour, hemoglobin 10 gm/dl, WBC 3.62 $\times$ 10^3/ml, hypergammaglobulinemia, reduced complement activity, and an ANA 1:640, speckled pattern, confirming the diagnosis of SLE.

Mucin is commonly found in microscopic amounts in the lesions of both DLE and SLE. The lesions resolved following therapy with chloroquine (500 mg/day) and avoidance of sun exposure. This grossly visible form of mucinosis in SLE has been reported in ten other patients since first being described by Gold in 1954. None of these patients had either paraproteinemia or dysthyroidism.

852   *Moral*:   If a biopsy comes back with mucin, look for lupus.

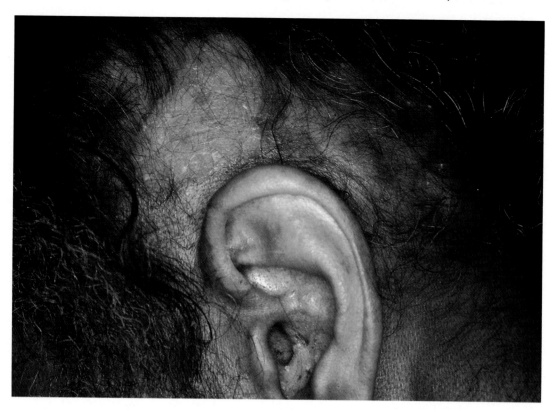

Rao BK, Coldiron B, Freeman RG, Sontheimer RD: Subacute cutaneous lupus erythematosus lesions progressing to **morphea**. J Am Acad Dermatol 1990; 23:1019–1022.

A 32-year-old woman had a 10-year history of annular scaling lesions with telangiectasia on the chest, arms, neck, and face. Histologically and serologically it was lupus erythematosus of the subacute cutaneous form. ANA was positive and anti-Ro and anti-La antibodies were present. C3 was low. Three years later studies again confirmed the diagnosis of subacute cutaneous lupus erythematosus.

However, hypopigmented **indurated lesions** appeared 2 years later. Histologic findings were those of morphea and very little of the epidermal changes of lupus. Three years after that, clinically obvious morpheaform plaques were present on the arms and chest. There was erythema, telangiectasia, cigarette-paper atrophy, and peripheral talangiectasia. A biopsy was compatible with morphea. There were minimal epidermal changes of inactive lupus erythematosus. The ANA was now negative.

A diagnosis was made of **morphea** as a sequence to slowly resolving lupus erythematosus.

For want of a biopsy, a diagnostician may be lost.
For want of a special stain, a pathologist may be lost.

Differential Diagnosis

Almeida L, Grossman M: Widespread **dermatophyte infections** that mimic collagen vascular disease. J Am Acad Dermatol 1990; 23:855–857.

A 19-year-old woman with a 2-year history of systemic lupus erythematosus experienced a marked exacerbation of the skin disease after a blistering sunburn in June, 1987. The continuing problem led to hospitalization in October when physical examination showed annular erythematous patches and plaques on the face, chest, and arms. In addition, she had a **boggy crusted scalp** with alopecia. Although some lesions improved during 2 weeks of hospital stay, others became more prominent.

The diagnosis of widespread fungous infection became evident once a **KOH** scraping was positive, a biopsy showed hyphae in the stratum corneum, a culture of the scalp and trunk grew *Microsporum canis*, and the patient told of her infected cat.

Griseofulvin (1000 mg/day) cleared the eruption in 10 days but induced an erythema multiforme drug eruption. Only after 8 months of subsequent ketoconazole (400 mg/day) therapy did the cultures of the hair and scalp become negative.

Here the diagnostic difficulty arose because of natural reluctance to make a second diagnosis in a lupus patient. Tinea faciei is a natural mimic and fools many into a **diagnosis** of discoid lupus erythematosus, dermatomyositis, Jessner's lymphocytic infiltrate, seborrheic dermatitis, granuloma faciale, granuloma annulare, idiopathic photosensitivity, polymorphous light eruption, acne rosacea, and even lupus vulgaris. In this patient it mimicked the anticipated photosensitivity reaction in a lupus patient.

Griseofulvin is one of the drugs poorly tolerated by lupus patients, and here is another example of this.

Cox NH, Tapson JS, Farr PM: **Lichen planus associated with captopril**: A further disorder demonstrating the "tin-tack" sign. Br J Dermatol 1989; 120:319–321.

The remarkable feature of this 58-year-old man's widespread scaling eruption was the "**tin-tack**" **sign.** When scales were mechanically detached, the undersurface showed many tacklike follicular plugs. This sign is well known as a characteristic of the scale in discoid lupus erythematosus and in pemphigus foliaceus, but in this patient the eruption evolved into clinically and histologically classic lichen planus. The putative cause proved to be **captopril**, since the eruption that had become chronic began to fade within days of stopping this drug.

Paramsothy Y, Lawrence CM: "Tin-tack" sign in **localized pemphigus foliaceus**. Br J Dermatol 1987; 116:127–129.

The presence of **small horny plugs** attached to the undersurface of a scale removed from a lesion has long been revered as a diagnostic sign of discoid lupus erythematosus. Here, however, are two patients with erythematous scaling lesions of the tip of the nose. Each had the tin-tack (carpet tack) sign indicative of discoid lupus erythematosus, but histologic immunofluorescent studies proved that they both had pemphigus foliaceus.

Dodd HJ, Sarkany I, Sadrudin A: **Reticular erythematous mucinosis syndrome**. Clin Exp Dermatol 1987; 12:36–39.

Redness of the central area of the chest and upper back that became raised and itchy upon sun exposure was the chief complaint of a 29-year-old woman.

Examination showed reticulate maculopapular erythema with an irregular but well-defined border. Skin biopsy confirmed the clinical diagnosis of **reticular erythematous mucinosis (REM)**, with a perivascular and periappendageal infiltrate of lymphocytes and plasma cells, and positive alcian blue staining of fibrillary deposits in the dermis.

This condition, also known as plaque-like cutaneous mucinosis, resembles lupus erythematosus in its photosensitivity, sex incidence, and good response to antimalarials. The absence of immunofluorescent deposits in REM normally distinguishes it from LE. In this case, however, direct immunofluorescence of lesional skin showed the unique feature of granular basement membrane zone IgM, IgA, and C3.

Cohen MG, Kevat S, Prowse MV, Ahern MJ: Two distinct **quinidine-induced rheumatic syndromes**. Ann Intern Med 1988; 108:369–371.

Quinidine may cause either a **lupuslike syndrome** with positive ANA or isolated polyarthropathy with no detectable antinuclear antibodies. Rashes and serositis appear to be less common than with procainamide and hydralazine-induced lupus erythematosus.

Pavlidakey GP, Hashimoto K, Heller GL, Daneshvar S: **Chlorpromazine-induced lupus-like disease**; Case report and review of the literature. J Am Acad Dermatol 1985; 13:109–115.

This 51-year-old black woman had numerous erythematous **maculopapular lesions of the forehead** and cheeks that had been present for a year. She had associated diffuse scalp hair loss with follicular plugging and bogginess. For 5 years she had noted hyperpigmentation of the cheeks. The fingertips were painful and tender. On questioning it was found that for the past 5 years she had taken chlorpromazine (Thorazine) 400 mg every day.

Laboratory studies were highlighted by an ANA titer of 1:640, a white cell count of 3100, and a biopsy characteristic of lupus erythematosus with significant deposits of mucin to explain the bogginess. A diagnosis of **lupus erythematosus-like disease due to chlorpromazine** was made. On cessation of the drug, dramatic improvement occurred in 2 weeks.

The **list of drugs** inducing lupus erythematosus–like disease keeps enlarging. It centers on the cardiovascular, antihypertensive, antimicrobial, anticonvulsant, and antithyroid groups with a sprinkling of miscellaneous drugs ranging from lithium to contraceptives. A list of 44 is provided in this reference. Interestingly, many examples show no cutaneous signs, unlike systemic lupus erythematosus in which more than 70% have skin lesions.

Palestine RF, Su WPD, Liesegang TJ: **Late-onset chronic mucocutaneous and ocular candidiasis and malignant thymoma**. Arch Dermatol 1983; 119:580–586.

This 56-year-old man had had a pruritic, erythematous, **scaling eruption** of the forehead and neck for over a year. It had been interpreted on the basis of a biopsy and immunofluorescent studies as being **lupus erythematosus**. Despite systemic corticosteroid therapy his condition worsened, the eruption extended into the trunk, and he developed corneal ulceration. For at least 6 years he had had oral moniliasis.

On examination the lesions were annular, polycyclic, scaling plaques that were **KOH positive** and that on culture grew out *Candida albicans*. All 20 nails were thin, dystrophic, and crumbly and showed both *C. albicans* and *Trichophyton rubrum* on culture. *C. albicans* was also grown out from corneal scrapings of the left eye, which was found on slit lamp to harbor a corneal abscess.

A diagnosis of **chronic mucocutaneous candidiasis** of late onset was made and a search undertaken to discern underlying malignancy. A right hilar mass on chest roentgenogram proved on transthoracic needle biopsy to be a malignant thymoma.

Other tumors reported in association with such late-onset chronic mucocutaneous candidiasis include lymphoma, oral carcinoma, and pancreatic islet cell carcinoma. Significantly, these patients may have other disorders. This patient had had ulcerative colitis requiring colectomy and ileostomy 5 years prior. Other patients have been reported to have myasthenia gravis, myositis, pancytopenia, and hepatitis as well as impaired cell-mediated immunity. The last is usually limited to yeast and fungal antigens.

The original diagnosis in this patient of lupus was not confirmed on more detailed repeated immunofluorescent studies.

Ketoconazole therapy improved the oral candidiasis within a week and within 3 weeks induced a remission of the circinate lesions that covered 50% of his body. The nails were slow to respond. The thymoma was not resectable, so chemotherapy and irradiation were employed. A year later the thymoma remained stable.

Parodi A, Regesta G, Rebora A: **Chloroquine-induced neuromyopathy.** Report of a case. Dermatologica 1985; 171:203–205.

A 23-year-old woman professional gymnast developed alopecia, arthralgias, and photosensitive erythematous telangiectatic dermatitis of the face. Systemic lupus erythematosus was diagnosed. One year later, after she responded well to prednisone therapy, **chloroquine** phosphate (250 mg twice daily) was introduced. After 18 months of this therapy she noted thigh weakness. Creatine phosphokinase (CPK) levels were normal. **Dermatomyositis** was suspected as the proximal muscle weakness progressed, with electromyogram evidence of myogenic involvement in the quadriceps on both sides and slowly increasing CPK levels. Six months later, nerve conduction studies suggested primary axonal dysfunction, with abnormal sensory conduction in the sural nerves. Finally, a muscle biopsy (done 26 months after she started chloroquine therapy) showed vacuolar **myopathy** with numerous small granules within the muscle fibers, which incriminated chloroquine. The chloroquine was then stopped, and the return of muscle strength began 1 month later. After 3 months muscle function was normal, and repeat determinations of serum enzyme levels, electromyography, and sensory nerve conduction studies showed no signs of neuromyopathy.

Kopelman RG, Zolla-Pazner S: Association of **human immunodeficiency virus infection** and autoimmune phenomena. Am J Med 1988; 84:82–88.

Patients with systemic lupus erythematosus (SLE) and AIDS or AIDS-related complex (ARC) share several clinical and serologic features, and each disease should be included in the differential diagnosis of the other. Fevers, weight loss, lymphadenopathy, rash, renal dysfunction, and neurologic and hematologic disorders occur in SLE and AIDS. Anemia, leukopenia, hypergammaglobulinemia, elevated erythrocyte sedimentation rate, and antinuclear antibodies all may occur in AIDS, as well as in SLE. The **malar seborrheic dermatitis** of AIDS may be mistaken for the **butterfly rash of SLE**.

In one study of 151 consecutive patients with AIDS or ARC, 19 had low titer–positive antinuclear antibodies (1:20 to 1:160).

Moral: If you think your patient has SLE, also check for HIV antibodies.

Santa Cruz DJ, Uitto J, Eisen AZ, Prioleau PG: **Verrucous lupus erythematosus**: Ultrastructural studies on a distinct variant of chronic discoid lupus erythematosus. J Am Acad Dermatol 1983; 9:82–90.

Patients with the atrophic facial lesions of discoid lupus erythematosus may have concomitant hypertrophic, hyperkeratotic **verrucous lesions** on the arms and hands. Although clinically these lesions suggest a diagnosis of hypertrophic lichen planus or of keratoacanthoma, immunofluorescent and ultrastructural study reveals that they actually represent a distinct yet rare subset of discoid lupus erythematosus.

It is apparent that the wolf of lupus can thicken as well as thin the skin.

John MD, Gruber GG, Turner JE, Callen JP: **Lupus erythematosus hypertrophicus**. Two case reports and a review of the literature. Cutis 1981; 28:290–300.

This 54-year-old black woman with typical discoid lupus erythematosus lesions for many years has had wartlike growths developing in the old sites.

A biopsy of a typical lesion showed hyperkeratosis and acanthosis with a band of mononuclear cells just below the epidermis. A diagnosis of **lupus erythematosus hypertrophicus** was made.

Clinically the most important condition to rule out was squamous cell carcinoma, since it does develop in areas of chronic discoid lupus. Other conditions in the differential list include prurigo nodularis, verruca, and keratoacanthoma. These can be eliminated on histologic if no other grounds.

Finally, the most difficult diagnosis to rule out is hypertrophic lichen planus. Here again, the biopsy is the most helpful tool.

Provost TT, Ratrie H III: **Autoantibodies and autoantigens in lupus erythematosus and Sjögren's syndrome**. Curr Probl Dermatol 1990; II:151–197.

Aids to interpreting diagnostic aids from the laboratory:

ANA test is positive in systemic lupus erythematosus (SLE). It is the most useful screening test for SLE, but has very poor specificity, being positive in a variety of diseases such as dermatomyositis, scleroderma, infectious disease. (This is an ANA fluorescent test using human tissue culture cells for nuclear staining. It has totally replaced the lupus erythematosus cell test.)

Anti-nDNA antibodies are specific for SLE, and their presence favors the development of glomerulonephritis. They occur in no other disease and are a criterion for the diagnosis of SLE. (These are antibodies against native double-stranded [ds] DNA in the kinetoplast of the trypanosome *Crithidia lucilae*.)

Anti-ssDNA antibodies are found in patients with discoid lupus erythematosus and in SLE patients who have a negative ANA test. (These are antibodies against DNA in the form of a single strand (ss) as a result of denaturation that exposes purine and pyrimidine bases, the binding epitopes for these autoantibodies. In double-stranded native DNA they are spatially unavailable.

Anti-Sm antibodies are found only in patients with SLE and hence rank with anti-nDNA antibodies as a serologic criterion for diagnosing this disease state. (These are antibodies against extractable nuclear polypeptides first demonstrated in a patient named Smith, hence the Sm prefix. They are not against DNA or histone and are now known to be directed against small nuclear ribonuclear particles [sn-RNPs].)

Anti-Ro antibodies are specific for SLE and for Sjögren's syndrome. Most importantly, they may be positive in photosensitive lupus patients who have a negative ANA. They are commonly found in patients with SLE and in mothers of babies with neonatal lupus. Furthermore, these anti-Ro antibodies appear to be involved in immune complex–mediated glomerulonephritis of lupus. (These are antibodies against a cytoplasmic glycoprotein, and being present in much larger quantities than the anti-DNA antibodies they can be detected by gel double diffusion. They are also known as SSA.)

Anti-La antibodies, like anti-Ro antibodies, are indicative of SLE and Sjögren's syndrome. (These antibodies are directed against a cytoplasmic RNA protein and are also known as SSB. These and anti-Sm and anti-Ro antibodies as well as the anti-RNP antibodies are directed against small nuclear [snRNP] and small cytoplasmic ribonuclear protein [scRNP]).

Antihistone antibodies are detected in patients with a drug-induced lupus erythematosus syndrome as well as in idiopathic SLE, mixed connective tissue disease and rheumatoid arthritis. The drugs commonly responsible are procainamide, hydralazine, isoniazid, and quinidine. (These antibodies are directed toward histones that are basic proteins linked to DNA to produce chromatin.)

Anticardiolipin antibodies are present in patients with lupus who have venous thromboses and often accompanying thrombocytopenia. They are also associated with recurrent fetal deaths. (These are the antiphospholipid antibodies known as the lupus anticoagulant. They react with platelet factor 3 and interfere with the generation of prothrombin to produce a bleeding disorder. Paradoxically, they also produce venous thromboses, possibly by clumping of platelets. Their presence may explain recurrent venous thromboses of the legs, myocardial infarction, retinal artery occlusion, pulmonary emboli, as well as livedo reticularis. They may be present without any evidence of lupus.)

If you know the pattern of a disease, but the disease doesn't, diagnosis can be difficult.

Lymphadenopathy

The most common form of enlarged lymph nodes is that associated with infection. It may range from the occipital nodes of pediculosis capitis to cervical nodes from a sore throat. The most dramatic examples may be those seen with cat scratch infection or lymphogranuloma venereum. Another example in which the node also enters into the name of the disease is Kawasaki's syndrome (mucocutaneous lymph node syndrome). Add to that angioimmunoblastic lymphadenopathy, another recently described malady, which may remain benign, but usually transforms into lymphoma.

Systemic diseases such as syphilis, mycosis fungoides, and sarcoidosis are commonly associated with widespread lymphadenopathy. Rubella characteristically exhibits occipital and posterior cervical enlarged nodes. Similarly, infectious mononucleosis (glandular fever) has a highlight of bilaterally enlarged cervical and, at times, axillary and inguinal nodes.

Hypersensitivity reactions such as those from drugs or serum sickness typically show lymphadenopathy. But most feared of all are the signal nodes of cancer that have spread along the lymphatic chain, e.g., the supraclavicular node of lung cancer or the submental node of squamous cell carcinoma of the lip. Likewise feared is the sudden appearance of large lymph nodes in the neck as the first sign of Hodgkin's disease. Widespread nodes also can be the herald of leukemia or lymphoma.

The shadow of fear also covers the **generalized lymphadenopathy** that consistently accompanies erythroderma. Usually it is benign dermatopathic lymphadenopathy, but at times it hails the spread of the T-cell lymphoma, mycosis fungoides. Only the lymph node biopsy can tell.

Willems PJ, Gerritsen J, Mulder HD, Van Loon JM: Picture of the month: **Cat-scratch fever**. Am J Dis Child 1986; 140:57–58.

A skin pustule or papule (inoculation site) may be present up to 30 days following a cat scratch. Regional lymphadenopathy develops approximately 2 weeks after the scratch, and nodes remain painful and tender for 1 to 3 months. A positive skin test (Hanger-Rose) at 48 hours confirms the diagnosis. The disease can also develop after a dog or monkey bite or a scratch from a thorn or splinter.

Carithers HA: **Cat scratch disease**: An overview based on a study of 1,200 patients. Am J Dis Child 1985; 139:1124–1133.

The inoculation site (scratch, mosquito bite, puncture, bite of cat) becomes a papule 3 to 5 days after exposure to an immature healthy cat. The papule becomes vesicular and crusted and persists about 1 week.

Lymphadenopathy begins in 1 to 2 weeks and is usually single (85%). Nodes regress over weeks to months or suppurate (12%). Approximately 50% are axillary/epitrochlear, with the neck and groin less common. Measure the lymph nodes using a caliper with rubber tips (ECG type) or by placing your fingernails at the outer edges of the tumor with a transparent rule between. Also measure vertically.

Generalized aching, malaise, and anorexia are common, and two thirds have fever (greater than 39°C [102°F] in 9%).

Atypical symptoms (number of patients)
oculoglandular (48)   osteolytic lesion (2)
erythema nodosum (5)   thrombocytopenic purpura (1)
encephalopathy (3)   erythema marginatum (1)

Biopsy of a node or the skin inoculation site is not warranted (although you may see the organism with special stains). Use the skin test with CSD antigen made from aspirated pus only in complicated cases and to forestall surgery. The test site becomes red and indurated after 48 to 72 hours in almost all cases.

Causes of unilateral or regional nodes:

pyogenic infections	early Hodgkin's disease
cat scratch disease	early tuberculosis
atypical mycobacterial infections	

A chest x-ray and tuberculin test help to distinguish between these conditions.

Slater DN, Messenger AG, Bleehen SS, et al: Lymphadenopathy mimicking **lymphoma associated with cryoglobulinaemia and arteritis**. J Roy Soc Med 1982; 75:346–350.

Lymphadenopathy that clinically resembles malignant lymphoma can be caused by various **drugs**, viral infections, and autoimmune diseases. When cryoglobulins are also present, a lymph node biopsy is necessary to rule out a hemoproliferative disorder and determine if vasculitis of nodal vessels with deposition of immune complexes is present, as in the two cases presented.

A 58-year-old white woman with wheezing, myalgia, and Raynaud's syndrome had digital splinter hemorrhages and enlarged right cervical nodes adjacent to a cervical scar. Removal of an enlarged cervical lymph node 1 year previously had revealed reactive hyperplasia with increased eosinophils. Polyclonal IgG cryoglobulins were present, as were IgG immune complexes and increased IgG, IgA, and IgE, but the ESR was normal, and no paraprotein band was seen on electrophoresis. Two years later she developed peripheral edema with proteinuria (6 gm/day), cryoglobulinemia, glomerulopathy, and an ESR of 122 mm/hr (Westergren). The following year, massive cervical lymphadenopathy developed, followed by numerous episodes of urticaria and vague abdominal pain. She died following an "acute abdomen," and autopsy showed widespread **necrotizing arteritis**, characteristic of polyarteritis nodosa.

A 42-year-old carpenter had developed **cold-induced urticaria** of the hands, face, and lower legs 20 years previously, with the lesions at times being purpuric. The lesions cleared after low-dose prednisolone, but he then developed asthma, which was precipitated by temperature change. When the **cold urticaria** recurred, there was moderate enlargement of cervical and axillary nodes and the ESR was 127 mm/hr. Polyclonal IgG cryoglobulins were present along with circulating immune complexes and increased IgG and IgA, but no paraprotein band. Lymph node biopsy done to confirm suspected lymphoma showed instead necrotizing arteritis. A skin biopsy showed small-vessel vasculitis. During warm weather the cold urticaria improved and lymph nodes diminished in size.

Massive lymphadenopathy is also seen in **Kawasaki's disease**, which is possibly related to infantile polyarteritis nodosa.

Weston WL, Huff JC: **The mucocutaneous lymph node syndrome**: A critical reexamination. Clin Exp Dermatol 1981; 6:167–178.

In 1967 Tomisaku Kawasaki, a Japanese pediatrician, described 50 infants and children with this distinctive constellation of clinical features:

1. Fever 1 to 2 weeks, unresponsive to antibiotics
2. Conjunctival congestion

| 3. Dry red lips, strawberry tongue | 5. Polymorphous rash |
| 4. Red, swollen palms and soles | 6. Cervical lymphadenitis |

Within 10 years, more than 10,000 cases had been reported, and Kawasaki's disease became recognized worldwide. The recognition of this entity is a clinical tour de force. There is no laboratory test for it. From the differential point of view, Kawasaki's disease is indistinguishable from **erythema multiforme**. (One is reminded of two other pediatricians also coming upon erythema multiforme, with the result that it is also known as Stevens-Johnson syndrome.) The second condition with identical diagnostic features is the **dilantin eruption**.

Another half-dozen conditions also suggest the **diagnosis of** Kawasaki's disease. These include Epstein-Barr viral infection (infectious mononucleosis) and scarlet fever. However, both lack the distinctive edema of the palms and soles. Hepatitis also is similar at times in its presentation, but shows no cervical lymphadenitis. Periarteritis nodosa fails to produce the "red mouth"; neither do juvenile rheumatoid arthritis, leptospirosis, and Rocky Mountain spotted fever. Otherwise, all six are possible. Kawasaki's syndrome thus crosses the terrain of previously described febrile diseases characterized by fever, lymphadenopathy, a red rash, mouth, and eyes.

Kawasaki's contribution is less in identifying a serious morphe of febrile childhood disease, but more in pointing out that these children are at cardiac risk. All deserve **cardiac consultation**, since arrhythmias, coronary aneurysms, and even myocardial infarctions can ensue. They have a syndrome as dangerous as motorcycle riding.

Ikeda S, Ogawa H: **Subacute necrotizing lymphadenitis**. J Am Acad Dermatol 1990; 22:909–912.

This 48-year-old woman had an **erythematous papular skin** eruption of the trunk, neck, and upper arms. Present for 2 weeks, it was associated with a sore throat, cervical lymphadenopathy, fever, and arthralgia.

The white count was 20,000/mm^3, and the sedimentation rate was elevated (59 mm/hr). Tests for lupus, syphilis, and rheumatic disease were negative, as well as antibody evidence of *Toxoplasma*, Epstein-Barr and herpes simplex virus, and cytomegalovirus. The biopsy of the skin showed little other than capillary dilatation and a weak perivascular infiltrate of lymphohistiocytic cells. However, biopsy of a cervical lymph node did show evidence of **lymphadenitis** with lymphoreticular cell proliferation. A diagnosis was made of skin changes due to subacute necrotizing lymphadenitis. This is a recently described entity of a benign self-limiting nature that may result from a viral infection.

We wonder if the skin lesions result from inflammatory or necrotizing changes in the miniature "lymph nodes" that are present in skin.

Talmi YP, Cohen AH, Finkelstein Y, et al: *Mycobacterium tuberculosis* **cervical adenitis**. Diagnosis and management. Clin Pediatr 1989; 28:408–411.

Cervical adenopathy may be the sole clinical presentation of **tuberculosis** in children. Chest x-rays, sputum cultures, and PPD skin tests with 5 tuberculin units are indicated. Remember that the word scrofula is derived from the Latin for glandular swelling. The disease still exists.

Hall SM: **The diagnosis of toxoplasmosis**. Br Med J 1984; 289:570–571.

The best serologic means of diagnosing acute **acquired toxoplasmosis** is the **ELISA** (enzyme-linked immunosorbent assay) for detection of specific antitoxoplasma IgM. It is more sensitive and specific than the IgM immunofluorescent antibody test (IFAT). Single high titers of IgG antibody (measured by the Sabin-Feldman dye test and hemagglutinin tests) do not identify recent infection.

Laboratory diagnosis is also based on identification or isolation of the organism in body fluids or tissues and by finding cellular changes in lymph nodes. Presence of the organism in body fluids indicates acute infection. The diagnostic challenge lies in differentiating between acute and chronic infection. *Toxoplasma* antibodies are frequently present in the general population and may persist for years at high titers.

Patients with acute infection needing treatment include those with chorioretinitis, severe or systemic symptoms, pregnant women and their infected infants, and those with immunodeficiency. Uncomplicated lymphoglandular toxoplasmosis is self-limited and not usually treated.

A **cytologic tissue diagnosis** may be made via fine-needle aspiration of an enlarged lymph node. This is important to rule out lymphoma and granulomatous change in young adults with unexplained lymphadenopathy, who may also have fever, lethargy, and malaise.

Weiss LM, Hu E, Wood GS, et al: Clonal rearrangements of **T-cell receptor genes** in mycosis fungoides and dermatopathic lymphadenopathy. N Engl J Med 1985; 313:539–544.

Palpable lymphadenopathy in mycosis fungoides indicates a worse prognosis, regardless whether the nodes show mycosis fungoides or only dermatopathic lymphadenopathy (reactive lymphoid hyperplasia with intranodal melanin released from damaged epidermis).

In this study, histologically occult mycosis fungoides was detected in lymph nodes by DNA analysis of the T–cell receptor gene. Since more than 50% of patients with mycosis fungoides have some degree of peripheral lymphadenopathy at the time of diagnosis, detection of involved nodes is important. Nodes may act as reservoirs for tumor cells, which repopulate the skin after therapy directed only at the skin.

Steinberg AD, Seldin MF, Jaffe ES, et al: **Angioimmunoblastic lymphadenopathy with dysproteinemia**. Ann Intern Med 1988; 108:575–584.

Characterized by sudden onset of constitutional symptoms and **lymphadenopathy**, angioimmunoblastic lymphadenopathy may present with nonspecific skin rashes. Early in the disease, autoantibody production is evident, but later immune suppression occurs. This may explain the appearance at that time of opportunistic infections of the skin as well as the lesions of Kaposi's sarcoma.

Diagnosis rests entirely on **lymph node biopsy**. The disease is viewed as standing part way between benign lymphoid proliferation and clonal transformation to lymphoma. Prognosis is poor, with 75% of the patients dying within 2 years. Many features provide a resemblance to AIDS.

McCarthy JT: Achoo! Achoo! We all fall down. Cutis 1982; 29:409.

A nursery rhyme guide to the diagnosis of bubonic plague:

> Ring around the rosie,
> A pocket full of posies,
> Achoo! Achoo! We all fall down.

The ring of roses consists of the buboes encircling the neck, axillae, and groin. The posies are the pressed flowers and herbs (particularly garlic) carried to ward off the disease. The "achoo" is the sign of pneumonic plague. We all fall down, the fatal outcome.

Macules

Although macules have little standing in the kingdom of lesions, they can be guides to diagnosis. The hypopigmented hyposensitive macule of tuberculoid leprosy must be noticed and respected. The café au lait spot and the axillary freckles speak to us of neurofibromatosis, and we cannot ignore the ragged border of the macule that is the wayside sign of Albright's disease.

In the infant, the very first sign of tuberous sclerosis is the ash leaf macule of scant pigment, sometimes seen only under Wood's light. Slate-blue macules on the acne face may tell us that there are grains of bone beneath. The spots of blue we poetically call maculae ceruleae make the diagnosis of pediculosis.

Some macules tell us what they are only when slapped or scratched. The brown macule of urticaria pigmentosa will become a hive when so mistreated. And the pale macule of vitiligo reddens on trauma, whereas its mimic, nevus anemicus, shows no change. And the brown macule of the fixed drug eruption will soon redden and itch upon proper oral challenge.

Interestingly, some macules are never called macules. They have their own names: freckles, nevi, purpura, and stains. These are the aristocrats.

Sehgal VN, Shyam Prasad AL, Gangwani OP: Magnesium trisilicate induced **fixed drug eruption**. Dermatologica 1986; 172:123.

> Four oval **hyperpigmented macules** on the arms of a 50-year-old housewife were proven by challenge to be due to tablets of the simple **antacid** magnesium trisilicate. This substance is broken down in the stomach to magnesium ions and silicon dioxide. (No studies were done on the possible role of excipients or flavoring.)

Brodkin RH, Abbey AA: **Osteoma cutis**: A case of probable exacerbation following treatment of severe acne with isotretinoin. Dermatologica 1985; 170:210–212.

> A 24-year-old white woman with chronic cystic acne was noted to have scattered **blue-gray macules** that were clinically diagnosed as osteoma cutis.
>
> Six months after completing a course of isotretinoin treatment (100 mg/day for 5 months) she complained of marked bluish discoloration of the face. On examination she proved to have innumerable small blue-gray macules in such profusion that a bluish hue was cast over the skin of the face. On biopsy, a 1-mm discrete hard, gray granule was seen, and histologic examination confirmed the clinical diagnosis of **osteoma cutis**. Numerous osteoblasts, osteocytes, and a haversian canal were seen.
>
> It is assumed that the isotretinoin prescribed favored the development of osteoid metaplasia in the dermis.

Miller RAW. **Maculae ceruleae**. Int J Dermatol 1986; 25:383–384.

> Many **light-blue, red, oval macules** (0.5 to 1.5 cm) of the abdomen and anterior aspect of the chest of this 8-year-old boy had been viewed as a possible cutaneous sign of myeloproliferative disease.
>
> The actual diagnosis proved far less intimidating. The boy had maculae ceruleae, due to the bites of **crab lice**. But only one louse was found, and it was hanging by an eyelash.

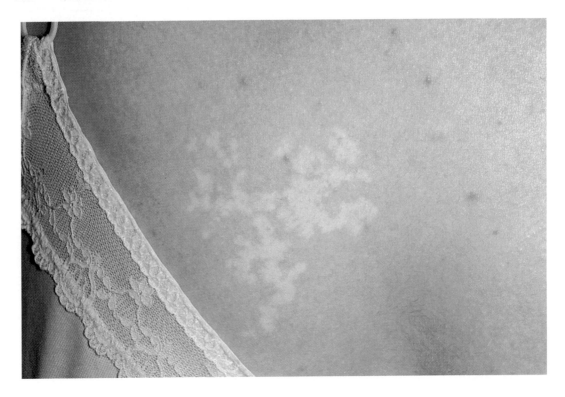

Mountcastle EA, Diestelmeier MR, Lupton GP: **Nevus anemicus**. J Am Acad Dermatol 1986; 14:628–632.

These **pale macules** and patches of varying size and shape are islands of skin where the cutaneous blood vessels are continuously constricted because of hypersensitivity to adrenergic stimuli.

Sympathetic block or injection of an alpha-adrenergic blocking agent (phentolamine 70 µg in 0.1 ml) reverses the skin to normal color. Beta-blockers (propranolol HCl 100 µg in 0.1 ml) have no effect. Histamine phosphate (10 µg in 0.1 ml) produced a wheal with diminished flare within the nevus anemicus.

The **differential diagnosis** includes nevus depigmentosus, vitiligo, tuberous sclerosis, and leprosy. Differentiation is easily accomplished by:

diascopy: Border disappears on pressure of glass slide.
Wood's light: This accentuates hypomelanotic macules, but has no effect on nevus anemicus.
mechanically: Stroking the area produces erythema in normal skin but not in nevus anemicus.
histologically: Nevus anemicus is histologically normal, whereas leprosy shows distinctive change.

Wilkin JK, Martin H: **Bier's spots** reconsidered: A tale of two spots, with speculation on a humerus vein. J Am Acad Dermatol 1986; 14:411–419.

The **Bier spot** is a white spot that appears on a cyanotic background during occlusion of the blood flow to the forearm. The spots are due to venoconstriction triggered by the ischemia-induced drop in skin temperature.

Tschen JA, Tschen EA, McGavran MH: **Erythema dyschromicum perstans**. J Am Acad Dermatol 1980; 2:295–302.

Look for asymptomatic **ash-colored macules** that sometimes have raised red

1- to 2-mm edges for a few months and later may have hypopigmented halos. The oval, irregular, polycyclic lesions slowly extend and can affect most of the body.

Although they are idiopathic, the persistence of fibrinogen at the basement membrane, even in longstanding lesions, suggests an inflammatory process. It may be a form of lichen planus pigmentosa, as there are histologic and immunofluorescent similarities.

Sehgal VN: **Inoculation leprosy.** Current status. Int J Dermatol 1988; 27:6–9.

Sign:

well-defined hypopigmented macule or plaque

Look for:

loss of pain, temperature, touch
loss of hair
local anhidrosis
proximal nerve thick, tender

Ask about prior:

dog bite
abrasion
vaccination
tattoo

Latent period: 15 days to 7 years

Do biopsy: tuberculoid form of leprosy, rare bacteria

Lepromin test: strongly positive

Differential diagnosis:

sarcoid reaction: no sensory deficit, no thickened nerves
lupus vulgaris: no thickened nerves

Recognition, not description, is the heart of diagnosis.

Mouth

The oral hunt for diagnostic leads and diagnoses calls for more than just having the patient open his mouth. You must not only look in, but also look out for specific lesions. This requires an alert inquiring mind as well as excellent lighting, a tongue blade for exposure, and the removal of any dentures. Don't skip the oral examination on the assumption nothing will be seen. You can be as amazed as a friend of ours whose child told him there was a giant snake in the back yard. After saying "You mustn't tell lies," the disbelieving father was dragged outside where he saw a gigantic boa constrictor. It had escaped from its owner in a nearby home.

Look at the **lips**. This is home base for recurrent herpes simplex and angular cheilitis, which can be missed unless the mouth is wide open. Are there any melanotic macules suggesting Peutz-Jeghers syndrome? Is the lip swollen and tender as in cheilitis glandularis? Look for the swelling of angioedema. What evidence is there of sun damage in the form of leukoplakia or actinic cheilitis? Do you see an erosion or any sign of squamous cell carcinoma? Are the submental nodes palpable? Is there scaling and inflammation suggesting factitial cheilitis? Patients will deny this, as well as excessive lip wetting. Direct evidence comes from questioning relatives. On one occasion our nurse by chance rode home on the same bus as the patient. She observed the patient in a continuous flow of ticlike lip biting on the entire ride.

The **tongue** shows its hairy brown papillae in patients taking antibiotics, as well as its patchy white coating in candidiasis. Most dramatic is the tectonic movement of the white continents seen in geographic tongue. Ulcers may be evidence of dental trauma or the dreaded squamous cell carcinoma. The white areas restricted to the sides of the tongue, called hairy leukoplakia, are a diagnostic sign of AIDS or other immunodeficiency states. The glossy smooth tongue of malnutrition also can be seen. Macroglossia may be of many causes.

Look at the **teeth**. Their malformation or delayed onset of appearance may reflect genetic disease. Caries, gingivitis, and pain are suggestive of focal infection, which can trigger the distant lesions of urticaria or psoriasis. The gums exposed by tongue blade add to the evaluation of dental care. They may be swollen and inflamed for many reasons, from pemphigoid to phenytoin.

Look about in the oral cavity for **pigmentation**. The most common form is the patchy melanosis seen in black patients. The rarest of rare is that of malignant melanoma.

Is the mouth dry? Could the patient be under tension? Could it be Sjögren's syndrome? Check tear production. Or is it the mundane side effect of a drug?

Most valuable of all is inspection of the **buccal mucosa**. Here are the murals of lichen planus and leukoplakia. Be sure not to miss the small ones by covering them with the tongue blade. And look at the labial mucosa. Throughout you may see the pinpoints of erythema, the erosions and the ulcers of aphthous stomatitis.

Look at the **hard palate** for the grouped erosions of herpes simplex. Watch for the speckled lesions of leukoplakia in the smoker.

Just before you leave, depress the extruded tongue to really visualize the **tonsils**. Here is the common focus of infection triggering guttate psoriasis. Here may be a chancre. And how is the **pharynx**? Is it inflamed, or is it coated with the mucus of pharyngitis?

When the patient closes his mouth, don't close your mind to the significance of what you have seen.

Silverman S Jr: Etiology and predisposing factors. *In* Silverman S Jr (ed): **Oral Cancer**, 2nd ed. New York, American Cancer Society, 1985, pp 7–36.

Precancerous factor: tobacco
Precancerous oral lesions:

    leukoplakia
    erythroplasia
    oral lichen planus

Silverman S Jr: Color Atlas of **Oral Manifestations of AIDS**. Philadelphia, BC Decker, 1989, 113 pp.

A comprehensive tour of what can happen to the immunosuppressed oral cavity.

Silverman S Jr: Diagnosis. *In* Silverman S Jr (ed): **Oral Cancer**, 2nd ed. New York, American Cancer Society, 1985, pp 37–49.

Early carcinomas may appear as small, apparently harmless areas of erythema, erosion, or keratosis, frequently leading the unsuspecting clinician into a false sense of security. Lesions that do not respond to therapeutic measures must be considered malignant until proven otherwise.

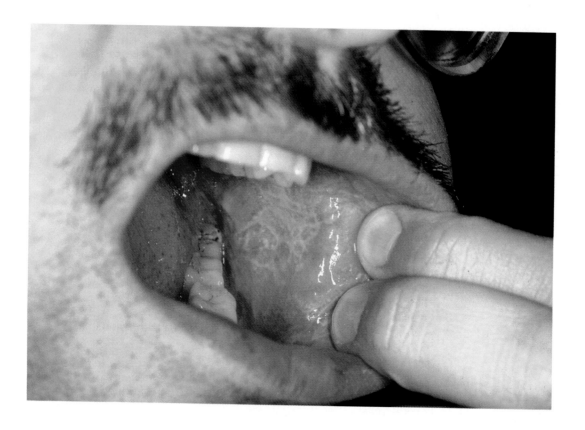

Cheilitis

Venable CE, Gaudio SA: **Persistent swelling** of the lower lip. Arch Dermatol 1988; 124:1706–1709.

Within 24 hours this 62-year-old woman developed painless edema of the lower lip for no apparent reason. Biopsy after 2 months of ineffectual therapy with compresses, antihistaminics, and erythromycin showed scattered non-caseating granulomas with an infiltrate of plasma cells and lymphocytes.

A diagnosis of **cheilitis granulomatosa (Miescher)** was made. The lip changes are usually of rapid onset and may involve the tongue and gingiva as well. The swelling is usually progressive.

This disorder is to be distinguished from the **Melkersson-Rosenthal** syndrome, which presents as a triad of facial swelling, facial weakness or paralysis, and fissured tongue. It too is of sudden onset with the lips the usual site of swelling. A common histologic picture suggests that cheilitis granulomatosa may be an abortive form of the Melkersson-Rosenthal syndrome.

In the search for causes the following have been considered:

recurrent oral or nasopharyngeal infection
recurrent infection, herpes simplex
food allergy
sodium silicate exposure
genetic factors

The differential diagnosis includes:

Crohn's disease of the oral cavity
sarcoidosis
tuberculosis
syphilis

Brenner S, Lipitz R, Ilie B, Krakowski A: **Psoriasis of the lips**: The unusual Koebner phenomenon caused by protruding upper teeth. Dermatologica 1982; 164:413–416.

A 54-year-old woman had thick **white plaques of the lips** for many years, which had developed in association with scattered plaques of psoriasis on the trunk. Psoriasis of the lips was confirmed by biopsy. Treatment with steroids, 5-fluorouracil, and surgical excision of the vermilion border was unsuccessful.

Attention was then paid to the protruding upper teeth, which caused pressure and friction on both lips. Once these teeth were replaced by a prosthesis with normal alignment, the lip psoriasis quickly disappeared. This woman's lip problem therefore represented a dental **Koebner phenomenon.**

Crotty CP, Dicken CH: **Factitious lip crusting**. Arch Dermatol 1981; 117:338–340.

Hemorrhagic crusting of the lips had been present for 3 weeks when this 16-year-old girl was admitted to the hospital for study. There was no history of a bleeding diathesis, melena, hematemesis, ulcers of the tongue or buccal mucosa, nor did she use lipstick or lip gloss. Furthermore, she had no history of photosensitivity, herpes simplex, or mucosal disease elsewhere. Health profile, clotting factors, x-ray studies of the upper gastrointestinal tract, patch tests, and a biopsy were nonrewarding.

Psychiatric consultation disclosed a trait of self-denial and an indication that the crusting was of psychogenic origin. Although the patient finally admitted to her parents that she had been picking at her lips, she continued to deny this to her physicians. The problem remained for months, and a diagnosis

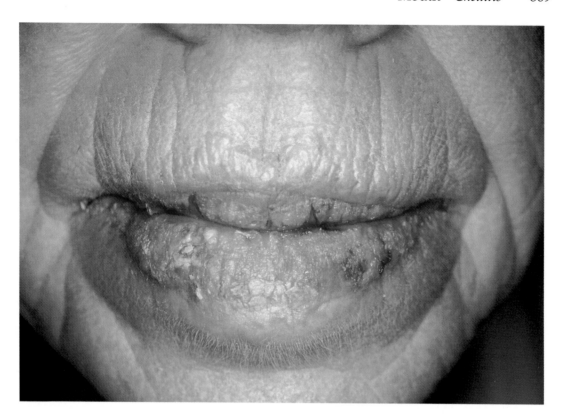

of **factitious lip crusting** was made when, on removal of the crusts, excoriations were seen.

Such a form of factitious cheilitis may present as dryness, scaling, fissures, or cracking of the lips as a result of biting or licking. The lips may become swollen or covered with thick, yellow, keratotic crusts. In some instances the patient may induce excessive dryness by protruding the lower lip for hours on end.

These cases must not be swept under the diagnostic rug of exfoliative cheilitis. They must be identified and **distinguished** from:

actinic cheilitis   cheilitis granulomatosis
contact dermatitis   *Candida* cheilitis
cheilitis glandularis

Picascia DD, Robinson JK: **Actinic cheilitis**: A review of the etiology, differential diagnosis and treatment. J Am Acad Dermatol 1987; 17:255–264.

Actinic cheilitis—usually lower lip

Acute:
edema, redness
congestion, fissuring, ulceration, vesicles, erosions
resolution: dryness, scaling associated with prolonged sunlight exposure

Chronic:
scaling, irregular hyperkeratoses
atrophy, white gray to brown
indistinct vermilion border
wrinkling of vermilion border
secondary infection, erosive ulcers

Differential:
squamous cell carcinoma
commonly missed unless biopsy done

Suspect when:
vermilion edge is indistinct, wandering, variegated, red and white
blotchy appearance
atrophy present with focal areas of whitish thickening
persistent chapping, local flaking, and crusting

Allergic contact cheilitis—usually upper and lower lip

dentifrices (bacterial agents, essential oils, preservatives)
mouthwashes
cosmetics: lipstick, lip salve, nail polish
foods: carrots, orange peel, coffee, menthol

Irritant contact cheilitis

Photosensitive cheilitis—polymorphous light eruption

Glandular cheilitis: thick, swollen

Angular cheilitis: only at angles of mouth

Factitial cheilitis: manipulation, biting, licking, bizarre hemorrhage

Exfoliative cheilitis: may be atrophic

Granulomatous cheilitis

progressive, relentless
granuloma on biopsy
enlargement
Melkersson-Rosenthal syndrome: if associated scrotal tongue and facial
nerve palsy

Plasma cell cheilitis: circumscribed plaques of erythema on lower lip in older
people

Drug-induced cheilitis:

isotretinoin   antineoplastics
antihistamines   diuretics
anticholinergics   narcotics
anticonvulsants

Fisher AA: **Chronic lip edema** with particular reference to the Melkersson-Rosenthal
syndrome (MRS). Cutis 1990; 45:144–146.

For the past 12 years this 29-year-old woman had had recurrent swellings
of the lips. Most of the flares occurred during her menstrual period. The
medical history disclosed that she had had three attacks of **facial palsy** at
4-year intervals during this time. Each had cleared spontaneously within a
couple of months.

Although she had consulted two allergists, an immunologist, and a dermatologist and had been treated with hormones, antihistamines, and intralabial
steroids, a diagnosis and therapeutic success had eluded all. None had looked
in her mouth.

Not only did she have firm, **solid edema of the lips**, especially the upper,
but on simply opening the mouth a deeply **furrowed tongue** came into view.
It was evident that she had the triad of the Melkersson-Rosenthal syndrome:
persistent lip edema, furrowed tongue, and a history of facial palsy. A biopsy
of the lip confirmed all this by revealing noncaseating epithelioid granulomas, resembling sarcoidosis.

It is important to point out the tongue in these patients is furrowed, not split (fissured), folded (lingua plicata), and certainly not deserving of the vulgar designation *scrotal tongue*. It is of normal appearance to the patient and not the source of symptoms. Hence, "a stick-out-your-tongue" request must come from the physician.

Any persistent lip edema calls for these **diagnostic thoughts**:

contact dermatitis
recurrent herpes simplex
erysipelas
lymphangiomas, hemangioma

facial edema with eosinophilia
hereditary angioedema
Crohn's disease

Biopsy for evidence of:

sarcoidosis
cheilitis glandularis
Miescher's cheilitis granulomatosa

Frankel DH, Mostofi RS, Lorincz AL: **Oral Crohn's disease**: Report of two cases of brothers with metallic dysgeusia and a review of the literature. J Am Acad Dermatol 1985; 12:260–268.

Think of **Crohn's disease** if you see:

aphthae that are persistent, deep, with hyperplastic edges
gingival, buccal, or labial swelling or bleeding
cobblestone appearance of focal areas of mucosal inflammatory hyperplasia and fissuring
polypoid or tag lesions of mucosae
indurated fissure on midline of lower lip
cheilitis, angular or granulomatous
pyostomatitis vegetans
metallic dysgeusia

Tatnall FM, Dodd HJ, Sarkany I: **Crohn's disease** with metastatic cutaneous involvement and granulomatous cheilitis. J Roy Soc Med 1987; 80:49–51.

A 15-year-old boy developed pronounced **lower-lip swelling**, which on biopsy showed chronic inflammation and epithelioid granulomas with Langhans' giant cells in the dermis. The swelling decreased spontaneously, leaving only residual thickening, and he was asymptomatic for 3 years until he developed weight loss, diarrhea, abdominal pain, an anal fissure, and purple crusted nodules on the lower legs. A skin biopsy from the leg showed noncaseating granulomas in the dermis and subcutaneous fat, vasculitis, and eosinophilic necrosis of collagen in the mid-dermis. **X-ray findings** of the large and small bowel favored a diagnosis of **Crohn's disease**.

Metastatic cutaneous Crohn's disease refers to skin lesions with granulomatous histology that are remote from the bowel. These are usually associated with colonic disease and take the form of ulcers, nodules on the extremities, or generalized lichenoid papules.

In the absence of bowel disease, **Crohn's cheilitis** may be difficult to distinguish from an incomplete form of Melkersson-Rosenthal syndrome.

Reilly GD, Wood ML: **Prochlorperazine**—an unusual cause of lip ulceration. Acta Derm Venereol 1984; 64:270–271.

For 3 months a 75-year-old English housewife had an **ulcer on the vermilion border** of the lower lip. She was a nonsmoker but had taken a phenothiazine-type medication (prochlorperazine) intermittently for 12 years for dizzy spells. The lesion began as a blister, which ulcerated. After little improvement with triamcinolone cream, she stopped the prochlorperazine, and within 3 weeks the lesion completely healed. Rechallenge with prochlorperazine (5 mg tid) produced a return of the lip ulcer within 3 days. Stopping the drug again led to prompt healing.

Presumably this is an ulcerative type of **fixed drug eruption**. Here is an anxiety drug that can give you something to be anxious about.

André J, Bernard M, Ladoux M, Achten G: **Larva migrans** of the oral mucosa. Dermatologica 1988; 176:296–298.

A 40-year-old Belgian woman had **migrant edema of the lower lip** for 3 months, associated with the feeling "like a mole was burrowing away underground." Right before this she had marked pharyngitis and gingivitis with white deposits, unresponsive to antifungals and antibiotics. Only an edematous mucosa could be seen on inspection.

After 1 week of systemic steroid therapy, reduction of the edema allowed visualization of a serpiginous, raised, white 3- to 4-mm wide track along the palate mucosa, leading to the clinical diagnosis of **larva migrans**. Although the nematode was not seen on biopsy, a 2-day course of oral thiabendazole (25 mg/kg bid) was curative.

It was assumed the patient had acquired the infection while on a recent trip to the West Indies. Sources of oropharyngeal infection could be polluted ground or sea water or the ingestion of contaminated food or infected animals or fish.

Note how the patient's history can clue you in to look for something "burrowing away."

Marshall RJ, Leppard BJ: Ulceration of the lip associated with "**calibre-persistent artery.**" Br J Dermatol 1985; 113:757–760.

For 5 months a 72-year-old woman had an enlarging **ulcer of the lower lip**, diagnosed as squamous cell carcinoma. However, wedge resection showed no evidence of carcinoma. Instead, an artery of abnormally large caliber (0.8 mm) ran immediately beneath the ulcer, parallel to the skin surface. The ulcer recurred 9 months later but healed spontaneously.

A **caliber-persistent artery** is a primary arterial branch that penetrates to the submucosa without dividing or losing caliber. They have been found in association with ulcers that appear to be **squamous cell carcinomas** in the stomach, jejunum, and lip. Presumably the atrophy of aging and solar damage brings the vessel close to the mucosal surface of the lip, interfering with normal capillary blood supply.

Laskaris GC, Nicolis GD: **Lupus vulgaris of the oral mucosa**: Report of 4 cases associated with asymptomatic pulmonary tuberculosis. Dermatologica 1981; 162:183–190.

Ulceration of the upper-lip mucosa was the presenting complaint of a 67-year-old Greek man. Examination showed extensive ulceration with an irregular periphery, sharp borders, and a granular base covered with a yellow-gray exudate. The regional lymph nodes were enlarged. **Lupus vulgaris** proved to be the correct diagnosis, as shown with a biopsy, positive Mantoux test, and complete healing within 1 month of starting antituberculosis therapy. It was never possible to demonstrate acid-fast bacteria in a smear, culture, or biopsy.

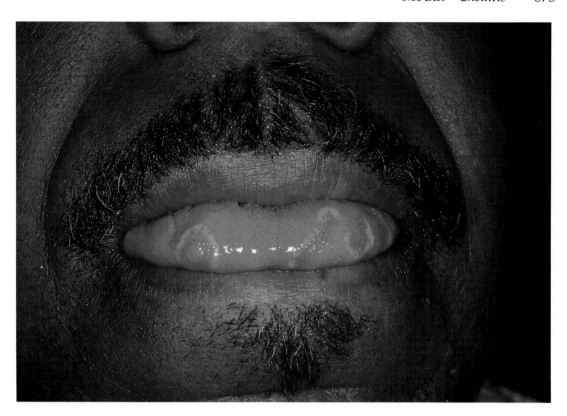

The importance of making the diagnosis in this man was underscored by finding asymptomatic unrecognized pulmonary tuberculosis on **x-ray** examination.

Walike JW, Bailey BJ: **Head and neck hemangiopericytoma**. Arch Otolaryng 1971; 93:345–353.

A 66-year-old black woman with quiescent pemphigus vulgaris and cushingoid appearance developed multiple **tan-appearing nodules** on the lower **lip**, tongue, and soft palate. These were slightly raised, nonulcerated, and less than 1 cm in diameter. Biopsy revealed **hemangiopericytoma**, which soon spread to the throat. She died 2 months after the initial nodules appeared.

A 16-year-old white boy fell and struck the right side of the mandible 2 years before being seen with a rapidly growing lump on the right jaw. The 6-cm, smooth **mass throbbed** with exertion and appeared as a plexus of small veins when the overlying skin and gingival mucosa were tensed. Histology showed a mixed type of hemangioendothelioma and hemangiopericytoma, most often seen in children and adolescents. He did well after surgery.

A **silver reticulin stain** is essential to identify the pericytes in this rare vascular tumor. Metastases occur in 50%, and local recurrences are common, necessitating lifelong follow-up.

Vincent RG, Marchetta FC, Nigogosyan G: Incidence of **cirrhosis in oral cancer**. NY State J Med 1964; 64:2174–2176.

In 106 patients with oral cancer, 45% had clinical evidence of liver damage. Similarly, histologic cirrhosis was found in 28% of 144 autopsies of patients with oral cancer.

Heavy alcohol consumption is probably an important factor in oral cancer, with liver dysfunction leading to abnormal metabolism of vitamin A and iron, both of which are important in maintaining integrity of the oral mucosa.

Lieberman J, Lynfield YL, Rosen P: **Noma.** Cutis 1987; 39:501–502.

Necrosis of the skin, mucosa, and deep tissues of the lower lip of a 72-year-old man had been present for just 1 week. Skin and blood cultures grew no organisms, but blood studies showed anemia associated with a white count of $13 \times 10^3/mm^3$, showing atypical monocytes. A diagnosis of preleukemia was made and the necrotic ulcer clinically diagnosed as **noma.**

Despite intensive care and antibiotic therapy, the ulceration enlarged progressively, and the patient died after a month of hospitalization.

Noma, classically seen in children, is rapidly spreading **orofacial gangrene** in a compromised host. It may destroy the entire cheek, as well as lip. Background contributors include malnutrition, blood dyscrasias, acatalasemia, febrile exanthems, steroids, and cytotoxic drugs. It is generally believed that given a compromised host, the normal oral bacterial flora become capable of invading and destroying the lip at a site of trauma. This is confirmed by the fact that antibiotic therapy has lowered the mortality rate of noma from 75% to 10%.

Gonçalves AP: **Paracoccidioidomycosis.** Cutis 1987; 40:214–216.

Also known as **South American blastomycosis**, this deep fungal infection is endemic in Central and South America.

Think of it:

with lesions having hemorrhagic spots
with chronic lesions around or in the mouth
with erosions, ulcers, abscesses, gummas, warty growth
with cheilitis, hoarseness
with profuse salivary flow

Look for the organism *Paracoccidioides brasiliensis*:

in touch, smears, biopsies
in inoculated mice (cultures rarely successful)

Look for pulmonary lesions

Unrecognized, it is a fatal disease. Because of its long incubation period, you must look for this patient profile—a man who has visited or lived in Latin America and who now has strange chronic sores in and around the mouth.

As a diagnostician you're gored, once you become bored.

Conant MA: **Hairy leukoplakia**. A new disease of the oral mucosa. Arch Dermatol 1987; 123:585–587.

Examine the **sides of the tongue** for:

poorly demarcated, white, filiform or hairy lesions
indistinct fine white vertical lines lying parallel and reminiscent of the representation of rain in Japanese woodblock prints
bold white clots, looking like billowing clouds

These are the clinical forms of **hairy leukoplakia**. They do not respond to nystatin, clotrimazole, or systemic ketoconazole, since they are due to Epstein-Barr virus (EBV) infection with the virus clearly apparent on electron microscopy.

These are the signs of an HIV infection and harbingers of AIDS. Thus, all of these patients deserve the following:

1. Tell the patient his tongue speaks of immunosuppression.
2. Look for other signs of immunosuppression:
   lymph node enlargement
   cutaneous infection: perianal candidiasis, molluscum, impetigo
3. Offer laboratory evaluation of immune state:
   white cell count
   sedimentation rate
   helper/suppressor T-cell ratio
4. If normal, biopsy tongue for more definitive diagnosis.
5. If helper/suppressor ratio is less than 0.9:1 and there are fewer than 500 helper T cells, tell the patient that there is immunosuppression and do an HIV antibody test.
6. If HIV test is positive, reassure the patient that this is not AIDS. Place him under rules of good health and medical surveillance.
7. Use Retin-A solution, applied with cotton-tipped applicator, once a day for suppression of lesions.

Alessi E, Berti E, Cusini M, et al: **Oral hairy leukoplakia**. J Am Acad Dermatol 1990; 22:79–86.

Whitish patches with a corrugated or hairy surface, most commonly located on the lateral margins of the tongue, are the sign of oral hairy leukoplakia. It represents a local **Epstein-Barr viral infection**. The virus could be found in the lesion in every one of the 59 cases reported here.

This form of leukoplakia is significant in that its appearance heralds the development of AIDS within a few months of its onset.

Syrjänen S, Laine P, Happonen R-P, Niemala M: **Oral hairy leukoplakia** is not a specific sign of HIV-infection but related to immunosuppression in general. J Oral Pathol Med 1989; 18:28–31.

A 32-year-old HIV-seronegative heterosexual man suffering from acute myeloblastic leukemia developed clinically and histologically typical hairy leukoplakia while receiving cytostatic therapy. Both lateral borders of the tongue showed corrugated, nonremovable **white lesions**.

Biopsy showed areas with characteristic ballooning cells, and hyphae of yeast were demonstrated with PAS stain. The in situ hybridization technique indicated that Epstein-Barr virus DNA with high copy numbers was present while human papillomavirus (types 6, 11, 16, 18) was not. The patient had no circulating antibodies to EBV, which may be considered a result of his immunosuppression.

Lamey P-J, Lamb AB: Prospective study of aetiological factors in **burning mouth syndrome**. Br Med J 1988; 296:1243–1246.

Patients with **burning mouth syndrome** (glossopyrosis, glossodynia, oral dysesthesia) have a normal oral mucosa. The burning is unremitting, either being present on waking and persisting the entire day or developing during the day and worsening as the day goes on. **Multifactorial** origins are important, as illustrated in this study of 150 consecutive patients with burning mouth syndrome, including 131 women with a mean age of 59 years. Approximately two thirds of the patients could be cured of their symptoms. At each visit, patients were asked to quantify their burning sensation on a scale of 1 to 10.

Laboratory and clinical investigations included:

Blood studies:
complete blood count
mean corpuscular volume and mean corpuscular hemoglobin
corrected whole blood folate
serum ferritin
vitamins B_1, B_2, B_6, B_{12}
Fasting glucose every 6 months and glucose tolerance test as indicated (abnormal in 8 patients).
Salivary gland stimulation with 1 ml of 10% citric acid using a Carlsson-Crittenden cup. The volume of saliva produced in 1 minute was measured, with less than 0.5 ml/min being abnormal (19 patients were greatly helped with artificial saliva).
Candidal isolation, done with a rinse technique in the mouth (*Candida* species were isolated in 40% of patients, with one-seventh helped by antifungal treatment).
Psychological investigation: Inquire about cancerophobia, stress, anxiety, and depression. Seek specific sources of anxiety: financial, social, marital, bereavement, housing, domestic upheaval. Also ask about sleep disorders, feelings of isolation and hopelessness, and depression (20% of patients were caring for handicapped relatives).
Obtain a specialist's opinion about denture design, particularly if denture removal eases symptoms. Features leading to overloading of denture-bearing tissues and tongue restriction are important. Acrylic allergy to dentures is very uncommon, but patch tests may be necessary. Tongue thrusting, jaw clenching, and teeth grinding are also important factors.
Patch tests to food-related products should be considered if symptoms of burning are intermittent and affect the tongue, soft palate, and throat. (Ascorbic acid, propylene glycol, benzoic acid, and cinnamon were causative factors, and dietary advice abolished symptoms.)
Ask about climacteric symptoms, such as facial flushing and night sweats (17 patients).
Ask about reflux esophagitis, with burning tongue on waking.

Overall, vitamin B supplements alleviated symptoms in 34 of 150 patients, while ferrous sulfate or cyanocobalamin helped 13 additional patients. New dentures helped 33 of 64 patients with inadequate denture design, and avoidance of tongue thrusting and jaw clenching helped 20 more. A tricyclic antidepressant (dothiepin) reduced symptoms in 27 patients.

McNeil JJ, Anderson A, Christophidis N, et al: **Taste loss** associated with oral captopril treatment. Br Med J 1979; 2:1555–1556.

Captopril, an angiotensin–converting enzyme inhibitor used in hypertension, caused **taste disturbances** in 3 of 16 patients. Sweet foods tasted salty, a bitter taste persisted, and loss of taste occurred. Oral zinc was not helpful, and normal taste returned only after the drug was discontinued.

Rippon JW, Arnow PM, Larson RA, Zang KL: **"Golden tongue"** syndrome caused by *Ramichloridium schulzeri*. Arch Dermatol 1985; 121:892–894.

During chemotherapy for acute lymphocytic leukemia, a 54-year-old woman developed a **golden-orange discoloration** of the dorsum of the **tongue**. It began as a 7- to 8-mm painful brownish-yellow tufted patch on the left side of the tongue.

Culture proved it to be a growth of *Ramichloridium schulzeri*, a saprophytic soil fungus that shows beautiful golden-orange growth on Sabouraud's agar.

There are three categories of **opportunistic fungi**, based on their frequency of occurrence:

1. Frequently encountered "first-line" organisms:

   Rhizopus oryzae: diabetic acidosis
   Aspergillus fumigatus: leukemia
   Cryptococcus neoformans: corticosteroid treatment
   Candida albicans: variety of conditions

2. Less frequently seen "second-line" infections, occurring with more severe immunosuppression and requiring a larger inoculum:

   Pseudoallescheria boydii
   Trichosporon beigelii: cancer
   Aspergillus flavus: cancer

3. Rarely seen "third-line" organisms, representing strain variants:

   Aspergillus terreus   *Sporothrix schenckii*

Adour KK, Byl FM, Hilsinger RL Jr, et al: The true nature of **Bell's palsy**: Analysis of 1000 consecutive patients. Laryngoscope 1978; 88:787–801.

The **tongue changes** show the neural inflammatory component of benign cranial polyneuritis secondary to herpes simplex virus. The fungiform papillae are inflamed bilaterally. The circumvallate papillae show unilateral inflammation when hypesthesia (numbness) of the glossopharyngeal nerve occurs. Without denervation, the papillae return to their normal pink fleshy state in 7 to 14 days; with denervation, atrophy develops.

Shelley WB, Shelley ED: The **dentate tongue** as a manifestation of tension. J Am Acad Dermatol 1986; 15:1289.

Scalloped indentations along the lateral margins of the tongue were seen in a 45-year-old man whose anxiety and psychic tension led to chronic forcing of the tongue against the teeth.

This dental imprint on an otherwise normal tongue provides objective evidence of a patient under stress.

Guinta J, Shklar G, McCarthy PL: **Diffuse angiomatosis of the tongue**. Arch Otolaryng 1971; 93:83–89.

Macroglossia may be associated with numerous pink, red, or purple papillary projections on the dorsal and ventral surfaces of the tongue and episodes of hemorrhage. Most cases are in females and begin in childhood. Lingual mobility is reduced, but speech remains relatively normal. Biopsy reveals vascular hamartomas.

If lesions occur elsewhere in the mouth or skin, Sturge-Weber disease should be considered.

Melmed S: **Acromegaly.** N Engl J Med 1990; 322:966–977.

Facial features coarsen, extremities enlarge, and soft tissues swell so insidiously that only one in ten patients consults a doctor about these changes. Accompanying skin changes, induced by a pituitary adenoma's excess secretion of growth hormone, are hyperhidrosis, macroglossia, and numerous acrochordons. The last may indicate the presence of precancerous colonic polyps.

Diagnosis is based on the demonstration that oral glucose fails to suppress the serum growth hormone level to below 2 μg/liter. Magnetic resonance imaging or computed tomography of the pituitary should reveal the adenoma. If none is found, consider ectopic secretion of growth hormone–releasing hormone. In this case magnetic resonance imaging allows superior contrast for visualizing the carotid arteries, cavernous sinus, and optic tracts.

Think of these studies when the glove or shoe size of the patient, either male or female, has enlarged. But the annual incidence is only three in one million. Hardly a diagnosis to be made in Montana.

Scherbenske JM, Benson PM, Rotchford JP, James WD: Cutaneous and ocular manifestations of **Down syndrome.** J Am Acad Dermatol 1990; 22:933–938.

The **Down syndrome,** described in 1860 by Langdon Down and later recognized as a consequence of having an extra chromosome 21 (trisomy 21), is a multisystem disorder. You recognize it by its manifestations, a very low IQ, typical **facies** (protruding tongue, epicanthal folds, upward slanting palpebral fissures), and a short broad neck. As you examine the patient you note the fissured tongue, the white specks in the iris (Brushfield's spots), the nystagmus, the dry skin (atopy, xerosis, ichthyosis), the wide space between the first and second toe.

In such a patient, **anticipate seeing** cheilitis, vitiligo, and alopecia areata. The patient is also susceptible to tinea pedis and Norwegian scabies. Some show widespread elastosis perforans serpiginosa, as well as syringomas.

Such a patient may have acrocyanosis and cutis marmorata, reflecting poor peripheral circulation and possible cardiac problems. Finally, hernias and cryptorchidism may be present.

Cristóbal MC, Aguilar A, Urbina F, et al: **Self-inflicted tongue ulcer:** An unusual form of factitious disorder. J Am Acad Dermatol 1987; 17:339–341.

A 9-year-old boy with a 5-year history of a chronic ulcer of the tongue had a 2-cm irregular crusted superficial ulcer of the left side of the tongue.

Exhaustive laboratory tests were normal, but psychiatric evaluation revealed a fragile personality structure with a psychotic base. A diagnosis of **factitial ulcer** was made, and psychotherapy led to immediate healing of the tongue. There has been no relapse in more than 1 year.

The **differential** diagnostic list included:

aphthous stomatitis
recurrent herpes simplex
eosinophilic ulcer of the tongue
Lesch-Nyhan syndrome
traumatic ulcer, as seen in epileptics

Greene RM, Rogers RS III: **Melkersson-Rosenthal syndrome:** A review of 36 patients. J Am Acad Dermatol 1989; 21:1263–1270.

Classically the **Melkersson-Rosenthal syndrome** is a triad of recurrent orificial edema, recurrent facial nerve palsy, and lingua plicata.

Note that orificial edema ranging from lower-lip swelling to bilateral facial swelling:

    occurs in every instance
    is the presenting sign in nearly half of the cases
    may be the only sign in nearly a third of the patients (monosymptomatic expression of syndrome)

Biopsy may show only nonspecific inflammation.

The facial paralysis is of sudden onset and identical to Bell's palsy. It may occur months to years after (or before) facial swelling. It generally clears, but tends to recur. Lingua plicata or the furrowed or scrotal tongue occurs in only half of the patients. The grooves are deep and on the dorsal surface, extending in all directions.

Differential diagnosis:

hereditary angioedema	lymphatic obstruction
recurrent erysipelas	sarcoidosis
facial edema with eosinophils	contact urticaria
Crohn's disease	

This is a difficult diagnosis to make because of its erratic appearance and disappearance of its signs.

Mier PD, van de Kerkhof PCM (eds): Textbook of **Psoriasis**. New York, Churchill Livingstone, 1986, 292 pp.

Geographic tongue involves only the dorsal lingual surface, whereas **annulus migrans** of the tongue, seen in generalized pustular psoriasis, involves the dorsal and ventral lingual mucosa as well as the gingival and buccal mucosa. The tongue is usually not sore, but is covered with discrete or confluent denuded red patches with slightly elevated white margins in annular patterns. Similar changes occur in Reiter's syndrome and acrodermatitis continua of Hallopeau.

Hubler WR Jr: Lingual lesions of **generalized pustular psoriasis**: Report of five cases and a review of the literature. J Am Acad Dermatol 1984; 11:1069–1076.

Both geographic tongue and fissured tongue occurred in association with repeated attacks of **pustular psoriasis** in five patients.

Each man had developed the characteristic asymptomatic furrowing of the tongue by the age of 4 years. Subsequent attacks of generalized pustular psoriasis were associated with the appearance of geographic tongue.

Geographic tongue is also known as benign migratory glossitis, stomatitis areata migrans, and annulus migrans. It presents as a gray-white advancing polycyclic band trailed by flat erythematous zones devoid of filiform papules. The fungiform papillae are not affected and stand out prominently. The advancing edge may travel several millimeters an hour. It usually remains only on the anterior surface of the tongue, but can cover the entire tongue and spread onto the floor of the mouth. The lips, gums, palate, and pharynx may be involved. It is ordinarily asymptomatic, but the patient may have the pain of glossodynia.

Fissured tongue exhibits numerous deep crevices, which appear by the age of 4 years and increase during puberty. In its severe form the term *scrotal tongue* is used. It often coexists with geographic tongue or one may precede the other.

Teeth

Leung AKC: **Natal teeth**. Am J Dis Child 1986; 140:249–251.

Superstition still clings to infants born with **natal teeth** (usually lower central incisors) or who have neonatal teeth erupt during the first 30 days. Among those "favored" by fate with natal teeth have been Hannibal, Napoleon, Richard III, and Louis XIV. Those "doomed" by fate with natal teeth may have associated cleft lip or palate or other syndrome. In a Canadian hospital over a 17-year period, natal teeth were found in 15 of 50,892 births (incidence 1 in 3392 births). Other anomalies were present in 5 of the 15, and 11 of the 15 were female.

A dental x-ray should be done to differentiate deciduous from supernumerary teeth, and loose teeth should be extracted to prevent aspiration.

Syndromes involving natal teeth:

Ellis-van Creveld syndrome (chondroectodermal dysplasia)
Jadassohn-Lewandowsky (pachyonychia congenita)
Hallermann-Streiff (oculomandibulofacial syndrome with hypotrichosis)
steatocystoma multiplex
adrenogenital syndrome

Fielding JE: **Smoking: Health effects and control** (first of two parts). N Engl J Med 1985; 313:491–498.

Cigarette, cigar, and pipe smoking greatly increase the **risk for oral cancer**, and alcohol ingestion has a synergistic effect. Smoking also increases periodontal disease and loss of alveolar bone. Chewing smokeless tobacco and dipping snuff increase the risk of oral cancer and induce changes in the hard and soft tissues of the mouth, discoloration and excessive wear of the teeth, periodontal destruction, and decreased ability to taste and smell.

Mimouni F, Mughal Z, Tsang RC, Feingold M: Picture of the month: **X-linked dominant hypophosphatemic rickets**. Am J Dis Child 1988; 142:191–192.

Mottled dental enamel and dental abscesses at the roots of the lower incisors are shown in a boy with bowing of the legs. Dental abscesses develop from direct microbial invasion into the pulp through tubular clefts in the abnormal dentin. Hypophosphatemia results from urinary phosphate loss due to poor phosphate resorption by the kidney. Altered vitamin D and mineral metabolism leads to rachitic bone changes.

Ruiz-Arguelles GJ: The lipstick-on-teeth sign in **Sjögren's syndrome**. NJ J Med 1986; 315:1030–1031.

Seeing a **lipstick smudge** on the teeth alerts you to the possibility of Sjögren's syndrome in which the dry mouth favors adherence of the lipstick to the teeth. Impaired salivation caused by drugs or dehydration is an alternate consideration.

Requena Caballero L, Liron de Robles J, Requena Caballero C, et al: **Tooth pits**: An early sign of tuberous sclerosis. Acta Derm Venereol 1987, 67:457–459.

Pits in the enamel of the incisors, at times filled with a bright white enamel "pearl," are yet another sign of tuberous sclerosis. They probably reflect defective amelogenesis and are smaller and less frequent in deciduous teeth than in permanent teeth.

Hyperplastic gingiva and 12 pits were observed incidentally in an 18-year-old man referred for dermabrasion of facial angiofibromas. He also had a

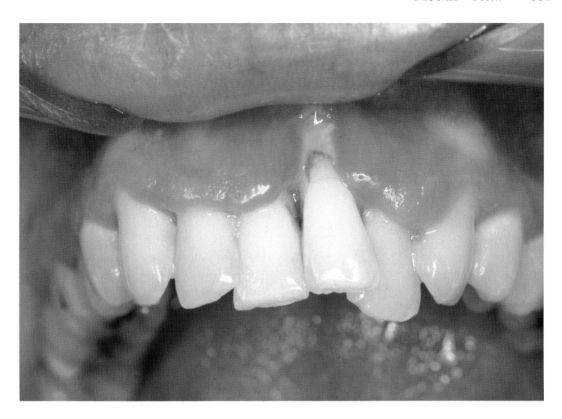

pedunculated gingival growth consistent with fibrous hyperplasia, shagreen patches on the back, and periungual fibromas. No hypopigmentation sites could be seen except under Wood's light in a totally darkened room, which revealed two white macules on the abdomen. He had had epilepsy since the age of 2 years and also mental retardation. Computed tomography showed periventricular calcification in the brain and tumors and hamartomatous cysts of the kidney.

The earliest marker for **tuberous sclerosis** is the ash leaf macule of hypopigmentation, since it appears at birth and remains a lifetime. Babies deserve a look in the dark.

Hill FJ, Winter GB: **The teeth in dermatological disease**. Rec Adv Dermatol 1986; 7:103–126.

Expect dental abnormalities in:

    epidermolysis bullosa: pitted enamel
    ectodermal dysplasia: hypodontia and microdontia
    incontinentia pigmenti: hypodontia, delayed eruption, malformed crowns

A touch of hope is worth more than a handful of diagnoses.

Pigmentation

Buchner A, Hansen LS: **Amalgam pigmentation** (**amalgam tattoo**) of the oral mucosa. A clinicopathologic study of 268 cases. Oral Surg 1980; 49:139–147.

Amalgam tattoos (localized argyria) result from the introduction of dental amalgam containing mercury, silver, and tin into soft tissue. They appear as isolated blue or black macules, most commonly on the gingiva, alveolar, or buccal mucosa. In half of the cases, biopsy reveals significant foreign body inflammation, sometimes resembling sarcoid with asteroid bodies.

Differential diagnosis:

focal melanosis
pigmented nevus
thrombosed varix
malignant melanoma

Horlick HP, Walther RR, Zegarelli DJ et al: **Mucosal melanotic macule, reactive type**: A simulation of melanoma. J Am Acad Dermatol 1988; 19:786–791.

Diffuse irregular **dark-brown spots** of hyperpigmentation had appeared in the last 10 days on the **buccal mucosa** of this 36-year-old black man. Although he had a lifelong history of patchy hyperpigmentation of the gums, he was concerned about this new pigment. He had not been exposed to any staining or irritating materials, and he took no medicine.

General studies, including determination of cortical and ACTH levels, were normal. The biopsy showed nests of pigmented dendritic cells in a spongiotic mucosa. A diagnosis of **reactive melanotic macule** was made. Within 3 months, 90% of the color had faded away.

Hyperpigmentation of the mucosa always deserves attention. The **differential diagnosis** includes:

malignant melanoma
racial characteristic
lentigo
nevus
amalgam tattoo
heavy metal poisoning
chemical stain
fixed drug eruption
postinflammatory hyperpigmentation, e.g., due to poorly fitting dental prosthesis; cigarette held in fixed position

Black spots in the mouth deserve a second look and an explanation.

Spann CR, Owen LG, Hodge SJ: The **labial melanotic macule**. Arch Dermatol 1987; 123:1029–1031.

Brown, irregularly **pigmented macules of the lower lip** in young adult women are best called labial melanotic macules. They do not darken with sun exposure and hence are not ephelides. They appear in whites and thus are not the melanoplakia seen on the mucosa of blacks. They are not preceded by inflammation and hence do not represent postinflammatory hyperpigmentation. They show no elongation of rete ridges on biopsy and are therefore not lentigines.

Goertz J, Goos M: **Traditional tattooing of the gingiva**: an Eritrean folk medicine practice. Arch Dermatol 1988; 124:1018–1019.

Soot introduced by multiple thorn pricks explained the puzzling **bluish-black discoloration** of the maxillary gingiva in a young woman. In her homeland,

Ethiopia, tattooing the upper gums was regularly done to enhance a girl's beauty. In boys, only the canine mucosal areas were tattooed.

Such tattooing is to be distinguished from foreign body discoloration due to amalgams, broken dental burs, fragments of carborundum discs or lead pencils, charcoal dentrifices, coal, or metal dust.

Systemic causes are headed by Addison's disease, yet most commonly patchy hyperpigmentation of the gums reflects the normal melanin patterning in black patients.

Nomachi K, Mori M, Matsuda N: Improvement of oral lesions associated with **malignant acanthosis nigricans** after treatment of lung cancer. Oral Surg 1989; 68:74–79.

This 70-year-old man developed darkening of the face and a dry cough. When seen for the first time a year later, he was found to have papillary hyperplasia, as well as large furrows and **pigmentation of the buccal mucosa.** The tongue was rough, fissured, and partially gray-white. The patient had lost his sense of taste. The lips had a rough texture and showed small papillary growths on the mucosal side. There were numerous nodules on the skin of the trunk as well as diffuse hyperpigmentation.

A radiograph revealed a mass in the right upper lung field that proved to be an **adenocarcinoma**. A diagnosis of acanthosis nigricans was made.

Diagnosis should go well beyond the chapter headings in a textbook. Don't stop at classification at the family level (urticaria), or at the genus level (urticaria due to food), or even at the species (urticaria due to beer). Look for the specific strain (urticaria due to Coors beer).

Dryness

Mitchell J, Greenspan J, Daniels T, et al: **Anhidrosis (hypohidrosis) in Sjögren's syndrome**. J Am Acad Dermatol 1987; 16:233–235.

A 6-month history of **heat intolerance** and a dry mouth as well as 2 years of dry eyes led to the diagnosis of Sjögren's syndrome in this 55-year-old man.

The patient showed virtually no sweat response to intradermal methacholine (0.1 ml, 1:500), and histologically the eccrine sweat glands were surrounded by a dense plasma cell infiltrate.

Other dermatologic causes of heat intolerance are:

congenital ectodermal defect
metal poisoning
miliaria profunda
dermatitis (lichen planus, atopic dermatitis, and psoriasis)

One must also look within:

multiple myeloma
diabetic neuropathy
damage to spinal cord or CNS

Newsom-Davis J: Lambert-Eaton myasthenic syndrome. Springer Semin Immunopathol 1985; 8:129–140.

In adults, **dry mouth** may be a very early symptom of the Lambert-Eaton myasthenic syndrome, along with fatigue, impotency, proximal muscle weakness with difficulty walking (waddling gait), and mild ptosis and bulbar weakness.

It is imperative to rule out oat cell carcinoma of the lung, which occurs in ⅔ cases. Affected patients frequently have other autoimmune problems such as thyroid disease and vitiligo and may have organ-specific antibodies to thyroid, stomach, and skeletal muscle. The primary defect involves impaired acetylcholine release, and patients may have IgG antibody to nerve terminal determinants.

To throw open the mind's door and allow all disease to enter into consideration each time that we are called to a bedside is foolish in the attempt and impossible in the performance.

RICHARD C. CABOT

Shelley WB: **Gingival hyperplasia** from dental braces. Cutis 1981; 28:149–150.

A 14-year-old black boy had noted an insidious **overgrowth of the gums** for the past year. It first became evident some months after orthodontic appliances had been put in place. There had been no change in toothpaste or brushing habits, and mouthwashes had never been used. The patient was in good health, had no history of epilepsy, had taken no hydantoin drugs, and had no skin signs of tuberous sclerosis. Previously he had had mild atopic dermatitis. However, his family history revealed that his father had had an idiopathic episode of gingival hyperplasia years ago that had required gingivectomy.

Examination revealed diffuse enlargement of the upper and lower gums, on both the labial and lingual side. The overgrown gum was firm and nontender and showed no petechiae or ecchymoses. The palate was not involved. There was no evidence of untreated caries or marked plaque formation.

General medical studies gave negative results, as did closed patch tests to both the dental brace and nickel sulfate. There was no evidence of malnutrition or growth retardation.

It was recommended that the metal **dental bands** be removed. This was done, and within 2 months the gum tissue had receded to its normal conformation and the teeth were no longer obscured by overgrowth.

The remarkable growth observed was true tissue hyperplasia, not the boggy, edematous, inflammatory response of gingivitis. The tissue was firm, resilient, and appeared as simply overgrown gum tissue. The prompt response to removal of the metal bands obviated the need for a biopsy and revealed the proximate cause—irritation by an orthodontic device.

Gingival hyperplasia is a response to a variety of stimuli or a manifestation or even a presenting sign of systemic disease.

Gingival hyperplasia is a manifestation of:

> Familial trait: idiopathic
> Hormonal change: puberty, pregnancy
> Nutritional state: scurvy
> Neoplasia: leukemia, lymphoma

A response to:

> Chronic irritation: orthodontic device, prosthetic device
> Drugs: antiepileptic, contraceptive

Associated with:

> Kinky hair disease
> Tuberous sclerosis
> Crohn's disease
> Melkersson-Rosenthal syndrome
> Anderson-Fabry disease

Rogers RS III, Sheridan PJ, Nightingale SH: **Desquamative gingivitis**: Clinical, histopathologic, immunopathologic and therapeutic observations. J Am Acad Dermatol 1982; 7:729–735.

> Presentation: Diffuse erythema and edema of marginal and attached gingivae with associated areas of vesiculation, erosion, and desquamation, usually in older patients. Always involves facial gingivae, may appear as paresthesias.

885

Nature: Reaction pattern that on study may prove to be cicatricial pemphigoid, lichen planus, pemphigus vulgaris, irritant reaction, hormonal disturbance, epidermolysis bullosa acquisita.

Specific diagnosis: Biopsy

Garioch J, Todd P, Lamey PJ et al: The significance of a **positive patch test to mercury** in oral disease. Br J Dermatol 1990; 123(Suppl 37):25–26.

Of 372 patients with oral disease who were patch-tested to mercury, only 29 reacted. The **mercury sensitivity** was thought to be relevant in 16 of these: 14 had lichen planus; the other 2 had recurrent aphthous dermatitis and gingivitis, respectively.

All 14 of the mercury–positive lichen planus patients improved significantly upon removal of mercury-containing amalgams or on avoidance of contact lens fluid containing thimerosal.

Shklar G, McCarthy PL: Oral lesions of **mucous membrane pemphigoid**. Arch Otolaryngol 1971; 93:354–364.

A review of 85 cases, with lovely photographs, stresses that the most characteristic lesion is **desquamative gingivitis**, with diffuse or patchy deep-red gingiva and white desquamation. Palpation also leaves erosive hemorrhagic areas, and lesions occur under ill-fitting dentures. Vesicles on the gingiva rupture, leaving irregular ulcerated areas. In other parts of the mouth vesicles and bullae are surrounded by a wide zone of erythema, and rupture leaves ragged ulcers with yellow suppuration from secondary bacterial infection. Vesicles develop quickly and may remain intact for 2 to 3 days because of the thick vesicle roof. Healing takes about 14 days.

Ocular lesions consist of conjunctivitis, which begins with redness, swelling, pain, and burning, usually without vesicles, erosions, or ulcers. Small fibrous adhesions gradually develop between superior and inferior palpebral conjunctivae and between palpebral and bulbar conjunctivae. Adhesions of eyelid to eyeball (ankyloblepharon) cause narrowing or obliteration of the palpebral fissure. Scarring and shrinking of the conjunctivae lead to inversion of the margins of the eyeballs (entropion), followed by trichiasis and corneal damage. Vascularization and opacity of the cornea result in blindness.

Desquamative gingivitis usually results from mucous membrane pemphigoid or erosive (bullous) lichen planus, but occasionally occurs in menopausal females or younger women following hysterectomy. A **biopsy** is needed to distinguish them. Bullous pemphigoid rarely affects the mouth, but may cause identical lesions. Gingivitis is very rare in pemphigus vulgaris and erythema multiforme.

Ellis CN, Vanderveen EE, Rasmussen JE: **Scurvy**: A case caused by peculiar dietary habits. Arch Dermatol 1984; 120:1212–1214.

A petechial rash, sore mouth, and lethargy led to the admission of this 9-year-old girl. On examination the skin showed follicular hyperkeratosis and **perifollicular hemorrhage**, especially on the legs and forearms. The gums were friable and eroded. She refused to walk and withdrew from all tactile stimuli. Her affect was depressed.

The history was remarkable in that for the past year this girl had lived on nothing but tuna fish, bread, and plain iced tea. All other foods were unpalatable.

The biopsy showed perifollicular hemorrhage, and the hemoglobin level was

10.5 mg/dl. A diagnosis of **scurvy** was made, although the serum ascorbic acid level was low normal.

Ascorbic acid (250 mg/day) therapy produced dramatic clearing of the gingival erosions and perifollicular hemorrhages. With continued vitamin C supplementation and a diet with fruit and vegetables, there has been no return of the problem.

Scheman AJ, Ray DJ, Witkop CJ, Dahl MV: **Hereditary mucoepithelial dysplasia**. Case report and review of literature. J Am Acad Dermatol 1989; 21:351–356.

Fiery-red` gums and mucosa were the diagnostic tip-off in this 16-year-old boy who sought attention for a pruritic eruption. Sparse scalp hair, dry rough skin, and visual loss as well as photophobia led to a diagnosis of **mucoepithelial dysplasia**.

Confirmation came with the finding on electron microscopy of a decreased number of dermosomes in the gingival biopsy. He also had the typical eosinophilia and keratitis, but had no history of recurrent infections.

This rare **hereditary** mucocutaneous disease is caused by a defect in epithelial cell junction. Involving the lungs as well as the mucosa, it can be responsible for fibrocystic disease, and the subsequent cor pulmonale may even prove fatal. It also predisposes to pneumothorax, pneumonia and repeated infections because of the loss of mucosal integrity. Finally, female patients must be acquainted with the fact that the Pap smear may be abnormal, but this is not necessarily an indication for hysterectomy.

Horan RF, Kerdel FA, Moschella SL, Haynes HA: Recent onset of **gingival enlargement**. Arch Dermatol 1986; 122:1436–1439.

Spongy, bluish-red masses of gingival hyperplasia had been present on the gums of this 36-year-old woman for a month. She had had low-grade fever and nightsweats for the same period, as well as nodules on the back. Tetracycline and penicillin had been without effect.

A biopsy of the gum lesions showed intense inflammation and vessels filled with fibrin thrombi. A biopsy specimen of a violaceous nodule on the back had the appearance of pyoderma gangrenosum.

The problem proved baffling, requiring hospitalization. The patient developed polyarthritis, myalgia, palpable purpura, and friable nasal mucosae. Purpuric vesicles arose at the sites of intravenous injection. After two gingival biopsies, three skin biopsies, a breast biopsy, a sacral nerve biopsy, a muscle biopsy, and a renal biopsy, the diagnosis was still not made until a retrospective review of one of the skin biopsies revealed the diagnostic **granulomatous angiitis of Wegener's granulomatosis**. The fires of inflammation had burned so violently as to destroy any evidence of the cause.

The banal appearance of the nodules that came on the face and trunk was misleading. The pathergy of trauma-elicited lesions explained the gum lesions, as well as the lesions at the sites of intravenous insertion and probably the nodules.

Wegener's granulomatosis rarely occurs as a gingivitis, but it can be the herald sign, as in this patient. Nonetheless, more common diagnostic possibilities for the gum lesions should include marginal gingivitis, pregnancy, trauma, drugs (Dilantin), scurvy, infectious agents, and leukemia, especially monocytic.

Worsaae N, Pindborg JJ: **Granulomatous gingival manifestations of Melkersson-Rosenthal syndrome**. Oral Surg 1980; 49:131–138.

Small distinct, bluish-red irregular edematous swellings were seen on the gingiva of 5 of 30 patients with complete or incomplete forms of Melkersson-Rosenthal syndrome. In some of these patients more extensive and diffuse edematous gingival swelling was present. Biopsy showed noncaseating epithelioid cell granulomas in all 5 patients, with lymphocytes and plasma cells interspersed and occasional Langhans type multinucleated giant cells.

Gingival symptoms may be the first manifestation of the disease.

Fitzpatrick R, Rapaport MJ, Silva DG: **Histiocytosis X**. Arch Dermatol 1981; 117:253–257.

Superficial ulcerating and **granulomatous lesions** of the right lower gum had troubled a 19-year-old woman for over a year. The lower molars on the same side were loose, and there was submental and anterior cervical lymph node enlargement. Small ulcerative lesions were also seen in the labial folds of the vulva. **Biopsy** of the mouth lesions revealed a heavy infiltrate of histiocytes suggestive of **histiocytosis X**. Corroboration of the diagnosis came from finding osteolytic lesions in dental roentgenograms and also demonstrating that she had diabetes insipidus (water deprivation and vasopressin tests).

Oral lesions are often the presenting sign of histiocytosis X, with initial involvement in the molar region. Because of the tendency to secondary infection, the patient may seek help for a foul breath or local tenderness of the mandible or maxilla. More advanced signs include purpura, swelling, necrosis, and ulceration of the gingiva and palate. X-ray findings of alveolar bone destruction and displacement of teeth (floating teeth) are virtually pathognomonic of histiocytosis X.

The diagnosis will be delayed when initial diagnosis centers on aphthous stomatitis, periodontitis, herpetic infection, or nonspecific chronic inflammation. Even the jaw lesions may be misconstrued as simple cysts, osteomyelitis, or malignant tumors.

Histiocytosis X in the skin may **mimic** seborrheic dermatitis, Darier's disease, lichen planus, or puzzling pustular or fluctuant nodules. Intertriginous lesions in adults, including simple intertrigo and granulomatous intertrigo, are not uncommon.

In these cases, a biopsy is your best friend.

Diagnosis is the art of bringing order out of chaos.

James WD, Lupton GP: **Acquired dyskeratotic leukoplakia**. Arch Dermatol 1988; 124:117–120.

A 38-year-old woman had **white plaques** on an erythematous base on the hard palate and a burning sensation on exposure to certain foods and liquids. The lesions resembled candidiasis, but did not respond to oral ketoconazole and topical nystatin therapy, could not be wiped off with gauze, were negative for mycelia on KOH examination and biopsy, and were negative on fungal culture. Furthermore, there was no history suggestive of tobacco, irritant, or functional-induced leukoplakia. New lesions appeared on the gingiva and lips as well as on the labia minora, causing burning pain after intercourse and during menstruation. The absence of lesions on the buccal mucosa and the negative immunofluorescent studies eliminated lichen planus as a possible diagnosis. Electron microscopy and DNA hybridization studies failed to reveal any evidence of viral infection.

Biopsies from all three sites showed dyskeratotic cells in benign-appearing mucosal epithelium, leading to consideration of hereditary white sponge nevus, hereditary benign intraepithelial dyskeratosis, and Darier's disease. However, all three were eliminated on closer examination of the family history and total skin surface. Therefore, the authors propose a distinctive new entity, acquired **dyskeratotic leukoplakia**.

Lesions of mucous membranes appear white because of a thickened epithelial layer or surface pseudomembrane. Induration should be assessed, and an attempt should be made to remove the white lesion by rubbing. A careful history should include familial occurrence, use of tobacco or drugs, exposure to someone with similar lesions, general health, and other concurrent skin lesions. A KOH preparation, biopsy, and serologic examination may be necessary.

The **differential diagnosis** of white spots in the mouth includes:

candidiasis	leukoplakia
carcinoma	lichen planus
condyloma acuminatum	lupus erythematosus
Darier's disease	oral hairy leukoplakia
hereditary benign intraepithelial dyskeratosis	pachyonychia congenita
Koplik spots of rubeola	secondary syphilis
leukoedema	white sponge nevus

The most common "white-spot diagnoses" are leukoplakia (induced by friction or tobacco), lichen planus, candidiasis, and leukoedema.

Jorgenson RJ, Levin LS: **White sponge nevus**. Arch Dermatol 1981; 117:73–76.

Bilateral white plaques had been present on the buccal mucosa of this 26-year-old man since birth. Located on the mucosa at the level of the plane of occlusion, they showed periods of exacerbation and remission. The salient feature in the history was the fact that his mother, half brother, and maternal aunt had the same type of lesions.

A biopsy showed an acanthotic mucosal epithelium covered by a parakeratotic cell layer. The underlying connective tissue showed no inflammation. A diagnosis of **white sponge nevus** was made.

Although white sponge nevus most commonly involves the buccal mucosa, it may appear on the labial mucosa, alveolar ridges, and the floor of the mouth. In the absence of a family history, cases may be labeled erroneously as traumatic keratosis of the mucosa, leukoplakia, or candidiasis. Other **mim-**

ics of white sponge nevus include hereditary benign intraepithelial dyskeratosis. One also has to rule out syphilis, lichen planus, lupus erythematosus, chemical burns, and tobacco. Darier's disease and pachyonychia congenita may produce similar lesions.

Waitzer S, Fisher BK: **Oral leukoedema**. Arch Dermatol 1984; 120:264–266.

Rough, asymptomatic **white patches** on buccal and labial mucosa of this 20-year-old man had been present as long as he could remember. A biopsy disclosed intracellular edema of the mucosal cells of an acanthotic epithelium consistent with the diagnosis of **leukoedema**.

Leukoedema is common, varying from a filmy opalescence that fades on stretching the mucosa, to a coarse granular or thickened plaque that cannot be scraped off. Tooth impressions may be seen. It is not related to smoking, nutrition, dental fillings, disease, or oral habits of thumb sucking, tooth grinding, or cheek biting.

Three oral lesions enter the differential diagnosis:

> Premalignant epithelial dysplasia:
> dyskeratotic cells on biopsy
> onset: older age group
> smoking, alcohol, irritation favors
> White sponge nevus:
> autosomal dominant inheritance
> onset in childhood
> may be in anogenital area also
> Papanicolaou's stain: orange staining, cytoplasmic condensates
> Morsicatio mucosae oris (cheek biting):
> white patches, alternating with erosions
> patient possibly unaware of habit; variable course

White JW, Olsen KD, Banks PM: **Plasma cell orificial mucositis**. Arch Dermatol 1986; 122:1321–1324.

The **analogue of Zoon's plasma cell balanitis** occurs in the mucous membranes of other orifices. Such plasma cell inflammatory changes occur in the lips, tongue, and gums. The diagnosis is not easily made, since contact or irritant dermatitis mimics this clinical condition. Extensive patch testing is required. Also in the differential is candidiasis, ruled out by culture and failure to respond to therapy.

The possibility of an extramedullary plasmacytoma is to be considered, but this shows a progressive course. The pathologist can also **rule out** a squamous cell carcinoma as well as erythroplasia of Queyrat and cheilitis granulomatosis. Another consideration is plasmacytoma, but this appears as a tumor. Finally, syphilis must be ruled out as a cause of any plasma cell response.

Burnett JW: Dermatology days. Cutis 1990; 45:155–158.

Factitial cheilitis and moniliasis can mimic contact dermatitis of the lips. Candidiasis of the palate in patients with oral prostheses can mimic contact allergy dermatitis. Eczematous dermatitis overlying a pacemaker may be a pressure phenomenon rather than an allergic reaction.

Burdon J, Bell R, Sullivan J, Henderson M: **Adriamycin-induced recall phenomenon** 15 years after radiotherapy. JAMA 1978; 239:931.

A 65-year-old man had radiation (3235 rads) for localized reticulum cell sarcoma of the palate. Fifteen years later he developed metastatic small cell carcinoma of the lung and was treated with a combination of doxorubicin, cyclophosphamide, vincristine sulfate, and high-dose methotrexate with folinic acid rescue. Two weeks later he had extensive **ulcerative stomatitis** with monilial superinfection in the previously irradiated areas.

This **radiation "recall phenomenon,"** in which a quiescent tissue response to radiation is reactivated by a chemotherapeutic agent, has been reported with dactinomycin (actinomycin D) and doxorubicin hydrochloride (Adriamycin).

Hogan DJ, Murphy F, Burgess WR, et al: **Lichenoid stomatitis associated with lithium carbonate**. J Am Acad Dermatol 1985; 13:243–246.

Erosive long white plaques had been present on the buccal mucosa of this 41-year-old man for 2 months. They interfered with eating and drinking. A diagnosis of oral lichen planus was made on the basis of the biopsy and direct immunofluorescent studies.

However, the cause was found to be the **lithium carbonate** capsules he had been taking for the past 5 months. The ulcers healed within 1 week of discontinuing the lithium, and by 3 weeks the plaques had decreased in size by one half. Challenge brought on a flare within hours, and a new ulcer as well as enlargement of the plaques was seen on the third day.

Again, stopping the lithium treatment resulted in complete healing of the stomatitis by 3 weeks. He is currently taking desipramine, and he has experienced no further lichen planus–like lesions.

Laskaris GC, Nicolis GD: **Erythroplakia of Queyrat** of the oral mucosa: A report of 2 cases. Dermatologica 1981; 162:395–399.

A 53-year-old man had **soreness of the right cheek** for 3 months. An erythematous velvety plaque with white speckles and irregular borders occupied the mucosa of the right cheek and ipsilateral half of the palate. Cultures and smears for *Candida albicans*, *Histoplasma capsulatum*, and acid-fast bacilli were negative. Biopsy showed carcinoma in situ, making the diagnosis speckled **erythroplakia of Queyrat**. Despite surgical excision, an invasive squamous cell carcinoma developed 2 years later in the area. It spread to the lymph nodes and distant sites, and death came 6 months later.

Whether small or large, smooth or granular, homogeneous or speckled, red plaques in the mucosa call for biopsy and close surveillance.

Kinney RB, Burton CS, Vollmer RT: **Necrotizing sialometaplasia**: A sheep in wolf's clothing. Healing as a diagnostic test. Arch Dermatol 1986; 122:208–210.

A 63-year-old merchant marine man had two symmetrical 1.2-cm midline deep **ulcers of the hard palate**, which exposed underlying bone. They began 2 weeks earlier with a burning sensation on the roof of the mouth followed by blisters on the hard palate and then ulcers. He was a heavy cigarette smoker and had intermittent alcohol abuse. Biopsies over a period of $1\frac{1}{2}$ weeks revealed submucosal salivary glandular tissue with severe acute and chronic inflammation and extensive deep squamous metaplasia and granulation tissue. All cultures were negative, and the ulcers healed in approximately 4 months.

This painless ulcerative condition of the hard palate clinically and histologically suggests squamous cell carcinoma. Actually it is a **benign infarct** of the minor salivary glands that will heal spontaneously in a few weeks to months. Photographs at 2-week intervals are important to document the subtle evidence of healing and avoid confusion with carcinoma and vasculitis. If no healing occurs in 2 weeks, the diagnosis of necrotizing sialometaplasia should be suspected, and an incisional or wedge biopsy should be taken from the ulcer margin.

Aphthous Ulcers

(See chapters on aphthous ulcers and Behçet's disease)

Arbesfeld SJ, Kurban AK: **Behçet's disease**. New perspectives on an enigmatic syndrome. J Am Acad Dermatol 1988; 19:767–779.

Recurrent, painful, **oral mucosal erosions** and ulcers are the index sign in **Behçet triple symptom complex**. The other manifestations are genital ulcers and a wide range of inflammatory lesions of the eye, with uveitis a central finding.

The lesions are transient and nondiagnostic per se. However, over half of the patients do show a unique predilection to form self-healing, sterile pustules at the sites of venipuncture or scratches. The phenomenon is called **pathergy** and resembles diminutive pyoderma gangrenosum. Strangely, the injection of but a drop of sterile saline provokes a tuberculin reaction at 48 hours.

The **aphthous stomatitis** of Behçet's syndrome presents as an erythematous circular area evolving into a round or oval ulcer in 48 hours. The ulcers may be single or come in crops not only on the buccal mucosa, but also the tongue, gums, and lips. Indeed, the larynx may also develop these ulcers. The ulcers are distinctive in being painful and having a yellow base and an erythematous border. In a week or two they heal, leaving no scar. But new lesions continue to develop at irregular intervals.

The **differential diagnosis** of oral ulcerations must always be considered. This includes:

aphthous stomatitis
pemphigus
lupus erythematosus
Reiters disease
syphilis
herpes simplex
Stevens-Johnson syndrome

The second part of the Behçet triad is the presence of **genital ulcers**. They are deeper than those of aphthous stomatitis, and produce scarring. This evidence of prior episodes remains. More painful in men than in women, these ulcers in a woman may be asymptomatic and found only by the physician who examines for them. They occur on the vulva, in the vagina, and in the perianal area. In a man, these deep painful ulcers are very much in evidence on the glans penis and scrotum.

The third member of the triad, at times missing, is **eye involvement**, again more severe in men. Typically, these lesions are recurrent painful attacks of uveitis, iridocyclitis and hypopyon, leading to blindness. Any part of the eye may be involved so that one sees conjunctivitis, scleritis, keratitis, and optic neuritis. The veins, not the arteries, show occlusive change.

Behçet's syndrome accounts for an ever-expanding range of **disabilities**. Arthritis of a joint such as a wrist, ankle, or elbow may occur, but it is non-deforming and self-limiting. Some few patients show central nervous system involvement. Such changes as meningomyelitis are ominous, leading to quadriplegia or even fatal brain stem involvement. Confusional states occur and even severe dementia in other patients. Intracranial hypertension has also been reported, and here the cause is central vein thrombosis.

A third of the patients have **thrombophlebitis**. Caput medusae may be the dermatologist's sign of hepatic vein occlusion. Nor are these patients exempt from arterial thrombosis. Arterial puncture for diagnostic or therapeutic reasons is a risk, since false aneurysms may ensue. Moreover, spontaneous arterial aneurysms may appear, possibly as a result of a vasculitis affecting the vasa vasorum.

In Behçet's syndrome, **vasculitis** is the common denominator for a host of pulmonary, cardiac, gastrointestinal, renal, muscular, and hematologic disorders. Nothing can be unexpected in the Behçet patient. The palate may perforate, the pylorus stenose, and the pancreas become inflamed. Again back to the skin, Behçet's syndrome can explain papules, vesicles, pustules, folliculitis, pyodermas, acneiform eruptions, and erythema nodosum–like bluish nodules on the legs.

It is an awesome disease, and you can only hope that your patient has but its forme fruste—aphthous ulcers only.

Duffy JH, Driscoll EJ: **Oral manifestations of leukemia**. Oral Surg 1958; 11:484–490.

Methotrexate and 6-mercaptopurine, used to treat leukemia, cause a characteristic stomatitis that closely resembles aphthous ulcers. The lesions are 1 to 5 mm in size with white centers and inflammatory margins.

Other oral lesions seen in 38 cases of leukemia included:

> candidiasis
> nonspecific gingivitis
> hypertrophic gingivitis
> Vincent's gingivitis
> frank bleeding
> ulcerations (not due to antimetabolite drugs)
> petechiae
> ecchymoses

Most patients with leukemia have oral findings, particularly due to leukemic infiltration of the gingival tissues, with concurrent gingivitis. Only very young patients and edentulous patients are spared these problems. Mouth irritation often comes from interdental calculus formation, so that good oral hygiene is particularly important.

Ballo FS, Camisa C, Allen CM: **Pyostomatitis vegetans**. Report of a case and review of the literature. J Am Acad Dermatol 1985; 21:381–387.

Four months of **oral ulcerations** in this 39-year-old woman had led to avoidance of solid food and dehydration for over a month. No diagnosis had been made by several oral surgeons, and therapy with oral antibodies, acyclovir, and topical corticosteroids had been ineffective.

Clinically the patient had a yellow, pustular, coated, and friable eroded gingival, labial, and buccal mucosa. A biopsy was consistent with the diagnosis of **pyostomatitis vegetans**, showing as it did eosinophil-laden microabscesses and intercellular IgG and IgA.

The critical determinant of the problem was found in the patient's history. She had had a 15-year history of daily rectal bleeding in association with abdominal cramping and diarrhea. The inflammatory bowel disease proved on visualization and biopsy of the colon to be **ulcerative colitis**. The response to systemic steroid treatment was rapid and dramatic.

Miliary abscesses of an erythematous hyperplastic oral mucosa point to inflammatory bowel disease.

We see not what we look at, but (what) we look for.
WILLIAM BENNETT BEAN

Mycosis Fungoides

The longer the patches of unexplained dermatitis remain, the more likely the explanation is that it is mycosis fungoides. The prelude to the T-cell lymphoma we call mycosis fungoides is measured in decades. Repeated biopsies down through the years yield nothing of diagnostic help. The unexplained itch persists, dampened by topical and systemic steroids. In some patients the presentation resembles patches of radiodermatitis. It may answer to the call of poikiloderma vasculare atrophicans. Others may be labeled large plaque parapsoriasis.

The eczematous, pigmented pruritic phase ends when the malignant clone of T cells overcomes the years of suppression. They become recognizable to the pathologist, who then pronounces the disease to be mycosis fungoides. The future course is fearsome, with a slow, yet unrelenting, progression to tumors in the skin and later within. Staging of the mycosis fungoides is indicated and directs the regimen of chemotherapy.

Just as leukemia may be acute, there is an acute form of mycosis, the tumor d'emblée type. Here the first sign is the fungating nodular tumor, instantly recognized histologically.

With the common chronic eczematous form, knowing that the diagnosis will be mycosis fungoides is a lot easier than knowing when the diagnosis is mycosis fungoides.

Samman PD: **Mycosis fungoides** and other cutaneous reticuloses. Clin Exp Dermatol 1976; 1:197–214.

Think of mycosis fungoides with:

1. Chronic patches of scaly or nonscaly erythema of the trunk, irregular in size and shape, variable in color. These must be differentiated from discoid eczema (usually more vesicular) and parapsoriasis en plaque (patches more uniform in size, shape, color, and often oval or fingerlike).
2. Plaques resembling chronic radiodermatitis (poikiloderma vasculare atrophicans). These are large but few in number and show a network pattern of erythema, telangiectasia, pigmentation, and atrophy.
3. Induration of plaques or the appearance of tumors
4. Any erythroderma

Edelson RL: **Cutaneous T cell lymphoma**: Mycosis fungoides, Sézary syndrome, and other variants. J Am Acad Dermatol 1980; 2:89–106.

Staging of cutaneous T cell lymphoma (CTCL):

T = Skin

T_0	Suggestive lesions
T_1	Limited plaques, papules, or eczematous patches covering less than 10% of the skin surface
T_2	Widespread plaques, papules, or erythematous patches
T_3	Tumors
T_4	Erythroderma

N = Lymph nodes

N_0	Negative
N_1	Clinical lymphadenopathy, but negative histologically
N_2	No clinical evidence, but pathology positive for CTCL
N_3	Clinical adenopathy and pathology positive

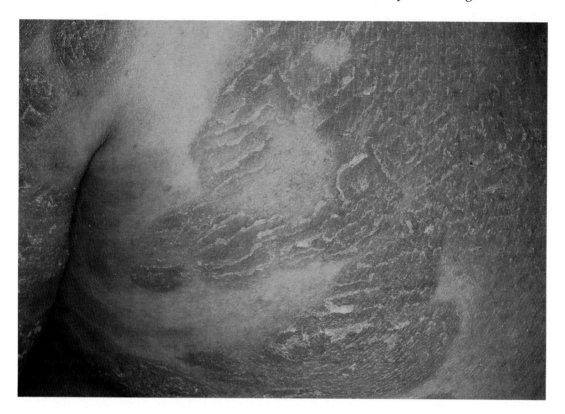

B = Peripheral blood
    B_0 No atypical lymphocytes
    B_1 Atypical cells present (>5%). Record total WBC, total
                    lymphocyte counts, and percent of atypical lymphocytes.

M = Viscera
    M_0 No organ involvement
    M_1 Organ involved with pathology confirmation

Antecedent skin changes are poorly defined, but include parapsoriasis, poikiloderma, alopecia mucinosa, lymphomatoid papulosis, and contact dermatitis. The interval between antecedent nonspecific skin disease and definitive histologic diagnosis of mycosis fungoides is nearly 4 years on the average.

T-cell lymphoma enters the diagnostic arena for any skin change that persists for years and won't heal. Look for it in the biopsy, and when you find it, "stage it."

Fransway AF, Winkelmann RK: Chronic dermatitis evolving to **mycosis fungoides**: Report of four cases and review of the literature. Cutis 1988; 41:330–335.

Five to nine years after verifiable nonspecific long-term chronic dermatitis was documented in four patients, clinical and histologically proven mycosis fungoides had evolved. In two patients, sensitivities were documented to nickel, potassium dichromate, and formaldehyde.

It is concluded that chronic antigenic immunostimulation, as by contact allergens, can induce clones of malignant lymphocytes that eventuate in T-cell lymphoma. In other studies of mycosis fungoides, elevated IgE levels and positive patch tests to nickel, chromium, paraphenylenediamine, and cobalt have been common. Patients with contact allergies to metal seem to be particularly at risk for developing mycosis fungoides, especially if employed in petrochemical, textile, or machinery industries.

Schwartz JG, Irvine Clark EG: Fine-needle aspiration biopsy of **mycosis fungoides presenting as an ulcerating breast mass.** Arch Dermatol 1988; 124:409–413.

A 44-year-old woman had had generalized persistent **pruritic erythroderma** with occasional ulcerating plaques for 10 years. Numerous skin biopsies were read as psoriasiform dermatitis, drug eruption, nonspecific dermatitis, and poikiloderma vasculare atrophicans. Excisional biopsy of an inguinal lymph node suggested Hodgkin's lymphoma, but a staging laparotomy showed no internal involvement.

She now had a 6-month history of an ulcerating breast mass (6 by 3 by 1.5 cm) with rolled edges and a shaggy denuded center covered by fibrinous exudate. A firm ill-defined nonmovable mass was palpable beneath the ulceration. She also had a similar mass on the scalp associated with alopecia, generalized lymphadenopathy, and erythroderma with plaques.

Fine-needle aspiration biopsies were secured from the ulcerative breast tumor using a 22-gauge, 3.8-cm needle attached to a 20-ml syringe by extension tubing. The aspirate was smeared on slides, alcohol fixed, and stained, using a modified Papanicolaou's stain, revealing convoluted cells consistent with mycosis fungoides. Some of the aspirated material was placed in glutaraldehyde fixative for transmission electron microscopy, which revealed lymphocytes with cerebriform nuclei and large nucleoli suggestive of mycosis fungoides. Rare binucleate Reed-Sternberg–like cells were also seen. Their presence in the midst of variable numbers of reactive lymphocytes, benign histiocytes, eosinophils, and plasma cells is diagnostic of **mycosis fungoides**.

Briffa DV, Warin AP, Calnan CD: **Parakeratosis variegata**: A report of two cases and their treatment with PUVA. Clin Exp Dermatol 1979; 4:537–541.

A striking eruption of reticulated **brownish-red scaly papules** covered most of the skin of a 55-year-old woman from Iran. The eruption was pruritic and began on the thighs, then slowly spread over a 20-year period. Biopsy showed patchy parakeratosis, epidermal edema, upper dermal infiltrate of mononuclear cells, abnormal mononuclear cells with a degree of epidermotropism, and marked pigmentary incontinence in the dermis. A diagnosis of parakeratosis variegata was made.

This exquisitely striking and chronic form of **mycosis fungoides**, so dramatic in its reticulate or zebra-like pigment patterning, has deserved and kept its special name. It is probably synonymous with parapsoriasis lichenoides. The patterning, pigment, and pruritus led to this diagnosis.

Mandojana RM, Helwig EB: **Localized epidermotropic reticulosis (Woringer-Kolopp disease).** J Am Acad Dermatol 1983; 8:813–829.

Presentation: solitary *ringed* lesion on an extremity. Scaly erythematous psoriasiform plaque with moderately elevated, circinate, verrucous margin surrounding a central clear or normal area

Clinical diagnosis: usually misdiagnosed as:

mycosis fungoides	basal cell carcinoma
granuloma annulare	iododerma
verruca	necrobiosis lipoidica
elastosis perforans serpiginosa	Kaposi's sarcoma

Histopathologic diagnoses made by referring pathologists included:

malignant melanoma: lentigo maligna, acral lentiginous melanoma
mycosis fungoides
chronic nonspecific dermatitis
intraepidermal carcinoma
lymphomatoid papulosis
arsenical keratosis

Histology: focal infiltrate of T lymphocytes into lower epidermis

Armed Forces Institute of Pathology diagnosis: localized epidermotropic reticulosis (Woringer-Kolopp)

Course: benign, chronic

Treatment: excision or radiotherapy

The pathologist may be as puzzled as the clinician by this rare growth that appears to be an intraepidermal T-cell lymphoma. The clinician's way out is through the ring!

Kardaun SH: **Pseudomalignant lymphomatoid skin reactions** due to drugs. Br J Dermatol 1988; 118:834–836.

Pseudolymphoma syndrome consists of the triad of fever, lymphadenopathy, and a generalized rash, sometimes accompanied by eosinophilia and arthralgia. It is almost always due to anticonvulsant drugs, particularly diphenylhydantoin.

Five patients are mentioned who had localized and/or generalized skin rashes showing the histologic picture of mycosis fungoides (epidermotropism, cerebriform mononuclear cells, Pautrier microabscesses). All patients showed prompt disappearance of the lesions once the causative drug was stopped. In four patients the causative drugs were not anticonvulsants (actual drugs are not listed).

Remember: Drug rashes can mimic malignant lymphomas.

Although pathologists hate to admit it, biopsy specimens are, on occasion, processed under the wrong patient name.

Nails

The nail unit is a four-part complex, so that diagnosis may rest on changes in one or more of these parts.

Congenital defects center on the germinal center, i.e., matrix. These defects may be the cause of abnormally small or large nails or in the case of complete absence of matrix, anonychia. With fragmentation or displacement of the matrix, patients present with nails that may be malaligned, onychogryphotic, or ectopic. Strangely, the index finger is particularly susceptible as indicated in the eponym COIF (congenital onychodysplasia of the index finger).

Congenital nail findings should lead to a search for congenital ectodermal dysplasias. Are the teeth, hair, and bones normal? A defect in the thumbnails may point to the nail patella syndrome with its bone, eye, and renal lesions. Absence of all the nails may be the alerting sign for a diagnosis of the DOOR syndrome (*d*eafness, *o*nycho-*o*steodystrophy, *r*etardation).

The **nailbed** is also responsible for congenital nail changes. Interestingly, when it is short, a false impression of onycholysis results because the nail plate adheres only to the bed. In these instances in which the nailbed produces too much keratin the plate curves over it, producing the analogue of an animal hoof. This gross hyperkeratosis is known as pachyonychia congenita. An unrelated congenital disease, epidermolysis bullosa, may produce so many blisters that the resultant scarred matrix elaborates a defective nail plate.

Once the history establishes the acquired nature of a nail problem, we look again at the components of the nail unit. The most common problem is paronychia usually caused by a wet work environment favoring the growth of yeast and bacteria, which thrive in the furrows. These organisms infect by entering tears in the **nail fold**. Commonly this occurs when the cuticle is pushed back or when the ingrown toenail occurs.

Next comes the **change in the plate** itself. The most common acquired alteration is the longitudinal ridging of age. The older matrix can no longer turn out a smooth polished plastic. Matrix failure also occurs with psoriasis, pityriasis rubra pilaris, and alopecia areata. In this instance the focal damage in the matrix results in pits and lacunae in the plate. Other diseases may produce more marked defects such as in the case of lichen planus. Here the nail plates may be very thin, ridged, or even present a winged adherence of the proximal nail fold, which attaches to the plate and is drawn out to give a pterygium. In more severe examples of lichen planus, transient or permanent anonychia may occur. Above all, chronic eczema of the nail area produces all kinds of dystrophic change, ranging from coarse pits, cross ridges, and pachyonychia to hypoplasia.

Brittle nails, another common complaint, is usually due to chemical damage from work or the use of detergents and strong shampoos. In its more evident form, onychoschizia, the terminal plate breaks in a manner suggesting isinglass. Again, this can reflect the repeated use of nail polish or organic solvents, or wet work environment.

Nail plate production is dramatically inhibited by serious illness or drug allergies. The result is a temporary transverse depression, known as Beau's lines. More dramatic are the white tufted waves of nail defect seen in drug erythrodermas.

We have called this shoreline nail. A longitudinal trough signals impingement of a synovial cyst on the nail matrix resulting in an atrophic band in the nail plate.

The usual nail complaint that brings the patient to the office is **fungal infection**. No matter what the origin of the dystrophy, ringworm of the nails is often the patient's diagnosis. Interestingly, the common fungal infection of toenails is interpreted by the patient as due to an injury but not as tinea. He also usually interprets the accompanying tinea pedis as "dry skin."

In the fingernails fungal infection is unusual; however, the diagnosis must be dismissed by KOH examination. A Gillette Super Blue Blade subsection of a white spot will quickly show hyphae if present. Be sure to discard the top normal-appearing plate. Go deep enough to secure a sample of the nail that has been digested by the fungi, leaving air pockets that reflect the light. Sometimes the diagnosis is difficult. White spots may be absent, and removal of the entire thickened nail may be required for identification of hyphae deep in the proximal nail. Always a culture aids. When both are negative and onychomycosis is still suspected, "diagnoses by therapy" may be made. Diflucan, 100 mg/day for 3 weeks, will induce a new thin band of normal nail in true onychomycosis.

Color change in the absence of dystrophy usually makes the diagnosis of leukonychia. The scattered or patterned white spots are indicative of former physical injury to the matrix. Manicurists who push the cuticle back at regular intervals may cause row on row of transverse white bands. Nonetheless, leukonychia trichophytica occurs rarely without much gross damage. A chalky white nail portends cirrhosis. Longitudinal white stripes are seen in Darier's disease, whereas black stripes are a sign of nevus cells in the matrix. But beware of the transformation into malignant melanoma or of its de novo appearance. Nail matrix biopsy may be necessary.

Finally, the **nailbed** accounts for many complaints, the most common of which is **onycholysis**. It may result from psoriasis, in which the immature thick stratum corneum provides no adhesion for the plate. Indeed, it is these tiny papules of subungual origin that give the optical illusion of an oil spot, so characteristic of psoriasis. Always, onycholysis calls for study of the patient's habits of cleansing. She may lift the nail away to clean out dirt. It can result from such injury, or it may reflect systemic disease such as hyper- or hypothyroidism. Commonly, in the summer onycholysis can be due to a photosensitivity reaction to a drug such as thiazide being taken orally.

More insidious are the growths of the nailbed that loosen and lift the plate up. Although the commonest is the wart, cancer and a variety of other skin tumors must be suspected.

Be sure to look at the nails even when the patient doesn't mention them as his problem. You may see the diagnostic periungual fibromas that tell of tuberous sclerosis. You may see the ragged telangiectasias of scleroderma or lupus erythematosus. And you may see the nicotine stain of the smoker or the chemical stain of his occupation or his medication.

The more you study and look at nails, the more you will learn and know about your patient.

General

Norton LA: **Nail disorders**: A review. J Am Acad Dermatol 1980; 2:451–467.

Notable onychopathic diagnostic associations:

Onychomycosis	*T. rubrum*, often
Pits, oil spots, leukonychia, grooves, crumbling, onycholysis, splinter hemorrhages	Psoriasis
Thinning, ridging, pterygium, red dots, streaks, subungual hyperkeratosis absence	Lichen planus
Pigmented bands	Nevus, chemotherapy
Yellow nail	Lymphedema
Spoon nails (koilonychia)	Iron deficiency
Atrophic, brittle	Genetic syndromes
Tumors	Exostosis, osteochondroma, enchondroma, inclusion cyst and glomus tumor

Nails deserve to be looked over rather than overlooked.

Greene RA, Scher RK: Nail changes associated with **diabetes mellitus**. J Am Acad Dermatol 1987; 16:1015–1021.

INFECTION

Paronychia–get culture and sensitivity tests
Onycholysis–due to bacteria; if colonized with *Pseudomonas*, the nail plate becomes greenish black
Yeast
Dermatophytes

VASCULAR

Beau's lines–transverse depression from ischemia
Hypertrophic thickening
Pterygium–fusion of undersurface of nail fold to nailbed and matrix
Pterygium inversum unguis–epithelium of distal nailbed remains attached to under surface of nail plate
Arterial emboli–see as 2 to 3 mm round hemorrhagic spots on hyponychium
Linear splinter hemorrhages–may suggest emboli; look for underlying atrial fibrillation, subacute bacterial endocarditis, mitral stenosis
Yellow nails–may be yellow-green, slow growing

NEUROPATHY

Loss of pain, temperature, vibratory and proprioceptive sensation
Onycholysis–from chronic pressure
Onychogryphosis–from chronic pressure

MISCELLANEOUS

Rosenau's depressions: small pitted craters on nail plate surface
Ingrown nails (onychocryptosis), entrapment of a spicule of nail in distal part of lateral nail fold.
Onychomadesis–nail plate separates proximally, caused by lesion of matrix. Can be result of diabetes, hemiplegia, neuritis, thrombosis, frostbite, poisoning, and exanthems.

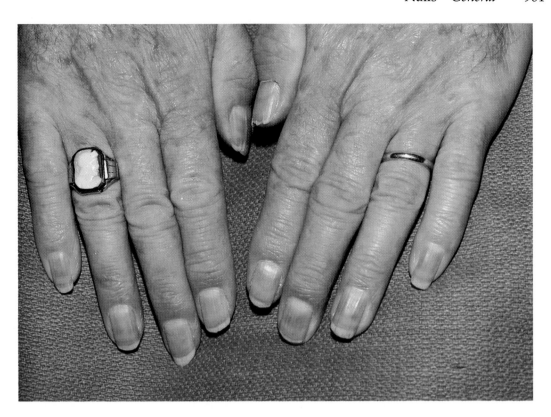

Leukonychia
    White spots in nail plate
    Leukonychia punctatum
    Small lesions
    May have small hyperchromic halo
    Indicate sites of parakeratosis—also seen with infection, nutritional, and
        cardiovascular disease.

Daniel CR, Scher RK: **Nail changes** secondary to systemic drugs or ingestants. J Am
    Acad Dermatol 1984; 10:250–258.

Onycholysis: rule out tetracycline photosensitivity, cancer chemotherapy

Pigmentation: rule out cancer chemotherapy, antimalarials

Lubach D, Cohrs W, Wurzinger R: Incidence of **brittle nails**. Dermatologica 1986;
    172:144–147.

The prevalence of **brittle nails** in 1584 persons examined was approximately
20%. Women were affected twice as often as men. The cause is the dehydration of the nail plate following damage from alkaline liquids, acetone, and
organic solvents. Brittle nails are not a common sign of internal disease but
may reflect anemia and nutritional disturbances.

If you can name it, you can claim it.

Diagnostic Procedures

Shelley WB, Wood MG: The **white spot target** for microscopic examination of nails for fungi. J Am Acad Dermatol 1982; 6:92–96.

Microscopic examination of dystrophic fingernails and toenails for pathogenic fungi can be greatly facilitated by the following steps:

1. Sample the area of whitish discoloration. This may lie well beneath the surface of the nail, so that the top layer of uninfected nail plate needs to be removed first.
2. Secure a thin slice of friable material within the white spot by employing a Gillette Super Blue Blade.
3. Immerse the specimen in xylene for instant clearing and viewing.

Kechijian P: **Nail biopsy** vignettes. Cutis 1987; 40:331–335.

FUNGAL INFECTION OF NAIL UNIT

Nailbed

If patient has been on a local or systemic antimycotic, discontinue and wait 1 month before examination.

Remove overlying nail plate with clippers. Scrape nailbed with scalpel or curette. Place scrapings on glass slide, add drop of 10% potassium hydroxide in dimethylsulfoxide and coverslip.

Examine for hyphae. If negative, repeat on three separate occasions.

Additional scrapings are placed on Sabouraud's dextrose agar both with and without cyclohexamide and chloramphenicol.

Nail plate

Nail clippings or nail plate can be sectioned and stained by the periodic acid Schiff reaction. Nail plate may be removed and similarly examined after occlusive dressing of 40% urea paste has been in place for several days.

DIAGNOSTIC NAIL BIOPSY

Instructions for Patient

Biopsy may not yield specific diagnosis, treatment, or cure.

Surgical infections can occur.

Permanent defect in plate may develop (grooving, thinning, splitting, irregularities, and onycholysis).

Instruct patient that malignant tumors may masquerade as warts, fungal infections, dystropic nails, paronychia, pigmented stripes, and onycholysis.

If circulatory impairment is present or patient has prosthetic cardiac valves, or if nail unit is infected or inflamed, give erythromycin (1 gm/day) for week before surgery. Because of stasis, heat, and humidity, toenail biopsies call for similar prophylaxis.

Give lidocaine (2%) digital block by injection at base of digit or local injection in nail folds and hyponychium. Use 30-gauge needle. Do not use epinephrine in lidocaine or more than 5 ml of lidocaine.

Wait 15 to 20 minutes for total anesthesia.

Secure 3-mm punch specimen of plate and underlying bed. Bed biopsy is facilitated by first taking 5-mm specimen of nail plate and then 3-mm specimen of bed. This is called the "double punch" technique. The firm connective tissue of the nailbed makes the plate-bed specimen far more difficult to obtain than that from the matrix, where connective tissue is soft.

Send specimen to a laboratory experienced in orienting, sectioning, and staining of nails.

Ingram GJ, Scher RK, Lally EV: **Reflex sympathetic dystrophy** following nail biopsy. J Am Acad Dermatol 1987; 16:253–256.

Two days after a nail biopsy of the left index finger, this 44-year-old man came to the emergency room with **intense pain** in the finger. There was a large bulla over the dorsum of the finger. This and the pain subsided within 2 weeks with use of compresses and steroids.

A diagnosis of **reflex sympathetic dystrophy** was made, which was confirmed a year later by the finding of a cold, sclerodermatous left hand, typical of end-stage reflex sympathetic dystrophy. Although systemic steroids for 6 months restored the normal function, the sclerodactyly remained. This striking entity, known formerly as causalgia, Sudeck's atrophy, or shoulder-hand syndrome, results from nerve injury. The range of injuries that can trigger it includes:

fracture
myocardial infarction
bullet wounds
surgery
head injury

It exhibits a spectrum of

intense prolonged pain
vasomotor changes
delayed functional recovery
trophic change

Although the mechanism remains obscure, certainly overstimulation of the sympathetic nerve forms a component. Systemic steroids are markedly helpful, suggesting the presence of a persistent postinjury inflammatory change.

Griffiths WAD: **Nail-blanching**: A new cutaneous sign indicating mechanical and functional impairment of the finger pulp. Br J Dermatol 1990; 123(Suppl 37):30.

The **nail blanch sign** is positive when the nailbed blanches upon extension of the fingers. It indicates rigidity of the digital skin and is seen in atopic hand eczema as well as psoriasis and keratoderma. It is a prelude to painful fissures of the fingertips.

Scher RK: **Acro-osteolysis** and the nail unit. Br J Dermatol 1986; 115:638–639.

In **acro-osteolysis**, destruction affects the distal phalanx and sometimes the middle and proximal phalanges as well, with resulting abnormalities of the nail. The most valuable diagnostic test for the patient with a strange nail deformity of obscure origin is an **x-ray**. Look for neoplasm, infection, inflammation, and hereditary conditions of the underlying bone and joint.

Kemp SS, Dalinka MK, Schumacher HR: **Acro-osteolysis**. Etiologic and radiologic considerations. JAMA 1986; 255:2058–2061.

X-ray evidence of a destructive process involving one or more terminal phalanges calls for a diagnosis of **acro-osteolysis** and a **search for the cause**. It may explain an overlying nail problem. The garden variety is associated with arthritis of all types, including psoriatic arthritis and polymyositis. A more exotic form preceded by Raynaud's phenomenon is seen in as many as 3% of workers exposed to vinyl chloride fumes. Any interference with blood supply, such as in scleroderma, diabetes mellitus, frostbite, or septic shock, likewise may induce acro-osteolysis.

Disturbances in bone metabolism such as hyperparathyroidism also lead to this problem, as does trauma to the fingertips, whether from guitar playing or impaired sensation (leprosy, tabes dorsalis, syringomyelia). The problem also may be familial (Hadju-Cheyney syndrome) or simply idiopathic.

Fairris GM, Rowell NR: Acquired **racket nails**. Clin Exp Dermatol 1984; 9:267–269.

A 32-year-old man undergoing intermittent hemodialysis for hypertension and proteinuria noted that his **fingernails** had become **short** and had broadened and flattened over a 2-year period. The ends of his fingers also had gradually shortened and become broader. The toenails were normal. Racket nails were diagnosed and x-rays of his fingers revealed the cause. The nail plate was conforming to a progressive severe erosive shortening of the terminal phalanges, due to tertiary **hyperparathyroidism**.

Racket nails are generally congenital or familial. They may involve only the thumbs or may involve all nails, sometimes exempting the thumbs. Often there are no underlying bony changes.

Racket nails must be distinguished from clubbing of the fingers (just as one should distinguish a racquet from a club).

Sometimes you have to make up an imaginary diagnosis for which there is a real treatment.

Lubach D, Strübbe J, Schmidt J: The **"half and half nail"** phenomenon in chronic hemodialysis patients. Dermatologica 1982; 164:350–353.

Half of 164 chronic hemodialysis patients showed **reddish-brown discoloration** of the distal half of the nailbed. However, only 11% qualified for the true **"half and half nail,"** with a band covering the entire outer half of the nail bed. The cause of the discoloration is not known, but the color reverts to normal within a few weeks of renal transplantation.

Half of the appeal of the half and half nail is its name. The other half is its value as a clue to chronic renal failure.

Feldman SR, Gammon WR: Unilateral **Muehrcke's lines** following trauma. Arch Dermatol 1989; 125:133–134.

Crush injury of the left arm of this healthy 30-year-old man led to marked edema for weeks. At 3 months, narrow (2 mm) **white lines** could be seen traversing the nails of the left hand only. They became obscured by blanching the nailbed and accentuated by suffusion of the nailbed with blood by proximal constriction (**Terry maneuver**).

Five weeks later as the edema receded, the lines remained in the same position but were less distinct. Therefore, the band is not within the plate. It is logical to assume that the lines represent transverse linear bands of nail bed edema with relative lines of separation of the nail plate from the bed.

Such a separation of the plate and the underlying bed likewise accounts for the whiteness of the lunula.

Rao VR: A difficult diagnosis. Lancet 1964 2:46.

Hemorrhages under the nails occurred in a 34-year-old woman with normal heart sounds but enlarged supraclavicular nodes and a left lung mass. One day later she had a stroke, and subsequently **subacute bacterial endocarditis** was diagnosed, with a mitral diastolic murmur and aortic systolic murmur. Bronchial carcinoma and acute bacterial endocarditis were found at autopsy.

DeCoste SD, Imber MJ, Baden HR: **Yellow nail syndrome**. J Am Acad Dermatol 1990; 22:608–611.

Yellow, thickened, opaque slow-growing **nails** suggest the presence of lymphedema, idiopathic pleural effusions, chronic bronchiectasis, or chronic sinusitis. There would appear to be a causal relationship, yet in this report two patients showed clearing of the yellow nail syndrome with no change in their respiratory infections.

Biopsy studies showed for the first time that primary subungual stromal sclerosis had produced **lymphatic obstruction** and this independently accounted for the yellow nail.

Gupta AK, Davies GM, Haberman HF: **Yellow nail syndrome**. Cutis 1986; 37:371–374.

Yellow, thickened fingernails and toenails had been present for many years in a 48-year-old woman, who was dyspneic and had bilateral nonpitting edema of both legs. A mass in the left breast proved at mastectomy to be infiltrating ductal carcinoma, and 70 cc of fluid was aspirated from the right pleural cavity at open lung biopsy. Her breast tumor recurred, requiring melphalan and steroid therapy over the following 2 years. During this period her fingernails returned to normal color and thickness. The patient thus had

905

the full triad (yellow nails, lymphedema, and pleural effusions) seen in yellow nail syndrome.

Such patients require a careful search for **underlying malignancy** or overt internal disease. A variety of malignant tumors have been responsible, and elimination of them, as in this patient, has been followed by disappearance of the yellow nail syndrome. Likewise, the syndrome may herald chronic pulmonary infections or bronchiectasis or endocrine or connective tissue disease. In some cases, penicillamine has been the cause.

The **differential diagnosis** for the yellow nail itself includes stains (picric acid, fluorescein) and drugs (tetracycline). The true yellow nail syndrome is always an interesting diagnostic puzzle.

Olsen TG, Jatlow P: Contact exposure to elemental iron causing **chromonychia**. Arch Dermatol 1984; 120:102–103.

The **orange-brown discoloration** of this 35-year-old woman's toenails appeared as soon as she moved from the city out to a farm. The color could be scraped off; mycologic as well as bacteriologic studies offered no clue as to the cause.

Finally, the color was traced to the **well water**, which contained at least six times the normal amount of iron. Her nails, in turn, proved to contain three times the normal amount of iron as determined by atomic-absorption spectrophotometry.

Six weeks after installation of a water purifier, her toenails were again normal in color.

Koch SE, LeBoit PE, Odom RB: **Laugier-Hunziker syndrome**. J Am Acad Dermatol 1987; 16:431–434.

A 34-year-old Hispanic woman had noted bands of pigment appearing in her nails for the past 10 years. Initially there was but a single band of pigment of the right index finger. At the time of examination, discrete **longitudinal bands** had appeared on eight fingernails and six toenails. In addition, multiple hyperpigmented macules were seen on the lower lips. Later, a macule of pigment appeared on the gingival mucosa.

The conjunction of these three sites of patchy hyperpigmentation made the diagnosis of Laugier-Hunziker syndrome. However, the following diagnostic **possibilities** were ruled out:

Racial characteristic–77% of blacks over age of 20 have longitudinal bands
of pigment in the nails
Radiation therapy
Malnutrition
Infection
Drugs
   minocycline
   antimalarials
   chemotherapy
     bleomycin
     cyclophosphamide
     doxorubicin
     melphalan
Toxic
   fluoride
   arsenic
   Addison's disease

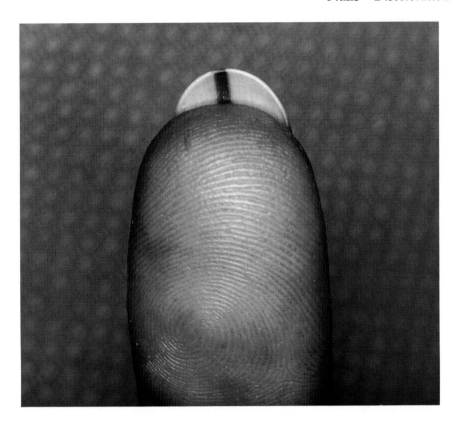

Peutz-Jeghers syndrome—autosomal dominant pigment appears at birth or in early childhood

Interestingly, although the pigmented nails may occur in neurofibromatosis and in Albright's syndrome, focal mucosal hyperpigmentation does not occur with these entities.

Boiko S, Kaufman RA, Lucky AW: **Osteomyelitis** of the distal phalanges in three children with severe atopic dermatitis. Arch Dermatol 1988; 124:418–423.

Unique wedge-shaped **subungual black macules** in one or more fingernails were followed by edema, erythema, and pain of the distal phalanges in three children with lifelong infected atopic dermatitis. An initial diagnosis of cellulitis (felon) caused delayed recognition of underlying destructive **osteomyelitis** of the distal phalanges, seen on x-ray. Cultures grew *Staphylococcus aureus* from both bone and skin in two children, while *Streptococcus viridans* grew from one child's nailbed. Presumably, extension of infection from skin to bone was favored by intense scratching of the infected skin and subsequent development of distal subungual microabscesses, as well as by depressed immunity in atopic patients.

Note the absence of fever and an elevated ESR, the traditional signs of hematogenous osteomyelitis.

Furth PA, Kazakis AM: Nail pigmentation changes associated with azidothymidine (zidovudine). Ann Intern Med 1987; 107:350.

A 36-year-old black woman noted a darkened bluish appearance at the base of all 10 fingernails 6 weeks after starting AZT for treatment of AIDS. Cyanosis was ruled out, with arterial blood gas pressures being normal. The same discoloration appeared in her toenails 4 weeks later. Ultimately, she had a 3-mm transverse pigmented band in all fingernails, which progressed distally.

A 38-year-old black male developed similar nail findings starting 2 weeks after he began taking AZT.

Patients taking AZT should be warned about possible **nail discoloration**, which may result from stimulation of matrix melanocytes by the drug.

Other drugs inducing nail hyperpigmentation include:

bleomycin	methotrexate
doxorubicin	nitrogen mustard
fluorouracil	nitrosoureas
melphalan	

Baran R: **Frictional longitudinal melanonychia**: A new entity. Dermatologica 1987; 174:280–284.

Longitudinal melanonychia of the toes initiated by trauma from footwear was found in 14 patients. Its recognition helps in ruling out brown streaks caused by malignant melanoma.

Melanonychia also calls for thinking about:

Adrenal failure	Malnutrition–B_{12} deficiency
Drugs	Nevus or lentigo (Peutz-Jegher)
Hematoma	Porphyria cutanea tarda
Irradiation	Pregnancy
Lichen planus	*Proteus mirabilis* or fungal infection

Chapel TA, Adcock M: **Pseudomonas chromonychia**. Cutis 1981; 27:601–602.

The possibility of a subungual malignant melanoma brought a hurried consultation request from an internist who had noted a progressive **black discoloration** of the right great toenail of his 67-year-old male patient.

Examination confirmed the finding of a greenish-black discoloration of the nail plate; removal of the discolored nail plate revealed a normal nailbed. The plate did not fluoresce on Wood's light examination. A KOH examination of the plate showed hyphae, which on culture proved to be *Trichophyton rubrum*. Aerobic bacterial cultures grew out *Pseudomonas aeruginosa*, whereas anaerobic cultures were negative.

A diagnosis of **Pseudomonas chromonychia** and onychomycosis was made. The pseudomonas organisms produce both a blue-black pigment (pyocyanin) and a yellow-green pigment (fluorescein). Their presence is favored by paronychia, working in a wet environment, or contact irritants. Their presence always raises the possibility of hematoma, nevus, or malignant melanoma.

Colver GB, Milard PR, Dawber RPR: Atypical **malignant melanoma** of the nail apparatus. Br J Dermatol 1986; 114:389–392.

A 40-year-old white man presented with a **longitudinal pigmented streak** of the right thumbnail, present for 2 years. Two prior biopsies failed to reveal evidence of a malignant melanoma. However, at this time a formal 3-mm wide **deep longitudinal nail biopsy** extending over the nail matrix and entire plate did show the responsible **malignant melanoma**.

Lessons learned:

1. Limited biopsies are hazardous.
2. Ulceration, pigmentation, nail loss, and pain may suggest infection, ingrown toenail, or trauma; however, do not forget that these are also the signs of malignant melanoma.
3. Be doubly suspicious of melanoma when the pigment extends to the periungual tissue (Hutchinson's sign).

   Moral—The presence of an acquired longitudinal pigmented band in a Caucasian must be regarded as a malignant melanoma until proven otherwise.

Daniel CR 3rd: **Nail pigmentation** abnormalities: An addendum. Cutis 1982; 30:364–370.

This and the preceding original article (Cutis 1982 30:348–360) list examples of **abnormal nail pigmentation**:

83 due to diseases
41 due to drugs
86 due to chemicals and local agents
32 due to named nail entities

Should you ever wonder "what could have colored that nail?" look here.

Rudolph RI: Subungual basal cell carcinoma presenting as longitudinal **melanonychia**. J Am Acad Dermatol 1987; 16:229–233.

A 3-mm **brown streak** along the left thumb nail had persisted for 15 years in this 59-year-old white woman. Removal of the nail plate twice had had no effect, and a course of griseofulvin produced no change.

A longitudinal biopsy of the nailbed and matrix revealed the cause: a superficial **pigmented basal cell carcinoma** extending from the matrix on through the proximal nailbed. At the time of operation the pigment could be seen in the matrix and nailbed itself.

The major **differential diagnosis** of concern was an acral lentiginous malignant melanoma. Other causes of longitudinal melanonychia of many years' standing are lentigo, nevus, and lichen planus.

Overindulging in laboratory tests is a sign of diagnostic insecurity.

Lunula

Shelley WB: The spotted lunula. A neglected nail sign associated with **alopecia areata**. J Am Acad Dermatol 1980; 2:385–387.

Spotty absence of the normal gray color of the lunula may be seen in patients with alopecia areata. Three patients are described who also had alopecia totalis. The sharply circumscribed spots are pink, are unaffected by pressure, and do not move out with the growth of the nail. In one patient they disappeared transiently during a short course of steroid therapy.

Other **nail changes in alopecia areata** may include fine pitting, brittleness, loss of surface smoothness and sheen, pale yellow color, striations, onycholysis, and total shedding.

Green ST, Natarajan S: Bilateral first-rib hypoplasia: A new feature of the **nail patella syndrome**. Dermatologica 1986; 172:323–325.

Bilateral dystrophic thumbnails present since birth led a 19-year-old nurse to seek dermatologic help. The ulnar halves of both thumb nails were absent, and the lunulas of the other fingernails showed an abnormal triangular shape. The toenails were normal. She had always been in excellent health but noted that she could never fully extend her elbows.

Radiologic study showed:

> radial dislocation at the elbows
> hypoplasia of the patellae
> loss of curvature of the clavicles
> hypoplastic first ribs
> iliac horns

A diagnosis of the **nail-patella syndrome** was made. Since no other family members were affected by this autosomal dominant disease, it was probably due to spontaneous gene mutation.

This syndrome is more than a strange hypoplasia of bones and thumbnails, and more than failure of the head of the radius to fully develop, leading to subluxation of the elbow. It is one in which a membranous nephropathy develops in 40% and leads to chronic renal failure and death by the fourth decade in 8% of cases. The presenting renal sign of proteinuria was present in this patient. One family has also been described with colonic cancer and the nail-patella syndrome.

Verdich J: **Nail-patella syndrome** associated with renal failure requiring transplantation. Acta Derm Venereol 1980; 60:440–443.

During treatment of a plantar wart, the lunulae of this 15-year-old girl's fingernails caught the physician's attention: every single one was V-shaped. Furthermore, all of the nails, both finger and toe, showed a mild degree of ridging, splitting, and dysplasia. The next step was **palpation of the patellae**. They were small, making the diagnosis of nail-patella syndrome.

Confirming this diagnosis of hereditary osteo-onychodysplasia was the observation of an **increased carrying angle of the elbows**. Extension was limited by 15° and supination by 30°. The patient's mother was then shown to have similar defects of the nails and elbow. As a rare yet significant autosomal dominant disease of the connective tissue, it alerts the observant clinician to the fact that **renal disease** may be present in as many as half of these patients.

In this case it proved to be a diagnosis made after the fact. This girl had had proteinuria since age 7. By age 14 her renal function had become impaired and she was severely hypertensive. A renal transplant was finally necessary.

Might we say that for want of a nail a patella was lost, and for want of a patella a kidney was lost.

And remember, a V-shaped lunula may point to the nail-patella syndrome.

Jorizzo JL, Gonzalez EB, Daniels JC: **Red lunulae** in a patient with rheumatoid arthritis. J Am Acad Dermatol 1983; 8:711–714.

For over 5 years this 63-year-old woman had noted a **dusky redness** of the nailbed in the area of the **lunula** of each fingernail. This erythema blanched on pressure and showed mottling with areas of discrete telangiectasia and also hypopigmentation. The cuticle, nail fold, and nail plate were entirely normal and the toenails showed no abnormality.

Detailed studies indicated that the red lunulae were associated with the classical **rheumatoid arthritis** she had suffered for the past 12 years.

Other **examples of red lunulae** have been associated with:

> alopecia areata
> psoriasis
> heart failure (Terry's red half moons)
> systemic lupus erythematosus
> dermatomyositis

The red lunulae most closely resemble the red palms seen in rheumatoid arthritis, but the pathogenesis remains unknown. They join the host of vascular lesions known to appear **in the rheumatoid arthritic**:

> macular erythema
> purpura, palpable
>> pigmented purpuric eruption
> vasculitis
> urticaria
> nail fold telangiectasia
> digital pulp nodules
> segmental hyalinizing vasculitis
> erythema multiforme
> erythema elevatum diutinum
> erythema nodosum
> digital infarcts
> gangrene

Finally, the yellow nail may be another in the color spectrum seen in these patients.

Hendricks AA: **Yellow lunulae** with fluorescence after tetracycline therapy. Arch Dermatol 1980; 116:438–440.

Diagnose patient compliance by shining a Wood's light on the fingernails. The ones faithfully taking tetracycline (1 gm/day for 3 weeks or more) will show lunulae that fluoresces yellow.

If it isn't quite right for any diagnosis, it may be a drug eruption.

Atrophic

Kitayama Y, Tsukada S: **Congenital onychodysplasia**: Report of 11 cases. Arch Dermatol 1983; 119:8–12.

Clinical

Anonychia, micronychia, or polyonychia
Both index fingers but not toes
Congenital but not hereditary
No bone or joint abnormalities

Associated Findings

Hypoplasia of finger
Syndactyly

Possible Etiology

Local ischemia, embryonic episode

Colver GB, Dawber RPR: **Multiple Beau's lines** due to dysmenorrhoea? Br J Dermatol 1984; 111:111–113.

Regularly spaced Beau's lines across each of the fingernails in four women (ages 16 to 19 years) proved to be **menses markers**. Each patient had severe dysmenorrhea, a form of illness that temporarily inhibits the normal mitotic activity. Nail plate thinning occurred during each menstrual period, much as occurs sporadically with illness or the use of cytotoxic drugs.

Really listen when the patient says, "This may sound funny, but. . . ." for it is then that you may hear the answer.

Lembo G, Montesano M, Belato N: Complete **pterygium unguis**. Cutis 1985; 36:427–429.

A 62-year-old man had had severe **onychodystrophy** of all 20 nails for 30 years. Pain, darkening, and onycholysis of the proximal nail plate began in two fingers and led to shedding of the nail plates. All nails were involved over the next 2 years and never grew back normally. Some nails were lacking, while others consisted of small nail plate remnants on scarred beds. His family history was negative, and there were no other significant skin findings.

Presumptive diagnosis: lichen planus (not confirmed by biopsy).

Handfield-Jones SE, Kennedy CTC: Nail dystrophy associated with **iron deficiency anemia**. Clin Exp Dermatol 1988; 13:54.

For 2 years, a 31-year-old woman had white flaky changes in various nails adjacent to the nail folds, followed by **shedding** of the affected nail leaving a red granulating surface proximally. New nail plate would then regrow. Although only two nails were presently affected, several fingernails and toe-nails had been involved previously.

She gave a history of menorrhagia and looked pale, and her hemoglobin was found to be 6.0 gm/dl. This returned to 13.2 gm/dl with oral iron therapy and at the same time her nails reverted to normal.

Hamann K: **Onychotillomania** treated with pimozide (ORAP). Acta Derm Venereol 1982; 62:364–366.

This 70-year-old woman was referred for evaluation of nail disease of 5 years' duration. She stated that her nails hurt and broke off. She had been using a curved heavy-duty nail scissors to remove the diseased nail plate. On the feet only the great toenails were affected. Her sister had a similar nail disease that she treated with a hobby knife.

Examination showed **exposed nailbeds** where the plate had been cut and plucked away piecemeal. A diagnosis of **onychotillomania** and of *folie a deux* was made.

Oral pimozide therapy resulted in considerable healthy nail regrowth in 3 months and by 7 months all the nails were normal. Her sister had an equally good result from pimozide therapy.

When you don't see disease and the patient does, it may be time for a trial of pimozide.

Colver GB: **Onychotillomania**. Br J Dermatol 1987; 117:397–399.

Nails with bizarre hollows, gouges, depressions, or scratches suggest that the patient may have an acknowledged or denied "hobby" of **nail carving**. Cuticle scissors, razors, and knives are used to attack minor nail flaws or remove presumed pathogens or pathologic nail tissue. Indeed, patients may pluck out the entire plate using pliers. The periungual tissue is usually normal.

Onychotillomania is to be contrasted with **onychophagia**, in which the teeth are the tools used. Nail biting is not a marker of psychiatric disturbance.

Sait MA, Reddy BSN, Garg BR: **Onychotillomania**. 2 case reports. Dermatologica 1985; 171:200–202.

In this rare psychocutaneous disorder, patients have an irresistible desire to rub, pick, or tear the nails, resulting in gradual destruction and mutilation. Both cases presented are men in India with depressive disorders.

One 55-year-old farmer had intense itching of all toenails and 9 fingernails in 2-week cycles, starting on the day of the new moon. He rubbed the nails vigorously against the ground, and after one year had a **19-nail dystrophy** with thin nail plates, pterygium formation, and periungual depigmentation. Fungal culture and KOH examination of nail clippings were normal. The conspicuous sparing of the right thumb nail was believed by the patient to be God's gift enabling him to protect himself against thorn pricks.

The other man, an 84-year-old retired weaver, had **delusions** of minute red-colored insects inhabiting his fingernails, eyebrows, and scalp. In an effort to get rid of them he plucked the hair on the eyebrows and scalp and continuously rubbed his fingernails against each other. His eyebrow hair was sparse and broken and four fingernails had gross dystrophic changes with normal KOH examination and fungal culture.

Put some "how come?" in your diagnoses.

Feinstein A, Friedman J, Schewach-Millet M: **Pachyonychia congenita**. J Am Acad Dermatol 1988; 19:705–711.

A survey of 168 cases of this rare autosomal dominant disease allowed the following classification of **pachyonychia congenita** and its associated findings. The percentages indicate frequency.

Type I   56%
   Hypertrophy of nails
   Palmoplantar hyperkeratosis
   Follicular keratosis
   Leukokeratosis in the mouth

Type II   25%
   Clinical findings of type I plus bullae of palms and soles.
   Hyperhidrosis of palms and soles
   Natal or neonatal teeth
   Steatocystoma multiplex 25%

Type III   12%
   Clinical findings of types I and II plus
   Angular cheilosis
   Corneal dyskeratosis
   Cataracts

Type IV   7%
   Clinical findings of types I, II, III plus
   Hoarseness, laryngeal lesions
   Alopecia and hair abnormalities
   Mental retardation

Just because you have a diagnostic handle on a disease doesn't mean you can handle it.

Dysplastic

Griffiths WAD: "**Curly nails**"—an unusual side effect of etretinate. J Dermatol Treat 1990; 1:265–266.

A 35-year-old woman with chronic pustular psoriasis of the left sole was given etretinate (0.25 mg/kg/day for 3 months). This cleared the psoriasis, but a month later three of her fingernails were found to be misshapen.

The **nail plates** were **curved** in their free portion, giving them an S-shaped curly appearance. It was believed that retinoid effect observed was the result of a wave of growth modulation within the matrix. Comparison is made with the kinky hair induced in some patients by retinoids.

Millman AJ, Strier RP: **Congenital onychodysplasia** of the index fingers. Report of a family. J Am Acad Dermatol 1982; 7:57–65.

Nine patients from one family showed the autosomal dominant **congenital onychodysplasia of the index finger** (COIF).

Six **variants** of COIF are presented:

micronychia
rolled micronychia
polyonychia
hemionychogryphosis
malalignment
anonychia

Look for underlying osseous changes:

Y-shaped bifurcation lateral view
narrowing of distal phalanx on A-P view
shortening of middle phalanx of 5th finger (brachydactyly)
syndactyly

The differential includes:

onychoheterotopia, i.e., ectopic nail
polyonychia–in congenital skin disease and in syndactyly
micronychia

Feingold M: Picture of the month: Syndromes associated with **nail dysplasia**. Am J Dis Child 1985; 139:425–426.

Dysplasia of the fingernails and toenails in association with absent or sparse hair, but normal facies and teeth suggests hidrotic ectodermal dysplasia. The sweat glands are normal in this autosomal dominant condition.

The presence of small, narrow dysplastic nails that split easily—especially on the thumb and index finger—calls for examination of the patellas. If the patellas are absent or hypoplastic, look for scoliosis, elbow anomalies, iliac horns, and glomerulonephritis. The **nail-patella syndrome** is an autosomal dominant with variable expressivity.

A short woman with a short webbed neck should be examined for dysplastic nails, lymphedema of the dorsal hands and feet, and lack of secondary sexual characteristics. A search for ovarian dysgenesis and congenital heart disease will help confirm **Turner's syndrome**.

Horn RT, Odom RB: Twenty-nail dystrophy of **alopecia areata**. Arch Dermatol 1980; 116:573–574.

Minute opalescent pits and longitudinal ridges on all 20 nails of this 15-year-old boy led to the diagnosis of **20-nail dystrophy**. The changes had developed during an attack of alopecia areata and had persisted for 6 years. The alopecia areata had not been clinically evident for 5 years following a remission induced by steroid injections.

The dull, thin, fragile ridged nails of the 20-nail dystrophy represent a reaction pattern. The primary disease may be occult. Look for a **background** of lichen planus, psoriasis, alopecia areata, or eczema.

Zaias N: **Psoriasis** of the nail, a clinical-pathologic study. Arch Dermatol 1969; 99:567–579.

Pits are punctate or irregular depressions that may form a pattern or may be randomly spaced on the surface of the nail plate. Although they are the most common lesion of nail psoriasis, they are not specific, being seen in a variety of dermatoses affecting the nail matrix and proximal nail fold.

Look for them in alopecia areata as well as with hand dermatitis. They are the result of desquamation of foci of incomplete keratinization, i.e., parakeratotic cells that are poorly adherent.

At a time when medicine is becoming more and more controlled by exact methods of counting, measuring, weighing, and chemical analysis, let us rejoice that in dermatology there is a large field in which the clinical eye, artistic intuition, cannot be disregarded.

H. HAXTHAUSEN

Ridging

Baran R, Dawber R: **Twenty-nail dystrophy** of childhood: A misnamed syndrome. Cutis 1987; 39:481–482.

Twenty-nail dystrophy (**trachyonychia**) is an acquired nonspecific nail dystrophy in which all the child's nails are uniformly and simultaneously ridged excessively, with loss of luster. The skin and ectodermal derivatives are otherwise normal.

In one type the nail is lusterless and rough, appearing as though the ridge had been produced by longitudinal sandpapering. It is most frequently associated with alopecia areata. In the second type the ridged nails are shiny and opalescent. In both types, lichen planus, psoriasis, atopic dermatitis, or alopecia areata may be associated or the nails may be the only expression of disease. In one instance, graft-vs-host disease may have been the determinant since the affected newborn had had an exchange transfusion.

Twenty-nail dystrophy of childhood is a diagnosis in search of one of 20 causes.

Kechijian P: **Twenty-nail dystrophy** of childhood. A reappraisal. Cutis 1985; 35:38–41.

Twenty-nail dystrophy of childhood is defined as a self-limited, noncongenital nail plate dystrophy with an onset early in childhood. The child is born with normal nails, but in months or years the dystrophic changes occur. It usually **clears by adulthood**. The nails show excess longitudinal ridging as a hallmark of the disease. The plates are thin, fragile, dull, and opalescent. Layering and notching are present as well. The thumbnails may be quite thick, yellow, and rough. Alternatively, the nails may be described as vertical striated sandpaper nails, or trachyonychia (trachy, rough).

The **differential diagnosis** includes onychomycosis, lichen planus, alopecia areata, eczema, and psoriasis. Only the aficionados of the nail will pursue diagnosis to the point of biopsy.

Brodkin RH, Bleiberg J: **Cutaneous microwave injury**. A report of two cases. Acta Derma Venereol 1973; 53:50–52.

Two women (ages 50 and 56 years) who operated a microwave oven in a department store snack bar developed **fingernail problems** at about the same time. This coincided with malfunctioning of the microwave oven, which resulted in burning of food. Nail changes consisted of severe but nonpainful transverse dystrophic ridging which began proximally in the nail plates of several fingers. The paronychial areas were normal. No soft tissue or bony abnormalities were present on x-ray. In both patients the lesions began to improve after the microwave unit was removed.

Microwaves (10 to 100,000 megacycles/sec) fall between very high-frequency radio waves and infrared waves. When absorbed, as by foods or human tissue, they produce thermal, electrical, and magnetic effects. They may produce thermal burns in deep tissue, such as the nail matrix, without causing a sensation of heat.

Shelley WB, Shelley ED: **Shoreline nails**: Sign of drug-induced erythroderma. Cutis 1985; 35:220–224.

Drug-induced erythrodermas produce an interruption in nail plate synthesis. Initially, this is evidenced by a white leukonychial band. Late, the nail plate fractures away, leaving a ragged, torn edge. The appearance of this resembles a **wave breaking at the shoreline**, and hence the name. Repeated attacks of

918

erythroderma produce similar "waves" in all of the nails, heightening the analogy with the shoreline.

Although nail matrix arrest occurs in all erythrodermas, such arrest is shorter in drug-induced erythroderma because here the drug is identified and stopped abruptly. As a result, nail matrix function is rapidly resumed before the old plate is shed, thus forcing the old distal and discontinuous nail plate to become elevated and resemble a wave.

Examples are shown of such **shoreline nails** in patients sensitive to cephalosporin, codeine, and allopurinol. In one patient, the nails exhibited four "waves," each the result of successive episodes of drug-induced erythroderma during the half year of fingernail growth.

Shoreline nails are not seen in the erythrodermas of atopy, psoriasis, or lymphoma, since these are not reversed rapidly enough to induce new nail, lifting up the old.

Beau's lines are to be distinguished by the fact that they are transverse depressions in the nail plate, not jagged discontinuities.

The most brilliant diagnosticians of my acquaintance are the ones who do remember and consider the most possibilities.

LOGAN CLENDENING, M.D.

Koilonychia

Hellier FF: **Hereditary koilonychia**. Br J Dermatol 1950; 213–214.

Koilonychia was found in 16 members of one family, inherited as a simple dominant. One little boy had so much **concavity** in the great toenails that they caught in his shoes and made walking difficult.

Familial koilonychia has also been **associated with** monilethrix, leukonychia, and dental abnormalities.

Dawber R: **Occupational koilonychia**. Clin Exp Dermatol 1977; 2:115–116.

Spoon fingernails were noted in 3 automobile mechanics, who attributed the depressed nails to constant immersion in oils. Interestingly, 5 of 94 mechanics who were surveyed showed this same koilonychia, whereas none was present in 128 manual laborers who had no contact with oils. It appears likely that the koilonychia reflects nail softening by oil and subsequent re-shaping by the mechnical pressures of work.

Differential diagnosis:

iron deficiency anemia
peripheral arterial disease
hereditary type
normal temporary change in childhood

Smith SJ, Yoder FW, Knox DW: **Occupational koilonychia**. Arch Dermatol 1980; 116:861.

Spoon-like depressions of the nails of the three middle fingers of the right hand had been noted for 6 months by this 45-year-old woman. Study revealed the problem to be koilonychia caused by her work as a coil winder, which required firm pressure of her fingers on the wire as it was being coiled.

Automobile mechanics, mushroom growers, cabinet makers, and others sustaining intermittent trauma and consequent ischemia also may develop occupational koilonychia. Organic solvents may also cause **occupational spoon nail**.

But phonetically, who could ask for more than a case of koilonychia from coiling wire?

Feit H: **Koilonychia**. Society Transactions. Arch Dermatol Syphilol 1935; 31:122–123.

Dr. A.C. Cipollaro stated that **occupational koilonychia** is most often due to exposure to strong alkalis or acids. Koilonychia may also be due to syphilis and thyroid disease.

Pedersen NB: Persistent **occupational koilonychia**. Contact Dermatitis 1982; 8:134.

A 55-year-old man had **koilonychia** of both thumbnails for 20 years associated with sore thumb tips. He worked as a plate smith for the Danish state railways, producing threaded pins and screwing them through metal jackets in steam engines. He cooled the pins with **mineral oil** poured on his bare hands and also removed metal chips from the pins with the tips of his thumbs. He had performed this job for over 20 years, and after stopping it the nail changes persisted.

Koilonychia may occur after exposure to oils, organic solvents, and mechanical stress.

Staberg B, Gammeltoft M, Onsberg P: **Onychomycosis** in patients with psoriasis. Acta Derm Venereol 1983; 63:436–438.

The classic changes seen in psoriatic nails are pitting, thickening, discoloration, onycholysis, and subungual hyperkeratosis. These tend to blind the clinician to the fact that about 15% of **psoriatics** have a **dermatophyte infection** of the toenails or a **yeast infection** of the fingernails.

Only by **KOH** examination and culture can you recognize these.

Kalter DC, Hay RJ: **Onychomycosis** due to *Trichophyton soudanense*. Clin Exp Dermatol 1988; 13:221–227.

Since *T. soudanense* is endemic to central and western Africa, it may be the cause of nail dystrophy in a patient who has traveled to Ghana or Nigeria. This infection is morphologically distinctive, with hyperpigmented, thickened fingernails having multiple transverse ridges, surface pitting, and lamellar splitting. *T. violaceum* is the other endothrix-type infection that causes similar nail changes. Presumably, **endothrix fungi** are more successful at penetrating keratin, and their keratolytic ability would explain proximal nail changes leading to ridging, diffuse mild thickening, and **distortion of the nail plate**. Contrast this with nails infected by *T. rubrum* or *T. mentagrophytes*, which have distal subungual hyperkeratosis and crumbling of the opaque nail plate.

Always, the fungal culture provides the true differentiation, but gross inspection allows us to perceive the varying capabilities of fungi to infect the nail plate and the nailbed.

Rollman O, Johansson S: *Hendersonula toruloidea* **infection**: Successful response of onychomycosis to nail avulsion and topical ciclopiroxolamine. Acta Derm Venereol 1987; 67:506–510.

A year of oral griseofulvin had no effect on the fingernail dystrophy of a 30-year-old man from Nigeria. The **nail changes** consisted of onycholysis, yellow-brown discoloration, partial irregular loss of the nail plate, subungual hyperkeratosis, and painful paronychial swelling. The nail was KOH positive and a PAS-stained nail biopsy showed mycelia in the upper plate. Culture on Sabouraud's agar showed fungal growth in 3 days, and by 1 week the Petri dish was filled with gray mycelia that soon became black. Nothing grew on the medium containing cycloheximide.

The fungus was identified as *Hendersonula toruloidea*, well known to be insensitive to griseofulvin, ketoconazole, and glutaraldehyde.

It is likely that this infection is missed since:

1. The clinician views it as a run-of-the-mill KOH positive dermatophyte nail infection.
2. Culture may be done on cycloheximide media, on which it will not grow.
3. Rapid, luxuriant growth deceives the mycology lab into viewing it as a contaminant mold, so that precise identification is never made.

Moral: If your KOH is positive and the onychomycosis fails to respond to internal treatment, look to the **culture** with and without cycloheximide for a better diagnosis.

Norton LA: Self induced trauma to the nails. Cutis 1987; 40:223–227.

Before one makes a diagnosis of psoriasis, lichen planus, or fungous infection of the nails, it is necessary to rule out **self-induced trauma** if there is no disease elsewhere. By compulsive picking, digging, and manipulating the nail unit, patients can induce changes that easily pass for psoriasis, lichen planus, or onychomycosis. In these instances, the cuticle is absent and the nail folds traumatized.

Lesser trauma to the nail produces simply the partial, transverse **ridging** of the thumbnail or fingernail seen in the habit tic. In this tic the patient constantly strokes or scratches his 2nd or 3rd nail across the thumb plate. Or conversely, the thumbnail may be the "tool" responsible for ridging on the other nails. Think of the habit tic nail when the lunula is very large, the nail folds are injured, the cuticle is absent and the most pronounced changes are on the dominant side.

Again, one of the common causes of **onycholysis** is the patient's well-meaning efforts to remove dirt and debris from under the nail. Unwitting self-induced trauma to the toenails produces ingrown toenails. Thus, wearing ill-fitting but stylish footwear, cutting the corners of the nails, and pulling hangnails are examples of pathogenic forces unwittingly exerted by the patient.

Onychopathomimia is the rarely used designation of self-induced trauma to the nails that the patient attributes to an occupational contactant or injury. Such misinterpretation gives rise to a number of compensation claims.

Puzzling over these can sometimes induce onychophagia in the physician.

Look for the second cause of a disease.

Kechijian P: **Onycholysis** of the fingernails: Evaluation and management. J Am Acad Dermatol 1985; 12:552–560.

Separation of the nail plate from its bonding to the terminal epidermal nailbed is **onycholysis**. The diagnosis is evidenced by the failure of light to be reflected by the freed nail and hence its opacity in a wider than usual band on the terminal part of the nail.

Although the causes are legion, one should initially approach the problem of finding a cause with just three suspects in mind:

> trauma
> maceration
> chemical injury, especially from nail care products

Is there a history of tearing or crushing? Is there a history of compulsive mechanical cleansing and debridement under the nail? Did hair, dirt, or a splinter become wedged under the nail plate, causing separation?

Did the nail become "unglued" by prolonged maceration, work in a wet environment, swimming, or hyperhidrosis?

Can the cause be occupational- or hobby-related exposure to gasoline, print remover, thioglycolate, nail enamel polish or base coats, hardeners, or artificial nails?

If these avenues are unrewarding, think:

> Microbial cause:
>> *Candida albicans* is the number one suspect; reserve KOH, culture scrape nailbed
>> Dermatophytes are also a cause and require some diagnostic maneuvers–KOH, culture
>> Bacteria are not a cause but are opportunistic invaders of the subungual space.

> Drug cause:
>> Usually phototoxic reaction as with tetracyclines, contraceptives, chlorpromazine
>> May be non-photoinduced, e.g.,
>>> 5-fluorouracil
>>> bleomycin
>>> doxorubicin

> Dermatologic cause:
>> Psoriasis
>>> Look for associated pitting, oil drop sign, subungual hyperkeratosis, splinter hemorrhages, crumbling of nail. May need biopsy to confirm.
>> Lichen planus
>>> Usually lesions elsewhere
>>> Requires biopsy
>> Nailbed dermatitis
>> Pachyonychia congenita
>> Congenital ectodermal defect
>> Lichen striatus
>> Neoplastic–warts, pyogenic granulomas, squamous cell carcinoma
>> Systemic disease cause:
>>> Pulmonary problems
>>> Thyroid disease
>>> Syphilis
>>> Porphyrias

Despite all this, some examples of onycholysis remains idiopathic, and even more of them remain refractory to treatment.

Logan RA, Hawk JLM: **Spontaneous photo-onycholysis**. Br J Dermatol 1985; 113:605–610.

Whenever a 40-year-old man visited tropical climates, he noted pain under his fingernails 10 days after arrival. The distal nail plate became discolored and **distal onycholysis** developed, affecting the middle three fingers of the right hand and the left ring finger, but not the toenails. The onycholysis resolved several months after he returned home. The usual causes of onycholysis were ruled out (psoriasis, hypothyroidism, trauma, burns, infection, drugs). Porphyrin studies were negative.

A diagnosis of onycholysis due to **sun exposure** was made. Since only UVA radiation can penetrate the nail plate, sensitization to this wave length is presumably responsible. Application of opaque plastic adhesive strips to the distal nail plate prevented the photo-onycholysis.

Two additional cases are presented in men who developed similar photo-onycholysis every summer. In one case the toenails were also affected.

Baran R: Acute **onycholysis** from rust-removing agents. Arch Dermatol 1980; 116:382–383.

Sudden acute pain in the tip of this cleaning woman's right index finger developed when a hole in her rubber glove permitted contact with the rust-remover solution (hydrofluoric acid) she was using. A throbbing pain persisted the next day until oral corticosteroids were administered.

By one month, **onycholysis** had developed in the distal half of the nail with a proximal border of dark erythema. Not until 6 months later did the nail plate completely reattach.

Any patient presenting with onycholysis must be questioned concerning **chemical contacts**. The following are known to be pathogenic:

    enzyme-containing detergents
    nail cosmetics
        base coat
        nail hardeners (formaldehyde)
        plastic nails, sculptured nails
    hair cosmetics
        dicyandiamide strengthener
        epilating agents
            thioglycolate

Baran R, Badillet G: **Primary onycholysis** of the big toenails: A review of 113 cases. Br J Dermatol 1982; 106:529–534.

Onycholysis, i.e, the separation of the nail plate from its bed, usually produces a nail of whitish color on the distal or lateral border. However, it may vary from gray or yellow to even black. The plate remains of normal surface, contour, and thickness, the color change being due to the presence of air and keratinous debris under the end or sides of the nail. Such onycholysis is usually of cosmetic concern only, although a black color occasionally calls for investigation of a possible melanoma.

The usual cause of onycholysis of the great toes is **trauma**. Although dermatophytes and potentially pathogenic bacteria were found in the lesions, they are commensal only.

In view of the role of trauma, therapy rests on avoidance of high heels, and narrow, slanting shoes. Further therapeutic intervention centers on arch supports to counteract the normal aging processes involving loss of plantar fat and joint flexibility, as well as flattening of the plantar arch.

If the shoe fits, wear it; if not, suffer onycholysis of the big toe.

Hogan DJ: **Subungual trichogranuloma** in a hairdresser. Cutis 1988; 42:105–106.

Any hairdresser with psoriatic onycholysis is at risk of having hair clippings become embedded under the nail plate. This may lead to inflammatory papules subungually at the site of implantation.

Penetration of short, sharp hair clippings within the skin itself also causes interdigital trichogranulomas and sinuses in hairdressers, particularly those who cut men's hair. A small shallow pit, inflammatory papule, or infected sinus results from a foreign body reaction to hair keratin in the dermis.

Onycholysis may also be the result of **subungual hair penetration**.

If you can diagnose everything you see, you probably can walk on water, too.

Subungual Lesions

Keeney GL, Banks PM, Linscheid RL: **Subungual keratoacanthoma**: Report of a case and review of the literature. Arch Dermatol 1988; 124:1074–1076.

For 6 weeks this 36-year-old man had treated what he thought was a painful **periungual infection** of his left middle finger. Incision and drainage as well as bacterial cultures were nonproductive except for friable gray-white material.

X-ray of the finger showed a cup-shaped lytic lesion of the distal phalanx. Curettage of the nailbed permitted a histologic diagnosis of **keratoacanthoma**. Anxiety on the part of the patient led to amputation of the distal phalanx.

The differential diagnosis of this subungual growth rested between subungual keratoacanthoma and squamous cell carcinoma. Although the young age of the patient, the rapid course, and the cup-shaped pattern of bone resorption seen on x-ray favored the diagnosis of subungual keratoacanthoma, ultimately the diagnosis had to be made histologically.

Mikhail GR: **Subungual epidermoid carcinoma**. J Am Acad Dermatol 1984; 11:291–298.

The initial manifestations of **subungual epidermoid carcinoma** are swelling, erythema, and localized pain of the nail layer. As the tumor slowly grows it becomes hypertrophic and ulcerated and the overlying nail plate becomes dystrophic or may be shed. After this the lesion looks verrucous, scaly, and crusted. It may become ulcerated and bleed or become infected.

Initially, the lesions fool the clinician into thinking that the patient has an inflammatory condition or an infection, either bacterial or fungal. Later, the lesions may **simulate** verruca vulgaris, pyogenic granuloma, subungual exostosis, glomus tumor, keratoacanthoma, malignant melanoma, and nail dystrophies.

All chronic recalcitrant lesions of the nailbed must be biopsied. First remove the nail plate; second, incise down to periosteum to detect invasive tumors.

A scant **biopsy** gives scant information. Go deep for in-depth understanding.

Milgraum SS, Headington JT: A **subungual nodule** of recent onset. Arch Dermatol 1988; 124:429–432.

A barefoot stroll by a 30-year-old physician on the sandy bank of the Carrao River in Venezuela was followed 3 days later by a **painful white pea-sized papule** on the tip of the second toe. Excision revealed a gravid female chigoe flea (*Tunga penetrans*). Untreated, tungiasis may lead to severe itching and inflammation, pyoderma, gangrene, tetanus, and amputation.

Think of this penetrating sand flea to explain painful papules in people coming back from a Caribbean holiday or the sandy beaches of Central and South America, the Seychelles, Africa, Pakistan, and India.

And remember, it is not the chigger but the chigoe lady that fashions an "egg house" in your skin. The ova are shed back to the sand, where the larvae molt several times and by the 17th day are adults (1 mm long). They hop about, ready to bite (male) or burrow (female) into the next tourist, gorilla, dog, cat, mouse, or rat that comes along.

Morimoto SS, Gurevitch AW: **Unilateral pterygium inversum unguis**. Int J Dermatol 1988; 27:491–494.

A 50-year-old man had a "fungal infection" of the nails on the right hand and right foot, noted 8 years previously following a cerebrovascular accident that left him with right-sided paresis. Due to pain from minimal pressure on the nails and bleeding when he attempted to cut the nails, he had allowed the nails to grow very long. Examination revealed atrophy of the tips of the fingers and toes, and **abnormal adherence** of the distal nailbed to the nail plate, with loss of the subungual groove. Potassium hydroxide scrapings and culture for fungus were negative.

Pterygium inversum unguis was diagnosed. In this nail disorder, the distal nailbed adheres to the ventral surface of the nail plate, resulting in subungual extension of the hyponychium and obliteration of the normal groove. Such an unusual winged nail may reflect atrophy of the digit tip with loss of the normal separation of the distal nail plate and nailbed. A similar pterygium is common in Raynaud's phenomenon and scleroderma. Most patients and physicians mistakenly view it as a fungus infection. We vote for a name change to subungual pterygium.

Two biopsies are better than one—and two pathologists better than one.

Neonates and Infants

Newborn skin usually arrives well-born; with ill-born skin, look to the mother. Could she have given her baby's skin the spirochete of syphilis, the mask of lupus, or the virus of herpes or AIDS? Look to the parents and their parents. Could they have provided the spotted DNA of hereditable disease? Do they have atopic skin, ichthyosis, epidermolysis bullosa? Or does their DNA transmit a disease of later years such as psoriasis, rosacea, and dysplastic nevi? Are the parents consanguineous? Should you expect a heightened expression of recessive gene defects? Is there a history of congenital ectodermal defects?

Newborn skin is delicate. Its fragile epidermal scarf comes loose with easy blister formation not seen with the same diseases later in life. Its moist warm folds play host to bacteria and yeast, with folliculitis and dermatitis common consequences. Witness the diaper dermatitis.

A difficult passage down the birth canal may not only lead to edema but also to fat necrosis.

As newborn skin ages and becomes infant skin, it acquires the capacity to mount immediate immune defenses. Many of these are directed to protein food antigens that slip through the infant's permeable gut. The result can be the common atopic dermatitis. No other disease provides a wider spectrum of incessant itch and the consequent dermatitis. Its symmetry and favored locales of the popliteal and antecubital fossae as well as the face favor its easy recognition.

Atopic dermatitis is not the only infantile itch to be seen in your office. Look to scabies with its mask of secondary infection and eczema. Look for the burrow and look for the source of the mite in the baby's family, relatives, and friends.

Some rarities are so unique and distinctive that once seen they are unforgettable. These include the pigmented macules of mastocytosis that become nodules on stroking (Darier sign). Equally memorable are the whorled streaks of incontinentia pigmenti, the bullae of epidermolysis bullosa, and the perioral dermatitis of acrodermatitis enteropathica. The telangiectatic flushed cheeks of congenital photosensitivity and the thick nails of pachyonychia congenita are unforgettable sights.

No scan of the infant's skin for a diagnosis must neglect the commonplace infectious diseases of childhood. Knowing the current epidemic will greatly aid in spotting that unusual example of varicella or measles.

All in all, the infant is a little person with his own set of dermatologic problems. Learn to recognize these diseases of young skin.

Red Scaly Baby

Spraker MK: **Pediatric dermatology**. Progress in Dermatology 1989; 23(3):1–7.

The **red scaly baby** is usually suffering from atopic or seborrheic dermatitis. If, however, the dermatitis is associated with a failure to thrive, a diagnosis of Leiner's disease may be made by exclusion. To be precise, such a diagnosis should be accompanied by evidence of a yeast opsonization defect.

Recently, the diagnostic reach has been extended to (1) the hyperimmunoglobulin E syndrome; (2) cystic fibrosis with deficiencies of essential fatty acids, proteins, and zinc; and (3) amino acid deficient diets used to treat rare amino acid metabolic defects.

Sometimes it's not what is there, but what is not there that makes the diagnosis.

Skin Color

Nanda A, Kaur S, Bhakoo ON, et al: **Pityriasis (tinea) versicolor** in infancy. Pediatr Dermatol 1988; 5:260–262.

Hypopigmented lesions on the neck of a normal healthy male were considered to be postinflammatory hypomelanosis. At 4-month follow-up he had numerous hypopigmented scaly lesions on the trunk, arms, and face, as well. Scrapings made the diagnosis of **pityriasis versicolor**.

Watch for it on the face and in the diaper area.

Elhassani SB, Feingold M: Picture of the month: **Kernicterus**. Am J Dis Child 1986; 140:247–248.

A "premie" infant with **neonatal jaundice** should be watched for opisthotonos and downward deviation of the eyes ("setting sun" sign), which signals kernicterus. Fever, seizures, dyspnea, and pulmonary hemorrhage follow. Those who survive the Rh isoimmunization develop spasticity, choreoathetosis, sensorineural deafness, and vertical gaze palsy.

Schumacher RE, Thornbery JM, Gutcher GR: **Transcutaneous bilirubinometry**: A comparison of old and new methods. Pediatrics 1985; 76:10–14.

The T.A. Ingram **icterometer** is a strip of transparent plexiglass on which are painted five yellow transverse stripes of precise and graded hue. When the plexiglass is pressed against a baby's skin, the color of the skin is compared with the yellow stripes to assign a jaundice score. This $10 instrument compared well in efficacy with the $2000 Minolta Air-Shields jaundice meter presently in use to detect infants in need of serum bilirubin screening. The icterometer has proved useful in white, Oriental, and black newborn populations.

Ashley JR, Littler CM, Burgdorf WHC, Brann BS IV: **Bronze baby syndrome**. Report of a case. J Am Acad Dermatol 1985; 12:325–328.

Twenty-four hours after phototherapy for neonatal jaundice this infant's skin began to turn **grayish brown**. It continued to darken. The phototherapy was discontinued on day 9. Although a biopsy revealed no cause for the color, spectrophotometry of the serum revealed the presence of a distinctive yet unidentified pigment. Within several months the skin color had returned to normal. A diagnosis of **bronze baby syndrome** was made.

A dusky hue in any newborn skin calls for a **differential**:

Cyanosis responds to O_2 inhalation
Jaundice is yellow-brown, not gray-brown
Carbon baby syndrome (universal acquired melanosis)–biopsy shows hyperpigmentation of all epidermal layers.

Gray baby syndrome
  Due to chloramphenicol overdosage
  Actually cyanosis due to shock
Bronze baby syndrome–due to hepatic dysfunction with accumulation of products from phototherapy; wanes with time

Purcell SM, Wians FH Jr, Ackerman NB, Davis BM: Hyperbiliverdinemia in the **bronze baby syndrome**. J Am Acad Dermatol 1987; 16:172–177.

Jaundiced babies who are given **phototherapy** for their hyperbilirubinemia may acquire a **"bronzed" look** in a few days. The pigment responsible for

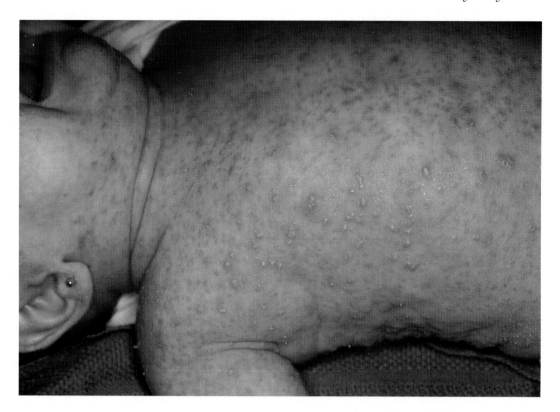

producing this transient gray-brown color in skin, serum, and urine is not known. Although the pigment is nontoxic and possibly is a photoxidation product of bilirubin, the appearance of the bronze baby syndrome suggests the presence of severe underlying liver disease.

In this report the baby's skin became bronzed while the serum became olive-green in color as a result of biliverdin (green bile pigment) accumulation. It is postulated that the bronze color was imparted by the complementary colors, green (serum) and red (erythrocytes).

Hyperbiliverdinemia can result from hepatitis due to indomethacin or from a genetic defect in biliverdin reductase with a resultant green jaundice in adults or bronzed skin in infants.

Cueto JM: **Mongolian spots** mistaken for child abuse. Cutis 1987; 40:308.

A mistaken diagnosis of child abuse in this case of a Mongolian spot in a 7-month-old baby produced a case of "parent abuse" until corrected.

To see more, keep asking yourself, What more is there to see?

Figurate Lesions

Cox NH, McQueen A, Evans TJ, Morley WN: An **annular erythema** of infancy. Arch Dermatol 1987; 123:510–513.

Four days after birth this baby girl developed papular enlarging lesions of the face and feet. Each lesion had a cycle of development from papule to a 3- to 4-cm **annular arciform or plaque form** over a few weeks. The lesions had wide round firm erythematous borders, were asymptomatic, and resolved without residue after a month. Multiple lesions were present at all times, predominantly on the face and trunk. A wide range of therapeutic trials has had no effect. The problem has persisted for 2 years.

The following **diagnoses** were dismissed:

Urticaria–disappears in 24 hours
Urticarial vasculitis–resolves with residual bruising
Erythema chronicum migrans–usually single lesion following tick bite
Erythema marginatum rheumaticum–rash is transient; occurs in older children with rheumatic fever
Neonatal lupus erythematosus–usually does not last beyond 6 months, photosensitive, anti-Ro antibody positive
Familial annular erythema–fades in 4 days with residual brown pigmentation
Erythema gyratum atrophicans–lesions have central atrophy
Annular erythema of infancy–lesions disappear in 2 days
Persistent annular erythema of infancy–central scaling; tissue eosinophilia
Erythema annulare centrifugum–usually seen in adults; eosinophilia
Erythema gyratum perstans–vesiculation and scaling
Erythema multiforme–patient shows evidence of infection, drug intake; connective tissue disease, food hypersensitivity

Thus Cox et al. view their little patient as a distinct entity, meriting further study.

Toonstra J, de Witt FE: "Persistent" **annular erythema of infancy**. Arch Dermatol 1984; 120:1069–1072.

Large, irregularly shaped **annular lesions** with red urticarial borders had been present on the face, back, and distal extremities of an 8-month-old girl for 2 months. The patient initially developed a red raised lesion on her right temple. This had enlarged into an annular lesion with a raised border covering the entire right side of the face. Similar new lesions began to appear on the arm and elsewhere. There was no vesiculation and no scaling peripherally.

Biopsy showed a nonspecific perivascular infiltrate; a diagnosis of **erythema gyratum perstans** was made. No treatment was prescribed, and all the lesions vanished without a trace 11 months after the initial presentation.

The reported examples of erythema gyratum perstans in youngsters form a heterogeneous group. The lesions persist for years, ranging from 3 to over 15 years, although individual rings fade in days or a few weeks.

The authors prefer the simple designation of annular erythema but distinguish it from erythema marginatum rheumaticum and erythema chronicum migrans.

Hebert AA, Esterly NB: **Annular erythema** of infancy. J Am Acad Dermatol 1986; 14:339–343.

This 7-month-old baby girl had recurrent asymptomatic **arcuate and annular** skin lesions since the age of 6 weeks. Cyclic attacks occurred, with single lesions usually involuting within 2 to 3 days. There were no associated constitutional signs.

The initial impression was that this represented erythema annulare centrifugum induced by the presence of oral thrush. However, a biopsy suggested a possible diagnosis of eosinophilic cellulitis or an insect bite reaction.

The child remained in good health and by the age of 14 months her skin showed no further attacks. A diagnosis of **annular erythema of infancy** was made, but only after **ruling out**:

> erythema annulare centrifugum on histologic grounds
> familial annular erythema, negative history
> erythema gyratum atrophicans, no atrophy
> urticaria, persistent
> erythema multiforme, no target lesions
> neonatal lupus erythematosus, not in sun-exposed areas
> erythema chronicum migrans, no tick exposure

Peterson AO, Jarratt M: **Annular erythema** of infancy. Arch Dermatol 1981; 117:145–148.

Annular and arcuate erythematous lesions had been appearing for 3 months in this 6-month-old baby boy. These nonpruritic lesions were generalized, each one disappearing without a trace at the end of 36 to 48 hours. No vesiculation, scaling, central puncture, or postinflammation hyperpigmentation was observed. The infant had not had contact with pets or traveled, or taken any medication, either by prescription or over the counter.

A biopsy showed only a mononuclear and eosinophil infiltrate. The epidermis was normal and immunofluorescence studies were negative. These findings ruled out the following **diagnoses**:

> erythema annulare centrifugum
> familial annular erythema
> erythema gyratum atrophicans
> erythema multiforme
> erythema chronicum migrans
> urticaria

The diagnosis made was the simple descriptive one of **annular erythema** of **infancy**. True to its name, it entirely disappeared as soon as infancy disappeared. Now a boy of 2 years, he has had no attacks since age 11 months.

Kettler AH, Stone MS, Bruce S, Tschen JA: **Annular eruptions of infancy** and neonatal lupus erythematosus. Arch Dermatol 1987; 123:298–299.

All cases of annular eruption in infancy call for an **Anti-SSA/Ro antibody** level. This antibody is the specific marker for neonatal lupus erythematosus which can present as an annular erythema. It is found in 100% of cases whereas the ANA is positive in only a third of the cases.

Comment is directed to a half dozen cases of ill-defined annular erythema in the literature in which an anti-Ro antibody determination might have provided a specific diagnosis of **neonatal lupus erythematosus**.

McCune AB, Weston WL, Lee LA: Maternal and fetal outcome in **neonatal lupus erythematosus**. Ann Intern Med 1987; 106:518–523.

Infants with **neonatal lupus erythematosus** have either subacute cutaneous lupus or third degree congenital heart block, or both. Most infants with skin lesions are female. Skin lesions resolve at about 6 months of age, and infants with skin manifestations alone have a good prognosis.

Infants with **congenital heart block** may die in infancy, but those who survive do well in early childhood, often wearing pacemakers. The long-term prognosis is unknown, although a few cases have eventuated in systemic lupus erythematosus.

Neonatal lupus is associated with the transplacental passage of anti-SSA/Ro antibodies, present in over 95% of affected infants.

In this large series of 21 families with 24 cases of neonatal lupus, 10 had skin lesions only, 12 had heart block only, 2 had both findings, and 3 died during the neonatal period. Most mothers (18/21) eventually developed signs of collagen disease but did not have a higher risk of spontaneous abortion. There was a 25% risk of having a second child with neonatal lupus.

Kikuchi I, Ogata K, Inoue S: **Pityrosporum infection** in an infant with lesions resembling erythema annulare centrifugum. Arch Dermatol 1984; 120:380–382.

This 2-month-old baby girl had erythematous round and **gyrate lesions** on her face, trunk, arms, and legs. There was central clearing with a suggestion of central atrophy. Two older siblings who had similar eruptions, one requiring hospitalization, had been diagnosed as having eczema.

A scraping showed *Pityrosporum ovale* organisms which were subsequently cultured on Sabourard-olive oil medium. A diagnosis of generalized tinea versicolor was made. Although clotrimazole ointment produced a cure in 2 weeks, postinflammatory annular depigmentation was still to be seen in the sites 7 months later.

The **differential diagnosis** included:

Erythema annulare centrifugum–Can be id reaction to tinea
Erythema gyratum atrophicans transiens neonatale–May be variant of erythema annulare centrifugum
Annular erythema of infancy–Cycles from erythematous papules to rings in 48 hours
Neonatal lupus erythematosus–Mother has lupus

Kalter DC, Griffiths WA, Atherton DJ: Linear and whorled **nevoid hypermelanosis**. J Am Acad Dermatol 1988; 19:1037–1044.

A few days after birth this infant girl developed brown streaks on her ankles. The hyperpigmentation spread, stabilizing at 1 year at which time it involved most of her body asymmetrically. There was no preceding inflammatory change at any time nor did she exhibit abnormalities of teeth, hair, or dermatoglyphics. The mucous membranes, eyes, palms, and soles were spared.

When she was 6, examination revealed **patterned streaks and whorls** of hyperpigmentation following Blaschko's lines. The streaks were made up of clusters of 1- to 5-mm light-brown macules. Biopsy showed basal cell hyperpigmentation. A diagnosis of linear and whorled **nevoid hypermelanosis** was made.

Note that the pigment was not distributed in a zosteriform fashion nor was it dermatomal. Rather it brought to mind the lines of Blaschko. This reticulate pigmentary disorder must be **distinguished from**

incontinentia pigmenti–preceded by bullous or even verrucous phase
epidermal nevi–become papillomatous and hyperkeratotic
hypomelanosis of Ito–reverse pattern showing "marble cake" leukoderma.

Also shows associated genetic anomalies of hair, teeth, eye, muscle, central nervous system

Chimerism—indicates melanocytes from two different zygotes, i.e., cell lines. May present in flaglike rectangular pattern, round café au lait lesions, striate patterns.

Blaschko's lines were a pragmatic derivative of painstakingly mapping out on a doll the patterns seen in 83 patients with linear nevoid anomalies. They are not a cutaneous representation of nerve, vessel, or lymphatic distribution. There was no relation to Langer's or Voigt's lines. They are not based on known anatomic landmarks but rather on the patterns of clinical experience.

Fox JD, Briggs M, Ward PA, Tedder RS: **Human herpesvirus 6** in salivary glands. Lancet 1990; 336:590–593.

Roseola infantum (exanthem subitum) is a special herpetic infection of infancy. It is caused by the **human herpesvirus 6 (HHV6)** and antibodies to it are found in nearly all adults.

This paper shows that the causative virus replicates in salivary tissue, persisting into the adult life of a previously infected individual. In turn, the disease is passed from these individuals to infants under the age of a year. Their sporadic shedding of virus explains why roseola infantum does not come in epidemics but rather as sporadic cases.

Herpes 6 joins Herpes 1 and 2 as fellow viruses who travel kiss-wise.

Better diagnosticians are better clinicians.

Vesiculobullous

Frieden IJ: **Blisters and pustules** in the newborn. Curr Prob Pediatr 1989; 19:551–614.

Blisters and pustules on newborn skin are scary and get our attention. This is the best guide we have seen. It reminds you not to forget that pustules may lead to a diagnosis of:

miliaria
neonatal acne
acropustulosis of infancy
histiocytosis X

eosinophilic folliculitis
incontinentia pigmenti
hyperimmunoglobulin E syndrome

When you see bullae you are reminded to think of:

bullous impetigo
congenital syphilis
sucking blisters

mastocytosis
protein C deficiency

When you see erosions you are reminded to think of:

scalded skin syndrome
streptococcal infection
epidermolysis bullosa

congenital syphilis
aplasia cutis

And it has a differential list of 37 diagnoses with 182 references to help you think more.

Guill MA, Aton JK, Rogers RB: **Neonatal herpes simplex** associated with fetal scalp monitor. J Am Acad Dermatol 1982; 7:408–409.

On the fifth day of life this infant girl was noted to have a grouped vesicular eruption of the crown of the scalp.

The vesicles were at the exact site that a spiral intrauterine fetal heart rate monitor had been screwed into her skin during delivery.

Culture of the vesicular fluid revealed herpes simplex type II. The child recovered without any dissemination of the infection.

Harris HH, Foucar E, Andersen RD, Ray TL: **Intrauterine herpes simplex infection** resembling mechanobullous disease in a newborn infant. J Am Acad Dermatol 1986; 15:1148–1155.

Scars and bullae covered 60% of the skin surface of this infant boy at the time of his birth by cesarean section. The bullae showed no evidence of herpes simplex virus infection by Tzanck smear, culture, or biopsy.

Clinically, the depressed scars with well-defined borders suggested a diagnosis of epidermolysis bullosa or aplasia cutis congenita. However, on day 3 new bullae appeared which showed **herpes simplex virus type II** infection (Tzanck smear for multinucleated giant cells and a frozen section of vesicle were both positive with monoclonal antibody stain for herpes simplex antigen). The viral culture was also positive.

A diagnosis of **intrauterine herpes simplex infection** was made. The infection could be precisely dated to the 14th week of gestation when the mother had noticed grouped erythematous vesicles of the vulva, shown on culture to be caused by herpes simplex type 2. There was an associated malaise, myalgia, and dysuria. The infection was acquired at that time rather than perinatally, since delivery was made by cesarean through intact membranes at a time when the mother had no lesions and a negative viral culture of the cervix.

The initial failure on day 1 to demonstrate the infant's herpes suggests that the lesions were old and hence sterile.

Blatt J, Kastner O, Hodes DS: Cutaneous vesicles in **congenital cytomegalovirus infection**. J Pediatr 1978; 92:509.

A newborn black infant, who had hepatomegaly and icterus at birth, had two **vesicles**, 2 mm in diameter, on the forehead.

Bacterial cultures of vesicle fluid were negative, but **viral cultures** on WI-38 cells (human fibroblasts) produced characteristic cytopathic effects of **cytomegalovirus**. Positive CMV cultures were also obtained from saliva and urine. The infant's complement fixation CMV titer was 1:128, while the mother's CMV titer was 1:64. HSV titers were 1:8 in both the infant and the mother.

CMV infection should be considered, along with herpes simplex infection, in neonates who have vesicles.

Laude TA, Rajkumar S: **Herpes zoster** in a 4-month-old infant. Arch Dermatol 1980; 116:160.

Grouped vesicles on an erythematous base had been present for 3 days in this 4-month-old baby boy. The lesions were seen only on the right side of the chest and were in the T6 and T7 dermatomes.

A diagnosis of **herpes zoster** was made. Confirmatory evidence included the fact that his varicella-zoster virus antibodies rose from an initial level of less than 1:4 to one of 1:16 at 18 days. Treatment was withheld and the lesions healed after 2 weeks.

The unique feature here was the fact that the infant had no prior history of having had **varicella**. However, the mother had had varicella in the 6th month of her pregnancy. It is likely the infant had at that time "fetal" varicella and his immature immune system failed to provide him with the usual lifelong immunity. Accordingly, a trigger factor such as the upper respiratory infection he had had at the initial visit accounted for his "infantile" herpes zoster.

Some things can come too early in life.

Bonifazi E, Rigillo N, DeSimone B, Meneghini CL: **Acquired dermatitis** due to zinc deficiency in a premature infant. Acta Derm Venereol 1980; 60:449–451.

At 2 months of age this premature infant developed what looked like a burn in the diaper area. Bacteriologic and mycologic studies were negative. Multivitamin and iron therapy had no effect. Within 10 days these well-marginated **burnlike lesions** spread down the thighs and appeared on the elbows and knees. Later, the backs of the fingers and toes, as well as the corners of the mouth and eyes, were involved.

It became a diagnostic puzzle. Zinc deficiency was considered, yet the child was taking a zinc-enriched milk formula and had no alopecia or diarrhea. Only after a plasma zinc level proved to be low (80 μg/100 ml vs a normal of 108 ± 15 μg/100 ml) was the diagnosis of **zinc deficiency dermatitis** made.

Zinc sulfate (15 mg tid) therapy led to a dramatic convincing resolution of the lesions within 48 hours.

Getting a zinc level will raise the level of your competence in dealing with an unusual dermatitis in premature babies, alcoholics, and the malnourished.

Leung A: **Toxic epidermal necrolysis** associated with maternal use of heparin. JAMA 1985; 253:201.

A newborn baby boy was erythematous with **superficial blisters** on the face and trunk. His skin peeled after 48 hours and a Nikolsky sign was positive.

Bacterial, fungal, and viral cultures were negative. Heparin was thought to be the cause of the necrolysis as his mother had received intravenous **heparin** for 2 weeks before his birth to treat an iliofemoral venous thrombosis.

Hashimoto K, Burk JD, Bale GF et al: **Transient bullous dermolysis** of the newborn: Two additional cases. J Am Acad Dermatol 1989; 21:708–713.

Within 2 days of birth this healthy newborn had numerous **vesicles and bullae** on the chest and hands. New blisters appeared with decreasing frequency over the next 4 months. Complete healing followed with hypopigmentation but no scarring.

A biopsy showed a subepidermal blister that on periodic acid Schiff staining showed the basement membrane in the roof of the blister. Under electron microscopy, unique stellate inclusion bodies were found within vesicles in the basal cell layer of keratinocytes.

The limitation of the process to the first few months of life made the diagnosis of **transient bullous dermolysis of the newborn**.

Benson PF, Rankin GLS, Rippey JJ: An outbreak of **exfoliative dermatitis** of the newborn (Ritter's disease) due to *Staphylococcus aureus*, phage-type 55/71. Lancet 1962; 1:999–1002.

During a 5-day period in January in a maternity ward, 4 newborn infants developed **Ritter's disease (pemphigus neonatorum)**, which began with erythema and **peeling of the fingers** in 3 infants. Erythema then appeared elsewhere (no definite pattern) followed by generalized desquamation, which appeared first in areas of friction such as the heels. Large sheets of skin could be peeled off easily with gentle pressure, leaving red glazed areas (Nikolsky's sign). In the 4th infant, bullous impetigo of the face, neck, and ears was followed within 24 hours by generalized exfoliation and a positive Nikolsky's sign. **Bullous impetigo** also occurred in 5 other infants, conjunctivitis in 2 infants, and paronychia in 1 infant. The **causative organism**, *Staphylococcus aureus* phage-type 55/71, was isolated from 15 of 49 infants (31%), including umbilical and nasal carriers. It was first detected in the milk of a mother with mastitis 2 weeks before the epidemic.

Gupta AK, Rasmussen JE, Headington JT: Extensive **congenital erosions and vesicles** healing with reticulate scarring. J Am Acad Dermatol 1987; 17:369–376.

Nearly the entire skin surface of this 8-year-old boy was covered with extensive **reticulate scarring**. Only the face, palms, and soles were exempt. Even the upper surface of the tongue was scarred.

The history disclosed that at birth he was covered with vesicles and erosions that healed in a few weeks, leaving this residue. Patients such as he (now numbering five) suffer heat intolerance due to an associated **anhidrosis**. Fevers of 40°C were not uncommon and were simply the result of hot weather.

The uniqueness of this congenital dermatosis of unknown origin was evident in considering the **differential**:

> Dermal hypoplasia (Goltz) syndrome—patients show linear areas of hypoplasia, not scars
> Poikiloderma congenitale (Rothmund-Thomson)—face involved, dyschromia
> Dyskeratosis congenita—reticular pigmentation
> Acrodermatitis chronica atrophicans—over extremities, spirochaetal cause
> Atrophoderma of Pasini and Pierini
> Linear scleroderma

Aplasia cutis congenita–sharply marginated, raw defects present at birth–gives sharply demarcated scar

Bart's syndrome–congenital aplasia of skin of extremities

Kamei R, Honig PJ: **Neonatal Job's syndrome** featuring a vesicular eruption. Pediatr Dermatol 1988; 5:75–82.

A **vesicular rash** on the hands and feet of this newborn led to a 3-week course of acyclovir and antibiotics despite negative Tzanck smears and negative bacterial and viral cultures. The rash continued as single grouped and confluent clear vesicles on inflamed skin. It progressed to involve the face. The only diagnostic clue was persistent eosinophilia (as high as 4750/mm^3).

Hospitalization at 7 weeks of age and 8 months of age for fever, diarrhea, otitis externa, hepatosplenomegaly, and a weeping vesicular rash of the scalp permitted the diagnosis of **hyperimmunoglobulinemia E**, or **Job's syndrome**.

When he was 11 months of age, his IgE levels were above 10,000 IU/ml and *Staphylococcus aureus* specific IgE antibody was markedly elevated (50% of total radioactivity where normal is less than 10%).

At 2 years he had to be treated with intravenous cefuroxime for a pulmonary abscess. At that time his IgE levels was 65,000 IU.

Job's syndrome was named after the biblical Job, who was cursed by Satan to have boils from head to toe. It is difficult to make the diagnosis early, but remember that vesicles may be the presenting sign. Thus it should enter your **differential** of herpes simplex, varicella, histiocytosis X, and incontinentia pigmenti.

Mascola L, Pelos R, Blount JH et al: **Congenital syphilis** revisited. Am J Dis Child 1985; 575–580.

In 1982, 50 cases of early **congenital syphilis** were reported in Texas. Approximately 60% were symptomatic at birth, with 40% having either skin lesions, prematurity, low birth weight, or hepatosplenomegaly. Jaundice, snuffles, and mucous patches were infrequent.

Screening tests:

quantitative serum test for syphilis	x-rays of long bones
serum IgM	darkfield microscopy
CSF VDRL	

Fenske NA, Lober CW, Pautler SE: **Congenital bullous urticaria pigmentosa**. Treatment with concomitant use of H$_1$- and H$_2$-receptor antagonists. Arch Dermatol 1985; 121:115–118.

A baby boy was born covered with **bullae, erosions, and hyperpigmented macules** over all body surfaces. His eyelids were swollen and blisters were seen even on the palms and soles. Denuded blister bases were also present. A positive **Darier's sign** suggested the diagnosis of **urticaria pigmentosa**, which was promptly confirmed by a skin biopsy showing a dense infiltrate of Giemsa-stained mast cells throughout the dermis.

In his first year of life, episodes of *Staphylococcus aureus* septicemia and seizures necessitated multiple hospitalizations. Subsequently, it was found that concurrent cimetidine and cyproheptadine therapy gave good clinical control.

Patients with this massive leukemic-like cutaneous infiltrate of mast cells are at risk for hypotension, shock, and convulsions due to **histamine release**. This may be particularly true during the trauma of delivery.

Fisher GB, Greer KE, Cooper PH: Congenital self-healing (transient) **mechanobullous dermatosis**. Arch Dermatol 1988; 124:240–243.

When a newborn baby develops **blistering of the skin** from mechanical trauma, the diagnosis is usually either epidermolysis bullosa or bullous mastocytosis. However, at times this classification is not so clear-cut, as demonstrated in a case presumptive of dystrophic epidermolysis bullosa with spontaneous remission after 4 months. Awareness of the existence of this condition is important since it offers the hope of a future with blister-free skin.

A 5-day-old boy had erosions and blisters of the arms, legs, and face, as well as denudation of the tongue and gingivae. Dystrophy of a few nails and scarring of the right leg and foot were also noted. Minimal trauma produced more blisters. Skin biopsy was consistent with the recessive form of **dystrophic epidermolysis bullosa**, and electron microscopy revealed subepidermal separation below the basal lamina. Conservative supportive treatment with zinc oxide ointment, antibiotic ointment, a mist environment, and low-dose phenytoin (15 mg/day) was followed by healing with fine reticulate scarring and milia. After age 4 months the skin remained blister free, although the nails remained dystrophic and the tongue denuded.

This boy's problem is viewed as self-healing **mechanobullous dermatosis**, which most likely falls within the scope of dystrophic epidermolysis bullosa. The absence of skin at birth probably represents blister formation and epidermal shedding in utero. A number of other examples are cited from the literature. Sometimes it may represent a dominantly inherited disorder (**Bart's syndrome**).

Tamaki K, Igarashi A, Nakamura K-i, et al: **Bullous pemphigoid** of childhood: Immunofluorescent investigation. J Dermatol 1988; 15:400–404.

A 4-month-old healthy Japanese girl had the sudden onset of **vesicles** and **bullae** over her hands, forearms, and feet. Some of the lesions were grouped. Treatment with topical steroids cleared the disease after 3 weeks.

Skin biopsy revealed a subepidermal bulla with mononuclear cells and eosinophils in the blister space. In addition, there was a moderately dense superficial perivascular infiltrate of lymphocytes and eosinophils. Direct immunofluorescence revealed linear IgG and C3 along the basement membrane zone of peribullous skin. There was no IgA or IgM present. Indirect immunofluorescence revealed circulating IgG anti-basement membrane zone antibodies at a titer of 1:180. Serum from her mother was negative for autoantibodies.

Further investigation after epidermal separation with NaCl showed that the immunofluorescent antigen localized on the epidermal side of the skin (characteristic of **bullous pemphigoid** antigen), not on the dermal side as with epidermolysis bullosa antigen.

Detlefs RL, Frieden IJ, Berger TG, Westrom D: **Eosinophil fluorescence**: A cause of false positive slide tests for herpes simplex virus. Pediatr Dermatol 1987; 4:129–133.

Two neonates with **vesicular eruptions** were erroneously diagnosed as having herpes simplex infections because of false-positive results of the new immunofluorescent slide test. The infants proved to have vesicular lesions of **incontinentia pigmenti** and **histiocytosis X**, respectively.

In such cases the multiple eosinophils in the lesions were the source of the error. The basic proteins of eosinophil granules bind with the fluorescein-labeled herpes antibody giving a nonspecific, hence false-positive, reading.

Elpern DJ: **Infantile acropustulosis** and antecedent scabies. J Am Acad Dermatol 1984; 11:895.

Seven cases of **infantile acropustulosis** in nonwhite infants and young children were really examples of **scabies**, confirmed in five cases by either positive scrapings or a positive family history.

Babies with pustules of the hands and feet often are "babies with scabies."

Okada DM, Chow AW, Bruce VT: **Neonatal scalp abscess** and fetal monitoring: Factors associated with infection. Am J Obstet Gynecol 1977; 129:185–189.

Direct **fetal heart rate monitoring** with a spiral electrode in the scalp is associated with **scalp abscess** in about 5% of neonates. The abscess is usually a 5-mm fluctuant mass from which pus can be expressed. The infection tends to be polymicrobial, containing both aerobes (*Staphylococcus epidermidis, Streptococcus*) and anaerobes (*Peptostreptococcus, Peptococcus, Bacteroides*).

In this study of 929 neonates who were monitored in Los Angeles, the major factors associated with scalp infection included prematurity and the duration of monitoring (6 hours, compared to 4 hours in the noninfected group).

Kahana M, Schewach-Millet M, Feinstein A: Infantile acropustulosis—report of a case. Clin Exp Dermatol 1987; 12:291–292.

A 10-month-old boy in Israel had 5 months of recurrent bouts of a pruritic **vesiculopustular rash** on the palms and soles. The crops came every 2 to 3 weeks and lasted 1 to 2 weeks. Biopsy showed an intraepidermal subcorneal pustule filled with neutrophils. By the age of 16 months the attacks were milder and less frequent.

Impetigo was ruled out by negative cultures, negative Gram stain, and no response to antibiotic therapy. Scabies was eliminated by negative skin scrapings and failure to respond to scabicide therapy. Dyshidrotic eczema is rare in infants and would have shown vesicles—not subcorneal pustules—on biopsy.

The diagnosis was **infantile acropustulosis**, a disease of unknown etiology but benign course that spontaneously remits at 2 to 3 years of age. It is unresponsive to antibiotics, scabicides, and mild topical steroids but does improve with dapsone (2 mg/kg/day).

Vignon-Pennamen M-D, Wallach D: **Infantile acropustulosis**. A clinicopathologic study of 6 cases. Arch Dermatol 1986; 122:1155–1160.

Little pustules on little hands and feet suggest the syndrome of **infantile acropustulosis**.

Crops of tiny **pruritic red papules** of the hands and feet (palms, soles, dorsal surfaces) within hours become papulovesicles filled with neutrophils and/or eosinophils, but no bacteria. Cultures of all types are frustratingly negative. New crops appear every 2 to 3 weeks for a few years, after which the process abates.

Skin biopsies reveal an intraepidermal pustule that progresses to a subcorneal pustule and then an intracorneal pustule. The **differential diagnosis** is daunting:

Scabies (skin scrapings positive)

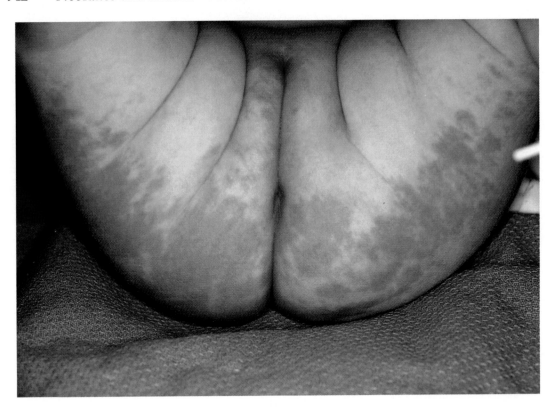

Dyshidrotic eczema (deep-seated vesicles)
Impetigo (gram-positive)
Candidiasis (PAS-positive)
Erythema neonatorum toxicum (first 2 weeks of life, usually on trunk, lasts only a few days, no relapse)
Transient neonatal pustular melanosis (present at birth, occurs on face and back, resolves spontaneously by age 3 months)
Subcorneal pustular dermatosis (rare in children)
Pustular psoriasis (psoriasis usually present elsewhere)
Pustular bacterid (not seen in children)

Newton JA, Salisbury J, Marsden A, McGibbon DH: **Acropustulosis** of infancy. Br J Dermatol 1986; 115:735–739.

Intensely pruritic papules, vesicles, and pustules may appear in crops on the hands and feet of black baby boys during the first year of life. Histologically, one finds an intraepithelial or subcorneal neutrophilic pustule, at times also showing an eosinophil infiltrate.

The eruption is of unknown origin and tends to spontaneously resolve within a year or two. Sulfapyridine is helpful. Always, scabies must be ruled out because of its similarity.

Bilinski DL, Ehrenkranz RA, Cooley-Jacobs J, McGuire J: **Symptomatic zinc deficiency** in a breast-fed, premature infant. Arch Dermatol 1987; 123:1221–1224.

At age 6 months, this premature infant girl developed an erythematous,

erosive plaque in the perioral and perinasal area. There was serous exudate and crusting. Peripherally, fine scaling and satellite pustules were present. Small vesicles of the dorsa of the fingers and toes were seen as well as friable white plaques of the tongue and buccal mucosa. Within 5 days the rash extended to involve the nail folds and perineal skin.

A diagnosis of **zinc deficiency dermatitis** was confirmed by a serum zinc level of 2.3 μmol/liter (normal 8.4 to 22.9 μmol/liter). Within 48 hours of administration of 5 mg zinc orally twice/day, there was noticeable improvement in the rash. The skin had completely returned to normal within one week.

This child's gestational age of 25 weeks is similar to that in 8 previously reported cases of transient zinc deficiency in breast-fed premature infants. These infants are in negative zinc balance for 2 months. Furthermore, they have a decreased ability to absorb zinc from the gut. Although breast milk provides adequate zinc for the normal infant, the premature infant needs zinc supplementation.

Note that the dermatitis usually appears at the age of 2 to 3 months. All were cleared within one week of zinc therapy.

The concentration of zinc in human milk falls throughout lactation. The previously reported cases were associated with maternal breast milk zinc levels that were low. However, this patient's mother's milk had normal zinc levels.

Lavoie A, Rottem M, Grodofsky MP, Douglas SD: Anti-*Staphylococcus aureus* IgE antibodies for diagnosis of **hyperimmunoglobulinemia E-recurrent infection syndrome** in infancy. Am J Dis Child 1989; 143:1038–1041.

Since 3 weeks of age, this black female neonate had had a **papular** and **pustular eruption** over her face as well as a diaper rash. By 6 weeks of age, the eruption had spread to her scalp and back as oozing crusted eczematoid dermatitis. Cultures of the scalp lesions revealed the presence of *S. aureus* and streptococci. Blood studies showed eosinophilia. Although dicloxacillin therapy partially allayed the dermatitis by 6 months, the pruritic papulovesicular eruption was in full force.

At this time her IgE level was 19,200 μg/liter (normal below 24 μg/liter) and her anti-*Staphylococcus aureus* IgE antibodies were also high (binding 24%, normal less than 10%).

The elevated eosinophil count could help make the diagnosis; the markedly elevated IgE levels in a child with multiple infections confirmed the diagnosis of the **hyperimmunoglobulin E recurrent infection syndrome**. The elevated anti-*S. aureus* IgE antibodies have not been detected in atopic dermatitis, parasitic infections, or in chronic or recurrent staphylococcal infections in normal individuals.

Delayed recognition is better than no recognition at all.

Papular or Nodular

Burns BR, Lampe RM, Hansen GH: **Neonatal scabies**. Am J Dis Child 1979; 133:1031–1034.

A 26-day-old girl had a papular rash on the anterior chest, associated with poor feeding and failure to gain weight. At 5 weeks of age she was very agitated and had an erythematous papulosquamous eruption of the entire trunk arms, legs, perineum, neck, and face. **Numerous pustules** were present on the trunk and proximal extremities, with cultures yielding *Staphylococcus aureus*. Despite treatment with oral dicloxacillin, the rash progressed to involve the palms, soles, cheeks, nasolabial folds, and postauricular areas. The perineum was cracked and peeling. A Gram stain again disclosed gram-positive cocci, and the baby was hospitalized to be given intravenous antibiotics. **Scrapings** disclosed adult scabies mites and eggs. History then revealed that both parents had a pruritic papular eruption several months before the birth of the child, and scrapings were positive from papules on the mother's wrist. Three applications of crotamiton sulfate over 3 weeks were needed for cure.

Similar lesions were seen in four other young infants with consistent involvement of the face, neck, scalp, palms, and soles. Erythematous papules, nodular crusts, and pustules were associated with poor feeding and failure to gain weight.

Examination of **close contacts**, including parents, siblings, housekeepers, and babysitters always revealed others with scabies. A careful history should also help lead to the correct diagnosis.

Ogino A, Ishida H: Spontaneous regression of generalized **molluscum contagiosum** turning black. Acta Derm Venereol 1984; 64:83–86.

Approximately 650 tiny pearly delled papules covered the back and buttocks of a 15-month-old Japanese male infant who also had mild atopic dermatitis. **Molluscum contagiosum** was diagnosed and treatment was begun with 5% sulfadiazine paste. In the ensuing 3 months the papules became more numerous but showed local inflammatory changes with erythematous halos. The central dell turned black, and then each black molluscum papule flattened and disappeared. Four months after the initial visit almost all of the papules had regressed, leaving slightly elevated scars.

This **cell-mediated involution** was considered similar to the hyperacute rejection of a kidney transplant. The black color was indicative of necrosis of the infected keratinocytes, which occurred along with thrombosis of small dermal blood vessels and hemorrhage into the lesions.

Even as with warts, the "black sign" is a good sign.

Lee CW, Park MH, Lee H: Recurrent cutaneous **Langerhans cell histiocytosis** in infancy. Br J Dermatol 1988; 119:259–265.

A 9-month-old baby girl developed approximately 40 **brown papules** on her abdomen and back at the age of 4 months, which involuted within 3 weeks leaving slightly atrophic white spots. A new crop of reddish-brown papules, vesicles, and crusts developed 5 months later. Histologic, immunochemical, and electron microscopy studies confirmed the diagnosis of **Langerhans cell histiocytosis (LCH)**. Numerous studies failed to reveal any internal disease, and within a few months the lesions had cleared completely. She remained well at follow-up after 22 months. A similar case is presented in a 4-month-old baby girl, who remained well after 24 months.

This is a benign form of histiocytosis X, which remains localized to the skin.

It is a member of the Langerhans cell proliferative disease family (Letterer-Siwe disease, Hand-Schüller-Christian disease, and eosinophilic granuloma) which affect not only the skin but also the internal organs.

It is comforting to realize that for every malignant disease there is a mimic that is benign.

Kapila PK, Grant-Kels JM, Allred C et al: Congenital, spontaneously regressing **histiocytosis**: Case report and review of the literature. Pediatr Dermatol 1985; 2:312–317.

A 1-day-old girl had been born with numerous widespread small purpuric indurated red to **purple papules and nodules** scattered over the face and scalp, with a less dense distribution over the trunk, extremities, and soles. Some lesions had fissuring and erosions, and a 1.0 × 0.5 cm deeply ulcerated area with a raised beefy border was present in the left groin. There was no lymphadenopathy or hepatosplenomegaly. The lesions regressed spontaneously without scarring and had completely disappeared by age 3 months. Skin biopsy revealed **histiocytosis X**.

The diagnostic criteria for self-healing histiocytosis X include:

1. Congenital or perinatal brown or dusty red nodules that resolve spontaneously.
2. Dermal infiltration of large histiocytes with eosinophilic cytoplasm containing PAS-negative, diastase-resistant inclusions.
3. Mixed dermal infiltrate containing eosinophils.
4. Electron microscopy showing Langerhans granules in 10 to 25% of the large atypical cells.

Messenger GG, Kamei R, Honig PJ: **Histiocytosis X** resembling cherry angiomas. Pediatr Dermatol 1985; 3:75–78.

A 4-month-old white boy with failure to thrive developed multiple 1 to 3 mm erythematous papular lesions resembling **cherry angiomas** with little scaling on his trunk. Initially he was thought to have diffuse neonatal hemangiomatosis. However, skin biopsy revealed **histiocytosis X**. Over several days more typical lesions of histiocytosis X appeared. No treatment was given except for nasogastric supplementation, and at 1 year of age the skin lesions had resolved. A second similar case is also presented. Capillary hemangiomas thus join the long list of skin lesions in histiocytosis X.

Pujol RM, Lloveras B: A newborn with a **solitary nodule** on the scalp. Arch Dermatol 1987; 123:1392–1395.

A solitary firm, erythematous **rubbery nodule** of the right side of the scalp was noted when this healthy baby boy was born.

Excision of the tumor when he was 2 months old showed histologically that it was an example of infantile **myofibromatosis**.

This tumor is a benign overgrowth of the contractile myofibroblast. It is usually solitary, occurring in the first 2 years of life. Although spontaneous regression has been described, surgical excision is generally done; the rate of recurrence is low.

Jensen AR, Martin LW, Longino LA: **Digital neurofibrosarcoma** in infancy. J Pediatr 1957; 51:566–570.

These innocuous-appearing nontender **pea-sized firm nodules**, which are glistening and skin-colored, appear on the fingers or toes in the first few months of life and grow very slowly. Usually multiple, they are located on the dorsal or lateral surface of the distal phalanx. Recurrence after excision is common, and histologically they closely resemble **dermatofibrosarcoma protuberans**.

Avril MF, Mathieu A, Kalifa C, Caillou C: **Infantile choriocarcinoma** with cutaneous tumors: An additional case and review of the literature. J Am Acad Dermatol 1986; 14:918–927.

This newborn girl had lesions over her entire skin. Some were pink papules, others black necrotic papules, and others were **crusted nodules**.

Examination of the placenta had shown a large white growth on the uterine surface. This gave clue to the newborn's problem; on biopsy it was a choriocarcinoma. Biopsies of the infant's skin tumors confirmed the presence of **metastatic choriocarcinoma**. As suspected, her serum human chorionic gonadotrophin level was very high (350,000 IU/L). Widespread metastasis led to the baby's death within the month, despite chemotherapy.

Neff FC, Tice G, Walker GA, Ockerblad N: **Adrenal tumor** in female infant with hypertrichosis, hypertension, overdevelopment of external genitalia, obesity, but absence of breast enlargement. J Clin Endocrinol Metab 1942; 2:125–127.

A 16-month-old girl developed **acne**, hypertrophied labia, and generalized hypertrichosis beginning at age 8 months. Hair growth was heaviest over the back, shoulders, axillae, and genitalia. Her blood pressure was 200/110. A **tumor mass palpable** above the left kidney was a 6 cm medullary tumor (chromaffinoma or **pheochromocytoma**), and its removal led to clearing of her problems within 3 months.

Medullary tumors usually cause paroxysmal hypertension, and cortical tumors cause precocious male characteristics. Cortical tumors occasionally cause feminization with gynecomastia, atrophy of penis and testes, loss of libido, and obesity.

Every diagnosis you make increases the diagnostic capability of your intracranial computer.

Rogers M, Kan A, Stapleton K, Kemp A: **Giant centrifugal miliaria profunda**. Pediatr Dermatol 1990; 7:140–146.

Rapidly enlarging **white plaques** developed on the hands, feet, and ankles of this 4-month-old boy during hospitalization for respiratory distress. Each lesion was at the site where adhesive tape had been applied for several days.

As the lesions grew, the center became depressed and yellowish, evolving into large doughnut-like lesions. Massive in size, 2 or 3 lesions spanned the dorsum of the hand or foot. There was a peripheral zone of erythema. By 3 weeks the lesions became crusted and sooner or later exfoliated, leaving normal skin. There were no recurrences despite a second hospitalization for bronchiolitis at age 13 months.

The finding of **miliaria profunda–like changes on biopsy** led to the diagnosis of giant centrifugal miliaria profunda. It has not been previously described but points up another hazard of adhesive tape for infant skin.

Rudolph RI: **Facial sporotrichosis** in an infant. Cutis 1984; 33:171–178.

A solitary 2.5 cm **crusted red plaque** was present on the **forehead** of this 18-month-old boy. It had begun 6 weeks before as a "blind pimple" which showed no response to systemic erythromycin or topical steroids. No satellite lesions were present nor were any lymph nodes palpable. There was no known trauma to the area.

A KOH preparation showed "spaghetti-like" hyphae suggesting a diagnosis of fungal infection. However, oral antifungal therapy was without effect as the lesion grew and became granulomatous.

On biopsy, yeast forms were sighted in the PAS-stained section. A **culture** of *Sporotrichum schenkii* was then grown, making the diagnosis of **sporotrichosis**. Three months of saturated solution of potassium iodide (5 drops 3 times a day) cleared the lesion.

The mother's memory was focused by the diagnosis; she remembered that her son had **stopped to smell the roses** in her garden a few months before. It was there his little bobbing head had obviously met a fungal-tipped thorn.

You will get the best history when you scatter cues, hints, and suggestions all along your patient's memory lane.

Induration

Norwood-Galloway A, Lebwohl M, Phelps RG, Raucher H: **Subcutaneous fat necrosis** of the newborn with hypercalcemia. J Am Acad Dermatol 1987; 16:435–439.

Generalized induration of the skin was noted at the time of birth of this baby boy. By 2 weeks, prominent indurated plaques were seen on both thighs. These were surmounted by fluctuant erythematous nodules, which on aspiration produced sterile viscous, white fluid. A biopsy showed necrotic adipocytes, needle crystals, and foreign body giant cells. On the basis of these findings, a diagnosis of subcutaneous fat necrosis was made.

There was a gradual resolution, but at 2 months a health profile showed a serum calcium of 17.0 mg/dl. Intensive therapy for the hypercalcemia centered on intravenous fluids, furosemide, calcitonin, low-calcium diet, and avoidance of vitamin D. The calcium levels returned to normal and at 11 months the skin was essentially normal.

Subcutaneous fat necrosis is a rare disease in the newborn that requires monitoring for calcium. The necrosis may express itself as but a few painless, sharply circumscribed nodules or plaques over bony prominences, cheeks, arms, shoulders, buttocks, and thighs. The lesions are symmetric and may be red or purple in color but are not warm to the touch.

The differential diagnosis centers on

sclerema neonatorum   sclerema edematosum   scleroderma

The hypercalcemia sometimes seen associated with fat necrosis always demands attention because clinically it accounts for the infant showing irritability, hypertonia, and failure to thrive as well as nausea and vomiting.

Chen TH, Shewmake SW, Hansen DD, Lacey HL: **Subcutaneous fat necrosis** of the newborn: A case report. Arch Dermatol 1981; 117:36–37.

Widespread **erythematous plaques** appeared on the trunk and thighs of this 3-day-old infant. They were bright red, tender, and blanched completely on pressure. The subcutaneous tissue in the affected areas felt firm and had a woody consistency. It was not attached to the overlying skin. Within a few days fluctuant nodular areas were seen to develop. There was an antecedent history of intrauterine asphyxia.

A biopsy from an erythematous plaque revealed focal areas of fat necrosis, with fat cells containing needle-shaped crystals. A diagnosis of **subcutaneous fat necrosis of the newborn** was made. The differential diagnosis included scleredema neonatorum; however, clinically this is manifested by a distinctive generalized hidebound, indurated skin. Joint movement and facial expression is compromised, as well.

The subcutaneous fat necrosis experienced by this baby showed the typical spontaneous involution. By 3 weeks there had been an 80% resolution.

Heilbron B, Saxe N: **Scleredema** in an infant. Arch Dermatol 1986; 122:1417–1419.

The appearance of tight, shiny **bound-down skin** in a month-old premature infant was associated with the presence of bronchopneumonia and with proven cytomegalovirus infection.

The nonpitting edema present was shown on biopsy (using 0.05% cetylpyridinium chloride fixation) to be caused by deposition of acid mucopolysaccharides in the dermis. Strangely, these polysaccharides were not found on ordinary formaldehyde fixation.

A diagnosis of **scleredema** was made; the prognosis was considered good because of the association with a respiratory tract infection.

The cracked, peeling skin raised the possibility of congenital ichthyosis. However, the major problem was differentiating the scleredema from sclerema neonatorum. Sclerema neonatorum is frequently associated with prematurity and this patient was premature. However, a biopsy is critical for demonstration of needle-shaped clefts in the fat cells, the distinctive sign of sclerema neonatorum.

Subcutaneous fat necrosis is a problem much more focal, with violaceous nodules of fat necrosis. Finally, another look-alike, scleroderma, can also be ruled out histologically.

Fretzin DF, Arias AM: **Sclerema neonatorum** and subcutaneous fat necrosis of the newborn. Pediatr Dermatol 1987; 4:112–122.

Sclerema neonatorum presents as hard smooth white skin. It is an extremely rare entity affecting premature or debilitated infants during the first week of life. Any older infant who develops it will surely be suffering from severe systemic disease. The boardlike stiffness of the skin is due to rapid solidification of the subcutaneous fat. It begins on the calves, and rapidly spreads to involve almost the entire skin, exempting only palms, soles, and scrotum. It may be fatal, ending with septicemia.

The **differential diagnosis** centers on scleredema neonatorum and scleroderma of the newborn. Scleredema neonatorum also occurs in the premature infant or in feeble neonates with congenital cardiac and other anomalies. However, here the skin is edematous, distended, and waxy. Scleroderma is a disease of adults, being quite rare in infants. The **biopsy** quickly produces the correct diagnosis, sclerema being a subcutaneous disease, scleredema being a mucopolysaccharide-generated edema, and scleroderma being collagen disease with sclerosis of collagen replacing the fat.

Finally, **subcutaneous fat necrosis** of the newborn poses no diagnostic difficulty, since an affected full-term baby develops firm red to violaceous nodules in discrete sites on the buttocks, thighs, arms, or face. The masses, although of variable size, are symmetrical, freely movable, and often begin several weeks after a difficult labor as plaques of edema. Abscesses may form with drainage, yet the prognosis is good, with gradual resolution in a few months. From the differential standpoint, this subcutaneous fat necrosis may be mimicked by poststeroid panniculitis. Such panniculitis can be distinguished by obtaining a history of long-term, high-dose steroid administration to a child, which is ended abruptly.

Hironaga M, Fujigaki T, Tanaka S: **Cutaneous calcinosis** in a neonate following extravasation of calcium gluconate. J Am Acad Dermatol 1982; 6:392–395.

In a 6-day-old baby girl with tetany, **extravasation of 10% calcium gluconate** into the right dorsal hand led to localized purpura several hours later and swelling and erythematous induration the next day. Two weeks later, firm, well-marginated erythematous induration appeared, followed by small eschars that sloughed, revealing necrotic bases with tiny calcium deposits. **X-ray examination** revealed extensive platelike or linear calcification along fascial planes and vascular channels. Treatment with gauze debridement and EDTA soaks resulted in resorption of calcium and healing.

The irritant reaction to an inadvertent unobserved extravasation of intravenous 10% calcium gluconate is **easily misdiagnosed as cellulitis** or an abscess. With massive extravasation, there is marked swelling, erythema, soft tissue necrosis, eschar formation, and eventual calcification. Radiographs are of no help in diagnosis until 1 to 3 weeks later, when the radiolucent calcium solution becomes a radiopaque calcium phosphate precipitate.

Aplasia and Dysplasia

Frieden IJ: **Aplasia cutis congenita**: A clinical review and proposal for classification. J Am Acad Dermatol 1986; 14:646–660.

Aplasia cutis congenita is a clinical diagnosis made on the basis of the absence of localized or widespread areas of skin at birth. Thus it includes a heterogeneous group of disorders.

Categorization centers on descriptive findings.

1. Limited to scalp

   86% occur in this site
   Tremendous range in size and depth
   May extend to meninges
   Hazards: hemorrhage, thrombosis, meningitis
   May see prominent dilated scalp veins
   Shape: round, oval, rhomboidal, stellate, linear
   May be erosion or deep ulcer, scar, keloidal
   Can have appearance of blister when covered with membranous epithelium
   Hair is absent but adjacent skin may show hypertrichosis
   Spontaneous resolution usually occurs in infancy
   Isolated anomalies may also be found
         Cleft lip, tracheoesophageal fistula, mental retardation, cutis marmorata telangiectasia congenita
   Inheritance: autosomal/dominant

2. Scalp lesions with associated limb abnormalities

   Distal phalanges, hypoplastic or absent
   Distal limb absence
   Polydactyly, syndactyly

3. Associated with nevi

   Organoid nevi of scalp
   Epidermal nevi

4. Associated with underlying embryologic malformations

   Meningomyelocele
   Malformed spinal cord
   Occult spinal dysraphia

5. Associated with placental infarcts or fetus papyraceus

   Fetus papyraceus representing death of twin in utero in second trimester resulting in thrombosis problems for surviving twin
   Placental infarction
   Fibrous bands

6. Associated with epidermolysis bullosa

   Four forms of epidermolysis bullosa have been reported
   Mechanical trauma from fetal movements such as kicking may explain localization on legs (Bart's syndrome)

7. Localized to extremities but no blistering

   Could be example of placental infarct or fetus papyraceus

8. Caused by teratogens or infection

   Herpes simplex intrauterine infection
   Congenital varicella infection from mother at 15 weeks
   Methimazole, taken by mother to control thyrotoxicosis

9. Associated with syndromes of malformation

Trisomy 13
4p-syndrome
Ectodermal dysplasia
Ectrodactyly-ectodermal dysplasia syndrome
Miscellaneous dystrophies of all types
Early amniotic membrane rupture giving amniotic bands

In all cases of aplastic cutis congenita

Check placenta
Examine other family members
Check hair, teeth, nails, central nervous system
Check eyes, extremities
Give genetic counseling

Levin DL, Nolan KS, Esterly NB: **Congenital absence of skin**. J Am Acad Dermatol 1980; 2:203–206.

A 5-day-old girl had been born with **crusted stellate defects** of the vertex of the scalp and large linear defects that zigzagged across the sides of her chest. Congenital absence of skin was diagnosed. Follow-up at 5 months showed complete healing with scar formation.

Although usually involving the midline of the scalp near the vertex, other sites may also be involved. The defects are circular, elongated, and stellate or triangular, and present as an ulcer, bulla, or scar, sometimes covered with a tough transparent membrane. Lesions are usually symmetrical and limited to skin but occasionally involve muscle and bone. Fearsome **complications** include hemorrhage, meningitis, and secondary infection.

An isolated scalp ulcer also may represent trauma from a scalp electrode placed during labor. Trauma from an adherent amnion or true aplasia is another possibility. In this patient, the defect was probably of **vascular origin**, since the placenta showed an infarct and only one placental artery.

Glover MT, Atherton DJ: **Congenital infection** with herpes simplex virus type I. Pediatr Dermatol 1987; 4:336–340.

At birth this full-term baby boy exhibited large areas of **atrophy and erythema**. The scarring gave the skin a wrinkled appearance. Not until the fifth day of life was the diagnosis made. At this time a cluster of small vesicles appeared at the edge of an area of scarring.

Electron microscopy revealed herpes particles. A diagnosis of **herpes simplex** was made and treatment with acyclovir orally for 9 days aborted further lesions.

Later, HSV type I was cultured from clusters of tiny papular erythematous lesions. The scarring has remained, but early diagnosis averted progression and possible death.

It is important to note that herpes simplex can **scar in utero**. And how did the virus get into the uterus? Apparently, the mother had a primary oral herpetic infection between the eighth to tenth week of pregnancy.

Van Dijke CP, Heydendael RJ, De Kleine MJ: Methimazole, carbimazole, and **congenital skin defects**. Ann Intern Med 1987; 106:60–61.

A newborn baby had three sharply marginated **skin defects** covered with moist membranes at the center of the scalp. They closed spontaneously within 6 weeks and at 3 months only one bald patch remained. The baby's mother had taken **methimazole** (Tapazole) and thyroid hormone extract during pregnancy for treatment of hyperthyroidism.

Despite earlier reports linking methimazole with aplasia cutis, these authors prove statistically that the drug is not hazardous during pregnancy.

Bronspiegel N, Zelnick N, Rabinowitz H, Iancu TC: **Aplasia cutis congenita** and intestinal lymphangiectasia. Am J Dis Child 1985; 139:509–513.

Two brothers in Israel with **aplasia cutis congenita** had nonpitting edema of the legs at birth. One baby with a large defect of the parietal bones died of sagittal sinus hemorrhage at age 2 months. The other boy at age $3\frac{1}{2}$ years had generalized edema, diarrhea, and fatigue along with a 5×6 cm oval hairless cicatricial area over the vertex.

Intestinal lymphangiectasia causes hypoproteinemia, transient edema (periorbital, scrotal, legs), and lymphopenia. The diagnosis is confirmed with a barium swallow, jejunal biopsy, and increased fecal excretion of chromium 51-labeled albumin.

This article includes a table of congenital malformations associated with aplasia cutis congenita.

Magid ML, Prendiville JS, Esterly NB: **Focal facial dermal dysplasia**: Bitemporal lesions resembling aplasia cutis congenita. J Am Acad Dermatol 1988; 18:1203–1207.

A $4\frac{1}{2}$-month-old Mexican-American infant had congenital bilateral **atrophic areas over the temples**, without other facial anomalies. His family history was negative for similar lesions. One week previously he had developed an enlarging head due to bilateral subdural hematomas, probably from accidental trauma. The scars were sharply demarcated, atrophic, and slightly hyperpigmented. It was not aplasia cutis congenita, since there was no prior ulceration, and it was not due to child abuse with an injury such as a cigarette burn, since the biopsy showed no scarring but only atrophic skin with absence of adnexae.

Congenital bilateral depressed focal scarring of both temples has its own nosologic niche: **focal facial dermal dysplasia**. It has previously been described with diverse titles: hereditary symmetrical systematized aplastic nevi, congenital ectodermal dysplasia of the face, familial focal facial dermal dysplasia, and bitemporal aplasia cutis congenita. It is hereditary, being autosomal dominant in some families and probably autosomal recessive in others. Sometimes other facial anomalies are associated.

Shuttleworth D, Marks R: Epidermal dysplasia and skeletal deformity in **congenital poikiloderma** (Rothmund-Thomson syndrome). Br J Dermatol 1987; 117:377–384.

At age 3 months a baby girl developed an **erythematous rash of her face**, which within weeks spread to her arms, legs, and buttocks. By 6 months of age the erythematous skin was clearly poikilodermatous. The scalp hair density was reduced and the eyebrows were sparse, but her teeth and nails were normal. Her growth was retarded and she was below the third percentile for height and weight. At age 3 years bilateral deafness was noted in association with cholesteatoma. By age 4 years keratotic lesions had developed on her feet, knees, and elbows, making walking difficult. They recurred after curettage, and histology showed massive hyperkeratosis, acanthosis, "budding" of the basal epidermis, and bizarre dyskeratotic cells in the granular layer with large keratohyalin granules. Light testing showed no photosensitivity.

A sister showed similar changes as well as hypoplastic thumbs and an asymmetrical skull due to stenosis of the right coronal suture. Both girls represented the **Rothmund-Thomson syndrome**, an autosomal recessive disease. The parents were normal and not consanguineous.

These patients remain at risk for malignant change in the warty lesions, as well as the development of osteogenic sarcoma.

Ray M, Hendrick SJ, Raimer SS, Blackwell SJ: **Amniotic band syndrome**. Int J Dermatol 1988; 27:312–314.

Here's what can happen when a pregnant woman falls or suffers abdominal trauma: The **amniotic sac ruptures**, so that part or all of the fetus lies outside the amniotic cavity. Fibrous strings of amnion then encircle parts of the fetus, interfering with growth and producing abortion, limb amputation, or constrictive bands with severe edema distal to the band. These bands may also cause atypical syndactyly of the distal digits (acrosyndactyly), clubbed feet, craniofacial anomalies, cleft palate, and cleft lip, which do not follow normal embryologic lines. Alopecia may occur at sites of band attachment.

Compression of the fetus due to loss of fluid (oligohydramnios) by increased chorionic absorption may also cause visceral and neural tube defects, scoliosis, and infarcts.

Known as the **ADAM complex** (*amniotic deformity, adhesions, mutilations*), this syndrome occurs in about 1 in 10,000 births. It is usually misdiagnosed as a genetic or teratogenic congenital deformity. It is important to recognize this strange complex, since parents can be advised of its nongenetic significance and unlikelihood of affecting future offspring.

In the 17th century physicians believed that intrauterine amputation occurred as a result of the pregnant mother seeing a crippled person. Strangely, they could have been right, if the mother fell in a faint.

Burgdorf WHC, Doran CK, Worret W-I: Folded skin with scarring: **Michelin tire baby syndrome**? J Am Acad Dermatol 1982; 7:90–94.

The **Michelin tire baby** (**MTB**) is a clinical diagnosis basis exclusively on the presence of **excess folds of skin** in an infant. The folds are made up of fat that extend into the arms. The prognosis is for gradual involution.

The example reported here was unique in that there was striking stellate scarring of the trunk. This may have resulted from a very traumatic delivery associated with a persistent posterior occiput presentation.

Felding IB, Björklund LJ: **Rapp-Hodgkin ectodermal dysplasia**. Pediatr Dermatol 1990; 7:126–131.

When a boy with congenital anhidrotic or hypohidrotic ectodermal defect has a cleft palate, midfacial hypoplasia and hypospadias, his condition probably is the **Rapp-Hodgkin syndrome**.

But, discouragingly, hereditary ectodermal dysplasia has over a hundred faces.

Leggett JM: **Laryngo-tracheal stenosis** in frontometaphyseal dysplasia. J Laryngol Otol 1988; 102:74–78.

Prominent supraorbital ridges may be part of a syndrome that includes conductive deafness, agenesis of the frontal sinuses, underdeveloped mandible, and splayed metaphyses of long bones leading to flexion contractures. The mode of inheritance is uncertain.

In the family reported here, upper airway obstruction due to **laryngotracheal stenosis** was also a feature of the syndrome.

Rafaat M: **Hypertrichosis pinnae** in babies of diabetic mothers. Pediatr 1981; 68:745–746.

Congenital hypertrichosis of the external ears is seen in babies with XYY syndrome, as well as some of the populace of Pacific islands.

It is also seen in most babies born to diabetic mothers. These babies also have puffy plethoric facies resembling patients who have been receiving corticosteroids (cushingoid or tomato facies).

Arlette JP, Johnston MM: **Zinc deficiency dermatosis** in premature infants receiving prolonged parenteral alimentation. J Am Acad Dermatol 1981; 5:37–42.

Prolonged total parenteral nutrition in a group of 10 premature neonates induced **hypozincemia**. Trigger factors included bacterial sepsis. The characteristic skin changes, which mainly involve seborrheic areas, appeared at the age of 3 months and consisted of:

> **red-brown patches in the neck folds** and cheeks
> taut shiny skin with maceration and crusting of the neck fold
> well-defined borders
> dry scaling dermatitis of the buttocks

When examining these infants, be sure to pull back the neck skin; if this is not done, their dermatitis may remain completely hidden.

Tanita Y, Tagami H: **Pericervical granuloma** in a child due to constricting rubber bands. Arch Dermatol 1984; 120:709.

This 1-year-old boy baby had a **band of erythema** around his neck for the past month. It exhibited erosions and granulomatous nodules. Neck movement was sharply limited. The diagnosis remained in doubt until a piece of partially decayed rubber band was extruded from an area of ulceration. A diagnosis of **foreign body granuloma** was made, and total excision of the cord-like indurated scar was done. At that time another strangulating thin rubber band was found, penetrating down to the sternocleidomastoid muscle.

The penis and finger are typical sites for such a ring granuloma, but here the baby had chosen to wear the rubber bands as a necklace.

Tong TK, Andrew LR, Albert A, Mickell JJ: **Childhood acquired immune deficiency syndrome** manifesting as acrodermatitis enteropathica. J Pediatr 1986; 108:426–428.

At 14 months of age this infant girl was hospitalized because of failure to thrive, as well as an **orofacial rash and diarrhea**. An initial diagnosis of acrodermatitis enteropathica was entertained. Zinc supplementation cleared the rash, but the diarrhea and poor weight gain persisted.

Repeated infections and pneumonia required further hospitalizations. The pneumonitis and hepatosplenomegaly was believed to be due to bronchopulmonary dysplasia. However, the past history of blood transfusions in the first months of life led to a serum test for AIDS. This was positive; HTLV III was isolated and grown from the infant's serum. The mother's test was negative. It was concluded that the infant's depressed immunity permitted an opportunistic organism such as *Cryptosporidium* or *Giardia* to induce the diarrhea, which, in turn, led to zinc loss and the orofacial rash. The correct diagnosis thus proved to be an **AIDS-induced zinc deficiency** dermatitis and not acrodermatitis enteropathica as first thought.

Küster W, Lombeck I, Frosch D, Goerz G: Skin eruptions caused by **nutritional zinc deficiency** due to infant formula. Z Hautkr 1990; 65:147–153.

Two newborn infants developed **scaly erythematous eruptions** on their faces and fingers at the 4th and 10th week after birth. Both children had been fed on **hypoallergenic formulas** since birth. Treatment with local steroids, antibiotics, and antifungal agents, as well as systemic nystatin and erythromycin, had no significant effect.

Serum levels of zinc were then proved to be low: 0.4 and 0.2 mg/liter, respectively (normal 0.6 to 1.0 mg/liter). A diagnosis of **zinc deficiency dermatitis** was made. The rash completely cleared a few days after the addition of zinc sulfate (10 mg/day).

Heyl T, Raubenheimer EJ: Sucking pads (sucking calluses) of the lips in neonates. A manifestation of **transient leukoedema**. Pediatr Dermatol 1987; 4:123–128.

Hyperkeratotic lesions on the innermost vermilion border of the **lips** of neonates are known as sucking pads. They are an adaptive response to the frictional forces of sucking, disappearing when breast-feeding ends.

Sucking blisters are easily distinguished as blisters that result from sucking in utero. They occur on the thumbs or arms, i.e., areas easily accessible to the baby's mouth.

Leukoedema is a diffuse opalescent nonscaling lesion of the buccal or labial mucosa. It may appear at any age.

There is always another step you can take to arrive at a diagnosis.

Diaper Area

Cavanaugh RM Jr, Greeson JD: *Trichophyton rubrum* **infection** of the diaper area. Arch Dermatol 1982; 118:446.

A 9-month-old baby girl had a **rash** that began in the **diaper area** and had spread to the thighs and to the right side of the face.

Initially, a diagnosis of diaper rash had been made, but the eruption failed to respond to steroid creams. Next a diagnosis of candidiasis was made; nystatin therapy was without effect. Weeks later the lesions became arcuate, with distinct raised borders. Although a scraping showed no fungi, dermatophyte infection was suspected. Topical miconazole therapy induced complete clearing well before the laboratory found the **culture** to be positive for *T. rubrum*.

Goldblum OM, Brusilow SW, Maldonado YA, Farmer ER: **Neonatal citrullinemia** associated with cutaneous manifestations and arginine deficiency. J Am Acad Dermatol 1986; 14:321–326.

A **perioral dermatitis** as well as marked scaling and erythema of the diaper area appeared when this infant boy was a month old. It was a striking part of a generalized erosive scaling exfoliative dermatitis, which on biopsy showed little of diagnostic import.

Although the skin lesions resembled the "flaky paint" dermatosis of **kwashiorkor**, there was none of the peripheral edema, muscle atrophy, and wasting seen in this disease. A normal serum zinc level excluded acrodermatitis enteropathica; the possibility of a drug eruption was not supported by the biopsy or clinical course. Again, there was a resemblance to necrolytic migratory erythema, but glucagonomas have not been reported in anyone under the age of 19 years.

The **plasma amino acid determinations** provided the answer. The infant had markedly elevated citrulline levels 1617 μmol/liter (normal 28 ± 8) with a concomitant low arginine level, 7 μmol/liter (normal 62 ± 9). Moreover, there was hyperammonemia (83 μmol/liter, normal 11–35).

This all was indicative of a diagnosis of **neonatal citrullinemia**. In this condition, there is an enzymatic failure in the Krebs urea cycle resulting in an accumulation of the amino acid citrulline due to a failure in the enzyme arginine–succinic acid synthetase. The precursor ammonia also accumulates, whereas the end product arginine falls below normal.

Supplemental arginine, 4 mmol/kg/day in this infant's diet, resulted in marked improvement in the skin in 48 hours. Within 2 weeks the skin had virtually returned to normal, and the plasma levels of arginine were normal. The citrullinemia, however, persisted.

It is assumed that the infant's skin lesions were the result of a deficiency in the essential amino acid arginine. Noteworthy in this regard is the fact that 16% of epidermal keratin is arginine.

Rasmussen HB, Hagdrup H, Schmidt H: **Psoriasiform napkin dermatitis**. Acta Derm Venereol 1986; 66:534–536.

Psoriasiform diaper dermatitis occurred in 18 infants; in half of them, *Candida albicans* was found on culture. Follow-up observation over 7 to 15 years revealed that 2 developed psoriasis and 2 have atopic dermatitis.

This condition is also known as **dermatitis psoriasiformis Jadassohn**. It presents as a psoriasiform rash in the diaper area surrounded by satellites of psoriasis-like papules, which may spread to the trunk, limbs, scalp, and face. It usually lasts 6 to 8 weeks.

Lovell CR, Atherton DJ: Infantile gluteal granulomata—case report. Clin Exp Dermatol 1984; 9:522–525.

Firm oval **purple nodules of the pubic** area developed in an 8-month-old infant boy within a month after he had been treated for diaper dermatitis with topical steroids, antibiotics, and nystatin. The nodules subsequently had resisted all therapy; biopsy of a nodule showed an intense granulomatous infiltrate. He also had mild intertriginous eczema of the axillae and neck. An intradermal skin test to *Candida albicans* antigen was negative, and serum precipitins to *C. albicans* and *C. parapsilosis* were absent.

Given the history, clinical findings, and biopsy, a diagnosis of **infantile gluteal granuloma** was made. Characteristically, uniform oval purple nodules occur on the convexities of the napkin area, with their long axes parallel to the skin creases. They persist for several weeks and regress spontaneously, sometimes with atrophic scars. The cause is unknown but probably includes chronic exposure of occluded skin to a variety of microbial antigens. Interestingly, the same condition has been encountered in incontinent elderly women.

Hansen RC, Lemen R, Revsin B: **Cystic fibrosis** manifesting with acrodermatitis enteropathica-like eruption: Association with essential fatty acid and zinc deficiencies. Arch Dermatol 1983; 119:51–55.

A **ringworm-like dermatitis of the diaper area** which then spread to the perioral area as well as the arms and legs was the presenting problem in this $7\frac{1}{2}$-month-old baby boy. The infant had failed to thrive, and topical preparations used for the past $2\frac{1}{2}$ months were without effect.

On examination the buttocks, legs, arms, and face were covered with interconnected erythematous sharply marginated scaling patches. There was pitting edema of the arms and legs as well. KOH examinations were repeatedly negative. The biopsy showed a nonspecific picture of spongiotic dermatitis with an inflammatory cell infiltrate. Extensive laboratory testing, including urinary amino acid chromatography, serum glucagon, and alpha-antitrypsin levels, was unrevealing.

The daunting **differential** included:

    acrodermatitis enteropathica
    seborrheic dermatitis
    atopic dermatitis
    psoriasiform dermatitis
    necrolytic migratory erythema
    histiocytosis
    Leiner's disease
    infantile biotin deficiency syndrome

The failure to thrive and a recent onset of diarrhea and mild cough lead to assessment of sweat chloride values. These showed high levels (>65 mmol/liter) diagnostic of **cystic fibrosis**. Moreover, the serum zinc level as well as linoleic acid and proteins proved abnormally low.

Within 10 days of initiating nutritional supplementation and zinc, the infant's skin was normal. The pitting edema disappeared and the infant has been thriving for the past 12 months with no recurrence of his dermatitis.

The dermatitis here was the index sign of cystic fibrosis, but it is not known whether the dermatitis reflected a zinc deficiency, an essential fatty acid deficiency, a protein deficiency, or all types.

A "why" diagnosis beats a "what" diagnosis.

Nevi and Melanomas

Nothing is more common than a gathering of melanocytes that we call a melanocytic nevus and the patient calls a mole. They are easy to recognize. They have been present as long as the patient can remember and they are not showing any change. We see so many of them, hundreds every day, that they become subliminal diagnoses. We see so many that we can recognize and name a score or more of different melanocyte assemblies.

There is the congenital nevus, a gathering from the day of birth. We know the junctional nevus that rests within the epidermis, and we can actually feel the hordes of melanocytes that make up the compound nevus. When the crowd is spotty we call it nevus spilus. If the group is in a cluster of hairs, we call it a hairy nevus. We can also name vast gatherings by where they are held, e.g., in the trigeminal area (nevus of Ota), shoulder (nevus of Ito), and in the sacral area (Mongolian spot).

If the crowd is wearing more red than brown, we think of the Spitz nevus and the red nevus of the redhead. Not surprisingly, the crowd deep down wearing blue is called the blue nevus. With no color at all we have the amelanotic nevus, and when they gather in the center of a white circle, 'tis the halo nevus. Most disquieting of all is the seething crowd that mills about and hops the police barricade. This is the dysplastic nevus. As the years pass, all these crowds quietly fade away, and in the old patient none are found or seen.

These crowds come and go, but the crowd to fear is the one that grows and grows and changes into black. This is the killer mole of malignant melanoma. It is our job to tell when the crowd has become that mole.

How we do fail? We fail when:

  we don't excise a nevus that is showing change in color, size, or shape that suggests a melanoma.
  we do not have the patient return for further observation of suspicious lesions.
  we do not encourage the patient to tell us about new spots, bumps, or sores.
  we examine the patient in poor light.
  we don't have histologic examination of essentially everything we excise.
  we forget that there are amelanotic malignant melanomas.
  we ignore a new black band in the nail bed because nail biopsies are deforming.
  we don't instruct and regularly follow patients with the dysplastic nevus syndrome.
  we don't insist that our receptionists give immediate appointments to anyone calling who is worried about a mole or black spot.

It is easy to know a nevus. But **to know a melanoma takes suspicion and excision**, and remember that close observation can help prevent a lentiginous lesion from becoming a "litigenous" one.

Steiner A, Pehamberger H, Wolff K: Improvement of the diagnostic accuracy in pigmented skin lesions by **epiluminescent light microscopy**. Anticancer Res 1987; 7:433–434.

In a study of 318 small (≤10 mm) pigmented lesions suspected to be melanomas, the clinical diagnosis made with the naked eye was correct in 61%. This improved to 85% when **epiluminescent light microscopy** (ELM) was used.

ELM involves covering the pigmented lesion with immersion oil and a glass slide, which renders the epidermis translucent and allows observation of the dermal-epidermal junction zone. A WILD M650 binocular surface microscope (objective 91-mm working distance, magnifications 6, 10, 16, 25, and 40) was used to examine the lesions. Criteria used to differentiate various types of nevi from dysplastic nevi and melanoma in situ included examination of the pigment network at the dermal-epidermal junction, a subtle network of brownish lines along this zone.

Kelly JW, Crutcher WA, Sagebiel RW: Clinical diagnosis of **dysplastic melanocytic nevi**: A clinicopathologic correlation. J Am Acad Dermatol 1986; 14:1044–1052.

It is important to identify the patient with **dysplastic nevi**, since that person has a lifetime risk of developing malignant melanoma that is more than 25 times that of a person having common melanocytic nevi. Should there be a family history of melanoma and dysplastic nevi, the lifetime risk for developing melanoma among family members approaches 100%.

Be prepared to identify dysplastic nevi and instruct the family appropriately. Examination calls for (1) a strong light directed tangentially; (2) examination of entire skin surface, including scalp areas, between toes and buttocks, as well as under breasts; and (3) stretching nevus to perceive erythema and irregularity of pigmentation.

The major clinical features of dysplasia are:

ill-defined border	erythema
irregularly distributed pigmentation	pebbly skin surface
diameter over 5 mm	

One in every 20 patients you see will have these aberrant dysplastic nevi.

Hamm H, Happle R, Bröcker E-B: Multiple **agminate Spitz naevi**: Review of the literature and report of a case with distinctive immunohistological features. Br J Dermatol 1987; 117:511–522.

Since the age of 3, a 13-year-old girl had developed an 18 × 14 cm sharply demarcated area on the right lumbar region that was studded with approximately **200 nodules and plaques**. The lesions were partly merging and varied in color from red to dark brown. The red tumors were smooth, while the darker lesions were papillomatous, and an area of leukoderma surrounded the entire lesion. The lesion was excised for cosmetic reasons.

Histopathology revealed a mixture of Spitz nevi and compound nevi with mild architectural dysplasia but no cellular atypia. However, monoclonal antibody staining revealed malignancy-associated melanocytic antigens seen in malignant melanomas and halo nevi (HLA-DR, PAL-MI, A-I-43, and A-10-33) in a large percentage of cells. These antigens are only rarely found in common nevi.

Agminate Spitz nevi usually behave in a benign manner, sometimes regressing completely. They may be triggered by sunburn, sun exposure, trauma, intralesional injection, radiation therapy, and excision of a solitary Spitz nevus. No provoking factors were evident in this case.

959

Sun C-C, Lü Y-C, Lee EF, Nakagawa H: **Naevus fusco-caeruleus zygomaticus.** Br J Dermatol 1987; 117:545–553.

Bilateral dark-grayish brown spotted **pigmentation over the cheek bones** was studied in 110 Chinese patients. Usually appearing in women after puberty, and sometimes familial, the pigment varies from grayish brown or blue to dark brown and does not involve the sclera. Biopsy shows elongated melanocytes dispersed between collagen fibers in the upper dermis.

Contrast this with the **nevus of Ota** (naevus fusco-caeruleus ophthalmomaxillaris), which is confluent, usually unilateral, and rarely familial. It commonly appears at birth or during the first year and is associated with ocular and palatal pigmentation.

Nicholls DSH, Mason GH: Halo dermatitis around a melanocytic naevus: **Meyerson's naevus.** Br J Dermatol 1988; 118:125–129.

A 21-year-old atopic man from New Zealand developed a 12-mm pruritic eczematous halo around a 3-mm pigmented nevus on the right medial calf. The lesion was excised, revealing psoriasiform hyperplasia of the epidermis with spongiosis, benign nevus cells in the dermis, and perivascular eosinophils, lymphocytes, and histiocytes.

A pigmented nevus may develop a **halo of dermatitis** for no apparent reason. It is benign and subsides spontaneously in a few months with no regression of the nevus, in contrast to the halo nevus of Sutton (leukoderma acquisitum centrifugum). Multiple nevi are usually involved over time. Biopsy consistently shows an eosinophilic infiltrate around a melanocytic nevus.

A halo of depigmentation may also be seen around a malignant melanoma, so that depigmentation does not necessarily bespeak benignity.

Warin AP: **Cockarde naevus.** Clin Exp Dermatol 1976; 1:221–224.

Two girls, ages 7 and 13, had junctional nevi, each consisting of a pink, slightly **raised papule in the center of a "target"** with an inner ring of normal skin and outer ring of macular pigmentation. The lesions were 0.5 to 1 cm in diameter. Previously described in two other young people as a **cockarde (rosette) nevus** or **target nevus**, this lesion is benign. In some instances the annular outer ring is a junctional nevus.

The literature records one example of a clinically recognizable **malignant melanoma** occurring in the center of an identical target with the outer ring being hyperpigmented. The lesion was a hemorrhagic nodule occurring in the center of a brown senile lentigo in a 79-year-old woman. These lesions differ from the **Sutton's halo nevus** in not undergoing involution and not involving leukoderma or any evidence of lymphocytic infiltration.

Uhle P, Norvell SS Jr: Generalized **lentiginosis.** J Am Acad Dermatol 1988; 18:444–447.

Multiple lentigines beget multiple **acronyms** stressing the multiple systems that can show multiple genetic defects:

LEOPARD SYNDROME	LAMB SYNDROME
Lentigines	Lentigines
ECG abnormalities	Atrial myxomas
Ocular hypertelorism	Mucocutaneous myxomas
Pulmonic stenosis	Blue nevi
Abnormal genitalia	
Retardation of growth	
Deafness	

TAY SYNDROME	NAME SYNDROME
Lentigines	Nevi
Mental retardation	Atrial myxomas
Skeletal defects	Mucoid neurofibromas
Short stature	Ephelides
Vitiligo	
Hypersplenism	
Café-au-lait spots	
Premature gray hair	

What a pleasure to read of the 20-year-old red-haired white man in this report who, upon careful study by a variety of specialists, proved to have absolutely no abnormalities except for extensive lentigines. The skin lesions varied from 1 mm to 2 cm and were dark brown to almost black. They covered his entire body, sparing only his tongue, buccal mucosa, and soles. Lesions were most abundant on his face, including the lips and conjunctivae. Similar lentigines were present in his 26-year-old maternal uncle, who was also healthy, with no signs of cardiac, ophthalmic, or other systemic problems.

Barker JNWN, MacDonald DM: Eruptive dysplastic naevi following **renal transplantation**. Clin Exp Dermatol 1988; 13:123–125.

Three months after receiving a renal transplant and consequent immunosuppression (prednisolone, azathioprine) a 12-year-old boy developed dozens of melanocytic nevi on his trunk. Eventually, over **100 nevi** were present on the trunk, proximal limbs, and scalp; many were asymmetrical with irregular edges and color variation from dark brown to brick red. Biopsy of three nevi showed that two were dysplastic and one was a benign compound nevus. Prior to the transplant he had not had excessive nevi, and there was no family history of either multiple nevi or melanoma.

These **eruptive nevi** must be distinguished from the benign eruptive melanocytic nevi that may arise during puberty or adolescence, pregnancy, or ACTH therapy. Eruptive dysplastic nevi occur also as a form of the familial or sporadic dysplastic nevus syndrome, without known immunosuppression.

It appears that **immunosuppression** is accountable for these dysplastic nevi and puts the renal transplant patient at risk for malignant melanoma, making close surveillance mandatory.

Duvic M, Lowe L, Rapini RP, et al: Eruptive dysplastic nevi associated with **human immunodeficiency virus infection**. Arch Dermatol 1989; 125:397–401.

Seven patients are reported who suddenly developed **multiple new nevi** in the same year that they developed symptomatic **HIV infection**. Although they had had no previous dysplastic nevi, these new nevi appearing in crops were histologically dysplastic nevi.

The dramatic appearance of dysplastic nevi may thus be another index marker for AIDS.

Rasmussen SA: **Obsessive-compulsive disorder** in dermatologic practice. J Am Acad Dermatol 1985; 13:965–967.

A 28-year-old accountant became obsessed with whether or not various nevi had become malignant. He would check himself over and over for irregular margins, color change, or alterations in the size of his nevi. He received five "**second opinions**" from physicians and dermatologists that his nevi were perfectly benign.

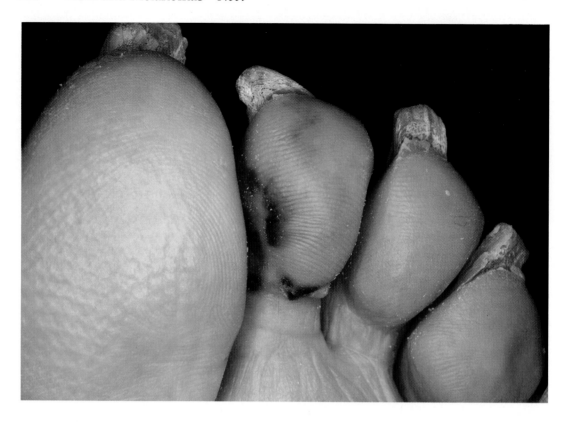

The diagnosis of **obsessive-compulsive disorder** was confirmed when an astute questioner elicited the fact that he was also consumed by the thought that the electrical outlets and gas connections in his home had been installed unsafely. He felt compelled to check the outlets and wiring for up to 10 hours a day.

One could then surmise that it was not the house wiring that was defective but rather the wires in his brain.

Like office visits, more than one biopsy may be required.

Melanomas

Sober AJ, Fitzpatrick JB, Mihm MC Jr: **Primary melanoma** of the skin: Recognition and management. J Am Acad Dermatol 1980; 2:179–197.

Early warning signals that a pigmented lesion may be a melanoma:

1. Variegate color

    Shades of red, white, and blue appearing in a brown or black lesion
    Irregular pigment distribution

2. Irregular border

    Angular indentation
    A notched edge

3. Increase in size or change in color

    Irregular elevation, best seen in oblique light

Clinical forms of primary melanoma of the skin:

1. Superficial spreading melanoma

    Begins as small brown-black lesion showing slight focal bluish discoloration
    Enlarges by centrifugal spread (radial growth)
    May show areas of regression resulting in irregular shape
    Exhibits spectrum of colors
    Nodules, i.e., vertical growth, may ensue when size reaches 2.5 cm months or years later

2. Nodular melanoma

    Begins as a blue-black lesion that patient (or physician) mistakes as a blood blister or hemangioma
    Grows rapidly to uniformly blue-black papule or nodule; can be polypoid or simple dome-shaped; can be purple, red-brown, or amelanotic

3. Lentigo maligna melanoma

    This is a nodular melanoma arising in the premalignant lentigo maligna.
    The premalignant stage (lentigo maligna): May last for 5 to 50 years
      Occurs in sun-exposed areas
      Begins as freckle-like irregular pigment change
      Onset late in life
      Color changes occur with reticulate patterns, black flecks
      Areas of regression occur with resultant white-gray and bluish zones
      Radial growth finally converts to vertical growth with malignant nodule

4. Acral lentiginous melanoma

    Arises in flat, usually uniformly pigmented lesions of palms, soles, nailbeds, and mucous membranes
    More common in blacks and Orientals

General observations:

  At least 6% of patients with malignant melanoma have a family history of malignant melanoma.
  Congenital nevi pose a risk of fatal melanoma developing before age 10.
  Amelanotic melanomas escape clinical detection and are found only by histologic examination of every single lesion removed from the skin.
  Metastatic melanomas may be preceded by a spontaneously disappearing mole; residual hypopigmentation is best detected by Wood's light examination.

Ho VC, Sober AJ: Therapy for **cutaneous melanoma**: An update. J Am Acad Dermatol 1990; 22:159–176.

Diagnostic guide:

OBSERVATION	SUSPECT MELANOMA
Lesion color	Variegation of red, pink, gray, white, blue in a brown or black lesion
Configuration	Irregular border, notching, asymmetry
Topography	Surface irregularly raised (use side-lighting)
Depigmentation (use Wood's light)	Suggests immunologic destruction of melanocytes and/or melanoma cells
NOTE IN RECORD	
Lesion location	Exact site
Lesion size	Greatest two dimensions at right angles
In-transit lesions	Inspect and palpate around lesion and over lymphatic drainage for satellite lesions
Lymph nodes	Palpate for tumor
Dysplastic/congenital nevi	Increases risk for melanoma presence

And don't forget to record family history of melanomas when risk assessing.

McLean DI, Lew RA, Sober AJ, et al: Erythema in the primary lesion of **superficial spreading melanoma** is not of prognostic importance. Br J Dermatol 1982; 107:339–342.

In 163 patients the presence of erythema in superficial spreading melanoma lesions failed to show any correlation with the level of invasion, size of lesion, location, metastasis, or prognosis.

The presence of white depressed areas also does not correlate with prognosis.

These red and white "flags" only indicate that a host-tumor battle is in progress, with a lymphoid cell response and areas of fibrosis in the battleground.

Howell JB: Spotting **sinister spots**. A challenge to dermatologists to examine every new patient at increased risk for signs of early melanoma. J Am Acad Dermatol 1986; 15:722–726.

"Skin scan" all who

sunburn easily
have a large number of nevi
have a large congenital nevus
have family history of melanoma

Look for the ABCDs

Asymmetry
Border irregularity
Color variation
Diameter over 6 mm

Make melanoma a word of warning, not a sentence of death.

Taylor B, Frumkin A, Pitha JV: Delayed reaction to "lead" pencil simulating **melanoma**. Cutis 1988; 42:199–201.

An enlarging, firm 1.4 cm **dark-gray nodule** of the right shin in a 74-year-old man was thought to be a malignant melanoma. The nodule had arisen in the past year within a dark-gray macule at the **site of a lead pencil** injury when he was a lad of 15. Other diagnoses considered were pigmented dermatofibroma, subepidermal calcified nodule, blue nevus, and lead pencil granuloma. Skin biopsy revealed many dark particles, presumably carbon, in macrophages and surrounded by foreign body giant cells, consistent with lead pencil granuloma.

The amazingly long lag period of 58 years indicates that graphite, like silica, can remain dormant in the skin for long periods.

Bruce DR, Goette DK: **Pseudomelanoma** in a black patient. Cutis 1985; 36:73–74.

In the course of examining this 62-year-old black male, a **black, slightly verruciform macule** 2 × 3 cm in diameter was noted on the palmar side of the left index finger. The lesion was not tender and not indurated and had been present for many years.

The patient forced the attending staff to run through a **differential** of:

superficial spreading malignant melanoma
acral lentiginous melanoma
lentigo maligna
lentigo senilis

Not until then did he reveal that the black lesion was a **skin graft** of abdominal skin placed there 20 years ago.

One of our patients with an abdominal skin graft of the right palm was not so fortunate. Twenty years after the grafting, he was unable to make a fist. The obesity he had acquired over the years was expanding his waist line while shrinking his grasp. He now had not only a beltfull but also a palmfull of fat.

Not all skin is created equal.

A brilliant diagnostician can still be a stupid therapist.

Nodules

Every clinician has a mental photo file of nodules he can recognize with assurance. This includes the **commonplace**: acne cysts and wens, synovial cysts and ganglions, xanthomas, lipomas, and rheumatoid nodules, as well as seborrheic keratoses. It extends to the pruritic nodules of prurigo nodularis, the tender nodules of erythema nodosum, and the rapidly growing nodules of keratoacanthoma.

Many other nodules have to be diagnosed or surmised **in context**. These include the nodules of sarcoidosis, metastatic carcinoma, leukemia, and gout. Nodules over traumatized knuckles or in a line of a cat scratch suggest multicentric reticulohistiocytosis. Sun-damaged skin may exhibit thickenings due to elastotic change.

A very few can be suspected because of their **distinctive behavior** or symptoms. We expect a hydrocystoma to vary in size in relation to sweating. We know that the nodule of mastocytoma will swell and flush on stroking (Darier's sign). A neuroblastoma will show blanching when palpated, since its complement of cells release catecholamines rather than histamine. Listen when the mother says, "The bumps become white when rubbed." The rubbing of the towel may produce pain with eccrine spiradenomas and cooling may produce a leiomyoma-induced pain.

Yet after all, some nodules will reveal their secret only to the pathologist. Only on biopsy can an adnexal tumor be identified. We turn to the biopsy to see the acid-fast bacterial swarms of lepromatous leprosy. Only on biopsy can the worm of dirofilariasis be viewed. It is only the pathologist who can look under the rug and tell us it was only a marble we stepped on.

Vainsencher D, Winkelmann RK: **Subcutaneous sarcoidosis**. Arch Dermatol 1984; 120:1028–1031.

Several **subcutaneous nodules** had been present on a patient's left forearm for 2 months. The lesions were painless, pink to skin colored, 1 to 2 cm in size, and freely movable above the fascia.

A clinical diagnosis of dermatofibromas proved on biopsy to be wrong. The patient had subcutaneous lesions of sarcoidosis. There was no evidence of systemic disease, and within the year the lesions disappeared spontaneously. A 33-year follow-up showed no recurrence.

Formerly known as **Darier-Roussy sarcoid**, these lesions are rarely seen in systemic sarcoidosis.

Samadaei A, Hashimoto K, Tanay A: **Insulin lipodystrophy**, lipohypertrophic type. J Am Acad Dermatol 1987; 17:506–507.

Large subcutaneous masses may develop at sites of repeated insulin injections. These "insulin tumors" represent lipohypertrophy and usually result from using pork insulin.

Raymond JZ, Goldman HM: An unusual **cutaneous reaction** secondary **to allopurinol**. Cutis 1988; 41:323–326.

A 60-year-old man developed a **reddish purple nodule** of the left temple and a score of erythematous papules and plaques on his abdomen and back. The lesions had been present 6 weeks and the nodule on the face was clinically and histologically lymphocytoma cutis. However, a true lymphoma could not be ruled out. Because the eruption had appeared just 2 weeks after allopurinol therapy was started for control of uric acid, the medication was stopped, and within days all lesions faded. The patient has subsequently had no recurrence.

Lymphocytoma cutis thus joins the lengthening list of cutaneous reaction patterns, and illustrates the old axiom, "Look *behind the diagnosis!*"

Spencer PS, Helm TN: **Skin metastases** in cancer patients. Cutis 1987; 39:119–121.

Autopsy data from 7518 patients with internal cancer at Roswell Park Memorial Institute showed **skin metastases in 9%**, a much higher figure than those reported in previous series. This included 26.5% of women with breast cancer, 5.9% of patients with lung cancer, and 6.6% of patients with kidney and ureter cancer. The **most common tumor metastasizing to skin** was malignant melanoma, seen in 36.6% of patients with melanoma.

Skin metastases usually resemble the primary tumor in color and consistency and are often freely movable cutaneous or subcutaneous nodules that are discrete, hard, indolent, skin-colored, or erythematous. **Unusual presentations** include cicatricial morphea-like plaques and alopecia neoplastica (circumscribed hair loss on the scalp). Other skin metastases can look like a lipoma, lymphoma, cylindroma, neurofibroma, Kaposi's sarcoma, or pyogenic granuloma

So if it looks like an "oma" and the patient's in an old people's "homa," think of metastatic "carcinoma" and do a biopsy. So ends our "poema."

Brown MD, Ellis CN, Billings J, et al: Rapid occurrence of nodular cutaneous T-lymphocyte infiltrates with **cyclosporine therapy**. Arch Dermatol 1988; 124:1097–1100.

Erythematous papules appeared on the face of a 58-year-old man just 10

days after initiation of cyclosporine therapy for psoriasis and by 14 days had become nodular. Skin biopsy showed a benign lymphocytic infiltrate, viewed as a cyclosporine-induced T-cell infiltrate. When the cyclosporine was stopped, the papules and nodules cleared completely within 3 weeks. The same eruption reappeared 5 months later without a cyclosporine challenge, and biopsy again showed a **benign T-cell infiltrate**. The lesions completely cleared without treatment after 3 months.

Other cutaneous side effects of cyclosporine include paresthesias, hypertrichosis, and gingival hyperplasia. However, it is nephrotoxicity that is most serious and requires continued monitoring.

Ohno S, Yokoo T, Ohta M, et al: **Aleukemic leukemia cutis**. J Am Acad Dermatol 1990; 22:374–377.

Numerous round, **violaceous nodules** had been rapidly appearing during the past 3 months over the entire skin of this 39-year-old man. Only the scalp, palms, and feet were spared. All blood counts and clinical studies were normal, but the bone marrow showed 21.5% monocytes. The skin biopsy showed a dense monocytic cell infiltration, proved by peroxidase staining. Staining by surface markers was negative for reticulum cells (OKT6), T lymphocytes (OKT11), and B lymphocytes (B1). Biopsy of an enlarged lymph node in the left inguinal region revealed an infiltrate of abnormal monocytes. A diagnosis was made of **monocytic leukemia cutis** in an aleukemic patient.

Such aleukemic leukemia cutis is rare and indicates an invasion of the skin by leukemic cells before their appearance in the peripheral blood. The skin findings could easily be misinterpreted as a lymphoma.

Following chemotherapy this patient developed the classic blood pattern of monocytic leukemia. He died the following year.

Patients with cutaneous infiltrates suggesting a lymphoma must be continually **monitored for lymph node enlargement** and for changes in the blood count.

Andersen BL, Brandrup F, Petri J: **Lymphocytoma cutis**: A pseudomalignancy treated with penicillin. Acta Derm Venereol 1982; 62:83–85.

This 72-year-old woman was referred to the dermatology clinic for evaluation of a radioresistant malignant lymphoma of the dorsum of her right hand. Examination showed a **massive purple mass** of the dorsum of the hand extending along the dorsa of the first three fingers.

Her history revealed that over a year ago she had initially been reviewed as having a ganglion of the second right finger. However, the histologic picture was one of massive lymphocytic infiltrate. The patient attributed the lesion to a thorn bush injury, but no evidence of sporotrichosis was found.

The mass grew, extended, and became purplish. The present diagnosis reflected a recent biopsy interpreted as a **malignant lymphoma**. Radiation therapy (2 courses of 10 Gy each) had no effect.

Review of the histology by a dermatopathologist failed to confirm the presence of malignancy. A diagnosis of **lymphocytoma cutis** was made.

Two weeks of penicillin therapy was completely curative.

Gupta AK, Billings JK, Headington JT: **Multisystem crystalline deposits**. Arch Dermatol 1989; 125:551–556.

Erythematous indurated nodules had been present for two months on the legs of this 30-year-old man. A key clinical clue was the history of 10 years of **recurrent renal calculi**.

Polarized light examination of an H and E stained slide of a biopsy gave the diagnosis. The distinctive **birefringent calcium oxalate** crystals were seen in the dermis. The diagnosis of **primary hyperoxaluria** had already been made by an analysis of his renal stones, which showed calcium oxalate. His urinary phosphate excretion was 10 to 15 times normal.

Significantly, the problem was a **multisystem** one. An endocardial biopsy specimen was taken to determine the cause of a heart block cardiac arrhythmia. Again, oxalate crystals were seen. His oxalosis was also the explanation of a loss of both sensory and motor function he was experiencing. Other complications include vascular ones. The skin may show livedo reticularis as a result of oxalate deposits in and around blood vessels. With arterial involvement, ischemia and gangrene may ensue.

This patient had a primary oxalosis that was due to an inherited enzymatic deficiency, either of a critical carboxylase or dehydrogenase. Were this not the case, one would have to explore for the following **causes of a secondary oxalosis**:

large doses of vitamin C
pyridoxine deficiency
methoxyflurane anesthesia
ethylene glycol poisoning
glycerol infusion
hyperabsorption of dietary oxalate (intestinal disease)

All of these are associated with hyperoxalemia, but a localized dystrophic form recurs as a result of oxalate deposition in altered tissue.

Asking about the family and about kidney stones can widen your diagnostic horizon in lesions ranging from nodules to livedo reticularis.

Samlaska CP, Levin SW, James WD, et al: **Proteus syndrome.** Arch Dermatol 1989; 125:1109–1114.

Proteus (old man of the sea) was a Greek god who could change shape at will to avoid capture. Today the patient with the ***Proteus syndrome*** has a mesoderm that can come in multiple malformations. From the skin standpoint, the index change is the unforgettable cerebriform masses covering the palms or soles. The patient may also show epidermal nevi, subcutaneous masses, and single fingers and toes that are greatly enlarged and lengthened. Add to this, hemihypertrophy and a host of bizarre defects in skin and bones.

The constellation of *Proteus* is to be **distinguished from**:

neurofibromatosis (indeed, the famed elephant man may well have had Proteus syndrome and not neurofibromatosis)
Klippel-Trenaunay-Weber syndrome
enchondromatosis
Maffucci's syndrome (enchondromatosis with cavernous hemangiomas)
Bannayan syndrome

Although **digital gigantism** may point to any one of these five entities, the mammoth convoluted masses pushing out from the palm or sole point another finger to the Proteus syndrome. Unlike the Greek god, this Proteus is recognized and captured because of its many shapes.

Want a quick diagnosis? Ask someone who recognizes it!

Infective

Welch RG, Inman P, Cooke RT: **Swimming-bath granuloma**. Lancet 1964; 2:42.

An 11-year-old boy grazed the bridge of his nose on the side of a swimming pool filled with chlorinated sea water. The lesion healed in 2 weeks but broke down 2 weeks later into a nonhealing **ulcer** associated over the next 3 months with enlarged right preauricular and submandibular nodes. Two small nodules appeared beneath the right eye and near the right side of the nose. Lymph node aspiration revealed fluid from which **acid-fast bacilli** were detected on Lowenstein-Jensen medium at 37°C in 3 weeks. The Mantoux test converted from negative (4 months after injury) to positive (5 months after injury).

Lober CW, Mendelsohn HE, Datnow B, Fenske NA: Clinical and histologic features of **Orf**. Cutis 1983; 32:142–147.

Lesion

> Erythematous spot initially. Vesicle evolves into nodule that is umbilicated. Despite appearance of being distended with fluid, little comes out on aspiration. By 1 to 2 weeks target lesion appears; has a red center, white rings in middle, and red halo. By 3 to 4 weeks lesions become dry. By 6 weeks resolution.

Location

> Hands, forearms, rarely face; never on covered skin.

History

> Exposure to infected sheep, goats, and farmyard work.

Systemic signs

> Rare fever, leukocytosis.

Unusual presentation

> Generalized papulovesicular eruption, generalized bullous lesions, and erythema multiforme.

Laboratory diagnosis

> Biopsy: necrosis of epidermis. Viral culture, virions on electron microscopy. Antibody studies, e.g., C.F.

de Moragas JM, Prats G, Verger G: **Cutaneous alternariosis** treated with miconazole. Arch Dermatol 1981; 117:292–294.

A 45-year-old Spaniard had a bizarre 20 × 15 cm indurated **keloid-like lesion** with interlacing indurated inflammatory cords on the right knee. Following **minor trauma** he sustained as a grain harvester 10 years before, it began with an erythematous papule that enlarged peripherally and developed a central crust. This was followed by development of a 3-cm fibrotic nodule over the course of 1 year. Satellite lesions appeared after treatment with topical steroids and occlusion, along with multiple crusted shallow ulcerations.

Biopsy revealed a hyperplastic epidermis with polymorphonuclear leukocyte abscesses and a mixed inflammatory infiltrate in the upper dermis. Giant cells were seen containing PAS-positive round structures and long filaments. **Cultures** of ulcers and punch biopsy specimens grew out *Alternaria*, leading to a diagnosis of **alternariosis**. The lesions responded to intralesional (but not intravenous) miconazole therapy. Although *Alternaria* species are considered to be saprophytes, in this patient the fungus was an opportunistic pathogen that produced an insidious granulomatous disease.

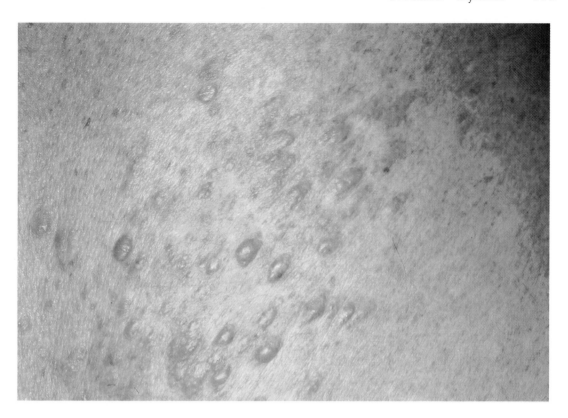

Chapel TA, Prasad P, Chapel J, Lekas N: Extragenital **syphilitic chancres**. J Am Acad Dermatol 1985; 13:582–584.

A firm crusted reddish-brown **nodule** had been present on the right side of this patient's **chin** for 6 weeks. There was an associated single, firm, movable, nontender submental lymph node.

Serologic tests for syphilis confirmed the diagnosis of an **extragenital chancre**. There was complete resolution within 2 weeks of treatment with intramuscular penicillin G benzathene (2.4 million units). The diagnostic Herxheimer of chills, fever, myalgias, headache came a scant 6 hours following the injection.

Extragenital chancres constitute one in every 20 chancres and usually appear on the arms or lip. The other sites include finger, nipple, eyelid, tongue, and tonsils. The syphilitic chancre should be brought into the differential of any papuloulcerative lesions with regional lymphadenopathy. This differential must also include

tularemia	sporotrichosis
cat scratch disease	tuberculosis

Hay RJ, Mackenzie CD, Guderian R, et al: **Onchodermatitis**—correlation between skin disease and parasitic load in an endemic focus in Ecuador. Br J Dermatol 1989; 121:187–198.

The classical presentation of **onchocerciasis** consists of large palpable subcutaneous nodules. These indicate the presence of the adult worm *Onchocerca volvulus*.

Far more subtle are the changes induced by the microfilariae, which swarm in the skin and incidentally provide the means whereby the biting black fly transmits the disease person to person. Microfilarial-induced skin lesions can be grouped under the term *onchodermatitis*. The following specific examples were each associated with the presence of microfilariae as shown in "**skin snip**" **biopsies**.

papules, papulopustules
atrophic hypopigmented scars (leopard skin)
unilateral lichenified plaques (Sowda), especially on the shins
pruritus, often severe, is a cardinal sign

The most common site is the gluteal region.

Diagnosis is achieved by thinking of onchodermatitis in patients traveling or living in the endemic areas of Africa, Central and South America, and the Arabian peninsula. Without the snip biopsy to show the microfilariae, the diagnostician would fall back on such terms as:

insect bites   ichthyosis
prurigo   neurodermatitis
anetoderma   idiopathic pruritus

But don't forget that these patients often have concurrent impetigo, tinea, or scabies.

With 50 million people suffering from onchocerciasis, and with the new specific treatment ivermectin, it behooves us to think onchodermatitis when we see the seemingly banal or commonplace in a patient coming from a tropical place.

Vermeer BJ, van der Kaay HJ: **Loiasis**: A case report. Acta Derm Venereol 1982; 62:78–79.

Shortly after returning home to the Netherlands from a year in Nigeria, this 27-year-old woman noted **transitory swellings** on her forearms. The swellings would last several days; 6 months later similar swellings began to appear on her eyelids.

A presumptive diagnosis of **Calabar swellings** was made, but no microfilariae could be found in the blood. She did, however, have eosinophilia (2400 × 10^6/liters) and serum antibodies to microfilariae were found. The diagnosis of loiasis prompted therapy with diethylcarbamazine. Within 2 days the patient developed 2 red edematous swellings of the upper arm and upper leg, respectively. Incision of their wormlike central silhouette allowed traction removal of 2 adult loa-loa nematodes.

Noteworthy in this patient was the history of having been in an endemic area of **loiasis**, viz., West and Central Africa. She no doubt had been bitten by an infectious mangrove fly, which had deposited infective larvae in her skin. By 18 months the adult worms were present, and as they migrated, induced local transitory subcutaneous swellings (Calabar swellings). She may well have thought she had arthritis. The absence of microfilariae in the blood is to be anticipated because several years may pass before they appear.

To find a case of loiasis, look for patients who have been in Africa the last year or two and who present with swellings that come and go, but who exhibit a persistent eosinophilia. The easiest diagnosis is made when the worm swims into view under the conjunctiva. It's then a true **eyeball diagnosis**.

Swerlick RA, Cooper PH, Mackel SE: Rapid enlargement of **pilomatricoma**. J Am Acad Dermatol 1982; 7:54–56.

A 21-year-old white man had an 8-week history of a **painful raised** tumor that had grown rapidly on his left temple. The lesion was a 1 × 1 cm blue-red translucent nodule that was movable and slightly tender.

The differential diagnosis included hidrocystoma, eccrine spiradenoma, mixed tumor, and pilomatricoma. Biopsy revealed a hematoma in a unilocular cystic **pilomatricoma** showing typical "shadow cells."

A "tumor" that comes out of nowhere in 14 days is best thought of as a hematoma.

Lesher JL Jr, Guill M: A tender **blue cyst** on the leg. Arch Dermatol 1988; 124:937–940.

A 2-cm firm, blue, **painful cystic lesion** had been slowly growing for 3 years on the lateral aspect of the left leg of a 47-year-old man. Possible clinical diagnoses included epidermal inclusion cyst, mucoid cyst, and eccrine or apocrine hidrocystoma.

On biopsy it proved to be an **eccrine hidrocystoma**. This tumor usually presents as a firm dome-shaped, bluish cystic lesion on the face, head, or trunk. The surface is smooth and shiny and the cyst may appear blue, clear, translucent, or pearly.

Apocrine hydrocystomas tend to be larger, darker blue, and less likely to be periorbital than eccrine hydrocystomas.

Shelley WB, Wood MG: A zosteriform network of **spiradenomas**. J Am Acad Dermatol 1980; 2:59–61.

A tortuous **network of irregular, firm, bluish nodules** had been present since infancy on the left side of the neck of a 41-year-old woman. Clinical diagnoses included nevi, fibromas with angiomatous elements, and neurofibromas. The zosteriform distribution that respected the midline spoke of a neural origin. Biopsies revealed **eccrine spiradenoma**.

Kozminsky ME, Bronson DM, Barsky S: **Zosteriform connective-tissue nevus**. Cutis 1985; 36:77–78.

Soft, flesh-colored **cobblestone-like plaques** present since childhood in a 23-year-old Nigerian woman suggested a connective tissue nevus. The distribution was unique, encompassing the left side of her back, left shoulder, and left arm. Routine histologic study showed apparently normal skin, but an elastic tissue stain revealed sparse fragmented elastic fibers in the mid-dermis. A trichrome stain for collagen was normal.

Zosteriform connective tissue nevus was diagnosed. Such lesions are benign and of unknown origin, although this one suggests the possibility of neural influences.

Lucky AW, McGuire J, Komp DM: **Infantile neuroblastoma** presenting with cutaneous blanching nodules. J Am Acad Dermatol 1982; 6:389–391.

A 2-month-old baby girl had a score of firm nontender, slightly **blue nodules** of her legs and trunk. On palpation the nodules developed **unique blanching** with a surrounding halo of erythema. The blanching persisted for up to an hour, followed by a refractory period of several hours. Excisional biopsy revealed **neuroblastoma**, which went on to produce hepatomegaly, retrobulbar masses, skeletal metastasis, and bone marrow infiltration. She did well with chemotherapy but had one recurrence of a subcutaneous mass at age 15 months.

973

The diagnostic blanching sign of this tumor results from release of catecholamine (vasoconstrictor) granules from the neuroblastoma cells during palpation.

Two other distinctive manifestations of neuroblastoma are raccoon eyes (periorbital purpura) and heterochromia iridis. Nodules that turn white on rubbing may be the first sign of neuroblastoma, the most common malignancy of childhood.

Barnes L, Mimouni F, Lucky AW: **Solitary nodule** on the arm of an infant. Arch Dermatol 1986; 122:89–93.

A firm brownish-red, well-defined 1.5 cm **nodule** with a central yellow crust was observed at birth on the posterior left upper arm of an infant boy. Excision revealed **infantile myofibromatosis**, with spindle cells having features of both smooth muscle and fibroblasts. Electron microscopy provided the ultimate diagnosis. It presents as a solitary lesion of the skin or muscle but can be multicentric, involving the gastrointestinal tract or long bones. The prognosis is good; the solitary tumors rarely recur after excision. Osseous lesions may spontaneously regress. Deaths have occurred in infants with multicentric visceral tumors.

With fibrous tumors in infants think of:

infantile myofibromatosis (solitary or multicentric)	fibromatosis colli
hyaline fibromatosis	intravascular fasciitis
digital fibromatosis	fibrous hamartoma of infancy
	calcifying aponeurotic fibroma

Other names for infantile myofibromatosis include:

congenital fibrosarcoma
congenital generalized fibromatosis
multiple mesenchymal hamartomas

Kim JH, Hur H, Lee CW, Kim YT: **Apocrine nevus**. J Am Acad Dermatol 1988; 18:579–580.

A 68-year-old white woman with multiple seborrheic keratoses, neurofibromas, and café-au-lait spots had a reddish-brown dome-shaped mammillary **nodule** 13 × 16 mm on the right side of the chest. Histopathology of the entire lesion revealed numerous well-differentiated mature apocrine elements. Carcinoembryonic antigen (CEA) staining was positive in the luminal spaces of eccrine and tumorous apocrine glands, indicating a benign **sweat gland hamartoma**.

Other apocrine nevi have presented as:

a fleshy mass in the axilla
a well-defined plaque in the axilla
a nodule of the neck
a red nodule of the scalp
multiple papules of the sternum

Hashimoto K, Mehregan AH, Kumakiri M: **Tumors of skin appendages**. London, Butterworths, 1987, pp 193–204.

1. Learn to recognize clinically the following adnexal tumors:

Eccrine poroma of the foot
Trichofolliculoma with white hair
Syringocystadenoma papilliferum of the scalp with its exudative and verrucous surface
Eccrine spiradenoma as a tender nodule
Trichilemmal cyst of scalp

2. Learn to suspect

Pilomatricoma—hardness on palpation
Clear cell hidradenoma—cystic fluctuation
Eccrine spiradenoma—pain on palpation

3. Think malignancy

Rapid growth
Inflammation
Erosion, abscess
Bleeding
Pain

4. Consider differential

supernumerary nipple
    acanthotic hyperpigmented epidermis
    central invagination
umbilical polyp
    remnant of omphaloenteric canal
mucinous syringometaplasia
    hyperkeratotic growth on sole
metastatic carcinoma to skin from breast, thyroid, digestive tract

5. Be aware of possible associations

nevus sebaceous in mid-face
    may show mental deficiency, seizures, nonfunctioning venous sinuses
sebaceous and eccrine carcinomas, clinically more malignant than suggested by histology
sebaceous adenomas
    may be marker for adenocarcinoma of colon or multiple carcinomas (Muir-Torre syndrome)
nevus comedonicus
    may show central nervous system disorders, myelitis, ocular changes
trichilemmomas in facial location
    marker for Cowden's disease or for neoplasms
pilomatricomas, multiple
    may be associated with myotonic muscular atrophy
trichoepitheliomas
    may be associated with lupus erythematosus. Familial form may show atrophoderma, basal cell carcinoma
follicular hamartomas
    may occur with myasthenia gravis
syringomas
    more often in Down's, Ehlers-Danlos, or Marfan syndromes
eccrine poroma
    may occur with hidrotic ectodermal defect

Raimer SS, Sanchez RL, Hubler WR Jr, Dodson RF: Solar elastotic bands of the forearm: An unusual clinical presentation of **actinic elastosis**. J Am Acad Dermatol 1986; 15:650–656.

The appearance of a band of **coalescing papules and nodules** on the flexor surface of both forearms in a 63-year-old Texas farmer was puzzling. The lesions were flesh- to yellow-colored and asymptomatic. A diagnosis of amyloidosis was considered; however, on biopsy the bands proved to consist of elastotic fibers.

A diagnosis of **solar elastosis** was made, which was consistent with his lifelong history of sun exposure and the presence of other signs of actinic damage, including actinic purpura.

This presentation of sun-induced deposits of abnormal amorphous fibrillar material can be compared with:

Cutis rhomboidalis nuchae
   yellow, furrowed, thickened skin
Actinic comedonal plaques
   thick yellow plaques on forearms surmounted by comedones
Nodular elastosis (Favre-Racouchot syndrome)
   yellowish plaques around lower eyelids with follicular cysts and open comedones
Elastomas
   discrete focal yellow plaques of neck, anterior chest, dorsum of nose. On the ears they may look like basal cell epithelioma, chondrodermatitis nodularis helicis, amyloidosis
Collagenous plaques of the hands
   (Keratoelastoidosis marginalis) groups of discrete or confluent yellowish hyperkeratotic papules at the juncture of dorsal and palmar skin
Colloid milia
   flesh-colored papules on face or backs of hands
Actinic granulomas
   annular, serpiginous nodular lesions with atrophic center
Colloid degeneration
   yellow deep-seated nodules; some may be pink, brown, or orange; rubbery to firm; widespread distribution

Posner DI, Guill MA, III: **Cutaneous foreign body granulomas** associated with **intravenous drug abuse**. J Am Acad Dermatol 1985; 13:869–872.

Tender, firm, 1 to 4 cm **nodules** had been developing on the forearms of a 22-year-old man for 2 years. They were not attached to tendons but were localized near veins. Biopsy showed a **foreign body granuloma** with diffuse birefringent crystals on polarized microscopy. X-ray spectrophotometer studies showed that the crystals contained magnesium, phosphorus, and silica, suggestive of talc (hydrous magnesium silicate).

When confronted with this information, the patient admitted to injecting drugs such as **heroin and amphetamines**, which often contain talc as a filler. He continued to develop new nodules up to 2 years after his last injection. His chest x-ray and pulmonary function tests were normal. Presumably, however, he was at risk for developing systemic talc-induced granulomatosis, which may develop after a long latent period.

The best histories are taken by the one who knows the diagnosis.

Aldridge RD, Main RA, Daly BM: The Koebner's response in **multicentric reticulohistiocytosis**. Cutis 1984; 34:78–80.

Numerous skin **nodules** had been appearing for over 16 years in a 41-year-old man; they were proven to be reticulohistiocytosis. When a row of nodules was observed in this patient's skin, it was postulated that physical trauma may have determined the localization of lesions. Confirmation came by means of a test involving scratching his skin with a pin. At the end of 6 weeks, new papules appeared at the sites of the scratches. Biopsy of the papules revealed **reticulohistiocytosis**, thus illustrating the Koebner phenomenon.

This probably explains the common localization of reticulohistiocytosis on the knuckles, which are subject to many knocks and bruises.

Also known as lipoid dermatoarthritis, this "multicentric" condition may involve fat, skeletal muscle, and the gastric mucosa. Patients should be apprised both of the hazards of trauma and the systemic aspects of the disease.

Rowland Payne CME, Wilkinson JD, McKee PH, et al: **Nodular prurigo**—a clinico-pathological study of 46 patients. Br J Dermatol 1985; 113:431–439.

Nodules: Split pea–size or larger, extremely pruritic, firm, lichenified, pink, dome-shaped, with an excoriated summit and halo of postinflammatory pigment. They are usually symmetrical and grouped and vary from 1 to 100. The intervening skin was often xerodermic and leathery. Lesions resolved with hypopigmented macules and scars. Lichenified plaques and lichen simplex chronicus were also seen in patients with eczema.

Location: Distal extensor arms and legs, but no area exempt.

History: Lesions were preceded by insect bites in 20% and on occasion by folliculitis, venous stasis, and nummular eczema. The pruritus is episodic, triggered by heat and anxiety, and persistent for months to years (average 9 years).

Look for:

Anemia	Eosinophilia (73%)
Iron deficiency	Elevated IgE (43%)
Hepatic disease	Intestinal parasites
Myxedema	Psychosocial disorders
Uremia	

Jorizzo JL, Gatti S, Smith EB: **Prurigo**: A clinical review. J Am Acad Dermatol 1981; 4:723–728.

Acute prurigo (papular urticaria) consists of papules, vesicles and/or urticarial lesions that are seasonal and caused by insect bites in young children. Lesions often persist for one week and are usually located on the extremities and trunk. They do not become confluent and resolve with postinflammatory pigmentation. Pediculosis, scabies, and dermatitis herpetiformis enter into the **differential diagnosis**.

Subacute prurigo occurs mainly in middle-aged women and consists of papules which are symmetrical on the trunk and extensor surfaces of the extremities. These patients often are atopic and usually show dermographism. In addition to insect bites and dermatitis herpetiformis, transient acantholytic dermatosis must be considered as an alternative diagnosis.

Chronic prurigo (prurigo nodularis) consists of hemispheric nodules (0.5 to 3.0 cm) which are often irregular with horny crateriform surfaces and are usually located on the backs of the forearms and thighs. The lesions persist and may form plaques with excoriations and pigmentation. The skin between the lesions is usually normal. Gluten hypersensitivity and uremia are occasionally associated, and hypertrophic lichen planus also must be considered in the differential diagnosis.

Doyle JA, Connolly SM, Hunziker N, Winkelmann RK: **Prurigo nodularis**: A reappraisal of the clinical and histologic features. J Cutan Pathol 1979; 6:392–403.

In 14 patients at the Mayo Clinic, the nodules were discrete and widespread, with verrucous hyperkeratotic surfaces that were often excoriated, bleeding, and crusting. They were set in normal skin. Individual nodules lasted months to years. In 2 patients skin trauma preceded some of the nodules (e.g., razor cut, venipuncture).

Skin biopsies revealed a vascular acanthomatous mass with perivascular lymphocytes, epidermal mast cells, and often hair follicles in the center of the nodule. Dermal nerves showed mild hyperplasia but no neuroma formation.

977

Boer J, Smeenk G: **Nodular prurigo-like eruptions** induced by etretinate. Br J Dermatol 1987; 116:271–274.

Nodular prurigo that was intensely pruritic developed on the back and buttocks of two women in their fifties who were being treated with etretinate (75 mg/day) for persistent hyperkeratotic eczema of the palms and soles (eczema tyloticum). The eruption promptly faded when the dose of etretinate was reduced to 25 mg/day.

Shelnitz LS, Paller AS: **Hodgkin's disease** manifesting as **prurigo nodularis**. Pediatr Dermatol 1990; 7:136–139.

Fourteen months of **pruritus** in this 15-year-old girl led to hospitalization. The pruritus had initially begun as pruritic papules of the ankles. The lesions progressed to involve the entire body, except for the head and neck. The itch resisted all attempts with antibiotics, steroids, antihistamines, lindane, antidepressants, and psychotherapy. Even a previous hospitalization with ultraviolet light and occlusive corticosteroid was to no avail. The skin biopsy showed typical prurigo nodularis.

After a year of incessant pruritus and scratching, palpable cervical lymph nodes were noted and a dry cough with wheezing developed. A diagnosis of asthma was made and a metaproterenol inhaler prescribed.

At the time of this admission, physical examination revealed a pale nervous teenage girl who had lost 10 pounds of weight in the last 6 months. Her skin was covered with hyperkeratotic erythematous nodules, many of which had ulcerated purulent centers. There was bilateral, nontender, movable adenopathy of the anterior cervical lymph nodes. A chest radiograph (the first she had had!) disclosed a large lobulated anterior mediastinal mass compressing her trachea. A cervical lymph node biopsy showed nodular sclerosing **Hodgkin's disease**, the explanation for the pruritus and asthma.

Within a month of chemotherapy all her pruritus had disappeared and by 4 months the lesions had gone.

Hodgkin's disease often stalks its prey with only an unremitting itch.

Borradori L, Rybojad M, Verola D, et al: Pemphigoid nodularis. Arch Dermatol 1990; 126:1522–1523.

A widespread pruritic papular and nodular eruption of 8 months' duration in an 83-year-old woman appeared to be prurigo nodularis. However, immunohistologic studies proved it to be a rare variant of bullous pemphigoid.

Attaching a diagnosis to a baffling disease often leads to a patient attached to you.

The skin suffers as much as the stomach from a lack of nutrition. Its fat disappears. Its color fades. Its hair falls. The starved skin is not healthy. And it was in the skin that the lack of specific nutritional elements was first recognized. The stories of sailors' scurvy and of sharecroppers' pellagra are part of our medical heritage. From them came the knowledge that calories alone are not enough. The skin needs the vitamin C of fruits and the nicotinic acid of grains.

With the discovery of **vitamins**, the diagnostic horizon of nutritional deficits widened. No longer were we limited to spotting the perifollicular petechiae, the bruise purpura, and the gingivitis of vitamin C lack. We could reach beyond the diagnosis of the photosensitivity dermatitis of niacin deficit. We were able to perceive that there is seborrheic dermatitis due to inadequate levels of B_6, angular cheilitis from low B_2, and rough skin from absent vitamin A. No less diagnostic was the edematous skin of no vitamin B_1. We sensed the alopecia of biotin lack. The diagnostic pictures were not specific but spoke to a selective starvation of the skin.

Soon came the awareness of our need of those **fatty acids** that the skin could not synthesize. Again, the picture of a nonspecific dermatitis—especially in infants—pointed to a diagnosis of nutritional lack of linoleic and linolenic acid.

The need for **mineral supplements** came with a look at the anemic skin of iron deficiency and the myxedematous skin of iodine-deprived individuals. The vital role of zinc in skin nutrition came with the astonishing discovery that a zinc supplement would erase the ravages of acrodermatitis enteropathica. A lack of zinc can result in seborrheic dermatitis and eczematous dermatitis of the anogenital and scrotal area, as well as nonhealing ulcers. Zinc is the driving force for over 70 enzymes.

What should you look for to support a diagnosis of nutritional deficiency dermatitis? There are many avenues to explore. The most obvious is that of country-wide famine. Here we find the diagnosis of kwashiorkor. The lack of calories may be just as real for the poor, the homeless, and those on crash diets. A social history may be far easier to secure than an accurate dietary history. Is the patient an alcoholic whose major caloric intake is vitamin-free ethanol? This may be difficult to answer in the case of the female socialite whose solitary drinking is known only to her.

To support the diagnosis of a dietary dermatosis, continue to search for evidence of anorexia nervosa. Do the hands show the stigmata of repeated dental trauma in the course of induction of emesis? Gently inquire for specific menus. One girl was found to have lived exclusively on bread and peanut butter for over a year. A diet of large amounts of raw eggs will induce the alopecia of biotin lack by means of the biotin antagonist avidin, present in the uncooked egg. The pathologic avoidance of essential foods must be recognized in those individuals who believe they are allergic to multiple foods.

Look to disease as a cause of malnutrition. Patients with Crohn's disease may develop pellagra. Chronic diarrhea may also favor the appearance of nutritional deficiency states. Absorption of essential vitamins also is impaired in those who are taking cholestyramine or mineral oil regularly. Absorption of nutrients is also altered in patients who have had bypass surgery. Long-term antibiotic therapy produces nutritional problems by reason of its elimination of the gut bacteria, which normally synthesize essential elements.

Again, patients dependent on hyperalimentation or parenteral feedings may well develop the skin lesions of vitamin or mineral deficiencies if their specific formulation is deficient.

Screen for **inborn errors of metabolism**. Especially in infants, metabolic deficits may account for pigmentary and keratinization errors. Testing for phenylketonuria, B_6 and B_{12} levels may provide significant diagnostic information.

Nutritional dermatitides may also result from drugs—contraceptives and isoniazid may act as antagonists to pyridoxine and vitamin B_6.

For diagnostic insight into that puzzling dermatitis, learn what goes into the gut and what the gut does with it. When the diet or the gut is wrong, the skin is wronged.

Miller SJ: **Nutritional deficiency** and the skin. J Am Acad Dermatol 1989; 21:1–30.

<hr>

CLINICAL DATA

Signs	Nutritional deficiency
Xerosis	Vitamin A, biotin
Dermatitis	Biotin
Alopecia	Biotin
Hyperpigmentation	Vitamin B_{12}, niacin
Seborrheic dermatitis	Riboflavin, pyridoxine
Perioral dermatitis	Zinc
Scrotal dermatitis	Riboflavin
Intertriginous erosions	Essential fatty acids
"Enamel paint" spots (dark burnished waxy papules over pressure sites)	Protein
Flag sign hair	Protein
Perifollicular hemorrhages	Vitamin C
Pellagra	Niacin

LABORATORY DATA ON NUTRITIONAL STATUS

Nutrient	Deficient values
Vitamin A	<20 μg/dl
Riboflavin (RBC glutathione activity coefficient)	>1.2
Pyridoxine (pyridoxine-6-phosphate)	<20 ng/ml
Niacin (fluorometric assay of urinary metabolites) (2-pyridone/N' methyl ratio)	<2.0
Biotin (microbiologic assay)	<200 pg/ml
Vitamin B_{12} (microbiologic or radioassay)	<150 pg/ml
Vitamin C (serum assay)	<0.1 mg < 7 mg/dl
Vitamin D (radioimmunoassay 25-vitamin D_3)	<5 mg/dl
Vitamin K (prothrombin time)	<2 sec above control
Protein (plasma/serum albumin)	<2.5 gm/dl
Copper (plasma ceruloplasmin)	<125 μg/dl
Zinc (plasma)	<70 μg/dl
Essential fatty acids (GLC of RBC membrane) (triene: tetraene ratio)	>0.4

<hr>

McLaren DS: Skin in **protein energy malnutrition**. Arch Dermatol 1987; 123:1674–1676.

In Ghana it was long the custom to depose the baby from breast feeding once the mother knew she was pregnant again. Left to the scant, nutritionally inadequate, starchy family fare, the child often developed "**kwashiorkor**," the native phrase for "the disease the first child gets when the second is on the way." Zinc deficiency, as well as protein deficiency, is probably a major factor.

Depigmentation is the basic skin change in kwashiorkor, with early circumoral pallor and pallor on the legs and localized pigment loss following trauma. Distinct bands of light-colored hair correlate with periods of malnutrition, resulting in the "flag sign" seen in scalp hair (alternating light and dark bands). Hair bulbs are depigmented and speckled and show a marked shift toward telogen, with atrophy and shaft constriction of anagen hairs.

Other signs of malnutrition:

> In fair-skinned children, erythema (an early sign) followed by small dusky purple patches that don't blanch.
> "Enamel paint" spots (dark burnished waxy papules over pressure sites).
> "Crazy paving" or "flaky paint" dermatosis (due to desquamation).
> Peeling and erosions (suggestive of burns or zinc deficiency).
> Linear fissuring (flexural folds, base of pinna, edge of foreskin, toewebs, central lip).

Angular cheilitis (suggestive of riboflavin deficiency).
Sparing of the neck, hands, and forearms (pellagra not present).

In true starvation (**marasmus**), none of these changes occur. The skin is dry, wrinkled, and loose due to loss of fat ("monkey face" develops when buccal fat pads fade). The hair gets thin, nails split, and follicular hyperkeratosis (keratosis pilaris) develops in adults (but not infants). Downy lanugo hair may cover the entire body of the infant with marasmus.

Surgeons use the prognostic nutritional index (PNI) in evaluating patients with malnutrition. The four indicators (combined into a formula) include:

triceps skinfold thickness
serum albumin
serum transferrin
skin tests of cell-mediated immunity

Although this index does not differentiate between marasmus and kwashiorkor, it does help predict surgical outcome.

Stimson WH: **Vitamin A intoxication** in adults. N Engl J Med 1961; 265:369–373.

The only frequent neurologic sign in adults is **headache**, while children and adolescents develop increased intracranial pressure with neurologic signs and papilledema.

A 32-year-old woman denied taking vitamins until her husband reminded her that she had been taking 100,000 IU of vitamin A daily for 5 years, originally prescribed for acne. After $3\frac{1}{2}$ years she developed intermittent abdominal pain, anorexia, nausea, fatigability, bone pain (low-back, hip, tibial), hepatosplenomegaly, and leukopenia (WBC 3200). Her eyes were prominent, and **scalp hair was sparse** over the anterior crown, having recently come out rapidly. Her lips were very dry and she described painful lumps along the tongue margin. Serum vitamin A was 250 IU/100 ml (normal 50 to 200). Within 3 days after she stopped taking vitamin A the **bone pain** disappeared and she no longer required a daily nap; after 7 months she felt entirely well, although her eyes remained exophthalmic.

Among the seven previously reported cases, the smallest vitamin A dose producing symptoms was 50,000 IU daily for 18 months. The shortest duration of treatment before onset of symptoms was 6 weeks with a dose of 275,000 IU daily. A dose of 600,000 IU daily gave symptoms after 12 months, while a dose of 500,000 IU daily gave symptoms after 5 months. There is always a **latent period** of weeks to months, somewhat dose related.

In the Arctic, liver from certain animals is poisonous. **Polar bear liver** contains 13,000 to 18,000 IU of vitamin A per gram, and eating it induces severe symptoms within a few hours, including abdominal pain, nausea, vomiting, headache, dizziness, sluggishness, irritability, and a strong desire to sleep. Full recovery occurs in a few days, accompanied by generalized peeling of the skin.

Too much of a good thing is not good.

Vitamin Deficiencies

Sydenstricker VP: The syndrome of **multiple vitamin deficiency**. Ann Intern Med 1941; 15:45–51.

The presence of signs of any of the avitaminoses is indicative of multiple deficiency. An **unbalanced diet** causes prolonged partial deficiency with functional and organic changes in the digestive tract that interfere with absorption and utilization of vitamins. Few patients present all the signs of a single avitaminosis but almost every patient shows signs of several.

Gastric **achlorhydria** interferes with extraction of all water-soluble vitamins, while **biliary obstruction** with lack of bile in the upper bowel prevents adequate absorption of the fat-soluble group. Vomiting and diarrhea cause loss of ingested vitamins; edema of the gastrointestinal tract prevents absorption. Liver disease interferes with vitamin A synthesis and vitamin B group formation and utilization.

Acute vitamin deficiency results from sudden large requirements for vitamins—substituting alcohol for food, dextrose maintenance, and severe febrile disease.

Thiamin deficiency	Tenderness of nerves and calf muscles
	Hyper- and hyporeflexia
	Muscular weakness and edema
	Sensory disturbances and loss of motor function
	Heart failure—edema and tachycardia
Nicotinic acid deficiency	Symmetrical dermatitis
	Glossitis with atrophy of lingual papillae
	Lesions of buccal mucosa or genitalia (ulcerative dermatitis)
	Mental changes
Ariboflavinosis	Cheilosis and glossitis
	Superficial vascularizing keratitis
	Seborrheic dermatitis
Scurvy	Gingivitis
	Hemorrhages into mucous membranes, skin
	Plasma ascorbic acid level of zero
Vitamin A deficiency	Follicular keratosis
	Xerosis of skin and cornea
	Delayed dark adaptation
	Low vitamin A and carotinoids in blood
	Photophobia
	Blurring of vision
	Poor vision in dim light
	Night blindness
	Rapid visual fatigue
	Irritation of eyes
Vitamin D deficiency	X-ray, loss of calcium from bones
	Abnormal phosphatase levels in blood

Selective treatment in pellagra has identified the cause of the following symptoms:

Thiamin deficiency		
	Paresthesias	Tachycardia
	Neuritic pains	Anorexia
	Decreased tendon reflexes	Flatulence
	Edema	Constipation

983

Nicotinic acid deficiency	Psychic manifestations	
	Hearing loss	Red atrophic tongue
	Appetite loss	Stomatitis
	Nausea	Esophagitis
	Diarrhea	Dermatitis
	Genital and rectal mucosa lesions	
Riboflavin deficiency	Keratotic comedones	
	Fissuring of commisures	
	Seborrheic dermatitis of face and neck	
	Sore mouth and tongue with redness and burning	
	Eye symptoms (photophobia, burning and itching, keratitis, dimness, superficial vascularization)	

Sydenstricker VP: The clinical manifestations of nicotinic acid and riboflavin deficiency (**pellagra**). Ann Intern Med 1941; 14:1499–1517.

Since the B group of vitamins occurs together in natural sources, deficiencies usually affect the whole group. In **pellagra** the signs and symptoms are attributable to deficiencies of riboflavin, thiamin, and nicotinic acid. Skin lesions occur especially after sun exposure, heat, friction, or chemical irritation. Look for:

Dermatitis with symmetrical erythema of the dorsal hands, neck, upper chest, malar areas, forehead, elbows, forearms, feet, genitalia, and knees; lesions may be vesiculobullous

Thickening and hyperpigmentation of these same areas without dermatitis

Balantitis or vaginitis

Decubitus ulcers from the rapid necrosis of skin over the dorsal hands, elbows, knees, feet

"Sharkskin" eruption–follicular keratoses of the sebaceous glands of the forehead, nose, malar eminences, chin

Seborrheic dermatitis–ears, cheeks, alae nasi, chin

Lips that are painful, red, desquamating, and fissured at the commissures

A tongue that is sore, bright red, atrophic, fissured, ulcerated, or geographic; it may also be magenta and pebbled with mushroom-shaped papillae

Mackie TT, Eddy WH, Mills MA: **Vitamin deficiencies** in **gastrointestinal disease**. Ann Intern Med 1940; 14:28–41.

Vitamin A deficiency causes dry, scaly skin with keratotic plugs in the hair follicles. Epithelial atrophy is followed by metaplasia and the development of stratfied squamous epithelium.

Vitamin B₁ (Thiamin) deficiency causes beriberi and peripheral neuritis.

Riboflavin deficiency causes oral changes with red shiny lips, maceration, and fissures at the corners of the mouth, and a magenta tongue with flattened mushroom-shaped papillae. Seborrheic accumulations may occur at the nasolabial folds and corneal opacities may develop from capillary ingrowth into the cornea.

Nicotinic acid deficiency causes pellagra with acute glossitis, stomatitis, and enteritis. Acute dermatitis of sun-exposed areas is followed by pigmentation and atrophy (thin, parchment-like skin), and similar changes occur in the perianal area, scrotum, vulva, and vagina.

Vitamin C deficiency causes weakened vascular walls and increased capillary fragility with red blood cell extravasation.

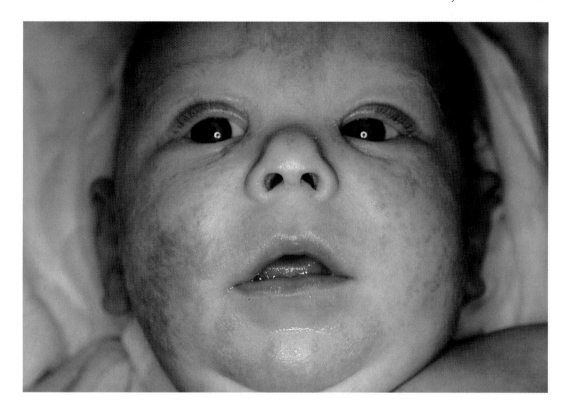

Wolf B, Feldman GL: The **biotin-dependent carboxylase deficiencies**. Am J Hum Genet 1982; 34:699–716.

There are four known human biotin-dependent enzymes:

> acetyl CoA carboxylase (fatty acid synthesis)
> pyruvate carboxylase (gluconeogenesis)
> propionyl CoA carboxylase (amino acid and fatty acid catabolism)
> beta-methylcrotonyl CoA carboxylase (leucine catabolism)

Deficiencies of these enzymes may occur separately or together and cause ketolactic acidosis, organic acidemia, hyperammonemia, and urine that smells like cat urine.

In the late-onset (age 3 to 6 months) form of multiple carboxylase deficiency patients have a skin rash, alopecia, candidiasis, conjunctivitis, ataxia, and developmental delay. Serum and urinary biotin levels are low.

Gompertz D, Draffan GH, Watts JL, Hull D: Biotin-responsive **β-methylcrotonylglycinuria**. Lancet 1971; 2:22–24.

A 5-month-old boy was hospitalized with persistent vomiting and an extensive **erythematous rash** that began on the buttocks and neck at age 6 weeks and gradually spread to all flexures despite treatment with topical steroids and nystatin. He was found to have severe metabolic acidosis and ketosis. His urine was negative for protein, sugar, and amino acids but had a peculiar odor reminiscent of male cat urine. This led to analysis of the urine for volatile fatty acids by steam distillation and gas chromatography, with the finding of beta-methylcrotonylglycine and beta-hydroxyisovaleric acid and recognition that the enzyme beta-methylcrotonyl CoA carboxylase was impaired. Treatment with biotin, the coenzyme of the carboxylase, led to rapid improvement of his condition and clearing of the skin rash.

McClain CJ, Baker H, Onstad GR: **Biotin deficiency** in an adult during home parenteral nutrition. JAMA 1982; 247:3116–3117.

A 36-year-old man with regional enteritis for 17 years developed **dermatitis** around his eyes, nose, and mouth. For the past 3 years he had been on parenteral nutrition (2500 calories/day/venous catheter). The dermatitis was similar to that he had experienced 5 years ago. This had been due to zinc deficiency and responded promptly to zinc supplementation.

This time intravenous zinc as well as fatty acid supplementation was ineffective. The patient experienced paresthesias of the feet and lethargy and progressive loss of both hair color and hair itself. A diagnosis of **biotin deficiency** was entertained and proven by addition of 60 μg of biotin to his formula. Within 2 weeks his skin lesions had improved. By 3 months the skin had returned to normal and he had no paresthesias.

Diagnosis is the genius of seeing order in the randomization of disease.

Gupta MA, Gupta AK, Haberman HF: Dermatologic signs in **anorexia nervosa and bulimia nervosa**. Arch Dermatol 1987; 123:1386–1390.

The deceitful dietary history of patients who eat too little or too much is a dangerous diagnostic trap. Learn to look beyond the diet described and think of **anorexia nervosa** in the thin adolescent girl who complains of:

diffuse alopecia	increased lanugo body hair	dry skin
brittle hair and nails	swollen ankles (edema that pits)	yellow palms

Learn to look beyond the dietary habits claimed and think of **bulimia nervosa** in the woman with:

calluses or abrasions of the dorsal hands (Russell's sign: due to frictional injury from the teeth as the patient induces vomiting by manual stimulation of the gag reflex)
enlarged parotids
laboratory findings of elevated serum amylase and hypokalemic alkalosis.

Learn to think of eating disorders in patients with:

acne excoriée	finger clubbing due to laxative abuse
hand dermatitis	complaints, but no signs
from compulsive washing	surreptitious use of diet pills, laxatives,
trichotillomania	emetics, and diuretics
dermatitis artifacta	

Learn to think of malnutrition in any patient who is failing to cope with life. Learn to be suspicious when the diet history doesn't match the current weight.

Herzog DB, Copeland PM: **Eating disorders**. N Engl J Med 1985; 313:295–303.

Most anorectic and bulimic patients are white females from middle or upper socioeconomic environments. Excessive physical activity to achieve weight loss may be the earliest sign.

Anorexia nervosa begins as an overweight young teenager tries to lose weight and then becomes preoccupied with being thin. She either severely restricts caloric intake or alternates this with binge eating that is terminated by self-induced vomiting or the use of laxatives and diuretics. Amenorrhea and osteoporosis result from estrogen depletion, and the "euthyroid sick syndrome" with decreased peripheral conversion of thyroxine to triiodothyronine may cause dry skin and hair, cold intolerance, bradycardia, hypercarotenemia, and slowed relaxation of reflexes. Hypotension, arrhythmias, azotemia, renal calculi, edema, constipation, elevated liver enzymes, and anemia largely reflect starvation, dehydration, and electrolyte imbalance. Major depression is common, and the patient is usually isolated and asexual.

Bulimia begins in late adolescence after many reducing diets have been tried without success. The patient becomes aware that self-induced vomiting or laxative use may control weight and alternates these with solitary daily binges of junk food high in carbohydrates. After eating she feels guilt, shame, and low self-esteem. She is usually outgoing, heterosexual, and may have other impulsive behaviors such as alcohol or drug use. Menstrual irregularities, weight fluctuations, and hypokalemia are common, and repeated vomiting may induce parotid enlargement, dental enamel erosion, and esophagitis with rupture. Patients often have a low frustration tolerance for therapy that does not produce immediate relief of symptoms.

Eating disorders are increasingly common and need to be recognized by physicians through careful history-taking, physical examination, and laboratory evaluation. Although patients and their families tend to deny the illness, they need to be guided into psychiatric treatment.

Occupational Disease

Making a diagnosis may be easy—finding the cause, difficult. To aid in the search for a cause, learn as much as you can about your patient's work. You may make a diagnosis of paronychia, but until you know of your patient's work in a wet environment the cause is hidden. You may make a diagnosis of miliaria, but until you find out that your patient works in the tropical environment of a boiler room, the cause remains puzzling.

In the case of allergic contact dermatitis, you can direct your patch testing only when you know the chemical exposures at the workplace of your patient. Is there an airborne allergen such as formaldehyde, pesticides, and chromium dust? Is that hand dermatitis due to rubber contactants, epoxy resins, or chrysanthemums encountered in their work? Could that chapped skin or facial flush result from low humidity in a sealed-off office building? Is that folliculitis due to cutting oils? Could a photosensitivity be the result of your beautician patient working in a perfume- or aerosol-laden room under a bank of fluorescent lights?

The list of insights goes on. Could the nurse or dental hygienist's fingertip herpes simplex be due to her occupation? Could her positive HIV test be of occupational origin? Could the construction worker's itch be due to sensitization to the oils of chromates? Could the housewife's eczema be due to sensitization to the citrus fluids she squeezes?

At times, it is not easy to obtain an adequate **history** of the patient's exposures at work or at play. The violinist with contact dermatitis may not tell you of his rosin dust. The pruritic secretary may not know of the fumigants used in her office last Saturday. And the cleaning woman with "vitiligo" may not mention the new phenolic disinfectant issued for her use last month. The gentleman farmer with orf may not recall petting his lambs. Nor can you be sure the hobby shop owner with a mycobacterial granuloma will tell you of his tropical fish. Learn to question evocatively.

You may have to turn from history taking to actually visiting the **workplace**. Make an appointment. Go when the full work force is there working. Look for the inapparent. Find out if there are others with the same problem, such as "Halowax acne." Learn if there are new factors such as a change in ventilation, manufacturing equipment, or cleansing routines. Listen to other workers for ideas. Workers in nursing homes, for example, know of occupational scabies.

Take time out some afternoon for an in-depth study of your most challenging patient's workplace. It will be an instructive divertissement. Whether or not you find the ultimate cause, your afternoon will do wonders for your patient-physician rapport, as well as win the admiration of the patient's co-workers. Remember, detectives rarely solve cases by simply sitting in their office.

Calnan CD: Prosser White Oration 1977. **Dermatology and industry.** Clin Exp Dermatol 1978; 3:1–16.

Samples of diagnostic sleuthing in industry:

Visit the factory:

In a gold and silver jewelry unit, a special cleaning solution (kept away in a corner) was the cause of chromate dermatitis.

Know the chemistry:

Transformers containing a paratertiary butylphenol formaldehyde resin were baked overnight, releasing phenol that accounted for vitiligo in the single worker in that room.

Question the data:

Independent chemical analysis showed isopropyl-aminodiphenylamine to be present in rubber fingerettes, despite claims of the manufacturer that it was not added to the rubber. It was this compound that accounted for dermatitis in workers.

Look for impurities:

Failure of precise control of temperature and pressure during the manufacture of lauryl ether sulfate resulted in trace amounts of halogenated sultones being formed. This led to an epidemic of severe dermatitis in individuals using this normally safe domestic detergent.

If synthetic soluble oils are used in machines, **contact dermatitis** is usually of the irritant type and attributable to emulsifiers or surface active agents in the oils. Skin eruptions consist of two main patterns: red papular lesions on the forearms and papulo-vesicular lesions on the hands and fingers. Two other less common presentations include chronic lichenified and fissured eczema of the fingers and a discoid eczema pattern on the dorsum of the hands and fingers.

Thiboutot DM, Hamory BH, Marks JG Jr: **Dermatoses** among floral shop workers. J Am Acad Dermatol 1990; 22:54–58.

One out of every four employees in a large floral company had **hand dermatitis**. A leading cause of their plant sensitization was the flower *Alstroemeria*. Workers may handle it for as long as 3 years before becoming sensitized. Interestingly, the amount of allergen (tuliposide A) varies with not only the species but with hundreds of cultivars. Furthermore, the amount of allergen varies among the bulb, leaf petal, stem, and phase of growth. This can easily lead to failure in recognizing exposure.

Stoner JG, Rasmussen JE: **Plant dermatitis**. J Am Acad Dermatol 1983; 9:1–15.

Diagnostic puzzles:

Plantar papules	Cactus needle granulomas after walking barefoot in an Arizona desert.
Stomatitis	Chewing on house plant leaves containing the irritant calcium oxalate. The reaction may be so intense as to result in massive tongue edema and loss of voice. Hence, the common name "dumb cane" for one of the offending house plants, Dieffenbachia.
"Photodermatitis"	Ragweed resin (sesquiterpene lactones, not the pollen) but involving upper retroauricular and submental areas, in addition to light-exposed areas.
Fingertip fissuring, scaling, erythema	Handling hyacinth bulbs.
Hemorrhagic papular eruption of covered areas of body	Plant mite bites.
Dermatitis followed by intense hyperpigmentation	Phytophotodermatitis due to contact with plant followed by UVA exposure; may appear in streaks (dermatitis bullosa striata pratensis).

Think plants when you see farmers, nursery men, florists, grocers, hunters, botanists, gardeners, and house plant enthusiasts.

Feldman LR, Eaglstein WH, Johnson RB: **Terminal illness**. J Am Acad Dermatol 1985; 12:366.

Redness, burning, and itching of the backs of the hands and the distal forearms was related to his work by this 33-year-old man. The problem had developed 2 weeks after starting work at a computer terminal over a year ago. The affected areas were directly under emissions from the visual display unit. His symptoms markedly lessened on weekends when he was away from work. Furthermore, when he covered one hand with duofilm while at work this site remained clear.

Detailed hospital studies revealed no cause for his problem other than long-term exposure to his computer display screen. Patch and photopatch tests to 41 work-related compounds were negative. Challenge by exposure to his office environment sans computer display unit led to disappearance of the redness, burning, and itching. When he resumed use of the visual display unit, his rash returned within a week.

A diagnosis of VDU dermatitis was made.

Hodgson MJ, Parkinson DK: Diagnosis of **organophosphate intoxication**. N Engl J Med 1985; 313:329.

Increased salivation and diarrhea occurred in all five office workers in a cement bunker within one hour after an exterminator applied chlorpyrifos and methylcarbamic acid to their building. An increase in red cell cholinesterase levels confirmed organophosphate pesticide poisoning.

Jacobs PH: **Dermatophytes** that infect animals and humans. Cutis 1988; 42:330–331.

Think tinea if your patient is a:

veterinarian or assistant	zoo keeper
farmer or farm hand	pet shop worker
horse trainer	pet owner
stable worker	infant
jockey	research animal handler
animal shelter employee	

Don't forget to ask about the pet llama, monkey, or hedgehog. Also remember that humans can transmit zoophilic mycoses to animals. In the small pet category, dogs have harbored 13 different dermatophytes, while cats have had 7 types, and birds have had 3 types.

Dermatophytes implicated include 7 species of *Microsporum* and 10 species of *Trichophyton*. The most frequent infections include:

Microsporum canis–cats, dogs, sheep, monkeys, horses
       "   *distortum*–sheep
       "   *gypseum*–dogs, rabbits, rodents
       "   *nanum*–pigs
Trichophyton gallinae–birds
       "   *erinacei*–hedgehogs
       "   *equinum*–horses
       "   *mentagrophytes*–dogs, rabbits, rodents, monkeys
       "   *simii*–birds, monkeys
       "   *verrucosum*–cattle

Doğanay M, Bakir M, Dökmetas İ: A case of **cutaneous anthrax with toxaemic shock**. Br J Dermatol 1987; 117:659–662.

Shortly after slaughtering a dying cow, a 16-year-old shepherd boy in Sivas, Turkey, noted a small pruritic papule on the left side of his neck, which enlarged and became edematous. Within one week, he developed high fever,

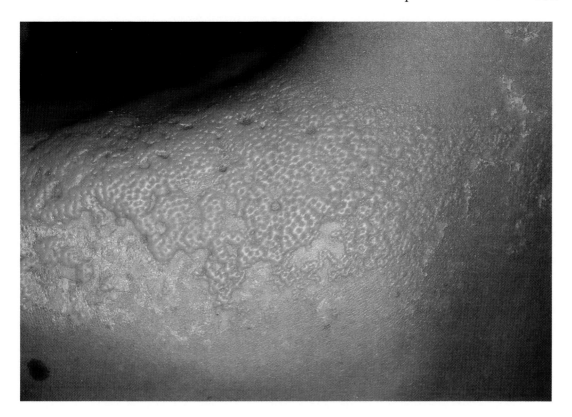

extensive erythema, and massive nonpitting edema of the face, neck, and thorax, leading to hospitalization. A 2 cm **necrotic black eschar** on the left neck showed gram-positive encapsulated bacilli on smear, suggesting anthrax. Treatment with penicillin (5 million units every 4 hours), led to complete recovery by 2 weeks.

In **anthrax**, a toxic protein produced by *Bacillus anthracis* induces increased vascular permeability with resulting extensive edema. It also causes hemorrhage due to platelet thrombi, stasis, and venous thrombosis and obstruction. Circulating toxins can lead to rapid death. Penicillin is the therapy of choice, since no antitoxin is available.

Anon: **Human cutaneous anthrax**—North Carolina, 1987. JAMA 1988; 260:616.

A 42-year-old maintenance man in a textile yarn mill in North Carolina developed a small **red, pruritic papule** on the right forearm. Over the next week it became vesicular and then necrotic, with a depressed black eschar and surrounding edema. He was then hospitalized with worsening edema, pain, fever, and chills and responded rapidly to intravenous ampicillin and cephalosporins. A diagnosis of **cutaneous anthrax** was made based on clinical observation, despite negative blood and wound cultures. It was confirmed by an electrophoretic transblot assay for antibody to anthrax antigens, with a titer of 512 to anthrax protective antigen and lethal factor.

The source of the infection was identified by finding *Bacillus anthracis* on five samples of **cashmere goat hair** within the mill. This cashmere had come from western Asia (Afghanistan or Iran), an endemic area for anthrax. This is the first case of anthrax reported in the United States since 1984 and only the ninth case in the last 10 years. The low incidence reflects the success of vaccination of workers who have to process imported animal products and of the decline in use of fibers of animal origin.

Think of anthrax when evaluating skin lesions in veterinarians and agricultural workers who handle infected animals or even bone meal fertilizer.

Rüdlinger R, Bunney MH, Grob R, Hunter JAA: **Warts in fish handlers**. Br J Dermatol 1989; 120:375–381.

No, Virginia, you do not catch warts from handling frogs, fish, poultry, or meat, whether it be fresh, frozen, or fried. Frogs, fish, chickens, and cows have their own species-specific papilloma viruses. But if you work as a fish monger or a butcher boy all day, your hands are macerated, fissured, and traumatized. Your skin is wide open to welcome the ubiquitous human wart virus, HPV_7 being the most popular one.

Warts, thus, may be an occupational disease when the occupation sets the stage, but the bad actor is the virus.

Rimmer S, Spielvogel RL: **Dermatologic problems of musicians**. J Am Acad Dermatol 1990; 22:657–663.

Fiddler's neck	Area of lichenification at site of chin rest just below jaw on left side of neck; may see edema, erythema, inflammatory papules, pustules, folliculitis, hyperpigmentation, even cysts, lymphadenopathy, and scarring
Guitar nipple	Inflamed cystic swelling at base of nipple due to edge of sound box being pressed against nipples. Such a mastitis usually appears in young girls playing an adult-sized guitar.
Guitarist's groin	Varicosities and venous thrombosis from compression of long saphenous vein
Cellist's chest	Pressure of cello on xiphoid process produces pain and tenderness of sternal area
Cello knee	Erythema, scaling, hyperpigmentation, calluses of medial knee from pressure of cello
Cello scrotum	Scrotal dermatitis
Harpist's fingers	Paronychia and calluses, onycholysis, subungual hemorrhages
Violinist's thrombosis	Axilla-subclavian vein thrombosis (**Paget-Schroetter syndrome**) due to pressure on brachiocephalic, external jugular, axillary, and subclavian veins; manifests as edema, erythema, and pain of upper arm; diagnosis of phlebography
Violinist's knuckles	**Garrod's pads**–thickened skin over interphalangeal joints from intense flexion of tendons of fingers during playing
Violinist's hand	Contact dermatitis due to rosin hypersensitivity
Clarinetist's cheilitis	Eczematous dermatitis of median lower lip at point of contact with reed
Flutist's chin	Inflammation, pustules, papules, hyperpigmentation at center of chin

Musicians, both amateur and professional, also suffer from **contact dermatitis** to the wood, metal, or plastic in their instrument or to cleansers or polish. Special dermatologic problems that can be disabling to wind players are:

mucosal fissures	xerostomia
herpes simplex	hypersalivation

For all musicians, palmar hyperhidrosis can be devastating. Your own performance on the clinical stage demands that you know not only your patient's vocation but his avocations as well.

Odor

Odor comes into our office in two ways. Some patients bring us a problem wherein odor is a diagnostic aid for us. Other patients bring their odor to us as the primary problem. In the first instance, we must be alert to the odor of bacterial infection, to the odor generated by a foreign body inserted into the nose or vagina, and to the odor of the inherited metabolic defects. Bacterial production of volatile fatty acids accounts for many of the 10,000 odors our nose can perceive, but which we cannot name. Possibly, the most common odors brought to our office are the odor of the alcoholic and the odor of sweaty feet.

When the infant's urine or diaper smells strange, it is well to do an amino acid screen for metabolic aberrations such as phenylketonuria or maple syrup urine disease. When the patient smells like rotten fish, look for trimethylaminuria. A choline challenge will cause marked accentuation of the odor, and gas chromatography will confirm the diagnosis. It should be noted that hospital and clinical laboratories do not provide this service. It is necessary to contact a special center for these "laboratory orphans."

Contact Marjorie A. Brewster, Ph.D., Director, Metab Lab Ark, Children's Hospital, Little Rock, AR 72202 or Paul V. Fennessy, Ph.D., Director of the Clinical Mass Spectrometry Research Resource, Medical School, University of Colorado, 4200 9th Avenue, Denver, CO 80262. Contact them for details on acidifying and freezing urine sample for mailing. They also have the capability of detecting and measuring other malodorous volatile compounds such as sulfides.

Much more challenging is the patient who comes with the primary problem of odor that is not there. A typical example is the delusional patient, also known as dysmorphic, who describes having an offensive odor that neither you nor his family senses. Known as **phantosmia**, such an error of perception may be erased by prescribing pimozide or an antidepressant; however, before closing the door to further etiologic thought, consider and review the possibility of rhinitis, sinusitis, solvent exposure, head injury, or brain tumor being responsible. Look to the tonsils and teeth and secure sinus films and possibly a CT scan of the head.

The possibility that such patients may simply be hyperosmic also crosses our mind. Such **hyperosmia** occurs in workers exposed to solvents and in cystic fibrosis patients. We must realize that any patient who could achieve the sensory level of the canine nose would be disturbed by his new world of overpowering odors.

Nonetheless, the patient who appears in your office with undocumented and unperceived odor must be viewed as having a problem other than odor. Recall that adaptation to odor is so quick and powerful that the patient who really has an odor is usually unaware of his problem. He has adapted.

Lockman DS: **Olfactory diagnosis**. Cutis 1981; 27:645–647.

The problem: "**Smelling like sour pickles** for 3 to 4 weeks" in a 40-year-old white man.

He did not have unusual dietary habits or eat large amounts of onions, curry, garlic, or pickles. The odor improved with bathing but returned in 3 to 4 hours. He did not use deodorant and had a pungently sweet odor emanating from the axillae.

The diagnosis: **Axillary bromhidrosis** due to failure to use deodorant.

The cure: Topical clindamycin (Cleocin). The problem resolved after 2 weeks.

The article has a table of 15 additional diagnostic odors, eight of these being in newborns with metabolic errors:

Diabetic ketoacidosis (breath)

Liver failure (fetor hepaticus–breath, urine)
Anaerobic infections (breath, wound)
Cutaneous infections (disease site)
Bromhidrosis (axillae, feet)
Foreign bodies (nasal, vaginal)
Fetor oris (halitosis)
Inborn errors of metabolism (urine, sweat, breath):
    Phenylketonuria (stale sweat)
    Maple syrup urine disease (caramel, maple syrup)
    Oasthouse syndrome (dried malt, hops)
    Odor of sweaty feet (Types I & II)
    Odor of cat syndrome (cat's urine)
    Fish odor syndrome (trimethylaminuria–dead fish)
    Rancid butter syndrome (rancid butter)

Knox, JDE: The **nose in diagnosis**. Lancet 1983; 1:292.

A day in practice:

an alcoholic sucking on peppermints to keep his disease incognito but forgetting that the alcohol odor comes out through sweat and skin.

the smell of wintergreen as the first diagnostic sign of spinal metastasis in a patient with bronchogenic carcinoma. He was using it in a liniment for his recent onset of back pain.

the premonitory unpleasant odor of an unrecognized bowel carcinoma

a house call to an indigent whose room had the musty smell of fleas, the unpleasant smell of bedbugs, and the aroma of the unwashed sweat of yesterdays.

and finally, the faint sweetish, slightly fecal smell of death in a DOA case.

Liddell K: **Smell** as a diagnostic marker. Postgraduate Medical Journal 1976; 52:136–138.

Diagnostic insights:

Infants with unexplained odors may have metabolic disease.
    Maple syrup urine disease
    Phenylketonuria
    Leucine disturbance in metabolism
    Methionine disturbance
    Oasthouse syndrome
Ulcers that become malodorous may harbor malignancy.
Patients may hide carcinomas of breast, penis, or ear to the point at which malodor makes them societal outcasts.
Odor may reflect systemic disease, uremia, diabetes, hepatic failure, bladder and bowel sphincter failure.
Odor may result from poor hygiene or special food intake (garlic, curry).
Schizophrenics may have a unique pungent odor.
In "bad breath," look beyond the mouth to bronchiectasis, lung abscess.
Check patients not only for how they smell but also for how well they can smell. Unilateral anosmia suggests a frontal lobe tumor. An olfactory aura of strong smell may be a prelude to an epileptic convulsion.

Smith M, Smith L, Levinson B: The use of **smell in differential diagnosis**. Lancet 1982; 2:1452–1453.

More diagnostic smells:

sweet	marijuana
cigarette smell	smoker

foul	bromides
musty	penicillin
cheesy	abscess
mousy	*Proteus* infection
rotten apple	*Clostridium* gas-gangrene infection
grapelike	*Pseudomonas aeruginosa*
burned tissue	Darier's disease
garlic	dimethylsulfoxide (DMSO) use

A glossary of odors:

Pleasant	*Neutral*	*Unpleasant*
fruity	alcoholic	pungent
spicy	yeastlike	caustic
sweet	grapelike	sweaty
floral		musty
		amino-like
		burnt
		cheesy
		buttery
		foul
		putrid

Kanda F, Yagi E, Nakajima K, et al: Elucidation of chemical compounds responsible for **foot malodour**. Br J Dermatol 1990; 122:771–776.

The scent of **smelly feet** can be reproduced by an in vitro 10-day incubation of sweat and surface lipids from subjects with foot malodor. In the case of samples from subjects without foot odor, addition of hydrochloric acid resulted in the sudden generation of foot odor by release of free fatty acids.

Short-chain fatty acids are responsible for the pungent foot odor of some individuals; specifically, **isovaleric acid** plays a major role.

Scott AE: Clinical characteristics of **taste and smell disorders**. Ear Nose Throat J 1989; 68:297–315.

Parosmia occurs when there is an abnormal or distorted perception of an odorant stimulus. By contrast, **phantosmia** is the perception of an odor in the absence of any odorant.

Any patient with either problem should be checked for these possible causes:

    hypothyroidism
    upper respiratory tract infection
    rhinitis
    sinusitis
    solvent exposure
    medication, e.g., streptomycin
    head trauma

Zilstorff K, Harbi IDO: **Parosmia**. Acta Otolaryngol 1979; Suppl 360:40–41.

The distorted perception of an odor is known as parosmia. It may arise centrally:

    Illusions of smell in premenstrual, pregnant, hemicrania, and neurotic patients.
    Olfactory hallucinations in psychotic patients, especially schizophrenics.
    Uncinate seizures with a large olfactory component.

Or it may arise peripherally:

A foul smell (cacosmia) due to sinusitis, rhinitis, tonsillitis.
May follow flu or cranial injury.
Often of unknown cause.

Selective anesthesia of the olfactory receptors is achieved by dropping anesthetic in saline solution into nostril. This is done while the patient is supine with his head bent way back so ear canal and chin are in the same plane. He remains in this position for 30 seconds. Treatments twice a week may prove curative.

Kare MR, Mattes RD: A selective overview of the **chemical senses**. Nutr Rev 1990; 48:39–48.

Individuals display innate differences in their ability to perceive certain odors. Such absence or diminished ability to detect selected odors is termed *specific anosmia* or *selective hyposmia*, respectively. It is remarkable that only 10% of individuals can sense the medicinal odor of the compound iodocresole.

Androstenone, which is in axillary secretions and has the odor of urine or a woody smell, cannot be detected by 45% of individuals. Of the women who could sense it, 72% found it offensive and the others found it pleasant.

With **trimethylamine**, the gas responsible for the rotten fish odor of those with trimethylaminuria, a full 6% of individuals were unaware of its malodor.

It is apparent that the doctor who disavows the patient's complaint of personal odor may be testifying only to his own selective anosmia.

Wysocki CJ, Dorries KM, Beauchamp GK: Ability to **perceive androstenone** can be acquired by ostensibly anosmic people. Proc Natl Acad Sci 1989; 86:7976–7978.

Nearly half of adults cannot perceive an odor from **androstenone**, a volatile steroid found in axillary sweat, bacon, and celery. Twenty individuals with this specific olfactory deficit sniffed androstenone for 3 minutes three times a day for 6 weeks. At the end of this time, 10 subjects had acquired the ability to smell androstenone.

Such induction suggests the acquisition of hyperosmia in patients who complain of odors the physician fails to sense.

Henkin RI: **Hyperosmia and depression** following exposure to toxic vapors. JAMA 1990; 264:2893.

A 45-year-old woman developed a **hyperacute sense of smell** one week after using a chemical paint stripper that contained toluene, methyl alcohol, and methylene chloride. Even pleasant smells became intolerable. This proved to be a prominent factor in the initiation of a depressive state that developed a few weeks later. Treatment with antidepressants was soon followed by her return to a normal sense of smell. It was concluded that the inhalation of those organic solvents contributed to her hyperosmia.

Description of olfactory symptoms may be classified as follows:

hyposmia
loss of smell function

phantosmia
sensing a smell without evidence of stimulant vapor

aliosmia
abnormal sensing of a stimulating vapor as an obnoxious smell

a. cacosmia–perception of a rotten or decayed odor arising from a pleasant aroma

b. torquosmia–perception of a chemical, burned, or metallic odor from a pleasant aroma

Shelley ED, Shelley WB: The **fish odor syndrome**: trimethylaminuria. JAMA 1984; 251:253–255.

For 6 months the nurses who attended this 31-year-old institutionalized man reported that he frequently gave off the **odor of rotten fish**. Not only the patient but also his urine exhibited this repulsive smell.

Gas chromatographic assays proved the odor to be due to **trimethylamine**, a malodorous volatile amine produced in the gut by bacterial action on choline-containing foodstuffs. Normally this compound, which is actually responsible for the odor of rotting fish, is converted by the liver to the nonodorous trimethylamine oxide.

The diagnosis of fish odor syndrome, i.e., trimethylaminuria, was made and dietary reduction of choline proved beneficial.

Leopold DA, Preti G, Mozell MM, et al: **Fish-odor syndrome** presenting as dysosmia. Arch Otolaryngol Head Neck Surg 1990; 116:354–355.

A 36-year-old woman complained of a **bad taste in her mouth** that had been progressively worsening since its onset 20 years ago. Three years of medical consultation with five physicians had failed to define a cause.

Selective anesthesia demonstrated her problem was not one of taste but rather smell. Pinching the nose shut eliminated the bad "taste." In the search for the internal odorant, the patient was asked to bring a fresh morning sample of sputum. This had a strong, fishlike odor, suggesting the diagnosis of trimethylaminuria, i.e., the fish odor syndrome.

This diagnosis was confirmed by demonstrating a climb of the urinary trimethylamine concentration to 10.28 mg/mg creatinine after choline bitartrate challenge. The normal value would have been 0.66 mg. By avoiding choline-containing foods such as beans, eggs, and fish, her problem was reduced.

Making the diagnosis for this patient freed her from not only the bad taste in her mouth but also the bad taste of seeing doctors who perceived her as psychoneurotic.

Resource centers for study of odor:

1. Olfactory Referral Center
   State University of New York Health Sciences Center
   750 E Adams St
   Syracuse, NY 13210
2. Analytical Core Facility
   Monell Chemical Senses Center
   3500 Market St
   Philadelphia, PA 19104

Pain

What diagnostic entry point does cutaneous pain provide?

Acute **unilateral pain** is the herald of herpes zoster. It may be severe, and prior to the objective signs of redness and vesicles it can be misinterpreted as migraine, a "coronary," pleurisy, appendicitis, or renal colic.

Burning pain of the feet relieved by cold or by nonsteroidal anti-inflammatory agents signals a diagnosis of erythromelalgia. Similar burning pain and redness of the hands of a child strongly suggest a diagnosis of acrodynia, with the need to search for exposure to mercury.

A painful site on a finger can be your entry point for considering a foreign body, glomus tumor, or a synovial cyst.

Tender, **painful papules** at the site of former injury suggest a neuroma, whereas the papule that hurts when chilled is often a leiomyoma in which the cold-induced smooth muscle contraction causes the pain. Painful nodules of the scalp suggest a proliferating pilar tumor, and we have seen simple wens produce headaches. In the case of a painful purplish area appearing after cold exposure, one has to consider chilblains (possibly better thought of as chill pains).

Idiopathic pain suggests a neuropathy, often metabolic. We see this in the painful feet of diabetics or in the cutaneous pain experienced by patients with Fabry's disease. Look for the glycosuria and look for the angiokeratomas.

Cold can relieve the torture of erythromelalgia; however, strangely, in the rare syndrome of painful cold erythema, it is the very trigger for intense pain.

Pain can be the cry of the skin for oxygen. An infarct, as in atrophie blanche, can produce exquisite pain. Again, pain is a diagnostic lead-in for arterial disease. In delayed pressure urticaria with its interleukin-mediated deep edema, pain is also a sign. Patients with the painful bruising syndrome, often of factitial origin, also relate that they have pain in their (battered) skin.

One of the most intriguing of all sources of almost unbearable pain is that due to **trauma** to a major nerve trunk. Known since Civil War bullets produced it, this pain has been termed causalgia. More popularly today it is labeled reflex sympathetic dystonia to indicate an etiologic role for the vasoconstrictive autonomic nerves.

The classic lightning pains of tabes dorsalis have now all but gone, eliminated by penicillin therapy. The pain presumably originated with sensory neuron firing during axon degeneration. Today one looks to leprosy to explain such severe pain.

Many examples of pain are recognized by the public. They expect the throbbing pain of a felon or furuncle or cellulitis. More subtle, but valuable as a diagnostic sign, is the tenderness exhibited by actinic keratoses as they become cancerous.

Sometimes it is the **absence of pain** that creates diagnostic thoughts. The child with burns that are unexplained until congenital absence of pain is discerned and the unfelt cigarette burns that suggest leprosy or neurologic disease are examples that make us think of the absence of pain in our diagnostic approach.

Michiels JJ: **Erythromelalgia and erythermalgia**. Lancet 1990; 336:183–184.

Both erythromelalgia and erythermalgia patients come to you complaining of burning pain and redness of the hands and feet.

The **erythromelalgia** patient finds:

warmth intensifies the discomfort
a single dose of aspirin gives complete relief for several days

The patient has a chronic myeloproliferative disease with thrombocythemia. Platelet clumping can lead to thrombi in the small vessels, with resultant acrocyanosis and finally necrosis. The dramatic action of aspirin results from its irreversible inhibition of the platelet cyclo-oxygenase activity, with resultant inhibition of platelet clumping.

The **erythermalgia** patient experiences the same redness and burning pain of the extremities brought on by heat or exercise but by contrast finds:

    no response to aspirin
    no progression to necrosis

It is not a platelet-mediated disease and hence the absence of aspirin relief. It is seen in children as well as in a secondary form in adults with gout, rheumatoid arthritis, cryoglobulinemia, endarteritis obliterans, or systemic lupus erythematosus. It is also the term to use in describing the painful red hands and feet of diabetics, of patients with neurologic disease, and those receiving vasoactive drugs. Again, aspirin is no help in either the primary or secondary form of erythermalgia.

Watch your vowels or you'll get the diagnosis wrong.

Mehle AL, Nedorost S, Camisa C: **Erythromelalgia**. Int J Dermatol 1990; 29:567–570.

A 55-year-old man had a 3-month history of **severe burning pain** of the right foot that was relieved only by cold. He was known to have had essential thrombocythemia for the past 2 years.

On examination the right foot and ankle were warm, swollen, and red. A biopsy was nondiagnostic. A diagnosis of erythromelalgia was made. One naproxen tablet (250 mg) every 4 days has kept him symptom free.

Garrett SJ, Robinson JK: **Erythromelalgia and pregnancy**. Arch Dermatol 1990; 126:157–158.

This 31-year-old woman suddenly developed numerous small, **tender, erythematous macules** over the thenar eminences and fingertips as well as the soles and toes. They had appeared about 10 days prior to delivery of a premature baby boy. By the fifth postpartum day, the pain was so severe that she could not bear weight or hold objects. Leg elevation and ice compresses afforded some relief.

A diagnosis of **erythromelalgia** was made, based on the presence of the triad of intense burning pain, increased temperature, and redness of the hands and feet. Three other conditions with the same findings were ruled out. It was not reflex sympathetic dystrophy, since there was no history of trauma. It was not shoulder-hand syndrome. There had been no cerebrovascular accident, myocardial infarction, or other reflex neurovascular response. Finally, it was not causalgia, since no lesion of the peripheral nerve was found.

It is possible that the administration of the vasodilator **nifedipine** just after the onset of symptoms did act as an aggravating factor by shunting more blood into the skin. Nifedipine, as well as bromocriptine, has been reported to initiate and induce erythromelalgia. In other patients there may be an association with **other diseases**. These include myeloproliferative diseases, lupus erythematosus, rheumatoid arthritis, hypertension, diabetes mellitus, gout, syphilis, astrocytoma, lichen sclerosus et atrophicus, multiple sclerosis, and hereditary nephritis.

Prostaglandin may be the ultimate mediator, since inhibition of prostaglandin synthesis by aspirin has proven to be a sovereign remedy.

Michiels JJ, van Joost T, Vuzevski VD: **Idiopathic erythermalgia**: A congenital disorder. J Am Acad Dermatol 1989; 21:1128–1130.

Since the age of 2 years, this 17-year-old girl had been experiencing **burning pain of the feet** after exercise or exposure to sunlight or warmth. Rest or cooling provided relief, but by the age of 14 the symptoms were so intense that she slept with her feet immersed in ice water. Aspirin and a variety of analgesics were ineffective. Her mother had suffered the same problem, also since childhood.

All studies were normal. There was no neuropathy, and the biopsy showed only a nonspecific inflammatory process. As a result, a diagnosis of primary or idiopathic erythermalgia was made.

Erythermalgia is distinguished from erythromelalgia by more than spelling. The classic example of erythromelalgia is due to thrombocythemia and the resultant platelet-mediated inflammatory vascular and circulatory changes. In all of these patients a cardinal diagnostic sign is the prompt 3 days of relief afforded by a single low dose of aspirin. This is attributable to irreversible inhibition of platelet cyclo-oxygenase activity induced by the aspirin.

Shelley WB, Caro WA: **Cold erythema**. A new hypersensitivity syndrome. JAMA 1962; 180:639–642.

Ever since the first month of life, this 5-year-old boy had **screamed with pain** and turned bright red in any area of skin that was chilled. Drinking cool liquids invariably caused vomiting. His fear of anything cold matched his fear of contact with an open flame.

Examination revealed a normal child with no skin abnormalities evident. However, 5-second contact with a 5-mm fragment of ice produced 8 cm of spreading erythema and intense local pain. The pain was so severe as to induce muscular rigidity for more than 5 minutes, the erythema fading over the next half hour. No urticaria was seen.

The problem is reported as a new syndrome of painful **cold erythema**. The child remains healthy and pain free in warm sunny southern California.

Stephens CJM, McGibbon DH: **Algodystrophy** (reflex sympathetic dystrophy) complicating unilateral acrodermatitis continua. Clin Exp Dermatol 1989; 14:445–447.

During an assault, the wedding ring was ripped off the left hand of this 65-year-old female alcoholic. She developed a rash at the site of injury that later involved the entire hand. The associated **pain** was so severe that she immobilized the arm. Because of a fear that the problem was cancer, she did not see a physician for an entire year and a half.

On initial examination, the dorsum and palm were studded with **pustules** on an erythematous base. The presumed diagnosis by her physician was an infective process, but repeated cultures for bacteria and viruses proved the pustules were sterile. Dermatologic consultation provided the diagnosis of pustular psoriasis. This was confirmed on biopsy. Negative immunofluorescence excluded the diagnosis of pustular pemphigus. X-ray of the bones as well as a bone biopsy revealed marked osteoporosis.

The persistent severe pain, the loss of joint movement, and focal osteoporosis all led to a diagnosis of **algodystrophy**. This condition, which represents an alteration in the sympathetic nervous system, has an extensive synonymy. Indeed, more names are known for it than explanations for its cause. Thus it has been labeled reflex sympathetic dystrophy, shoulder-hand syndrome, post-traumatic sympathetic atrophy, and Sudeck's atrophy.

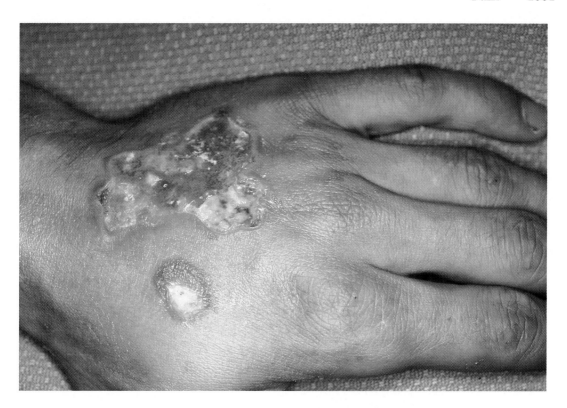

The benefit this patient received from a sympathetic ganglion block supports the theory that an abnormal sympathetic reflex is responsible.

Finally, the diagnosis of **acrodermatitis continua of Hallopeau** provides more precision. It can be considered a specific form of pustular psoriasis that begins on the fingers or toes following trauma. Rare, persistent, and painful, it continues to extend proximally. Untreated, it can lead to algodystrophy, as seen in this patient.

Shelton RM, Lewis CW: **Reflex sympathetic dystrophy**: A review. J Am Acad Dermatol 1990; 22:513–520.

Unbelievably severe, constant, **burning pain** of an arm or leg that has sustained an injury is the cardinal sign of reflex sympathetic dystrophy. Recognized for more than 100 years, it sails through our literature under a dozen other diagnostic flags, causalgia being a favorite. The injury may be so minor and the pain so intense that the patient may be erroneously viewed as having a hypochondriacal or emotional reaction. It can be triggered by as little as an air current, the lightest touch of the physician's hand, or even certain words.

This first sign of reflex sympathetic dystrophy appears a few days to a few weeks after the **injury**. This injury may range from a fracture to frostbite, from a sprain to myocardial infarction, and from cervical disc disease to a nail biopsy. The injury is nonspecific and of a varied nature, but it accounts for a period of sympathetic loss for about 1 month. During this time, there is not only the hyperesthesia of neuralgia but also vasodilation following absence of sympathetic control. The skin becomes erythematous, at times in a strange hand-in-glove pattern, in other instances simply as red knuckles.

In the second stage, lasting a half-year, there is evidence of **sympathetic**

overactivity. Now there is vasoconstriction and hyperhidrosis. The extremity is cool and cold intolerant. The skin is edematous, mottled with cyanotic and whitened areas. The pain may be even more severe and extensive.

Finally, in the third stage, which lasts for years, there is **atrophy**. Pain may have disappeared or still be intractable. Subcutaneous atrophy and tender contracture are common, along with tapered fingers. Bullae may appear. Unilateral osteoporosis of disuse may be found as the extremity is no longer used.

Throughout all of this, the physician has to be restrained from making a diagnosis of **factitial dermatitis** or feigned illness. The geometrically marginated erythema not overlying the dermatome of any sensory nerve, the patterned hyperesthesia, and the pain presumed to be inappropriate, all tend to divert the physician from realizing that the patient has trauma-induced reflex sympathetic dystrophy. Aside from x-rays in the later stages, objective laboratory evidence is never present.

Erythermalgia is ruled out, for it is bilateral. It has a pain that is episodic. Other conditions that may cross the diagnostic horizon are herpes zoster, rheumatoid arthritis, gout, ischemia, phlebitis, and the lightning pains of tabes dorsalis.

Truly the patient with reflex sympathetic dystrophy is an orphan patient if his physicians do not make the diagnosis.

Saland G: **Acute occlusions of the peripheral arteries**; clinical analysis and treatment. Ann Intern Med 1941; 14:2027–2036.

Sudden arterial occlusion is due to either **embolism or thrombosis**. Heart disease (especially atrial fibrillation) and lung infection predispose to emboli, whereas concurrent peripheral vascular disease favors thrombosis. The symptoms and signs are the same.

Analysis of 31 cases showed that a **sudden sharp pain** or sudden onset of numbness in the limb was followed rapidly by pallor and grayish cyanosis, coldness of the limb, and loss of sensation and motion of the distal part of the extremity. The superficial veins were collapsed, and pulsations of the main arterial vessels were absent, often above as well as below the site of occlusion. Pulsation was sometimes lost in the opposite limb because of reflex vasomotor spasm.

Wallace HJ: **Anderson-Fabry disease** (AFD). Br J Dermatol 1974; 91(suppl 10):72–74.

At the age of 8 years this patient first complained of **burning pains** in the feet. Seven years later he began to experience pains in the hands. The attacks lasted from minutes to days and at times were caused by heat or exercise.

Examination disclosed a few small **angiectases** around the umbilicus, on the upper arms, and scapulae. A presumptive diagnosis of **Fabry's disease** was confirmed by showing a low level alpha-galactosidase in the leukocytes and finding diagnostic lamellar bodies on electron microscopy of the urinary sediment.

Diphenylhydantoin (100 mg/day) gave relief of the pain.

Symmers WS: **Exotica**: A further miscellany of clinical and pathological experiences. New York, Oxford University Press, 1984; pp 150–157.

This 20-year-old woman began to note **pain in the tip of the left index finger**. The finger became so sensitive that the slightest pressure or temperature change induced marked pain. There was no apparent cause, and x-rays showed no foreign body or lesion in the bone.

As the months passed, the site of the pain became sharply defined. Close inspection showed a minute break in the papillary ridge pattern. It was at this point that 4 years prior she stapled herself accidentally. The **staple** had been easily removed and the incident forgotten until now.

Biopsy of the area revealed the cause of the pain. She had developed a **tactile neuroma** in the area. Its removal provided a complete cure.

Brooke RI: **Atypical odontalgia**: A report of 22 cases. Oral Surg 1980; 49:196–199.

The cause of the **dental pain** in these patients eluded all studies. The teeth and gums were in excellent health. These 22 patients had no evidence of ear, eye, or sinus problems. The conclusion was that a **depression** was responsible, and indeed half of these patients obtained permanent relief from the pain by use of antidepressants or tranquilizers.

The more treatments undertaken, the more problems that appeared. In those patients in whom a tooth restoration was done, fruitless root canal therapy, apicectomy, and finally extraction followed without help. The dentist must be firm in overriding the demand of these patients to *do something*.

Rasmussen OC: **Painful traumatic neuromas in the oral cavity**. Oral Surg 1980; 49:191–195.

Dental extractions may be followed by **severe, longstanding pain**. It is of a burning or paresthetic nature and can routinely be elicited or exaggerated by local pressure. Dentures are troublesome; also, jaw movement may induce attacks.

Excision reveals the cause to be a small papule that, histologically, is a **neuroma**. Its removal spells cure.

Lazarus GS, Goldsmith LA: Diagnosis of skin disease. Philadelphia, F.A. Davis, 1980; p. 217.

Painful skin papules and **papulonodules**:

Angiolipoma
Chondrodermatitis nodularis chronica helicis
Eccrine spiradenoma
Glomus tumor
Leiomyomas
Neuroma

The biopsy is often the greatest diagnostician.

Panniculitis

The deeper the lesion, the more shallow the diagnosis. Panniculitis is an example. It is an inflammation in the nether region of the skin, the subcutis. We sense it well as deep tender inflammatory nodules, but its monomorphic clinical presentation allows little for the clinician in the way of taxonomy. It's a disease covered over by skin. It is this blanket that limits our ability to classify. We must search other than with our eyes for a taxonomy.

We listen to the history. Could it be due to cold? Could it be the Popsicle panniculitis of the pediatric patient or the thinly dressed equestrian in the northern clime? Could it be from trauma at work or following an accident? We listen intently. Could it be factitial? Was something injected? Is the story consistent with the paradigm of panniculitis, viz., relapsing febrile nodular nonsuppurative panniculitis? With the associated findings of malaise, arthralgia, and fever, we can call this paradigm the Weber-Christian syndrome. We can sense a couple of subdivisions here. It may be the liquefying form in which the lesions become fluctuant and drain an oily fluid. Or it may be the nonfebrile form.

Might we call it poststeroid panniculitis, such as occurs in children days or weeks after oral prednisone is stopped? Does the history help us label it pancreatic panniculitis by alcoholism, pancreatitis, or the pain of pancreatic cancer? Is there a history of recurrent streptococcal infection that might localize in traumatized fat such as over the shin? Does the patient have a history of renal disease or evidence of hyperparathyroidism that could lead us to think of calcifying panniculitis?

To help us further in classification we turn to the **laboratory**. We ask for lupus screens to see if the patient has lupus panniculitis. We order determinations of amylase, trypsin, and lipase levels to see if the label of pancreatitis panniculitis is possible.

We order the health profile for evidence of hyperparathyroidism and its calcifying panniculitis. Finally, we order an alpha$_1$-antitrypsin level. If it is low, the patient is susceptible to trauma, since he has no buffer against the destructive protease enzyme release from the injured panniculum. He has the antiprotease deficiency panniculitis.

We then turn to the **pathologist** for help in classification. He will see if we have missed the classic septal pannulides such as erythema nodosum, polyarteritis nodosa, and necrobiosis lipoidica. He will tell us if our panniculitis is the lobular type of panniculitis, truly involving the fat lobules. He will help us with histologic classifications, such as cytophagic histiocytic panniculitis. He may detect the panniculitis of foreign body origin, as in the patient with sclerosing lipogranuloma of the penis or scrotum suffering from petrolatum injected years before. And he will protect us from simply labeling nodular vasculitis as panniculitis.

If you really dig into panniculitis, your final diagnosis won't be so shallow.

Hendrick SJ, Silverman AK, Solomon AR, Headington JT: α$_1$-Antitrypsin deficiency associated with panniculitis. J Am Acad Dermatol 1988; 18:684–692.

A 24-year-old American Indian construction worker fell into an 8-foot-deep excavation site, landing on his buttocks. The next day a large ecchymotic area developed on the left buttock, which became painful, indurated, and nodular. **Noduloulcerative lesions** rapidly ensued, and these, as well as new lesions on the thigh, ankle, right buttock, abdomen, and arms, failed to respond to systemic antibiotics given over the next 4 months. The **differential** diagnosis included erythema nodosum, deep fungal infection, and Weber-Christian disease. At that time, he had intermittent swelling of both legs and multiple erythematous subcutaneous nodules and draining sinuses on the buttocks and thighs. Eventually he had massive enlargement of the left leg, anasarca, and disseminated subcutaneous draining nodules. Accidental trauma to the left arm initiated a new violaceous indurated draining lesion. Repeated hospitalizations for exhaustive testing failed to reveal the cause or nature of the panniculitis, but a 3-week course of dapsone (400 mg/day) resulted in complete healing.

When seen 8 years later, he had severe emphysema, cirrhosis, and recurrent deep-venous thromboses in the legs. He was also found to have an **alpha$_1$-antitrypsin deficiency**, which accounted for the skin lesions. Lack of this antiprotease in serum permitted proteases released by trauma (such as collagenase and elastase) to produce an uncontrolled inflammatory cascade, with destruction of the dermis and fibrous septa of the subcutis. There was no fat cell necrosis, in contrast to the panniculitis of pancreatitis, in which high serum levels of pancreatic lipase destroy the fat cells.

The cutaneous lesions of alpha$_1$-antitrypsin deficiency are frequently mistaken for **bacterial cellulitis**, but do not respond to a parade of antibiotics and are exacerbated by corticosteroids. The lesions do respond to dapsone. In the past these cases have been reported as Weber-Christian disease, a reaction pattern that includes widespread panniculitis, fever, pancreatitis, thrombosis, pulmonary embolism, fat necrosis, and anasarca.

If "cellulitis" does not respond to antibiotics or steroids, check the following:

serum alpha$_1$-antitrypsin level
deep incisional elliptical biopsy (pathognomonic: extensive liquefactive necrosis of the dermis and fibrous septa of the subcutis, with separation of fat lobules)
history of trauma precipitating lesions
response to dapsone
presence of emphysema and cirrhosis

Two other cases of this rare entity are included:

A 7-year-old boy had multiple, firm, **warm skin nodules**, the oldest of which was draining. He then developed acute swelling of the right foot and left knee, with soft tissue swelling and an effusion of the left knee. The lesions cleared with nafcillin treatment, but 5 years later his sister developed liver disease and was found to have alpha$_1$-antitrypsin deficiency. He was screened and had an alpha$_1$-antitrypsin level of 55 mg/dl (normal 200 to 400).

A 33-year-old woman developed painful swelling and redness of the right forearm. Three days later she suffered trauma to this arm. A chest x-ray showed emphysema. Despite antibiotics the **cellulitis** persisted, and tender erythematous plaques and draining nodules developed on the right buttock, thighs, vulva, and inguinal areas. An ANA titer was 1:160 (speckled). A deep skin biopsy showed liquefactive necrosis of the midreticular dermis and collagenolysis of the fibrous septa of the subcutis. The alpha$_1$-antitrypsin level was 72 mg/dl. Dapsone (150 mg/daily) controlled the lesions.

Smith KC, Pittelkow MR, Su WP: Panniculitis associated with severe α_1-antitrypsin **deficiency**. Treatment and review of the literature. Arch Dermatol 1987; 123:1655–1661.

Hot, tender, **red nodules that drain and ulcerate** are the cardinal sign of an alpha$_1$-antitrypsin deficiency. The nodules appear at sites of trauma or at random on the buttocks, thighs, groin, arms, and trunk. The patient is often febrile, and the clinical picture is that of **Weber-Christian syndrome**.

Since alpha$_1$-antitrypsin levels are genetically determined, the patient's relatives should be tested and counseled appropriately. Partial deficiency (phenotype MZ) occurs in 1 of 50 people in the United States, whereas severe deficiency (phenotype Z) afflicts 1 in 2500. Associated **internal problems** include emphysema, hepatitis, and cirrhosis, while additional skin problems include vasculitis, cold contact urticaria, angioedema, and severe psoriasis.

The treatment of choice is **dapsone**. The patient must also avoid smoking, (which lowers the alpha$_1$-antitrypsin level and favors emphysema) and drinking alcohol (to prevent alpha$_1$-antitrypsin noninfectious hepatitis and cirrhosis).

Alpha$_1$-antitrypsin is a glycoprotein antienzyme produced in the liver that is responsible for more than 90% of the proteolytic inhibitory activity of the blood. It is needed to reduce tissue damage caused by the release of proteolytic enzymes (neutrophil elastase, pancreatic elastase, collagenase, cathepsin G, leukocyte neutral protease, trypsin, chymotrypsin, factor VIII, and kallikrein). Accordingly, alpha$_1$-protease inhibitor is a more scientific designation, but alpha$_1$-antitrypsin remains its generic name.

Beacham BE, Cooper PH, Buchanan S, Weary PE: **Equestrian cold panniculitis** in women. Arch Dermatol 1980; 116:1025–1027.

Tender, indurated, erythematous **violaceous nodules** had recently appeared on the upper lateral aspect of both thighs of this 22-year-old woman. The history revealed that not only had they appeared this February, but during the past two winters similar lesions in the same sites had also puzzled her. They began as small red pruritic areas, becoming painful, raised, and violaceous and clearing in 3 weeks. New lesions kept coming throughout the winter, with complete resolution during summer and fall.

The diagnostic clue came from awareness that she was an equestrian who rode daily for hours despite the winter cold. Riding apparel of tight-fitting pants gave little protection from the cold. On investigation for cold sensitivity, cryoglobulins and cryofibrinogen were not found, but histologic study showed panniculitis, and the diagnosis of **cold panniculitis** was made.

This condition is more common in children, appearing as painful facial plaques after they have been out in the cold. **Challenge with ice cube** contact for 2 minutes often will reproduce the lesion, which then may persist for several weeks.

Popsicle panniculitis is a popular pediatric presentation.

Winkelmann RK, Barker SM: **Factitial traumatic panniculitis**. J Am Acad Dermatol 1985; 13:988–994.

Hard purple-red, **painful subcutaneous masses** developed on both legs of this 47-year-old woman. Within 2 months they had resolved but recurred. A biopsy showed nodular panniculitis, and studies revealed a persistent mildly elevated serum amylase level (131 to 492 U/liter, normal 20 to 110). A diagnosis of **pancreatic fat necrosis** was made.

After a year of recurrent lesions, the patient was hospitalized, and a Robert Jones occlusive dressing put in place. Within a week the lesions on the legs disappeared, but for the first time new lesions developed on the forearms.

The diagnosis of **factitial panniculitis** became apparent when a nurse observed the patient hitting herself on the forearms. Psychiatric evaluation revealed no disorder other than her anger at being widowed at the age of 46. The anger was focused on a lawsuit against the physician who took care of her husband the day of his fatal pulmonary embolus.

Traumatic factitial lesions to the skin are usually recognizable. One form—

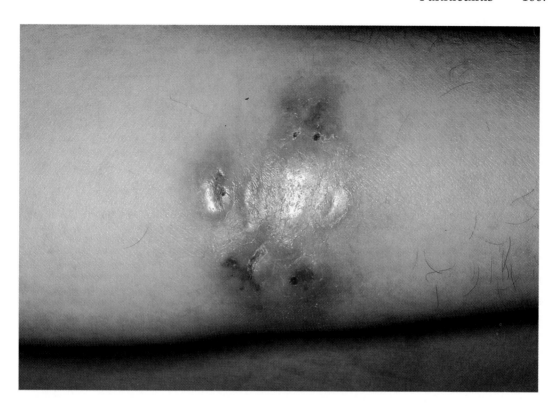

Secrétan's syndrome (l'oedeme bleu)—is a factitial edema and/or hemorrhage of the dorsum of the hand. Usually unilateral, the recurrent episodes produce chronic edema, fibrosis, and contractures. These patients are usually seen by the orthopedic surgeons.

Factitial panniculitis is more difficult to recognize, since it simulates pancreatic fat necrosis, as in this case, or Weber-Christian disease or thrombophlebitis. One may even see **factitial erythema nodosum**.

This patient used the simplest "**do-it-yourself**" method of producing panniculitis, viz., use of the fist. Others, however, inject feces, urine, milk, or drugs in the hope of creating a more puzzling clinical picture than that of simple traumatic bruising.

Diagnosis of these factitial panniculides is facilitated by finding remarkable involution once the affected area is occluded. The appearance of new lesions in new uncovered sites also points to a diagnosis of a factitial panniculitis. Ideally the diagnosis is most easily made by observing the patient "in the act" or finding the "paraphernalia" in the hospital room.

Interestingly, the referring physician may develop a **folie à deux** relationship with the patient (or prefer not to admit he was deceived) and will resist accepting the diagnosis as much as the patient does.

Mason J, Apisarnthanarax P: **Migratory silicone granuloma**. Arch Dermatol 1981; 117:366–367.

Small subcutaneous **nodules** of the inner aspect of the left upper arm of this 38-year-old woman were diagnosed as **factitious panniculitis**. The histologic basis for such a diagnosis was the biopsy finding of granulomatous panniculitis that suggested the injection of foreign lipid material. Cultures had been negative for acid-fast bacteria as well as fungi. Nor did complete laboratory studies reveal any abnormality.

Reevaluation of the diagnosis was made months later when the nodules coalesced to form a tender, firm, subcutaneous plaque on the arm, and a second plaque developed on the left upper chest area, extending onto the left shoulder. The patient continued to steadfastly deny injection of any material.

An x-ray of the chest showed **bilateral breast implants**, and the patient confirmed that she had had silicone implants put in place over 3 years ago. Furthermore, 4 months before the nodules first appeared, she had sustained a wrenching injury of the left arm. The diagnostic trail was followed by demonstration by xeromammograms that the left implant was smaller than the right. Moreover, free radiopaque material was seen in the left breast.

A xeroradiograph showed the material was tracking into the deltoid region. A diagnosis was then made of a **migratory foreign body granuloma** due to a ruptured breast implant. Cure came with excision of the ruptured implant and dissection of the fibrotic masses that released silicone from a track extending along the pectoral fascia down into the left upper arm.

Moral: Ladies with implants shouldn't wrestle, whereas physicians should wrestle with diagnostic problems until they have the right answer.

Izumi AK, Takiguchi P: **Lupus erythematosus panniculitis**. Arch Dermatol 1983; 119:61–64.

This 26-year-old woman had had a firm, freely movable nontender subcutaneous **plaque** in the right deltoid region for 1 year. She had multiple complaints of fatigue, myalgia, arthralgias, and enlarged lymph nodes.

On biopsy the deltoid plaque proved to be massive **lobular panniculitis**. Direct immunofluorescence showed a linear stain of the basement membrane zone of the epidermis and follicular epithelium with deposition of IgM and C3. Although the ANA and anti-DNA antibody studies were negative, antibodies to ENA (extractable nuclear antigen) were strongly positive (1:12,500 dilution, normal < 100).

A diagnosis of **lupus erythematosus panniculitis** was made. The plaque completely resolved with 3 months of chloroquine therapy.

Lugo-Somolinos A, Sanchez JL, Méndez-Coll J, Joglar F: Calcifying panniculitis associated with **polycystic kidney disease and chronic renal failure**. J Am Acad Dermatol 1990; 22:743–747.

Tender erythematous, **indurated plaques** on the distal third of the right leg and ankle of this 48-year-old woman had been diagnosed as cellulitis. She denied specific trauma or injections in this area, nor did she have a history of abdominal pain or fever. However, the history did reveal the critical fact that she was in end-stage renal disease as a result of having polycystic kidneys. She had been undergoing peritoneal dialysis for months.

The serum calcium proved to be 8.5 mg/dl and the serum phosphate 6.3 mg/dl. Urinalysis indicated 3+ albumin, and the urine was loaded with RBCs, WBCs, and bacteria.

A skin biopsy showed the process to be **calcifying panniculitis**. This was consistent with the presence of a renal disease induced secondary to hyperparathyroidism. In these patients the high concentrations of parathyroid hormone reflect concurrent hypocalcemia and hyperphosphatemia as shown by the serum calcium × phosphorus product being 53.6. The high parathyroid hormone level promotes the deposition of calcium in any area traumatized, such as a bruise, or at sites of antibiotic or heparin injections. It also occurs in patients with pyelonephritis, the nephrotic syndrome, or other forms of renal failure. The process is known as calciphylaxis and can be reproduced experimentally. It is important to measure the serum **parathyroid hormone** level. In the second patient reported, the value was 77 pg/ml (normal 4 to 19 pg/ml).

This condition must be distinguished from **metastatic calcification** of skin, as well as pancreatic panniculitis. Metastatic calcification also occurs with renal failure, but in this entity there is no panniculitis. The calcium deposition appears in the dermis only, so that the biopsy findings are definitive. The pathologic calcification occurs not only in the skin, but in the lungs, heart, and kidney.

Pancreatic panniculitis is associated with evidence of pancreatitis. Commonly, these patients have abdominal pain and arthralgias. The amylase and lipase levels are also elevated, and computed tomography is often positive. Note, however, that amylase levels are high in renal disease because of failure of the kidneys to clear this enzyme.

Burket JM, Burket BJ: **Eosinophilic panniculitis**. J Am Acad Dermatol 1985; 12:161–164.

Two **subcutaneous nodules** on the right side of the trunk and one in the left popliteal fossa called for biopsy in this 31-year-old woman. She had had an episode of palpable purpura of the lower legs several months before. This had shown leukocytoclastic vasculitis on biopsy and cleared with short-term systemic antibiotic and steroid therapy.

The histologic picture was that of eosinophilic cellulitis, mainly localized in the subcutis. There were numerous eosinophils, flame figures, and some thrombosis of the small vessels. A diagnosis of **eosinophilic panniculitis** was made and the analogy to eosinophilic cellulitis drawn.

The histologic findings clearly ruled out erythema nodosum and steroid-withdrawal panniculitis.

Although the findings did resemble those of allergic granulomatosis (Churg-Strauss), the absence of findings in other organ systems spoke against this diagnosis. Hypereosinophilic syndrome was ruled out, since there was no eosinophilia. Likewise, the absence of drug intake gave no support for drug sensitivity panniculitis.

The solitary clue as to possible cause was a positive streptozyme test in association with pharyngitis she had the month before the initial episode of palpable purpura. The streptozyme test (formalin-treated erythrocytes coated with group A streptococci) has a 90% specificity for detection of recent streptococcal infection. It is postulated that this patient's eosinophilic panniculitis was the result of **streptococcal sensitivity**.

Abildgaard WH Jr, Hargrove RH, Kalivas J: **Histoplasma panniculitis**. Arch Dermatol 1985; 121:914–916.

Erythematous nodules suddenly appeared on the arms, legs, and torso of this 65-year-old woman. She had felt sick, was febrile, and had lost weight during the past 2 months.

A biopsy showed panniculitis with the remarkable feature of numerous spores of ***Histoplasma capsulatum*** present in the macrophages. A biopsy culture for fungi showed *H. capsulatum*.

The clinical picture suggested erythema nodosum, that is, hypersensitivity-type panniculitis, but here the organisms causing the panniculitis actually were seen.

Haber RM, Assaad DM: Panniculitis associated with a **pancreas divisum**. J Am Acad Dermatol 1986; 14:331–334.

A tender, firm, **erythematous nodule** in the left forearm and one on the right upper arm in this 67-year-old man proved to be well-demarcated granulomatous panniculitis with fat necrosis.

Because of the fat necrosis, a search was made for pancreatitis or pancreatic carcinoma. Laboratory study revealed normal amylase, lipase, and urinary amylase levels. The pancreas was normal on examination by ultrasound and computed tomography.

However, during the next 2 months new nodules of **fat necrosis** appeared on the chest, abdomen, and legs. He was readmitted to the hospital where endoscopic retrograde cholangiopancreatography showed a ventral pancreas, viz., **pancreas divisum**. At laparotomy it was found that the entire major pancreatic duct emptied into the duct of Santorini and a congenitally constricted orifice. A cure was obtained by sphincterotomy.

The patient has not developed any new nodules, and associated diarrhea and abdominal pain have gone.

Histologically it was possible to rule out the other major clinical diagnostic considerations of erythema induratum, Weber-Christian disease, lupus panniculitis, and factitial panniculitis. However, the features of granuloma rather than inflammation and the absence of calcification were not those of the classic fat necrosis of pancreatitis. Furthermore, this patient had none of the antecedents of pancreatitis, such as alcoholism, trauma, cholangitis, or pancreatic stones. Again, the laboratory finding of increased amylase and lipase was absent.

Only by persistent attention to the gastrointestinal symptoms, and finally laparotomy, was the "embryologic" defect found and corrected and the skin cured.

Kwee D, Fields JP, King LE Jr: **Subcutaneous Whipple's disease**. J Am Acad Dermatol 1987; 16:188–190.

Multiple, mildly tender **nodules** on the neck, arms, and legs of this 37-year-old black man showed nonspecific panniculitis. It was not until **PAS staining** was done that a diagnosis of **Whipple's disease** was made on the basis of finding the same intracellular inclusions as are seen in the gut biopsy of this disease. Electron microscopy revealed the inclusions to be double-walled bacteria in varying states of degeneration.

This study shows the value of looking beyond the H & E stain.

Aronson IK, West DP, Variakojis D, et al: Fatal panniculitis. J Am Acad Dermatol 1985; 12:535–551.

A review of 52 patients with fatal panniculitis revealed:

Cutaneous portrait:

   lesions usually on extremities and buttocks
   overlying skin color normal, pink, erythematous, purple, bluish, brown
   mild scale in some
   flat or raised, discrete or diffuse, well circumscribed or abscess-like
       irregular

soft, fluctuant, firm, hard, indurated

usually nodules, may coalesce to form 20-cm indurated plaques

indurated cords extending outward

singly or in crops

persist or regress over a period of weeks

healing followed by localized depression and/or hyperpigmentation

ulceration developed in half of the patients

biopsy site may drain for months

rarities: mucous membrane lesions, palpable abdominal masses of inflamed adipose tissue, small-bowel perforation

Systemic portrait:

fever, malaise

nausea, vomiting, pain, diarrhea

headaches, seizures, ataxia

weakness, weight loss

night sweats

hepatosplenomegaly

lymphadenopathy

Course: Half died within 2 years with relentless persistent course.

Trigger factors: trauma, drugs, infection

"I can see nothing," said I, handing it back to my friend. "On the contrary, Watson, you can see everything. You fail, however, to reason from what you see."

SHERLOCK HOLMES (SIR ARTHUR CONAN DOYLE)

Papules

Umbilicated	Erythematous
Pedunculated	Blue
Warty	Brown
Patterned	Yellow
Pruritic	White
Flesh colored	

Some papules are known to every clinician. Such are the umbilicated papules of molluscum contagiosum, the rough-surfaced papules of warts, and the smooth ones of nevi.

Some are known for their **color**, such as the yellow xanthoma, the blue nevus, and the white milium. Others are known for their symptoms, the pruritic papules for Fox-Fordyce disease or prurigo, and the painful papules, leiomyoma. Yet others are recognized by their location—persistent pearly papules of the penis and fibrous papules of the nose and ears. A few papules may be recognizable because by palpation you can make them instantly disappear (neurofibromatosis) or instantly appear by having the patient stand (piezogenic pedal papules). Others lose their designation as a primary lesion, i.e., papule, and become a diagnosis when seen in the context of other changes. The beadlike string of papules in lichen ruber moniliformis, the inflamed papules of acne, and the excoriated papules of lichen simplex chronicus are typical examples of this.

Yet in the presence of some papules, the clinician can only guess or surmise, knowing that a biopsy is necessary. He can only ask, Is it a lymphoma, an insect bite reaction, or metastatic carcinoma? Of questions papules ask, there is no end.

Shelnitz LB, Esterly NB: **Umbilicated papular eruption** on the extremities of a child. Arch Dermatol 1986; 122:933–936.

A 3-year-old girl exhibited 2- to 4-mm flesh-colored **papules** over the elbows, knees, ankles, hands, and feet. Many had the distinctive finding of central umbilication with scale. Some were described as having been pustular and vesicular. Lesions progressed from small erythematous papules to larger papules with yellow centers resembling pustules, finally discharging a clear viscous fluid. The eruption had been present for a year before a biopsy revealed the diagnosis of **perforating granuloma annulare**.

Simply glancing at the umbilicated lesion can lead to a **misdiagnosis** of molluscum contagiosum. Careful analysis demands that other perforating disorders be ruled out, including perforating collagenosis, perforating folliculitis, and elastosis perforans serpiginosa.

In children, we favor trauma, insect bites, and hidden foci of infection as the major causes for granuloma annulare. The prognosis is better than most of the treatments employed, since these granulomas slowly resolve.

Okamoto H, Horio T, Izumi T: **Micropapular sarcoidosis** simulating lichen nitidus. Dermatologica 1985; 170:253–255.

Glistening skin-colored **pinhead-sized papules** over the upper back of a 28-year-old Japanese woman had been present for 6 months. Most had a flat surface, and some exhibited central depressions. Clinically and histologically the lesions appeared to be lichen nitidus. However, biopsies of a nodule on the left elbow and the lung proved the underlying disease to be **sarcoidosis**. The chest x-ray showed bilateral hilar lymphadenopathy, and she had had one episode of clouded vision from anterior uveitis 8 months previously.

Sarcoidosis comes in many "oid" forms:

hypopigmentation	erythroderma
psoriasiform	ulcerative
ichthyosiform	

and in this patient, it was lichenoid!

Patterson JW: **The perforating disorders**. J Am Acad Dermatol 1984; 10:561–581.

It is the patients with chronic renal failure or long-term diabetes who will present to you a strange set of lesions. They will show you papules and **keratotic papules** that may look like prurigo nodules but that are actually spots in the skin where the dermis is being extruded through the epidermis or hair follicle.

The prototype is **Kyrle's disease**. It manifests itself as widespread keratotic papules that may coalesce into plaques. Clinical inspection makes one also think of:

> hypertrophic lichen planus
> prurigo nodularis
> keratoacanthomas, eruptive
> Darier's disease
> keratosis pilaris
> keratosis follicularis contagiosa of childhood
> phrynoderma

The perforating nature is evident on histologic study. Once perceived, the three other perforating disorders must be considered in the **differential**: 1013

perforating folliculitis:
>   hairy extensor, limited to follicles; look for hair or white keratotic core in lesion; promoted by frictional forces such as rubbing of clothing

elastosis perforans serpiginosa:
>   symmetric serpentine patterns
>   elastic tissue being extruded

reactive perforating collagenosis:
>   umbilicated papules resembling molluscum contagiosum
>   may resemble perforating granuloma annulare
>   usually in children, exposed sites subject to trauma or insect bites
>   shows Koebner phenomenon

Although Kyrle in 1916 named his disease hyperkeratosis follicularis et parafollicularis in cutem penetrans, the present-day concept of the dynamics reverses the flow to transepithelial elimination rather than the epidermis entering and penetrating the dermis. In any event, his lengthy designation of the disease assured him that we would call it by his name, rather than by the name he gave it.

The process of transepithelial elimination is not restricted to the big four primary **perforating diseases** but at times occurs in a variety of well-known entities. Thus, portals of exit may be seen as crusted or umbilicated papules and nodules arising in:

>   granuloma annulare
>   pseudoxanthoma elasticum
>   amyloidosis
>   calcinosis cutis
>   chondrodermatitis nodularis chronicus helicis
>   necrobiosis lipoidica

Those bumps you see may simply be something in the skin saying, "I want out."

Hood AF, Hardegen GL, Zarate AR, et al: **Kyrle's disease** in patients with chronic renal failure. Arch Dermatol 1982; 118:85–88.

Hyperkeratosis follicularis et parafollicularis in cutem penetrans (Kyrle) presents as papules or nodules, each with a pale central, depressed keratin plug. The lesions may be single or grouped in plaques or linear streaks.

The **differential diagnosis** varies.

>   The early lesions suggest:
>   follicular eczema
>   lichen nitidus
>   pityriasis rubra pilaris
>   perforating folliculitis

>   Later, one must consider:
>   prurigo nodularis
>   elastosis perforans serpiginosa
>   keratoacanthoma

Each can be distinguished on biopsy.

The pathogenesis of Kyrle's disease is unknown, but in this report nine examples were found in a population of patients with renal failure.

The diagnostic process can vary from exhilarating to maddening.

Miller OF III, Tyler W: **Cutaneous bronchogenic cyst with papilloma** and sinus presentation. J Am Acad Dermatol 1984; 11:367–371.

This 5-year-old boy had a flesh-colored **pedunculated papule** on the upper chest at birth. Initial evaluation on the first day of life suggested it was a midline skin tag representing a midline dermoid or a thyroglossal duct cyst and sinus. At 5 weeks, another consultant considered the accompanying seepage to be from a branchial cleft.

Shortly thereafter, there was no further drainage, and when the boy was 5 years old, a diagnosis was made of a simple skin tag without any relation to any congenital cyst or fistula. However, during excision of the "tag," an underlying **sinus** and sac were found.

On biopsy the sinus tract was lined with ciliated respiratory epithelium. A diagnosis of bronchogenic cyst was made.

It is noteworthy that although these cysts or draining sinuses usually present in the suprasternal notch or over the manubrium sterni, they have been found on the shoulder or scapular area, presumably because of **embryologic migration**. They are always single and may have an opening only pinpoint in size. In this patient, only by pulling back the polypoid flap could one discern an opening.

The **differential diagnosis** included:

teratomas: embryologically derived tissue from sites other than the tracheobronchial tree
bronchogenic cysts: biopsy shows only respiratory tract epithelium
epidermoid cyst: keratinizing epithelial lining
thyroglossal duct cyst: thyroid tissue present
heterotopic salivary gland tissue: appears typically along border of sternocleidomastoid muscle
branchial cleft anomaly: usually present laterally and higher up on the neck

A **congenital drainage site** around the neck or sternum calls for excision to solve both diagnostic and therapeutic problems. It may represent sequestered lung, thyroid, salivary gland, mesoderm, or skin tissue. If ignored, it is always an avenue for infection.

Simply imagining that the patient is very much older or very much younger can provide additional diagnostic insight.

Warty

Grattan CEH, Hamburger J: **Cowden's disease in two sisters**, one showing partial expression. Clin Exp Dermatol 1987; 12:360–363.

A 40-year-old woman sought advice concerning flat-topped verrucous papules of the forearms and dorsal aspect of the hands, as well as numerous **follicular papules** with central keratotic plugs on the forehead, nose, and neck. Biopsy of a forehead lesion revealed **trichilemmoma**, marker of this syndrome, while a forearm lesion showed a simple squamous papilloma. She also had diffuse verrucous hyperplasia of the gums. Past history revealed a left ovarian cyst seen at hysterectomy for uterine fibroids.

In a busy practice, it is well to stop when you see "warts" of the face and arms and ask yourself if the poor complexion reflects the presence of trichilemmomas. Look at the **gums**. If they are verrucous, and you return to the skin to find subtle fibromas, lipomas, lymphangiomas, or angiomas, **Cowden's disease** is the diagnosis, not acrokeratosis verruciformis.

These banal, easily overlooked changes stand alone for the recognition of Cowden's disease, since there is no known biochemical defect or diagnostic test for this systemic hamartoma that can involve the skin, thyroid, breast, gut, and genitourinary and skeletal systems. Cowden's disease presages **breast carcinoma** in one out of five cases and thyroid carcinoma in others.

Remain alert to the early danger sign of the "warty" gum.

Lazarus GS, Goldsmith LA: Diagnosis of Skin Disease. Philadelphia, F.A. Davis, 1980, pp 189–216.

Multiple chronic **warty scaly papules**:

Warts
Actinic keratoses
Seborrheic keratoses
Darier's disease
Lichen amyloidosus
Lichen myxedematosus
Lichen planus
Psoriasis
Pityriasis rubra pilaris
Lupus erythematosus
Prurigo nodularis
Elastosis perforans serpiginosa
Epidermal nevus
Kyrle's disease
Multiple keratoacanthomas
Pemphigus foliaceus
Perforating folliculitis
Perforating collagenosis

All diagnoses are provisional formulae for action.
LORD COHEN

Watkins DB, Hoeffler DF: Confluent and reticulated **cutaneous papillomatosis**: Report of a case and commentary. JAMA 1960; 174:1153–1156.

For 2 years this 22-year-old black patient had noted a **progressive papular eruption** of his trunk, shoulders, and extremities. On examination, numerous round-to-oval papulosquamous lesions 0.5 to 2.0 mm in size were seen. They tended to follow the lines of cleavage, giving the skin a striate appearance. Around the neck and upper chest the papules became confluent, with varying degrees of pigment producing a reticulate pattern. Many glistening small papules were seen on the hard palate.

No fungi could be demonstrated on scrapings. A biopsy showed hyperkeratosis and acanthosis, as well as changes consistent with a clinical diagnosis of cutaneous papillomatosis of **Gougerot and Carteaud**. It is to be distinguished from acanthosis nigricans.

Pitt AE, Ethington JE, Troy JL: Self-healing **dystrophic calcinosis** following trauma with transepidermal elimination. Cutis 1990, 45:28–30.

This 18-year-old woman was thrown from a car, landing on asphalt and sustaining multiple bruises and **abrasions**. Two weeks later she developed multiple pruritic erythematous papules. The lesions were linear and annular at the sites of the trauma. The biopsy showed amorphous particles of calcified material that did not polarize. The von Kossa stain was positive for calcium. Normal phosphorus and calcium levels attested to the fact that she had **dystrophic calcinosis cutis** due to trauma. Within 2 months, self-healing had occurred.

Various forms of trauma may be associated with **calcinosis**. These include incisions, heel pricks for blood samples in infants, and using the knee as a fulcrum for bending water pipes. It is seen outside the skin, as in the shoulder of seamstresses—the so-called Milwaukee shoulder. Calcium nodules also occur in chronic leg ulcers and burns and from extravasated calcium gluconate. Abrasions in **miners** wading in 3.5% calcium chloride water have been associated with calcinosis cutis, as has the exposure of farmers to saltpeter fertilizer.

Kennedy CTC, Sanderson KV: **Corymbose secondary syphilis**: Occurrence as a solitary group of lesions. Arch Dermatol 1980; 116:111–112.

A group of **brownish-red**, slightly scaly **papules** over the right scapula was the solitary finding on routine examination of this 27-year-old homosexual man. In the center the papules were confluent; at the periphery, each discrete. The overall diameter was 5 cm, each papule being about 3 mm in size. The patient gave a history of having had syphilis successfully treated with penicillin more than 4 years previously.

In view of the corymbose lesion (Greek for "cluster of fruit or flowers," i.e., confluence in center, satellites at edge), a diagnosis of **secondary syphilis** was made. Such brownish-red corymbose lesions are remarkably diagnostic of syphilitic relapse or reinfection. Confirmation came with a strongly positive STS battery.

Rongioletti F, Rebora A, Crovato F: **Acral persistent papular mucinosis**: A new entity. Arch Dermatol 1986; 122:1237–1239.

Flesh-colored papules had been present for 5 years on the backs of the hands of this 41-year-old woman. A biopsy revealed them to be mucin deposits, mainly hyaluronic acid. Detailed studies of thyroid function showed no abnormalities.

It is to be distinguished from lichen myxedematosus, mucinosis with thyroid disease, and self-healing juvenile cutaneous mucinosis. Other **mucinoses** are the follicular mucinosis of the hair follicle, mucoid cysts, cutaneous myxoma. 1017

Pruritic

Fawcett HA, Miller JA: Persistent **acantholytic dermatosis** related to actinic damage. Br J Dermatol 1983; 109:349–354.

Ten male patients aged 38 to 63 years are described as having a chronic **itchy papular eruption** of the upper trunk. All had evidence of considerable solar damage. Biopsies showed the typical changes of Darier's disease.

The diagnosis coined by the authors is persistent **acantholytic dermatosis**. This entity is to be contrasted with **Grover's** disease, i.e., transient acantholytic dermatosis, which is an acute reaction to sun exposure that fades spontaneously within days or weeks. Both present with pruritic papules of the trunk, and both have the same Darier-like histology.

Buslau M, Marsch WC: **Papular eruption in helminth infestation**—A hypersensitivity phenomenon? Report of four cases. Acta Derm Venereol 1990; 70:526–529.

For the past 2 weeks this 13-year-old girl had had a strongly itching papular eruption of the face, trunk, and extremities. On examination, numerous red, slightly **scaling papules** were present along the skin tension lines, giving a pityriasis rosea–like appearance. No herald patch was seen. The blood showed 11% eosinophils. The feces showed neither worms nor eggs. However, an adhesive strip applied to the anal ring revealed masses of embryonated eggs of *Enterobius vermicularis*.

Therapy with oral mebendazole (100 mg twice a day, 1 day only) caused a flare in the pruritus as well as the appearance of new papules. By 1 week the itch, papules, and eosinophilia were gone.

A diagnosis of a **pinworm hypersensitivity** papular eruption was made with note of the Herxheimer reaction occurring as a result of the therapy.

Other examples of papular eruptions due to infestations with dwarf tapeworm (*Hymenolepis nana*) and whipworm (*Trichuris trichiura*) are detailed.

Barker JNWN, MacDonald DM: **Hamartoma moniliformis**: A case report. Clin Exp Dermatol 1988; 13:34–35.

A 25-year-old Jamaican woman had a pruritic eruption of the arms, shoulders, and upper back. The clinical diagnosis was florid **keratosis pilaris** or trichostasis spinulosa. No biopsy was secured until she returned 2 years later with beads of flesh-colored papules lying in rows. Biopsy showed large sebaceous glands, perifollicular fibrosis, and pigmentary incontinence.

A diagnosis of **hamartoma moniliformis** (Latin *monile*, necklace) was made. A similar problem, juxtaclavicular beaded lines, is limited to the clavicular area. Also in the **differential** is infundibulofolliculitis. This was ruled out by the absence of folliculitis histologically.

Diagnosis is not made by a committee but by a committee member who recognizes the problem.

James WD, Redfield RR, Lupton GP, et al: A **papular eruption** associated **with** human **T cell lymphotropic virus Type III disease**. J Am Acad Dermatol 1985; 13:563–566.

A 24-year-old black homosexual man presented for evaluation of chronic lymphadenopathy. In the course of examintion, he was found to have numerous asymptomatic **skin-colored papules** covering the forehead and the sides of the neck. They had been present for a year. The lymph node biopsy showed only follicular hyperplasia; the skin lesion, a nonspecific perivascular, mononuclear cell infiltrate. However, HTLV-III antibodies were found in the serum, and the HTLV-III virus was isolated from the blood leukocytes.

On the basis of observation of this patient and experience with the same distinctive chronic papular eruption in six other HTLV-III–infected patients, **HTLV-III papular eruption** is recognized as a new disease entity. The cause is unknown but the condition is sufficiently distinct and frequent to be recognized clinically as a cutaneous sign of human retrovirus infection.

The **differential diagnosis** includes:

papular granuloma annulare	secondary syphilis
papular mucinosis	viral exanthem
folliculitis	drug eruption

Kaaman T, Torssander J: **Dermatophytid**—a misdiagnosed entity? Acta Derm Venereol 1983; 63:404–408.

Twenty-six patients with clinical signs of tinea pedis and a diagnosis of dermatophytid were subjected to careful study. Only ten proved to have a verifiable, proven **dermatophytid**, i.e., a lesion that could be reproduced by a skin test to trichophytin in patients who had a culturally demonstrated dermatophytic infection elsewhere.

In nine of the ten proven examples of dermatophytid, a *Trichophyton mentagrophytes* infection of the feet was present. In one, the primary infection was *Epidermophyton floccosum* of the groin. In this instance the id was a papular eruption of the trunk. In seven, the dermatophytid presented as a **vesicular eruption of the hands**. In the last two patients it was a scaling erythematous rash of the hands and/or extremities.

In the 16 patients in whom a dermatophytid was originally suspected, study revealed a variety of **correct diagnoses**. These included:

Staphylococcus aureus and/or *beta-hemolytic streptococcus* infection, atopic dermatitis, contact dermatitis, erythema multiforme

To diagnose dermatophytid on clinical grounds alone is to be on shaky ground.

Brenner S: **"Pediculid"**: An unusual id reaction to pediculosis capitis. J Am Acad Dermatol 1985; 12:125–126.

Twenty per cent of patients with **pediculosis capitis** develop a fine, skin-colored papular rash on the back and arms. Some papules coalesce into plaques. Histologically there is a perivascular mononuclear cell infiltrate.

This eruption has been called a **pediculid**, since it disappears 3 days after treatment of only the pediculosis capitis. Furthermore, it reappears in the event of reinfestation.

Sensitization to the louse, even as to the fungus, accounts for these id reactions, well-named pediculid and **trichophytid**.

1019

Friedman SJ, Butler DF: **Syringoma** presenting as milia. J Am Acad Dermatol 1987; 16:310–314.

Ordinarily **syringomas** are small, firm, flesh-colored or tan papules on the infraocular skin. They may also appear in the genital or acral areas and be unilateral, solitary, linear, or even inapparent in examples of hair loss. Some mimic lichen planus, and others have been clinically confused with nevi, trichoepitheliomas, and even basal cell carcinomas.

In the present report, two patients had syringomas that presented as white papules, read clinically as **milia**. On biopsy, keratin-filled cysts were found, but beneath these were the classic ductal structures of syringoma.

Reymond JL, Stoebner P, Beani JC, Amblard P: **Buschke-Ollendorf syndrome**. An electron microscopic study. Dermatologica 1983; 166:64–68.

Since early childhood these identical twins exhibited firm, skin-colored papules grouped into plaques. The changes were largely confined to the trunk and the upper arms and thighs.

A biopsy revealed an increase in elastic tissue, making the diagnosis of juvenile elastoma. **X-ray** of the feet showed small spots of density in the tarsal bones, revealing that the children suffered from the Buschke-Ollendorf syndrome, also known as dermatofibrosis lenticularis disseminata with osteopoikilosis. Actually it represents an elastoma of the skin coupled with osteopoikilosis.

Clinically one thinks of **connective tissue nevus** until the biopsy and bone study are done.

Finlayson LA: **Hunter syndrome** (mucopolysaccharidosis II). Pediatr Dermatol 1990; 7:150–152.

A scapula full of **flesh-colored papules** was the tip-off to the diagnosis in this young boy. A urinary serum test for mucopolysaccharidoses was positive, showing he had mucopolysaccharidosis in which the fibroblasts of the skin were making and storing excessive amounts of mucopolysaccharides. A specific diagnosis of type II, i.e., **Hunter's syndrome**, was made by showing on fibroblast assay that the critical lysosomal enzyme, iduronate sulfatase, was low in concentration.

The **index sign** of flesh-colored papules over the scapulae is typical of Hunter's syndrome. These papules are asymptomatic and noninflammatory, developing in the second or third year of life. They may coalesce and form reticular or linear patterns. They are also seen on other areas of the chest and thighs where the fibroblast is present in great amounts.

The **facies** become coarse. There is frontal bossing, a saddle nose, hypertelorism, and a thickened tongue, all from storage of dermatan sulfate and heparan sulfate. Once the child begins to walk, there is a diagnostic shoulder hunch and kyphosis arising from what is known as dysostosis multiplex. This child can be expected to develop frequent upper respiratory tract and ear infections, mental retardation, and hydrocephalus. Heart failure is a cause of death, since the heart valves malfunction because of accumulation of the mucopolysaccharides. This may come in the first or second decade.

Hunter's syndrome is the only one of the **mucopolysaccharidoses** to be X linked. There are seven other types. Although type I characteristically is seen by the ophthalmologist because of corneal clouding (Hurler, Scheie syndromes) Hunter's patients show no clouding. The other classes, including Morquio's (type IVB), generally exhibit the skeletal abnormality of dysostosis multiplex as well as spleen and liver enlarged by storage of the mucopolysaccharides. Typically, it is only the Hunter's syndrome patient who comes to the dermatologist.

Today, amniocentesis or chorionic villus sampling permits prenatal diagnosis of this set of syndromes.

Flowers SL, Cooper PH, Landes HB: Acral persistent **papular mucinosis**. J Am Acad Dermatol. 1989; 21:293–297.

This 42-year-old woman had a 6-year history of a slowly progressive eruption of **discrete asymptomatic papules**. They first appeared on the dorsa of both hands. After 4 years they began to appear on the forearms and knees.

Examination revealed about 40 flesh-colored to erythematous firm, smooth papules on the areas cited. Health profile studies were normal, including thyroid tests. On biopsy the dermis was filled with hyaluronic acid. A diagnosis of **acral persistent papular mucinosis** was made.

It would appear to be an acral form of papular mucinosis or lichen myxedematosus. The numerous lesions distinguish it from the solitary focal mucinosis deposits such as focal cutaneous mucinosis and the digital myxoid cyst. The follicular location makes follicular mucinosis distinctive.

The puzzle remains. Why did some of this lady's fibroblasts decide to become "mucinoblasts?"

Carney JA, Headington JT, Su WPD: **Cutaneous myxomas**. A major component of the complex of myxomas, spotty pigmentation, and endocrine overactivity. Arch Dermatol 1986; 122:790–798.

Harmless-looking, smooth little **papules of the eyelids**, ears, or nipples should have a biopsy. If they prove to be **myxomas**, obtain a detailed cardiac review, since they may herald a cardiac myxoma, a potentially lethal cardiac neoplasm.

The **association** is even more likely in young patients with spotty pigmentation (lentigines or blue nevi). Endocrine problems may also be associated, such as Cushing's syndrome, Sertoli cell tumor of the testis, and acromegaly.

Cutaneous myxomas are usually multiple asymptomatic, smooth-surfaced papules smaller than 1 cm. Their color varies from opalescent and white to flesh color, dusky-pink, or blue. They may be sessile, pedunculated, or subcutaneous and have a cystic appearance. They appear any time from infancy to early adult life and often recur after excision. Rarely, they are very large, up to 7.5 cm. Histologic distinction must be made between cutaneous myxomas, focal dermal mucinosis, and benign myxoid tumor of the nerve trunk.

Sperling LC: **Congenital cartilaginous rests of the neck**. Int J Dermatol 1986; 25:186–187.

Two asymptomatic bilateral papules had been present at the base of the anterior aspect of the neck of this 13-year-old girl since birth. The "papules" were not in the skin but just beneath it. They were firm yet stringy, suggesting cartilage.

Excision revealed the lesions to be yellowish nodules that extended deep, blending with the platysma. Histologic study showed mature hyaline cartilage.

These congenital cartilaginous rests are malformations resulting from the abnormal development of the embryonic branchial apparatus. In that way, they are related to the more common branchial cysts and sinuses of this area.

Erythematous

Martinez MI, Sanchez JL, Lopez-Malpica F: **Peculiar papular skin lesions** occurring in hepatitis B carriers. J Am Acad Dermatol 1987; 16:31–34.

Asymptomatic recurrent erythematous papular lesions on the upper arms were seen in 12 adult patients in the chronic phase of hepatitis B virus infection. They call to mind the **papular acrodermatitis of childhood**, long associated with hepatitis.

Ariza J, Servitje O, Pallares R, et al: Characteristic cutaneous lesions in patients with **brucellosis**. Arch Dermatol 1989; 125:380–383.

Only 6% of 436 patients with brucellosis showed skin changes due to the disease. The most common finding in these was a widespread violet-red **papulonodular eruption**. Also seen were examples of erythema nodosum. These lesions developed during the initial phases of the disease when blood cultures were on occasion positive for *Brucella melitensis*. Indeed in two of four such patients, the skin cultures were positive for *B. melitensis*.

Horlick HP, Silvers DN, Knobler EH, Cole JT: **Acute myelomonocytic leukemia** presenting as a benign-appearing cutaneous eruption. Arch Dermatol 1990; 126:653–656.

During the past 2 months, **hundreds of pink to** violaceous 2- to 4-cm dome-shaped **papules** had appeared over the entire body of this 62-year-old woman. They were nonpruritic. She described them as stress related, showing a waxing and waning course. Indeed, the lesions were transient, coming in crops. Clinically the **eruption suggested** the possibility of a drug eruption, a viral exanthem, urticaria, secondary syphilis, atypical pityriasis rosea, sarcoidosis, or atypical lymphomatoid papulosis.

A skin biopsy showed a diffuse infiltrate of atypical mononuclear cells in the upper half of the dermis. The picture was suggestive of metastatic carcinoma, leukemia, or lymphoma. Immunoeperoxidase studies showed the common leukocyte antigen indicative of the hematopoietic origin of the cells. Next, the monoclonal antibody studies suggested an atypical T-cell lymphoma with positive Leu-1 and Leu-9 staining. The blood studies were normal. Only by **bone marrow aspiration** was the definitive diagnosis of acute myelomonocytic leukemia made. After this, an expanded panel of monoclonal antibodies confirmed the myeloid origin of the skin infiltrate.

Leukemia can present solely as a cutaneous eruption that looks benign and nonspecific. **Monoclonal antibodies** must be used to distinguish the rare myeloid malignant cells from the common lymphocytic malignant cells.

Baden TJ, Woodley DT, Wheeler CE Jr: **Multiple clear cell acanthomas**. Case report and delineation of basement membrane zone antigens. J Am Acad Dermatol 1987; 16:1075–1078.

Erythematous puncta on the surface of slow-growing, dome-shaped papules alert one to a rare, distinctive epidermal tumor, the clear cell acanthoma. These puncta are the vessels of the dermal papillae showing through. They and the erythema can be blanched on diascopy. The growths themselves are asymptomatic, sharply demarcated, and completely benign. They may reach 4 cm in size and are usually on the lower extremities. Examples have been reported on the face, forearm, trunk, or even scrotum. Not only is one's suspicion aroused by the patient's complaint of bleeding from the lesion following minor trauma, but also the presence of a **collarette of scale** or a wafer scale covering the lesion is another diagnostic characteristic.

Incidentally, the **vascular element** of the growth may be so striking as to give the appearance of a granuloma pyogenicum or hemangioma. Others may mimic psoriasis or epitheliomas. The name comes from its component, the clear, pale cells, rich in glycogen.

Haynie LS, Taylor RM: **Blue papules** on the chest. Arch Dermatol 1988; 124:1103–1106.

Multiple nontender, firm, **blue** asymptomatic **papules** on the anterior aspect of the chest of a 33-year-old woman for 2 years proved to be **eruptive vellus hair cysts**. These benign and at times familial papules can be blue, yellow, or reddish-brown with a predilection for the anterior aspect of the chest and extremities. They are usually not brought to the attention of the physician. The cyst may resolve spontaneously by transepidermal elimination.

Lazarus GA, Goldsmith LA: Diagnosis of Skin Disease. Philadelphia, F.A. Davis, 1980, p. 176.

Blue to **blue-black** papules:

Blue nevus
Giant comedone
Malignant melanoma
Acne comedones, open
Lichen planus
Lymphoma, leukemia, mycosis fungoides
Foreign body in dermis
Osteoma cutis

Compressible blue vascular lesions:

Venous lakes
Blue rubber bleb nevus syndrome
Kaposi's sarcoma

Sometimes blue vascular lesions:

Angioma, cherry
Fabry's disease
Hemangioma
Glomus tumor

Slightly bluish papules:

Angiolipoma
Eccrine spiradenoma
Eccrine hidrocystoma
Apocrine hidrocystoma

You can be a very good clinician without knowing one T cell from another, and you can be terribly clever with keratinocytes and not know that the best therapeutic agent is to get up, as the patient enters the room, shake his hand and hang on to his hand until he is firmly in his chair. Anyway, he cannot then complain if you have kept him waiting.

DAVID I. WILLIAMS

Requena L, Sanchez Yus E: **Pigmented spindle cell naevus**. Br J Dermatol 1990; 123:757–763.

The typical presentation, as seen in 22 patients (5 to 34 years in age), is **heavily pigmented papules** on the legs of young patients. The diagnosis is based on finding numerous spindle-shaped pigmented melanocytes in large junctional nests.

The diagnosis represents a distinctive benign acquired melanocytic nevus that in the past has been missed as a malignant melanoma or an atypical Spitz nevus.

Wheeland RG, Roundtree JM: **Calcinosis cutis** resulting from percutaneous penetration and deposition of calcium. J Am Acad Dermatol 1985; 12:172–175.

Multiple millimeter-sized, light-brown follicular papules covered the backs of the hands and fingers of this 38-year-old male **oil-field worker**. They had been present for several years and did not concern the patient, since his fellow oil-rig workers also had them.

Biopsy revealed clumps of basophilic material in the upper dermis that on von Kossa staining proved to be calcium. Serum calcium and phosphorus levels were normal and thus did not explain the **calcinosis cutis**.

The origin of the calcium was traced to the **drilling fluid** ("mud") he used at work. It contains calcium (oxide, carbonate, nitrate) as well as bentonite (porous volcanic rock that swells or slakes in the presence of water). In addition, the mud contains caustic soda, cottonseed hulls, mica, and graphite, all to facilitate oil-well drilling, prolong the drill-bit life, and inadvertently promote absorption of calcium through the follicle.

Similar **calcinosis cutis** has been reported in:

> farmers using a calcium nitrate fertilizer, which results in antecubital fossa involvement and lesions simulating pseudoxanthoma elasticum
> coal miners exposed to calcium chloride present on the walls of the mine, which rubs off, entering abrasions
> infants receiving intravenous calcium chloride, which produces calcification of the superficial scalp veins
> patients undergoing electroencephalography, hard nodules of the scalp being produced after prolonged contact with the paste that is used, which contains a saturated solution of calcium chloride

Winkelmann RK, Peters MS, Venencie PY: **Amyloid elastosis**: A new cutaneous and systemic pattern of amyloidosis. Arch Dermatol 1985; 121:498–502.

Yellow-brown papules and nodules had been appearing on the trunk and extremities of this 56-year-old man for the past 5 years. Clinically the diagnostic **possibilities** were pseudoxanthoma elasticum, connective tissue nevus, and dermatofibrosis lenticularis perstans.

Remarkably the skin biopsy showed amyloid selectively deposited on the elastic fibers.

The elastosis was not limited to the skin but was found in other organs, and it led to a chronic lethal course.

Rongioletti F, Clavarino M, Gortan C, Rebora A: Papules on the lower limbs of a woman with **cervical lymphadenopathy**. Arch Dermatol 1988; 124:1422–1425.

Irregular plaques of **reddish-brown papules** of the dorsum of the feet and

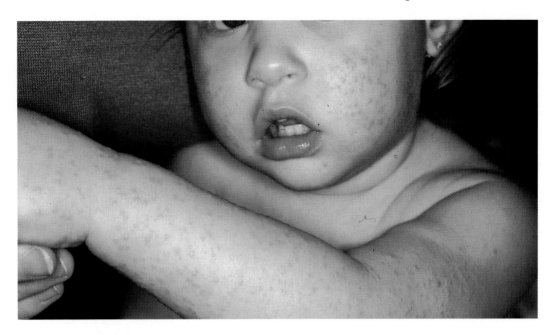

the lower legs had been present for 2 months, according to the history of this 77-year-old Italian woman. She also had similar papules scattered on the trunk. Her general medical problem was fatigue, fever, and weight loss. The dominant physical finding was bilateral cervical lymphadenopathy.

Although the biopsy of a papule showed a noncaseating granuloma, the diagnosis of **lichen scrofulosorum** was not made until cultures of the lymph node biopsy specimen showed *Mycobacterium tuberculosis*.

The lesions result from a cutaneous immune response to hematogenous dissemination of the bacilli. The smaller lesions of these sterile tuberculids are called lichen scrofulosorum, whereas the larger are labeled papulonecrotic tuberculids.

The **differential diagnosis** centers on lichenoid sarcoidosis, but also includes:

lichenoid drug eruption   keratosis pilaris
lichen nitidus   secondary syphilis

Hudson PM: **Tuberculide (lichen scrofulosorum)** secondary to osseous tuberculosis. Clin Exp Dermatol 1976; 1:391–394.

Mildly itchy, **small brown papules** with slight scales scattered on the trunk and arms of a 36-year-old Indian woman proved to contain tuberculoid granulomas with central caseation but no demonstrable organisms. The primary locus of tuberculosis was a painful 5-cm cyst at the medial end of the left clavicle, which showed bony destruction on tomography. Treatment with streptomycin, isoniazid, and rifampicin cleared the skin lesions in 6 weeks.

She was thought to have **lichen scrofulosorum**, a tuberculid seen especially in association with caseous lymphatic glands and osseous tuberculosis. Other **tuberculids** include erythema induratum, erythema nodosum, and papulonecrotic tuberculid, which all share the characteristic absence of demonstrable bacilli.

Horney DA, Gaither JM, Lauer R, et al: **Cutaneous inoculation tuberculosis** secondary to "jailhouse tattooing." Arch Dermatol 1985; 121:648–650.

Two weeks after having been tattooed by a fellow prisoner using a staple and burnt candy wrappers, this 24-year-old man noted a pruritic papular eruption in the **outline of the tattoo**.

A punch biopsy 2 months later showed a nonspecific lymphohistiocytic infiltrate. Granulomas were not seen. The eruption persisted, and a second biopsy 2 months later showed granulomas, but no organisms on special staining.

The diagnostic knot was untied when the first biopsy specimen was then stained by the **Ziehl-Neelsen technique**. It showed numerous acid-fast bacilli. Meanwhile, culture of the second skin biopsy grew ***Mycobacterium tuberculosis***. Finally, the tattooist was discovered to have untreated cavitary pulmonary tuberculosis. His sputum culture was positive for *M. tuberculosis*, which had a biochemical profile identical to the patient's.

The patient's problem was thus the result of a "**spit-and-pigment**" tattoo.

Gee-Lew BM, Nicholas EA, Hirose FM, et al: Unusual skin manifestations of **brucellosis**. Arch Dermatol 1983; 119:56–58.

Multiple small, **subcutaneous papules** appeared on the trunk, arms, and legs of this 29-month-old girl. Of only 2 weeks' duration they had been preceded for several weeks by an erythematous macular rash that faded to leave hyperpigmentation. The child had had unexplained intermittent fevers, night-sweats, and abdominal pain for the past 6 months. Just 1 month ago the family had migrated from Mexico to the United States.

Biopsy of a papule showed a granulomatous inflammatory process in the fat, but multiple stains for bacteria and organisms were negative. The answer came from the blood **culture**, which grew out gram-negative coccobacilli identified as *Brucella melitensis*.

Subsequently, culture of a biopsy specimen from another papule grew out *Brucella melitensis* on sheep's blood agar plates. *B. abortus* antibodies were also found in the serum at a level of 1:640. A diagnosis of brucellosis was made.

Brucellosis can exhibit an unbelievably wide array of cutaneous changes. These include erythema nodosum, purpura, scarlatiniform eruption, psoriasiform lesions, and papular or even vesicular changes.

Think of it when not only the skin but also the patient is sick.

Diagnosis is a species of guesswork in which the experienced physician has the advantage.

SIR JOHN BLAND SUTTON

Kumar P, Marks R: **Sebaceous gland hyperplasia** and senile comedones: A prevalence study in elderly hospitalized patients. Br J Dermatol 1987; 117:231–236.

Yellowish or skin-colored **papules** are a common manifestation of sebaceous gland hyperplasia in the elderly. Twenty-six per cent of 286 elderly patients (age range 65 to 102 years, mean 82 years) exhibited these papules on the face. They were not a result of sun exposure.

Lazarus GS, Goldsmith LA: Diagnosis of Skin Disease. F.A. Davis Co., 1980, pp 184–188.

Definitely **yellow lesions**:

Eruptive xanthomas	Focal dermal hypoplasia (Goltz syndrome)
Noneruptive xanthomas	Lupus vulgaris
Necrobiosis lipoidica diabeticorum	Nevus lipomatosus
Pseudoxanthoma elasticum	Nevus sebaceus
Sebaceous hyperplasia	Xanthogranuloma

Sometimes **yellow** lesions:

Amyloid	Gout
Sarcoid	Calcinosis cutis

du Vivier A: Atlas of Clinical Dermatology. Philadelphia, W. B. Saunders Co., 1986, pp 17.10–17.11, pp 17.5–17.6.

Myriads of small firm yellow papules on the **buttocks** are typical of **eruptive xanthomas**. They occur in patients with diabetes mellitus who have either type IV or type V hyperlipidemia. Discrete yellow papules on the face, scalp, and trunk in a *young child* require a biopsy to rule out **Letterer-Siwe disease** (histiocytosis X).

Braun-Falco O, Plewig G, Wolff HH, Winkelmann RK: Dermatology. New York, Springer-Verlag, 1991, pp 548–550, 1109, 1113–1115.

Numerous **yellowish**-whitish closed **cyst-like comedones** on the **sun-exposed areas** of the face are characteristic of nodular elastosis with cysts and comedones (**Favre-Racouchot syndrome**). The nose, zygomatic arches, and periorbital areas are particularly involved. Symmetrical soft **yellowish transparent papules** containing gelatinous material on sun-exposed areas are typical of **colloid milia**. They are rare and may be intermixed with actinic elastosis, and sometimes coalesce into yellowish plaques.

Acrokeratoelastoidosis consists of thickly aggregated white or ivory-colored indented hard papules that appear yellow on diascopy. Located on the thumb and metacarpal I, they involve the sharply demarcated transition zone from the palm to the back of the hand. It is a rare familial problem. In *pseudoxanthoma elasticum* solid yellowish, orange, violet, or whitish papules resemble **plucked chicken skin**. The surface is soft, flabby, irregular, and inelastic. Look between the fingers and examine the axillae, elbows, groin, and popliteal fossae.

Bright yellow smooth round *dome-shaped papules* on the head and extensor surfaces of the extremities in young children are typical of **juvenile xanthogranuloma** (nevoxanthoendothelioma). A very small erythematous margin may be present. They are not uncommon and usually involute within 6 months to 3 years.

Yellowish brown papules in a *baby* or adult should be rubbed to see if they urticate, typical of **urticaria pigmentosa**.

In adults **yellow-brown papules** that slowly enlarge into dome-shaped nodules may represent **multicentric reticulohistiocytosis**. Mutilating polyarthritis develops at the same time.

Shimizu H, Kimura S, Harada T, Nishikawa T: **White fibrous papulosis of the neck**: A new clinicopathologic entity? J Am Acad Dermatol 1989; 20:1073–1077.

White papules on the neck of elderly individuals appear to be an entity. The papules are round or oval, clearly marginated, unrelated to hair follicles, and asymptomatic. There may be as many as 100, but they do not appear before the age of 40 years. Histologically each papule represents an area of thickened collagen bundles.

The differential diagnosis includes:

Acrochordon	Pigmented, pedunculated
Anetoderma	Shows elastolysis on biopsy
Trichodiscoma	Shows thick-walled vessels
Dermatofibrosis lenticularis disseminata	Yellowish papules; often osteopoikilosis present
Postinflammatory scars	Preceded by lesions
Connective tissue nevi	Rarely on neck, appear earlier in life
Pseudoxanthoma elasticum	Color
Eruptive vellus hair cysts	Location
Milia	Appearance
Eruptive xanthoma	Color
Perifollicular elastolysis	Atrophy; follicular location

Ive FA: **Follicular molluscum contagiosum**. Br J Dermatol 1985; 113:493–495.

Numerous large, **deeply situated waxy papules** were present for 2 months under the chin of a 20-year-old man. Some were surmounted by coarse facial hairs, but the overlying epidermis was neither umbilicated nor broken. Biopsy revealed molluscum bodies in the dermis in a follicular arrangement, with some molluscum cells passing right up to the follicle mouth. Molluscum bodies could be expressed, but this required considerable force.

This type of **"deep" molluscum** occurs mainly in adults, particularly those with atopic dermatitis. The small pearly, semitranslucent white papules would seem to resemble milia.

Wilson BB, Dent CH, Cooper PH: **Papular acne scars**. Arch Dermatol 1990; 126:797–800.

More than half of the patients with a history of acne have small asymptomatic, **hypopigmented follicular papules** on the upper trunk. Biopsy reveals perifollicular or parafollicular lesions in which both elastic and collagen fibers are reduced in amount.

It is proposed that they be labeled **papular acne scars**, recognizing the previous more cumbersome synonymy: perifollicular elastolysis, postacne anetoderma–like scars, and papular elastorrhexis.

Tsuji T, Kadoya A, Tanaka R, et al: **Milia induced by corticosteroids**. Arch Dermatol 1986; 122:139–140.

Nine elderly patients had numerous **milia** that formed in areas of atrophy and telangiectasia secondary to prolonged use of topical steroids. These whitish globoid, firm lesions were 1 to 3 mm in size and occurred on the neck, upper chest, and upper arms. They looked like kernels of rice lying beneath a thin translucent layer of tissue. Histologic study showed features of epidermal cysts that were connected with hair follicles and often contained cut portions of hair shafts in the lumen.

Skin changes **induced by prolonged use of topical corticosteroids** include:

skin atrophy
telangiectasia
milia
purpura
striae atrophicae
delayed healing of ulcers
florid facies
steroid acne
infection
perioral dermatitis
hypertrichosis
hyperpigmentation
hypopigmentation
skin blanching
granuloma gluteale infantum
allergic contact dermatitis
photosensitivity
stellate pseudoscars
nodular elastoidosis with cysts and comedones (Favre-Racouchot syndrome)

Ribera M, Servitje O, Peyri J, Ferrandiz C: **Familial syringoma** clinically suggesting milia. J Am Acad Dermatol 1989; 20:702–703.

Milia of the eyelids may prove on biopsy to be **syringomas**.

Neild VS, Marsden RA: **Pseudomilia**: Widespread cutaneous calculi. Clin Exp Dermatol 1985; 10:398–401.

This 9-year-old girl had had self-healing white spots on the knees, wrists, and thighs for the past 4 years. Each spot was a firm, white papule 1 to 3 mm in diameter that, over a period of weeks, would become inflamed, form a scab, and then disappear.

Although these lesions resembled milia, biopsy revealed large masses of calcified material in the dermis. Each was defined by a border of epithelial cells. A diagnosis of **cutaneous calculi** was made. The cause of the calcium deposits remained unknown. Serum and urinary calcium levels were normal. The possibility remains of the calculi being related to a neuroectodermal defect, since the child was mildly mentally retarded and exhibited an odd facies, hypertelorism, and a large café au lait spot on the abdomen.

Intern: Is there any other finding you would wish to draw to my attention?
Sherlock H.: Yes, to the curious findings in the laboratory.
Intern: But they were absolutely normal.
Sherlock H.: That was the curious finding.

Parapsoriasis

Parapsoriasis is the square diagnosis that doesn't fit into any of the round holes. Parapsoriasis **is that something that isn't quite that**. It isn't psoriasis, yet it may come as scaly macules (guttate parapsoriasis). It isn't lichen planus, yet it may come as lichenoid papules (pityriasis lichenoides). It isn't lymphomatoid papulosis, yet it may come as crusted, necrotic, or hemorrhagic papules (pityriasis lichenoides et varioliformis acuta, i.e., Mucha-Habermann disease). It isn't mycosis fungoides, yet it may come as brownish plaques that persist for years (parapsoriasis en plaques). It isn't radiodermatitis, yet it may appear as patches of atrophy, dyschromia, and telangiectasia (poikiloderma vasculare atrophicans, retiform parapsoriasis). It is obviously the square peg disease that fails to quite fit the nice round holes that accommodate the things it looks like.

No disease has a richer or a more daunting **synonymy** than parapsoriasis. To read its literature, have a thesaurus close by. Remember that pityriasis (meaning scale) is a major synonym, regularly qualified by the term *lichenoides* to distinguish it from other totally unrelated "pityriasis." Then recall that this has an acute form that exhibits inflammatory necrotic, even vesicular, lesions that come in crops and scar. It also has a chronic form that resembles psoriasis or syphilis. The other major variant is the plaque-type parapsoriasis, in which the brown-to-yellow lesions come in small and large versions. The large version carries the prognosis of possible eventual conversion to mycosis fungoides.

If chronicity is the hallmark of parapsoriasis, whether it be the pityriasis lichenoides chronica or the plaque-type parapsoriasis, **diversity** is certainly its form. But wherefore this astonishing diversity and mimicry of many diseases? From our vantage point today, we see it as a manifestation of the body's defense against clones of malignant T cells. In its mildest form the battleground may be only a postinflammatory plaque of brown. More vigorous battles bring necrosis and scarring, appearing on the grand scale as poikiloderma vasculare atrophicans. In some patients the enemy T cell can be recognized histologically and the malignant nature identified, as in lymphomatoid papulosis. Should the body lose, the cutaneous T-cell lymphoma (mycosis fungoides) appears as the histologically and clinically recognized victor.

Parapsoriasis is thus the diagnosis of T-cell wars.

Lambert WC, Everett MA: The **nosology** of parapsoriasis. J Am Acad Dermatol 1981; 5:373–395.

For nearly a century this group of uncommon dermatoses has suffered 100 or more designations. What a relief to have them reduced to the triad of lichenoides, small plaque and large plaque!

1. **Pityriasis lichenoides:** Generalized erythematous or brown scaly papules and small macules, often hemorrhagic, that persist or show periodic exacerbations and occur predominantly over the trunk and flexural surfaces of the extremities.

    Acute pityriasis lichenoides: Lesions appear within a few days and last a few weeks to months. Stages of evolution include vesicular, pustular, necrotic (varioliform), and scarring.

    Chronic pityriasis lichenoides: Lesions are more chronic with no necrotic or varioliform type. They may last for years with exacerbations and remissions.

2. **Small plaque parapsoriasis:** Well-defined oval, round, slightly scaly, erythematous to yellow-brown macules. These are mostly less than 5 cm in diameter, nonatrophic, and nonindurated, and occur predominantly on the trunk and proximal surface of the extremities.

"digitate dermatosis" variant: digitate, elongated, pallisading lesions
  xanthoerythrodermia perstans variant: identical to digitate dermatosis,
    but yellow

3. **Large plaque parapsoriasis** (atrophic parapsoriasis): Large ill-defined,
   irregularly shaped erythematous to brown macules or plaques. They are
   often 10 cm in diameter on the buttocks, breasts, thighs, and flexural
   surfaces. Lesions have characteristic pigmentary changes, telangiectasia,
   and widespread fine scaling.

   Retiform parapsoriasis variant: 1- to 2-mm flat-topped scale-covered
     papules that coalesce into a netlike, retiform pattern associated with
     prominent epidermal atrophy. Widespread lesions may blend with
     typical large plaque parapsoriasis lesions.

Parapsoriasis synonyms:

  parapsoriasis en plaques: small and large plaque parapsoriasis
  parapsoriasis guttata: pityriasis lichenoides
  parapsoriasis lichenoides: large plaque parapsoriasis
  poikiloderma vasculare atrophicans: large plaque and retiform parapso-
    riasis together

Poikiloderma vasculare atrophicans is a reaction pattern consisting of mottled hyperpigmentation and hypopigmentation, telangiectasis, and progressive atrophy. Almost all cases will be found to have an underlying cause. It
occurs in many diseases:

large plaque parapsoriasis	poikiloderma congenitale
mycosis fungoides	(Rothmund and Thomson)
lupus erythematosus	arsenic ingestion
scleroderma	polycyclic hydrocarbon exposure
atrophic lichen planus	radiation
xeroderma pigmentosum	cold exposure
dermatomyositis	

Shelley ED, Shelley WB: **Chronic dermatitis** simulating small plaque parapsoriasis due
to cyanoacrylate adhesive used on fingernails. JAMA 1984; 252:2455–2456.

For $1\frac{1}{2}$ years this 66-year-old woman had had a **scaly, mildly pruritic eruption**. Initially it had involved the breasts, but later it spread to the abdomen,
scapular area, and thighs. It had been diagnosed as **parapsoriasis en plaques**,
based on its clinical and histologic appearance. A second biopsy 6 months
later was interpreted as possible **mycosis fungoides**.

On inspection, sharply circumscribed 5- to 15-cm pink, barely palpable
plaques were seen on the trunk. Clinically, it was thought to be small plaque
parapsoriasis. Review of the biopsy slide added nummular eczema and contact dermatitis to the differential.

An in-depth history disclosed that the patient strengthened her brittle fingernails with tea bag paper glued onto each nail plate with an ethyl cyanoacrylate adhesive (**Krazy Glue**). A patch test to dried Krazy Glue gave a 3+
vesicular reaction at 48 hours, whereas 29 other contact allergen patch tests
were negative.

Stopping the use of the cyanoacrylate adhesive was followed by complete
clearing of the dermatitis. A diagnosis of **parapsoriasis-like contact dermatitis** was made.

Guin JD, Baker GF: **Chronic fixed drug eruption** caused by acetaminophen. Cutis
1988; 41:106–108.

A 45-year-old black woman had a 7-month history of a **dusky erythematous**

scaly eruption of the left upper back, left arm, and dorsal aspect of the right index and middle fingers. **Parapsoriasis en plaques** was suspected, but not supported by biopsy, which showed focal parakeratosis, spongiosis, and mild perivascular lymphocytic infiltrate. Topical steroid therapy had led to hypopigmentation and atrophy. Since the patient was taking nine oral medications, the possibility of a **fixed drug eruption** was explored.

Acetaminophen, which she took many times daily, was the culprit, as its elimination was followed by complete disappearance of the eruption within 3 months. Inadvertent challenge with acetaminophen 3 months later produced a recrudescence of dermatitis in some of the old sites, as well as new lesions. Again, discontinuation of acetaminophen cleared the eruption. Patch tests with acetaminophen on both normal and previously involved skin were negative. Avoidance of the drug produced total clearing, as there had been no pigmentary incontinence leading to hyperpigmentation.

Other fixed eruptions to acetaminophen have been more acute, hyperpigmented, and mucocutaneous. Both acute and chronic forms have a tendency to "wander," clearing in some sites while appearing in others, apparently due to a refractory state in some locations.

Longley J, Demar L, Feinstein RP, et al: Clinical and histologic features of **pityriasis lichenoides et varioliformis acuta** in children. Arch Dermatol 1987; 123:1335–1339.

Clinical features in five children:

A *synchronous life cycle* of individual lesions that can number into the hundreds:

    erythematous spot
    erythematous papule: reddish-tan, violaceous puncta in some
    vesiculation, hemorrhage, necrotic crust
    hypopigmented macule or scar

These changes occur in a single lesion within a time window of 2 or 5 weeks. However, the evolution of a given lesion may abort at any time with rapid resolution.

The patient thus presents **scores of lesions** in varying stages of evolution. They localize on the anterior trunk and proximal rather than distal aspect of the extremities. The face, scalp, and mucous membranes were exempt in all. This **symptomless disease**, even as a single lesion, may abort spontaneously or persist for several years.

For diagnosis, a high index of suspicion is needed. It must be considered in any case of:

Scabies	Note absence of itch in pityriasis lichenoides et varioliformis acuta
Insect bites	Exposure history
Varicella	Involves scalp; no new lesions after 1 week
Gianotti-Crosti syndrome	No necrosis occurs; presents acrally; has associated lymphadenopathy
Erythema multiforme	Involves mucous membranes

Willemze R, Scheffer E: Clinical and histologic differentiation between **lymphomatoid papulosis and pityriasis lichenoides**. J Am Acad Dermatol 1985; 13:418–428.

Eighty-two patients with acute and chronic **pityriasis lichenoides** (parapsoriasis lichenoides et varioliformis acuta, Mucha-Habermann disease, and pityriasis lichenoides chronica) were compared clinically with 26 patients with lymphomatoid papulosis.

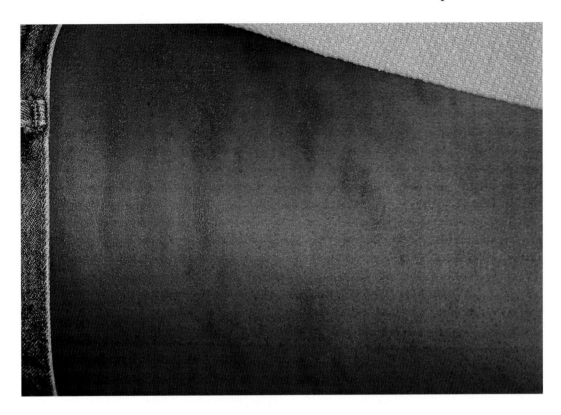

In both conditions, crops of scattered papular and papulonecrotic lesions appeared, **disappearing spontaneously** in a month or so. Resolution of the large nodules and plaques in lymphomatoid papulosis took months rather than weeks. The ultimate distinction remained histologic.

Sina B, Burnett JW: **Lymphomatoid papulosis**. Case reports and literature review. Arch Dermatol 1983; 119:189–197.

Clinical	Mucha-Habermann look-alike
	Grouped lesions resembling pityriasis lichenoides
	Lesions begin as scaling or necrotic papules evolving into macules
	May become ulcerative or show infiltrative plaque-like mycosis fungoides
	Self-healing with life cycle of lesion 1 to 3 months.
Histologic	"Bark is worse than bite;" looks malignant, but acts benign.
Course	many years; crops keep reappearing.
Prognosis	guarded: 10% evolve into malignant neoplasms— lymphoma (T cell, lymphocytic, histiocytic), reticulum cell sarcoma, and Hodgkin's disease.

Sanchez NP, Pittelkow MR, Muller SA, et al: The clinicopathologic spectrum of **lymphomatoid papulosis**: Study of 31 cases. J Am Acad Dermatol 1983; 8:81–94.

Here is a **clinically benign, histologically malignant dermatosis**. It is benign because it is self-healing. Its erythematous papules and nodules do heal, despite being hemorrhagic, pustular, and ulcerative. It is malignant histologically because under the scope the tissue looks like malignant lymphoma.

The clinical course is benign but protracted and recurrent. The individual lesions, which resemble those of Mucha-Habermann disease (pityriasis lichenoides et varioliformis acuta), last for weeks, eventually scarring.

As clinicians, we marvel that the fearsome histologic picture these cases present is clinically benign. And yet there is a cloud over all of these patients. If followed long enough, some cases veer off into a clinically malignant course. The patients have lost the battle, and their disease is no longer benign but rather is now the full-fledged clinical and histologic malignancy of **lymphoma**.

Thomsen K, Wantzin GL: **Lymphomatoid papulosis**. A follow-up study of 30 patients. J Am Acad Dermatol 1987; 17:632–636.

Recurrent crops of dark-red papules and nodules with occasional bullae occur on the trunk and extremities in this provocative disease. It is provocative, since one in ten will evolve into a true malignant disease. **Biopsy surveillance** remains at once the diagnostic and prognostic tool. Use it.

Rongioletti F, Rivara G, Rebora A: **Pityriasis lichenoides et varioliformis acuta** and acquired toxoplasmosis. Dermatologica 1987; 175:41–44.

In a 50-year-old woman who had recently moved to a country farm, crops of papular, papulonecrotic, and hemorrhagic lesions appeared over a 15-day period. The clinical diagnosis of **pityriasis lichenoides et varioliformis** was confirmed histologically. She had slight cervical lymphadenopathy and the liver was palpable 2 cm below the costal arch.

She had serologic evidence of recent acute toxoplasmosis, with tests for *Toxoplasma gondii* showing:

> Indirect hemagglutination (IHA) test for total IgG: 1:512
> Enzyme–linked immunosorbent assay (ELISA) for IgG: positive
> ELISA for IgM: positive
> Indirect fluorescent test for IgM (IgM-IFA): positive 1:16

These serologic results, and the rapid clearing of the patient's skin lesions with antitoxoplasma therapy (Spiramycin 2 gm/day for 2 months), favor the view that **toxoplasma infection** played a major etiologic role.

Muller SA (ed): **Parapsoriasis**: Proceedings of the First International Parapsoriasis Symposium. Mayo Foundation, Rochester, Minnesota, 1990; 117 pp.

A summary of how 33 international authorities look at the multifaceted nature of nomenclature and diagnosis of this kaleidoscopic entity called parapsoriasis.

*Clinical diagnosis oscillates between assurance, hopeful guessing,
and frank bewilderment.*

Paresthesias

While the specific branch of medical knowledge needed to solve a dermatologic problem is not always evident, the patient with numbness, tingling, prickling, burning, or crawling sensations requires expertise in the area of neurology.

Paresthesias have as many different causes as dermatitis, but they all reflect damage to the sensory nervous system, particularly the peripheral nerve fibers. Commonly the strange sensations result from demyelination of small myelinated fibers that carry the sensations of pain, temperature, and touch. Careful testing may reveal a sensory deficit in the area of paresthesia. While sometimes the neuropathy is axonal in nature, it may also reflect biochemical alterations in the milieu of the nerve endings.

Always the sensory pathway goes up the spinal nerve, through the dorsal root synapses, up the anterolateral fasciculus of the spinal cord to the thalamic nuclei, and onto the postcentral cortex for sensory processing. Paresthesias of the face and head pass through trigeminal nerve pathways to the pons, merging with spinothalamic pathways in the midbrain, and then traveling to the thalamic nuclei and finally the somatic postcentral sensory cortex. These pathways point to the many sites of potential interference in the processing of sensory messages from the skin.

Practically one must search in a systematic fashion for known causes of paresthesias:

Physical injury
Chemical damage
Systemic disease
Neurologic disease
Psychiatric problem

Physical Injury

Schiller F: Sigmund Freud's meralgia paresthetica. Neurology 1985; 35:557–558.

Perhaps the most famous patient to have suffered **meralgia paresthetica** was Sigmund Freud. In 1895 he reported that for more than 7 years he had had a funny sensation, a feeling of alien skin on the outer surface of the right thigh. Walking made it worse, but otherwise little could be discerned as to its etiology. **Compression of the lateral femoral cutaneous nerve**, usually by the overlying inguinal ligament, is now recognized as the cause.

Weber PJ, Poulos EG: **Notalgia paresthetica**. Case reports and histologic appraisal. J Am Acad Dermatol 1988; 18:25–30.

Sensory mononeuropathies have been described and named:

meralgia paresthetica (lateral cutaneous femoral nerve; *mer* = thigh)
  synonyms: puzzling posterior pigmented pruritic patches; peculiar spotty pigmentations; hereditary localized pruritus
notalgia paresthetica (posterior rami of the second through sixth dorsal spinal nerves; *nota* = back)
incisura scapulae syndrome (suprascapular nerve)
cheiralgia paresthetica (radial nerve–derived hand pain)
gonalgia paresthetica (saphenous nerve; *gony* = knee)
other nerves occasionally involved:

auriculotemporal	cutaneous branch of obturator
digital	sural
ulnar	calcaneal

In two cases of **notalgia paresthetica** reported here, there was a brown patch over the right scapula. A 66-year-old woman had had intermittent pruritus for several months, whereas a 50-year-old woman had a localized partial deficit of touch, pinprick pain, and temperature. A 60-year-old man also had intermittent pruritus, tingling, and burning of the right upper back for 10 years. Although the skin appeared normal, there was a sensory deficit for touch, pinprick pain, and temperature. Histologically, amyloid was not seen in any of the three patients, although each showed some necrotic keratinocytes.

The findings of **11 additional patients** with notalgia paresthetica are summarized, with complaints of pruritus, burning, tingling, crawling sensations, and hyperalgesia. Only two showed asymptomatic brown patches. Sweating was found to be reduced in others. Excoriations were not seen. Electromyography demonstrated paraspinal denervation from T-4 to T-10. It is likely that the dorsal roots of T-2 through T-6 are easily damaged, since they travel a unique 90-degree course through the multifidus spinae muscles.

The clinical and historical anatomic location of notalgic parasthetica may be verified by electromyographic studies, as well as starch–iodine sweat tests.

The **differential diagnosis** of a brown patch or plaque with altered sensation on the back includes:

notalgia paresthetica	fixed drug eruption
lichen simplex chronicus	postinflammatory hyperpigmentation
macular amyloidosis	Hansen's disease
lichen amyloidosis	

Awareness of this innocuous yet persistent problem may save your patient from an ominous misdiagnosis such as multiple sclerosis and from unnecessary surgical maneuvers such as laminectomy.

Good DC, Couch JR, Wacaser L: **"Numb, clumsy hands"** and high cervical spondylosis. Surg Neurol 1984; 22:285–291.

In 13 patients with **numb, clumsy hands** and associated tingling and paresthesias, myelography demonstrated cervical spondylosis with spinal cord compression. Numbness and paresthesias were present in the lower legs of four patients. Surgical intervention (laminectomy) gave complete relief to seven patients.

Greenhouse AH, Page K: **Scuba diver's thigh**. West J Med 1986; 145:698–699.

The 30-pound lead belt worn by a young woman during a 50-minute scuba dive at 80 feet produced an immediate pressure neuropathy of the left lateral femoral cutaneous nerve. The **numbness of the left thigh** persisted several months and reappeared when she used the same equipment 6 months later.

Other causes of similar meralgia paresthetica include:

    an expanding abdomen (ascites, obesity, pregnancy)
    stretch due to pelvic tilt
    tight pants, corset, truss
    tourniquet
    parachute harness
    heavy wallet

Jarrell HR: **Vegas neuropathy**. N Engl J Med 1988; 319:1487.

Sixteen continuous hours of leaning on the right elbow at the gaming table in **Las Vegas** resulted in a **sensory deficit** of a man's right hand due to ulnar compression neuropathy. This persisted for more than 2 months and on electromyography was shown to be associated with local denervation of several muscles. (It is to be hoped that the winnings covered the medical expenses!)

Ryan EL: Breast weight and **hand paraesthesiae**. Med J Aust 1988; 148:320.

Thirteen women with **paresthesias of the hands and forearms** were found to be wearing bras that produced a mean downward strap force on each shoulder of 3.1 kg. In the control group without paresthesias, the mean downward strap force was 1.7 kg. Generally the **bra strap pressure** was directly proportional to the breast weight. The paresthesias promptly remitted once the excessive strap pressure on the shoulder was eliminated.

Nelson GA, Puhl RW, Altman MI: **Superficial dysesthesias** secondary to epidermoid cyst of the foot. J Foot Surg 1985; 24:269–271.

A 48-year-old man was cured of a constant **burning** and tingling sensation of the dorsolateral aspect of the right foot by excision of a **keratinous cyst** just proximal to the area of dysesthesia. The cyst had formed at the site of an old fracture that had developed osteomyelitis.

Grace DM: **Meralgia paresthetica** after gastroplasty for morbid obesity. Can J Surg 1987; 30:64–65.

Three morbidly obese patients developed severe hip pain and **numbness** immediately after gastroplasty. Although the differential diagnosis included thrombophlebitis, osteoarthritis, and lumbar disc protrusion, the cause was found to be compression of the lateral cutaneous nerve of the thigh by the **Gomez retractor** used in surgery. All of the symptoms of this meralgia paresthetica resolved spontaneously within 3 months.

Flanagan WF, Webster GD, Brown MW, Massey EW: **Lumbosacral plexus stretch injury** following the use of the modified lithotomy position. J Urol 1985; 134:567–568.

Within hours after surgery, two patients developed **paresthesias of the right foot and right knee**, respectively. Each had surgery requiring several hours of modified **lithotomy positioning** on the table. The paresthesias were shown to be due to stretching of the sciatic nerve during the period the hip was kept in hyperabduction. Such nerve stretching produces epineural injury with pseudoneuroma formation and perineural rupture. Electromyography is helpful in the diagnosis. The paresthesias, as well as associated muscle weakness, persisted for several months, but the overall prognosis was good.

Aranoff SM, Levy HB, Tuchman AJ, Daras M: Alopecia in **meralgia paresthetica**. J Am Acad Dermatol 1985; 12:176–178.

Two men with longstanding **meralgia paresthetica** exhibited **local alopecia** in the area supplied by the lateral femoral cutaneous nerve. Whether the paresthesias or the neuropathy itself caused this nonscarring alopecia is not known, although both may have contributed. Herpes zoster and Hansen's disease were ruled out as a cause of the meralgia and hair loss.

Nordin M, Nyström B, Wallin U, Hagbarth K-E: **Ectopic sensory discharges and paresthesiae** in patients with disorders of peripheral nerves, dorsal roots and dorsal columns. Pain 1984; 20:231–245.

Tungsten microelectrodes inserted into cutaneous nerves permitted the recording of ectopic **antidromic nerve impulses** when **paresthesias** were induced by the following:

1. Eliciting Tinel's sign in a patient with entrapment of the ulnar nerve at the elbow
2. Elevation of the arm in a patient with thoracic outlet syndrome
3. Straining with a chin-chest maneuver in a patient with a herniated lumbar disc
4. Straight-leg raising test (Lasègue's sign) in a patient with an S-I syndrome due to root fibrosis
5. Neck flexion elicitation of Lhermitte's sign in a patient with multiple sclerosis

If you feel uncertain about the diagnosis, you probably don't have the right diagnosis.

Freed DLJ, Carter R: Neuropathy due to **monosodium glutamate intolerance**. Ann Allergy 1982; 48:96–97.

A 54-year-old doctor's 5-year struggle with **paresthesias of the hands** and **feet** ended once he eliminated foods containing **monosodium glutamate** (MSG). After 9 months of freedom from symptoms, he was given a challenge dose of MSG in a pork pie. Within 10 minutes he experienced tachycardia and glove-and-stocking paresthesias, which were maximal at 45 minutes and faded away after 3 hours. He remained irritable and in a bad temper for 6 days, after which there was brisk diuresis and recovery of his usual equability.

Noteworthy is the fact that attacks of paresthesias had previously been triggered in this patient by influenza vaccine and house dust mite injections.

Fishman HC: **Notalgia paresthetica**. J Am Acad Dermatol 1986; 15:1304–1305.

A persistent **itch** of the right scapular region, present for many years, disappeared once **saccharin** (a sulfa compound) was eliminated from a man's diet. The itch returned 10 years later despite the patient's avowal he had continued to avoid saccharin. However, he had started drinking low-calorie beverages with the sugar substitute aspartame (NutraSweet), assuming it was safe. But it wasn't safe. Close label reading revealed that the drinks all contained saccharin as well as aspartame. Removing these drinks from his diet again resulted in a cure.

(We can cite two patients who had severe persistent paresthesias of the feet and lower legs due to the artificial sweetener cyclamate.)

Lutz EG: **Restless legs, anxiety, and caffeinism**. J Clin Psychiatry 1978; 39:693–698.

Unpleasant creeping sensations in the lower legs are the cardinal symptom of the restless legs syndrome, first described graphically in 1685 as "Anxietas tibiarum" by the great neurologist, Thomas Willis:

Wherefore to some, when being a Bed they betake themselves to sleep, presently in the Arms and Leggs, Leapings and Contractions of the Tendons, and so great a Restlessness and Tossings of their Members ensue, that the diseased are no more able to sleep, than if they were in a place of the greatest Torture.

Today, the cause of these unpleasant **nocturnal creeping sensations** and the resulting irresistible need to move the legs appears to be caffeine. In the 62 patients in this study, **elimination of caffeine-containing** medications and beverages (coffee, tea, cola, cocoa) gave measurable relief. The first description of this problem occurred in the period when coffee and tea were introduced into the British Isles.

Young JJ, Brownlee HJ, Delaney R: **Caffeine and burning feet**. Drug Intell Clin Pharm 1982; 16:779–780.

For 3 years a 51-year-old man experienced **burning sensations** on the soles of both feet, particularly the toes and distal aspects rather than the heels. The burning paresthesias of the feet began in the early afternoon and resolved by the next morning. He was in good health but smoked two packs of cigarettes daily and consumed 10 to 12 cups of coffee daily. He worked in an office and denied chemical exposures. Neurologic examination was normal, and there was no evidence of peripheral vascular disease. The foot 1039 temperature was normal, despite the sensation of burning. All laboratory studies were normal, as were x-rays of the feet. No cause of the burning was discerned by the physician.

The patient learned by chance that his older sister had had burning feet until she stopped drinking caffeinated beverages for unrelated reasons. The patient then **eliminated caffeine** consumption, with complete resolution of the problem in 5 days. Later the burning recurred after he drank caffeinated cola beverages. Likewise, blind challenge with caffeine (200 mg on day 1, 400 mg on day 2) produced burning feet sensations that persisted for 24 hours after the caffeine was taken.

Le Quesne PM: **Neuropathy due to drugs**. *In* Dyck PJ, Thomas PK, Lambert EH, Bunge R (eds): Peripheral Neuropathy, 2nd ed. Philadelphia, W. B. Saunders Company, 1984, vol 2, pp 2162–2179.

The following **drugs** are neuropathic and may **induce paresthesias** along with other neurologic findings:

chloramphenicol	doxorubicin
clioquinol	ethambutol
dapsone	gold
phenytoin	isoniazid
disulfiram	misonidazole
nitrofurantoin	perhexiline
platinum	thalidomide
glutethimide	vinblastine
vincristine	vindesine

Koller WC, Gehlmann LK, Malkinson FD: **Dapsone-induced peripheral neuropathy**. Arch Neurol 1977; 644–646.

Dapsone (50 mg/day increasing to 200 mg/day) was given to an 18-year-old man with severe cystic acne. After 5 weeks he noted **numbness and weakness** of both feet, and 10 days later he had difficulty walking, with an unsteady gait and dragging of the feet. He could not stand on the heels or toes or perform tandem gait. There was marked decrease of vibration sense in the feet, particularly in the toes. One week after stopping dapsone he noted subjective improvement, and 2 months after the dapsone had been discontinued only mild motor and sensory deficits were demonstrable.

He was shown to be a slow acetylator of isoniazid, which is metabolized by the same enzyme (*N*-acetyltransferase) as dapsone. The glucose-6-phosphate dehydrogenase (G6PD) level was normal.

Dapsone-induced peripheral neuropathy is rare and reversible. Although mainly of the motor type, involving arms or legs, sensory changes may also occur. The neurotoxicity is apparently not dose dependent.

Porter IH: **Isoniazid neuropathy**. Handbook of Clinical Neurology 1982; 44:648.

Paresthesias and numbness of the fingers and toes may be an early complication of **isoniazid therapy**. If treatment continues the paresthesias extend over the hands and up the legs, becoming painful and burning. This is followed by distal weakness and calf tenderness.

The conjoint administration of pyridoxine with isoniazid prevents the appearance of paresthesias. However, pyridoxine is of no therapeutic benefit once paresthesias have developed. If isoniazid is discontinued early, the symptoms fade in a few weeks, but if it is continued for more than a few weeks after onset of symptoms, recovery may take more than 1 year, being eventually complete.

Two interesting points:

1. Patients in whom isoniazid is acetylated (inactivated) slowly develop high blood levels of the drug and are prone to neuropathy.
2. Isoniazid increases the excretion of pyridoxine, so that pyridoxine should be given prophylactically to prevent neuropathy. Pyridoxine has no effect on the speed of recovery of established neuropathy.

Macdonald JB: Muscle cramps during treatment with nifedipine. Br Med J 1982; 285:1744.

Paresthesias of the right arm and both legs developed in a 55-year-old woman after 2 weeks of treatment of angina with nifedipine (10 mg tid). Doubling the dose intensified the painful paresthesias to the point where she was bed-bound and unable to sleep. The serum potassium was normal, and she was not taking diuretics. Stopping the **nifedipine** led to disappearance of all paresthesias and also associated leg cramps within 24 hours.

Although angina may cause arm paresthesias and hypokalemia may induce leg paresthesias, neither factor was operative here, and "looking behind the diagnosis" paid off!

Ramilo O, Kinane BT, McCracken GH: **Chloramphenicol neurotoxicity**. Pediatr Infect Dis 1988; 7:358–359.

A 12-year-old boy had severe progressive **paresthesias** in a stocking distribution, along with decreased visual acuity.

The cause was traced to **chloramphenicol**, which he had been taking for 2 months for multiple cerebral abscesses caused by *Streptococcus intermedius*. Stopping the chloramphenicol therapy, along with starting oral administration of vitamins B_6 (500 mg bid) and B_{12} (0.5 mg daily) was followed by resolution of both the paresthesias and the optic neuritis within 6 weeks.

Lokich JJ, Moore C: Chemotherapy-associated **palmar-plantar erythrodysesthesia syndrome**. Ann Intern Med 1984; 101:798–800.

Within weeks of receiving protracted daily infusions of **fluorouracil** or doxorubicin for malignant disease, 18 of 300 patients developed **tingling of** the **hands and feet** that progressed over 3 to 4 days to pain on holding objects and walking. The palms and soles become swollen and erythematous, with tenderness of the distal phalanges and periungual erythema and swelling. With continued therapy the swelling and erythema progress, and a central pallor develops on the tufts of the fingertips and toes and the soles. Nearly half of the patients also had associated stomatitis. Once the drug was discontinued, the paresthesias and skin changes resolved, with desquamation of palms and soles in the final stage. Restarting the drug treatment led to reappearance of the same signs and symptoms.

Williams AC, Cullen MH, Haynes IG: **Cisplatin neuropathy** with Lhermitte's sign. J Neurol Neurosurg Psychiatry 1986; 49:1326.

Chronic **tingling of the feet** developed in a 38-year-old man during a course of **cisplatin** therapy for an undifferentiated teratoma in the anterior mediastinum. The paresthesias remained for more than a year, and his feet would become numb and unsteady after he ran about 100 yards. An associated **Lhermitte's sign** (sudden electric-like shocks on bending the head forward) faded within a few weeks. This sign is nonspecific for posterior column dysfunction.

Windebank AJ, McCall JT, Dyck PJ: **Metal neuropathy.** *In* Dyck PJ, Thomas PK, Lambert EH, Bunge R (eds): Peripheral Neuropathy, 2nd ed. Philadelphia, W. B. Saunders Company, 1984, vol 2, pp 2142–2147.

A 39-year-old man had **burning pain** in the soles, calves, and hands for 1 year, associated with weakness. In the hospital he showed signs of pneumonia and mental confusion and also had peeling and hyperkeratosis of the palms and soles. His condition improved, but relapsed after he returned home. Later, examination revealed diffuse areas of hyperpigmentation and depigmentation on the trunk, blotchy red feet, and transverse white striate lines (**Mee's lines**) on the fingernails. There was generalized muscle atrophy, particularly in the distal limb muscles, and weakness was most marked in the lower limbs. Glove-and-stocking sensory loss was present to the elbows and midthighs, and tendon reflexes were absent.

Exhaustive studies were for nought until an arsenic level in the urine was found to be somewhat elevated. The hair and nails also contained large amounts of arsenic. It was then shown that his **wife had been dusting his food with arsenic.** Today, most cases of arsenic neuropathy are no longer iatrogenic, but represent attempts at murder or suicide. Still, there are a few cases of iatrogenic origin.

Peabody CA: **Trazodone withdrawal** and formication. J Clin Psychiatry 1987; 48:385.

A 65-year-old black man had the sensation of **bugs crawling** over the skin of the right hand and arm, as well as the face and neck, starting a few days after long-term trazodone antidepressant medication was reduced from 300 mg/day to 200 mg/day. Increasing the dose back to 300 mg/day led to disappearance of the symptoms within few weeks. The patient resisted further attempts to decrease the trazodone.

The specific sensation of insects crawling over the skin (**formication**) is well known in the following settings:

schizophrenia
cocaine use
amphetamine use
delirium tremens
somatosensory seizure
inhalation of gasoline (lead encephalopathy)
azathioprine therapy
dynorphin therapy
lesion in the posterior columns of the spinal cord
Parkinson's disease
postmenopausal syndrome

Smith HV, Spalding JMK: Outbreak of paralysis in Morocco due to **ortho-cresyl phosphate poisoning.** Lancet 1959; 2:1019–1021.

In the month of September, 1959, 10,000 Moroccans developed **paresthesias** and loss of superficial sensation in the stocking-glove distribution. This was followed within a few days by weakness of the lower legs and subsequently of the hand. Victims could be recognized by their ungainly high-stepping gait. Recovery required at least a year.

The cause was traced to ingestion of a product sold as "**olive oil,**" which appeared dark like old motor oil. Analysis revealed that it contained not only vegetable oils but also large amounts of aircraft jet engine oil. The outdated discarded oil, which the food manufacturer had added in the interest of cost control, contained neurotoxic cresyl phosphates in a concentration of nearly 3%.

Morton-Kute L: Rubella vaccine and **facial paresthesias**. Ann Intern Med 1985; 102:563.

A 35-year-old woman noted **numbness** in the left maxillary area 9 days after receiving **rubella vaccine** (human diploid cell culture). Over the next 2 weeks, numbness involved the ophthalmic and mandibular branches of the left trigeminal nerve. The paresthesias faded slowly over 4 months and were interpreted as being due to a vaccine-induced neuritis.

Brachial neuritis, carpal tunnel syndrome, pain in the knee with a crouching gait, and nocturnal paresthesias are also known to occur in children following rubella vaccination.

Knox JM II, Tucker SB, Flannigan SA: **Paresthesia** from cutaneous exposure to a synthetic pyrethroid insecticide. Arch Dermatol 1984; 120:744–746.

Chrysanthemums elaborate powerful neurotoxic agents (pyrethrins) as their form of "Star Wars" against invading insects. Man has synthesized analogues of these compounds for commercial use in controlling insects attacking man and animals, as well as food and fiber products. These lipophilic compounds penetrate human skin and damage the rich supply of fine nerve endings, causing paresthesias in farm workers and others occupationally exposed to the synthetic **pyrethroids**. Microgram quantities of the commonly used pyrethroid fenvalerate (phenyl acetate ester of pyrethroid alcohol) applied to the skin of volunteers produced **numbness, itching**, burning, tingling, and warmth after a latent period of about an hour. The paresthesias peaked at 3 to 6 hours and faded after 24 hours.

The next time you see a patient who feels bugs crawling over him, find out about exposure to dried or fresh chrysanthemums, as well as synthetic pyrethroids. The flower may be what's bugging him!

Fisher AA: **Paresthesia of the fingers** accompanying dermatitis due to methylmethacrylate bone cement. Contact Dermatitis 1979; 5:56–57.

Contact with the liquid monomer of bone cement places orthopedic surgeons at risk of developing not only dermatitis, but also persistent **burning sensations**, tingling, and numbness of the fingertips. These paresthesias may continue for months after the dermatitis has healed. The liquid monomer, **methylmethacrylate**, is a unique hazard, since it readily penetrates rubber gloves. Similar paresthesias have been associatedwith industrial dermatitis from benzene.

Sometimes an old patient needs a new diagnostician and a new diagnosis.

Systemic Disease

Nass R, Chutorian A: **Dysaesthesias and dysautonomia**: A self-limited syndrome of painful dysaesthesias and autonomic dysfunction in childhood. J Neurol Neurosurg Psychiatry 1982; 45:162–165.

An 11-year-old boy complained of generalized pruritus, followed by symmetrical painful **burning dysesthesias** of the feet, which ascended to involve the arms and caused self-imposed immobilization. Symptoms began 1 day after he experienced an afebrile upper respiratory infection. No motor or reflex abnormalities were present. Hypertension (155/125) developed within the week of onset and responded to propranolol (30 mg tid). The paresthesias gradually descended and receded, involving only the ankles after 2 months, and disappearing after 4 months.

Two other children had similar syndromes, believed to be a variant of acute **polyneuritis** involving both sensory and autonomic systems. Although similar dysfunction occurs in the Guillain-Barré syndrome, this diagnosis is precluded by the complete absence of motor system involvement. Excessive adrenergic function was considered to be the cause of the pain and hypertension, and the dysesthesias improved in one case when propranolol was started.

McLennan HG, Oats JN, Walstab JE: Survey of **hand symptoms** in pregnancy. Med J Aust 1987; 147:542–544.

Numbness, tingling, pain, and **burning of the hands** was a complaint in 35% of women in the **third trimester of pregnancy**. This study of 1216 pregnancies did not reveal a specific cause, although the paresthesias did correlate with the complaint of tight rings. In 19% "carpal tunnel syndrome" was present, with paresthesias resulting from compression of the median nerve between the flexor retinaculum and the carpal bones. Ulnar nerve neuropathy was seen in 12% of patients, and generalized nerve distribution in the hand was affected in 69%. This has previously been called the four-finger syndrome, with edema presumably affecting digital nerve function in both the median and ulnar distribution.

Lambrianidis T, Molyvdas J: **Paresthesia** of the inferior alveolar nerve caused by periodontal-endodontic pathosis. Oral Surg 1987; 63:90–92.

Numbness of the buccal gingiva on the right side of the mandible and the right half of the lower lip in a 22-year-old woman proved to be due to a **periapical abscess** of the right mandibular first molar, which compressed the inferior alveolar nerve. Surgical treatment was followed by disappearance of the paresthesia in 2 months.

Half the cases of facial numbness are due to dental problems. Of these, the most common is postinjection paresthesia due to either intraneural hemorrhage or needle contamination with a chemical disinfectant.

Byrne E, Henderson K, Jelinek M: **Burning feet** complicating cardio-pulmonary bypass. Aust NZ J Med 1984; 14:686–687.

Coronary artery vein graft surgery in a 43-year-old man was followed 3 days later by intense **painful paresthesias** of the feet. Sensory and motor testing showed only depressed pinprick sensation. The paresthesias persisted for more than 12 months and were assumed to be due to small nerve fiber injury from ischemia, which occurs in a patient as extracorporeal circulatory support is alternately used and discontinued.

Nickel SN, Frame B: Nervous and muscular systems in myxedema. J Chron Dis 1961; 14:570–581.

Every single patient in a series of 25 patients with **myxedema** complained of **paresthesias**! Numbness of the hands and feet with pricking and tingling were the most common, and burning sensations of the hands and feet occurred in about 10% of cases. Myopathy was also common, with muscle weakness in the proximal shoulder girdle and hip muscles and aching and spasm in the calves and low back. Pinching of the muscles or percussion of muscles with a reflex hammer caused transient localized swelling (myo-edema, mounding) which was very distressing.

Victor M: **Polyneuropathy** due to nutritional deficiency and alcoholism. *In* Dyck PJ, Thomas PK, Lambert EH, Bunge R (eds): Peripheral Neuropathy, 2nd ed. Philadelphia, W. B. Saunders Company, 1984, vol 2, pp 1899–1940.

The **burning feet syndrome** was seen in thousands of World War II prisoners as a distinctive **nutritional deficiency disease**. The specific etiology was unknown but was probably a vitamin B deficiency. It began as a severe metatarsal ache "like a toothache," followed soon by tingling, prickling, electric shocks, pins-and-needles feeling, coldness, stabbing pains, and sensations of heat and burning. Beginning on the soles, the problem extended over the dorsal aspect of the feet and eventually involved the entire legs. Hyperhidrosis of the soles, cyanosis, and reddening of the feet were common. Symptoms were worse at night, and patients often soaked their feet in ice water. Prisoners named the disorder hot feet, happy feet, painful feet, and jittery legs.

Burning feet are also common in alcoholic neuropathy, beriberi, and pellagra.

Asbury AK: **Uremic neuropathy**. *In* Dyck PJ, Thomas PK, Lambert EH, Bunge R (eds): Peripheral Neuropathy, 2nd ed. Philadelphia, W. B. Saunders Company, 1984, vol 2, pp 1811–1825.

Uremic patients commonly experience protean **distal dysesthesias**:

Painful, tingling, or electric feelings of the feet and hands
Unpleasant raw sensations resulting from mild cutaneous stimulation of the fingers or toes
Bandlike constrictive feelings around the feet and ankles
Aberrant sensations of swelling and turgidity of the fingers or toes
Feelings of the distal extremities being twisted into bizarre positions
Burning of the soles

The restless legs syndrome and muscle cramps of the distal extremities are also seen frequently in uremic patients. The diagnosis of uremic neuropathy rests on the presence of chronic renal failure with symptomatic uremia (several months' duration) and the absence of other drugs, toxins, and metabolic states that may cause neuropathy. **Nitrofurantoin** (Furadantin, Macrodantin) is a major cause of **neuropathy**, especially in patients with renal impairment and should not be used in azotemia. Lead intoxication, polyarteritis nodosa, multiple myeloma, lupus erythematosus, and diabetes mellitus may also cause renal dysfunction and neuropathy.

Paller AS: **Fabry's disease** (angiokeratoma corporis diffusum universale). Dermatol Clin 1987; 5:242–243.

Paresthesias of the hands and feet are the most characteristic and often the **first symptom of Fabry's disease**, and these are associated with episodes of severe pain and fever. Attacks are triggered by exercise, temperature change, fatigue, and emotional stress. They reflect the deposition of glycosphingolipid within cutaneous nerves, resulting from an X-linked genetic deficiency of alpha-galactosidase. Hypohidrosis, slow facial hair growth associated with delayed puberty, decreased fertility, and periorbital edema are also found occasionally.

Cohen DM, Reinhardt RA: **Systemic sarcoidosis** presenting with Horner's syndrome and mandibular paresthesia. Oral Surg 1982; 53:577–581.

In a 59-year-old white woman with sarcoidosis, a noncaseating granuloma of the right mandible led to a loose second molar. After extraction of the tooth, the socket failed to heal, and she developed **paresthesias** and pain in the right lower quadrant of the mouth. It masqueraded as periodontal disease with bony destruction and evaded detection until a biopsy was obtained.

She also had Horner's syndrome with ptosis of the right eyelid and a constricted right pupil (miosis). Originally thought to be due to metastatic breast carcinoma, it was later found to be due to **sarcoid** involving the cervical sympathetic nerves.

Dyck PJ: **Neuronal atrophy and degeneration** predominantly affecting peripheral sensory and autonomic neurons. *In* Dyck PJ, Thomas PK, Lambert EH, Bunge R (eds): Peripheral Neuropathy, 2nd ed. Philadelphia, W.B. Saunders Company 1984, vol 2, pp 1557–1599.

Burning feet are common in hyperalgesic **neuropathies** (diabetic, alcoholic, toxic) and in the **aged**. However, there is a dominant hereditary version that appears during the second decade of life. The discomfort is made worse by walking, relieved by cooling, and can be almost crippling.

Bodner L, Oberman M, Shteyer A: **Mental nerve neuropathy** associated with compound odontoma. Oral Surg 1987; 63:658–660.

A 42-year-old man had a "strange feeling" in his left lower lip for 6 months, leading to total **numbness** and anesthesia. A panoramic radiograph showed a radiolucent lesion in the left mandible. This was excised and proved to be an **odontoma**, which had been pressing on the mental nerve. Sensation returned gradually, starting 3 months after surgery. Odontomas are benign tumors composed of odontogenic cells that produce enamel, dentin, cementum, and pulp, laid down in a disorderly pattern.

Numbness of the lower lip suggests trauma, surgical procedures, dental treatment, infection, and benign or malignant lesions in the mental nerve area. Rapid onset points to infection, surgery, or malignancy. Anesthesia of the lower lip calls for a panoramic radiograph and careful examination of the mandibular canal integrity.

Brooks D: Clinical presentation and treatment of **peripheral nerve tumors**. *In* Dyck PJ, Thomas PK, Lambert EH, Bunge R (eds): Peripheral Neuropathy, 2nd ed. Philadelphia, W.B. Saunders Company, 1984, vol 2, pp 2236–2251.

A professional violinist found that after a half-hour of playing she experienced **paresthesias in the median nerve** distribution of the right hand. The severity increased to the point that she was forced to resign from a well-known orchestra. Consultants agreed that her problem was psychogenic. Finally a neurologist discovered that he could reproduce the paresthesias by simply compressing the proximal third of her right forearm. At operation a typical well-encapsulated **schwannoma** was discovered lying between the two heads of the pronator teres muscle.

A **schwannoma** is by far the most common nerve tumor, with a peak incidence between ages 20 and 30 years. It usually presents as a painful swelling, and palpation causes shooting pains and paresthesias in the distribution of the nerve (a diagnostic sign). Neurofibromas are painful swellings that are not encapsulated and do not cause shooting pains or paresthesias upon palpation. They are more likely than schwannomas to be associated with motor and sensory deficits.

Remember that **any type of tumor** can be responsible for paresthesias—often with absence of sensory loss or motor paralysis (to the dismay of the neurologist). Direct pressure on the skin may reproduce painful symptoms and point to the location of an unsuspected nerve tumor.

McLeod JG, Walsh JC: Peripheral neuropathy associated with lymphomas and other reticuloses. In Dyck PJ, Thomas PK, Lambert EH, Bunge R (eds): Peripheral Neuropathy, 2nd ed. Philadelphia, W.B. Saunders Company, 1984, vol 2, pp 2192–2203.

Paresthesias of the extremities occur in 10 to 20% of patients with **polycythemia vera**. It is believed that increased blood viscosity leads to ischemia of the peripheral nerves with resulting axonal degeneration affecting myelinated and unmyelinated fibers.

McLeod JG: **Carcinomatous neuropathy**. *In* Dyck PJ, Thomas PK, Lambert EH, Bunge R (eds): Peripheral Neuropathy, 2nd ed. Philadelphia, W.B. Saunders Company, 1984, vol 2, pp 2180–2191.

Carcinomas, small or large, can produce **sensory neuropathy**. It presents as numbness, dysesthesias, and paresthesias of the extremity, commencing distally and spreading proximally. Unsteadiness of gait and aching pains in the limbs may also be present. Symptoms usually precede discovery of the primary tumor by 6 to 15 months but occasionally by as many as $3\frac{1}{2}$ years. In the vast majority of cases the tumor is an oat cell carcinoma in the lung. Rare instances of remission of the paresthesias following excision of the tumor have been reported.

Foss RD: Early detection. J Am Dent Assoc 1986; 113:126.

In any patient who has **paresthesias of a branch of the trigeminal nerve**, look for metastatic or primary **malignant disease**. Examples are cited of maxillofacial metastatic breast carcinoma and glioblastoma multiforme.

I wouldn't have seen it if I hadn't believed it.
An old geologist's saying

Neurologic Disease

Wilberger JE, Abla A, Maroon JC: **Burning hands syndrome** revisited. Neurosurgery 1986; 19:1038–1040.

While playing a saxophone at a football game, a 14-year-old girl fell to the ground, striking her head and momentarily losing consciousness. She awakened with **burning, tingling, and numbness** of the hands and subsequently had diffuse neck pain and marked cervical muscle spasms. Cervical spine films and computed tomography were normal, but magnetic resonance imaging showed widening of the spinal cord from C-4 to C-7, indicating that the paresthesias were due to a contusion with **edema of the spinal cord**. There was no evidence of cervical fracture or displacement. A Philadelphia collar reduced the cervical spasm during the 3 weeks of recovery.

The burning pain reflects involvement of pain-mediating fibers located superficially in the spinothalamic tract of the anterolateral quadrant of the spinal cord. In most cases the burning hands syndrome of spinal cord injury is associated with an outright cervical fracture or dislocation. However, children and adolescents with burning hands may have **ligamentous instability**, leading to excessive spinal mobility and spinal cord injury, despite normal x-ray studies.

Fisher CM: **Pure sensory stroke** and allied conditions. Stroke 1982; 13:434–447.

This is a review of 135 patients with acute or persistent **attacks of numbness and paresthesias**, many of which resulted from an **occlusive cerebrovascular lesion** involving the thalamus. The numbness was unilateral, usually involving the face, arm, and/or leg and was not associated with muscle weakness or paralysis.

The pure sensory stroke may represent a true **thalamic infarct** with symptoms lasting more than 24 hours or a transient ischemic attack with numbness lasting less than 24 hours. The **differential diagnosis** includes migrainous attacks, cervical disc disease, and thrombosis of a posterior cerebral artery. Florid paresthesias were also found in a woman with thrombocythemia (platelet count 1.5 million), with reduction in platelets being curative.

In **migrainous attacks**, paresthesias last about 30 minutes and march gradually from one area to another over 10 to 20 minutes. Bilateral numbness strongly suggests migraine. Paresthesias involving only one limb suggest cervical or lumbar disc disease. If other neurologic symptoms occur with the paresthesias, occlusion of the posterior or middle cerebral arteries or the internal carotid artery should be suspected. In pure sensory stroke, paresthesias may also change to dysesthesia (e.g., feelings of tightness, pulling, constriction, swelling, stiffness, woodenness, cold, stone-like) or to feelings of thalamic pain (e.g., soreness, hurting, unpleasant sensation, burning, hotness).

Kostulas VK, Henriksson A, Link H: **Monosymptomatic sensory symptoms** and cerebrospinal fluid immunoglobulin levels in relation to multiple sclerosis. Arch Neurol 1986; 43:447–451.

Tinglings, **feelings of pins and needles**, and hypoesthesias (impaired sensation) are common first manifestations of **multiple sclerosis**.

Look to the spinal fluid for more evidence. This study showed that over half of 53 patients with unexplained paresthesias had oligoclonal IgG bands in the cerebrospinal fluid, consistent with an inflammatory process. Within 5 years, nine of these patients developed multiple sclerosis.

Bucci MN, Farhat SM, Papadopoulos SM: Ipsilateral **sensory symptoms** caused by a temporal lobe glioma. Neurosurgery 1985; 17:332–334.

A 48-year-old man had personality change, confusion, and the complaint of foul odors not perceived by others. This was followed by transient left-sided headache and **paresthesias** and numbness of the left upper and left lower extremities. Computed tomography revealed a left temporal lobe mass, which at resection proved to be a grade III **astrocytoma**. After surgery the dysosmia and paresthesias resolved. However, recurrence a year later resulted in death.

The complexities of sensory perception are reviewed to explain the unusual ipsilateral symptoms of this glioma.

Blumenkopf B, Gutierrez J, Bennett W: **Primary leptomeningeal gliomatosis and "numb, clumsy hands"**: A case report. Neurosurgery 1986; 18:363–366.

A 48-year-old right-handed man noted difficulty in writing and eating, as well as numbness and weakness of the right hand for 2 months. This was followed by diffuse **paresthesias** in the right hand and paresthesias in the fourth and fifth (ulnar) digits of the left hand. He also had weakness of the right arm. Evaluation revealed a high cervical cord lesion, which on exploration proved to be primary leptomeningeal **gliomatosis** without a parenchymal component. Radiotherapy halted the progression of the disease.

With the numb, clumsy hand syndrome, look for high cervical myelopathy.

Reaching a diagnosis may call for a ride with the patient in an untidy carriage over unmarked roads for an uncertain period.

Psychiatric Disease

Blau JN, Wiles CM, Solomon FS: **Unilateral somatic symptoms** due to hyperventilation. Br Med J 1983; 286:1108.

In 12 patients, mysterious short attacks of unilateral **paresthesias** and numbness were proven to be due to **anxiety-induced hyperventilation**. Other simultaneous symptoms included dizziness, lightheadedness, tightness in the chest, and difficulty in taking a deep breath. The paresthesias could be reproduced regularly by voluntary hyperventilation. This simple diagnostic test ruled out **previous diagnoses** of migraine, epilepsy, transient ischemic attacks, multiple sclerosis, and malignant disease.

Cotterill JA: Dermatological non-disease: A common and potentially fatal **disturbance of cutaneous body image**. Br J Dermatol 1981; 104:611–619.

Burning and itching of the scalp, face, or perineum may alert you to a patient who is depressed, possibly suicidal, or schizophrenic. These patients may be anxiously preoccupied with their skin, or truly deluded. They are frequently depressed, with dysmorphophobia (disturbed body image).

They may also complain of too little hair on the scalp (with a morbid fear of baldness) or too much hair on the face, with neither being any more apparent to the clinician than the basis for their paresthesias.

Male patients with perineal symptoms usually complain of an uncomfortable **red and inflamed scrotum** with symptoms extending to the upper anterior thighs. Symptoms often begin after trauma to the area or frank or imagined exposure to infection or venereal disease. Patients tend to be unresponsive to treatment.

Kuffer R: Les paresthésies buccales psychogènes (stomatodynies et glossodynies). Ann Dermatol Venereol 1987; 114:1589–1596.

The oral mucosa and **tongue** are a common site for **psychogenic paresthesias**, as seen in this report analyzing close to 2000 cases. It remains four times more common in women than men.

Lindenbaum J, Healton EB, Savage DG et al: Neuropsychiatric disorders caused by **cobalamin deficiency** in the absence of anemia or macrocytosis. N Engl J Med 1988; 318:1720–1728.

Paresthesias of the extremities were the most common finding in 40 patients with **low** serum **vitamin B$_{12}$** levels. The most common physical finding was diminished vibration sense, but patients also commonly had abnormalities of joint-position sense, cutaneous touch, pain sensation, reflexes, and gait. Ataxia, memory loss, limb weakness, and psychiatric disorders were other common symptoms. Not one had the classic diagnostic signs of anemia or macrocytosis, and all of them benefited from vitamin B$_{12}$ given parenterally.

It is apparent that a serum B$_{12}$ determination is warranted in anyone with unexplained paresthesias.

Lombard J, Levin IH, Weiner WJ: **Arsenic intoxication** in a cocaine abuser. N Engl J Med 1989; 320:869.

An 18-year-old male cocaine abuser developed nausea, vomiting, and profuse diarrhea after a "crack" binge. Two weeks later, while he continued to use **cocaine**, he developed **painful paresthesias** of the distal aspect of the lower extremities with motor weakness, absence of deep tendon reflexes, and a dense loss of sensory reactions to pain, vibration, and temperature change in the distal surface of the upper and lower extremities. No skin, hair, or nail lesions were present.

Electromyographic studies showed a diffuse demyelinating axonal neuropathy. Heavy metal screening was positive for urinary arsenic (>360 μg/liter, reference range 5 to 50) and arsenic in the hair (10.8 μg/gm, normal < 1). He also had normocytic anemia, leukopenia, and burr cells on a peripheral smear. Liver enzymes were mildly increased, but tests for hepatitis, human immunodeficiency virus, mononucleosis, cytomegalovirus, syphilis, and mycoplasma were all negative.

Cocaine may often be "cut" with compounds containing arsenic. Nausea, vomiting, diarrhea, and the presence of a symmetrical sensorimotor neuropathy in a cocaine abuser may indicate **arsenic intoxication**.

Leonard JC, Tobin J O'H: **Polyneuritis** associated with cytomegalovirus infections. Q J Med 1971; 40:435–442.

Cytomegalovirus (CMV) infection is described in detail in nine patients who had **paresthesias of the hands and feet** that developed 1 to 2 weeks after a mild upper respiratory infection associated with aching of the limbs and general malaise. Proximal muscle weakness of the limbs developed along with the paresthesias and remained severe for several weeks. Complete recovery took at least 3 months. The cranial nerves were often involved also. The diagnosis was made by isolating CMV from throat swabs or urine cultures or by finding rising complement–fixing antibody titers to CMV over 2 to 4 months.

Ho DD, Rota TR, Schooley RT et al: Isolation of HTLV-III from cerebrospinal fluid and neural tissues of patients with neurologic syndromes related to the **acquired immunodeficiency syndrome**. N Engl J Med 1985; 313:1493–1497.

The HTLV-III virus is neurotropic and capable of causing AIDS-related acute and chronic dementia and spinal cord degeneration with peripheral neuropathy. It was isolated from the CSF of 24 of 33 patients with **AIDS-related neurologic syndromes**.

Snider WD, Simpson DM, Nielsen S et al: Neurological complications of **acquired immune deficiency syndrome**: Analysis of 50 patients. Ann Neurol 1983; 14:403–418.

Peripheral neuropathy occurred in 8 of 50 patients with **AIDS**. Most patients had painful dysesthesias with symmetrical distal sensory loss in a stocking-and-glove distribution. Electromyography and nerve conduction velocity studies showed evidence of demyelinating distal sensorimotor neuropathy.

Samarasinghe PL, Oates JK, MacLennan IPB: **Herpetic proctitis and sacral radiomyelopathy**—a hazard for homosexual men. Br Med J 1979; 2:365–366.

Continuous burning rectal pain, constipation, malaise, fever, and paresthesias and aching of the buttocks and upper thighs were common symptoms in 11 **homosexual men**. Micropurulent rectal discharge and proctitis were present, but only four had herpetic ulceration. Associated urinary dysfunction lasted up to 3 weeks. Herpes simplex virus was isolated from swabs of the rectal mucosa in seven patients, and three patients had repeated positive cultures and bouts of proctitis. A lumbosacral radiculopathy or localized sacral meningomyelitis probably caused the symptoms.

Photosensitivity

The diagnosis of photosensitivity may be as elementary as a simple affirmation of what the patient already knows. It appears within minutes or, at most, 2 days after sun exposure. And it appears precisely in the exposed areas, with the anatomically shielded areas exempt. It shadow-skips the upper eyelids, the under chin, and retroauricular areas, as well as skin creases of the neck.

So far so good. So when do we need diagnostic prowess in recognizing a photosensitivity dermatosis? We need it when the problem is chronic, and sunlight is a distant, forgotten trigger. We need to search back in the history of the long-ago sunburns that preceded that inscrutable erythroderma the patient has. We need to question and probe for the early repeated phototoxic or photoallergic reactions that come before the lymphoma-like mask of actinic reticuloid.

We need prowess in maintaining a high index of suspicion for light sensitivity when the eruption looks like a commonplace dermatitis. Is that dermatitis of the exposed areas an airborne contact dermatitis, or can we see shadow-skipped areas on the under chin? Is that dermatitis of the face and hands a photocontact dermatitis or simply a contact dermatitis? Photopatch tests will tell. Are those blisters from photosensitivity or are they those of lupus erythematosus? A biopsy will help. Be sure to test for the anti-Ro and anti-La antibodies if the ANA test and the biopsy are negative. They sometimes are the only laboratory sign of lupus.

Are those blisters from sunlight or from frictional trauma, as in epidermolysis bullosa? Their presence in nonexposed areas favors the latter. Is that eruption photosensitivity or erythema infectiosum? Time will soon tell.

We need prowess to think of photosensitivity as a cause of isolated changes. Is that onycholysis due to sunlight in a patient taking Minocin? The same question of photosensitivity must be raised in patients with prurigo. We need to think of the possible role of sunlight and lipstick or lip balm in cheilitis. Nor should we forget sunlight as a cause of the dermatitis of pellagra. Ask about the patient's nutrition. Equally demanding of the diagnostic mind are examples of pruritus, acne excoriée, and dermatitis of just the tips of the nose or the ears, which on study prove to be true photosensitivity states.

We need prowess to perceive the role of sunlight in promoting or maintaining an underlying disease that itself is photosensitive. These conditions include seborrheic dermatitis, rosacea, lupus erythematosus, lichen planus, pityriasis rubra pilaris, and atopic dermatitis. Even flushing shows this pattern. An informed patient will direct you to the adjuvant role of sun exposure, if you listen.

We need prowess in finding out causes of photosensitivity. Is it simply a phototoxic contactant such as tar or a psoralen-containing fruit or vegetable? Is it a photoallergic compound such as a fragrance in a perfume or after-shave lotion? is it simply a drug such as quinine, hydrochlorothiazide, furosemide, or amiodarone? Take a complete drug history. Or is it the patient's altered metabolism elaborating the intrinsic photosensitizer family of porphyrins? Do a complete study of serum, red cell, and urine and stool porphyrin status. Finally, is the photosensitivity a genetic flaw in the repair of sunlight-damaged DNA? Onset in infancy, a history of a photosensitivity trait, and fibroblast culture studies all point the way to a diagnosis of a DNA excision repair defect, as is seen in the Cockayne syndrome.

1052   Sometimes photosensitivity is the easiest to diagnose and sometimes the hardest.

Hölzle E, Plewig G, Hofmann C, Roser-Maass E: **Polymorphous light eruption**: Experimental reproduction of skin lesions. J Am Acad Dermatol 1982; 7:111–125.

Polymorphous light eruption, as seen in 180 patients in the Munich Skin Clinic, comes in five distinctive forms, each pruritic:

1. Papular type (common): papules and vesicles
2. Plaque type: erythematous urticarial plaques
3. Erythema multiforme type: bullous lesions
4. Hemorrhagic type (rare): hemorrhagic papules
5. Insect-bite–type: urticarial papules topped by tiny vesicle, but lacking central pinpoint hemorrhage of true insect bite

Although these light reactions embrace a polymorphic set, they are monomorphous in any given patient. They appear within hours or days following intense sun exposure. They persist for a few days, regressing spontaneously without scarring.

The **sites of predilection** are the cheeks, the area of the neck and chest, the backs of the hands, the extensor aspects of the arms, and in women, the lower legs.

The disorder is usually seen in **spring or early summer**, since hardening occurs, resulting in sun-induced attacks being less frequent. Insufficient sun exposure in the winter accounts for the rarity of polymorphous light eruptions during this season. Such sun sensitivity may remain for years, but finally resolves spontaneously. The **differential diagnosis** includes solar urticaria, porphyria, photoallergic dermatitis, lupus erythematosus, or any sunlight-provoked eruption.

The clinical lesions can be **elicited** by exposing the patient to UVA (50 to 100 J/cm^2). The sunburn spectrum must be excluded, and the testing is best done at the end of the winter, using a large area and a site previously involved.

A UVA-blocking sunscreen is the best preventive, since these patients are not sensitive to UVB.

Leenutaphong V, Hölzle E, Plewig G: Pathogenesis and classification of **solar urticaria**: A new concept. J Am Acad Dermatol 1989; 21:237–240.

Itching, erythema, and whealing that occur immediately after exposure to sunlight are recognized as **solar urticaria**. The trigger is blue-violet light (400 to 500 nm), which forms a photoallergen to which the patient is sensitive.

Injection of **irradiated serum reproduces the disease**. If such urticaria results only when the patient's own irradiated blister fluid, serum, or plasma is injected, the solar urticaria is called type I. In contrast, type II solar urticaria is diagnosed when irradiated samples from a normal person produce an urticarial response in the patient. It is unlikely in these days of HIV that many examples of solar urticaria will be subclassified into type I or II on the basis of serum injections.

Kalivas L, Kalivas J: **Solar purpura**. Arch Dermatol 1988; 124:24–25.

Sun exposure for an hour produced **multiple petechiae** on the legs of a 33-year-old woman, as well as her sister. The lesions appeared on the day after sunning, but were not associated with sunburn. Petechiae had been noted in early summer for each of the last 5 years, but disappeared after several weeks and stayed away until the following summer. A **Rumpel-Leede** 1053 (tourniquet) test on the arm was negative, and an ANA determination, platelet count, and blood-clotting studies were normal. Four minutes of irradiation with UVA yielded numerous petechiae without any erythema the next day, whereas UVB (1.5 MED) produced erythema with only a few petechiae.

Solar purpura appears to be an inherited photosensitivity disorder whose main expression is on the legs. In addition to UVA exposure, fragile capillaries and/or high hydrostatic pressures may be needed to produce the minute hemorrhages.

Lim HW, Buchness MR, Ashinoff R, Soter NA: **Chronic actinic dermatitis**. Study of the spectrum of chronic photosensitivity in 12 patients. Arch Dermatol 1990; 126:317–323.

Chronic photocontact dermatitis, persistent photosensitivity to systemic agents, persistent light reactivity, photosensitive eczema, and actinic reticuloid should be considered as entities along a continuum, best described by the all-encompassing term **chronic actinic dermatitis**. Seen even in dark skin, these five subsets represent an eruption in a photodistribution, consisting of erythematous, hyperpigmented papules and plaques, excoriations, erosions, and lichenification.

Chronic **photocontact dermatitis** is distinguished by a positive photopatch test. Persistent photosensitivity to a systemic agent is the analogue of systemic contact dermatitis. Persistent light reactivity is essentially the same, while photosensitive eczema is associated with negative photopatch tests and heightened sensitivity to UVB. Finally, actinic reticuloid can be characterized by the extensive lichenification and the distinctive presence of atypical mononuclear cells in the epidermis and dermis.

Unfortunately, in all of these examples of chronic actinic dermatitis, elimination of a known cause does not eliminate the sensitivity to sunlight.

Toonstra J, Henquet CJM, van Weelden H et al: **Actinic reticuloid**: A clinical, photobiologic, histopathologic and follow-up study of 16 patients. J Am Acad Dermatol 1989; 21:205–214.

Actinic reticuloid is the epitome of the chronic photosensitivity state. Look for it in middle-aged and elderly men.

Presentation: usually severely pruritic infiltrated papules and plaques of light-exposed skin, yet nose and ears may be exempt; may extend to covered areas; often associated with episodes of erythroderma

Light testing: sensitive to entire spectrum of ultraviolet *and* visible light

Biopsy: predominance of suppressor T cells on immunophenotyping of infiltrate

Patch testing: may have sensitivity to contact allergens, especially air borne

Course: chronic, for decades

Differential:

    photosensitive eczema
    sensitivity confined to UVB
    chronic photosensitivity dermatitis: histologic picture is dermatitis
    persistent light reaction: histologic picture is dermatitis
    mycosis fungoides: histologic pattern distinctive

Any chronic photosensitivity state may evolve into actinic reticuloid, so precision in taxonomy is elusive.

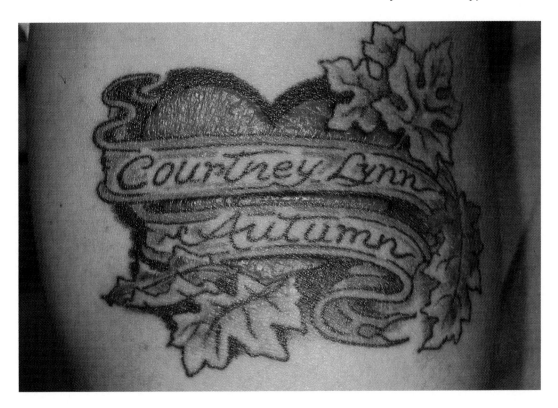

Thomsen K: The development of Hodgkin's disease in a patient with **actinic reticuloid**. Clin Exp Dermatol 1977; 2:109–113.

An extremely pruritic, lichenoid skin eruption of the face, neck, and backs of the hands in a 53-year-old salesman evolved over a period of a year into an infiltrated scaly **erythroderma**. Skin biopsy showed a dense perivascular infiltrate of lymphocytes, polymorphonuclear leukocytes, eosinophils, and reticulum cells with prominent nucleoli, and increased mitoses. Eosinophilia (30% eosinophils) was the only blood abnormality. A severe flare developed after the patient mowed the lawn, and marked photosensitivity was confirmed with phototesting. Soft, 1- to 2-cm axillary and inguinal nodes were palpable; histologically, they were dermatopathic lymphadenopathy.

Six years after the diagnosis of **actinoid reticuloid** was established by biopsy and study, he developed weight loss and enlarged lymph nodes. **Malignant lymphoma** (Hodgkin's disease) was proven by lymph node histology.

Clinical case presentation meetings are the practice greens for diagnostic swings. Use them.

Sonnex TS, Hawk JLM: **Hydroa vacciniforme**: A review of ten cases. Br J Dermatol 1988; 118:101–108.

Umbilicated vesicles and crusted round plaques on the face are the typical lesions of **hydroa vacciniforme**, which appear in March or April and persist through October. Lesions may also appear in winter with exposure to exceptionally bright sunlight or snow reflectance. Girls with fair complexions are most commonly affected, starting at age 1 to 3 years. Sometimes the problem resolves by adolescence.

Less than an hour of sunlight exposure induces the following sequence of lesions on exposed areas in these young children:

1. Erythema, pruritus, stinging, swelling (15 min to 24 hr)
2. Tender red papules with burning pain (1 to 24 hr)
3. Vesiculation with umbilication and hemorrhage (5 hr to 3 days)
4. Crust formation with loss of pain (2 to 7 days)
5. Depressed persistent pock scarring, at times with telangiectasia (1 to 6 weeks)

All of these patients have normal urinary, fecal, and erythrocyte porphyrins. It is essential to determine these levels, especially the erythrocyte porphyrin level, since erythropoietic protoporphyria and other forms of porphyria produce a similar photodermatosis in children. Xeroderma pigmentosum should be excluded by DNA repair studies. Aminoaciduria and Hartnup's disease, previously reported to be associated with hydroa vacciniforme, should also be excluded by urinary amino acid screening.

Photosensitive children need **porphyrin and amino acid screens** as well as sunscreens!

Eramo LR, Garden JM, Esterly NB: **Hydroa vacciniforme** diagnosis by repetitive ultraviolet-A phototesting. Arch Dermatol 1986; 122:1310–1313.

An 8-year-old boy gave a 3-year history of developing vesicles within minutes of sun exposure. These lesions were followed by **scarring**. He was in good health, had no porphyria disorder, and was exposed to no known photosensitizers.

The diagnosis of **hydroa vacciniforme** was made and confirmed by reproduction of the lesions and subsequent scarring, using repetitive UVA (40 J/cm^2) irradiation. Multiple exposure to UVB (60 mJ/cm^2) irradiation had no effect.

Hydroa vacciniforme is easily distinguished from hydroa aestivale and the vesicular form of polymorphic light eruption, since these never scar. The entire family of sunlight sensitivities due to porphyrins can be ruled out by laboratory study. These include erythropoietic protoporphyrin and porphyria cutanea tarda. Finally, bullous lupus erythematosus yields to a biopsy.

Czarnecki DB: **Hepatoerythropoietic porphyria**. Arch Dermatol 1980; 116:307–311.

Since the first year of life this little girl had experienced erythema and **blistering** within minutes of being in sunlight. It was associated with severe pruritus and burning. The hands were most seriously affected. There was no family history of photosensitivity. At the time of examination, the patient was 8 years of age and had mild scarring of the dorsum of the hands and on the forehead. There was an increased amount of fine dark hair on the temples and cheeks.

Porphyrin assays showed greatly increased amounts, respectively, of uroporphyrin in the urine, coproporphyrin in the feces, and protoporphyrin in the red cells. The liver was considered to be the source of the uroporphyrin and the bone marrow the source of the protoporphyrin. A diagnosis of **hepatoerythropoietic** porphyria was made.

Only seven other examples of this rare hereditary disorder have been reported. It is a photosensitivity state that must be distinguished on biochemical grounds from erythropoietic porphyria and erythropoietic protoporphyria. However, there are clinical clues. **Erythropoietic porphyria** is characterized by more severe scarring and by red urine, often the first manifestation in an affected baby. The prognosis for these patients is poor, death coming in the second or third decade. By contrast, the hepatoerythropoietic porphyria patient shows little scarring, rarely has red urine, and spontaneous improvement occurs with age. At times, patients may show sclerodermoid features. Interestingly, nearly all porphyric patients show some anemia.

Erythropoietic protoporphyria is dominantly inherited and again develops in infancy. It is photosensitivity much milder in form, rarely showing blisters, scars, or facial hypertrichosis.

In the **laboratory**, hepatoerythropoietic porphyria patients show increased red cell, urinary, and fecal porphyrins of both type I and type III isomers, whereas in erythropoietic porphyria, type I isomers predominate. In erythropoietic porphyria, no porphyrins are found in the urine, but the red cells and, at times, the feces have raised protoporphyrin levels.

The porphyrins are the photosensitizers that, if kept in the red cell away from the epidermis or kept in low concentration in the tissue fluids, bespeak a milder, gentler disease.

Lim HW, Poh-Fitzpatrick MB: **Hepatoerythropoietic porphyria**: A variant of childhood-onset porphyria cutanea tarda: Porphyrin profiles and enzymatic studies of two cases in a family. J Am Acad Dermatol 1984; 11:1103–1111.

Two young brothers, ages 7 and 9 years, began developing **vesicles** on the face and dorsum of the hands when they were 3 and 4 years old. Both showed facial hypertrichosis and many 3- to 4-mm shallow, hyperpigmented scars on the forehead, periorbital area, and cheeks. A few 2- to 4-mm vesicles and crusted erosions were present on the dorsum of the hands, the skin of which was sclerodermoid.

Under Wood's light the **teeth** of both boys showed red **fluorescence**. The older boy showed hepatosplenomegaly, which had been first detected when he was 4 years old. A skin biopsy from each child showed a subepidermal bulla and deposition of PAS-positive material around the thickened capillary walls. A diagnosis of photosensitivity was made and porphyrin studies ordered.

Under the fluorescence microscope many slightly fluorescent erythrocytes were seen. The erythrocyte porphyrin levels were dramatically elevated, as were the plasma, urine, and feces porphyrin levels. The plasma porphyrins were at a level seen in congenital erythropoietic porphyria and 4 to 10 times higher than in porphyria cutanea tarda.

The **differential diagnosis** in these patients included:

    erythropoietic porphyria (Günther's disease)
    erythropoietic protoporphyria
    porphyria cutanea tarda (childhood onset)
    hepatoerythropoietic porphyria

The porphyrin profile excluded congenital erythropoietic porphyria, since this condition shows a predominance of uroporphyrin in the erythrocytes, whereas these patients showed a predominance of protoporphyrins. Furthermore, fluoroblasts classically seen in congenital erythropoietic porphyria were not spotted in fluorescence studies of the peripheral blood of these two boys. Likewise, erythropoietic protoporphyria was eliminated, since it is associated with free protoporphyrin in both erythrocytes and plasma, whereas in these boys, although the predominant porphyrin in the red cells was protoporphyrin, the predominant porphyrin in the plasma was uroporphyrin.

The high porphyrin levels in these boys were not consistent with a diagnosis of porphyria cutanea tarda, although the plasma and urinary porphyrin profiles were compatible with that diagnosis.

The best diagnostic fit was the rare variant of porphyria cutanea tarda, **hepatoerythropoietic porphyria**. Only nine cases had been previously reported. All patients had the onset of photosensitivity within the first few years of life. All had mild to severe scarring of the light-exposed skin, and many had facial hypertrichosis. All had porphyrin profiles like these boys, and all cases, including those reported here, were due to an enzyme defect. All showed uroporphyrinogen decarboxylase enzyme activity less than 10% of the normal level in erythrocytes. This same enzyme deficiency is seen in porphyria cutanea tarda, suggesting that hepatoerythropoietic porphyria is simply a severe early-onset porphyria cutanea tarda. It is porphyria cutanea *non* tarda, if you will.

Without a **porphyrin laboratory**, you cannot shed much light on the nature of your patient's congenital photosensitivity.

Norris PG, Elder GH, Hawk JLM: **Homozygous variegate porphyria**: A case report. Br J Dermatol 1990; 122:253–257.

Since infancy, this 14-year-old girl has experienced recurrent **small blisters**, erosions, and crusts in sun-exposed areas. They usually occurred in the summer months.

On examination, she was found to be mentally retarded. The face, backs of hands, and the knees were dry and showed scars and milia, as well as crust and erosions. She did not have hypertrichosis or sclerosis, but clinodactyly was present.

The photosensitivity proved to be due to porphyria. The urinary and stool porphyrin excretion rates were high, as was the level of porphyrins in the erythrocytes. The basic defect proved to be diminished protoporphyrin oxidase, critical in the biosynthesis of heme. On the basis of this, a diagnosis of **homozygous variegate porphyria** was made.

The parents had no abnormality in porphyrin excretion but were identified as having heterozygous variegate porphyria, since both had low protoporphyrin oxidase levels.

The variable expression of **variegate porphyria** must explain the absence in this patient of the classic extracutaneous signs of acute abdominal and neuropsychiatric episodes.

Mathews-Roth MM: The consequences of not diagnosing **erythropoietic protoporphyria**. Arch Dermatol 1980; 116:407.

Patients with **erythropoietic protoporphyria** are at risk of developing life-threatening **liver disease**. In the last decade, 16 fatal cases have been reported. Awareness of the early reversible stages such as liver disease may come only with the diagnosis of erythropoietic protoporphyria. Hence, every photosensitive patient should be screened for elevated protoporphyrin levels in erythrocyte, plasma, and stool samples. Simply ordering determination of urinary porphyrins is worthless, since protoporphyrin is not excreted in the urine.

Once identified as protoporphyric, these patients must embark on a strict **lifetime avoidance** of alcohol, barbiturates, sulfonamides, and birth control pills. Such patients also merit regular surveillance of liver function and protoporphyrin levels. Attempts to lower the protoporphyrin level have included the administration of cholestyramine.

The consequence of not diagnosing erythropoietic protoporphyria can be deadly.

"Perhaps I have trained myself to see what others overlook. If not, why should you come to consult me?"

SHERLOCK HOLMES (SIR ARTHUR CONAN DOYLE)

Contactant and Drug Induced

Wojnarowska F, Calnan CD: **Contact and photocontact allergy** to musk ambrette. Br J Dermatol 1986; 114:667–675.

A 46-year-old Indian dentist developed acute **weeping dermatitis** of the face and forearm after use of a new after-shave lotion while visiting sunny Los Angeles. Patch testing revealed marked sensitivity to **musk ambrette**, which was in his soap as well as his after-shave lotion. The dermatitic patch on the forearm was then recognized as a site of contact with the beard of his dental patients. Avoidance of this exposure as well as all musk ambrette–containing perfumes, lotions, sprays, and soaps by both his wife and himself was curative, except for disfiguring postinflammatory hyperpigmentation.

Note that musk ambrette is a common sensitizer. This report details the findings in 34 patients with lesions involving various areas, including the dorsum of the hands, fingernails, arms, trunk, legs, and axillae. It is also a photocontactant, and 10% of all positive photocontact patch tests result from sensitivity to musk ambrette. Continued use invariably leads to the picture of chronic **actinic dermatitis**.

Williams HC, Du Vivier A: Strimmer season is here again. Br Med J 1990; 301:188.

This 42-year-old man developed a severe **bullous eczematous eruption** of the face, neck, and exposed areas of the arms. It resulted from his use of a garden tool (the strimmer), which **trims weeds** by means of a high-speed rotating nylon cord. Weed fragments and copious amounts of irritant plant pieces containing psoralens had been propelled onto and into his exposed skin. The summer sun then produced this variant of phytophotodermatitis.

It is apparent that those who use strimmers must not be strippers. Clothing is one's best protection.

Addo HA, Ferguson J, Frain-Bell W: **Thiazide-induced photosensitivity**: A study of 33 subjects. Br J Dermatol 1987; 116:749–760.

The **most common photosensitizing drugs** are:

    chlorothiazide, hydrochlorothiazide
    phenothiazines (chlorpromazine)
    nonsteroidal anti-inflammatory drugs
    quinine, quinidine
    sulfonamides and derivatives (furosemide)
    tetracyclines
    amiodarone
    nalidixic acid

Thiazide eruptions may simulate subacute lupus erythematosus, lichen planus, or a petechial eruption. Itching, burning, and an erythematous reaction occur on the exposed skin sites: forehead, balding scalp, back and sides of the neck, V of the neck, earlobes, and backs of the hands and wrists. There is sparing under the chin and earlobes. Sometimes the eruption becomes edematous, papular, or dermatitic. In three subjects the covered skin was also involved with variable pigmentation, including reticulate patterning in one case.

The eruption can be induced by sunlight transmitted through window glass, with the precipitating action spectrum UVA and/or UVB. The reaction is phototoxic but does not lead to a persistent light reactor state. Clearing may require 1 to 6 months once the photoactive drug is discontinued.

Chlorothiazide and hydrochlorothiazide are derivatives of the sulfonamides, which thus also must be avoided.

Ferguson J, Addo HA, Johnson BE, Frain-Bell W: **Quinine-induced photosensitivity**: Clinical and experimental studies. Br J Dermatol 1987; 117:631–640.

Photosensitivity in elderly patients is usually drug related, and inquiry should include questions about **quinine sulfate**, commonly taken for leg cramps. Four cases are presented.

A 69-year-old man developed an **acute itching edematous erythema** of the exposed skin of the face, neck, ears, bald scalp, dorsal area of the hands, and forearms, followed by leukoderma and hyperpigmentation simulating vitiligo. Two months earlier he had started taking **quinine sulfate** (200 mg daily) for muscle cramps. Phototesting revealed abnormal delayed erythema in the UVA spectrum, which faded after he stopped the drug. When he resumed taking quinine sulfate, the eruption returned and could not be blocked with sunscreens.

A 75-year-old woman suddenly developed **pruritic erythema** and edema of the face, neck, dorsal area of the hands, and forearms after prolonged sun exposure on the golf course. She was also taking **quinine sulfate** for muscle cramps. Phototesting revealed abnormal delayed erythema with the longer wavelength UVA spectrum (365 ± 30 nm). Use of a broad-spectrum sunscreen (zinc oxide 5%, cinnamic ester 10%) enabled her to continue taking the quinine sulfate.

An 83-year-old woman abruptly developed **burning erythema** of the dorsal area of the hands, which spread over a few days to her forearms, face, back, neck, and earlobes. She had been taking **quinine sulfate** (300 mg/day) for 6 months. Phototesting revealed abnormal delayed erythema in the UVB, UVA and visible wave bands. The photosensitivity slowly decreased over several months after she stopped taking quinine.

In an 83-year-old woman taking quinine sulfate (200 mg daily), violaceous papules with Wickham's striae developed on the light-exposed areas of the dorsal aspect of the hands, forearms, calves, and neck, but not on the face. These were histologically confirmed as **lichen planus**. Within 1 month of the stopping of quinine, the eruption cleared and the abnormal delayed erythema monochromator phototests returned toward normal.

After withdrawal of quinine, the **photosensitivity persists** but gradually improves over several months and is not the same as the persistent light reaction that follows photocontact dermatitis. Individual metabolic variations may result in idiosyncratic high concentrations of the drug or a photoactive metabolite in the skin.

Westwick TJ, Sheretz EF, McCarley D, Flowers FP: **Delayed reactivation of sunburn** by methotrexate: Sparing of chronically sun-exposed skin. Cutis 1987; 39:49–51.

A 60-year-old white man with bladder carcinoma who had been receiving weekly intravenous methotrexate had second-degree burns (erythema, confluent vesicles, and bullae) on both legs. Two weeks earlier he had gone fishing and been exposed to 2 to 3 hours of early afternoon sun on the legs with only transient erythema. The following day he received intravenous methotrexate (75 mg) followed by leucovorin rescue. One week later the **methotrexate treatment** was repeated, and over the next 2 days erythema and bullae developed on the legs.

The **sunburn recall phenomenon** is not well understood; it has occurred with other chemotherapeutic drugs, producing erythema and pigmentation in previously irradiated skin. These drugs may also reactivate symptoms of previously dormant scabies and contact dermatitis.

Flax SH, Uhle P: **Photorecall-like phenomenon** following the use of cefazolin and gentamicin sulfate. Cutis 1990; 46:59–61.

A 21-year-old woman hospitalized for cefazolin and **gentamicin** therapy of a urinary tract infection developed a photodistributed eruption on the fifth day. The diagnostic feature in the history was a **sunburn** she had experienced **a month ago**.

A diagnosis of **photorecall drug eruption** was made. Her eruption "recalls" the dermatitis that chemotherapeutic drugs can elicit, which is precisely limited to the skin sites of prior radiation injury. In this patient the prior radiation was sunlight and the drug not a chemotherapeutic one but rather an antibiotic.

It behooves one to explore prior as well as recent sun exposure in patients with photosensitivity. We wonder if topical photosensitizers can also elicit the recall phenomenon.

There's a time to biopsy and there's a time to wait for the time to biopsy. . . .

Fitzpatrick JE, Thompson PB, Aeling JL, Huff C: **Photosensitive recurrent erythema multiforme**. J Am Acad Dermatol 1983; 9:419–423.

Erythematous papules and plaques with some typical **target lesions** of erythema multiforme had been appearing in crops on the dorsa of the hands, the extensor surface of the upper arms, and the tips of the ears of this 31-year-old man for the past year. Initially the process was viewed as tinea, but antifungal therapy had no effect. Although the lesions were in sun-exposed areas, the patient could not correlate their appearance with sun exposure. Nor had he noted any correlation with attacks of "cold sores" on the lips. Occasionally some lesions had appeared on non–sun-exposed areas such as the palm and the scrotum.

Despite no support from the patient's history, a diagnosis of **photosensitive erythema multiforme** was made. Although sun avoidance and sunscreen were prescribed, the patient continued to have episodic attacks that he now could identify as following sunlight exposure.

The definitive proof of the correctness of the diagnosis came with the **elicitation** of an erythema multiforme lesion 72 hours after a 10-second exposure to ultraviolet light (UVA, UVB) from a Burdick UV 800 hot quartz lamp. Biopsy of this showed the same perivascular lymphohistiocytic infiltrate as in the initial biopsy.

Usually erythema multiforme localizes in sites of trauma such as the skin over palms, soles, genitalia, and joints as well as the extensor surfaces. In this instance the presumed viral immune complexes lodged in sun-damaged cutaneous vessels. **Subclinical recurrent herpes simplex** appears to have been the source of the antigen. Photoreproduction of the disease was possible only at times of circulating complexes.

Always in a patient with recurrent papules, plaques, and target and annular lesions the differential includes photoallergic drug reactions, polymorphous light eruption, lupus erythematosus.

Each of these was ruled out in the present case.

One leaves this patient with a greater awareness of the interplay of sun and virus in the pathogenesis of skin diseases.

Herrero C, Bielsa I, Font J et al: **Subacute cutaneous lupus erythematosus**: Clinico-pathologic findings in thirteen cases. J Am Acad Dermatol 1988; 19:1057–1062.

Subacute cutaneous lupus erythematosus shows a variety of recurrent photosensitive, nonscarring lesions. They stand in sharp contrast to the fixed chronic scarring lesions of discoid lupus erythematosus.

The cutaneous lesions of this subacute group are **erythematous scaly** papules and plaques that evolve into an annular or psoriasiform pattern with widespread and symmetrical distribution.

Look also for **Raynaud's phenomenon**, periungual telangiectasia, nonscarring thinning of scalp hair, as well as aphthae. More than half of these patients have antibodies to the Ro(SS-A) antigen as well as antinuclear antibodies. Three out of four show the specific human leukocyte antigen (HLA-DR3) phenotype.

The **annular lesion** or pattern was far more common than the papulosquamous presentation. Usually appearing on the sun-exposed areas, the lesions may occur on the trunk. Small vesicles and crusts on the active edge of the ring were observed at times. The lesions regressed to leave pigmentation and telangiectasia but no scarring. Photosensitivity was a common finding.

Some of the patients complained of arthralgias, fever, and malaise, but seri- 1063 ous systemic disease was not seen. Thus this subset of lupus erythematosus bridges the gap between strictly cutaneous discoid lupus erythematosus and the systemic lupus with its fleeting nonspecific erythema.

Barranco VP: Multiple **benign lichenoid keratoses simulating photodermatoses**: Evolution from senile lentigines and their spontaneous regression. J Am Acad Dermatol 1985; 13:201–206.

Numerous red pruritic **lichenoid plaques** had been present on the dorsal aspects of the arms, hands, legs, and upper trunk of this 59-year-old woman for 3 months. She also had numerous actinic (senile) keratoses in the sun-exposed areas.

The plaques were diagnosed as **cutaneous lupus erythematosus**, and the histologic pattern on H and E staining was consistent. However, immuno-fluorescent studies failed to confirm the presence of lupus erythematosus, nor did the blood studies. She had a negative ANA test and a normal blood count.

Use of steroid cream for 2 weeks resulted in clearing of the lichenoid change, leaving underlying faintly pigmented lentigines.

A diagnosis of **multiple benign lichenoid keratoses** was made. It is important to recognize that such lesions can simulate a photosensitivity reaction or lupus.

Braddock SW, Davis CS, Davis RB: **Reticular erythematous mucinosis** and thrombo-cytopenic purpura. Report of a case and review of the world literature, including plaque-like cutaneous mucinosis. J Am Acad Dermatol 1988; 19:859–868.

This 75-year-old farmer complained of a rash he had had for 3 years. It first appeared on the sun-exposed areas of the shoulders, was worse in summer, and more recently had spread to the chest, abdomen, arms, and groin.

On examination, he had an **erythematous reticular, maculopapular eruption** that blanched on pressure. It was most prominent in the sun-exposed areas of the chest and arms. The role of the sun was dramatically underscored by the absence of the rash under the strap lines of his undershirt.

On biopsy the presence of large quantities of mucin attested to the diagnosis of **reticular erythematous mucinosis** (REM).

Fifty-three cases of REM are now in the world literature since it was first identified by Steigleder in 1974. Noteworthy observations on it include:

> presents as a photosensitivity
> unique feature: network of erythema
> may have palpable border
> twice as common in women as in men
> mimics lupus erythematosus

Vassileva S, Pramatarov K, Popova L: **Ultraviolet light–induced confluent and reticu-lated papillomatosis**. J Am Acad Dermatol 1989; 21:413–414.

Dark-gray, flat, pin-sized, confluent papules with a slightly hyperkeratotic surface appeared on the abdomen and back of this 16-year-old girl 2 weeks **after sunbathing**. The confluent and reticulate pattern as well as the histo-logic findings supported a diagnosis of **Gougerot-Carteaud** papillomatosis.

Noteworthy is the fact that sun exposure determined a localization of lesions dissimilar to the typical inflammatory and interscapular sites of the Gougerot-Carteaud syndrome.

Weinstock MA, Olbricht SM, Arndt KA, Kwan TH: Well-demarcated **papules and plaques in sun-exposed areas**. Arch Dermatol 1987; 123:1073–1076.

Discrete oval, tan lesions 0.5 to 2 cm in diameter scattered over the lateral aspect of the arms, upper torso, and anterior surface of the thighs had been appearing for 9 years in this 39-year-old woman. They were asymptomatic, did not involute, and were darker in the summer. Most of the lesions were plaques with increased skin markings, while a few were flat or depressed with a cigarette-paper appearance.

It took a biopsy to make the diagnosis of **multiple large-cell acanthomas**, i.e., a form of actinic keratosis. Histologically the lesion is made up of keratinocytes twice as large as normal. Clinically the lesions are sharply circumscribed, lightly pigmented, slightly hyperkeratotic plaques on erythematous bases.

One should distinguish them from seborrheic keratoses, actinic keratoses, and lentigines.

Bernhard JD: **Photosensitivity**. *In* Lebwohl M (ed): Difficult Diagnosis in Dermatology. New York, Churchill Livingstone, 1988, pp 405–417.

Disorders that can be **precipitated, provoked,** or **exacerbated by light**:

acne vulgaris
atopic eczema
bullous pemphigoid
Darier-White disease
erythema multiforme
Hailey-Hailey disease
herpes simplex labialis
   (recurrences)
lichen planus
lupus erythematosus
pemphigus erythematosus
pemphigus foliaceus
pemphigus vulgaris

physical occlusion of skin (increased
   susceptibility to sunburn)
pityriasis alba
pityriasis rubra pilaris
pseudoporphyria
psoriasis
reticular erythematous mucinosis
   syndrome
rosacea
seborrheic dermatitis
transient acantholytic dermatosis
   (Grover's disease)
viral infections of the skin
vitiligo

You ask the cause of your disease? I suspect it is due to a misspent youth.

RICHARD PYE

Pityriasis Rosea

Physicians' minds leap up with diagnostic joy at the sight of the Christmas tree of pityriasis rosea ornaments. It is the one image they all retain from their student days in the dermatology clinic. Confidently, they look for the singular scaling patch that preceded and heralded all of this.

But step back and ask yourself:

Could this be secondary syphilis? If so, there should be a brownish tint to the lesions, generalized adenopathy, mucosal and palmar lesions, a positive STS, or even a faded chancre.

Could this be a drug eruption? Search for such offending drugs as arsenicals, barbiturates, and captopril to start the alphabetic query.

Could this be a papular "id"? Is there tinea pedis, pharyngitis, or dental abscess?

Could this be tinea or tinea versicolor? A scraping will tell!

Could this be the lesions of cleavage line–oriented psoriasis or seborrheic dermatitis? Look for the scalp lesions, the family history, and the recurrence of psoriasis. Look for the greasy scale and the facial lesions of seborrheic dermatitis.

If the patient has none of these signs, you can proceed to instruct him to take the ornaments off the pityriasis rosea Christmas tree with steroid creams.

Imamura S, Ozaki M, Oguchi M, et al: **Atypical pityriasis rosea.** Dermatologica 1985; 171:474–477.

The **"Christmas-tree" patterning** of disseminated ovoid, papulosquamous macules on the trunk and proximal surface of the extremities makes typical pityriasis rosea one of the "diagnosis-at-a-glance" dermatoses. Any doubt is quickly resolved by the history of a "herald" plaque.

But the **uncommon presentation** of this common disease must also be recognized. By using its 1- to 2-month course and histologic clues (extravasated red blood cells in dermal papillae, dyskeratotic cells in the epidermis), six examples of atypical pityriasis rosea were identified:

1. Scaly reddish-brown macules of the legs and dorsal area of the hands and feet in a 25-year-old woman. Only a few lesions were present on her back.
2. Scaly erythematous macules on the groins of a 14-year-old boy who also had a slightly sore throat. Ten days later he developed similar 1.5-cm lesions on the dorsal area of the feet, axillae, palms, and lower abdomen. An STS was negative.
3. Erythematous macules of the upper chest and face in a 46-year-old man. He had common cold–like symptoms before the eruption developed.
4. Pruritic, erythematous, scaly macules of the left surface of the waist and proximal aspect of the extremities in a 27-year-old woman.
5. Annular scaly erythema of the chest, abdomen, and back in a 47-year-old woman.
6. Scaly erythematous macules on the left thigh, neck, and lower legs in a 34-year-old man. Just prior to the eruption he had common-cold–like symptoms.

"Hark the herald angel sings" . . . The Christmas tree is soon to come. This may be true for many—but not all—cases of pityriasis rosea. Histologic examination is very helpful in atypical cases.

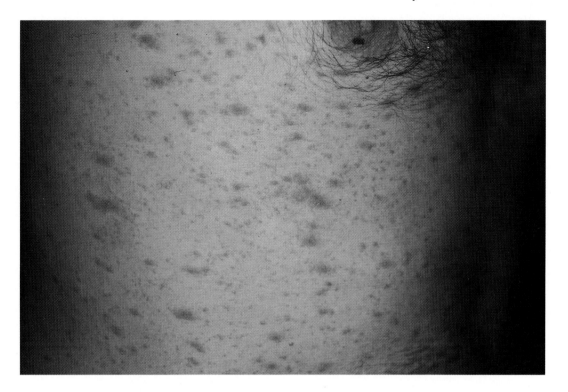

Verbov J: **Purpuric pityriasis rosea**. Dermatologica 1980; 160:142–144.

A 20-year-old woman had a discrete macular, **purpuric eruption** of the trunk for 2 weeks, exhibiting the typical distribution pattern of pityriasis rosea. This diagnosis was confirmed by biopsy findings and subsequent clearing 4 weeks later.

Pityriasis rosea, like ice cream, may come in different flavors. This example was purple.

Crovato F, Nazzari G, Gambini C, Massone L: Meyerson's naevi in pityriasis rosea. Br J Dermatol 1989; 120:318–319.

This 19-year-old man developed atypical herald plaque of pityriasis rosea. It was followed 3 weeks later by small asymptomatic erythematous oval lesions that largely **localized around the nevi** on the chest and back. Biopsy showed the junctional nevus activity and an underlying lymphocytic infiltrate.

A diagnosis was made of **Meyerson's phenomenon**, i.e., the appearance of a halo of dermatitis around melanocytic nevi. In this instance the halo was the "rosy scale" of pityriasis rosea.

Bork K: Cutaneous side effects of drugs. Philadelphia, W. B. Saunders Co., 1988, p 169.

Drugs that may cause **pityriasis rosea-like** eruptions:

Barbiturates	Isotretinoin
Beta-blockers	Ketotifen
Bismuth compounds	Methoxypromazine
Captopril	Metronidazole
Clonidine	Organic arsenicals (obsolete)
Gold compounds	Penicillin
Griseofulvin	Tripelennamine

The typical "herald patch" is absent and the distribution of lesions may not follow the classic pityriasis rosea pattern.

Pregnancy

For many women the first sign of pregnancy is fingernails that grow faster and harder. It is a time for growth. Skin tags and angiomas flourish, nevi enlarge and darken, and hair becomes luxuriant and long. The mask of pregnancy appears, and dark lines of demarcation become more evident. Sooner or later, in many women, comes the pruritus of pregnancy. We deem it the sign of an autoimmune sensitivity to progesterone.

More severe examples of this progesterone sensitivity may develop, presenting as the pruritic urticarial papules and plaques of pregnancy or the vesicles and bullae of herpes gestationis. Pregnancy is also the stage of a wide spectrum of scratch-induced papules. Acneiform lesions may appear, but most dreaded is the generalized pustular psoriasis of pregnancy. This will be encountered in the literature under the nom de plume of impetigo herpetiformis. We prefer its real name of pustular psoriasis.

Finally, since pregnancy is a time of immunosuppression, anticipate flares of disease that normally are kept in check immunologically. Thus, candidiasis may become rampant. For other women it may be a time of remission for cutaneous ailments. Possibly the elevated cortisone levels may be responsible for this. It is more rewarding to listen to what the pregnant patient tells you than to predict.

Pregnancy is indeed a time of growth, and nothing attests more to the growth within than the striae distensae that appear.

Lawley TJ, Hertz KC, Wade TR, et al: **Pruritic urticarial papules and plaques** of pregnancy. JAMA 1979; 241:1696–1699.

A 26-year-old woman in the 38th week of her first pregnancy noted the onset of intensely pruritic urticarial plaques on the abdomen. Many small erythematous papules with peripheral blanching were also present. Within days the eruption spread to cover much of the thighs and buttocks. Scattered lesions were also seen on the arms and legs.

A biopsy specimen showed an inflammatory infiltrate of lymphocytes and histiocytes. Immunofluorescent studies were negative. Within 7 days of parturition the eruption abated. On the basis of these findings and similar observations in six other women in their third trimester, these authors coined the diagnosis of **pruritic urticarial papules and plaques of pregnancy**. It is to be distinguished from the other pruritic dermatoses of pregnancy:

Herpes gestationis: may see vesicles and bullae; onset, any time during pregnancy or postpartum period

Prurigo gravidarum: associated jaundice

Papular dermatitis of pregnancy; excoriated papules; widespread

Prurigo gestationis (Besnier): excoriated papules; extensor surfaces

Shornick JK: **Herpes gestationis.** J Am Acad Dermatol 1987; 17:539–556.

This rare vesiculobullous disease characteristically appears as intense pruritus in the second or third trimester of pregnancy. However, it may have an explosive onset within hours of delivery. The apparent time frame extends vertically from conception to 3 days post partum.

The formidable pruritus may go for days, or even weeks, before the characteristic **papular, erythematous, or urticarial plaques** are seen studded with vesicles or bullae. The preferred site is the abdomen, but the legs or arms may be an initial site. The face is generally exempt.

1068

Resolution may occur as inexplicably as onset. Moreover, this disease may appear for the first time in any pregnancy. Once it appears, anticipate that further attacks will be more severe and occur early in the course of the pregnancy. Postpartum involution may take several months and is slower in successive pregnancies. Indeed, persistent menstrual flares may continue for months post partum. A few women will experience **recurrences** when treated with contraceptives. Note that the newborn infant may have a mild form of the mother's affliction, but it usually fades in a matter of weeks.

For us personally, herpes gestationis is simply an example of autoimmune progesterone sensitivity in the pregnancy setting.

Winton GB: **Skin diseases** aggravated by pregnancy. J Am Acad Dermatol 1989; 20:1–13.

Pregnancy is a mild state of immunosuppression, to wit:

Vaginal candidiasis is 10 to 20 times more frequent.

Condyloma acuminatum may grow rapidly, even to the point of blocking the birth canal.

Leprosy may flare.

Dermatomyositis may worsen.

Acrodermatitis enteropathica flares as serum zinc levels drop.

Pseudoxanthoma elasticum may worsen, leading to gastrointestinal bleeding.

Neurofibromas may enlarge and invade vessel walls, inducing rupture.

Congenital and dysplastic nevi may undergo malignant transformation.

James WD, Meltzer MS, Guill MA, et al: **Pigmentary demarcation lines** associated with pregnancy. J Am Acad Dermatol 1984; 11:438–440.

This 24-year-old woman complained of asymptomatic **dark streaks** down the **posterior aspect of the legs**. They had been present since the latter part of her pregnancy, persisting into the post partum period. A diagnosis of pigmentary demarcation lines was made.

Ninety per cent of **pregnant women** show **darkening of the linea nigra**, areolae and nipples, and genitalia, as well as of nevi and freckles. These demarcation lines are but a rare example of darkening of a streak of melanocytes otherwise inapparent. The present patient's lines correspond to those **lines of Voigt**, i.e., delineating boundaries of the areas supplied by the main cutaneous nerve stems. They do not correspond to the lines of Blaschko that mark the distribution of linear nevoid conditions. Nor do they match the lines separating dermatomes.

Ott F, Krakowski A, Tur E et al: **Impetigo herpetiformis** with lowered serum level of vitamin D and its diminished intestinal absorption. Dermatologica 1984; 164:360–365.

A 26-year-old woman with Crohn's disease developed a severe generalized rash in the third month of her third pregnancy. It consisted of grouped pustules on an erythematous base, brownish-red papules, plaques, and circinate lesions, all covered with fine silvery scales. She was febrile and felt sick. The dermatitis was identical to previous eruptions she had experienced in the ninth month of her first and fifth month of her second pregnancy.

The **pustules** were sterile and showed Munro abscesses and pustules of Kogoj on biopsy. The serum calcium level (8.0 mg/dl) was low, as were serum 25-hydroxyvitamin D (the major circulating metabolite of vitamin D) and 24,25-dihydroxyvitamin D (a renal metabolite). The intestinal absorption of

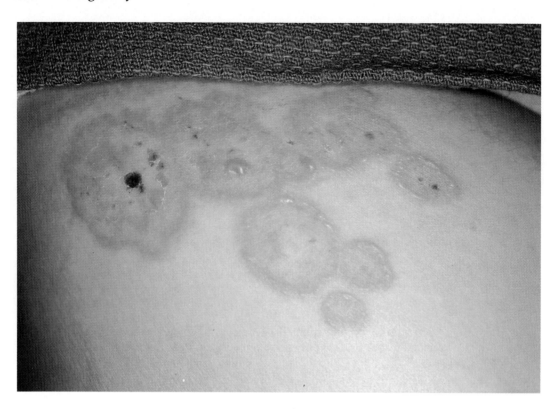

vitamin D was also decreased. Serum parathyroid hormone and alkaline phosphatase levels were normal.

Treatment with systemic antibiotics, steroids, calcium, vitamin D, plasma, and dapsone did not significantly help. Fetal death occurred at 31 weeks' gestation, and some days after delivery the patient's skin cleared completely.

Hypocalcemia in pustular psoriasis and **impetigo herpetiformis** may be due to a very short albumin half-life (4 days instead of 11 days), as calcium is bound to albumin. Endogenous vitamin D_3 production in the skin may also be decreased.

Farrag OA, Al-Suleiman SA, Bella H, Al-Omari H: **Behçet's disease** in pregnancy. Aust NZ J Obstet Gynecol 1987; 27:161–163.

A 29-year-old Egyptian woman living in Saudi Arabia developed a 1.5-cm shallow **painful ulcer on the right labium** majus, along with multiple infected ulcers in the anterior vaginal wall and cervix. She was 32 weeks' pregnant and had negative tests for syphilis, gonorrhea, herpes, monilia, and trichomonas. Biopsies showed nonspecific chronic inflammation, with no granulomas or Donovan bodies.

Behçet's disease was diagnosed on the basis of the history, which revealed an episode of severe mouth ulcers 1 year previously, followed by three ulcers on the left labium majus and anal area 8 months later. Her first pregnancy, 3 years before, had been uneventful.

Treatment with prednisolone (25 mg every other day) resulted in almost complete healing within 2 weeks, but when the dose was reduced to 10 mg/day the ulcers recurred more vigorously. She also developed a painful round, sharply demarcated mouth ulcer with a yellowish floor and bright-red areola. Cultures from both ulcers revealed group B **beta-hemolytic streptococci**; she was treated with long-acting penicillin.

She was delivered at term of a normal infant by cesarean section because of the multiple infected ulcers. Prednisolone was continued postnatally, with complete healing of the ulcers within 10 days. Withdrawal of the prednisolone over 2 months did not result in recurrence of lesions, and she remained free of lesions at a 1 year follow-up.

The **dramatic healing** of the genital ulcers immediately **after pregnancy** suggests a hormonal role in the disease, possibly progesterone withdrawal. Sensitivity to progesterone has been postulated in aphthous ulcers, and some patients have obtained relief of oral and genital ulcers with oral contraceptives.

Hamza M, Elleuch M, Zribi A: **Behçet's disease** and pregnancy. Ann Rheum Dis 1988; 47:350–352.

In Tunis, a study of 21 pregnancies in eight women with Behçet's disease showed that the **influence of pregnancy was variable** between patients and also in the same patient. This confirms previous reports.

Remission occurred without any treatment during 12 pregnancies, while there was exacerbation in 9 pregnancies, despite treatment with prednisone (10 to 15 mg/day). Painful genital ulcers during the third trimester were the main type of exacerbation during pregnancy.

HLA-B5 was present in five of six patients tested.

Put a drop of tincture of optimism in your diagnosis.

Pruritus

General Background
Types
External Causes
Internal Causes

Of course you made the diagnosis of pruritus. He told you, or you watched him scratching, or you saw the dermographism, if not the excoriations. But why does he itch?

If you see nothing at all, think of **overbathing** as the cause. Lubrication and abstinence can quickly confirm or eliminate that diagnosis. Expect itching in pregnancy, in uremia, in hepatitis, in biliary cirrhosis, and in thyroid disease. An early **health profile** is an essential guide and will save later embarrassment.

Next, a history of medications is very useful, for herein may be the answer to an intractable itch sine dermatosis. Likely suspects are the drugs producing hepatotoxicity with cholestasis. Are the conjunctivae yellow? Does the patient take vitamins? Thiamine and vitamin A are troublemakers.

Next, the **medical history**. Patients with AIDS and patients undergoing dialysis are common victims of daily itch. Add to this the patients with leukemia, lymphomas, and other malignant diseases. Check for hidden lymph nodes and secure a chest x-ray and stools for occult blood. Is the patient an atopic individual with a history of asthma? His itch may be just the tip of an iceberg of atopy. Secure an IgE determination.

Finally, **simple inspection** of the skin may show the answer to why this patient itches. Most commonly, you will see contact dermatitis. Here, itching is the sine qua non of diagnosis. But many dermatitides itch—some unexpectedly, such as psoriasis. Often the skin change, and not its essential itch, is the patient's complaint. This is true for urticaria. In others, such as atopic dermatitis, lichen planus, prurigo, and insect bites, the itch is the raison d'etre for seeing you.

For the fiercest itch of all, one that burns, think first of **dermatitis herpetiformis**. You may see nothing but excoriations. The vesicles have been torn away. Teach the patient to observe and preserve a primary lesion for biopsy.

For the itch at night and the itch that is shared with the family, think **scabies**. Search for the burrow and secure a stratum corneum biopsy for immediate microscopic confirmation. Or scrape the scratch areas for sighting a wandering mite. Even if you fail, the patient enjoys the immediate alleviation of his itch. If no scybala, ova, or mites are found, have the patient come back after one whole week of not bathing. This greatly enhances your chances of finding the primary lesion. Alternatively, a therapeutic diagnostic trial with Kwell may be indicated.

Now, for that itch that has no lead-ins of dry skin, drug intake, systemic or skin disease, you must do more than scratch your head. First, have another look at the **history**. Does the patient work with fiber glass? Does he have exposure at work or at home to birds, dogs, cats that could be the source of mites that bite and run? Could he give you a history of some episode or other symptom of neurologic disease such as multiple sclerosis? Is there a history of diarrhea (Giardia sensitivity) or of vaginitis (yeast allergy)?

Next, have the patient remove his shoes and socks. Look for **tinea pedis**. Sensitization to fungi on the feet is one of the most commonly missed causes of stubborn idiopathic pruritus.

Finally, is the itch the itch of a **depressed** patient? Keep looking for a cause, or the itch will be that of a depressed diagnostician.

Denman ST: A review of **pruritus**. J Am Acad Dermatol 1986; 14:375–392.

Making the diagnosis is easy; looking behind the diagnosis for a cause is the hard part.

First, be sure you haven't missed these **diseases** hidden in the scratches:

dermatitis herpetiformis   insect bites
scabies   overbathing
fiber-glass dermatitis

Next, **screen for**:

uremia   cholestatic liver disease
hyperparathyroidism, secondary   polycythemia vera
hyperphosphatemia

Look for:

Hodgkin's disease or malignancy
thyroid disease—hyperthyroidism or hypothyroidism
multiple sclerosis

Order:

complete blood count, differential count   liver panel
chest x-ray   determination of serum BUN,
stool for occult blood   calcium, phosphorus, iron
thyroid panel

Lober CW: Should the patient with **generalized pruritus** be evaluated for malignancy? J Am Acad Dermatol 1988; 19:350–352.

Yes, and here is what you do:

examination of patient's lymph nodes, liver, spleen, as well as pelvic and
    rectal area as part of a comprehensive physical examination
complete blood count and blood chemistry
chest x-ray
stool for occult blood

And do it again if the pruritus persists.

Koblenzer CS: The **dysmorphic syndrome**. Arch Dermatol 1985; 121:780–784.

This 49-year-old woman spent $12,000 in a $4\frac{1}{2}$-year search for relief of **itching**, paresthesias, and transient swellings of the face. Within a month of their onset, her skin "fell apart," the facial muscles drooped, and she developed severe scalp pain. She attributed these to toxic fumes at her workplace.

On examination she was an attractive woman with healthy skin. It became evident that she suffered intensely, both from **delusions of physical disfiguration** and from **intolerable sensations** in the skin. The only appropriate diagnosis was **dysmorphic syndrome**. It represents the patient's distortion of his or her body image and is usually accompanied by dysesthesias, burning numbness, and pain. The delusions may include those of odor, wrinkles, holes in the skin, glossodynia, and vulvodynia. The symptoms become all-consuming, but there are no objective changes. For this reason the dysmorphic syndrome has also been termed *cutaneous nondisease*.

It is a serious disease with a serious prognosis, but at least this patient derived benefit from haloperidol (1 mg bid).

Sheehan-Dare RA, Henderson MJ, Cotterill JA: Anxiety and depression in patients with **chronic urticaria and generalized pruritus**. Br J Dermatol 1990; 123:769–774.

A study of 34 patients with chronic idiopathic generalized pruritus revealed that one out of three was depressed.

Wouldn't you be?   1073

Types

Hazelrigg DE: **Paroxysmal pruritus**. J Am Acad Dermatol 1985; 13:839–840.

For 9 months a 72-year-old woman had daily attacks of sudden intense itching, as though red ants had been dumped on her skin. There were no primary lesions. She would scratch the skin until bleeding or ulceration occurred, but she never felt pain. The attacks ended as abruptly as they began, shortly after her invalid husband died.

The cause remained unknown, but the diagnosis was **paroxysmal pruritus**.

Heyl T: **Brachioradial pruritus**. Arch Dermatol 1983; 119:115–116.

Clinical

> itch of external elbow
> no skin change
> recurs in summer, disappears in winter

Best treatment

> long sleeves

Etiology

> may represent nerve damage associated with degenerative change in cervical spine
> role of sunlight unknown, other than favoring physical exercise

Walcyk PJ, Elpern DJ: **Brachioradial pruritus**: A tropical dermopathy. Br J Dermatol 1986; 115:177–180.

Severe episodic bursts of **pruritus of the flexor surface of the elbow** or elbows appear to represent a **photosensitivity reaction**. It has been called brachioradial pruritus, since it localizes at the site of concurrence of the brachial and radial nerves. Although the pathogenesis may reflect peripheral nerve injury, as in neuralgia paresthetica and notalgia paresthetica, its unique localization merits diagnostic distinction. Localization to one small area and not an entire dermatome speaks against a neuropathy, although it might be a photoneurologic disorder.

Forty-two patients are presented with this solar pruritus as seen in Hawaii. The episodic symptoms were described as "crawling under the skin" or "pins and needles itch sensation." Pruritus preceded the skin lesions, which consisted of marked xerosis and also variable mild erythema, flesh-colored papules, lichenification, and occasional excoriations. In Florida this condition has been called **solar pruritus of the elbows**.

Shapiro PE, Braun CW: **Unilateral pruritus** after a stroke. Arch Dermatol 1987; 123:1527–1530.

In a 72-year-old woman, pruritus of specific areas of the left side of the body appeared a few days after a stroke. Computed tomography indicated a small **infarct in the right parietal lobe**. The areas of **left-sided pruritus** were on the face (ear, cheek, ala nasi, upper lip), neck, upper back, and knee. There were no other paresthesias. Although sensory and motor functions partially returned, the pruritus continued. Two years after the stroke she had two poorly circumscribed hyperpigmented macules (5 cm and 8 cm in length) at the sites of pruritus on the left upper back.

Amitriptyline (20 mg qhs) was successfully prescribed to block the uptake of serotonin at synapses and thereby enhance its action in the medulla. This suggests that the unilateral pruritus resulted from interruption of an undefined descending pathway involving the medulla.

Rycroft RJG: **Occupational dermatoses** from warm dry air. Br J Dermatol 1981; 105 (Suppl 21):29–34.

A small group of men talking together over morning coffee each brought out bottles of an identical antihistaminic. It was their first awareness that they had the same problem with **itching and wheals** for which their individual doctors had prescribed Chlor-Trimeton.

They worked in an air-conditioned new international telephone exchange building. The symptoms were predominantly on the covered areas of their bodies, were worse at the end of the day, and abated on weekends.

The problem was subjected to intense study with elimination of the following possible causes: inhaled and ingested allergens, glass fibers from air conditioner filters, powder from cables, and fear of loss of job.

A total of 28 individuals of the 500 in the building proved to have the same problem. All of them, both men and women, worked on the third or fourth floor.

Cure came when the room **humidity was raised from 35 to 50%**. Dry warm air can cause not only pruritus and wheals but also burning redness and scaling of the face. In another factory, such problems were dismissed as rosacea, menopausal hot flashes, trichlorethylene vapor, alcohol for lunch. Again the problem vanished when the relative humidity was raised to 45%.

Dry skin, chapping, asteatotic eczema, itch, and wheal all must call for asking how dry the air is.

Bernhard JD: Nonrashes: 5. **Atmoknesis**: Pruritus provoked by contact with air. Cutis 1989; 44:143–144.

The Greeks provided a word for it: *atmos* ("air") and *knesis* ("itching"). **Atmoknesis** is the common complaint of patients—that they itch upon exposure of their skin to air after undressing. It is severe at times and unique in occurring precisely at the moment of undressing.

Often seen in patients with dry skin, the mechanism remains unknown. Possibly the epidermal nerve endings subserving itch are fired by static electricity, by friction, or the sudden temperature change.

Air must be joined with **water**, **sunlight**, **heat**, and **cold** as a **cause of the invisible itch**. It all adds up to a set of patients who must sleep in their clothes, never bathe, and stay indoors in a room at 68°F.

Bircher AJ: **Water-induced itching**. Dermatologica 1990; 181:83–87.

Although the trigger is the same pure water contact, there are three types of **aquagenic pruritus** when based on response to therapy. These are the essential aquagenic pruritus, responsive to bicarbonate baths; aquagenic pruritus of the elderly, responsive to emollients; and water-related itching in polycythemia rubra vera, which lessens with aspirin.

Only the **polycythemia rubra vera** will become evident on laboratory test. In these patients as many as half will itch. Although the itch may occur spontaneously, its appearance after a bath or sudden temperature change is characteristic.

Steinman HK, Greaves MW: **Aquagenic pruritus**. J Am Acad Dermatol 1985; 13:91–96.

Clinical:

> severe pruritus, prickling or stinging, burning, or buzzing sensation after contact with water, irrespective of its temperature

begins minutes after contact or only after end of water exposure and may
   last 10 minutes to 2 hours
no visible skin lesions seen
may be associated with emotional change during attack

Aquagenic pruritus is one of the herald signs of polycythemia rubra vera.
Check your patient's blood count.

Newton JA, Singh AK, Greaves MW, Spry CJF: **Aquagenic pruritus** associated with
idiopathic hypereosinophilic syndrome. Br J Dermatol 1990; 122:103–106.

A 61-year-old patient was found to have **eosinophilia** as an incidental finding.
Bone marrow studies showed hyperplasia of the eosinophil precursors.
Shortly after the diagnosis of idiopathic hypereosinophilic syndrome was
made, he developed **aquagenic pruritus**. No other symptoms or manifestations of the syndrome were present.

When the eosinophil count was reduced by prednisone and busulfan, the
pruritus faded. Later he became alcohol intolerant as a second clinical manifestation of the disease.

Leiferman KM, Ackerman SJ, Sampson HA, et al: Dermal deposition of eosinophil-
granule. **Major basic protein in atopic dermatitis**. Comparison with onchocerciasis.
N Engl J Med 1985; 313:282–285.

Major basic protein is an arginine-rich polypeptide localized to the eosinophil granule. It kills parasites, damages tissues, induces histamine release
from basophils, and provokes wheal-and-flare reactions in human skin. As
detected by immunofluorescence, it is deposited heavily in the dermis of
atopic dermatitis and onchocerciasis, diseases that share **intense pruritus**,
lichenification, increased IgE, and an abnormally large number of eosinophils in the peripheral blood. Despite the striking deposition of major basic
protein, few tissue eosinophils are found in the skin in these diseases. The
deposition pattern is fibrillar and closely resembles the pattern and location
of elastic tissue fibers.

Eosinophil involvement in cutaneous disease cannot be determined solely
by the presence of tissue eosinophils.

Lawlor F, Kobza Black A, Breathnach AS, Greaves MW: **Vibratory angioedema**: Lesion
induction, clinical features, laboratory and ultrastructural findings and response to
therapy. Br J Dermatol 1989; 120:93–99.

For 10 years this 28-year-old woman had noted development of **itching** and
erythema in any area of skin subjected to **vibration**. Within minutes of using
a power mower, the wrists and forearms tingled, itched, and became red.
Simply walking for 10 minutes resulted in itching and erythema of the anterior aspect of the thighs. As the walking continued the itch intensified, the
face flushed, and she felt a tightness of the chest.

Even more remarkable were the results of 5 minutes of **jogging**. A blotchy
erythema appeared on the thighs and abdomen, followed by generalized
pruritus and flushing. On resting, the symptoms disappeared within minutes.
Additionally, tight garments, waist bands, or sitting on a hard-edged chair
resulted in local pruritic erythematous lesions.

Using a vibrator (13 cps, amplitude of 1 mm, 7 min) as a standardized test,
it was possible to induce localized angioedema.

Although **plasma histamine levels** are known to increase during the vibratory
reaction, neither mast cell degranulation nor tolerance with repeated vibration could be demonstrated in this patient. Interestingly, the patient did
exhibit the typical clustering of physical urticarias in that she also exhibited
dermographism and delayed pressure urticaria.

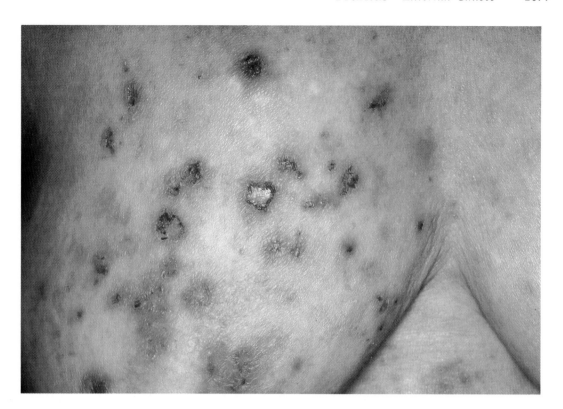

We can only wonder about the status of her eardrums during a rock concert.

Melino M, Toni F, Riguzzi G: Immunologic **contact urticaria to fish**. Contact Dermatitis 1987; 17:182.

This 48-year-old woman was seen in consultation because of **attacks of itching and burning**, as well as erythema and edema of the hands. She had also experienced attacks of angioedema of the lips and tongue. The common denominator was simple direct **contact with uncooked fish**, whether fresh or frozen. The symptoms began 10 minutes after exposure and persisted all day. A diagnosis was made of contact urticaria due to fish.

Twenty-minute patch tests to five different fresh fish showed a strongly positive reaction to three of them (cod, mullet, and anchovy). Reactions to tuna and pilchard were negative. Patch tests to the same five cooked fish were all negative. The patient was an atopic with a high IgE level (3900 U/ml). The radioallergosorbent test (RAST) was positive to cod, and the prick test to fish was a strangely positive local wheal reaction.

Contactants have to be considered as potential causes of **pruritus alone**.

Lempert KD, Baltz PS, Welton WA, Whittier FC: **Pseudouremic pruritus**: A scabies epidemic in a dialysis unit. Am J Kidney Dis 1985; 5:117–119.

The presumed index case in this **itch epidemic** was in a 57-year-old man whose extreme pruritus was assumed to be due to renal failure. No dermatologic examination was done. The intense unremitting itch finally led to his death by his withdrawal from a hemodialysis program that had been otherwise successful for the past 14 months.

Two other dialysis patients with recent pruritus were sent for dermatologic consultation, and **uremic pruritus** was the diagnosis. When a staff nephrologist and three dialysis nurses noted intense itching, worse at bedtime, the dermatologist diagnosed contact dermatitis due to laundry detergent used in washing of their new scrub uniforms. Next, family members became affected.

At this time, the diagnosis of epidemic **scabies** was made. When all of the staff was carefully examined, 25 cases of scabies were identified. This represented an attack rate of 36% for the staff and 20% for the dialysis patients.

Simply attributing the itch of the index case to the uremia of renal failure proved to be a costly case of cerebral failure.

Gupta AK, Billings JK, Ellis CN: **Chronic pruritus**: An uncommon cause. Arch Dermatol 1988; 124:1102–1106.

A sparrow's nest in the attic and a vent directly over the patient's bed resulted in 90 days of **itch** in a 30-year-old female physician. She thought she had scabies because of numerous erythematous pruritic papules scattered over her body, but lindane lotion had been of no help.

The mystery was solved when she brought in specimens of the hundreds of "insects" 0.5 to 1.0 mm in length that she noticed in the bed sheets. These were identified as northern **fowl mites** (*Ornithonyssus sylviarum*) that were infesting the attic sparrows. Although her lesions were only papules, in more sensitive individuals, vesicles, urticarial plaques, and even punctate hemorrhagic lesions may develop.

Avian mite dermatitis suggests insect bites more than scabies, since the face is often involved and there are no burrows or interdigital web involvement. However, like scabies, it is very pruritic at night and dermographism and urticarial lesions are common. The mite drops off after satisfying its thirst for blood and must be searched for elsewhere than on the patient. Look for its vector of vents, air conditioners, and windows. It is also an occupational disease of poultry workers and bird fanciers. The problem can spring from contact (direct or indirect) with sparrows, chickens, ducks, pigeons, starlings, robins, finches, and canaries.

Recall that pruritus is not the worst that can happen, as the bites may transmit encephalitis (St. Louis or Western equine) as well as other diseases.

Theis J, Lavoipierre MM, LaPerriere R, Kroese H: Tropical **rat mite dermatitis**: Report of six cases and review of other mite infestations. Arch Dermatol 1981; 117:341–343.

While playing on the patio of her home, a 15-month-old girl developed an **itch**. Later in the day, erythematous papules were noted on the child's shoulders and trunk. Clinically these were identified as bites of some kind.

The child continued to have new lesions whenever she played on the patio. The mystery of the "bites" was solved when the mother observed the family cat bringing a **dead mouse** over for its lunch on the patio. Examination of the mouse showed large numbers of mites crawling on its skin and these mites were also on the patio itself. These were identified as *Ornithonyssus bacoti*. The patio thus proved to be the lunchroom for not only the cat but also the mites. Other mite sites to be explored are attics or ceiling space— inhabited by the roof rat *Rattus rattus*.

Other hosts include bats, pet snakes, chickens, caged birds, or even the nests of birds to be found in gutters or windowsills. Persistent problems may need to be tracked to their source by professional rodent control assistance.

Don't forget that these mites are large enough to be seen with the naked eye. Don't just look at the bites, but look around the patient's skin and clothing. Even better, have the patient look at the site at the moment of feeling a bite. **A slap with Scotch tape** and he can "bring it in alive."

Chakrabarti A: **Pig handler's itch**. Int J Dermatol 1990; 29:205–206.

Of 46 people who handled two scabietic pigs in a veterinary school 30 experienced itching within a few hours of contact. They developed widespread papulovesicular and eczematous eruptions, but no burrows were seen, and the interdigital webs and genitalia were not affected.

Sarcoptes scabiei was recovered in 20 of 30 scrapings. A diagnosis of "**pig handler's itch**" was made. It proved to be self-limiting, disappearing within 2 to 3 weeks after the infected pigs were treated.

Such **acarine bites** also account for dairy man's itch, calvary man's itch, goat handler's itch, cat handler's itch, and buffalo man's itch.

Henwood BP, MacDonald DM: **Caterpillar dermatitis**. Clin Exp Dermatol 1983; 8:77–93.

It all begins with **pruritus**. The face and neck, arms, and hands are scratched, and next the patient notes pink macules, urticarial wheals, and later papules. The scratch marks may become evident as excoriations or as purpuric grouped, even linear, lesions. An attack lasts a week.

It is all due to contact with **toxin-containing hairs** from those innocent-looking larvae of butterflies and moths, i.e., the caterpillars. Look for it in farmers, gardeners, building contractors, entomologists, and children. Look for it when the caterpillars hatch out in the spring and summer. Look for it to be carried by pets, brush, and even breezes. The toxic pruritogen remains an irritant for years after being shed.

The most dramatic form is the **Caripito itch**, wherein ships docked at Caripito, Venezuela, are invaded by hordes of *Hylesia* moths. Soon the invaded vessel becomes a ship of fools who can do nothing but scratch.

Dinehart SM, Archer ME, Wolf JE Jr, et al: **Caripito itch**: Dermatitis from contact with *Hylesia* moths. J Am Acad Dermatol 1985; 13:743–747.

One evening in July the British oil tanker *Alvenus* docked at the port of **Caripito**, **Venezuela**, to take on crude oil. Not only did it take on oil but also hundreds of **thousands of moths**, attracted by the ship lights. By morning, a 5-inch thick carpet of moths covered the entire deck. Other moths swept through the ventilators and swarmed over the entire crew, who noted an immediate itch.

By 48 hours, 34 of the 35-man crew had an **intensely pruritic**, erythematous, papulovesicular eruption on the exposed skin areas. When the ship sailed into Lake Charles, Louisiana, later that week, all of the moths were dead, and the carpet had been blown away at sea. Yet the itch remained. The diagnostic possibilities of moth-borne mite bites and even an epidemic of scabies were considered. The ship was fumigated with lindane and methylbromide bombs, while the crew was treated with lindane lotion, antihistamines, and steroids. Still the dermatosis persisted.

Not until a month later, with the ship now under quarantine, was the definitive diagnosis made as a result of finding a moth hair (seta) in the specimen from a skin biopsy of one of the crew. The problem was then recognized as **Caripito itch**, a form of lepidopterism in which sharp fine hairs from the abdomen of the female moth of the *Hylesia* genus introduce a toxic pruritogenic substance into the skin. Interestingly, half of the crew even had palmar lesions where the spicules (moth hairs) had entered.

Thus the remarkable 4-week saga of this "**ship of itch**" was ended when the remaining dead moths were all "swept" overboard.

Internal Causes

Kendall ME, Fields JP, King LE Jr: **Cutaneous mastocytosis** without clinically obvious skin lesions. J Am Acad Dermatol 1984; 10:903–905.

Generalized **unexplained pruritus** had been the plight of this 46-year-old woman for more than 2 years. Numerous studies, including routine skin biopsies, did not reveal the cause of the pruritus and associated excoriations, erythematous macules, and papules, as well as postinflammatory hyperpigmentation.

It was not until **toluidine blue staining** was employed that the high population of dermal mast cells was found (20/high power field). Subsequent urinary histamine levels were elevated (182 µg/24 hr vs normal of <25) as well as a PGD_2 metabolite (6,160 ng/24 hr vs <400). All of this made the diagnosis of **clinically inapparent mastocytosis** the correct one and thus the cause of the years of itching and scratching.

Think of it in unexplained urticaria, flushing, and blushing as well, and ask for a toluidine blue stain.

Haustein U-F: **Adrenergic urticaria and adrenergic pruritus**. Acta Derm Venereol 1990; 70:82–84.

CASE 1

A 51-year-old business manager experienced **urticarial attacks** for 2 years. Their appearance correlated with episodes of high stress. Attacks could be produced also by coffee ingestion. Excessive and hot baths never provoked attacks. A clinical psychologist diagnosed high psycholability and the need for psychotherapy.

Examination revealed macules and papules (1 to 4 mm), some exhibiting white halos (3 to 5 mm). During attacks, plasma epinephrine, norepinephrine, dopamine, and prolactin levels were all elevated. The hives could be reproduced by intradermal testing with epinephrine (10 ng in 0.02 ml saline) and norepinephrine (5 ng). The hives elicited pharmacologically were 2 to 5 mm in diameter, surrounded by a white halo (1 to 4 mm). Control subjects showed no response. An increase in dose led to vasoconstriction and no hive. The hives could not be reproduced by acetyl β-methylcholine injections (5 times 10^{-4}M/liter), or nicotine acid tartrate (2 times 10^{-7}M/liter). They were not blocked by atropine sulfate (2 ml, 0.05 mg), but were blocked by intradermal propranolol (0.1 mg) as well as tolazoline (1 mg in an area 5 by 5 cm). A biopsy showed only edema.

A diagnosis of **adrenergic urticaria** was made. The white halo of the lesions sharply distinguishes it from the broad-brimmed red zone around the papule in cholinergic urticaria.

CASE 2

For 3 years this 34-year-old woman had suffered from **episodic pruritus** after emotional stress. The itching appeared within the hour, was generalized, and faded over the following 2 to 3 hours. There was no visible change in the skin. During attacks the plasma epinephrine, norepinephrine, and prolactin levels were elevated, but plasma histamine, serotonin, and dopamine values remained normal.

Local itching could be **reproduced by intradermal testing with epinephrine** and also norepinephrine in a manner as described in Case 1. Propranolol (25 mg bid) greatly lessened the severity of the attacks of pruritus. A diagnosis of **adrenergic pruritus** was made.

When patients say "It's due to my nerves," sometimes it actually is.

Berth-Jones J, Graham-Brown RAC: **Cholinergic pruritus, erythema and urticaria**: A disease spectrum responding to danazol. Br J Dermatol 1989; 121:235–237.

Episodic, increasingly **severe pruritus** had troubled this 19-year-old man for the past 3 years. The attacks were triggered at first by physical exertion but later by hot food, a hot room, or by being emotionally in a "hot spot." Eight different drugs were tried, but none proved successful in stemming the severe pruritus. Eventually he had to drop out of college because the pruritus proved incapacitating. Because of the trigger factors, a **diagnosis of cholinergic pruritus** was made.

Complete biochemical studies revealed no changes except for a low antiprotease level in the plasma (alpha$_1$-antichymotrypsin 0.2^a/liter [normal 0.3 to 0.6]). As a result, danazol, 200 mg tid was prescribed. Within 2 weeks the pruritus had almost completely resolved. By 2 months the level of the antiprotease (**alpha$_1$-antichymotrypsin**) had risen to 0.75 gm/liter, and a 5-month follow-up showed no further attacks of pruritus. Significantly, this same enzyme level is also low in cholinergic urticaria and responds as well to danazol therapy.

Although no skin changes had been seen in the first 3 years of this patient's pruritus, continuing surveillance during the 6 months prior to danazol therapy did show erythema appearing during the attacks, and finally a trace of cholinergic urticaria was observed during an exercise challenge. From this came the awareness of the **cholinergic triad** of pruritus, erythema, and urticaria. The dominant feature in this patient was the pruritus; in others it is the urticaria or the erythema.

Failure to diagnose cholinergic pruritus follows failure to elicit a history of the autonomic triggers or stress factors in patients with episodic or paroxysmal pruritus, and on that failure may rest therapeutic failure.

It is particularly gratifying to us to see the role of proteases reentering into the pathogenesis of pruritus. Our isolation and characterization of the protease mucunain as the active principle of itch powder first led to an awareness of the pruritogenic significance of the release of proteases from the keratinocytes and inflammatory cells.

Valsecchi R, Cainelli T: **Generalized pruritus**. A manifestation of iron deficiency. Arch Dermatol 1983; 119:630.

A 3-year history of treatment-resistant **generalized pruritus** in a 68-year-old man resulted in hospitalization for study. He was found to have **iron deficiency anemia** (hemoglobin 7.7 gm/dl, serum iron 27 μg/dl).

Within 10 days of his starting oral iron supplementation, the pruritus had completely disappeared.

Liautaud B, Pape JW, DeHovitz JA, et al: **Pruritic skin lesions**. A common initial presentation of acquired immunodeficiency syndrome. Arch Dermatol 1989; 125:629–632.

Intensely pruritic eruptions were seen in nearly every other one of a series of Haitian patients with **AIDS**. The lesions defied specific diagnostic categorization, nor could any specific cause or therapy be found. They began on the arms as papular and nodular lesions, spreading to the trunk, legs, and face. Vesicles were seen. The biopsy simply showed an inflammatory cell infiltrate.

The geographic restriction of these pruritic eruptions to tropical areas suggests insect bites or an allergen as the cause, but neither could be established.

In four out of five of the patients, these pruritic eruptions were the initial symptom of AIDS.

Duvic M: Staphylococcal infections and the **pruritus of AIDS-related complex**. Arch Dermatol 1987; 123:1598.

Severe pruritus is one of the most common problems seen in patients with **AIDS-related complex** (ARC). In a study of 100 such patients:

Twenty per cent had scabies (requiring 4 to 6 weeks of treatment).
Five per cent had *Demodex*-induced folliculitis (the papular rash of AIDS that requires Eurax therapy).
Thirty per cent had *Staphylococcal aureus* folliculitis.

Twenty-five ARC patients had staphylococcal infections of the axilla or groin that could not be distinguished clinically from candidiasis. Lesions were red and confluent with satellite pustules and represented atypical bullous impetigo. There were no *Candida* present, and the *Staphylococcus aureus* isolates were resistant to erythromycin. Dicloxacillin orally was remarkably effective.

Mühlendahl KEv: **Intoxication from mercury** spilled on carpets. Lancet 1990; 336:1578–1579.

A 3-year-old girl had had widespread **pruritic eczema** for the past 4 months. Noteworthy were sweaty, scaling, pink palms. The clinical picture included photosensitivity, anorexia, and weight loss. A diagnosis of **acrodynia** was made. Confirmation came with the finding of elevated mercury levels in the urine. Significantly, a 20-month-old sister exhibited severe prurigo of 2 months' duration. The third sibling was 7 years old, and he too showed a pruritic exanthem.

None had been knowingly exposed to mercury. The mystery was not solved until months later when the family recalled a **mercury thermometer** having **broken** in a small carpeted room where the children played.

The mercury could not be retrieved, and it was presumed that mercury vapor inhalation accounted for the acrodynia appearing 4 to 6 months later.

It is important to note that without the index case the **diagnosis of mercury poisoning** would have been a most difficult one. Yet the mercury did account for a widespread itch in all three. No history can ever be too complete in the search for the cause of idiopathic itch.

Schaffner F: **Cholestyramine**, a boon to some who itch. Gastroenterology 1964; 46:67–70.

Patients suffering from intense itching are constantly scratching, irritable insomniacs aggravating their basic disease because of inadequate rest, reduced appetite, and recurrent skin infections.

In **primary biliary cirrhosis**, unrelenting **itching** often precedes other signs and symptoms by months to years, driving the patient from general physician to dermatologist to psychiatrist.

Other diseases causing pruritus include extrahepatic biliary obstruction and intrahepatic cholestasis due to hepatitis, drugs, or cirrhosis. These have in common increased bilirubin, alkaline phosphatase, cholesterol, and bile acids, all of which come from bile. Pruritus is probably due to the increased blood bile acid levels (cholemia).

Kopelman H, Robertson MH, Sanders PG, Ash I: The **Epping jaundice**. Br Med J 1966; 1:514–516.

A medical student at St. Margaret's Hospital in Epping developed severe acute abdominal pain followed by **jaundice and pruritus**. Subsequently, 83 other persons in the area were similarly affected. Tests for mononucleosis, brucellosis, enteroviral infection, and leptospirosis, as well as ova and parasites in the stool, were all negative.

Whole-wheat brown bread from the local bakery was finally established as the cause. Contamination with 4,4'-diaminodiphenylmethane had occurred 16 days before in the delivery van when a plastic jar full of this compound had spilled its contents onto a sack of flour on its way to the bakery. This **aromatic amine**, which is a hardener for epoxy resin, is derived from benzene.

Similar poisonings with bread as the vector had been reported due to the alkaloids of *Senecio* seeds (Compositae family), fungicides, and the insecticides parathion and endrin.

Goldman RD, Rea TH, Cinque J: The **"butterfly" sign**: A clue to generalized pruritus in a patient with chronic obstructive hepatobiliary disease. Arch Dermatol 1983; 119:183–184.

Two years of **generalized pruritus** in this 59-year-old woman had led to diffuse generalized hyperpigmentation from the constant scratching. The unique feature was a large "butterfly" configuration of relative hypopigmentation over the unreachable areas of the back. This is the butterfly sign, a sign of long-term generalized pruritus.

Bilirubin and alkaline phosphatase levels were elevated. A biopsy of the liver was consistent with a diagnosis of biliary cirrhosis. Oral cholestyramine resin (4 gm qid) controlled the pruritus.

The **butterfly sign** is seen in a variety of conditions in which long-term generalized pruritus occurs. These include biliary cirrhosis, carcinoma of the bile duct, sclerosing cholangitis, scleroderma, renal and endocrine disease, and lymphoma.

Ryatt KS, Cotterill JA, Littlewood JM: **Generalized pruritus** in a baby as a presenting feature of the **arteriohepatic dysplasia syndrome**. Clin Exp Dermatol 1983; 8:657–661.

This 2-year-old infant had suffered with intense **unexplained itch since** birth. On examination there were numerous excoriations of normal-appearing skin. Notable was the absence of eczema.

Two significant diagnostic signs were present on general physical examination. The **facies** were abnormal, showing a prominent forehead, a straight nose, and a small, pointed chin. Secondly, the liver was palpable to 1 fingerbreadth below the costal margin.

The possibility of intrahepatic bile duct hypoplasia was explored as a cause of cholestasis and consequent pruritus. The alkaline phosphatase level was elevated, and the plasma 25-hydroxyvitamin D, low. Although the liver had been considered normal, a needle biopsy showed intrahepatic bile duct hypoplasia.

This finding with the unusual facies and a cardiologist's demonstration of **mild pulmonary stenosis** made the diagnosis of **arteriohepatic dysplasia**. Originally recognized as simple biliary hypoplasia, this congenital syndrome now is known to encompass dysplastic changes in the bones, eyes, and cardiovascular system, as well as the liver. A dramatic reduction in the presenting symptom of itch immediately followed cholestyramine (3 gm/day) therapy.

Itchy nonatopic babies with unusual facies need to be studied for liver dysplasias.

Kagen CN, Vance JC, Simpson M: **Gnathostomiasis**: Infestation in an Asian immigrant. Arch Dermatol 1984; 120:508–510.

Two weeks of **pruritus** of the abdomen associated with fleeting erythematous patches was the complaint of this 25-year-old Laotian woman. She provided the answer by bringing in a centimeter-long threadlike object she had removed from an excoriation. It was the **nematode** *Gnathostoma spinigerum.*

Removal of the worm was curative, since patients are infested with but one worm.

The definitive hosts for *Gnathostoma spinigerum* are the cat, dog, and the tiger. In fact, the nematode was first sighted in a stomach tumor of a tiger in 1836. It is from these tumors the ova pass out to *Cyclops*, a fresh-water crustacean, and become larvae. Once the infested *Cyclops* are eaten by secondary hosts such as fish, children, and pigs, the larvae encyst, and the uncooked infested meat becomes the vector for human infestation.

This patient probably became infested while **eating raw fresh-water fish** in Thailand. It is significant that symptoms did not begin until $2\frac{1}{2}$ years later.

Migratory intermittent swellings of the skin with pruritus or pain are the cardinal diagnostic signs. Another clue is the **eosinophilia** that occurs. Since the worm can migrate anywhere in the body, an unbelievable array of symptoms and signs can occur, mimicking anything from appendicitis to encephalitis. All this from one worm!

Human gnathostomiasis is another of the diseases endemic in Asia that can present in your office in Asian immigrants or in tourists with a fondness for the native uncooked food.

Rozenman D, Kremer M, Zuckerman F: **Onchocerciasis** in Israel. Arch Dermatol 1984; 120:505–507.

A mysterious unexplained **generalized pruritus** of 5 months' duration afflicted this 15-year-old boy from Ethiopia. Some depigmented scaly papular lichenoid lesions were present on the shins.

A **biopsy** of these nonspecific sites of excoriation revealed **coiled microfilaria** of *Onchocerca volvulus* in the upper dermis. Subsequent ophthalmologic examination showed microfilaria in the cornea and anterior chamber of the eyes. A diagnosis of onchocerciasis was made.

Treatment with diethylcarbamazine citrate produced a **Herxheimer reaction**. By 3 weeks the drug was stopped, the boy's itch was gone, and no microfilaria could be seen on slit lamp examination. He has remained cured.

Onchocerciasis produces severe pruritus without localization. Papules may occur on the elbows, knees, and chest. The onchocercomas are inflammatory infiltrates around the adult worms. Regional lymphangitis may occur as well. Ocular lesions arise late and can produce the dreaded river blindness. The slit lamp is an essential diagnostic tool, as is the skin biopsy. Noteworthy is **Mazzotti's test**, in which a flare of the eruption, arthralgias, and fever occur within 24 hours of administration of the vermicide diethylcarbamazine.

Look to this diagnosis in your pruritic patients who have traveled in Central and South America or in Ethiopia and Africa.

White JJ, Prevost JV: Weil's disease: Report of three cases, including the morbid anatomy of one case, and a brief review of the pertinent literature. Ann Intern Med 1941; 15:207–225.

A 46-year-old white man from New Jersey worked in a garage that became flooded after heavy rains. He sustained abrasions on his hands when he had to bail out a heater pit every day. Buildings in the area had no sewerage system, and numerous rats were around. He developed anorexia, weakness, malaise, chills, fever, mild prostration, and jaundice over a 7-day period. **Severe pruritus** resulted in hemorrhagic excoriations that bled freely, raised up in purple lumps, and had peculiar secondary inflammatory purple areolae. The temperature remained around 99°C to 100°C, and the liver was barely palpable. Darkfield examinations of blood serum and urine were positive for *Leptospira*. Guinea pigs inoculated with his blood and urine died after 10 days with evidence of *Leptospira* infection. The *Leptospira* agglutination test was negative. The patient recovered after 2 months.

For darkfield examination, serum is used from blood collected in a capillary tube that is sealed at one end and then centrifuged for 5 to 10 minutes. This test is recommended for all jaundiced patients. Look for spirochetes with tightly wound coils. They are quite active with an erratic course, rotation, and lashing movements of the last six to eight spirals of the motile end, which resemble chains of coccoid bodies. They stain with Fontana's silver stain.

Weil's disease is contracted from contaminated water in areas where soil is neutral or alkaline. Urine from rats or dogs may contaminate ponds, lakes, or swimming pools.

Serologic tests are not reliable because of antigenic variation of the many strains of *Leptospira*, which include *L. icterohaemorrhagiae* and *L. canicola* (which causes the milder canicola fever).

Spaulding HS Jr: Pruritus without urticaria in **acute giardiasis**. Ann Allergy 1990; 65:161.

The author of this paper experienced a sudden attack of **severe pruritus** a week after returning from a sheep hunt near Tok, Alaska. It did not respond to large doses of hydroxyzine. He had no gastrointestinal symptoms. He recalled frequently filling his canteen from mountain streams where sheep had been seen crossing.

Concern led him to consult a gastroenterologist, who tended to dismiss the possibility of underlying, recently acquired giardiasis. However, examination of a stool swab disclosed abundant cysts and trophozoites. The diagnosis of **giardiasic pruritus** was quickly confirmed when the itch disappeared completely after 36 hours of metronidazole therapy. There was no recurrence.

You don't become a great golfer by sitting in the clubhouse, or a great diagnostician by sitting in the lecture hall.

Psoriasis

Psoriasis is the diagnostician's delight. It has an honest, forthright portrait. There are none of the variable misleading guises of other diseases. Look at that distinctive silvery scale. Look at its lesions sharply cut off from normal skin. And look at the symmetrical involvement of the elbows and knees. You can't mistake it.

This portrait is consistent down to the very fingertips, where the pitted nails and subungual oil spots add authenticity to the diagnosis. Add to this the scaling plaques hidden in the scalp. Observe the figurate patterns that have appeared as the round lesions enlarge, fuse, and clear eccentrically. Look at the fissured, sharply marginated, red plaques on a palm "koebnerized" by trauma. And ask to see the family portraits, for it is a disease that runs in families.

You will know it's psoriasis, with itch or not. It is a disease that breeds true. But where are the slippery slopes of misdiagnosis? It comes sans scale in the intertriginous groin and gluteal cleft. Don't mistake it for seborrheic dermatitis. It comes sans scale in the treated patient who will always give the diagnosis if you but ask. It comes, at times, as dystrophic nails that look like the result of onychomycosis but fail to yield hyphae on scrapings. It may be mistaken for pityriasis rubra pilaris, but that disease's salmon color, skip spots, and keratin cast of the palms should save you clinical embarrassment. It may look like secondary syphilis, but the ham color, adenopathy, and palmar papules all point away from psoriasis. Indeed, psoriasis may become a component of other diseases, since the psoriatic patient can produce psoriasis scaling in any injured site. Poison ivy dermatitis, herpes zoster, and neurodermatitis are examples of skin disease that can evolve into psoriasis when the psoriatic is in the reactive (Koebner positive) phase.

The only blemish in the portrait of psoriasis is when it develops pustules. This we can see in pustular psoriasis of the palms and/or soles or in its fearsome form of generalized pustular psoriasis. It is as though psoriasis had a pox upon it. And maybe it does.

Fry L: **Psoriasis**. Br J Dermatol 1988; 119:445–461.

Look for:

Koebner phenomenon: In 1872, Heinrich Koebner reported psoriasis examples limited to skin damaged by saddle burns, suppuration, a horsefly bite, and a tattoo. He believed that the entire skin had a latent predisposition for producing chronic inflammation, and that therapy should be directed at reducing the vulnerability of the whole skin to a great many internal and local stimuli. Koebner-positive patients have a higher T helper/suppressor ratio in uninvolved skin compared with Koebner-negative patients. The Koebner response also correlates with the age of onset, being positive in 75% of patients with psoriasis starting before the age of 15 years and in only 5% of patients who got the disease after age 30.

Infections: Streptococcal infection is the major precipitating factor in guttate psoriasis. Streptococcal monoclonal antibodies bind to components of keratinocytes, possibly indicating cross-reactivity that might give rise to a self-perpetuating autoimmune state.

Heredity: One third of the patients have a family history of psoriasis. While some studies showed that every affected child had an affected parent, others concluded that inheritance was a simple autosomal dominant with 60% penetrance. A multifactorial inheritance was also postulated.

Stress: This precipitates and aggravates psoriasis, probably by affecting hormones and immunologic processes.

Drugs: Lithium, beta-blockers, indomethacin, and antimalarials may aggravate psoriasis. This may be an idiosyncratic response, as it does not occur in everyone taking these drugs.

Bernhard JD: **Auspitz sign** is not sensitive or specific for psoriasis. J Am Acad Dermatol 1990; 22:1079–1081.

Only 41 of 234 patients with psoriasis showed the **small bleeding points** Heinrich Auspitz found so characteristic of psoriasis lesions. Even more disconcerting for the beginning student is the fact that Auspitz's sign was present in some actinic and seborrheic keratoses as well as in Darier's disease.

It was all so easy when a sign was noted and studied in just one patient. Speaking of the **Auspitz sign**, we vividly recall a dermatologist's pallor when after eliciting the sign with his fingernail, his colleague at the meeting said, "Did you know that patient has AIDS?"

Miller RAW, Griffiths WAD: Pressure **inhibition of the Koebner reaction** by capillary occlusion. Acta Derm Venereol 1982; 62:331–333.

Scarifying the normal skin of a 38-year-old psoriatic induced the appearance of psoriasis in this exact site a month later when the psoriasis flared. The remarkable finding was absence of any lesions in the area that had been mildly **compressed** for just the 24 hours after the challenge trauma.

Clinically we see such an absence of the Koebner phenomenon in the area under a wristwatch band.

Ben-Chetrit E, Rubinow A: **Exacerbation of psoriasis** by ibuprofen. Cutis 1986; 38:45.

A 41-year-old nurse had psoriasis under successful control for 16 years with topical coal tar preparations and sunlight exposure at the Dead Sea. She developed wrist pain 3 months after such treatment and was given **ibuprofen** (1200 mg/daily). Two weeks later the wrist pain had lessened, but many new 1087

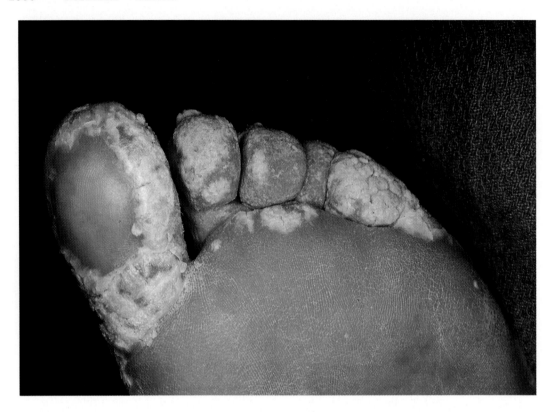

psoriatic lesions had appeared. After the ibuprofen was stopped and the psoriasis treated with coal tar and sunlight, the skin promptly cleared, but persistence of joint pain led to a challenge with ibuprofen 2 months later. Within 4 days, new psoriatic lesions appeared.

Alert your patients with psoriasis (as well as those with urticaria) to the hazard of responding to TV advertisements for Motrin, Advil, Nuprin, and the like. Whatever the name, they still contain ibuprofen.

Fisher DA, Elias PM, LeBoit PL: **Exacerbation of psoriasis** by the hypolipidemic agent, gemfibrozil. Arch Dermatol 1988; 124:854–855.

Within 2 weeks of beginning gemfibrozil (**Lopid**) treatment, a 64-year-old woman experienced explosive generalized pruritic guttate psoriasis. Two months before starting the medication she had noted scaly patches on the backs of her hands. The gemfibrozil was stopped, and the psoriasis largely cleared after a few weeks of topical clobetasol and coal tar gel therapy. Challenge with gemfibrozil 2 months later resulted in a pronounced flare.

Gemfibrozil, a fibric acid derivative in the same category as clofibrate, decreases production of very low density lipoprotein (VLDL). It joins the drugs known to **elicit or exacerbate psoriasis**:

beta-blockers	isotretinoin
antimalarials	chlorthalidone
nonsteroidal anti-inflammatory agents	lithium

Shiohara T, Kobayashi M, Abe K, Nagashima M: **Psoriasis** occurred predominantly **on warts**. Arch Dermatol 1988; 124:1816–1821.

Warts can get psoriasis! This 54-year-old man developed a guttate form of psoriasis limited essentially to preexisting warts on the hands.

Atherton DJ, Kahana M, Russell-Jones R: **Naevoid psoriasis.** Br J Dermatol 1989; 120:837–841.

Remarkable **bands of psoriasis** strictly limited to the left side of the body were seen in this 2-year-old boy. The plaques followed the lines of Blaschko with a sharp midline cutoff.

Although **nevoid psoriasis** has been a diagnosis in doubt, this is a true example. The clinical lesions as well as the biopsy were typical, as was the response to treatment and to sunlight. Indeed, the Koebner phenomenon was observed.

The alternative diagnosis focused first on invasion of an **epidermal nevus** by psoriasis as a result of the isomorphic phenomenon. This has been observed, but on treatment of the psoriasis the underlying nevus was revealed. In this child, normal skin appeared when the psoriasis was treated. The second differential diagnosis is the **inflammatory linear verrucous epidermal nevus** (**ILVEN**), which has a psoriasiform appearance. This condition is extremely pruritic, shows linear patterns of excoriated eczematous papules, has distinctive histology, and is amazingly refractory to treatment.

The swirling banded pattern of this little boy's psoriasis was reminiscent of the swirls we see in incontinentia pigmenti. It may reflect a **cutaneous mosaicism** for the genetic predisposition to psoriasis that is universally present in the skin of the ordinary patient with psoriasis.

Jacobs PH: **Psoriasis**—The numbers and the anguish. Cutis 1984; 33:140.

It takes but a glance to diagnose psoriasis, but it takes understanding and rapport to "diagnose" what is going on in the mind of the psoriatic patient.

Here is a sampling from letters written by patients who may have remained inarticulate in your office.

If only the doctor could cure me:

I could cut my bangs.
I could wear short sleeves and shorts.
I could go in the swimming pool without others leaving for fear of contagion.
I could use the team shower room without being laughed at.
I could stop smelling of tar.
I could plan on marriage.
I could stop my husband from thinking of me as repulsive.
I could stop thinking of suicide.

Cherchez la drogue.
Henri Gougerot

Differential Diagnosis

Griffiths WAD: **Pityriasis rubra pilaris**—an historical approach. Clinical features. Clin Exp Dermatol 1976; 1:37–50.

INITIAL LESION

Follicular hyperkeratosis presenting as an acuminate (pointed) cone of compact keratin at the mouth of the follicle with a small broken or dystrophic hair at the summit.

DIAGNOSTIC SIGN

Black dots on the dorsal surface of the proximal phalanges, representing acuminate plugged follicles. This sign is unreliable, inconstant, and not pathognomonic for pityriasis rubra pilaris (PRP). It may also be seen in ichthyosiform erythroderma, erythrokeratoderma (noncongenital), follicular ichthyosis, and follicular irritation from oils and other chemicals. The morphology of the papules changes, with perifollicular erythema and a flat caplike scale often present.

SEQUENCE

The intervening skin between the papules becomes erythematous and scaly, and the follicular papules coalesce and disappear. The erythema and scaling extend into large well-demarcated plaques or generalized erythroderma, with the color being red-brown. Islands of normal skin seen in the midst of the erythema are very suggestive of PRP, but not specific (seen in 10% of other erythrodermas). The scaling is fine, powdery, furfuraceous (resembling wheat bran), and most pronounced on the face and scalp. Most patients also develop diffuse yellowish hyperkeratosis of the palms and soles with painful fissures. Subungual hyperkeratosis, splinter hemorrhages, and longitudinal ridging are also common. Silvery, psoriasiform scaling of the elbows, knees, and shins appears as the disease progresses; it is often associated with pruritus, which is severe initially but tends to fade as the papules are replaced by sheets of erythema and scaling. Hair loss is rare, even when the scalp is involved.

MUCOSAL LESIONS

mouth: Look for a diffuse white ground-glass appearance, white spots and lines, white streaks on an erythematous base, or pale blue lines. The buccal mucosa, tongue, gingivae, and penis may be similarly affected.

eye: Lesions include corneal ulceration and opacification, conjunctival redness, pearly conjunctival papules, chemosis, hyperemia, interstitial keratitis, and pannus formation.

TRIGGER FACTORS

Burns of all types, especially sunburn
Trauma: cuts, bruises
Vaccination
Infections: scarlet fever, pertussis, mumps, diphtheria, varicella, sore throat, phlebitis, orchitis
Leg ulcer
Parturition

EXACERBATION

pregnancy
menses
sunlight

Course

The disease may start slowly or rapidly, and the patient may be febrile at the sudden onset. Lymphadenopathy occurs if the disease is widespread.

The disease may last a few months to a lifetime and may evolve into or from psoriasis. The Koebner phenomenon is commonly seen, and the relationship to psoriasis is very close.

Brodthagen H: **Pityriasis rubra pilaris** (with Köbner's sign). Acta Derm Venereol 1955; 35:243–244.

A 15-year-old girl, using a pin, superficially scratched the name Bent on the dorsum of the right hand, with no bleeding. One month later, by chance, she developed **pityriasis rubra pilaris**, beginning with a fine branny scaling of the scalp and face. The eruption spread down the extremities as follicular hyperkeratosis, and after 2 weeks the name Bent could be clearly read on the hand.

Thus, minor mechanical **trauma** 6 weeks before served to localize precisely the lesions of pityriasis rubra pilaris.

Yarbrough GK, Iriondo M: Diabetic patient with **crusted plaques**. Arch Dermatol 1987; 123:811–814.

For 13 months this 56-year-old diabetic woman had progressively worsening hyperkeratotic **papulosquamous plaques** that were asymptomatic. The others in her family had no skin problems. The **differential diagnosis** included psoriasis, eczema, drug eruption, and bacterial or fungal infection.

The diagnosis was made by biopsy of a crusted area, which revealed the mite *Sarcoptes scabiei*, high in the epidermis.

This variant, first described as **Norwegian scabies** in 1848 and now politely called crusted scabies, is an affliction most commonly seen in:

 patients with mental deficiencies and/or institutionalized patients who are either unable to express or respond to the infestation
 patients with disease-induced immunodeficiency such as this patient's diabetic state, patients with leukemia or tuberculosis, or individuals in a malnourished state
 patients taking immunosuppressant drugs, e.g., transplant patients (or patients with AIDS)

Note: This patient experienced no itch and her family experienced no scabies. Thus the diagnostician was robbed of his two most sensitive indices of scabies.

Wishner AJ, Lynfield Y: **Psoriasiform dermatitis** in a cachectic man. Arch Dermatol 1988; 124:1852–1855.

For 2 months this 43-year-old man had noted **patchy hyperkeratosis** of the **soles** as well as discrete papules and pustules of the palms. All of the toes and some of the fingers showed **periungual violaceous erythema** and scaling. Several nails had been lost, and all showed onycholysis. KOH examinations were negative.

Additional findings were erythematous scaly plaques of the inner thighs, lower back, and buttocks, as well as a 1-cm ulcer under the tongue and an enlarged left cervical lymph node. The history disclosed a dramatic weight loss of 40 pounds and associated anorexia. Biopsy of the tongue and the lymph node as well showed squamous cell carcinoma. Excision of the tumor and nodes was followed by rapid clearing of the rash.

This case is an example of **Bazex syndrome**, i.e., **acrokeratosis paraneo-plastica**. Its initial presentation is a psoriasiform eruption of the fingers and toes along with a scaling erythema of the nose and ears. It then extends to the palms and soles as the responsible neoplasm becomes symptomatic. Unless the neoplasm is treated, the third stage of lesions appears on the arms, legs, face, and scalp. Local treatment is of little avail, but resolution occurs when the tumor is successfully treated. Metastasis is signaled by recurrence.

One looks to the laryngopharyngeal region, the esophagus, and lungs as the common sites of the responsible cancer.

Prendiville J, Kaufman D, Esterly NB: **Psoriasiform plaque** on the buttock. Arch Dermatol 1985; 125:113–118.

Recently adopted from Bolivia, this 6-year-old girl had a sharply demarcated erythematous **scaling plaque** on the right buttock. It had a psoriasiform appearance and had been diagnosed as **tinea corporis**. Antifungal as well as steroid creams had had no effect, nor could any fungi be found on KOH examination or culture. A chest roentgenogram was normal.

On two occasions biopsies showed intraepidermal abscess formation, an intense inflammatory infiltrate, with a few multinucleated giant cells. Special stains for fungi and acid-fast organisms were negative on multiple sections. Fungal and mycobacterial cultures of two biopsy specimens were likewise sterile. However, later, using ATS medium, *Mycobacterium tuberculosis* was grown by inoculation of the second biopsy specimen. At this time, an intradermal tuberculin skin test was done (0.1 ml intermediate-strength PPD) and was strongly positive at 48 hours.

The diagnosis was thus **tuberculosis verrucosa cutis** and within a month of rifampin and isoniazid therapy the lesion began to involute. The full course required a year.

The **differential diagnosis** for this patient's lesion called for consideration of:

psoriasis
lichen simplex chronicus
hypertrophic lichen planus
atypical mycobacterial infection

sporotrichosis (fixed)
blastomycosis
chromomycosis

and, of course, "warty tuberculosis," as it painstakingly proved to be.

Mesquita-Guimaraes J, Azevedo F, Aguiar S: **Silica granulomas** secondary to the explosion of a land mine. Cutis 1987; 40:41–43.

A 36-year-old man developed erythematous nodules with scaly **psoriatic surfaces** of the left side of the face, neck, and left arm. The distribution was patterned: circinate on the face, linear on the neck, and zosteriform on the arm. Yellow miliary nodules with erythematous halos were intermixed, and black punctate incrustations were seen in numerous lesions. Fifteen years previously during war service in Mozambique he had stepped on a land mine that exploded, producing numerous wounds and burns with implantation of black particles. The lesions healed normally, but 3 years later inflammation developed around the particles, leading to purulent ulcers that eventually healed.

A diagnosis of **silica granuloma** was made by finding foreign bodies under polarized light and the presence of silica on x-ray spectroscopy.

The long latent period between implantation of silica and the development of visible lesions may mean that the patient cannot recall the responsible original accident (unless it be a land mine).

Ruiz-Maldonado R, Tamayo L, del Castillo V, Lozoya I: **Erythrokeratodermia progressiva symmetrica**: Report of 10 cases. Dermatologica 1982; 164:133–141.

Sharply marginated static, **erythematosquamous plaques** occur with perfect symmetry on the extremities, buttocks, and head. The palms and soles are involved, but not the chest and abdomen. Lesions begin in the first year of life, progress for 1 to 2 years, and then remain stationary. Itching occurs occasionally.

This was the largest series reported to date of this rare genetically determined disease that is apparently transmitted as an autosomal dominant. Skin biopsy reveals a psoriasiform pattern without Munro's microabscesses.

The **differential diagnosis** includes:

> psoriasis (may be asymmetrical and on thorax)
> erythrokeratodermia figurata variabilis (onset early in life with figurate lesions that keep changing and involve the chest and abdomen; biopsy shows hyperkeratosis and acanthosis)
> erythrokeratodermia en cocarde (Degos) (early onset of circular changing lesions with relapses; genetic transmission unknown; biopsy shows hyperkeratosis, focal parakeratosis, and acanthosis)
> ichthyosis (no erythema, squamous nature)

Boyd AS: **Lichen spinulosus**: Case report and overview. Cutis 1989; 43:557–560.

This 22-year-old man had had roughness of the elbows and knees since he was 11. It had waxed and waned and was mildly pruritic. He had been told it was psoriasis.

On examination, discrete well-demarcated plaques were seen on the elbows and knees. Within the plaques, which also involved the anterior surface of the legs, there were individual **follicular spines**.

A diagnosis of **lichen spinulosus** was made on the basis of the nutmeg-grater feel and the spinous appearance. This is a problem that may occur on almost any area. At times it may arise within patches of nummular eczema.

It is **distinguished from** keratosis pilaris by its spines. Miliary papular syphilis is ruled out by serologic tests. Lichen planopilaris is similar, but affects the scalp and hair-bearing areas exclusively. Finally, the frictional eruption of childhood shows flat lichenoid papules.

If the eruption has true spines, it is truly best to think of lichen spinulosus.

de Mare S, van de Kerkhof PCM, Happle R: Dithranol in the treatment of **inflammatory linear verrucous epidermal nevus**. Acta Derm Venereol 1989; 69:77–80.

Although **inflammatory linear verrucous epidermal nevus** appears to be a rare, very pruritic nevus, the rapid clearing in this patient to short contact therapy with dithranol cream (0.25%) suggests the true diagnosis may be linear psoriasis.

Ikai K, Uchiyama T, Maeda M, Takigawa M: Sézary-like syndrome in a 10-year-old girl with serologic evidence of human T-cell lymphotropic virus Type I infection. Arch Dermatol 1987; 123:1351–1355.

At age 6 months, this patient developed an erythematous, pruritic, scaling eruption of the scalp and face. It spread to other sites, and when she was 6 years old a diagnosis of **psoriasis vulgaris** was made.

The eruption became generalized, evolving into erythroderma with lymphadenopathy. Blood studies showed not only Sézary cells (2500/mm^3) but also a high titer of antihuman T-cell lymphotropic virus type I antibody. This anti-HTLV-1 antibody usually found in adult T-cell leukemia was also present in the mother's blood. Thus, **HTLV-1 infection** may be considered to have been responsible for this young girl's problem.

Yoshikuni K, Tagami H, Yamada M, et al: Erythematosquamous skin lesions in hereditary lactate dehydrogenase M-subunit deficiency. Arch Dermatol 1986; 122:1420–1424.

Circinate scaly, **erythematous lesions** and plaques with marginal scaling on the elbows and the extensor surfaces of the arms and legs were the cutaneous sign of an enzyme deficiency in this 18-year-old man. Associated keratosis pilaris was also noted.

Present since childhood, the lesions were worse each summertime. They had been neglected until the patient was studied because of fatigue and dark urine. He was found to have myoglobinuria after heavy exercise. This, in turn, was traced to a **lactate dehydrogenase (LDH) deficiency** as shown by low serum lactate–high serum pyruvate and but one isoenzyme band of LDH activity.

The skin lesions that serve as a marker for this condition could be ignored as strange dry skin. Others might consider it an example of **ichthyosis linearis circumflexa** or of **erythrokeratodermia variabilis**. The plaques on the elbow could too easily be dismissed as psoriasis. The scaly lesions of acrodermatitis enteropathica, necrolytic migratory erythema, and pellagra also enter the **diagnostic ring**. A biopsy helps by showing the presence of pale swollen keratinocytes as well as the hyperkeratosis and acanthosis.

Check the lactate dehydrogenase isoenzymes on that patient with dry scaly skin that gets worse with exercise or in summertime.

Rarities are rarely found by those who rarely look for them.

Ginsburg IH, Link BG: Feelings of stigmatization in patients with psoriasis. J Am Acad Dermatol 1989; 20:53–63.

Recognize that in your patients with psoriasis:

Strategies of concealment abound
Self-examination is endless
Embarrassment over appearance may govern their lives
Some may not feel that life is worth living

The diagnosis of psoriasis is easier than the diagnosis of its effects on the patient, his family, his employer, and his social contacts.

Look more for truth than beauty in your diagnosis.

Purpura

Purpura is **blood-stained dermis**. It is a stain of many colors and many origins. We can learn much by studying its color, size, and location. The fresh stain is the red of hemoglobin that has just escaped the confines of the vascular system. As its oxygen is lost, the purple becomes evident and then the sequence of yellow-green and blue of any "black-and-blue" mark. If the stained skin is swollen, we think of a hematoma, which begins when a large vessel is being torn or cut resulting in continued bleeding with no clotting to stop the staining. If the stain is palpable, we think of a vessel leaking its hemoglobin as a result of walls weakened by vasculitis.

Inspection may reveal the purpura of **aging** or atrophic skin in which minor—even inapparent—trauma tears fine capillaries that have long since lost their protective sheath of collagen. Or we may see the evidence of steroid atrophy with its unprotected fragile vessels. Are the stains but mere follicular spots? Check the gums for evidence of scurvy. In looking at the petechial and punctate stains of the lower legs we see the stains of **capillaritis**. The prototype is the progressive pigmented dermatoses of Schamberg with its cayenne pepper spots of hemosiderin. Variants may be discerned with annular and papular lesions, such as the purpura annularis telangiectodes (PAT) (Majocchi's purpura), the pigmented purpuric lichenoid dermatitis of Gougerot-Blum; and the golden lichenoid patches of lichen aureus. The heightened venous pressure of gravitational origin favors the appearance of all these capillary leak stains on the lower legs. But in all these types, there is an implied weakening of the capillary wall or a failure in the platelets to close the leaky endothelial gaps.

As much can be learned by listening to the patient as by looking at him. Is the purpura but the tip of the iceberg of a **systemic illness**? Is he acutely ill as with bacteremia, septic shock, or an incipient fasciitis? Is the progression of the purpura so rapid and alarming that the patient should be hospitalized? Is there the possibility of disseminated intravascular coagulation of acute lupus or, in a child, a protein C deficiency?

Question and cross examine for a **drug** history. We see explosive purpuras with drug sensitivity reactions; suspects include penicillin, sulfonamides, furosemide, allopurinol, and quinine. Is the patient receiving heparin or coumarin?

Does the patient have an air of belle indifference, as in the autoerythrocyte sensitivity syndrome? Are the lesions painful, as in an arterial disease? Could the purpura be of **factitial origin**?

Taking a careful, complete history can save laboratory tests. We recall that one of our healthy-appearing young women patients came to us with dozens of purpuric macules of just 24 hours' duration. She had no idea of their origin and, fearing a major problem, we ordered a battery of tests and a complete coagulogram. It was the phlebotomist who found the answer, even before she drew the blood. The patient had spent that weekend on her first white water rafting trip.

The **laboratory** is the third leg of the purple stool of diagnosis. Secure a health profile for finding out if the stain is for want of platelets. Look for an underlying leukemia. Order a coagulogram if hematomas are present. Ask for a cryoglobulin and cryofibrinogen determination, as well as serum protein electrophoresis. Macroglobulinemia often presents as a purpura. Check for lupus anticoagulant and do protein C levels.

If the origin of the purple stains is still unclear, your patient needs a good hematologist.

General

Taylor RE, Blatt PM: Clinical evaluation of patients with **bruising and bleeding**. J Am Acad Dermatol 1981; 4:348–368.

Easy bruising may be due to a **coagulation defect**, qualitative or quantitative **platelet defect**, or **abnormal connective tissue**. Petechiae signal platelet or blood vessel disorders and are evanescent, occur in crops, and regress over a period of days. Recurrent spontaneous bruises greater than 5 to 6 cm in diameter, particularly on the face and trunk, suggest a coagulation defect.

A bleeding history should include inquiries about:

congenital or acquired?
circumstances of bleeding (trauma, duration, frequency, distribution)?
other episodes of bleeding (epistaxis, hematemesis, melena, hematuria, hemoptysis)?
menstrual history?
postsurgical bleeding (during or afterward)?
blood or plasma transfusions (why, where)?
drug history (prescriptions, aspirin, over-the-counter)?
family history of bleeding symptoms?

The physical examination should emphasize:

the type, size, and distribution of hemorrhagic lesions
a careful search for telangiectasia (eyegrounds, mouth, nailbeds)
joint examination (deformity, hemarthrosis, extensibility)
skin elasticity and scar formation
body habitus (marfanoid)

An initial evaluation should include:

CBC	prothrombin time (PT)
peripheral blood smear	partial thromboplastin time (PTT)
platelet count	thrombin clotting time (TCT)
bleeding time (evaluates	tourniquet test
platelet function)	

Does your purpuric patient have:

low platelet count (drug induced)
platelet defect (drug induced)
sepsis
leukemia
hereditary problem
    Glanzmann's disease (thrombasthenia, prolonged bleeding time, poor clot retraction)
    Bernard-Soulier syndrome (giant platelets, prolonged bleeding time, defective prothrombin consumption)
vasculitis (drug induced)
immune complex disease
dysproteinemia
    cryoglobulinemia
    cryofibrinogenemia (look for metastatic malignancy)
    hyperglobulinemia (Waldenström)
    paraproteinemia (multiple myeloma, Waldenström's macroglobulinemia)
amyloidosis, systemic (vascular fragility, prolonged PT & PTT, acquired Factor X deficiency)
heritable connective tissue defect
    Ehlers-Danlos syndrome (vascular fragility)
    Marfan's syndrome
    osteogenesis imperfecta
    pseudoxanthoma elasticum
uremia (platelet dysfunction)

liver disease (platelet dysfunction)
collagen vascular disease (thrombocytopenia, circulating anticoagulants, autoimmune antibodies)
autoerythrocyte sensitization (painful ecchymoses)
disseminated intravascular coagulation (thrombocytopenia, prolonged PT, PTT, TCT)
scurvy (qualitative platelet defects)
congenital coagulation disorder
  hemophilia A (Factor VIII deficiency)
  von Willebrand's disease (Factor VIII deficiency)
  absent or abnormal fibrinogen

In practice, qualitative platelet disorders induced by drugs are the most common causes of bruising. If eliminating aspirin and other drugs does not help, call for the help of a hematologist.

Gentry RH, Fitzpatrick JE: A peculiar purple bruise. Arch Dermatol 1990; 126:816–820.

A 63-year-old diabetic noted a small blister on the medial aspect of his left thigh. Within hours it enlarged, as he developed nausea and malaise. Ten hours later in an emergency room he was noted to have a **large purplish bruise** with irregular borders. In 9 hours he was acutely ill, and ruptured hemorrhagic blisters were seen on the single well-defined purpuric area, encompassing half of his thigh. There was no lymphangitis or lymphadenopathy.

Diagnosis was made by a simple Gram stain of a **smear from a biopsy site**. Chains of gram-positive cocci indicated necrotizing fasciitis due to group A beta-hemolytic **streptococci**. The tissue Gram stain showed the same cocci.

At immediate surgical debridement necrosis extended to the muscle. Culture of the biopsy site yielded group A beta-hemolytic streptococci. The patient needed 6 weeks of intensive hospital care and skin grafting.

Necrotizing fasciitis is one of the **true emergencies** in dermatology, demanding immediate wide excision of the devitalized toxic tissue. Infection spreads along fascial planes, inducing thrombosis of blood vessels with gangrene and blistering of the overlying skin. Two significant features aid in its recognition. There is no lymphangitis and the biopsy site does not bleed. The necrotic tissue has lost its blood supply; intravenous antibiotics are of no help. So-called "cellulitis" that fails to respond to intensive antibiotics may be necrotizing fasciitis. It may develop in postoperative wounds, in a perirectal abscess site, around an ulcer, at sites of intravenous drug abuse, and even from an insect bite. Often, there is no antecedent event.

Diabetics are at the greatest risk for a lethal outcome, which occurs in nearly half of those with this frightening form of fasciitis. Your receptionist must be instructed that any patient with an unexplained rapidly enlarging bruise must be seen instantly. The bruise can be the purple mask of death.

Evarts CM: Diagnosis and treatment of **fat embolism**. JAMA 1965; 194:157–159.

If **petechiae** suddenly appear in the conjunctivae, axilla, or across the root of the neck 2 to 3 days after a fracture of the hip or long bone, suspect **fat embolism** and act quickly to give heparin. The petechial rash fades rapidly. Other signs include fever, tachycardia, tachypnea, and mental confusion. A skin biopsy of a petechia will reveal intravascular fat. Other laboratory findings include free fat in the urine (lipuria), increased serum lipase, decreased hemoglobin, and a "snowstorm" appearance on chest x-ray.

Fine J-D, Arndt KA: The **TORCH syndrome**: A clinical review. J Am Acad Dermatol 1985; 12:697–706.

The TORCH syndrome refers to the clinical findings of a group of clinically indistinguishable infections seen in the newborn. These infections are acquired in utero, and specifically they are: *t*oxoplasmosis, *o*ther infections, *r*ubella, *c*ytomegalovirus, *h*erpes).

Only by serologic and microbiologic study can the specific diagnosis be made, for clinically one sees a potpourri of:

petechiae	jaundice
purpura	"blueberry muffin" lesions
ecchymoses	

These latter represent **dermoerythropoiesis** and may occur anywhere on the skin, fading in a month or so.

Congenital herpes had one redeeming clinical diagnostic clue not seen in the others, viz., vesicles or vesiculopustules.

For specific laboratory differentiation:

toxoplasmosis—serial titres on antitoxoplasma gondii antibodies will rise
Rubella—virus can be cultured from nose and from urine
Cytomegalovirus—CMV specific IgM present; fresh urine sediment shows intranuclear inclusions in exfoliated cells; culture for CMV
Herpes—Tzanck smear shows multinucleated giant cells; culture vesicle fluid

Ordinarily, an acronym refers to a group of signs and symptoms in search of a diagnosis. In the case of TORCH, we have a group of diagnoses in search of a distinction.

Bowden JB, Hebert AA, Rapini RP: **Dermal hematopoiesis** in neonates: Report of five cases. J Am Acad Dermatol 1989; 20:1104–1110.

The "**blueberry muffin**" eruption of the newborn is characteristic of focal dermal hematopoiesis. It is associated with intrauterine viral infection or congenital hematologic dyscrasia. Clinically, the skin lesions are bluish-red macules or papules that fade soon after birth, leaving light-brown macules in the month-old infant.

The **differential diagnosis** includes other purpuric rashes such as in coagulopathies, thrombocytopenia, vasculitis, and drug eruption. Biopsy quickly distinguishes such mimics as histiocytosis, leukemia, and neuroblastoma.

Dermal hematopoiesis may signal either a contagious disease or an underlying disease. Its causes in the neonate center on:

congenital viral infection (TORCH)
twin transfusion syndrome
　　monochorionic pregnancy in which the placenta takes blood from one fetus and transfers it to the other, leaving the donor twin anemic and prone to hematopoiesis in the skin and the other, plethoric.
Rh hemolytic disease of the newborn
hereditary spherocytosis

In the adult, look for:

myelofibrosis
chronic myelogenous leukemia

Blueberry muffin syndrome sends you to the lab for:

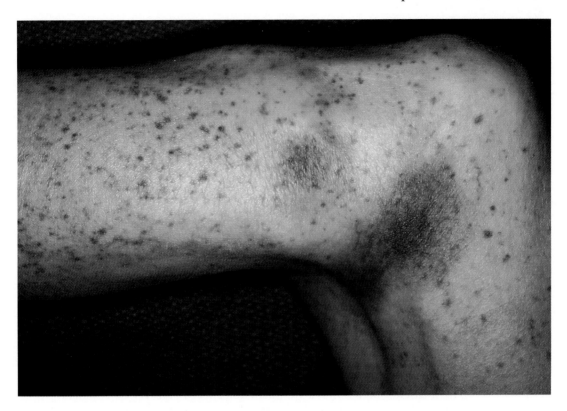

CBC, platelets, reticulocyte count, nucleated red blood cell count
Liver function tests
Cord blood quantitative IgM
TORCH IgG titres (*t*oxoplasmosis, *o*ther, *r*ubella, *c*ytomegalovirus, *h*erpes) in maternal and cord blood
rapid plasma reagin (maternal cord)
blood culture, bacterial
virus culture (nasopharynx, rectum, urine)
punch biopsy of cutaneous lesions

You won't see one of these "muffins" in a blue moon, but it is nice to be prepared.

Groark SP, Jampel RM: **Violaceous papules** and **macules** in a newborn. Arch Dermatol 1989; 125:113–118.

This female newborn exhibited scattered discrete **purple macules** and papules (2 to 10 mm). They did not blanch and were present at birth. The skin was jaundiced, and on examination the infant was found to have thrombocytopenia and hepatosplenomegaly.

A **biopsy** showed the lesions to be an example of **ectopic erythropoiesis**, occurring in the dermis. Known as blueberry muffin syndrome, it achieved recognition in 1964 when an epidemic of neonatal rubella occurred in which as many as half of the babies showed this purpura as evidence of red cell formation in the skin.

Today histologic evidence of dermal erythropoiesis sends the clinician in search of **three congenital infections**: rubella, cytomegalovirus, and toxoplasmosis. In this infant, the cause was shown to be cytomegalovirus by isolation of this virus in urine cultures. Also known to be associated with dermal erythropoiesis are the twin transfusion syndrome and hereditary spherocytosis.

The observation of purpuric macules and papules in the newborn in the absence of dermal erythropoiesis calls for **consideration of** the following:

neonatal sepsis
neonatal systemic LE
congenital leukemia
metastatic neuroblastoma

The true dermal erythropoiesis is most vivid as a blueberry muffin at 48 hours of life. It then "dries out" with a sequence of fading red to copper brown macules, with complete clearing by 6 weeks. By that time, the baby no longer needs an accessory myeloid system.

Caputo R, Ackerman AB, Sison-Torre EQ: **Acute hemorrhagic edema of the skin of the newborn** (Finkelstein's disease). *In* Pediatric Dermatology and Dermatopathology. Philadelphia, Lea & Febiger, 1990. Pp 81–88.

Its onset is heralded by fever, exquisitely tender symmetric edematous foci on face and extremities. These rapidly become **purpuric**. The climax lesion has a central hemorrhagic crust, a palpable ring, and a halo of redness. The lesions may show nummular, arciform, or polycyclic shapes; they appear in crops so that varying stages of development are present at one time. Although the child is in great distress, physical examination is normal aside from the skin.

It is a **disease of newborns or infants** and follows an upper respiratory infection by 2 weeks. Years ago the eruption commonly followed vaccination against smallpox.

Clinically, it is to be **distinguished from** Sweet's syndrome, erythema multiforme, and leukocytoclastic vasculitis. Sweet's syndrome does not involve the hemorrhage that Finkelstein's disease does. Erythema multiforme shows vesicles and bullae and a more striking target lesion. Henoch-Schönlein lesions do not usually occur on the face.

Finkelstein's disease fades in a week or so and does not recur. It is of unknown cause.

Look for **underlying infection**:

meningococcal meningitis
scarlet fever
diphtheria
pneumonia
syphilis

In newborns, causes of adrenal hemorrhage include prolonged labor, eclampsia, and congenital syphilis.

A diagnosis-oriented history is the most rewarding.

McConkey B, Fraser GM, Bligh AS, Whiteley H: **Transparent skin and osteoporosis**. Lancet 1963; 1:693–695.

Senile purpura occurred in 11 of 19 (58%) patients with transparent skin compared with only 7 of 33 (21%) patients with opaque skin.

Senile purpura alone does not correlate with osteoporosis, but 7 of 8 patients with senile purpura and transparent skin also had osteoporosis.

Rasmussen JE: Puzzling **purpuras** in children and young adults. J Am Acad Dermatol 1982; 6:67–72.

The **dark side of purpura** in children has the "colors" of infection, drug eruption, vasculitis, coagulation defects, and malignancy. The **light side of purpura** in children comes with the hues of a bruise caused by pressure (trauma) or a "pseudopurpura" caused by a harmless dye. These usually occur overnight in previously well patients and have a bizarre anatomic distribution with sharp margins and oval, circular, annular, or linear configurations. Skin biopsy, which is rarely needed except for legal implications, shows perivascular red blood cells in the upper dermis or the presence of dyes. A thorough history and physical examination are much more helpful than coagulation studies.

Be alert to the sudden appearance, unusual distribution, sharp margins, and bizarre shapes of purpura in children.

> **pants** pressure purpura (a purpuric band encircling the thigh due to tight pants, pantyhouse, or a plastic diaper cover).
> **opera glove** purpura (sharply marginated single arm purpura below the site of a venipuncture tourniquet or blood pressure cuff used the previous day when the child had an infection that compromised vascular integrity).
> **doughnut** purpura (a 3- to 6-cm ring at the site of impact of a hard ball used in squash or golf).
> **cough** purpura (occurs on the upper part of the body due to raised venous pressure; also seen with vomiting and childbirth, sometimes only on the cheeks and conjunctivae).
> **linear** and loop-shaped purpura (the imprint of grills, grates, or whips in the battered child).
> **palatal** purpura (a petechial circle on the soft palate caused by sucking hard candy or trauma from a hard object; consider possible child abuse or fellatio).
> **pseudobattering** (a Vietnamese treatment consisting of rubbing the chest and back with warm oil and then firmly stroking with the edge of a coin to produce broad purpuric bands parallel and perpendicular to the ribs.)
> **cupping** purpura (purpura on the chin and cheek due to sucking on a cup or mug slid over the chin; "coffee cup chin," "mug mouth").
> **passion marks** ("hickeys"–usually on the sides of the neck; often on the backs of the hands and forearms in the retarded).
> **suction cup** purpura (seen with children's crib toys and electrocardiograms).

Pseudopurpura is caused by topical dyes that localize in the depths of skin folds, skin lines, dermatoglyphics, and follicle ostia. It may mimic cellulitis. Diagnostic test: remove it with soap and water, mineral oil, alcohol, acetone, or Scotch tape.

Wilkin JK: **Benign parturient purpura**. JAMA 1978; 239:930.

Obstetric patients who vigorously "push" with **Valsalva maneuvers** during 1101 the second stage of labor may develop **petechiae on the face**, neck, upper chest, back, and arms. This reflects intermittent increased intravascular pressure in cutaneous blood vessels drained by the superior vena cava. The platelet count is normal. Coughing, vomiting, convulsions, and asthma may cause similar petechiae.

This must be distinguished from **disseminated intravascular** coagulation, particularly in preeclamptic patients, in whom generalized or acral petechiae or palpable purpura may be the presenting sign.

Alcalay J, Ingber A, Sandbank M: Mask phenomenon: **Postemesis facial purpura**. Cutis 1986; 38:28.

A 25-year-old woman headed for a hospital emergency room when she suddenly saw her face covered with hundreds of pinhead-sized red macules. It proved to be purpura brought on by vigorous **vomiting** 2 hours previously, associated with gastroenteritis. Blood studies were normal, and the macules disappeared within 3 days.

Whinnery JE: Comparative distribution of **petechial haemorrhages** as a function of aircraft cockpit geometry. J Biomed Eng 1987; 9:201–205.

High-speed turns in military aircraft subject the crew to **elevated G forces**, with resulting petechial hemorrhages on the legs, buttocks, and arms. The distribution of petechiae depends on cockpit configuration and can be blocked by wearing elastic bandages, stockings, and long-arm gloves to apply uniform counterpressure.

Mechanical purpura results from either an increased pressure inside the capillaries or a decreased pressure outside the capillaries. The purpura begins as small round, purplish spots (reduced hemoglobin) that change to yellow-green as the hemoglobin is broken down to bilirubin, and then tan-brown as the bilirubin gradually diffuses and is broken down to hemosiderin. Petechiae may be associated with an occasional mild pruritus following formation, which resolves in 24 to 48 hours. The dependent areas of the body are most susceptible to developing petechiae due to greater intravascular pressures.

In this type of purpura ("**high-G measles**") the exact mechanisms of formation are not yet known—whether it be capillary rupture, corrosive or ulcerative perforation, or diapedesis through the unruptured capillary wall. Increased capillary fragility has been observed with elevated venous vascular pressure, but whether it is fragility or permeability affected by high-G force is not known.

Lucia SP, Aggeler PM: Simply easy bruisability: **A pseudo-hemorrhagic diathesis** of probable endocrine origin. J Clin Endocrinol Metab 1942; 2:457–459.

Easy bruising without blood coagulation defects occurs in fair-complexioned women with thin skin who burn and freckle easily and are very sensitive to chemical irritants. Bruises smaller than 4 cm in diameter occur on the arms and legs after slight trauma, and at least one bruise is usually present. Bruising begins in childhood and increases during menstrual periods and at the menopause. Excessive bleeding may follow tonsillectomy or tooth extraction. Menstrual disorders, irritability, anxiety, fatigability, peripheral circulatory disturbances, and joint pains are common. A skin biopsy is not diagnostic, but results of thyroid tests may be low. Small doses of thyroid extract are helpful.

van Joost T, van Ulsen J, Vuzevski VD, et al: **Purpuric contact dermatitis** to benzoyl peroxide. J Am Acad Dermatol 1990; 22:359–361.

Irregular patches of **purpura** and erythematous papules suddenly appeared on the cheeks and chin of this 22-year-old woman. Clinically it looked like vasculitis. Actually it proved to be due to 5% benzoyl peroxide gel which she had been using.

Patch test validated the diagnosis of purpuric contact dermatitis. On biopsy the epidermis was completely normal. However, there was an eosinophil and mononuclear infiltrate around the vessels with evidence of obliteration of the capillary lumina resulting from endothelial swelling.

Significantly, primary **irritant contact dermatitis** from cobalt may express itself as a petechial eruption.

Nalbandian RM, Pearce JF: **Allergic purpura** induced by exposure to *p*-dihlorobenzene. JAMA 1965; 194:238–239.

A 69-year-old white man sat in a chair that earlier in the day had been treated with **mothball crystals of *p*-dichlorobenzene** by his wife. While seated, he experienced dyspnea, and 24 to 48 hours later he developed symmetrical purpuric lesions and numerous petechiae over the hands, forearms, feet, and legs, along with swelling of the hands and feet. He then developed acute glomerulonephritis and occult blood in the stool, all of which resolved following treatment with prednisone.

An indirect basophil degranulation test 5 months later was strongly positive, with 62% of basophils showing degenerative changes when tested with *p*-dichlorobenzene. The same test showed no sensitivity to aspirin, phenacetin, or caffeine.

Colver GB, Kemmett D: **Eruptive Capillary Hemangiomas**. Arch Dermatol 1991; 127:127–128.

The rapid onset of multiple petechial-like lesions can represent a benign eruptive form of angiomas known as eruptive capillary hemangiomas. They must be distinguished from petechiae as well as the pinpoint capillary angiomas of acute thyroid disease and angiokeratoma corporis diffusum.

Some diagnoses are made out of the corner of your eye, others out of the corner of your mind.

Drug

Capewell S, Reynolds S, Shuttleworth D, et al: **Purpura and dermal thinning** associated with high-dose inhaled corticosteroids. Br Med J 1990; 300:1548–1551.

Your asthmatic patient's purpura and thinned skin may simply reflect high-dose **inhalation of beclomethasone**.

McConkey B, Fraser GM, Bligh AS: Osteoporosis and purpura in **rheumatoid disease**: Prevalence and relation to treatment with corticosteroids. Quart J Med 1962; 55:419–427.

Osteoporosis and senile purpura are closely associated in rheumatoid disease, regardless of age or steroid treatment. They may be caused by similar collagen changes in bone and skin. Corticosteroid purpura closely resembles senile purpura. A high incidence of purpura correlated with an increased duration of **rheumatoid disease**.

Osteoporosis was found in approximately 30% (30/97) of patients who had rheumatoid disease and senile purpura. In rheumatoid patients with osteoporosis, senile purpura was seen in 55% (11/20).

Gafter U, Komlos L, Weinstein T, et al: **Thrombocytopenia, eosinophilia**, and ranitidine. Ann Intern Med 1987; 106:477.

A 57-year-old man with polycystic kidney disease, hypertension, and mild renal failure developed epigastric pain and was started on ranitidine hydrochloride (**Zantac**) for treatment of a duodenal ulcer. He was also taking aspirin and dipyridamole (Persantine) for antiplatelet aggregation treatment. Two weeks later he noted bilateral pedal hyperpigmentation. CBC showed hematocrit 40%, WBC 6500/mm^3, eosinophilia 13%, and platelets 70,000/mm^3. Two days after stopping ranitidine his platelet count was 170,000/mm^3, eosinophils were 17%, and no new purpuric lesions appeared. The purpura was probably due to drug hypersensitivity coupled with aspirin and dipyridamole.

Goldstein JB, McNutt NS, Hambrick GW Jr, Hsu A: Penicillamine dermatopathy with **lymphangiectases**: A clinical, immunohistologic, and ultrastructural study. Arch Dermatol 1989; 125:92–97.

Brownish-red hemorrhagic plaques had been appearing during the past 4 years over all of the bony prominences and areas of repetitive trauma (eyeglasses, phone receiver) in this 43-year-old man. Numerous cream-colored papules and areas of erosion and crusting were also prominent.

The biopsy showed thin collagen bundles, fragmented elastic fibers, prominent vascular channels, and small keratinous cysts. A history of 25 years of penicillamine for Wilson's disease revealed the cause and thus the diagnosis of penicillamine dermatopathy. **Penicillamine** by chelating the copper had on the one hand protected him from the hazards of copper storage of Wilson's disease and on the other hand gravely interfered with the synthesis of the vascular-supporting collagen and elastin.

Reducing his dosage of penicillamine from 2.5 gm a day to 1.0 gm a day was dramatically helpful.

This hemorrhagic dermatopathy is another example of the effect of chronic copper starvation.

Shelley WB, Sayen JJ: **Heparin necrosis**: An anticoagulant-induced cutaneous infarct. J Am Acad Dermatol 1982; 7:674–677.

A large, sharply marginated area of redness and hemorrhage developed on the lower abdomen of this 75-year-old man. Initially, it was viewed as an infected **hematoma** at one of the sites of the subcutaneous heparin injections he was receiving.

The area became indurated and within 5 days had developed a back eschar measuring 6 cm in diameter. At this point the other areas of injection on the thighs as well as on the abdomen showed large plaques of erythema, swelling and tenderness. The **eschar** was debrided leaving a deep ulcer, which healed over the next 6 weeks. The heparin injections were discontinued and skin tests done to determine whether or not the patient was sensitive to heparin. Intradermal skin tests to 5 different brands of heparin showed a positive erythematous response at 48 hours to all of them.

A definitive diagnosis was made of **heparin necrosis** due to intravascular clotting. This paradoxic reaction to an anticoagulant apparently results from the release of clotting factors from heparin sensitivity–induced platelet aggregates. This complication can not only involve the skin but also may arise from random thrombotic episodes leading to cerebral infarction or gangrene of an extremity.

The diagnostic laboratory prelude sign of such an event is a **dramatic fall in the platelet count**. Monitoring the platelet count can alert one to the nature of cyanotic sore toes in that patient receiving heparin therapy.

Gladson CL, Groncy P, Griffin JH: Coumarin necrosis, neonatal purpura fulminans, and **protein C deficiency**. Arch Dermatol 1987; 123:1701–1706.

In the yin and yang of blood coagulation, one of the powerful agents preventing intravascular clotting of the blood is **protein C**. Not identified until 1976, it now is recognized as a natural anticoagulant protease that blocks clotting Factors V and VIII and promotes fibrinolysis. Protein C is activated by an "ambivalent" thrombin, responsible for forming the fibrin clot. The action of protein C is enhanced by another vitamin K–dependent plasma protein, **protein S**.

The hereditary or acquired deficiency of either protein C or protein S allows clotting to proceed relatively unimpeded. Homozygous PC deficiency presents as neonatal purpura fulminans, with massive venous thrombosis of the skin and other organs in the first few days of life. Oral anticoagulants are an immediate necessity.

Paradoxically, the anticoagulant **coumarin** can occasionally cause focal clotting and skin necrosis in the first 3 to 5 days of administration. Coumarin inactivates both anticlotting and clotting factors that are vitamin K–dependent, permitting other clotting factors with much longer half-lives to become temporarily dominant.

Acquired deficiency of the PC pathway occurs in disseminated intravascular coagulation and possibly with diseases in which there is lupus anticoagulant, such as lymphoma and multiple myeloma.

Look for **protein C or protein S deficiency** in patients with:

> purpura
> ecchymoses
> hematomas
> necrosis
> gangrene
> thrombophlebitis (recurrent or familial)

There is a toad called uncertainty that often sits on top of our diagnoses.

Infection

Shelley WB, Zolin WD: Disseminate intradermal bacterial colonization presenting as palpable purpura in **lymphoblastic leukemia**. J Am Acad Dermatol 1983; 8:714–717.

This 68-year-old man, while in the hospital for chemotherapy of his lymphoblastic leukemia, suddenly developed scattered punctate, purpuric spots on his back. Over the next 5 days they became papular and spread over the entire skin.

The patient's white count had been 100 and 77/mm^3 while his platelets hovered around 1,000/mm^3. Although blood cultures were negative for bacteria, a biopsy of the skin showed numerous **clusters of gram-positive cocci**. Five days later the patient died of respiratory failure.

This terminal palpable purpura was construed as evidence that this patient's defenses against infection were totally gone. As a consequence, the dermis became a "vast gelatin plate" for growing bacteria.

Ashkenazi S, Mimouni M, Versano I: **Henoch-Schönlein vasculitis** following varicella. Am J Dis Child 1985; 139:440–441.

A 6-month-old boy developed a purpuric rash with small ecchymoses over the buttocks and extensor surfaces of both legs. His left ankle was swollen and tender. Scattered crusted lesions of **varicella** remained, which had started 10 days earlier as vesicles.

Garty BZ, Danon YZ, Nitzan M: Schönlein-Henoch purpura associated with hepatitis A infection. Am J Dis Child 1985; 139:547.

In an 8-year-old boy, pain, swelling, and dark discoloration of the right side of the scrotum appeared a few days before a purpuric rash on the penis, buttocks, and legs. His liver and spleen were enlarged, but there was no visible jaundice. His brother had had icteric **infectious hepatitis** 5 weeks earlier. Liver enzymes were elevated and an anti-HAV was positive.

These authors screen all Schönlein-Henoch patients for the following bacterial and viral infections:

streptococcal
upper respiratory tract
acute hepatitis A virus (HAV)

acute Epstein-Barr virus
influenza A

Ramilo AC, Jackson MR, Wise RD, Kaul A: *Mycoplasma* **infection** simulating acute meningococcemia. Arch Dermatol 1983; 119:786–788.

An acute purpuric petechial eruption of the trunk in a febrile, acutely ill 9-year-old boy resulted in hospitalization with a diagnosis of **acute meningococcemia**. However, cultures of blood, CSF, and needle aspiration of a petechial lesion disclosed no bacterial pathogen.

A chest roentgenogram showed pneumonic infiltrates in left lower and right middle lobe. Chloramphenicol therapy produced immediate clinical improvement and a resolution of the skin lesions within a week and a notable clearing of the lung changes. Acute and convalescent *M. pneumoniae* complement-fixing antibody titres provided a retrospective diagnosis of mycoplasma pneumonia. The initial level was 1:4 and the level at 14 days was 1:128.

This petechial eruption is a rare manifestation of a **mycoplasmic infection**, whereas it commonly occurs in meningococcemia. The usual cutaneous sign of the mycoplasma infection is erythema multiforme, but again this is an organism that can induce urticaria, a macular-papular morbilliform rash, as well as scarlatiniform and vesicular eruptions.

In the febrile patient with petechial and purpuric lesions, think first of meningococcemia. The simulators are less lethal.

Lesher JL: **Cytomegalovirus infections** and the skin. J Am Acad Dermatol 1988; 18:1333–1338.

The cytomegalovirus (CMV), a card-carrying member of the herpes family of viruses, has relatively little in the way of cutaneous credentials. Although it is the most common congenital viral infection known, there are no specific skin entities associated with its presence. It does not produce fever blisters, chickenpox, or zoster.

Its identity crisis comes from being placed in an acronymic syndrome that provides little in recognition of it other than its ability to make babies very sick. We refer to the TORCH syndrome, which covers the range of disease caused by *t*oxoplasmosis, *o*ther infections (syphilis, bacterial sepsis), *r*ubella, *c*ytomegalovirus, and *h*erpes simplex. Any one or all of these members of TORCH can cause:

hepatomegaly   microcephaly
splenomegaly   pneumonitis

with a cutaneous overlay of jaundice, purpura, and blueberry muffin lesions. The latter are violaceous, dark blue and red or magenta-colored infiltrative papules or nodules that represent temporary loci of extramedullary hematopoiesis in the skin.

Odd lesions recognized as being due to CMV on biopsy (large cell, intranuclear inclusion with halo) may include:

vesicles, bullae   perianal ulcers
papular acrodermatitis of infancy   indurated pigmented plaques
scleredema   vasculitis
mononucleosis with rubelliform rash

Immune-compromised and AIDS patients are particularly at risk for this virus.

Barrett-Connor E, Connor JD: Skin lesions and **shigellosis**. Am J Trop Med Hyg 1969; 18:555–558.

Two black sisters, ages 3 and 4 years, were hospitalized with fever, lethargy, dehydration, anorexia, watery diarrhea, cough, and multiple discrete petechiae (pinpoint to 2 mm) on the trunk and extremities. One child also had excessive tearing, while the other had severe photophobia, conjunctivitis, and a dendritic ulcer of one cornea. **Stool cultures** were positive in both for *Shigella sonnei*, and a blood culture in one child showed the same organism. Serologic tests were negative for measles and enterovirus in both children. Chest x-rays revealed bilateral pneumonitis in one girl and right lower lobe pneumonia in the other girl. Treatment with intravenous chloramphenicol was curative, and the corneal ulcer healed without scarring.

Skin manifestations in **shigella enteritis** are very unusual and may represent transient undetected bacteremia. Petechial lesions have also been reported with *Proteus* bacteremia. Extraintestinal complications of shigellosis, including pneumonitis, meningitis, and corneal ulceration, apparently may occur in the absence of bacteremia.

von Kuster LC, Genta RM: Cutaneous manifestations of **strongyloidiasis**. Arch Dermatol 1988; 124:1826–1830.

An acute generalized petechial and purpuric eruption in a 64-year-old man with lymphoma of the small bowel remained puzzling until a **biopsy** was done.

The microscopic examination of the purpuric skin showed not only red cell extravasation but also numerous **nematode larvae**. These proved to be live filariform *Strongyloides stercoralis* larvae, present in gastric aspirate, ascitic fluid, and urine, as well as bronchoalveolar lavage.

S. stercoralis is a nematode, unique in its ability to complete its life cycle in humans. Chronic infestation of the bowel may exist for decades without symptoms, or at least an unexplained eosinophilia with vague gastrointestinal symptoms.

In other instances the larvae may migrate to the skin, where its rapid movement through the dermis produces an intensely pruritic linear and serpiginous urticaria. Thus, the lesion may advance several inches while the patient sits in your waiting room. The buttocks, groin, and trunk are the usual sites for this form, called **larva currens** (racing larva). An attack may last but a few hours with intervals of weeks to months of freedom. The patient has difficulty in convincing the doctor of the reality of his problem. Some have been referred to a psychiatrist when the real need is for a stool examination. It is difficult to find the larva on biopsy since it is always well ahead of the visible urticarial track. Serpiginous urticarial lesions always call for ruling out zoonotic Strongyloides infections as well as ancylostoma (dog and cat hookworm) infections. In the latter only the epidermis is involved.

A second manifestation of Strongyloides is **chronic urticaria**. This presents as fixed urticarial wheals, lasting 1 to 2 days on the waistline and buttock. Again, one must look to the stool or a trial of thiabendazole.

The third form, exhibited by the patient described, is a rapidly progressive **petechial and purpuric eruption** of the trunk and proximal limbs. This usually reflects suppressed immunity and can be rapidly fatal. Indeed, the patient presented here lived less than a month after the petechiae appeared. The seriousness of dissemination and hyperinfection with Strongyloides demands that appropriate diagnostic (stool and serology) procedures be routinely undertaken before immunosuppressive therapy is instituted.

Finally, a few patients treated with systemic corticosteroids for dermatologic conditions ranging from pemphigus to lupus have also developed disseminated **strongyloidiasis** within a short time and died.

Thus, inattention to intestinal parasites can be hazardous to both the patient and your reputation as a diagnostician.

Benson PM, Lupton GP, James WD: **Purpura and gangrene** in a septic patient. Arch Dermatol 1988; 124:1851–1854.

Widespread ecchymoses, hemorrhagic bullae, and dry gangrene of the fingers and toes were the cutaneous signs of a pneumococcal sepsis in a 63-year-old woman who had had a splenectomy. Multiple blood cultures were positive for *Streptococcus pneumoniae*.

Such a purpura is labeled **purpura fulminans**. It has been reported with the following infections:

scarlet fever	varicella
Rocky Mountain spotted fever	rubella
leptospirosis	roseola

bacteremias:

streptococcal	meningococcal
staphylococcal	*Hemophilus influenzae*
pneumococcal	

fungal:

Candida sepsis

The **gangrene** results from disseminated intravascular clotting; similar occlusive changes may occur in the kidney, brain, lung, and gastrointestinal tract.

Removing the spleen increases the risk of sepsis, since these patients lack the ability to clear the blood of bacteria and they exhibit defective IgM.

The **differential diagnosis** of purpura fulminans is daunting:

> vasculitis (septic, allergic)
> thrombotic thrombocytopenic purpura
> coumarin or heparin necrosis
> circulating lupus anticoagulant
> macroglobulinemia (Waldenström)
> paroxysmal nocturnal hemoglobulinuria
> protein C deficiency (hereditary, acquired)

Stasko T, De Villez RL: **Murine typhus**: A case report and review. J Am Acad Dermatol 1982; 7:377–381.

A 72-year-old man was found in a debilitated state by his neighbors and referred into the hospital with a diagnosis of "**dermatitis and fever**."

He was lethargic, comatose, and had no purposeful speech. There was a diffuse purpuric eruption over the trunk and proximal extremities as well as the oral mucous membranes and scrotum.

Cultures of blood, spinal fluid, bone marrow, urine and skin aspirates were negative. Skin **biopsies** showed thrombosis of the superficial and deep blood vessels. Direct immunofluorescent studies showed numerous organisms reactive with **Rickettsia typhi** (*Rickettsia mooseri*).

Serologic data revealed a Weil-Felix reaction of OX-19 positive 1:320 and rickettsial indirect fluorescent antibodies positive at 1:512.

After a stormy course, including a gastrointestinal hemorrhage, the patient recovered. At that time he provided the history that 10 days prior to the onset of his illness he had been removing **dead rats** from traps.

Note that this patient's exanthem began on the trunk and spread peripherally, in contrast to the centripetal spread of the purpuric lesions of **Rocky Mountain spotted fever**. In both instances the purpura results from the growth of rickettsiae in the vascular endothelial wall with the ultimate destruction of the vessel wall.

This patient who was unable to give a history posed the problem of eliminating typhoid fever, virus infection, rat bite fever, drug eruption, and secondary syphilis as the cause of his purpura and fever.

Findlay GH: Dermatology of the **rickettsioses**. Recent Adv Dermatol 1983; 6:57–73.

The spots of Rocky Mountain spotted fever and the vesicles of rickettsial pox are due to the actual growth of minute gram-negative bacteria. These **rickettsiae**, introduced by the bite of an infected tick, flea, louse, or mite, live within the cells of the blood vessel wall. It is thus that they initiate the microthrombi, purpura, or vesiculopustules of diagnostic significance. Actually, full-thickness **gangrene** of the skin down to the muscle may occur. Both venous and arteriolar thrombosis have been seen. Likewise, the initial bite site may show local necrosis ("tache noire") or an eschar. And this entrance point may be the only skin sign of the disease. Typhoid fever can be distinguished because its rash is not hemorrhagic.

Fluorescent antibody staining of a small trephine biopsy will allow recognition of the pathogen. Do this immediately before any tetracycline therapy is initiated.

The larger the inoculum, the shorter the incubation period and the worse the course. Thus, ticks are the most harmful because they spend more time on the skin and introduce a larger inoculum.

Question your febrile purpuric patients for a history of travel and insect bites and recall that the average incubation period is 4 days.

Suleiman MNEH, Muscat-Baron JM, Harries JR, Satti AGO: **Congo/Crimean haemorrhagic fever** in Dubai. An outbreak at the Rashid Hospital. Lancet 1980; 2:939–941.

A 40-year-old Bengali man came to the emergency department with a 7-day history of sore throat, hoarseness, and slight oral bleeding, and was given antibiotics. The following day he returned very ill with fever, dyspnea, bleeding gums, markedly congested throat, and oral ulcerations. He then had a cardiopulmonary arrest with vigorous attempts at resuscitation, including mouth-to-mouth respiration by five medical staff personnel. Just before death he had massive fresh melena. Subsequently, five **secondary cases** developed among the medical staff, culminating in two deaths. Skin findings consisted of large ecchymoses on the flexor arms and forearms, including venipuncture sites, white spots on the buccal mucosa, and bleeding in the mouth.

The **virus** that causes **Congo/Crimean hemorrhagic fever** is widespread in Russia, Bulgaria, Yugoslavia, the Middle East, Pakistan, and East and West Africa. It is transmitted by infected cattle ticks of the *Hyalomma* spp. Insecticide dipping of the cattle might help stop spread of the disease.

When you are looking for the cause of disease, think food, bugs, and drugs.

Brauner F, Brenner W, Gschnait F: **Autosensitization** to DNA. Acta Derm Venereol 1980; 60:345–348.

Widespread, well-circumscribed **ecchymoses** of the arms, legs, and buttocks was the presenting complaint of this 45-year-old woman. The first attack had come 5 months ago with new lesions appearing every 2 to 3 weeks. There was no history of preceding trauma, each lesion arising spontaneously as a red tender patch. During the next few hours it either disappeared or enlarged peripherally, developing a blue ring-shaped periphery. Finally, numerous ecchymoses evolved and the lesions could be recognized as hematomas. There were no associated systemic signs or symptoms.

The **differential diagnosis** included the following:

amyloidosis Ehlers-Danlos syndrome
anaphylactoid purpura autoerythrocyte sensitization
pseudoxanthoma elasticum autosensitization to DNA

Biopsies showed the presence of marked edema and extravasation of red blood cells. Immunofluorescent studies were negative. The diagnosis was established by skin tests to autologous lymphocytes, as well as to calf thymus DNA. Both of these induced a pruritic pink plaque that had increased in size to 6 cm by 6 hours. Control subjects showed no response, nor was there any response to the injection of autologous red cells in this patient.

A diagnosis of **autosensitization to DNA** was made. Clinically, such a DNA sensitivity can be distinguished from erythrocyte sensitivity by virtue of its delayed appearance of ecchymosis. By contrast, in **autoerythrocyte sensitization** (**Gardner-Diamond syndrome**), the bleeding is the initial finding, followed later by swelling and tenderness. However, it is the skin tests that really reveal the antigen.

Alegre VA, Winkelmann RK: Histopathologic and immunofluorescence study of skin lesions associated with circulating lupus anticoagulant. J Am Acad Dermatol 1988; 19:117–124.

The presence of the lupus anticoagulant favors noninflammatory **thrombosis** of the small dermal vessels resulting in:

hemorrhage (ecchymoses, hematoma) ulcers
thrombophlebitis gangrene
necrosis

This lupus anticoagulant, first observed in patients with systemic lupus erythematosus, is a heterogeneous group of antiphospholipid antibodies that inhibit phospholipid-dependent coagulation tests.

Focal intravascular thrombosis alerts you to search actively for:

circulating anticoagulant thrombocythemia
protein C deficiency thrombocytopenic hematologic disorders
cryoglobulinemia

Diederichsen H, Sørensen PG, Mickley H, et al: **Petechiae and vasculitis** in asymptomatic primary biliary cirrhosis. Acta Derm Venereol 1985; 65:263–266.

A 65-year-old woman was hospitalized for study of recurrent **petechiae**, numbness, and burning sensations of the lower legs of 2 years' duration. Skin biopsy showed leukocytoclastic vasculitis with IgM, C3, and fibrinogen deposits in and around small vessels of the upper dermis. Circulating immune complexes were also found. However, it was the elevated liver enzymes and mitochondrial antibodies that led to a liver biopsy and the diagnosis of primary biliary cirrhosis.

1111

Asymptomatic liver disease can produce skin changes as part of its multisystem pathology. **Primary biliary cirrhosis** is classically associated with pruritus, hyperpigmentation, xanthelasma, maculopapular exanthems, thyroiditis, rheumatoid arthritis, mixed connective disease, and Sjögren's syndrome.

The liver is the root of much dermatologic evil. Think of it with vasculitis on the lower legs.

Rabiner AM, Joachim H, Freiman IS: **Hepatolenticular degeneration** (Wilson's disease) following splenectomy; inter-relationship of the reticuloendothelial and central nervous systems. Ann Intern Med 1941; 14:1781–1801.

A 23-year-old woman with mild parkinsonian coarse tremors of the arms for 4 years following typhoid fever gave a history of bleeding gums and a tendency to bleed excessively from slight wounds. The spleen was greatly enlarged (4 × normal) and liver was markedly cirrhotic. **Brownish-green pigmentation on the margins** of the cornea rapidly increased as her neurologic state deteriorated, and she died 3 months later.

A 25-year-old woman had frequent nosebleeds, easy bruisability, and excessive bleeding after tooth extractions. She began to tire easily and was found to be anemic and had marked **hepatosplenomegaly**. Following splenectomy, she developed tremors of the hands, fixed facial expression, and a circumcorneal ring of greenish pigmentation. The basal ganglia syndrome progressed and she died 2 years later.

Goette DK: **Unilateral palpable purpura**: A manifestation of septic emboli from an infected aortofemoral bypass graft eroding the jejunum. Arch Dermatol 1981; 117:430–431.

The title tells it all.

Kaplan RP, Grant JN, Kaufman AJ: Dermatologic features of the **fat embolism syndrome**. Cutis 1986; 38:52–55.

A 25-year-old Korean man fractured multiple bones in his right leg in a motorcycle accident. Initial laboratory tests indicated kidney damage (trace protein, 3+ glucose, 20 to 30 red blood cells/high-power field). He became febrile to 102°F the following day, following by increasing irritability, lethargy, and **petechiae of the conjunctivae**, head, neck, and upper torso on the 3rd day. His hematocrit fell from 39 to 24.6%, but coagulation studies were normal. He became hypoxemic, with chest x-rays on the 4th day showing patchy densities in the midlung fields. His urine became normal, with no signs of blood or fat. Skin biopsy showed distended dermal capillaries and extravasated red blood cells. No fat was detected, possibly due to Technicon processing. The petechiae disappeared by the 7th hospital day.

Signs of **fat embolism** include petechiae of the upper body, pulmonary insufficiency, and agitation, confusion, and stupor. Confirmation of the diagnosis may be made with frozen sections stained for fat, showing fat in the capillaries of skin in the petechial areas.

Causes of fat embolism include:

long bone fracture	extracorporeal circulation
carbon tetrachloride poisoning	external cardiac massage
pancreatitis	

Leone GE: **Spontaneous hemorrhage** into the suprarenals (suprarenal apoplexy). Ann Intern Med 1941; 14:2137–2142.

At 5 PM, a 43-year-old soldier who was getting over a mild drinking spree was admitted to the hospital with vomiting and epigastric pain. By 7 PM his temperature was 104°. At 4 AM a purpuric eruption was noted on the abdomen and extremities, which became generalized by 7 AM as a dark blue to black **petechial eruption**. He remained alert but seemed in shock, with no pulse or blood pressure. His temperature of 106° fell to subnormal shortly before 11 AM, when he suddenly died. At autopsy the entire skin, including palms and soles, was covered with bluish-red discrete purpuric macules varying in size from pinhead to 1 centimeter. The adrenal glands were hemorrhagic.

The purpuric eruption of **adrenal hemorrhage** is characteristic. Petechiae are bluish-red to purple and increase in size. They become generalized, including palms and soles, and coalesce around smaller joints, especially those of the hands.

Adrenal "apoplexy" causes sudden adrenal insufficiency with circulatory collapse and shock, generalized nonthrombocytopenic purpura, and marked pallor followed by cyanosis. Severe gastrointestinal disturbances accompany a high fever, which drops immediately before death. This picture may resemble acute hemorrhagic pancreatitis and splanchnic shock.

Before you request a test, you should first ask yourself what you are going to do if the result is positive, then ask yourself what you are going to do if the test is negative, and if the answers are the same, do not do it.

COCHRANE'S LAW

Syndromes

Roberts DLL, Pope FM, Nicholls AC, Narcisi P: **Ehlers-Danlos syndrome** type IV mimicking nonaccidental injury in a child. Br J Dermatol 1984; 111:341–345.

Extensive bruising of the arms, legs, and trunk of a 5-year-old girl resulted in hospitalization with the presumptive diagnosis of battered child syndrome. Poorly healed scars as well as bruises were seen in her skin, which had a transparent quality permitting ready visualization of the venous system. No abnormalities were found on hematologic study.

An electrofluoretogram of ^{14}C-labeled collagens produced on fibroblast culture showed a **type III collagen deficiency** diagnostic of **Ehlers-Danlos syndrome** type IV. Her brother and mother were then shown to have the same skin changes and an autosomal dominant hereditable defect in collagen III. Her mother also had premature aging of the skin of the face and extremities (acrogeria), pinched nose, and prominent eyes, which are features of this disease.

The "**battering**" this little girl suffered was from her parents, but not from their physical abuse. Thus, **Ehlers-Danlos syndrome** should be considered in all cases of undiagnosed easy bruising without a hematologic disorder, as the syndrome may be commoner than reported.

Alexander E, Provost TT: **Sjögren's syndrome**. Association of cutaneous vasculitis with central nervous system disease. Arch Dermatol 1987; 123:801–810.

Does your patient with palpable purpura of the lower extremities or urticaria-like lesions have **Sjögren's syndrome**—the dry eyes, dry mouth—or sicca syndrome?

Did you ask about a feeling of ocular grittiness, burning, itching, or foreign body sensation? Did you ask about photophobia or lack of tears? Did you ask if the patient is using eyedrops or increasing fluid intake to compensate?

Did you objectively check for xerophthalmia by measuring the 5-minute migration of tears along a strip of filter paper placed under the anesthetized lower eyelid? This is the Schirmer test; less than a 5 mm ring is abnormal.

Did you order a rose bengal dye test by the ophthalmologist to demonstrate punctate or filamentous keratoconjunctivitis sicca?

Did you ask about a dry mouth, increased dental caries, and recurrent swelling of the parotid gland? Did you ask about the use of sourball candies?

Did you look for saliva in the sublingual pool? Did you biopsy the lip for the presence of a lymphocytic infiltrate in the minor salivary glands?

If you made a diagnosis of Sjögren's syndrome, is it the primary form or is it secondary, i.e., associated with systemic lupus erythematosus, systemic sclerosis, or rheumatoid arthritis?

The basis for the cutaneous lesions of palpable purpura and urticaria-like lesions is **vasculitis**. Hence, some of your Sjögren patients may present with erythema multiforme, erythema perstans, erythema nodosum.

These are the patients who daunt the diagnostician who fails to hear or see the dry mouth or dry eyes. They have a "crock-full" of problems ranging through pneumonitis, hepatitis, glomerulonephritis, myositis, and thyroiditis. To top it off, they may have organic brain damage that precludes good history taking.

Schachne JP, Glaser N, Lee S, et al: **Hermansky-Pudlak syndrome**: Case report and clinicopathologic review. J Am Acad Dermatol 1990; 22:926–932.

This 45-year-old woman appeared to have a **bruising syndrome**. Even a venipuncture produced large ecchymoses. On query it was found that she had bleeding gums, postpartum hemorrhages, and her bleeding time had been shown to be prolonged.

She was a **Hispanic** from Puerto Rico but of notably lighter skin than her siblings. Her skin color and an associated photophobia was compatible with a diagnosis of albinism. The melanocytes proved to be tyrosinase positive, since although unexposed skin showed no pigment, on biopsy the sun-exposed freckled skin sample showed some pigmentation. This set the stage for making a diagnosis of **Hermansky-Pudlak** syndrome. It was confirmed by finding golden-brown granules in the macrophages in the papillary dermis. On ultrastructural studies this proved to be the pigment ceroid, completing the diagnostic triad of albinism, bleeding, and **ceroid deposition** that comprises the Hermansky-Pudlak syndrome.

Look for the **red-haired albino who is a bleeder**. This continuous deposition of ceroid through the body leads inexorably to the dyspnea of lung disease and also to the bloody diarrhea of granulomatous colitis.

Alegre VA, Winkelmann RK: **Histiocytic cytophagic panniculitis**. J Am Acad Dermatol 1989; 20:177–185.

The hallmark of this chronic entity is large inflammatory subcutaneous nodules or plaques of the arms and legs. In some patients the **panniculitis** is seen on the face, neck, and trunk as well. The lesions become **ecchymotic** and may ulcerate. Fourteen of the 19 patients reviewed were febrile and 9 had coagulation defects. In 13, the disease proved fatal, the other 6 responding to chemotherapy.

The clinical overlap is with **Weber-Christian disease** (chronic relapsing febrile panniculitis). Distinction is made histologically since these patients show on biopsy a benign histiocytosis with phagocytosis of red cells, leukocytes, and platelets alike.

It is, in essence, the **"hungry histiocyte" syndrome**.

If you don't have time to take a good history, the patient shouldn't take the time to see you.

Pustular Eruptions

The pustule is the hallmark of **infection**. Its classic expression is the impetigo of Bockhart, as well as sycosis barbae with its follicular pustules, a swarm of leukocytes in full attack on pathogenic staphylococci. Eosinophilic pustular folliculitis is a special form in which asymmetric patches of papulofolliculitis appear. Ordinary impetigo has its pustules also, but lacking follicular protection they are soon gone and replaced by crusts. One of the most characteristic pustular eruptions is that of candidiasis with its satellite pustules extending out from the primary intertriginous zone.

But the pustule is not always the sign of infection. One of the most persistent examples we see is the pustular eruption of the palms and soles. This may be a **bacterid** or the essential lesion of pustular psoriasis of that area. Far more alarming are the extensive explosive pustules arising on plaques of psoriasis in the generalized pustular psoriasis of von Zumbusch.

In the absence of psoriasis, the appearance of plaques of dermatitis studded with pustules is most likely a pustular **drug eruption**. These patients call for in-depth and repeated questioning regarding their intake of medicines, analgesics, vitamins, and cough syrups. When pustules appear in annular and circinate patterns, think of the subcorneal pustular dermatosis of Sneddon and Wilkinson.

In **pregnancy**, consider the diagnosis of impetigo herpetiformis, wherein the trigger is a sensitivity to the woman's own progestational hormone.

Look also to a history of **systemic disease**. The endotoxemia of ulcerative colitis, as well as that of the blind loop of bowel bypass surgery, may well induce macules and papules surmounted by pustules.

Recall that many **dermatoses** may show a pustular stage. Examples are miliaria rubra (which becomes miliaria pustulosis), dysidrosis, dermatitis herpetiformis, vasculitic syndromes, and contact dermatitis.

Pustules are hide-and-seek dermatology. The leukocytes are after something hidden in the epidermis and you must seek their prey.

Hoffmann TJ, Kettler A, Bruce S: **Acute acral pustulosis**. Br J Dermatol 1989; 120:107–111.

Numerous **pustules over the hands and feet**, as well as the forearms and lower legs, of this 32-year-old black patient had arisen overnight. The onset occurred just 4 days after a culturally proven **beta-hemolytic streptococcus** Group A **pharyngitis**. His only treatment had been a single intramuscular injection of benzathine penicillin for the sore throat.

On examination 4 days after the appearance of the pustular eruption, multiple hemorrhagic pustules and vesicles were seen on the palms and soles. A distinctive band of involvement covered the border between dorsal and plantar surfaces. The other areas showed only a few scattered pustules.

The patient showed no bacterial growth on culture of the pustules, nor were any hyphae seen on KOH examination. The blood showed an elevated antistreptolysin 0 titer (340 Todd units versus a normal of below 50). The Raji cell assay for **circulating immune complexes** was markedly elevated (220 μg AHG equivalents/ml versus a normal of less than 50). A skin biopsy showed an intraepidermal pustule filled with neutrophils. There was heavy fibrin deposition in the upper dermal vessels as well as a dense lymphoid cell infiltrate.

The eruption promptly subsided the following weekend, with no recurrence. A diagnosis of **acute acral pustulosis** was made with emphasis on the etiologic role of streptococci in inducing an immune complex–mediated disease. It thus may represent a true **bacterid**.

Waldman GD, Wise RD: **Miliary pustular syphilid**. Cutis 1984; 34:556–558.

A **generalized eruption of pustules** of 2-weeks duration brought this 25-year-old black woman to the doctor. On examination, she was found to have a temperature of 101.2°F. There were hundreds of discrete follicular pustules covering the entire body. The palms and soles exhibited copper-colored papules. The scalp revealed patchy alopecia. Smooth papilla-free macules were seen on the tongue. Cervical, posterior auricular, occipital, axillary, and inguinal **lymph nodes were enlarged** and firm. The labia minora presented numerous erosions.

It was the classic clinical picture of **syphilis**, strange only because of the pustules. A smear from the pustules showed only a Gram stain loaded with polymorphonuclear cells. On biopsy granulomata were seen. No spirochetes were found here, but transudates from the labial erosions were rich in **treponemes on darkfield examination**. The full battery of serologic tests for syphilis was positive. A diagnosis of secondary syphilis was made and confirmed by a **Herxheimer** response to penicillin therapy.

Big or little, flat or tall, pustuloderms call for serologic tests for syphilis.

Iwatsu T: **Cutaneous alternariosis**. Arch Dermatol 1988; 124:1822–1825.

Dark red plaques of the left cheek of this 77-year-old woman had been present for 5 years. They appeared to enlarge after she had topical and systemic corticosteroids. Clinically, the lesions were atrophic, sharply circumscribed, **infiltrated plaques** showing some scale, crust, and pin-sized pustules.

A biopsy showed **hyphae** in a granulomatous infiltration. Placing part of the biopsy specimen on potato dextrose agar without antibiotics and keeping it at room temperature permitted isolation, identification, and antimycotic drug sensitivity tests of *Alternaria tenuissima* at 5 days.

1117

The epidermal type of this **cutaneous alternariosis** is usually scaly infiltrated erythema or ulcers. The dermal form is usually plaques with papules, pustules, and crusts. The surface may be granular, atrophic, and vermiculate in appearance. Although immunodeficiency or severe debilitation predisposes to this condition, this patient was suffering only from hypertension and hyperlipemia.

Five years is a long time to wait for a diagnosis, but it is one that can be made only by biopsy.

Nunzi E, Parodi A, Rebora A: **Ofuji's disease**: High circulating titers of IgG and IgM directed to basal cell cytoplasm. J Am Acad Dermatol 1985; 12:268–273.

For 4 years this 64-year-old man had suffered an itching eruption. It began on the left calf and later spread to the back, chest, and thighs. Clinically, at the time of examination large polycyclic, brick-red, scaling plaques covered most of his body. Close observation revealed that the process began with erythematous follicular papules that coalesced into the sharply marginated plaques.

Noteworthy was the presence of:

follicular pustules at the edge of the plaques
thick scaling in certain plaques
cobblestone appearance of large papules in certain areas
loss of hair from affected follicles during healing

A complete blood count showed a **54% eosinophilia** with a white count of 9900/cu mm. *S. aureus* was grown from the pustules. Biopsy showed hair follicles destroyed and replaced by an eosinophilic infiltrate. There was a parakeratotic scale in the follicular pore.

A diagnosis of **eosinophilic pustular folliculitis** was made. It most closely resembles a diffuse pustular dermatophytosis, but scraping and cultures allow differentiation. The disintegration of the follicle as seen on **biopsy** distinguishes eosinophilic pustular folliculitis from follicular impetigo, pustular psoriasis, Sneddon-Wilkinson's subcorneal pustulosis, and nummular eczema.

Lewis JE: **Intestinal bypass dermatitis** occurring in a patient with a postoperative blind loop. Cutis 1988; 41:33–34.

A 57-year-old woman with Raynaud's disease developed over a 7-month period a series of hemorrhagic pustular nodules on her right thumb and index finger, resembling bullous pyoderma gangrenosum. Bacterial cultures showed no growth, but healing was rapid with oral metronidazole.

Four years previously she had undergone a hemigastrectomy and isoperistaltic antecolic gastrojejunostomy (Billroth II) procedure for a benign gastric ulcer. It is postulated that bacterial overgrowth in a blind loop of bowel led to circulating immune complexes of enteric origin, which then lodged in the compromised cutaneous blood vessels of her fingers.

Some dermatoses have to mature to be recognized.

Miyachi Y, Ikehata C, Imamura S: Localized pustular vasculitis in **rheumatoid arthritis**. Dermatologica 1982; 164:189–194.

A 46-year-old Japanese woman presented with multiple bean-sized groups of erythematous **papules** with **central pustule formation** that appeared suddenly on both shins. She had had rheumatoid arthritis for 10 years and was being treated with ibuprofen, indomethacin, and gold. Cultures of pustules were sterile. Skin **biopsy** showed a spongiform pustule with underlying leukocytoclastic vasculitis. Deposits of C3 were shown around blood vessels of normal skin 2 hours after an intradermal histamine challenge test (0.1 ml of histamine 0.01%) into normal skin. This suggests the presence of immune complexes, although no circulating immune complexes were found in the blood. Cryoglobulins were negative.

A diagnosis of **pustular vasculitis** was made. It is likely that nonspecific injury to the shins led to the trapping of circulating immune complexes within that skin and subsequent vasculitis.

Rouchouse B, Bonnefoy M, Pallot B, et al: Acute generalized exanthematous pustular dermatitis and **viral infection**. Dermatologica 1986; 173:180–184.

CASE 1

A 17-year-old woman with psoriasis of the knees and elbows for 5 years developed **generalized pustular erythema** on the trunk and limbs and erythema multiforme on the extremities one week after an episode of untreated pharyngitis. Numerous pustules 0.5 to 2 mm in diameter occurred in clusters and coalesced into large intraepidermal bullae on a background of scaling erythema. Her temperature was 38.5°C. Skin biopsy showed an intraepidermal non-necrotic bulla with neutrophils, parakeratotic crust, hydropic degeneration of basal cells, and a perivascular neutrophilic and eosinophilic infiltrate in the upper and mid dermis. Immunofluorescence revealed granular C3 deposits in upper dermal blood vessels. Extensive laboratory tests were normal except for erythrocyte sedimentation rate of 75 mm/h, 21,000 white blood cells mm^3 with 87% neutrophils, and IgM-neutralizing antibodies to **echovirus 30** positive at a titer of 128. The skin lesions healed in 10 days without treatment.

CASE 2

A 63-year-old man had generalized erythema, shivers, and fever of 40°C. Within a few hours a **scalded-skin appearance** resulted from the coalescence of pustules and erosions. He had had a sore throat 8 days earlier that was untreated, and 8 hours before the rash appeared he had taken 4 tablets of pristinamycin for a cut on his ankle. Skin biopsy showed eosinophilic subcorneal pustules, **leukocytoclastic vasculitis**, and intravascular C3. Routine laboratory studies were normal except for erythrocyte sedimentation rate of 60 mm/h, IgE level > 1000 IU/ml, and IgM-neutralizing antibodies to **coxsackievirus A9 positive** at a titer of 512. The fever disappeared in 2 days, and skin lesions cleared within 8 days.

CASE 3

A 52-year-old-woman with no history of psoriasis presented with widespread **pustular erythema** (sparing only the palms and soles) and fever of 40°C. She had experienced untreated pharyngitis 8 days earlier. Skin biopsy showed a spongiform neutrophilic and eosinophilic pustule, neutrophilic vasculitis, and intravascular C3. Laboratory studies were normal except for IgE 900 IU/ml and stool and urine cultures showing **echovirus 11**. Blood IgM- 1119 neutralizing antibodies to echovirus 11 were positive at a titer of 16. Skin lesions cleared spontaneously in 10 days.

This new clinical entity, first described in 1980, presents as an acute generalized exanthematous pustular eruption. The **diagnostic features** center on:

Generalized erythema with extensive, coalescent sterile pustules.
Erythema multiforme–like lesions.
Spontaneous healing in 10 days.
Fever.
Histology showing neutrophilic vasculitis and subcorneal, spongiform, eosinophilic pustules.

Each of the three patients reported here had untreated **pharyngitis** one week before the onset of the rash and evidence of infection with three different enteroviruses (echovirus 30, coxsackievirus A9, and echovirus 11). Only one patient had underlying psoriasis. Possibly, a transient viremia triggered the vasculitis, which then led to the pustules.

This entity must be **distinguished from**:

Generalized pustular psoriasis of von Zumbusch.
Pustular drug eruption.
Generalized pustular bacterid.
Pustulosis acuta generalisata (leukocytoclastic vasculitis).
Erythema multiforme with subcorneal pustules.

Most doctors when confronted with a diagnostic dilemma schedule visits further and further apart, whereas the master diagnostician schedules them more frequently.

Colver GB, Burge SM, Millard PR, Ryan TJ: **Dermatitis repens, Lapière and gener-alized pustular psoriasis.** Br J Dermatol 1985; 113:623–628.

A 3 × 4 cm indurated pustular plaque with lakes of pus beneath the crust appeared on the right calf of a 78-year-old woman with known psoriasis of the elbows since age 76. Skin biopsy showed large subcorneal pustules, and perivascular infiltrates indicated **dermatitis repens** (Crocker-Degos). She had had a previous plaque on that same calf, mistakenly thought to be met-astatic breast carcinoma and excised, which was also dermatitis repens. Der-matitis repens is a solitary **unilateral pustular plaque** that is recalcitrant and gradually enlarges to a huge size. Contrast this with **Hallopeau psoriasis** and **pustular bacterid (Andrews)**, which are bilateral and more acral.

Months later she developed an itchy red rash of the buttocks, arms, back, and thighs, resembling acute symmetrical annular erythema with active ery-thematous, slightly indurated margins, trailing scale, and central clearing, but only two pustules. Although toxic erythema was considered, biopsy again showed subcorneal pustules. Diagnosis was the Lapière-Milian type of an-nular **centrifugal psoriasis**. She also developed typical generalized pustular psoriasis, with many areas retaining an annular configuration.

In this patient the microscope gave witness to the unifying presence of subcorneal pustules in all three forms of her psoriasis: dermatitis repens, erythema annulare centrifugum, and generalized pustular psoriasis.

Oumeish OY, Farraj SE, Bataineh AS: Some aspects of **impetigo herpetiformis.** Arch Dermatol 1982; 118:103–105.

This 32-year-old woman developed a generalized erythematous rash with **pustules and fever** and malaise. The superficial pustules came in waves, with burning sensations. She was in her **34th week of a seventh pregnancy.** Her brother had had generalized pustular psoriasis of von Zumbusch.

Cultures were sterile and a biopsy showed spongiform pustules of Kogoj. A diagnosis of **impetigo herpetiformis** was made and the eruption controlled with prednisolone. At the 40th week, a full-term infant was born who lived only 48 hours. The patient's eruption completely faded with a subsequent 3-month course of tapered prednisolone.

Each of three subsequent pregnancies was associated with generalized **im-petigo herpetiformis**, requiring hospitalization.

The disease was then reproduced directly by **challenge with estrogens.** On the 40th day of contraceptive therapy (norgestrel 0.5 mg, ethinyl estradiol 0.05 mg) the impetigo herpetiformis reappeared. Discontinuing the hor-mones was followed by clearing. Once clear, the impetigo herpetiformis reappeared on the 36th day of challenge with norethindrone (5 mg/day). Significantly, 3 months of diethylstilbestrol (5 mg/day) later induced no rash.

The patient thus proved to be a veritable clinical laboratory for the study of this disease. She had a total of 10 pregnancies with attacks of impetigo herpetiformis in each of the last nine. There were 8 fetal deaths. Each suc-cessive attack began earlier during the pregnancy as her immune sensitivity heightened.

The family history of generalized pustular psoriasis of von Zumbusch in this patient supports the current concept that **impetigo herpetiformis** is a variant of **pustular psoriasis** triggered by progestational hormones and thus is often seen in pregnancy or with contraceptive hormones.

The role of pregnancy remains unquestioned as these authors observed the reappearance of the disease in nine successive pregnancies; Hebra, who first described and named impetigo herpetiformis in 1872, saw it in five pregnant women. And now the disease has appeared in the "pseudopregnancy" state of hormonal contraception.

Drug Eruption

Shelley ED, Shelley WB: The **subcorneal pustular drug eruption**: An example induced by norfloxacin. Cutis 1988; 42:24–27.

A 10-day generalized **exanthematic pustular eruption** in a 62-year-old man with a renal transplant 3 years previously proved puzzling. It began as erythema following 8 hours of sun exposure while fishing. Skin biopsy showed a subcorneal vesicle filled with neutrophils, suggesting impetigo, subcorneal pustular dermatosis (**Sneddon-Wilkinson disease**), or pustular psoriasis. He took multiple drugs, including cyclosporine, prednisone, prazosin hydrochloride, chlorthalidone, and most recently, norfloxacin for a urinary tract infection. Clinically, the **diagnoses favored** were pustular psoriasis, Sweet's syndrome modulated by cyclosporine, pustular miliaria, and drug eruption. Systemic steroids gave prompt clearing of the eruption, but shed no diagnostic light.

The diagnosis finally was made 2 months later when **norfloxacin** was prescribed again for a *Klebsiella pneumoniae* urinary tract infection. Within one hour of the first dose the patient saw five red pruritic papules on his right forearm. Following the second dose 7 hours later he developed erythroderma, which required hospitalization. Again, steroid therapy produced prompt clearing.

Norfloxacin is one of a **group of drugs** known to produce a distinctive subcorneal pustular eruption. Others include co-trimoxazole, furosemide, chloramphenicol, piperazine, carbamazepine, phenylbutazone, and pyrimethamine.

Although current monographs and texts do not acknowledge this class of drug eruption, it does occur and should be considered in cases of "idiopathic toxicoderma." You and your patient need not be ignorant of the true cause!

Shuttleworth D: A localized recurrent pustular eruption following **amoxycillin administration**. Clin Exp Dermatol 1989; 14:367–368.

A 3-year history of a recurrent **pustular eruption of the chin** in this 42-year-old woman was related to dental treatment. Further questioning revealed that because she had a congenital cardiac valve defect she was always given 3 grams of **amoxycillin** an hour before dental treatment. Within 12 hours her chin became irritated and erythematous; by 2 to 3 days later it was pustular. Resolution occurred within a week, with no scarring.

Cultures from the pustules were negative for fungi, bacteria, and viruses. The biopsy showed an intracorneal pustule filled with neutrophils. Repeated challenges with amoxycillin reproduced the eruption.

A diagnosis of a **fixed pustular drug eruption** was made, thus expanding our horizons as to the clinical presentations of a drug reaction in a fixed site.

Lauret PH, Godin M, Bravard P: **Vegetating iodides** after an intravenous pyelogram. Dermatologica 1985; 171:463–468.

Three days after an **intravenous pyelogram**, a 68-year-old woman with chronic renal failure developed fever and pustules over her face. Within a week the pustules became extensive soft, vegetating masses. Her face was swollen and she also had pustulous conjunctivitis. More pustules appeared on her legs as well as at a scratch site on the leg (Koebner phenomenon) and in a scar on her forearm. The **pustules** on the legs and knees showed inflammatory halos and soon become necrotic.

Bacterial and viral cultures of skin lesions were negative. Skin biopsy revealed acute necrotizing **vasculitis** with a heavy infiltrate of eosinophils. A diagnosis of iododerma was made. Recovery was complete by 6 weeks, has-

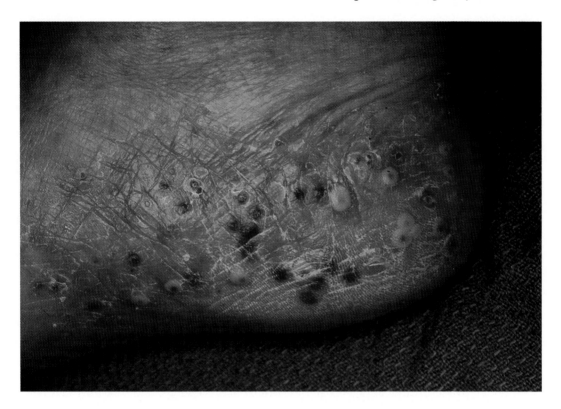

tened by a hemodialysis program with 2 sessions per week. After the first treatment her fever disappeared and no new pustules appeared.

Two factors contributed to this eruption: her chronic renal failure and the dose of radiopaque contrast dye (sodium diatrizoate) containing 30.4 gm of iodine. As a result, her serum iodine level climbed to over 14,200 μg/100 ml (normal 4 to 8 μg/100 ml).

Iodide-related eruptions have been reported in several renal failure patients, as well as normal individuals. The presence of fever and lesions on the face is of diagnostic significance. The range of lesions is great, simulating:

> vegetating pemphigus
> mycosis fungoides
> erythema multiforme
> acne
> pustular eruptions
> ulcers

Think of it not only with radiographic contrast media but also with iodine-containing drugs (Quadrinal, Calcidrine) and even povidone iodide (Betadine) irrigations.

Haste makes diagnostic waste.

Systemic Disease

Fenske NA, Gern JE, Pierce D, Vasey FB: **Vesiculopustular eruption** of ulcerative colitis. Arch Dermatol 1983; 119:664–669.

For 2 years this 32-year-old man had had diarrhea and dermatitis. The diarrhea was intermittent and watery. The dermatitis consisted of a generalized eruption of discrete **erythematous vesicles, pustules, and flaccid bullae**.

Biopsy showed neutrophil abscess formation within the epidermis. The immunofluorescent study was negative except for a slight band of IgG at the dermoepidermal junction. Cultures and stains for organisms were negative, as were stool cultures.

A barium enema disclosed mucosal ulceration, characteristic of **ulcerative colitis**. The lesions healed and the diarrhea lessened with sulfasalazine therapy (1 gm qid).

A diagnosis was made of vesiculopustular eruption of ulcerative colitis. The **differential** had included pyoderma, subcorneal pustular dermatosis, generalized pustular psoriasis, dermatitis herpetiformis, pemphigus, bullous pemphigoid, erythema multiforme, as well as papulopustular eruption of bypass surgery and drug eruptions.

Ulcerative colitis is well known for its dermatologic facies of pyoderma gangrenosum or erythema nodosum. However, numerous other dermatologic aspects may be **attributable to ulcerative colitis**. These include aphthous ulcers, urticaria, erythema multiforme, neurodermatitis, herpes zoster, and bacterial infections such as erysipelas and furunculosis vegetans. Rarely, pyodermatitis, dermatitis herpetiformis–like eruptions, and vasculitis may occur.

The ulcers of ulcerative colitis are indeed the portal of skin disease of all types.

Wright S, Phillips T, Ryan J, Leigh IM: **Intra-epidermal neutrophilic IgA dermatosis** with colitis. Br J Dermatol 1989; 120;113–119.

Multiple herpetiform, pus-filled vesicles and flaccid bullae were seen on the trunk and proximal limbs of this 73-year-old woman. Their onset was associated with an episode of bloody diarrhea. She had previously experienced a similar dermatosis that had healed spontaneously.

A biopsy of the skin showed a mid-epidermal bulla with a neutrophil and eosinophil infiltrate. IgA was detected in a suprabasal location. A rectal biopsy showed epithelial ulceration and, again, a heavy deposition of IgA in the mucosal epithelium. Circulating IgA could also be demonstrated using normal colonic epithelium, but not normal human skin.

A diagnosis of **intraepidermal neutrophilic IgA dermatosis** with IgA colitis was made. This is a unique, recently described form of bullous disease. It is to be distinguished from subcorneal pustular dermatosis by its pustular lesions being within the mid-epidermis rather than just above the stratum granulosum. It also showed a dramatic rapid response to dapsone, whereas subcorneal pustular dermatosis is more slowly responsive to dapsone therapy.

Ely PH: The bowel bypass syndrome: A response to **bacterial peptidoglycans**. J Am Acad Dermatol 1980; 2:473–487.

One in five patients having ileojejunal bypass surgery for obesity develops intermittent attacks of **neutrophilic dermatosis** associated with polyarthritis, tenosynovitis, malaise, fever, and cryoglobulinemia.

Skin lesions begin as 3- to 10-mm round or ovoid erythematous macules that evolve within 12 hours into palpable indurated insect bite–like papules, at times surmounted by vesicles. These become pustular, deep red, and indistinguishable from **gonococcal sepsis** in acral areas; many are tender or even painful. The legs may show tender red plaques and erythema nodosum–like nodules. Typically, lesions come in crops, fade over a week or so, and reappear monthly for several years.

The pathologist will call it "**Sweet's syndrome**" and the bacteriologist will report sterile pustules. After excluding flea bites and gonorrheal infection by history, the best diagnostic ploy is an **intradermal skin test.** *Streptococcus pyogenes* antigen (10^9 organisms/ml) reproduces the disease, with exacerbation of symptoms and induction of a papule with a central pustule. Absorption of bacterial antigens from an altered bowel in a sensitive patient is postulated as the cause.

The **bowel bypass syndrome** remains an "experiment of surgery" that teaches us to look for foci of infection in any patient having concurrent skin lesions and arthritis.

Dicken CH: **Bowel-associated dermatosis-arthritis** syndrome: Bowel bypass syndrome without bowel bypass. J Am Acad Dermatol 1986; 14:792–796.

The **bowel bypass syndrome** is a widely recognized complication of the jejunoileal bypass operation to treat marked obesity. The patients experience **crops of pustules** and papules appearing on the upper trunk and extremities. A panniculitis resembling erythema nodosum may also occur. These skin changes are accompanied by a flu-like episode of fever, chills, malaise, myalgia, and arthralgia. The illness lasts less than a week and may recur in a few weeks.

The **pustules are sterile** and reflect a circulating bacterial immune complex, the antigen being absorbed from the bacterial overgrowth in the surgical blind loop. Reversal of the bypass is curative and systemic antibiotics an alternate approach.

The same syndrome of papules, pustules, and febrile illness can occur in patients who have not had surgery but who have **bowel disease.** These include those with peptic ulcer, Crohn's disease, and ulcerative colitis.

Gonococcal sepsis mimics this syndrome; however, positive cultures quickly provide a diagnosis since the bowel syndrome lesions and blood are sterile on culture.

Grob JJ, Mege JL, Prax AM, Bonerandi JJ: **Disseminated pustular dermatosis** in polycythemia vera. Relationship with neutrophilic dermatosis of myeloproliferative disorders: Study of neutrophil function. J Am Acad Dermatol 1988; 18:1212–1218.

A 72-year-old man with the myeloproliferative disorder **polycythemia vera** developed a progressively severe widespread pustular eruption of 2 months' duration. The eruption was considered to be a manifestation of the polycythemia since careful study eliminated the following entities:

pustular psoriasis	dermatitis herpetiformis
drug eruption	bowel bypass syndrome
bromoderma	ulcerative colitis
folliculitis	

Thus, pustular dermatosis must be added to these well-known signs of polycythemia vera.

facial plethora	purpura
aquagenic pruritus	pyoderma gangrenosum
urticaria	

Pyoderma

The essence of clinical diagnosis is to discern form and order in the patient's presentation. For the diagnosis of pyoderma, however, one looks for disorder. By using the term pyoderma, we are recognizing the superficial crusted, erosive, even ulcerative lesions that often occur on a background of eczema, bites, and excoriations. It is the diagnosis of messy, junkyard skin. Although caused by pus-producing coccal bacteria, pyoderma has none of the morphologic integrity of other bacterial infections, such as furunculosis or staphylococcal scalded skin syndrome. But no term is more useful as a workhorse in daily clinical practice. Your next patient may well have this déshabillé dermatitis, whereas you may wait a year or more to see the crystalline diamond shape of erysipeloid.

But beware of dismissing the patient's problems as simply pyoderma. Look for background problems such as atopic dermatitis, scabies, insect bites, herpes simplex, contact dermatitis, or a faded impetigo.

Next, secure a culture. It will bring bacteriologic order into this diagnosis of disorder. Furthermore, sensitivity tests will direct your therapy.

Finally, explore the possibility that your patient's pyoderma is actually another entity in disguise. A fungal culture, blood count, and biopsy may widen your diagnostic horizon to include tinea, leukemia cutis, and familial benign chronic pemphigus. Nor should you forget to consider those namesakes pyoderma gangrenosum and pyoderma faciale.

Pyoderma is a workhorse diagnosis, but don't work it to death.

Coskey RJ, Coskey LA: Diagnosis and treatment of **impetigo**. J Am Acad Dermatol 1987; 17:62–63.

On culture of impetigo, 59 of 60 patients proved to have coagulase-positive *Staphylococcus aureus*, which was resistant to both penicillin and ampicillin. One patient had **beta-hemolytic streptococci** isolated, whereas six had mixed cultures of streptococci and *S. aureus*.

Tunnessen WW Jr: Practical aspects of **bacterial skin infections** in **children**. Pediatr Dermatol 1985; 1:255–265.

Streptococcal impetigo–Transient tiny vesicles soon rupture leaving expanding golden crusts with a little surrounding erythema. Local adenopathy common. Preceded by insect bites, abrasions, burns, lacerations. Watch for subsequent acute glomerulonephritis.

Staphylococcal impetigo–Cloudy intact bullae with no surrounding erythema; rupture to leave erythematous moist bases that dry quickly with a varnished appearance. May have thin collarettes of scale. No local lymphadenopathy.

Fehrs LJ, Flanagan K, Kline S, et al.: Group A beta-hemolytic streptococcal skin infections in a US meat-packing plant. JAMA 1987; 258:3131–3134.

During a 3 month period at an Oregon meat-packing plant, 32/69 workers had 44 episodes of pustular, draining, or inflamed lesions associated with hand lacerations. Meat is suspected as a vehicle of bacterial transmission; meat-packers have an occupational risk of infection.

Cultures from 50 lesions:

group A β-hemolytic *streptococcus* (38)
Staphylococcus aureus (12)
both (20)

Harnisch JP, Tronca E, Nolan CM, et al: **Diphtheria** among alcoholic urban adults. A decade of experience in Seattle. Ann Intern Med 1989; 111:71–82.

Look for **cutaneous diphtheria** under the guise of a *Staphylococcus aureus* or *Streptococcus pyogenes* **pyoderma**. You may think it simply ecthyma or a secondarily infected insect bite, bruise, or dermatosis. It has no pathognomonic features except a gray membrane around a skin ulcer.

You make the diagnosis on **culture**, and you enhance your ability to do so by asking the laboratory to culture on Loeffler or tellurite agar. In that way the "big bugs" are suppressed, allowing these lesser pathogens to be in full view in as short a time as 8 hours.

Cutaneous diphtheria is an important diagnosis to make, because without antitoxin and antibiotic therapy the patient is at risk for serious exotoxin-induced neurologic (Guillain-Barré) or myocardial lesions in a week or two. Cutaneous diphtheria and pyodermas are not the only skin problems of the **poor and unimmunized homeless**. Be alert for:

traumatic injury (shoe abrasions, purpura)
ectoparasites
intravenous and subcutaneous drug abuse
stasis dermatitis
AIDS
scurvy and pellagra

These are the diseases at home with the homeless.

Differential Diagnosis

Taylor J, Westfried M, Lynfield YL: **Pemphigus vulgaris** localized to the nose. Cutis 1984; 34:394–395.

A crusted lesion on the left ala nasi of a 65-year-old man resembled actinic keratosis and was read histologically as acantholytic actinic keratosis. However, the biopsy site failed to heal and enlarged with crusting and oozing, eventually covering his entire nose. Although a second biopsy came back "**actinic keratosis**," a third biopsy showed follicular acantholytic dyskeratosis.

Direct immunofluorescent studies revealed intercellular IgG in the epidermis, consistent with **pemphigus vulgaris**. The clinical diagnosis of pemphigus did not become more evident until 7 months later when classic intraoral erosions and erosions on the hair line and chest appeared.

Very early pemphigus may come to you as an **actinic keratosis** or **impetigo**. The diagnosis can remain in the dark until you turn on the immunofluorescent light.

Galimberti RL, Kowalczuk AM, Bianchi O, et al: **Chronic benign familial pemphigus**. Int J Dermatol 1988; 27:495–500.

Examples are presented that initially appeared to be:

impetigo	acanthosis nigricans
candidal intertrigo	seborrheic dermatitis of the scalp
tinea circinata	

Pruritus is a regular symptom, and the perilesional Nikolsky sign is generally positive. Skin biopsy shows a suprabasal vesicle with acantholytic fissures and villi, and the immunofluorescence is negative.

Powell FC, Muller SA: **Kerion** of the glabrous skin. J Am Acad Dermatol 1982; 7:490–494.

This is a report on four farmers and one veterinarian who had **boggy suppurative nodular lesions** on the forearm or chest. These were misdiagnosed as bacterial infections and unsuccessfully treated with incision, drainage, and antibiotics.

The correct diagnosis was made by **fungal culture**. Two were due to *T. verrucosum* and two due to *T. mentagrophytes*. In one the culture was negative despite a positive KOH examination. All responded to long-term griseofulvin therapy.

Infected cows exhibiting "**barn itch**" were the source, and inoculation by trauma the transfer mode. This type of dermatophytic infection is also known as **tinea profunda** or agminate folliculitis. It may be easier to recognize as an ectopic example of the scalp kerion so well known with tinea capitis.

Other conditions that this **kerion** of glabrous skin may **simulate** are sporotrichosis, blastomycosis, and mycobacterial infection. The key diagnostic key in these patients was their occupation.

Shum DT, Guenther L: **Metastatic Crohn's disease**. Case report and review of the literature. Arch Dermatol 1990; 126:645–648.

Small tender erythematous papules of the lower legs of this 24-year-old woman rapidly became draining **ulcerative nodules**. They appeared in episodes that coincided with flare-ups of her Crohn's ileocolitis, from which she had suffered for over 5 years.

Although the lesions appeared to be infectious, bacterial cultures were nega-

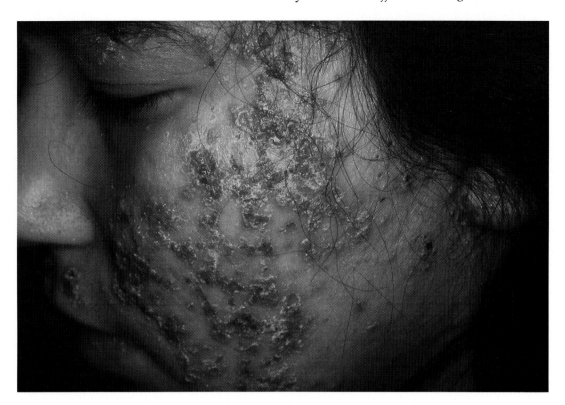

tive and treatment with antibiotics without benefit. Some lesions remained for as long as a year. A biopsy showed a sarcoidal granulomatous inflammatory picture identical to her bowel lesions. A diagnosis of **metastatic Crohn's disease** was made.

Twenty-three similar examples of "Crohn's lesions" at sites distant from the bowel are to be found in the literature. They have appeared on the penis, vulva, umbilicus, and face, as well as elsewhere.

Knowing your patient has Crohn's disease can help you make a diagnostic coup.

Pye RJ, Choudhury C: **Bullous pyoderma** as a presentation of acute leukemia. Clin Exp Dermatol 1977; 2:33–38.

In a 32-year-old woman, painless large purulent papules with brown crusts on the chin and wrist of 9 days' duration rapidly became bullous, with central ulcerations and necrosis. Despite systemic antibiotics, multiple new lesions appeared, along with a large white indurated lesion on the tip of her tongue. Neither laboratory studies nor biopsies provided a diagnosis, showing only intraepidermal bullae with a dense polymorphonuclear epidermal infiltrate. **Sweet's syndrome and pyoderma gangrenosum** were suspected. Within 2 weeks, however, blood changes showed **acute myelomonocytic leukemia**, Chemotherapy for 3 months led to complete disappearance of blast cells and healing of skin lesions; however, both reappeared later and she died of gramnegative septicemia 5 months after the onset of skin lesions.

Hemorrhagic **bullous lesions** suggestive of **pyoderma gangrenosum** have been reported in 15 other patients, including 7 with acute leukemia and one with metastatic adenocarcinoma. Other cases have probably been reported with the diagnosis of pyoderma gangrenosum or **Sweet's syndrome**.

Helander I, Aho HJ, Mäki J: **Lupus vulgaris** with Michaelis-Gutmann—like bodies in an immunologically compromised patient—cutaneous malacoplakia of tuberculous origin? J Am Acad Dermatol 1988; 18:577–579.

A 73-year-old woman had a sharply demarcated **oozing crusted area** of alopecia covering the entire crown of her scalp. Multiple skin biopsies showed only granulomatous inflammation with no organisms; however, Langhans type multinucleated giant cells containing spherical or elongated laminated or targetoid bodies were seen. Electron microscopy showed a concentric laminated intercellular Michaelis-Gutmann—like body and vacuolar intracellular spaces with myelin figures inside a multinucleated giant cell. The picture was consistent with **lupus vulgaris**.

Such bodies represent incomplete digestion of bacteria by macrophages and are characteristic of malacoplakia, a local inflammatory lesion that occurs usually with an immunosuppressive disease or treatment. This patient had a previous history of tuberculosis, positive PPD antibodies (ELISA), and newly diagnosed myelofibrosis with anemia and thrombocytopenia. She presumably had **malacoplakia of tuberculous origin**, which healed with scarring after antituberculous treatment.

Diaz LA, Sampaio SA, Rivitti EA, et al: **Endemic pemphigus foliaceus** (fogo selvagem). I. Clinical features and immunopathology. J Am Acad Dermatol 1989; 20:657–669.

Fogo selvagem is Portuguese for "wild fire"; indeed, these patients have not only a "burnt" appearance but also a "burning" pain in the lesions.

Clinical presentation

Superficial vesicles resembling impetigo, rupture easily leaving superficial erosions.
Always on head and neck and spreads acrally.
Positive Nikolsky sign.
Localized form:
  round oval keratotic plaques of seborrheic areas of face.
  yellow-brown or violaceous surface.
  looks and localizes like Senear-Usher syndrome.
Generalized forms:
  bullous exfoliative dermatitis.
  may develop fatal Kaposi's varicelliform eruption if exposed to herpes.
  also susceptible to scabies, tinea, warts.
  vesicles may form circinate, annular forms resembling tinea imbricata.
  exfoliative erythroderma with confluent crusted erosions.
  generalized keratotic plaques and nodules resembling prurigo nodularis.
Hyperpigmented form:
  during remission (in Portuguese, *aurora da cura*).
  dramatic increase in coloring (Caucasians look like mulattoes, mulattoes become black, black patients become gray-blue).
Incidence
  Endemic in Brazil; affects children, young adults, and families.
Biopsy
  Acantholytic intraepidermal vesicles in area of stratum granulosum.
Lab
  Autoantibodies to keratinocyte cell surface.
  No antinuclear antibodies (negative ANA, and the like).

Don't be puffed up with clinical pride. It goeth before a diagnostic fall.

Pyoderma Gangrenosum

There are ulcers and there are ulcers, but those of pyoderma gangrenosum are among the worst. They are ulcers that are deep, undermining, and necrotic. They are ulcers that bring excruciating pain. They are ragged ulcers that develop after minor local trauma, and progressively enlarge peripherally by the formation of satellite papules and ulcers along their margins. Healing occurs centrally with the formation of a thin atrophic scar, even as the disease rolls on with vegetative hypertrophic borders.

Although for grand rounds the resident's differential list of 20 diseases is an exercise in gamesmanship, the experienced clinician limits initial consideration to about three. In this case, he thinks of vasculitis, a deep fungal infection such as sporotrichosis, and factitial. A biopsy, fungal cultures, and personality assessment are his initial avenues for exploration. His history should rule out coumarin ulcers and his blood count, hemorrhagic purpura. A PPD will rule out tuberculosis, and the VDRL, the ulcers of tertiary syphilis.

And if it remains classic pyoderma gangrenosum occurring as it typically does on the legs in an adult, what window does it open to systemic disease? First and foremost, pyoderma gangrenosum is an entity in which bowel disease is a fellow traveler. Usually the patient has ulcerative colitis, but enteritis, gastritis, or vague abdominal symptoms somehow inter-relate with pyoderma gangrenosum. We personally suspect that episodic gram-negative bacteremia, such as from *E. coli*, with deposition of immune complexes in traumatized areas of skin, are involved in the pathogenesis of this disease. In that respect, pyoderma gangrenosum is a cousin of ecthyma gangrenosum, in which *Pseudomonas aeruginosa* bacteremia explains the necrotic black ulcers seen.

In the absence of a bowel disease association, look for blood dyscrasias such as leukemia, polycythemia vera, myeloma, or macroglobulinemias. Scan for hepatitis and also for HIV infection.

Often, such studies are noncontributory and you must return to the bowel because no disease reveals a gut-skin connection better than pyoderma gangrenosum. Ask your gastroenterologist for help in understanding it.

Schwaegerle SM, Bergfeld WF, Senitzer D, Tidrick RT: **Pyoderma gangrenosum**: A review. J Am Acad Dermatol 1988; 18:559–568.

Early lesions are small erythematous papules suggestive of erythema nodosum, erythema multiforme, folliculitis, or malabsorption and malnutrition. Rapid evolution leads to **tender pustules**, followed by necrosis and characteristic **ulcers with ragged undermined violaceous borders** and pus-covered centers. Exquisite pain and depigmented parchment-like scarring bordered by hyperpigmentation are **hallmarks of the disease**. **Factitial ulceration** and deep mycosis must be ruled out. Skin biopsy shows epidermal and dermal necrosis and ulceration with perivascular cuffing of lymphocytes and plasma cells, with or without vasculitis. The typical location is the **anterior leg**, but single or multiple lesions may occur at any site, possibly as a result of injury. **Exacerbations** parallel recurrences of bowel inflammation.

Look for associated diseases (not present in 25%):

Ulcerative colitis (50%)	Myeloma
Crohn's disease	Malignancy
Rheumatoid arthritis	Sarcoidosis
Hepatitis	

Wernikoff S, Merritt C, Briggaman RA, Woodley DT: **Malignant pyoderma or pyoderma gangrenosum** of the head and neck. Arch Dermatol 1987; 123:371–375.

The authors present a cogent argument that when pyoderma gangrenosum involves the face it should be recognized as such and not be given the diagnosis of **malignant pyoderma**.

They find no difference in the appearance, course, and response to therapy between malignant pyoderma and pyoderma gangrenosum. Both begin as pustular lesions that rapidly ulcerate with undetermined edges, have a recurrent, relapsing course, and finally heal with hypertrophic and cribriform scarring.

Malignant pyoderma refers only to the localization of lesions on the face. Such an anatomic feature would not appear to justify another diagnosis.

Wilson-Jones E, Winkelmann RK: **Superficial granulomatous pyoderma**: A localized vegetative form of pyoderma gangrenosum. J Am Acad Dermatol 1988; 18:511–521.

Twenty-five patients exhibited a superficial ulcerative and **vegetative pyoderma**, beginning with a single furunculoid purple abscess, nodule, or plaque that either discharged pus or was associated with pustules. Cultures were negative for bacteria, fungi, and mycobacteria. Lesions usually appeared on the back—sometimes along a scar—and often resembled **blastomycosis** and **dermatitis vegetans**, with crusted vegetative verrucous borders. **Sinus tracts** were often present. Healing took many months, even with antibiotics and steroids, and **cribriform scars** resulted.

This **subset of pyoderma gangrenosum**, identified retrospectively at St. John's Hospital (London) and Mayo Clinic, is probably a limited superficial granulomatous response to the pyoderma gangrenosum phenomenon. The ulcers were superficial and lacked the usual liquefying, rapidly advancing border of classic pyoderma gangrenosum. The ulcer base was also usually clean and granulating. None of the patients had gastrointestinal disease. Unusual histologic findings included giant cell granulomas, massive plasmacytosis, and tissue eosinophilia suggestive of allergic responsiveness to an antigen.

Draelos ZK, Hansen RC: **Hemorrhagic bullae** in an anemic woman. Arch Dermatol 1986; 122:1327–1330.

Large **hemorrhagic bullae** that became hemorrhagic crusts appeared first on the left ear then on the face, trunk, and lower extremities of this 33-year-old woman. She was anemic and had a history of a resection for a bowel infarct 2 years ago. The clinical appearance was nondiagnostic but brought forth the following **diagnostic sweep**:

bullous lupus erythematosus	coumarin necrosis
leukocytoclastic vasculitis	thrombotic thrombocytopenic purpura
pyoderma gangrenosum	purpura fulminans
Sweet's syndrome	paroxysmal nocturnal hemoglobinuria

The biopsy, which showed only thrombi occluding the arterioles and capillaries, quickly eliminated vasculitis, Sweet's syndrome, pyoderma gangrenosum, and lupus erythematosus.

The answer came when the patient was studied in depth hematologically to explain the anemia. There was increased hemoglobin in the serum and urine as well as hemosiderinuria. Her red cells showed a positive sucrose lysis test and the leukocytes showed an absence of alkaline phosphatase. These are the diagnostic findings of **paroxysmal nocturnal hemoglobinuria**.

Such hemolysis can be exacerbated by infection, drugs, trauma, emotional

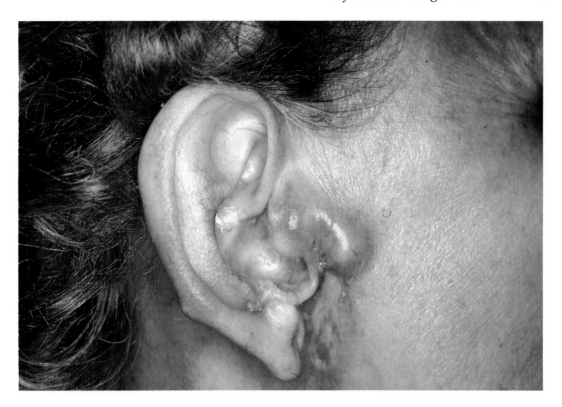

states, or transfusion reactions. Basically, the red cells are inordinately sensitive to complement but the nature of the critical feature of the thromboses remains unexplained.

Skin lesions in paroxysmal nocturnal hemoglobinuria are rare but dramatic. Think of them when the patient has a history of prior **infarcts**. Think of them with **bullae** that may present as black eschars with ulcers and with reddish blue spots, and think of them when the pathologist reports **thrombi**. They may occur on any area of skin from the tip of the nose to top of the toes.

Spiers EM, Hendrick SJ, Jorizzo JL, Solomon AR: **Sporotrichosis** masquerading as pyoderma gangrenosum. Arch Dermatol 1986; 122:691–694.

A negative report from special stains and cultures led to a 3-month delay in making the diagnosis of **sporotrichosis** in a 46-year-old man with nonhealing **ragged-edged ulcers** of the abdomen and thumb. The erroneous diagnosis of pyoderma gangrenosum was made when cultures showed no growth of aerobes, anaerobes, fungi, or acid-fast bacilli. Meanwhile, despite intensive steroid and dapsone therapy, the ulcer on the abdomen grew to 14 × 6 cm and the one on the thumb measured 2.5 × 1.5 cm, with violaceous undermined borders and extension deep into the fat.

Although the patient had been under care since September 1984, it was not until January 1985 that the **mycology lab** identified *Sporothrix schenckii*, noted originally in one of the cultures as an unidentified yeast. Historical cross-examination then revealed that the patient had trimmed a rosebush the preceding spring shortly before the onset of his problem. Six months of supersaturated potassium iodide therapy produced complete healing of the ulcers.

Norris JFB, Marshall TL, Byrne JPH: **Histiocytosis X** in an adult mimicking pyoderma gangrenosum. Clin Exp Dermatol 1984; 9:388–392.

Multiple painless ulcers (up to 3 cm in diameter) with purplish-red rolled edges and necrotic bases occurred on the back of a 58-year-old woman. She had had 2 similar ulcers of the breast $1\frac{1}{2}$ years previously, diagnosed clinically and histologically as **pyoderma gangrenosum**. No underlying disease had been found and the ulcers healed after 4 months of prednisolone therapy.

Although these ulcers appeared to be pyoderma gangrenosum, the **biopsy** revealed **histiocytosis X**. The mononuclear infiltrate proved on electron microscopy to be Langerhans cells filled with Birbeck granules. Review of the earlier biopsy of the breast disclosed the same cells, previously unnoticed in a sea of inflammation.

Skin biopsies of pyoderma gangrenosum should be examined with particular care, with a search for the characteristic Langerhans cells of histiocytosis X.

Lewis SJ, Poh-Fitzpatrick MB, Walther RR: **Atypical pyoderma gangrenosum** with leukemia. JAMA 1978; 239:935–938.

In two women, ages 42 and 32, pyoderma gangrenosum was the presenting sign of **acute myeloblastic leukemia**.

In one patient with fever, tenderness of the right buttock developed at an injection site and led to swelling, erythema, and edema which spread diffusely on the posterior thigh. A small central area of necrosis and purpura with a **bullous covering** then developed and rapidly enlarged, forming a 40 cm central **bulla on a necrotic base**. Cultures were negative and skin biopsy showed massive infiltration of neutrophils in the dermis and subcutaneous fat, with extravasation of RBC's and necrosis of the upper dermis, without vasculitis.

The other patient had three 5-cm **erythema nodosum-like nodules**, one on the left scapula and one on each shin. Three days later she had fever and chills, and the skin lesions had progressed to exquisitely tender, bluish-black necrotic indurated plaques with central bullae and erythematous halos. Cultures were negative and skin biopsy showed heavy neutrophilic inflammatory infiltrates without vasculitis.

Pyoderma gangrenosum lesions associated with **leukemia** are relatively superficial and form early central bullae, which rupture and continue to enlarge with wide bullous overhanging edges.

Cox NH, White SI, Walton S et al: **Pyoderma gangrenosum** associated with polycythaemia rubra vera. Clin Exp Dermatol 1987; 12:375–377.

Although **pyoderma gangrenosum** usually suggests the presence of ulcerative colitis or polyarthritis, it also may be associated with **hematologic disorders** (monoclonal gammopathy, myeloma, leukemia, polycythemia vera).

A 73-year-old man with **polycythemia vera** suffered six episodes of progressive painful ulcers with purple undermined edges and cribriform scarring following minor injury.

A 55-year-old man with **polycythemia rubra vera** had an **inguinal herniorrhaphy that failed to heal for 6 months**. Ulcerated lesions then developed at venesection sites and finally on the trunk and limbs. Antibiotics were of no avail; however, healing was achieved within 10 days of starting prednisolone (60 mg/day).

Massa MC, Doyle JA: **Cutaneous cryptococcosis** simulating pyoderma gangrenosum. J Am Acad Dermatol 1981; 5:32–36.

Multiple cutaneous ulcers and an area of **indurated cellulitis** on the right thigh of a 33-year-old man were associated with longstanding ulcerative colitis. Two skin biopsies confirmed a clinical diagnosis of pyoderma gangrenosum. However, a **silver methenamine stain** later revealed cryptococcal-like yeast forms and cultures from the ulcers all grew out *Cryptococcus neoformans*, confirming **cutaneous cryptococcosis**.

Pyoderma gangrenosum remains a clinical diagnosis that always requires the exclusion of specific diseases such as:

necrotizing vasculitis	syphilis
blastomycosis	atypical mycobacterial infection
sporotrichosis	synergistic gangrene
Behçet's disease	cryptococcosis
factitial disease	

It is well to think of pyoderma gangrenosum as a "first approximation" diagnosis, even in a patient with chronic ulcerative colitis. Pyoderma gangrenosum should be biopsied and special stains for fungi and bacteria should be done on all specimens.

Lerner EA, Kibbi A-G, Haas A: Calf ulcer in an **immunocompromised host**. Arch Dermatol 1988; 124:430–434.

In a 65-year-old man with a 30-year history of Crohn's disease, a large ulcer developed rapidly at the site of blunt trauma to the right calf. **Pyoderma gangrenosum** was diagnosed and he was admitted for intravenous antibiotic therapy, but the ulcer continued to enlarge and extended down into the muscle. Chest x-rays showed a nodule in the right lower lobe, and skin biopsy of the ulcer edge showed budding yeast forms typical of **cryptococcosis**. *Cryptococcus neoformans* was also **cultured** from the skin biopsy and cerebrospinal fluid. A serum cryptococcal antigen titer was 1:4096.

It is surmised that long-term prednisone therapy for Crohn's disease contributed to a primary focus of cryptococcosis in the **lung**, and that trauma permitted localization of circulating cryptococci in the skin. The usual source of infection is inhalation of *Cryptococcus* spores from pigeon droppings.

This patient illustrates how a very **reasonable morphologic diagnosis** (pyoderma gangrenosum) **can blind the clinician to the real disease**. His ulcer demanded consideration of the following diagnoses:

vasculitis	sporotrichosis
factitial ulcer	amebiasis
atypical mycobacterial infection	cryptococcosis
blastomycosis	

The *Cryptococcus* organism can usually be seen not only in biopsy but also on a KOH or Tzanck smear if the clinician is looking for it.

Note:

1. The culture medium must contain no cycloheximide since this compound is inhibitory.
2. India ink preparations dramatically display the capsule.
3. The disease was previously called torulosis (caused by *Torula histolytica*) and European blastomycosis.
4. All patients with cutaneous cryptococcosis must be carefully studied for disseminated disease (which is usually present).

This man's ulcer provided another example of the importance of looking beyond your diagnosis.

Radiation-Induced
Effects

Ionizing radiation kills. It kills the normal as well as the malignant cells and leaves its own scar of chronic radiodermatitis. Recognize this scar in patients who have had treatments years ago for acne, hirsutism, hand eczema, ringworm, and other benign conditions. They must be instructed that it is a precancerous scar.

The killing of cells produces a predictable acute and possibly chronic radiodermatitis. However, deep radiotherapy may explain the appearance of a variety of dermatitides. Be sure to ask about radiotherapy in your history taking. It may account for erythema multiforme, pemphigus, as well as a polymorphic dermatitis within weeks of the radiation. Might we call them radio-ids?

Radiation therapy may also be responsible for bullous pemphigoid (p. 393), vesiculobullous cutaneous lymphatic reflux (p. 419), and morphea (p. 1165).

Rosen T, Dupuy J, Maor M, Altman A: **Radiation port dermatophytosis**. J Am Acad Dermatol 1988; 19:1053–1056.

The puzzle was a **heavily crusted patch of dermatitis** on the left side of the neck entirely within the portal of radiation therapy being given this 50-year-old man for laryngeal carcinoma. The answer was in the positive KOH and *Microsporum canis* culture derived from the papulo pustules present.

It was assumed that the radiation induced a diminution in the local immunologic defense mechanism, although radiation trauma may have produced a locus minoris resistentiae. In any event, **tinea** must enter into the differential diagnosis of any radiation dermatitis.

Cochran RJ, Wilkin JK: Failure of **drug rash** to appear in a previously irradiated site. Arch Dermatol 1981; 117:810–811.

A dramatic perfect **rectangle of absolutely normal skin** was present on the right abdomen of this 12-year-old girl during a **generalized maculopapular drug eruption**. The explanation was not obvious until it was realized that this rectangle was the **entry portal for 4000 rads** given 6 years before in the treatment of a Wilms' tumor.

This same portal had been the site of radiodermatitis originally, but it had healed well, leaving the skin indistinguishable from the surrounding areas. Yet it can be assumed that subtle permanent vascular changes were induced by the radiation, which **"hardened" the skin to drug** reactions.

Perhaps the failure of the face and hands to be affected by many drug reactions results from a similar **protective effect** of lifelong radiation exposure to sunlight.

Rongioletti F, Pisani S, Rebora A: **Postradiation polymorphic dermatitis**. J Am Acad Dermatol 1990; 22:844–845.

After 22 external electron beam treatments, this 59-year-old man developed an edematous **papular eruption within the irradiated** area. Within hours it had spread to the arms and legs in an annular configuration.

Radiotherapy being given postsurgically for a pulmonary carcinoma was stopped, as well as the drugs he had been taking. Within a month the eruption had cleared. The oral medication was then resumed without incident.

A diagnosis was made of **polymorphic dermatitis due to deep radiation therapy**. It usually occurs in the form of **erythema multiforme** within 3

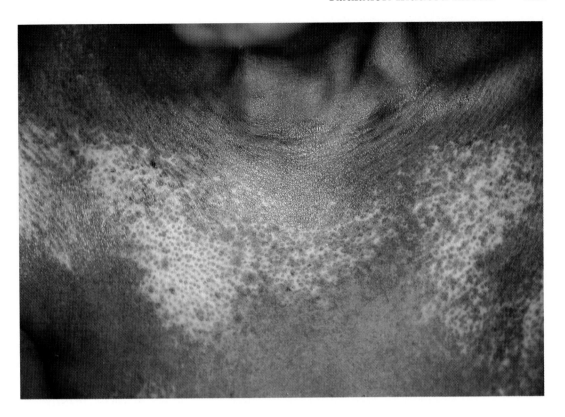

weeks of the radiation exposure. At times it may present as a pruritic urticarial or lichenoid eruption. It can also present as a papulovesicular bullous or purpuric change. Rarely, the problem becomes an exfoliative process, whereas often fevers and arthralgias accompany the skin change.

Even diagnostic x-rays may trigger a response 8 years after the primary episode. The patient truly becomes **sensitized to the irradiated cells**. Its presentation is so varied as to call for use of the name postradiation polymorphic dermatitis rather than lumping together all examples as postradiation erythema multiforme.

Do not expect to see it occurring often, as it is seen in only 1 in 5000 patients receiving deep radiation.

Kossard S, Commens CA: **Keratotic miliaria** precipitated by radiotherapy. Arch Dermatol 1988; 124:855–856.

Radiotherapy of an abdominal lymphoma in a 48-year-old man induced a monomorphous papular rash on a background of erythema precisely marking the radiation portal on his lower abdomen. It resembled **miliaria or pustular psoriasis** and appeared 3 weeks after the beginning of the radiation course (4000 rads in 20 fractions over 30 days). It subsided several weeks after the treatment was completed. Biopsy revealed lamellated keratotic plugging of the eccrine sweat pores and extensive keratinization of the entire eccrine apparatus.

This patient's eruption **differs from** the follicular comedones, digitate keratoses, and acneiform eruptions known to follow radiotherapy. It must also be distinguished from **neutrophilic eccrine hidradenitis**, which occurs in patients undergoing chemotherapy for lymphomas and consists of erythematous infiltrated plaques.

Salomon D, Saurat J-H: **Erythema multiforme** associated with radiotherapy. Dermatologica 1989; 179:110–111.

Look for a drug as the true cause, not an x-ray.

David M, Feuerman EJ: Induction of **pemphigus** by x-ray irradiation. Clin Exp Dermatol 1987; 12:197–199.

Radiotherapy (4000 rads) to a lymphoma of the retroperitoneum in a 70-year-old woman resulted in vesicles along the border of the irradiation field shortly thereafter. Within days, there were numerous flaccid vesicles and bullae over the abdomen, and lesions were also seen to a lesser extent on the chest, arms, and scalp. The Nikolsky sign was positive, and many brownish crusted erosions were present. Erosions were also observed on the buccal mucosa. Direct immunofluorescence of perilesional and uninvolved skin confirmed the diagnosis of **pemphigus vulgaris**. Circulating autoantibodies to the epidermal intercellular space were present at a titer of 1:80.

Pemphigus has also been reported to be induced by butazolidin, rifampicin, and *d*-penicillamine. Pemphigus-like antibodies also appear in burn cases.

Braun-Falco O, Plewig G, Wolff HH, Winkelmann RK: Dermatology. New York, Springer-Verlag, 1991, pp 379–380.

Acute radiodermatitis

Latent period: 6–12 days

First degree: Dark-red erythema followed by diffuse or spotty hyperpigmentation.
Transient alopecia begins 3 weeks after radiation, regrows in 4–12 weeks.

Second degree: Inflammatory erythema, edema, blister formation, exudation.
Permanent loss of hair, nails, sebaceous glands, and some sweat glands.

Third degree: Primary deep tissue necrosis leads to acute painful ulcerations that heal slowly.

Chronic radiodermatitis

Latent period: 2 years to decades; inevitable after second- and third-degree radiodermatitis; may occur after multiple smaller doses over long periods. Look for:

Poikiloderma: Atrophic and sclerotic smooth skin with telangiectases, mottled hyper- and hypopigmentation and loss of appendages.

Roentgen ulcer: Sharply defined central ulceration with a greasy yellow, firmly attached necrotic eschar. Very poor healing.

Roentgen keratoses: Horny, hard excrescences resembling actinic keratoses. Precursors of carcinoma.

Roentgen carcinoma: Hard infiltration palpable around a roentgen ulcer. Occurs in 20% of patients.

See your patients with difficult diagnostic problems in the morning and think about those problems the rest of the day.

Rosacea

Rosacea should be an easy diagnosis to make. It typically appears in a butterfly distribution over the cheeks and nose. Its signature is inflammation with redness, papules, pustules, and telangiectasia. It's usually seen in middle-aged women who have long been "blushers." Its course is insidious, on occasion leading to dramatic thickening of the skin of the nose known as **rhinophyma**. It often is accompanied by conjunctivitis and blepharitis, i.e., ocular rosacea.

But the diagnosis is not always easy—the **many forms** of this condition may deceive. In its earliest phase it may pass for a flush, seborrheic dermatitis, or photosensitivity. Its butterfly pattern may suggest **lupus erythematosus**. Its pustules call for a diagnosis of acne, and indeed one of its synonyms is rosacea conglobata, again making one distinguish it from acne conglobata. It may be viewed as a **gram-negative folliculitis** or a demodex-induced hypersensitivity reaction. Cultures and **demodex folliculorum** counts are necessary. It may be confused with tuberculosis, posing the question as to whether or not it is the rosacea-like tuberculid of Lewandowsky. In its fulminans expression it may have to be distinguished from pyoderma faciale.

Nor is it easy to distinguish morphologically from bromoderma or iododerma without benefit of history or serum levels of these halogens. Its granulomatous expression may be impossible to separate from **sarcoidosis** without biopsy. It may be confused with a papular syphilid in the absence of serology.

But with a diagnosis of rosacea, one of the most important things to do is to find out if it is a **steroid rosacea**. Long-term use of **fluorinated topical steroids** not only can worsen but actually induce rosacea. The wondrous daily remissions these steroids induce guarantee easy addiction in the uninformed patient. Furthermore, the use of these powerful steroids elsewhere can induce rosacea in ectopic sites such as the scrotum.

If the rosacea has appeared early in life, look for verrucous keratotic lesions elsewhere. With a family history of dry red facial skin and seborrheic keratosis, the findings point to **Haber's syndrome**.

The tendency of rosacea to slowly produce the hypertrophic skin of W.C. Fields is not limited to the nose. A whole spectrum of **facial "phymas"** may evolve singularly or in consort. These may show a predilection for the forehead (metophyma), the eyelids (blepharophyma), the ears (otophyma), or the jaw (gnatophyma). Beware of them and inspect closely. More than one physician has missed a **basal cell carcinoma** nestled unobtrusively and in full camouflage within these "phymas." Asymmetric focal growth, pearly or translucent appearance, as well as ulceration are your best clues. But as always, you often don't see what you are not looking for.

Fisher AA: **Steroid rosacea**: A friendly pharmacist syndrome. Cutis 1987; 40:209–211.

A 76-year-old woman's face had been covered with erythematous nodules for the past few years. Her history revealed that a "friendly" pharmacist had been regularly supplying her with **fluocinolone acetonide cream** for the past 5 years. Discontinuance of the cream was followed by prompt clearing of this nodular steroid rosacea.

Without benefit of history, one had to consider a **differential** of:

sarcoid	Jessner's lymphocytic infiltrate
lupus vulgaris	perioral dermatitis
granuloma faciale	polymorphous light eruption
tinea faciale	

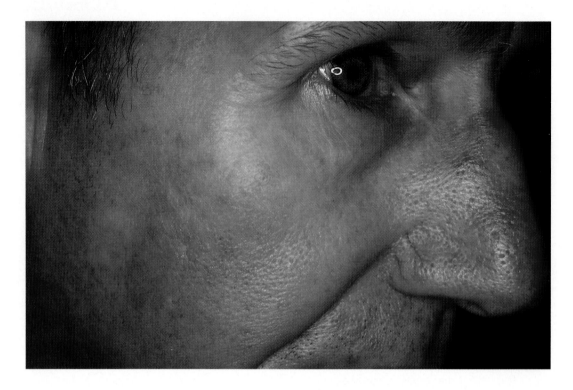

Shelley WB, Shelley ED, Burmeister V: Unilateral **demodectic rosacea**. J Am Acad Dermatol 1989; 20:915–917.

In any example of unilateral rosacea, scrape for *Demodex* mites.

If enormous numbers are found, they are the cause of the rosacea.

Rufli T, Mumcuoglu Y: The **hair follicle mites** *Demodex folliculorum* and *Demodex brevis*: Biology and medical importance. A review. Dermatologica 1981; 162:1–11.

Use the cyanoacrylate slide for a surface skin biopsy or take scrapings to look for an abundance of *Demodex* mites as a contributing cause of:

    rosacea
    blepharitis
    perioral dermatitis

Kikuchi I, Saita B, Inoue S: **Haber's syndrome**. Report of a new family. Arch Dermatol 1981; 117:321–324.

A 54-year-old Japanese man had **dry red skin of the face** and neck since boyhood, with a strong **burning sensation** aggravated particularly by wind exposure. All of his siblings suffered the same problem. His face showed areas of **orange peel–like induration** with enlarged follicular orifices and telangiectasia on a background of erythema and brown pigmentation. The anterior neck, axillae, and trunk had numerous 2- to 6-mm black papules, shown to be **seborrheic keratoses** on biopsy. Since age 40, he had developed dry brown scaly hyperkeratotic lesions on the elbows and dorsal feet, along with xerosis on the legs.

A diagnosis of **Haber's syndrome** was then possible, for this is a genodermatosis characterized by persistent rosacea-like facies and numerous verrucous lesions on unexposed areas.

A family history is the best clue about Haber's syndrome. Remember it to keep your own face from being red.

Sevadjian CM: **Pustular contact hypersensitivity** to fluorouracil with rosacea-like sequelae. Arch Dermatol 1985; 121:240–242.

Two days after beginning her third course of 1% fluorouracil cream for the treatment of actinic keratosis, this 51-year-old woman noted a weeping pustular reaction on her face. Although she stopped the cream at once, the eruption became more severe with edema, induration, and heavy crusting. It required systemic antibiotics and steroids to control and evolved into a rosaceal dermatitis.

Patch testing to **fluorouracil** (1% aqueous) produced a **pustular reaction** on the arm.

The eruption persisted with redness, flushing, and sweating of the face remaining for at least 2 years.

Day TW, Gibson GH, Guin JD: **Rosacea-like sporotrichosis**. Cutis 1984; 33:549–552.

This 64-year-old man had had the flushed appearance of rosacea of the nose and cheeks for the past 4 months. The unusual feature, however, was a crusted **advancing border** on the left nasolabial fold. His history disclosed he had been involved recently in extensive gardening and landscaping. Oral tetracycline as well as topical corticosteroids had been ineffective. A KOH examination had been negative.

The diagnosis came with the biopsy showing in PAS sections a number of budding yeast forms in a granulomatous setting. Study on culture showed *Sporothrix schenkii*, whereas cultures for bacteria were negative. The diagnosis was confirmed by the patient's rapid response to saturated solution of potassium iodide therapy.

The late onset, the crusting, and the failure to respond to tetracycline were all tips to the diagnostic mind to look for a better diagnosis than rosacea.

Swanbeck G, Bleeker T: Skin problems from **visual display units**. Provocation of skin symptoms under experimental conditions. Acta Derm Venereol 1989; 69:46–51.

Patients working with visual display units (VDUs) for long periods complain of a variety of skin problems ranging from pruritus to rosacea. A careful double-blind study with 30 such patients failed to show any effect of such electric or electromagnetic fields on the skin.

VDU dermatitis appears to be a **voodoo diagnosis**.

I love fixed ideas, but only if they can be changed.

FRANÇOIS JACOB

Scabies

If it itches and you don't know why, give scabies a try. Look for the epidemiologic trail of the mite as well as its **burrow**. Do others in the family itch? Often this is a better clue to scabies than the classical burrow. We usually see an erythematous skin covered with scores of scratch marks. More often than not the patient's fingernail has removed both the burrow and the mite, hence the value of microscopic study of subungual debris. Here you let the patient's fingernail do the scraping for you.

In the absence of burrows, we look for an intact **vesicle or papule** in the interdigital area. A subsection epidermal biopsy secured by transection with a Gillette Super Blue Blade provides an excellent specimen for study in xylene or oil. At the least, scybala or ova will be seen, but often the ghost-like outline of the mite comes into view. In an infant, the vesicles and burrows may be dramatic and obvious, especially on the soles. Again, the evidence of scabies is amplified in those babies who have been treated with steroids topically, thereby suppressing the immunologic defenses. Lacking confirmation, we ask the patient not to bathe for a week. Upon return, inspection of the elbows or elsewhere may well reveal an undisturbed burrow. Random multiple scrapings of itchy areas using a dull scalpel also can be rewarding.

Ultimately, one may have to resort to a **therapeutic trial** with lindane lotion or permethrin cream. But recall that for a cure everyone in the family or in the nursing home will have to be treated.

Dermatitis herpetiformis can present the same clinical picture of generalized excoriations. Here the response to dapsone clearly distinguishes dermatitis herpetiformis from scabies. Much less commonly individuals handling mite-infested animals or dried plant materials may show scabies-like lesions from bite and run mites. These acari do not stay on human skin nor do they burrow. The diagnosis here depends on finding the parasitized animal and effecting a cure by its removal.

We urge that the patient's entire skin be examined. One of us still recalls vividly the embarrassment suffered as a resident while presenting a young patient with a recalcitrant hand dermatitis, who had denied all skin lesions elsewhere. When the professor said, 'drop your trousers," classic **scabies of the penis** came into full view.

The longer scabies has been present the more difficult it is to make the diagnosis due to the inexorable eczematous changes, infection, and lichenification. It may even present as an **erythroderma**. Another special form of scabies includes nodules, seen especially on the penis and scrotum. In immunosuppressed or institutionalized individuals, scabies may take on a crusted hyperkeratotic form with involvement of the scalp and face, as well as elsewhere. Instead of a few mites being present as in ordinary scabies, thousands of mites roam and infest skin that shows little immunologic resistance. Keratotic (Norwegian) scabies is easily missed by those who have never seen it before.

In summary, think of scabies in those whose **itching** is more severe at night, in those in whom the face and scalp are exempt, in women with pruritic nipples, in men with itching papules of the penis and scrotum, and in those with itching shared by others. And think of a strange crusted keratotic scabies that also involves the face and scalp in transplant patients and in those with AIDS, leukemia, mongolism, and neurologic disorders.

If the hands are thickened, crusted, and fissured, reach for a blade with which to sample. The diagnostic and prophylactic rewards can be great.

Orkin M: Special forms of scabies. *In* Orkin M, Maibach HI (eds): Cutaneous infestations and insect bites. New York, Marcel Dekker, Inc., 1985, pp 25–30.

Scabies is "at once the easiest, and the most difficult diagnosis in dermatology" (JH Stokes, 1936). The **differential diagnosis** includes all pruritic diseases. Watch out for:

Scabies in the clean patient–ill-defined papular eruption without identifiable burrows. May include larval papules.

Scabies incognito–systemic or topical steroids may either ameliorate the symptoms and signs or cause the eruption to become much more extensive. Scabies may mimic other entities or be superimposed on other skin conditions.

Nodular scabies–reddish-brown pruritic nodules mimic lymphoma, clinically and histologically. Located on covered areas, particularly the male genitalia, groin, and axilla. Probably represent a hypersensitivity reaction.

Animal-transmitted scabies–puppies are the major source, with the external ears the most frequent site of predilection. May be acquired from 40 different hosts. Lesions occur commonly on the hands, but no burrows. Short incubation period. Excoriated papules occur at sites of contact with the infested animal.

Scabies in infants and young children–causes widespread secondary eczematous changes and bacterial infections with pustules, bullous impetigo, severe crusting, and ecthyma. Poor feeding results. Atypical distribution on head, neck, palms, and soles. Common in children adopted from foreign countries, who may have a recalcitrant dyshidrosiform or pustular eruption of the hands and feet.

Scabies in the elderly–severe itching, often blamed on dry skin. May lack inflammatory lesions. In bedridden patients, the back is frequently involved.

Crusted (Norwegian) scabies–generalized erythematous scaling eruption that is psoriasiform on the hands and feet with dystrophic nails. Highly contagious due to myriads of mites in exfoliating scales, resulting in epidemics in hospitals and other institutions. Favors the mentally retarded, physically debilitated, and immunologically deficient.

Venereal scabies–seen in VD clinics along with other sexually transmitted diseases. When genital lesions are present, look for gonorrhea and syphilis.

AIDS and scabies–crusted (Norwegian) scabies or scabies incognito associated with *Pneumocystis carinii* pneumonia points to AIDS.

Urticaria–widespread hives may overshadow inconspicuous scabies lesions.

Vasculitis–lesions on the lower legs may histologically show vasculitis and overshadow other scabies lesions.

Localized scabies–in solitary locations such as one axilla or the buttocks. Must examine household members and sexual contacts.

Acute glomerulonephritis—may occur if nephritogenic streptococci colonize scabietic lesions.

Shelley WB, Wood MG: Larval papule as a sign of scabies. JAMA 1976; 236:1144–1145.

The developmental or junior forms of *Sarcoptes scabiei* produce exquisitely **pruritic papules** that arise quickly in response to **larval mites** boring into the outermost epidermis. They do not form burrows but rather produce microchambers for molting, which surmount the papules. In a sensitized host the antigenic parasite calls forth a papule within hours. The patient's fingernails rapidly remove the acarus. Any mark, dot, or crust atop the papule probably means that the mite has been evicted.

It is important to biopsy an early papule in any pruritic eruption of unknown cause.

Arlian LG, Estes SA, Vyszenski-Moher DL: Prevalence of *Sarcoptes scabiei* in the homes and nursing homes of scabietic patients. J Am Acad Dermatol 1988; 19:806–811.

In a study of 37 cases of scabies, **live mites were found in dust samples** taken from 44% of the infested patients' homes. The density of live and dead mites ranged from 1 to 9 mites/m^2 of surface. Mites were recovered most often from bedroom floors, mattresses, and overstuffed chairs and couches. A person may thus become infested with dislodged mites in a contaminated home, school, or work environment. Sweeping the floors or doing the laundry in these areas could be hazardous.

In 5 nursing homes with scabies patients, only a small number of mites was recovered from beds, furniture, and floors. This suggested that mite-contaminated fomites may be less important in the transmission of scabies in nursing homes than in private homes.

Witkowski JA, Parish LC: **Scabies**: Subungual areas harbor mites. JAMA 1984; 252:1318–1319.

A 72-year-old woman with severe pruritus for 6 months had generalized dryness, punctate excoriations, scattered erythematous papules, and a few burrows on the fingers and elbows. Scrapings were positive for scabies mites. Treatment with lindane lotion cleared her symptoms after 5 days but generalized nocturnal pruritus occurred 6 days later.

Although her skin appeared clear, examination of **subungual keratotic debris** from several normal fingernails showed numerous mites. The nails were then cut and the subungual areas were scrubbed with a nail brush before application of the scabieticide. Although the pruritus cleared, it recurred in 10 days. Scrapings from beneath the nails of the right index finger and thumb showed a few mites and ova. The subungual areas were then compressed with lindane lotion for 2 days and the patient's condition then cleared.

Woodley D, Saurat JH: The **burrow ink test** and the scabies mite. J Am Acad Dermatol 1981; 4:715–722.

Gently rub a suspect papule with the underside of a **fountain pen** to cover it with ink. Wipe off the excess ink with an alcohol sponge. If a burrow is present it will be **vividly stained**. The burrow can then be removed with a superficial shave excision and placed on a glass slide for microscopic examination under a drop of immersion oil. Elevating the lesions with an 8-inch curved forceps prior to biopsy is especially helpful, particularly with interdigital lesions.

Highest yield sites are the medial hypothenar and wrist areas.

Vesicles and excoriations were omitted from this study as they are "low-yield" lesions for finding the mites, eggs, and feces.

Shelley WB, Shelley ED: Scanning electron microscopy of the scabies burrow and its contents, with special references to the *Sarcoptes scabiei* egg. J Am Acad Dermatol 1983; 9:673–679.

The **scabies burrow** is black, tortuous, threadlike, and slightly raised, measuring about 5 mm in length and 0.3 mm in width.

Serial transverse sectioning of a burrow, viewed under scanning electron microscopy, revealed a cluttered Lilliputian world crammed full of debris, including empty egg shells and large numbers of fecal pellets (scybala). The burrow winds from side to side and up and down within the stratum corneum. The mite continuously races against **desquamation** of the entire stratum corneum, which occurs every 2 weeks.

Blankenship ML: **Mite dermatitis** other than scabies. Dermatol Clin 1990; 8:265–275.

Mite bites should be suspected in any unexplained pruritic eruption. Most mites are rarely found on the patients, so that a clinical history is often the most important factor in detecting the causative agent. Mites are sought on the host or in the environment as indicated by the history.

Signs of mite dermatitis include:

erythematous macules	ecchymoses
papules	hyperpigmented macules
papule with central punctum	transient erythema
papulovesicles	angioedema
bullae	eczematous dermatitis
crusted papules	dermatitis herpetiformis–like
urticaria	varicelliform eruption
generalized pruritus	fine papular rash

Some mites bite at night to feed and then retreat to hide in warm concealed locations such as the backs of television sets, stoves, hot water pipes, heaters, radiators, baseboards, walls, and ceiling fixtures. The patient may complain of nighttime pruritus, irritability, and insomnia. Lesions often consist of groups of small hemorrhagic papules, vesicles, or urticarial papules. These mites may bite humans if their natural hosts abandon their nests (birds, rodents) or are killed off in extermination programs (mice, rats).

Look for:

   tropical rat mites (*Ornithonyssus bacoti*)
   northern fowl mites (*Ornithonyssus sylviarum*)
   tropical fowl mites (*Ornithonyssus bursa*–infest domestic poultry and wild birds such as the house sparrow)
   red mites of poultry (*Dermanyssus gallinae*–infest poultry, sparrows, starlings, pigeons)
   house mouse mites (*Liponyssoides sanguineus*)
   chicken mites (*Haemolaelaps casalis*)
   rat mites (*Hydroaspis fenilis*)

Mites that produce "grain itch" or "straw itch" feed on larvae of insects that infest grain and cause dermatitis, particularly at harvest time. They also infest seeds, plant stems, wood, and animal feeds. They are mainly *Pyemotes* mites. Agricultural workers are chiefly affected, although mites may also be encountered by sleeping on unsterilized straw or sitting on infested furniture.

Cheyletiella **mites** infest various mammals, causing "walking dandruff" on the back, with or without itching. The pet may be asymptomatic. Only one member of the household may be bitten, usually on the forearms, anterior thighs, breasts and abdomen where the pets are held and petted. Bites appear as pruritic small papules with pustules, crusts, and central necrosis. Cats, dogs, and rabbits are commonly affected, and treatment of their infestation is curative.

Gardeners, agricultural workers, and others who work around vegetation and orchards, as well as walk through grass, encounter mites predaceous on arthropod plant eaters. They bite humans incidentally, causing a stinging bite with a small hemorrhage and wheal. Some of these mites are large, fast moving, long-legged and bright red or orange ("whirligig mites"). Others are called "spider mites" due to their silk webs. Clover mites infest grasses and may migrate into houses during autumn.

Chiggers are the parasitic larval stage of trombiculid mites (harvest mites, red mites, red bugs). These six-legged red larvae hatch from eggs in the soil and lurk in the grass until a vertebrate host passes by, then crawl up the legs under tight clothing at the ankle, thigh or waist and engorge for 2 to 3 days on digested epidermis and lymph. No blood is taken. Itching begins 3 to 24 hours later, and an allergic reaction to the mite saliva causes extremely pruritic 3- to 6-mm erythematous papules that persist up to 3 weeks. There are 15 species of trombiculids around the world that cause trombidiosis (chigger bites). *Eutrombicula alfreddugesi* is the major cause of chiggers in the United States and Canada. In other parts of the world trombiculid mites are important vectors of rickettsial diseases such as scrub typhus. Host and mite populations occur in "mite islands" in widely diverse habitats, which shift locations over time and have wide variations in size.

Grocers, bakers, and others who handle stored food products encounter **mites which do not bite** but cause an allergic contact dermatitis. The allergens are located in the mite exoskeletons and feces. Dust with infested material may be a factor. Lesions consist of erythema with profuse minute papulovesicles and pustules on exposed skin areas such as the hands, forearms, face, and neck.

Look for:

Copra mites (*Tyrophagus putrescentiae*–dried coconut meat)

Wheat (pollard mites; *Suidasia nesbitt*)

Baker's itch (*Acarus siro*–cheese)

Dried fruit itch (*Carpoglyphus lactis*–dates, figs, prunes, feathers, skin)

Grocer's itch (*Glycyphagus domesticus*–hay, animal food, rotting food)

Coolie itch (*Rhizoglyphus parasiticus* and *R. hyacinthi*–onions, tea, plant bulbs)

House dust mites (*Dermatophagoides*) are free-living on the skin surface of mammals and birds and in skin detritus that accumulates in human habitats. They are also general feeders. Their allergens cause respiratory symptoms, but their role in atopic dermatitis remains to be proven.

Elgart ML: **Scabies**. Dermatol Clin 1990; 8:253–263.

Sarcoptes scabiei **mites** affect 40 different animal hosts belonging to 17 families. Pet owners, farmers, and animal handlers are at risk from dogs, cats, horses, goats, pigs, sheep, cattle, and lions. These mites cause mange with crusts and oozing on hair-bearing animals. Close personal contact is usually present, but the role of fomites in transmission of mites is unclear.

Canine scabies can affect any breed of dog. Inflammatory papules and crusts first appear near the ears after an incubation period of 4 to 6 weeks. They then spread to the axillae, groin, and midsternum, producing sarcoptic mange. Mites can easily be demonstrated in the crusts. If the condition is not adequately treated, the dog may die of secondary infection in a few months. Through direct contact with the dog, humans acquire bites most often on the arms, wrists, and anterior abdomen. Children tend to be most seriously affected and develop excoriated crusted papules with secondary infection. Itching occurs almost immediately after contact with the animal and subsides in several days after the dog is removed or treated.

Cat scabies, caused by *Notoedres cati*, is common in Czechoslovakia, India, and Japan but uncommon in Great Britain and the United States. Lesions affect the hands, legs, and face, especially in women. Cats also harbor the *Cheyletiella* mite.

Equine scabies used to be common, with lesions on the wrists and inner thighs of riders. The military variant was called cavalryman's itch. The lesions resemble those of canine scabies.

Arlian LG, Runyan RA, Achar S, Estes SA: Survival and infestivity of *Sarcoptes scabiei* var. *canis* and var. *hominis*. J Am Acad Dermatol 1984; 11:210–215.

Live mites affecting humans that were recovered from bed linen slept on by infested patients could still penetrate a host after 96 hours, even in alternating conditions of 12 hours of refrigeration and room temperatures.

At room conditions (21°C, 40% and 80% relative humidity) the human and canine-affecting varieties **survived** 24 to 36 hours off the host. The canine-affecting variety also survived 19 days at 10°C and 97% relative humidity, showing that lower temperatures and higher relative humidities favored survival.

Penetration required less than 30 minutes for all life stages and was accomplished by secretion of a solution that dissolves a minute depression on the host skin. The burrow in the stratum corneum then results from the digestion and consumption of dissolved tissue.

Hoefling KK, Schroeter AL: Dermatoimmunopathology of **scabies**. J Am Acad Dermatol 1980; 3:237–240.

The delayed host response (one month) in primary scabies coupled with the rapid (24-hour) host response in reinfection suggests a **hypersensitivity** mechanism. The histopathologic findings are compatible with an immune response, showing:

> acute eczematoid changes
> perivascular lymphocytes and eosinophils
> nodular form
>> dermal vasculitis
>> lymphoid hyperplasia

Direct immunofluorescence of scabies lesions in four patients showed a vasculitis-like pattern with IgM and C3 conjugates. IgM, IgA, C3, and fibrin were seen in the cornified layer of the epidermis, dermoepidermal junction, and papillary dermal vessels. The granular IgM and IgG deposits in the dermoepidermal junction resembled those found in lupus erythematous.

These findings support a humoral immune response secondary to scabies infestation. Previous studies had also demonstrated **IgE deposits** in vessel walls.

Dahl JC, Scwartz B, Graudal C, et al: **Serum IgE antibodies** to the scabies mite. Int J Dermatol 1985; 24:313–315.

In an effort to develop a specific serologic test for scabies, extracts were made from porcine scabies mites. Circulating IgE antibodies specific to these mites were found in 6 of 20 (30%) patients with scabies, as measured by the RAST test. However, they did not correlate with the duration of pruritus or total IgE levels.

The human scabies mite, *Sarcoptes scabiei* var. *hominis*, has **antigens in common** with other closely related mites. Immediate intracutaneous reactions and/or positive RAST reactions in scabies patients have been found with rat mite (*Notoëdres alepis*) and house mite (*Dermatophagoides pteronyssinus*) extracts. Immunologic reactions in scabies are quite variable and include types I to IV, indicating the presence of scabies-specific antibodies.

When it comes to scabies, a diagnosis in time saves nine.

Scalp

The scalp is the land of wens and dandruff. And it's a land hidden beneath hair. You have to painstakingly part the hair or use a hair blower to see the wart and the wen, the dermatitis, and the scale. And when this covering of hair is gone or going, the exposed crown becomes a site for the new problems of sunburn and actinic keratoses.

Aside from alopecia and hair breakage, which we review elsewhere, the most common problem of the scalp is **pruritus**. Look, really look, for nits and for pediculi. Remember, pediculosis capitis may be a second diagnosis—for example, in a patient with psoriasis of the scalp induced by the constant scratching. Consider the possibility of scabies "capitis" which remains untreated in the "from the neck down" treatment routine. However, the usual cause of pruritus of the scalp is **seborrheic dermatitis**. The diffuse redness may be all that you see, the tell-tale scale having been carefully shampooed out that morning by the "helpful" patient. Contact dermatitis due to shampoo, hair spray, hair tonic, or hair dye must be considered and the patient rigorously cross-examined. The range is from vitamin E creams to jojoba shampoos. Paresthesias of the scalp may occur, partially because the rich innervation of the 100,000 hair follicles of the scalp.

The **scale of dandruff** is the second most common diagnostic problem. Is it really the dandruff of seborrheic dermatitis? If the scaling comes from circumscribed well-defined patches, think psoriasis. If it is diffuse, contact dermatitis and atopic dermatitis in the differential. Patch tests may be necessary. In an adult, scaling of the scalp may be fungal in origin. A Wood's light, scrapings, and culture may make the diagnosis missed by others. Even kerions occur in adults. Don't mistake it for the boggy mass of bacterial infection.

The third major area of diagnostic interest is recalcitrant **infection**. Many patients suffer chronic staphylococcal folliculitis of the scalp. In its most insidious type, folliculitis decalvans, there is loss of hair and scarring. The infection may extend deep into the dermis and subcutaneous tissue as a dissecting cellulitis. Its boggy, inflammatory draining sinuses make it a fearsome entity of exquisite chronicity. And its name summons visions of the mythological age of slaying dragons. This dragon of a dermatitis is called perifolliculitis abscedens et suffodiens.

The scalp really is the land of wens and dandruff and dragons, too.

Elmros T, Hörnqvist R: **Infestation of scabies** in the **scalp area**. Acta Derm Venereol 1981; 61:360–362.

A 25-year-old woman had severe pruritus of the scalp for one month, with diffuse redness and scaling thought to be **seborrheic dermatitis**. Two months earlier she had had a pruritic vesicular interdigital eruption, self-diagnosed as scabies and successfully treated by herself, using a benzyl benzoate preparation. After 2 months of treatment with topical steroids, her scalp showed diffuse redness and excoriations, along with a 3- × 5-cm erythematous crusted scaly area. No burrows or vesicles were seen, but microscopic examination of the crust showed numerous scabies mites. Treatment with benzyl benzoate lotion both *above* and below the neck produced a prompt cure of her scalp problem.

Look for "**scabies capitis**" in pruritic scalp eruptions resistant to topical steroids. The mite can hide in crusts as well as in the stratum corneum.

Knight AG: **Pityriasis amiantacea**: A clinical and histopathological investigation. Clin Exp Dermatol 1977; 2:137–143.

A study of 71 patients with "**tinea amiantacea**" revealed:

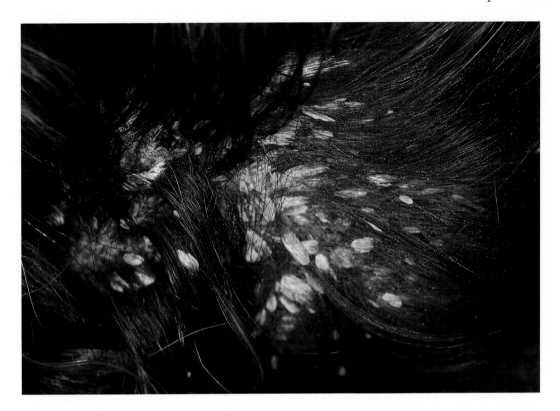

Thick heavy scales bind down tufts of hair.

The scales are shiny, silvery, and asbestos-like.

Usually there is associated temporary alopecia.

It is not due to bacteria or fungi (although *Staphylococcus aureus* was isolated in 4 cases).

It is not a manifestation of psoriasis.

Earlier studies suggested an infective etiology for this scalp problem. In 1917 Gougerot reported cases of impetigo transforming into pityriasis amiantacea, and in 1925 yeast cells were found in the scales. In 1929 a yeast organism was cultured from scales of 12 cases and inoculated into guinea-pigs, reproducing the disease.

Babel DE, Baughman SA: Evaluation of the adult carrier state in **juvenile tinea capitis** caused by *Trichophyton tonsurans*. J Am Acad Dermatol 1989; 21:1209–1212.

Cultures were taken from the scalp of asymptomatic parents or grandparents of children with *T. tonsurans* tinea capitis. One in every three grew *T. tonsurans*, suggesting an unrecognized source of reinfection.

Furthermore, **T. tonsurans** infection in the scalp can easily be **confused** with **seborrheic dermatitis** unless cultures are taken.

Conerly SL, Greer DL: **Tinea capitis** in adults over 50 years of age. Cutis 1988; 41:251–252.

For 2 months an 89-year-old woman had severe pruritus of her scalp, diffuse hair loss, and an excoriated pustular follicular dermatitis of the entire scalp. A boggy **kerion-type abscess** was present in the occipital region, and gentle plucking removed numerous hairs.

KOH examination showed endothrix hair invasion and 10 days later fungal culture showed **T. tonsurans**. Bacterial cultures of pustules revealed *Staphylococcus epidermidis*. Within 2 months of treatment with griseofulvin the scalp was healthy with excellent hair regrowth and negative mycological examination.

Family history revealed that 1.5 years earlier the patient's 6-year-old great-**granddaughter** had been treated for tinea capitis due to *T. tonsurans*.

Although this patient was in good health except for anemia, other examples of adult tinea capitis have occurred in immunosuppressed, diabetic, and debilitated patients. Listen for patient contact with children, especially children with hair loss problems.

Reque PG, Lorincz AE: Supravital microscopic fluorescent technique for the detection of **tinea capitis**. Cutis 1988; 402:111–114.

Add a drop of buffered 0.2 mM **acridine orange** solution (pH 7.2, citrate-phosphate buffer) to skin scrapings or hair clippings on a glass slide. Apply a glass coverslip and seal the edges with melted paraffin. Examine immediately using a fluorescent microscope (436 mm excitation filter, 490 mm barrier filter) for fluorescent hyphae, spores, or conidia. Sometimes exact species may be identified from characteristic macroconidia or microconidia. *Malassezia furfur* may also be identified.

A stock solution of 2.0 mM purified acridine orange in deionized water can be kept refrigerated for many months. A working solution is prepared by adding buffered filtered saline.

Stephens CJM, Hay RJ, Black MM: **Fungal kerion**—total scalp involvement due to *Microsporum canis* infection. Clin Exp Dermatol 1989; 14:442–444.

For 3 months, this 5-year-old girl had had generalized scaling of the scalp that was unresponsive to tar shampoo. It then rapidly evolved into a florid, foul-smelling **suppuration of the whole scalp**.

On examination the scalp showed boggy areas, weeping scaly plaques as well as numerous active tender discharging abscesses. The hair was matted in a thick yellow brown crust, with areas of **diffuse hair loss**.

A very faint green fluorescence of some sites and a scant number of round arthrospores were found surrounding the hair shafts. This confirmed the presence of an ectothrix fungal infection. However, it took a long period before cultures eventually grew out *Microsporum canis*.

The diagnosis of **kerion** was based on the extremely inflammatory response the child showed over the entire scalp. In such suppurative ringworm, the chance of finding the cause is enhanced by sampling fluorescent hairs and taking scrapings from areas of primary scaling.

Grattan CEH, Peachey RD, Boon A: Evidence for a role of local trauma in the pathogenesis of erosive pustular dermatosis of the scalp. Clin Exp Dermatol 1988; 13:7–10.

This chronic eruption of the scalp in elderly men and women consists of persistent well-defined **areas of crusting** and adherent keratinous debris, removal of which reveals moist superficial erosions and pus. Discrete pustules, open erosions, alopecia, and scarring are also common. Cultures frequently reveal *Staphylococcus aureus* or *Candida albicans*, but these are apparently **secondary invaders**.

In this series of 13 cases, **local trauma** to the scalp appeared to be an ante-

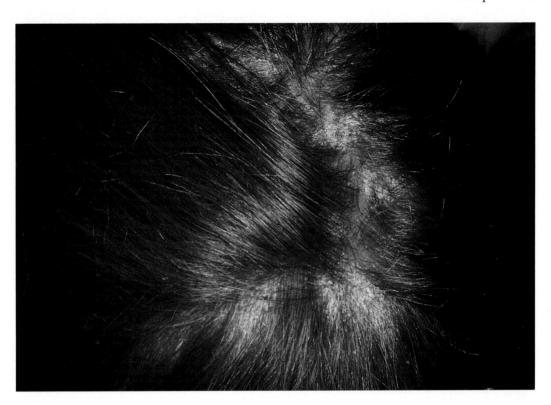

cedent factor in 12 patients. In half of the patients, the scalp was poorly protected by thin or absent hair. Six patients had herpes zoster in the ophthalmic division of the trigeminal nerve extending onto the frontal scalp. Others had preceding cuts, bruises, bumps, lacerations, sunburn, and marked actinic damage.

Ghorpade A, Ramanan C, Manglani PR: **Tuberculoid leprosy** on hairy scalp: A case report. Lepr Rev 1988; 59:235–237.

The **scalp** is considered to be one of the "**immune zones**" in leprosy because its **temperature is higher** than that acral areas. Lepromatous and tuberculoid leprosy involvement of the scalp is very rare and usually confined to bald or shaved areas.

In this case, a 45-year-old Indian man had had a well-defined erythematous dry anesthetic raised circular plaque 1 inch in diameter with sparse hairs on the occipital scalp for 6 months. Two similar larger plaques were present on the lower left leg and dorsum of the right foot. There was no nerve thickening, and slit-smear examination of skin lesions was negative for acid-fast bacilli. Scalp biopsy revealed **tuberculoid granulomas** with Langhans' giant cells.

Abdullah AN, Keczkes K, Wyatt EH: Skin necrosis in **giant cell (temporal) arteritis**: Report of three cases. Br J Dermatol 1989; 120:843–846.

In elderly patients **unexplained ulcerations of the scalp** may be due to **giant cell arteritis**. In some instances the ulcers may appear to be of factitial origin until the biopsy clearly shows an underlying arteritis.

The arteritis may involve only short segments of the vessel so that a single biopsy may fail to reveal its presence.

Dignostic clues present at times:

palpable tender arteries in temporal region and scalp
markedly elevated erythrocyte sedimentation rate
ulceration of face and tongue

Wyatt EH: **Cutis verticis gyrata**. Clin Exp Dermatol 1987; 12:293.

Thick folds developed over the entire scalp during 19 years of scratching and rubbing of vesicopapular lesions by a 41-year-old man. The skin showed **lichenification** as well as patches of "rubbed out" hairs and some epidermoid cysts. Scalp biopsies showed chronic inflammatory changes with folliculitis and epidermoid cysts with foreign body giant cell reaction.

A diagnosis was made of **cutis verticis gyrata** associated with atopic dermatitis. His serum IgE was greater than 1000 units/ml and he had multiple positives on RAST testing.

Ross JB, Tompkins MG: **Cutis verticis gyrata** as a marker for internal malignancy. Arch Dermatol 1989; 125:434–435.

This 56-year-old woman had noted gradually increasing **lumpiness of scalp** for the past year. On examination there were thickened indurated folds in the scalp extending from the anterior margin to the vertex. Biopsy showed minimal inflammatory change.

A diagnosis of **cutis verticis gyrata** was made. Five months later she complained of an occasional intermittent itch; examination revealed a firm immobile mass in the right lower quadrant. Laparoscopy disclosed a stage III **carcinoma of the fallopian tube** and widespread abdominal **metastases**.

Resection of the tumor and cisplatin therapy led to a cure and complete regression of the gyrate folds in the scalp. Cutis verticis gyrata thus proved in this patient to be a paraneoplastic disease and as such an indication for early CT scans.

Khare AK, Singh G: **Acquired cutis verticis gyrata** due to rotational traction. Br J Dermatol 1984; 110:125–126.

Cutaneous folds resembling **cutis verticis gyrata** were present on the scalp of a 70-year-old holy man of India, who also had scalp folliculitis, scaling, crusting, and left parietal alopecia. The **folds resulted from traction pull** on his hair, which he had plaited for 55 years. Due to lack of combing, washing, and cutting, the plaits became matted in time, requiring a new row of plaits that pulled up a new fold of skin. The force was tremendous because his hair was $6\frac{1}{2}$ feet long.

It should be noted that the hair itself had not grown to be $6\frac{1}{2}$ feet long, but rather the plaits resulted from "weaving" in of shed hairs. The **world record for long hair** is 26 feet, recorded in an Indian Sadhu.

There are two small holes in your skin to let diagnostic light enter your brain. Keep them both open.

Scar

A scar is rebuilt skin. It has been rebuilt by fibroblast carpenters who worked randomly in the absence of the original DNA architectural plans, which were destroyed by disease or trauma. It is a jerry-built collagen replacement without any elastin. Sometimes it is too thin, sometimes too thick. But it does help us diagnostically.

Here are scars that have left their mark on us:

Solitary dimple scar of an infant	Amniocentesis needle puncture
Bald, white stepping-stone scars of scalp	Pseudopelade
Small smooth, shiny scars of scalp	Folliculitis decalvans
Cobblestone aggregate scarring of occipital scalp	Folliculitis keloidalis
White atrophic, faintly pitted scars of concha of ear	Diagnostic for discoid lupus erythematosus
Conjunctival bands: symblepharon	Ocular pemphigoid
Bands of worm-eaten type scar, e.g., eyebrow	Atrophoderma vermiculatum, ulerythema ophryogenes
Scar encircled by tumor	Regressing basal cell carcinoma
Rolling-countryside scars	Acne
Large scars near hairline or in scalp	Acne varioliformis
Smooth white, slightly depressed	Varicella
Irregular, thick and thin with cords	Burn
A swarm of scars traveling in a band	Herpes zoster
Thickened red scar of sternal area	Keloid
Telangiectatic atrophic scars	Poikiloderma vasculare atrophicans, chronic radiodermatitis
	Excoriations
Multiple depigmented scars—arms, legs, or back	
Stretch mark scars	Striae atrophicans
Cigarette paper wrinkling scar	Mid-dermal elastolysis
Bizarre, geometric	Factitial
Soft depressible papules	Anetoderma
Multiple small scars of elbows	Papulonecrotic tuberculid
Thin, crinkled scars of knees	Ehlers-Danlos syndrome
Scar with papules	Sarcoidosis

A scar is a scar is a scar, and only a scar if you don't ask why.

Owen SM, Durst RD: **Ehlers-Danlos syndrome** simulating child abuse. Arch Dermatol 1984; 120:97–101.

Because this 6-year-old girl had had eight visits to the emergency room over the past four months for repair of lacerations, the attending physician considered her **scarred lacerated skin** could be the result of child abuse. When the parents failed to cooperate, a judge ordered a child abuse evaluation done by the child psychiatry department on an in-hospital basis.

Examination showed the child's skin to be soft, hyperelastic, and **paper-thin**. There were multiple scars and bruises in varying states of resolution. These scars had resulted from healing by secondary intention, with "railroad tracking" as evidence of the sutures that had been placed initially. The patient's head showed lop ears, epicanthic folds, and a crooked nose. The joints were hyperextensible, and near the right knee there was a molluscoid pseudotumor. Detailed studies of her general health, affect, and behavior over the $2\frac{1}{2}$ weeks of hospitalization revealed no other changes and no evidence of child abuse.

A diagnosis of **Ehlers-Danlos syndrome** type 1 or the gravis type was made. The patient's parents had initially failed to cooperate although fully aware of the nature of their daughter's india rubber skin. Their reluctance to co-operate reflected their fear that the father, who had the same skin problem, might lose his job if his employer learned of this disability.

Although this little girl had the prototypical type 1 Ehlers-Danlos syndrome, and certainly the most common form, there are at least 7 other well-defined **types**:

> II–mitis, milder
> III–largely limited to joint hypermobility, may have Barlow's syndrome of floppy mitral valve.
> IV–ecchymoses, rupture of large arteries, and even the bowel (Sack-Barbas type).
> V–laxity of joints limited to fingers. Skin stretchable but joints normal. This is X-linked recessive; all others are autosomal dominant (I, II, III, VIII) or autosomal recessive (IV, V, VI, VII).
> VI–retinal detachment, ocular rupture due to lysyl hydroxylase deficiency.
> VII–congenital dislocations due to protease deficiency.
> VIII–loss of teeth from severe periodontosis; fragile skin over shins.

Raimer SS, Raimer BG: **Needle puncture scars from midtrimester amniocentesis**. Arch Dermatol 1984; 120:1360–1362.

Two **dimple-like depressions** were noted on the back of a newborn baby girl. They were 2 mm scars of amniocentesis needle punctures she had sustained as a 16-week-old fetus.

Other infants have been observed to have linear scars rather than the typical dimple form. Indeed, the **amniocentesis needle** has been held accountable for blindness (corneal puncture), ileocutaneous fistula, ileal atresia, peripheral nerve injury, patellar disruption, gangrene of a limb, and a porencephalic cyst. Unfortunately, the fetus has no place to hide.

Wilson-Jones E, Winkelmann RK: **Papulonecrotic tuberculid**: A neglected disease in Western countries. J Am Acad Dermatol 1986; 14:815–826.

Clinical:	Symmetric inflammatory papules, pustules, and discrete crusted ulcers scattered over area of varioliform scars 2 to 8 mm.
	Distribution: elbows, knees, extremities, ears.
	Lesions involute slowly over weeks.
	May have history of having had tuberculosis.
Cardinal test:	Strongly positive tuberculin (PPD) test in all cases.
Pathology:	Immune vasculitis leading to infarct due to sensitization to blood-borne tubercle bacilli antigens but no mycobacteria found in biopsy.
Confirmatory:	Lesions completely heal within 1 to 3 months of isoniazid and para-amino salicylic acid therapy.
Differential	Necrotizing vasculitis
	Papulopustular syphilid
	Lymphomatoid papulosis
	Pityriasis lichenoides
	Perforating granuloma annulare
	Perforating collagenosis
	Churg-Strauss granuloma
	Miliary tuberculosis (patients gravely ill, tubercle bacilli seen and cultured on biopsy)

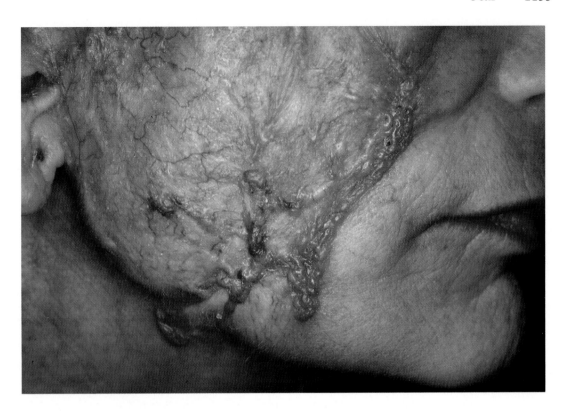

Think **tuberculin skin test** next time you see a chronic inflammatory papulopustular eruption. It will make the diagnosis for you when it reproduces the disease.

Frosch PJ, Brumage MR, Schuster-Pavlovic C, Bersch A: **Atrophoderma vermiculatum.** Case report and review. J Am Acad Dermatol 1988; 18:538–542.

A 9-year-old girl had had strange symmetrical **reticular scarring of her cheeks** since age 3. Her 39-year-old father was similarly afflicted. The scarring left a worm-eaten or honeycombed appearance and was without symptoms or prior lesions. Erythema, milia, and grouped horny plugs resembling comedones were also present.

This is typical of **atrophoderma vermiculatum**, which has scarred our dermatologic nosology with at least nine unwieldy synonyms. The most picturesque description is in astronomical terms, comparing the cribriform pattern of scarring with that of a telescopic view of the first quarter moon's surface.

It may involve the upper lip and helices as well as the ear lobes. **Ulerythema ophryogenes (keratosis pilaris atrophicans faciei)** is a variant involving the eyebrow area with alopecia.

Atrophoderma vermiculatum was the end stage of **chlor acne** in children exposed to 2,3,7,8-tetrachlorodibenzo-*p*-dioxin in the Seveso, Italy, chemical accident in 1976.

Heng MCY, Haberfeld G: **Thrombotic phenomena** associated with intravenous cocaine. J Am Acad Dermatol 1987; 16:462–468.

Bullous necrotic plaques over the thighs of this 35-year-old man proved to be due to **infarcts** as a result of intravenous **cocaine** given 8 hours earlier.

These infarcts were the result of vasoconstriction and thrombus formation induced by the cocaine. They healed slowly to leave bizarre depressed scars.

Bisaccia E, Scarborough DA, Carr RD: **Cutaneous sarcoid granuloma** formation in herpes zoster scars. Arch Dermatol 1983; 119:788–789.

Five months after this 52-year-old woman had had herpes zoster of the C5 through T2 dermatomes, she experienced firm, grouped papules appearing in sites of the healed zoster. On biopsy these proved to be **sarcoidal granulomas**.

Patchy pulmonary infiltrates were found on x-ray. A diagnosis of sarcoidosis was made and she showed an excellent response to oral prednisone.

It still remains a mystery of how and why **sarcoidosis develops in scars**, and at the sites of venipuncture or folliculitis. However, the second author of this paper should know. He comes from that area.

Rossis CG, Yiacoumettis AM, Elemenoglou J: **Squamous cell carcinoma** of the heel developing at site of previous frostbite. J Roy Soc Med 1982; 75:715–718.

During World War II, many Greek soldiers suffered severe **frostbite** in the mountains of Northern Greece. Old frostbitten areas **resemble burn scars** and eventually ulcerate if subjected to constant irritation and pressure. In 10 patients with old frostbite on the heel, low-grade well-differentiated squamous cell **carcinoma** also developed. Presenting signs included fungation, ulceration, induration, lack of marginal epithelialization, nodules, and general unresponsiveness to conservative management. Surgical excision was curative.

Frostbite thus joins **old burn scars** (**Marjolin's ulcer**) as a predisposing factor for development of squamous cell carcinoma.

Ahmed AR, Salm M, Larson R, Kaplan R: **Localized cicatricial pemphigoid** (Brunsting-Perry): A transplantation experiment. Arch Dermatol 1984; 120:932–935.

If you transplant some normal skin into an area of any of the following diseases, the **transplant will "catch" the disease surrounding** it:

Cicatricial pemphigoid
Morphea
Vitiligo
Fixed drug eruption
Lupus erythematosus
Keloid

Patients like certain doctors—rather than uncertain ones.

Scleroderma

Here's a **diagnosis you can feel**. Shut your eyes and make the diagnosis as you feel that immobile taut skin over the fingers, or the patch of thickened skin on the trunk or the linear band of hard skin running up a leg or arm. Open your eyes to the calcium deposits in this bony hard acrosclerosis of the hands. Look at the dilated nail fold capillaries, the shiny yellowish fingers in fixed contractures with fingertip ulcers, even gangrene. Note loss of hair and anhidrosis from follicles and glands pinched functionless by the grip of a collagen vice.

Look on the forehead for the saber scar furrow (**en coup de sabre**) of a skin enfolding down on an atrophic skull plate. Look on the trunk for the pigmentary "cloud" over a patch of hardened skin we call morphea. Look for the **speckled depigmentation** dotted with follicular pigment (salt and pepper) that is so diagnostic of widespread scleroderma of the upper chest. Look for the shiny plaques of ivory-colored depigmentation of large irregular areas of morphea. Look at the expressionless taut facial skin of a patient who has lost her once happy smile and whistle. Look at this prisoner, imprisoned in a shrinking cage of collagen.

Listen to her tell of her hands going purple and then white in the cold, a **Raynaud's phenomenon** that can lead to gangrene. Listen to her tell of her insidious loss of swallowing and bowel function, her dyspnea as the lungs and heart fibrose, her incessant joint pains, and ultimate arthrosis. Measure her blood pressure as it climbs to hypertension. Assay her renal function for failure and her eyes for retinopathy. No organ is beyond the grasp of this sclerosis.

Note that scleroderma may have **fellow travelers** such as Sjögren's syndrome, myasthenia gravis, thyroiditis, or progeria. Or a patch of scleroderma may be a part of another disease or syndrome. Thus, we see localized sclerodermatous change in Werner's syndrome, ataxia telangiectasia, Günther's porphyria, and rheumatoid arthritis, as well as mixed connective tissue disease.

Always, the **differential diagnosis** may add a twinge of doubt. Does the patient have scleredema adultorum? Look for the reassuring localization on the upper back, the onset after a sore throat, or the coexistence of diabetes mellitus. Does the patient have the stiff skin syndrome with its onset in infancy and its negative immunologic tests? Could it be the eosinophilic fasciitis of Shulman with its edematous erythematous thickened skin and guiding diagnostic star of eosinophilia? Can you rule out lupus erythematosus, that medical mime, by laboratory study? Could the finger atrophy be due to fluorinated steroid therapy? Could the ulcers be a sign of leprosy, even syringomyelia? Is the terminal atrophy of the arms that of scleroderma or acrodermatitis chronica atrophicans that follows a tick bite?

The diagnostic questioning continues with the localized form, i.e., **morphea**. Could it be lichen sclerosus et atrophicuns, the other major cause of "white spot disease" of years ago? Could it be a fixed drug eruption, or later could it be vitiligo, or but a scar? Finally, are you sure it isn't a morpheiform carcinoma?

You've made the "what it is" diagnosis of scleroderma. Now turn to the "why it is" diagnosis. Let history be your guide. Rule in or out the following proven causes of scleroderma.

1. Tryptophan, prolonged high dose
2. Penicillamine therapy
3. Bleomycin chemotherapy
4. Tick bite leading to *Borrelia burgdorferi* infection, often with an index sign of erythema chronicum migrans
5. Vinyl exposure, look for acro-osteolysis
6. Solvent exposure, e.g., trichloroethylene
7. Silica dust, occupational
8. Silicone breast implant
9. X-ray therapy, e.g., in mammary region
10. Graft versus host reaction, chronic form

Feel, look, and **listen** for the diagnosis of scleroderma.

General

Serup J: Clinical appearance of skin lesions and disturbances of pigmentation in localized **scleroderma**. Acta Derm Venereol 1984; 64:485–492.

A study of 58 patients with circumscribed scleroderma lesions favored the following classification:

1. Localized morphea (1 or 2 medium-sized lesions)
2. Generalized morphea (several large plaques in several regions)
3. Guttate morphea (numerous droplike lesions)
4. Linear scleroderma (one or a few linear bandlike lesions of the extremities or trunk)
5. En coup de sabre scleroderma (a linear form on the front of the scalp or forehead)

Noteworthy features of localized scleroderma:

A simple patch of redness may be the first evidence of morphea.

Fully developed morphea is white and indurated, with increased skin thickness.

Most patients show pigmented spots on the trunk, resembling atrophoderma of Pasini and Pierini.

Lesions tend to be symmetric, involve the midline, and have a linear patterning, except on the upper chest, lower abdomen, and lower face.

Lines are most similar to those Blaschko described for linear dermatoses but do not exhibit the V- and S-shaped patterns.

The lines do not correspond to the cleavage lines of Langer, the innervation fields of peripheral and cranial nerves, or the boundary lines of Voigt between the innervated fields.

A predisposing defect in crest cell migration during embryonal life may play a role in both morphea and linear scleroderma.

Krieg T, Meurer M: **Systemic scleroderma**. Clinical and pathophysiologic aspects. J Am Acad Dermatol 1988; 18:457–481.

The earliest signs of this disease are **Raynaud's phenomenon** and cutaneous findings, with later involvement of the heart, lungs, kidneys, and gastrointestinal tract. Initially, the fingers and hands appear swollen with nonpitting edema, making it impossible for the hand to lie flat. The skin appears thickened, edematous, and slightly erythematous. The face and often the frenulum of the tongue then begin to show edematous change. As **sclerosis** develops the hand feels hard; eventually ulcers and telangiectasia develop, with atrophy in the third stage. Hair is lost and sweating stops. The hand finally shows profound articular deformities. This and the beaked nose, radial furrowing of the lips, and **constricted oral orifice** make the diagnosis an easy one. The feet show lesser changes.

The tightening of the skin produces **telangiectasia**, common on the face, back and periungual areas. In the **CREST (Thibierge-Weissenbach) syndrome**, there is also marked calcinosis, Raynaud's phenomenon, and esophageal involvement. Marked hyperpigmentation resembling Addison's disease may occur, in addition to mottled pigmentation and focal hypopigmentation of the trunk.

As the months and years pass, the sclerosis grasps the forearm, the upper legs, the upper trunk, and finally the entire integument.

The **differential diagnosis** of systemic scleroderma includes:

Morphea	Shulman syndrome
Scleroedema generalized Buschke	Shoulder-hand syndrome
Mixed connective tissue disease	Pseudoscleroderma

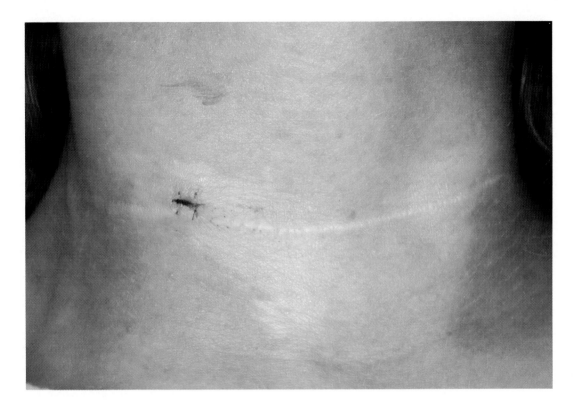

Pseudoscleroderma is seen with:

porphyria cutanea tarda   scleromyxedema
polyvinyl chloride disease   Werner's syndrome
toxic oil syndrome

In 1980, the American Rheumatism Association classification included the following **criteria** for scleroderma:

Major criteria: proximal scleroderma
Minor criteria: sclerodactyly
                  pulmonary fibrosis
                  digital pitting scars

By indirect immunofluorescence, circulating antinuclear antibodies (ANA) can be found in the sera of more than 95% of patients with systemic scleroderma. Their pathogenic significance is questionable, but some are highly specific for certain clinical features. There are 3 characteristic fluorescence patterns: nucleolar, centromere, and fine-speckled.

Antinucleolar antibodies. Mostly seen with diffuse scleroderma
Anticentromere antibodies. Mostly seen with CREST syndrome
and primary biliary cirrhosis with scleroderma.
Anti-Scl-70 antibodies. Highly specific for systemic scleroderma.

Your fingertips feeling her fingertips is better than a biopsy in diagnosing scleroderma.

Forms

Jawitz JC, Albert MK, Nigra TP, Bunning RD: A new skin manifestation of **progressive systemic sclerosis**. J Am Acad Dermatol 1984; 11:265–268.

This 49-year-old black man had a one-year history of arthralgia, sclerodactyly, and poikiloderma. Examination revealed diffuse sclerosis of his hands, arms, legs, face, chest, and back. X-ray studies of the esophagus showed atony of the distal esophagus. A diagnosis of **systemic sclerosis** was made.

The **distinctive features** were the pigmentary changes which were uniquely diagnostic.

1. Retention of perifollicular pigment in areas of loss of pigment on the chest, back, neck, and forehead.
2. Retention of pigment precisely over large superficial vessels, for example, the temporal artery.

The diagnostic follicular dots of pigment and wavy vascular patterns of pigment are thought to reflect the **higher skin temperature** in these areas. The follicle has a rich capillary network, and the skin overlying the temporal vessels was measured at a degree **warmer** than the adjacent depigmented skin.

A warm melanocyte is an active melanocyte. Look for these warm spots of pigment preservation to aid you in avoiding the diagnosis of vitiligo in black patients with scleroderma.

Jarratt M, Bybee D, Ramsdell W: **Eosinophilic fasciitis**: An early variant of scleroderma. J Am Acad Dermatol 1979; 1:221–226.

For 7 months a 58-year-old woman experienced induration and stiffness of the skin of her legs, as well as fever and ankle pain. The skin of the legs, arms and abdomen was firm, brawny, and indurated with a peculiar cobblestone appearance, and there was painful movement limitation and edema of the ankles. A biopsy of skin and muscle showed thick sclerotic fascia, and a complete blood count had 19% eosinophils, permitting a diagnosis of **eosinophilic fasciitis**.

The **skin tightness** progressed, leading to joint immobility and flexion contractures. Following steroid and azathioprine therapy the eosinophil count dropped to 1%, but another biopsy disclosed dense sclerotic dermal collagen and a dense lymphocytic infiltrate without eosinophils in the deep fascia. The diagnosis of **scleroderma** was made, leading to the realization that eosinophilic fasciitis may be an early inflammatory stage of scleroderma. She had been exposed to two herbicides but had no family history of rheumatic disease. She had no dysphagia or Raynaud's phenomenon.

A slice of life (or disease) may be quite different from the whole loaf! Today, the question to ask is, "Did you take **tryptophan**?"

Long PR, Miller OF III: **Linear scleroderma**: Report of a case presenting as persistent unilateral eyelid edema. J Am Acad Dermatol 1982; 7:541–544.

Recurrent swelling of the upper eyelids was the complaint of this 66-year-old woman. On examination she had edema and erythema of the left upper eyelid. The clinical impression by the ophthalmologist was blepharitis with possible angioedema. Dermatologic consultation suggested the alternative diagnosis of seborrheic dermatitis and contact dermatitis.

There was no response to topical steroids and a reduction in contactants. Blood studies had ruled out hypothyroidism as a cause.

Three months later on examination of her idiopathic lid edema, two areas of

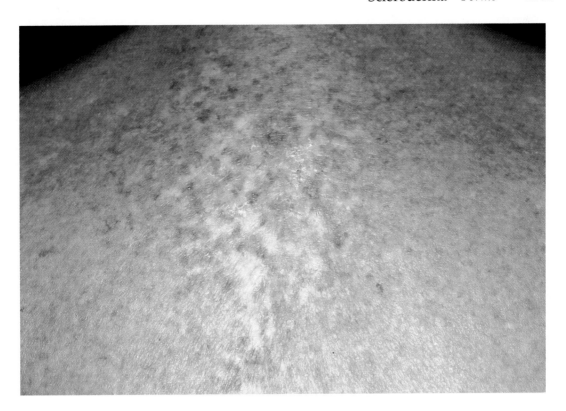

erythema were noted extending from the left eyebrow to the scalp. On palpation questionable **mild induration** was sensed. A biopsy failed to give the diagnosis. However, the process rapidly developed so that a definitive diagnosis of **linear scleroderma** was apparent. At that time, she exhibited marked induration, atrophy and alopecia of the left frontotemporal portion of the scalp in addition to the eyelid edema.

Our one and only personal experience with chronic unilateral idiopathic eyelid edema proved to be caused by hypothyroidism.

Ishikawa O, Nihei Y, Ishikawa H: The skin changes of **POEMS syndrome**. Br J Dermatol 1987; 117:523–526.

Thickened, dark skin and scattered hemangiomas may lead to the detection of an extramedullary plasmacytoma.

A 68-year-old woman presented with **Raynaud's phenomenon** and thickening and tightening of the skin of her arms, legs, and fingers. There was diffuse hyperpigmentation with hypertrichosis and edema of the lower legs. In fact, her whole body was diffusely hyperpigmented and there were multiple dark red dome-shaped nodules on her trunk and occiput. She had had no exposure to organic solvents.

A skin biopsy of the forearm showed scleroderma. A nodule from the back proved to be a hemangioma, with endothelial cell proliferation similar to intravascular papillary endothelial hyperplasia. Further study showed the presence of polyneuropathy, lymphadenopathy, a high estrone level, and an elevated monoclonal IgA protein. Bone marrow analysis revealed an increase in large plasma cells.

Thus the full **complement of changes** made the diagnosis of POEMS syndrome:

P–*Polyneuropathy*
O–*Organomegaly*
E–*Endocrinopathy*
M–*Monoclonal* protein
S–*Skin* changes

Tuffanelli DL: **Lymphangiectasis** due to scleroderma. Arch Dermatol 1975; 111:1216.

Multiple small papules with a digitate surface were seen on the hands and forearms of three patients with systemic scleroderma. All of these patients had well-demarcated, thick "**hidebound**" **skin** in these areas. Biopsy showed lymphatic vessel dilatation in the upper dermis, presumably due to obstruction by the sclerosing process.

James WD, Berger TG, Butler DF, Tuffanelli DL: **Nodular (keloidal) scleroderma.** J Am Acad Dermatol 1984; 11:1111–1114.

Patients with progressive systemic sclerosis can develop, within areas of sclerotic skin, well-defined papules and plaques that are true **keloids**. The same is true for morphea, in which the clinician may be puzzled by the appearance of nodules. Within the thickened skin studies show these to be true keloids, both on a clinical and histologic basis.

Monroe AB, Burgdorf WHC, Sheward S: **Platelike cutaneous osteoma.** J Am Acad Dermatol 1987; 16:481–484.

A hard mass in the right flank of this 85-year-old man proved to be cutaneous osteoma. It has been present for 30 years and was in a site of former morphea.

True bone formation in the skin suggests **Albright's hereditary osteodystrophy** (short stature, brachydactyly, elevated parathyroid hormone). In addition to this rare primary form, secondary bone formation occurs in areas of trauma, inflammation, neoplasms, and all sites of cutaneous calcification such as are seen in dermatomyositis, scleroderma, and morphea. Thus, these are potential sites for osteoblast activity with the subsequent genesis of spicules of true bone.

If it looks like something you've never seen before, try looking at a small part of it.

Aberer E, Stanek G, Ertl M, Neumann R: Evidence for spirochetal origin of **circumscribed scleroderma (morphea)**. Acta Derm Venereol 1987, 67:225–231.

Spirochetal organisms were cultured from the skin biopsy of one patient with **morphea**. Antibodies to the spirochete of Lyme disease (*Borrelia burgdorferi*) were found in 8 of 15 patients with morphea, and in three spirochetal organisms were seen on histologic sections. Further evidence to support the spirochetal origin of morphea is its response at times to penicillin and its clinical resemblance to acrodermatitis chronica atrophicans, a known component of **Lyme disease**.

Garioch JJ, Rashid A, Thomson J, Seywright M: The relevance of elevated *Borrelia burgdorferi* titres in **localized scleroderma**. Clin Exp Dermatol 1989; 14:439–441.

This 46-year-old man developed an erythematous rash on the flexor aspect of the right wrist. By the next day it extended up the arm, becoming painful and swollen. Within 2 weeks, the affected skin was **woody hard**. There was joint restriction and he experienced a reduced sensation in the right arm, the right side of his chest, and the right toes.

The patient was unemployed and lived in rural Scotland, had not traveled abroad, and noted no prior insect bite. There were sheep and horses in the field near his home but no deer.

A biopsy showed the changes of **localized scleroderma**. His general studies were all normal but he did have elevated *Borrelia burgdorferi* titres: IgG of 1/256 by indirect immunofluorescence and 54 units of ELISA. This suggested that his **scleroderma** was a **manifestation of Lyme borreliosis**, i.e., a *Borrelia burgdorferi* infection. However, the elevated titres were believed to be only a chance finding because:

1. No spirochetes were found on silver staining or on electron microscopy.
2. No spirochetes could be grown in modified Kelly's medium.
3. Antibiotics for 10 days were without effect.

Silver RM, Heyes MP, Maize JC, et al: **Scleroderma, fasciitis** and **eosinophilia** associated with the ingestion of **tryptophan**. N Engl J Med 1990; 322:874–881.

A 67-year-old man developed unexplained widespread pruritus. Study revealed an associated **eosinophilia of 30%**. When an initial course of prednisone was stopped 6 months later, he noted skin tightness. Most of his skin on examination was taut but there was no sclerodactyly. A skin biopsy showed changes consistent with **scleroderma**.

It was at this time that the cause was ascertained. He had begun taking **tryptophan**, 2.0 gm/day, just one month prior to the onset of his pruritus. Tryptophan is an essential amino acid commonly purchased over-the-counter to combat insomnia. Once the tryptophan was stopped, the tightening of the skin lessened.

A diagnosis of **tryptophan-induced scleroderma with eosinophilia** was made. Study of an additional eight patients with the same tryptophan ingestion syndrome disclosed variants of scleroderma, including the localized form, generalized morphea, morphea profunda, and eosinophilic fasciitis. In the latter instances deep biopsy revealed a thickened fascia with a dense inflammatory infiltrate. Other patients experienced a prominent myalgia associated with the tryptophan intake.

This is a new syndrome and one to be considered in all patients with sclerodermatous change and eosinophilia.

Kilbourne EM, Swygert LA, Philen RM, et al: Interim guidance on the **eosinophilia-myalgia syndrome**. Ann Intern Med 1990; 112:85–87.

The disease symptoms develop over several weeks, with myalgia and fatigue and sometimes arthralgia. The myalgia is intense and often incapacitating. Dyspnea and cough are common, as well as muscle weakness and swelling of the extremities. Ascending **polyneuropathy** is rare but may be fatal. Heart failure, pulmonary hypertension, and thromboembolic phenomena also occur. Steroid therapy is recommended in severe cases.

Common skin lesions include transient maculopapular, vesicular, or urticarial eruptions. A few patients have had sclerodermoid skin thickening.

CDC: **Eosinophilia-myalgia syndrome**—New Mexico. JAMA 1989; 262:3116.

On October 30, 1989, three cases of **eosinophilia and severe myalgia** in people who had been taking oral L-tryptophan were reported to the New Mexico Department of Health and Environment. On November 11, 1989, the FDA advised consumers to discontinue oral **L-tryptophan products**. By November 15, 1989, following media publicity, 154 cases in 17 states had been identified. Most of the illness started after July, 1989. L-tryptophan is an essential amino acid found in dietary protein. It has been used for **insomnia, depression, and premenstrual syndrome**.

This new clinical entity resembles the **toxic-oil syndrome** epidemic which occurred in Spain in 1981, with patients having severe myalgias and intense eosinophilia.

For surveillance purposes four criteria were developed to characterize the disease:

1. eosinophil count $\geq$ 1,000 cells/mm^3
2. generalized myalgia that has been incapacitating
3. exclusion of trichinosis by serologic tests or muscle biopsy
4. absence of infection or neoplasm

The differential diagnosis includes:

eosinophilic myositis	polyarteritis nodosa
eosinophilic fasciitis	trichinosis

CDC: Update: **Eosinophilia-myalgia syndrome** associated with ingestion of L-tryptophan—United States, as of January 9, 1990. JAMA 1990; 263:633.

By January 9, 1990, 1046 cases had been reported from 49 states and Puerto Rico. Patients ranged in age from 11 to 84 years. The median dose of L-tryptophan ingested was 1500 mg per day.

Flindt-Hansen H, Isager H: **Scleroderma** after occupational exposure to trichlorethylene and trichlorethane. Acta Derm Venereol 1987; 67:263–264.

A disabling **sclerodactyly and scleroderma** of the hands and forearms developed over 18 months in a 52-year-old man. On x-ray, there was osteolysis of the phalanges. It was suspected that his job of cleaning high-voltage cables was responsible, with regular exposure for 12 years to **trichlorethylene** and **trichlorethane** in spray form. Two additional patients are described with the same problem and same occupational exposure.

Miyagawa S, Yoshioka A, Hatoko M, et al: **Systemic sclerosis-like lesions** during long-term penicillamine therapy for Wilson's disease. Br J Dermatol 1987; 116:95–100.

The heavy metal chelator **penicillamine** is often used to treat systemic sclerosis. In this instance 11 years of D-penicillamine therapy (530 mg/day) resulted in a diffuse tightening and darkening of the skin of the fingers, hands, and forearms of a 14-year-old boy with **Wilson's disease**. The tightening also extended proximally from the wrists and ankles to include the shoulder girdles and hips, with flexion contractures of the elbows and knees. Histologic examination revealed typical changes of **scleroderma** on skin biopsy and C3 and fibrinogen deposits at the dermal epidermal junction. Pulmonary function was reduced with a decreased forced vital capacity and diffusion capacity, and antinuclear antibodies were present at a titer of 1:40 (homogeneous pattern). However, the autoantibodies specific for systemic sclerosis (antinucleolar, anticentromeric, anti-Scl-70) were not found.

Since morphea has also been reported to occur as a result of **penicillamine** therapy, one can question its use in treating scleroderma. Penicillamine may also induce autoantibodies, sometimes resulting in drug-induced lupus erythematosus.

Snauwaert J, Degreef H: **Bleomycin-induced Raynaud's phenomenon** and **acral sclerosis**. Dermatologica 1984; 169:172–174.

After 7 months of treatment with **bleomycin** (total dose 240 mg) for a seminoma, a 34-year-old man developed **Raynaud's phenomenon**. His fingers were sclerodermatous with onycholysis, pus formation, and eventually subungual necrosis and gangrene of several fingertips. Although he also had received vinblastine and cisplatin, bleomycin was blamed.

Skin toxicity should be expected in patients who have received more than 165 mg of bleomycin. Well before this, one may see **alopecia**, **stomatitis**, and **hyperpigmented brittle nails**. The unique sensitivity of skin (and skin tumors) to bleomycin stems from the **absence** of the inactivating enzyme **bleomycin hydrolase in the skin**. The sclerodermatous changes and Raynaud's phenomenon result from a direct stimulatory effect on fibroblasts.

Colver GB, Rodger A, Mortimer PS, et al: **Post-irradiation morphoea**. Br J Dermatol 1989; 120:831–835.

Nine patients developed **morphea after radiotherapy**, usually following mastectomy. In every patient it began within the irradiated area, and in four of them it spread beyond.

Be alert to this and avoid mistaking it for a sclerosing type of local tumor recurrence.

Graham-Brown RAC, Sarkany I: **Scleroderma-like changes** due to chronic **graft-versus-host disease**. Clin Exp Dermatol 1983; 8:531–538.

This 43-year-old man developed an acute toxic erythema 10 days after receiving a bone marrow transplant for his lymphoblastic leukemia. This persisted for nearly a month and was diagnosed as acute **graft versus host disease**.

This was followed shortly after by a widespread **lichenoid rash**, including **lichen planus–like** lesions within the oral mucosa. It gradually faded over the year, leaving reticulate pigmentary changes over the entire body.

By a year and a half post-transplant, he had gone from a mild stiffness of the shoulders to extensive thickening and binding down of the skin over the arms, legs, and lower trunk. Finger movement remained normal, but elsewhere the skin was smooth and shiny, as seen in morphea. The skin biopsy showed densely packed collagen and total loss of dermal appendages. A diagnosis of **chronic graft-versus-host scleredema-like skin** was made.

Friedman SJ, Doyle JA: Sclerodermoid changes of **porphyria cutanea tarda**: Possible relationship to urinary uroporphyrin levels. J Am Acad Dermatol 1985; 13:70–74.

Scleroderma in the V-shaped area of the neck, the presternum, and preauricular area of the face calls for an assay of the **urinary uroporphyrins**. Indeed, scleroderma in the light-exposed areas especially may be the first clinical sign of porphyria cutanea tarda. Intralesional calcification is an additional clue. Six patients are presented in whom the other cutaneous features of porphyria cutanea tarda did not appear for a year on average. In nine other patients the reverse was true, the scleroderma appearing on an average of 4 years after the typical lesions of porphyria cutanea tarda.

The **morpheiform lesions** do not herald systemic sclerosis. However, they are clinically and histologically identical with idiopathic scleroderma. The lesions disappeared in six patients and improved in four following phlebotomy treatment and avoidance of alcohol. Significantly, those patients who had been given antimalarial agents rapidly became ill with weakness, vomiting, and dark urine. This response to chloroquine is another way of making the diagnosis of scleroderma due to porphyria, but it is an awkward diagnostic tool.

Any example of **sclerosis of the skin calls for a porphyrin screen** since it may be indicative not only of porphyria cutanea tarda but also of erythropoietic protoporphyria, hepatoerythropoietic porphyria, variegate porphyria, and even subcutaneous injections of hematoporphyrin.

In the **differential diagnosis** of cutaneous sclerosis, one must consider carcinoid syndrome, bleomycin toxicity, vibration syndrome, and scleredema.

Haustein U-F, Ziegler V, Herrmann K, et al: **Silica-induced scleroderma**. J Am Acad Dermatol 1990; 22:444–448.

Ninety-three of these 120 male **scleroderma** patients had long-term exposure to **silica dust**. The interval between the beginning of exposure and the onset of scleroderma was 9 to 40 years. It is suspected that crystalline particles of silica less than 5 cm are phagocytosed by macrophages, which by releasing cytokines, activate fibroblasts to produce the collagen responsible for scleroderma as well as silicosis.

Rustin MHA, Bull HA, Ziegler V, et al: Silica exposure and **silica-associated systemic sclerosis**. Br J Dermatol 1989; 121(Suppl 34):29–30.

Miners exposed for years to **silica dust** may develop **systemic sclerosis**. This places silica with vinyl chloride, aromatic hydrocarbon solvents and epoxy resins as agents capable of producing occupational scleroderma.

A genetic susceptibility is suspected of entering into the pathogenesis of this problem as in so many others.

Spiera H: **Scleroderma** after **silicone augmentation mammoplasty**. JAMA 1988; 260:236–238.

Five years after **silicone breast implants**, this woman noted **thickening of** her **hands**, **upper arms**, and face. It was associated with intense pruritus and arthralgia. A biopsy confirmed the clinical diagnosis of **scleroderma**.

Although there was no inflammation or adenopathy, the breast implants were removed. She experienced a rapid improvement in her sense of well-being as well as the arthralgias. The skin hardness has slowly abated.

It is postulated that even without a tear, **silicone may escape** from the implant envelope. This silicone, once **converted to silica**, is well known to be

associated with the pathogenesis of certain examples of industrial scleroderma. The silica may serve as a stimulus for increased collagen synthesis
by the fibroblasts.

With 100,000 breast implants being done every year, it is important to ask
your patient about such surgeries.

Brozena SJ, Fenske NA, Cruse CW, et al: **Human adjuvant disease** following **augmentation mammoplasty**. Arch Dermatol 1988; 124:1383–1386.

This 60-year-old woman had noted a progressive tightening of the skin of
her hands, arms, upper thorax, and face. It had begun about a year ago and
was associated with mottled hyperpigmentation and decreased ability to
sweat, as well as complete hair loss on the arms. An ANA was positive at
1:640. A diagnosis of **progressive systemic sclerosis** was made. The history
revealed the cause: she had had **bilateral breast augmentation** with silicone
injection 25 years earlier.

Bilateral mastectomy was associated with a dramatic reversal of her scleroderma. The hair of the arms regrew and her ability to sweat returned. This
patient can be considered to have had **human adjuvant disease (HAD)**. It is
analogous to the inflammatory changes induced in animals by the injection
of Freund's adjuvant.

It is this version of the autoimmune spectrum of disorders that is associated
with implantation of silicone or paraffin. Fifty cases have been reported. The
usual association is with progressive systemic sclerosis, but one may **also see**
associated morphea, systemic lupus erythematosus, Sjögren's syndrome,
mixed connective tissue disease, thyroiditis, or primary biliary cirrhosis.

*A doctor who cannot take a good history and a patient who cannot
give one are in danger of giving and receiving bad treatment.*

PAUL DUDLEY WHITE

Differential Diagnosis

Venencie PY, Powell FC, Su WPD, Perry HO: **Scleredema**: A review of 33 cases. J Am Acad Dermatol 1984; 11:128–134.

The clue	Nonpitting edema or induration of skin
	Inability to wrinkle or pick up involved skin
	Difficulty in opening mouth or eyes
	Trabeculate indentations
The prior event	Sore throat 2 weeks before or diabetes mellitus for years
The location	Face, neck, back, arms
	Symmetric, gradual transition to normal skin
	Never hands or feet
The course	Prolonged for years (usually)
The differential	Edema–does not show as much induration
	Scleroderma–look for atrophy, hidebound hands, pigmentation change, calcification, telangiectasia
	Pseudoscleroderma (sclerodermoid)–look for other disease
	Scleromyxedema, look for mucin in biopsy

McNaughton F, Keczkes K: **Scleredema adultorum** and **diabetes mellitus** (scleredema diutinum). Clin Exp Dermatol 1983; 8:41–45.

An obese 58-year-old man with an 11-year history of diabetes was admitted for study of **thickened, hard skin on his back and shoulders**. It had been present and progressing for over a year. There was some resultant restriction of movement of his neck. A biopsy showed bundles of thickened, poorly cellular collagen fibers in the lower dermis. Because there was no mucin present, a diagnosis of **scleredema** was made.

Although most examples of scleredema, resolving in 8 to 10 months, follow a streptococcal or viral infection, some are associated only with diabetes mellitus, with no known antecedent infection. This type begins insidiously and progresses relentlessly for many years. Accordingly, it has been called **scleredema diutinum**.

Deffer TA, Goette DK: **Distal phalangeal atrophy** secondary to topical steroid therapy. Arch Dermatol 1987; 123:571–572.

A 62-year-old woman with a **shiny, firm, tapered right index fingertip** gave the history of having treated a paronychial infection there with 0.5% fluocinonide ointment four times/day for one month. Occlusive dressing had not been used.

Such a "**disappearing digit**" brings up the **differential** of scleroderma, occupational acro-osteolysis, and damage due to repetitive trauma. An x-ray revealed marked soft tissue atrophy but no bone changes.

A diagnosis of **steroid atrophy** was made; in this report a plea is made for the recognition of this special form of steroid-induced atrophy. Although it appeared in less than 30 days, it was still unchanged 4 months after the steroid was stopped.

Jablonska S, Schubert H, Kikuchi I: **Congenital fascial dystrophy**: Stiff skin syndrome — a human counterpart of the tight-skin mouse. J Am Acad Dermatol 1989; 21:943–950.

Since early infancy this man had had **stony-hand indurations of the skin** and deeper tissues of the buttocks and thighs. These had spread to involve the trunk and arms but spared the hands and feet. Joint mobility became limited and extensive contractures ensued.

When he was 17 years old a diagnosis of **scleroderma** was made, but not until 15 years later was stiff skin syndrome diagnosed correctly.

Stiff skin syndrome (congenital fascial dystrophy) is distinguished from scleroderma by the fact that it shows:

A genetic characteristic of onset in infancy.
No progression to visceral or muscle involvement.
No inflammatory or vascular changes.
No Raynaud's phenomenon.
No immunologic defects.
Rock-hard skin firmly bound to underlying tissue.
A localization to areas of abundant fascia.
Fascia four times thicker than normal.
No abnormally increased mucopolysaccharides in skin, urine, or tissue culture.

Three other stiff skin syndrome patients are presented in whom scleroderma and sclerodermatomyositis had been previously diagnosed.

Interestingly, there is an animal model for the study of this condition. It is an inbred mouse strain known as the **tight-skin mouse**. It too shows the same genetically programmed increase in dermal and fascial collagen.

Caputo R, Sambvani N, Monti M, et al: **Dermochondrocorneal dystrophy (François' syndrome).** Arch Dermatol 1988; 124:424–428.

A 45-year-old woman presented with **scleroderma-like** hands and numerous white-gray fibromatous papules and nodules on the face, auricles, and joints of the hands and feet. Her fingernails were convex, resembling a watchglass, with occasional subungual fibromas. A thick pterygoid vascularized conjunctival rim was seen in her eyes, along with oval subepithelial opacities in the corneas. Dental examination revealed severe diffuse gingival inflammation with edema, hyperemia, and localized **erythematous gingival enlargements**, along with carious teeth. X-rays of the hands and feet showed cysts and cortical erosions of the metacarpals, metatarsals, and phalanges. Laboratory tests were normal except for an erythrocyte sedimentation rate of 40 to 60 mm/hr and a twofold increase of urinary hydroxyproline. Skin biopsy of a recent lesion showed numerous bulky cells with light cytoplasm (PAS positive) and eccentric nuclei (spongiocytes). Older lesions were composed of compact fibrous tissue and few cells. **Gingival lesions showed fibroblast and plasma cell proliferation** with rich vascularization.

In this often familial disease (autosomal recessive transmission), hyperproduction of type III collagen by proliferation of faulty fibroblasts results in:

sclerodermoid hardening and thickening of the skin of the hands and wrists.
grayish nodular lesions of the face and hands.
osteochondral dystrophy with limitation of joint movement.
white or brown opacities in the cornea.
hyperplasia of mucous membranes.

The **following four entities must be ruled out**:

1. **Familial histiocytic dermoarthritis of Zayd** (similar skin and joint changes, but no corneal opacities. Eye changes include cataract, uveitis, and glaucoma).
2. **Multicentric reticulohistiocytosis** (polyarthritis and papulonodules of the

skin and mucous membranes, but no corneal lesions. Electron microscopy shows histiocytes with specific pleomorphic cytoplasmic inclusions).

3. **Fibroblastic rheumatism** (polyarthritis, sclerodactyly with retraction of
palmar aponeuroses, nodules on the extremities, and lung fibrosis, but
no corneal dystrophy).

4. **Juvenile hyaline fibromatosis** (dermal and subcutaneous nodules, flexion
contractures, osteolytic bone lesions, hypertrophic gingiva, and stunted
growth. Fibroblasts appear "chondroid" and are surrounded by an eosinophilic granular, fibrous, intercellular substance).

All of which shows the strange ways the fibroblast can immobilize us.

Badame AJ: **Progeria.** Arch Dermatol 1989; 125:540–544.

The ominous signs of progeria appear in infancy. The parents note first that
the skin around the hip region is becoming sclerodermatous. It is thick and
inelastic. By the age of 2 aging, wrinkled, saggy skin appears over the phalanges. Other skin sites become taut and shiny as the subcutaneous fat atrophies. The premature aging of the sweat glands and hair become evident
with a loss of sweat and hair. The nails as well as the skin thins. Eventually
one sees a diminutive old person. Along with this there is osteoporosis and
bone resorption, as well as aging atherosclerotic changes in the blood vessels
and cardiac hypertrophy. Yet throughout their shortened total life span of
10 to 15 years, there is no apparent aging of the brain and these children
remain keenly aware of their unique appearance.

Progeria (Hutchinson-Gilford syndrome) is usually diagnostic on its clinical
features by the second year of life. Significantly, in some individuals the
speed-up of the clock of aging does not start until they reach 15 to 30 years.
This is the Werner's syndrome (pangeria, progeria of adults). Again the sclerodermatous skin, the prematurely aged appearance, as well as sexual arrest
and cataracts allow a clinical recognition. Arteriosclerosis enters and most
die in their fifties.

Acrogeria is another version, appearing in early childhood but affecting
mainly the arms, legs, and face. The atrophy and subcutaneous wasting does
not involve the trunk. Hair growth remains normal. The child has an excellent prognosis for a normal life span since the vital heart and major vessels
are also spared.

The **Rothmund-Thomson** syndrome of poikiloderma congenitale also enters
into the differential. This strikes infants between the ages of 3 and 6 months,
producing the white, thinning hair of the elderly as well as cataracts. The
poikiloderma, however, makes it unique.

Lastly, **Cockayne's syndrome** may be confused with progeria, although here
premature aging and short stature are not evident until the teens. These
patients suggest a "Mickey Mouse" appearance with their protruding ears
and characteristic facies. They have long limbs as well and disproportionately
large hands and feet. They may come for help with cutaneous photosensitivity or because of ocular defects.

Within the chromosomes of these progeria patients lies an answer to the
riddle of what turns off our fountain of youth.

Dahl MGC, Malcom AJ: **Diffuse neurofibroma**—unrecognized and undertreated? Br J
Dermatol 1989; 121(Suppl 34):24.

Any patient with neurofibromatosis deserves a search for **diffuse neurofibromas**. They are seldom recognized clinically since they masquerade as

morphea, morpheiform basal cell carcinoma, and dermatofibrosarcoma. The clinical feature is a 3- to 8-cm sclerotic plaque with an irregular surface.

On biopsy, spindle cells are seen, which may be mistakenly identified as histiocytoma or fibromatosis. Special stains (S-100 antibody, Leu-7 antibody) and electron microscopy all confirm a neural origin for this diffuse neurofibroma.

The lesions extend well beyond their clinical borders and can undergo malignant transformation. Accordingly, a micrographic surgical removal is appropriate.

Murphy GM, Hawk JLM, Nicholson DC, Magnus IA: **Congenital erythropoietic porphyria** (Günther's disease). Clin Exp Dermatol 1987; 12:61–65.

It is easy to suspect **Günther's disease** in an infant with sunlight-induced blistering and **pink staining of the diaper**, but it is much more difficult to diagnose it in an adult. A 40-year-old man from Sudan presented with facial scarring with mottled hypo- and hyperpigmentation. The **skin was taut**, the nose beaked, and the teeth brown, without fluorescence under Wood's light. The exposed skin was fragile and the hands were clawed with sclerodermatous contractures and acro-osteolysis of the digits. His freshly voided urine was burgundy color. His lifelong history included multiple blisters appearing 24 to 40 hours after sun exposure and healing in 10 days with scarring and dyschromia.

Microscopy of the blood film with Wood's light showed the stable diagnostic fluorescence of **erythropoietic porphyria**. Both plasma and red cells showed elevations in uroporphyrin and coproporphyrin. High-performance liquid chromatography (HPLC) of urine demonstrated a porphyria excretion profile of predominantly Type I isomers. Enzyme studies showed depressed uroporphyrinogen and δ-amino-laevulinic acid synthases.

Jayson MIV, Black CM (eds): **Systemic sclerosis**: Scleroderma. John Wiley and Sons, New York, 1988, 341 pp.

A master reference on all aspects of this disease, which may affect all organs.

Cantwell AR Jr, Kelso DW, Rowe L: **Hypodermitis sclerodermiformis** and unusual acid-fast bacteria. Arch Dermatol 1979; 115:449–452.

Two patients are described as having localized, chronic, painful, scleroderma-like lesions of the lower part of the leg associated with venous stasis. This type of lesion, designated as hypodermitis sclerodermiformis, differs from scleroderma in that the vascular components are prominent. These include ankle edema, varicosities, pain, tenderness, and dyschromia.

If you've never seen Harry Smith, it's hard to identify him in a crowd, even using an algorithm.

Seborrheic Dermatitis

Location is everything in the diagnosis of seborrheic dermatitis. Here is a disease that knows its place and stays there. And it has the perfect symmetry of a Rorschach. Seborrheic dermatitis is the dermatitis of the **well-oiled skin**. It expresses itself on the scalp, the central area of the face, the eyelids, ears, presternal area, axilla, groin, and the unwashed folds. These are the sites hospitable to the causative lipophilic yeast, *Pityrosporum ovale*.

Seborrheic dermatitis lives on oil and won't go near the asteatotic extremities. It thrives when the patient, for example in the hospital, fails to wash the oil away. Leave one side unwashed, and you will see only half of the Rorschach. Increase oil production, as in Parkinson's disease or by androgens, and you will have magnified the seborrheic dermatitis. AIDS patients have it in spades. Conversely, it melts away in the summer sun.

Can there be a differential for seborrheic dermatitis that breeds so true? Yes, and it centers on psoriasis. It helps to know that psoriasis usually avoids the face, is not necessarily symmetrical, boasts of much thicker scales, and favors coming out in a band at the anterior hair line. Furthermore, psoriasis favors the intertriginous areas, where it may appear as a Koebner response to intertrigo. We suspect that much of what is called seborrheic dermatitis of the folds is actually intertriginous psoriasis with minimal scale and much erythema. On the scalp, psoriasis is random patchy dandruff, whereas seborrheic dermatitis is diffuse and uniform. Still, these two diseases are probably only half a gene apart. Frustration in distinguishing them has led to the "cop-out" diagnosis of "seborrhiasis."

When seborrheic dermatitis is limited to the perioral area, it is not surprisingly called **perioral dermatitis**. If you think you are seeing unilateral seborrheic dermatitis, do a scraping for tinea and demodex. When "seborrheic dermatitis" extends down on the neck and elsewhere in a baby, biopsy for histiocytosis X. Watch out for **pemphigus**, **pemphigoid**, and **Hailey-Hailey disease** simulating seborrheic dermatitis on the chest. And remember that especially severe seborrheic dermatitis in infants may lead to **exfoliative dermatitis**. Normally it is only cradle cap. Drug eruptions such as those from gold can trigger seborrheic dermatitis. Finally, **vitamin B–deficient diets** may be the cause of seborrheic dermatitis in a food faddist.

Knowing the cause of seborrheic dermatitis to be yeast permits us the luxury of a therapeutic diagnostic probe. In our experience, it isn't seborrheic dermatitis if it doesn't quickly fade when the patient takes ketoconazole (200 mg/day).

Seborrheic dermatitis has such a consistent expression in such an exact localization that we use it as our first lesson in diagnosis for medical students.

Saied NK, Schwartz RA, Hansen RC, Levine N: **Atypical familial benign chronic pemphigus.** Cutis 1981; 27:666–669.

A **large crusted, erythematous plaque** over the sternal area in this 29-year-old man suggested a diagnosis of **infected seborrheic dermatitis**. The axillae, neck, back, and groin were clear, although he had had recurring pruritic plaques at times on the back. The family history disclosed that his father and paternal grandfather had had eruptions in the axillae.

The correct diagnosis was easily made on **biopsy**. The patient had **familial benign chronic pemphigus**. Mentally transposing the lesion from the sternal area to the axilla would have greatly facilitated making the diagnosis clinically.

Sometimes seeing an acquaintance in a strange place hinders recognition.

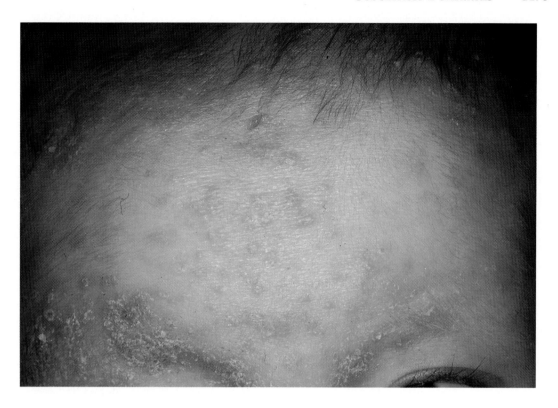

Horiuchi Y, Umezawa A, Kamimura K: Erythematous plaque **variant of transient acantholytic dermatosis**. Cutis 1986; 38:48–49.

A 58-year-old woman developed erythematous scaly plaques over the central area of the face following sun exposure while gardening. Each 1.5-cm plaque consisted of papules and a few papulovesicles in a circular pattern, located on the glabella, nose, perinasal area, and chin. A diagnosis of seborrheic dermatitis was made, but biopsy showed **Grover's disease** (suprabasal clefting with acantholysis, dyskeratosis, focal spongiosis). This self-limited vesiculobullous disease is usually located on the trunk and extremities. Actinic damage, excessive sweating, and nonspecific irritation may elicit it, but the basic cause remains unknown.

Kaplan MH, Sadick N, McNutt NS, et al: Dermatologic findings and manifestations of **acquired immunodeficiency syndrome** (AIDS). J Am Acad Dermatol 1987; 16:485–506.

Think **AIDS** when you see:

> **severe seborrheic dermatitis**
> ichthyosis
> herpes zoster in the young
> recurrent bacterial infections
> candidiasis
> molluscum contagiosum (confirm this, since cryptococcosis or histoplasmosis can mimic)
> Kaposi's sarcoma
> T-cell count below 100 cells/mm^3

Neumann C, Kolde G, Bonsmann G: **Histiocytosis X** in an elderly patient. Ultrastructure and immunocytochemistry after PUVA photochemotherapy. Br J Dermatol 1988; 119:385–391.

A confluent purpuric, reddish-brown, papular eruption with crusted yellow scaling of the anterior chest area of a 76-year-old man suggested seborrheic dermatitis. Lesions also involved the proximal flexures of the extremities and the temporoparietal scalp areas. He had no lymphadenopathy or hepatosplenomegaly. A diagnosis of **Langerhans' histiocytosis** was made **on biopsy**, but extensive medical studies failed to show systemic involvement. There was a prompt response to PUVA therapy, but relapse occurred when treatments were reduced, and he also developed palpable submandibular lymph nodes.

The eruption was similar to the Letterer-Siwe types of histiocytosis X occurring in early childhood, which usually includes hepatosplenomegaly.

Gibson JR, Pegum JS: **Favus**: A report of two cases. Clin Exp Dermatol 1983; 8:421–423.

Six months of **itchy red spots of the scalp** and dandruff brought this 8-year-old girl to medical attention. On examination there was scaling but no alopecia. On Wood's light examination, green fluorescence outlined the lower shaft of some of the scalp hairs. A specimen of hair and scale provided a growth of **Trichophyton schoenleinii** and thus the diagnosis of **favus**.

Examination of the mother's scalp revealed areas of **scarring alopecia** with yellow sulfur-cup crusts. Again, some of the hairs fluoresced and KOH examination showed hyphae that grew out to be *T. schoenleinii*.

The yellow crusts or scutula are a mix of fungal and epidermal debris centered at the orifice of the hair follicle. In the advanced forms of the disease, these crusts are diagnostic, but bear in mind that this fungal infection, which ultimately scars, may **exhibit no more than a trace of erythema and scaling at first**.

Groisser D, Bottone EJ, Lebwohl M: Association of **Pityrosporum orbiculare** (*Malassezia furfur*) with seborrheic dermatitis in patients with acquired immunodeficiency syndrome (AIDS). J Am Acad Dermatol 1989; 20:770–773.

Two patients with overt seborrheic dermatitis were treated for 2 weeks with 2% topical ketoconazole, with rapid clearing and a dramatic decrease in the number of *Pityrosporum* cells per keratinocyte.

This is a useful therapeutic diagnostic aid.

You look at lesions better when you photograph them.

Sporotrichosis

Look at that line of nodules moving up the arm. Feel for the swollen regional lymph node. Ask for the history of the rose thorn prick. Culture for the black mycelia of the deep fungus *Sporothrix schenckii*. One, two, three, four, and you have a diagnosis of sporotrichosis.

But it isn't always that simple. The initial nodule may simply ulcerate and remain the only lesion. This so-called **chancre** may appear in an unusual spot. Rather than on the hand or arm it can come on the face. It may not be a dusky red nodule, but rather a **papillomatous vegetative lesion**, or even a **rosacea**. It may look like a **granuloma** or a cold abscess. There may be no regional lymphadenopathy.

The history may trick you into thinking of **cat scratch disease**, for there is feline-transmitted sporotrichosis. The patient may deny all contact with vegetative material. He may not even know a gardener, florist, or farmer who is so much at risk. He may be only a child who finally remembers playing with sphagnum moss, or a high-school student building a brick wall. The history may be that of a skin graft that wouldn't take because the surgeon had unknowingly excised and grafted sporotrichotic ulcer. The biopsy supported his diagnosis of an idiopathic ulcer, since the tiny cigar-body spores are often never found histologically.

And sporotrichosis isn't simple to diagnose even when you see the nodules strung in line. Other organisms can travel up the lymphatic line, setting up focal lesions at lymphatic way stations. The atypical as well as the typical mycobacteria like this route. Cat scratch disease bacteria usually go swiftly to the major node itself, but can, at times, have more than the primary entrance papule. Other deep fungi such as *Blastomyces*, *Histoplasma*, and *Coccidioides* may give a sporotrichoid line of lesions, but their rarity gives you sound statistical support for your diagnosis while waiting for the culture findings. In these days of immunosuppression, remember to ask the laboratory to look for *Nocardia*. Both you and they will have to wait a month for it to grow.

Finally, don't forget that the guy who is doing drugs may have a line of nodules along his track of crack.

Read SI, Sperling LC: **Feline sporotrichosis**: Transmission to man. Arch Dermatol 1982; 118:429–431.

A 30-year-old woman veterinarian had a tender, **draining ulcerated nodule of the left palm**. This had been present for 2 months and was associated with a line of tender, linear, nonulcerated, subcutaneous nodules extending up the volar surface of the forearm. The epitrochlear and axillary nodes on that side were tender and enlarged.

A **biopsy** of the palmar nodule when stained with Gomori's methenamine silver stain showed ovoid and cigar-shaped forms compatible with *Sporothrix schenckii*. Fungal cultures confirmed the presence of *S. schenckii*. A diagnosis of sporotrichosis was made.

A search for the source of the infection did not lead to vegetation or soil, but, strangely, to a **cat**. The veterinarian had handled a sick cat that was under study for draining granulomatous nodules of the face, ears, forepaw, and at the base of its tail. These were proven by biopsy and culture to be sporotrichosis.

Further inquiry revealed that a student working in the veterinary clinic at that time had developed a tender nodule of the hand, shown on cultures to be sporotrichosis. Meanwhile, the cat owner had been seeing his dermatologist for tender, ulcerated lesions of the fingers, back, and abdomen. His son had similar sores on the back and legs. His wife and daughter developed tender nodules on their hands. All four were shown to have sporotrichosis. None of the six people who had contact with the cat had any knowledge of being bitten or even scratched. Complete resolution of all lesions was achieved with oral potassium iodide solution.

Cats have long been known to acquire sporotrichosis, but this is the first report of transmission of sporotrichosis from animal to man.

Cherchez le chat.

Schamroth JM, Grieve TP, Kellen P: **Disseminated sporotrichosis**. Int J Dermatol 1988; 27:28–30.

Three months of painless, slightly pigmented **nodules** appearing over the **entire body** brought a 56-year-old black woman to medical attention. A skin **biopsy with culture** brought a quick diagnosis of sporotrichosis. She also had pulmonary tuberculosis and a negative tuberculin test, but no evidence of systemic sporotrichosis on careful screening. The nodules resolved following 4 months of treatment with potassium iodide (300 mg tid), amphotericin B (50 mg/day IV), and oral ketoconazole.

She was then not seen for 8 months, at which time the sporotrichosis had returned in a **fulminant form** with generalized ulcers, plaques, and vegetations covering all body areas. Again, systemic infection was not evident, but she died 2 weeks later despite intensive therapy. On **autopsy** *Sporothrix schenkii* spores were seen in the tongue, liver, spleen, kidney, myocardium, and bone marrow. Presumably she had impaired cellular immunity, which allowed dissemination of the organism.

Tanaka S, Mochizuki T, Watanabe S: **Sporotrichoid pyogenic bacterial infection**. Dermatologica 1989; 178:228–230.

A 43-year-old male lumberjack **injured his right thumb**. Not only did the site fail to heal, but over the next 2 months he developed new nodules in a linear pattern over the dorsum of the thumb and hand. A presumptive diagnosis of sporotrichosis had been made.

On examination he had four ulcerative nodules showing a **sporotrichoid distribution** along the right thumb and hand. On biopsy, botryomycotic grains were seen within a subcorneal abscess. Biopsy cultures showed *Staphylococcus aureus* and group A streptococcus, but no fungi or mycobacteria.

A diagnosis of **botryomycosis**, i.e., pyogenic bacterial infection, was made. The nodules completely disappeared after 10 days of cefaclor therapy.

In any sporotrichoid patterned lesion, look for other than *Sporothrix schenkii*. The following **organisms** may be the responsible pathogen:

Mycobacterium marinum	*Leishmania tropica*
Pasteurella tularensis	*Nocardia brasiliensis*
Bacillus anthracis	*Pseudoallescheria boydii*

Any one of them can move up the lymphatics, leaving a trail of infected nodules.

Graham WR Jr, Callaway JL: Primary **inoculation blastomycosis** in a veterinarian. J Am Acad Dermatol 1982; 7:785–786.

A 31-year-old veterinarian cut the dorsum of his left index finger while doing a **postmortem examination on a beagle**. Two weeks later he noted a small swelling at the puncture site. His family physician incised and drained the lesion and prescribed amoxicillin. When the lesion showed no improvement

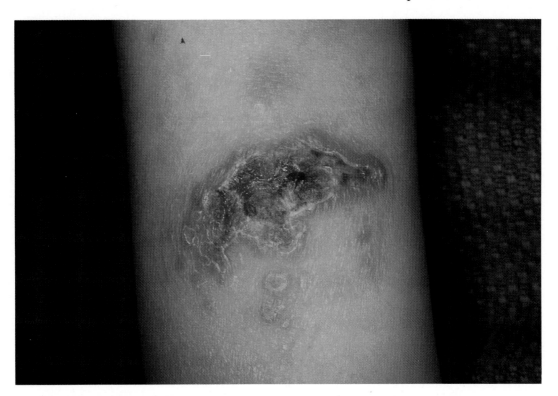

and a nodule appeared up the arm, a second physician prescribed erythromycin and then dicloxacillin.

By 6 weeks, examination revealed a 3-cm red, slightly tender swollen plaque over the left index finger as well as a nodule of the forearm. The **diagnostic spectrum** had now widened from a bacterial infection to include sporotrichosis, atypical mycobacterial infection, and inoculation blastomycosis.

A biopsy showed chronic inflammation only, but no fungi. Cultures for mycobacteria and for bacteria were negative. However, a **fungus culture** grew out *Blastomyces dermatitidis*, permitting the diagnosis of blastomycosis.

Making the diagnosis could have been facilitated had note been made of the fact that the **beagle's lung**, which the veterinarian was "sectioning" along with his finger, was culture positive for *B. dermatitidis*. But that report remained hidden in the state laboratory files.

Higgins EM, Lawrence CM: Sporotrichoid spread of *Mycobacterium chelonei*. Clin Exp Dermatol 1988; 13:234–236.

A 65-year-old woman with chronic active hepatitis and chronic paronychia of the right fourth finger had been treated for 12 years with oral prednisolone. She then developed a painful red nodule on the right wrist, followed by deep tender nodules with surrounding erythema in **a linear pattern** along the ulnar border of the right arm. Sporotrichosis was suspected, but biopsy showed a dermal and subcutaneous abscess and foreign body giant cell formation with many Ziehl-Nielsen–positive bacteria, identied as **M. chelonei**, which grew out in culture in 4 days.

M. chelonei is a saprophyte in soil and water and only rarely is a human pathogen, usually following penetrating trauma. Presumably, in this case the portal of entry was the **chronic paronychia**. Resistance to standard antituberculous drugs is usual, and determination of sensitivities is crucial. In immunosuppressed patients, an estimated 9% of infections become fatally disseminated.

Moral: All that spreads along the lymphatics is not sporotrichosis.

Wlodaver CG, Tolomeo T, Benear JB: **Primary cutaneous nocardiosis** mimicking sporotrichosis. Arch Dermatol 1988; 124:659–660.

A 74-year-old man had a 6-week history of linear nodules and pustules of the dorsal aspect of the right hand and wrist. The first lesion appeared 2 weeks after he abraded the area while working in his **rose garden**, and subsequent nodules "marched" up the arm. The medial aspect of the forearm had subcutaneous, cordlike, erythematous induration. He also had non-Hodgkin's lymphoma and was taking chlorambucil (8 mg/day). Gram stain of purulent drainage showed no organisms, but *Nocardia asteroides* grew on Sabouraud dextrose agar on the fifth day of incubation. Treatment with sulfamethoxazole (800 mg) and trimethoprim (160 mg) produced prompt response with complete clearing at 1 month.

The **differential diagnosis of "sporotrichoid" lesions** includes sporotrichosis, nocardiosis, mycobacterial infection, tularemia, leishmaniasis, and deep fungal infection.

Always alert the laboratory if the search is for *Nocardia*, since up to 4 weeks' incubation at 39°C may be required.

Kalb RE, Kaplan MH, Grossman ME: **Cutaneous nocardiosis**: Case reports and review. J Am Acad Dermatol 1985; 13:125–133.

An erythematous, weeping ulcer of the right hand of this 73-year-old mason developed within days after a **puncture wound**. Oral cephalosporin and intravenous nafcillin therapy failed to prevent the appearance of lymphangitis and axillary lymphadenopathy. Four nodulopustules soon appeared on the forearm in a sporotrichoid pattern.

Gram stain showed gram-positive branching organisms. X-rays of the wrist and hand showed no osteomyelitis. Cultures from the wound permitted eventual isolation of *Nocardia brasiliensis*.

This was an example of the gram-positive bacterial infection that presented as a chancre with a spread up the lymph vessel, which was suggestive of sporotrichosis. Treatment with sulfisoxazole intravenously for 2 weeks and orally for 2 months effected a cure.

Think of **nocardiosis** with:

cellulitis, abscess, ulcers, or mycetoma granulomas that do not respond to systemic antibiotics
puncture wounds in farmers or gardeners
sporotrichoid ascending lesions. Recall that same pattern is seen with sporotrichosis, blastomycosis, tularemia, mycobacterial infections, coccidioidomycosis, and lymphatic tumors.

Common **diagnostic missteps**:

failure to secure culture
failure to plate on medium free of *Nocardia* growth–inhibiting antibiotics
failure to alert laboratory that culture must be kept for more than 2 weeks, since *Nocardia* is very slow growing

Sweet's Syndrome

Rare but recognizable, Sweet's syndrome is an acute, alarming presentation of **tender red nodules or plaques**. It is a disease that deserves an immediate diagnosis and immediate steroid therapy.

Acute febrile neutrophilic dermatosis is Sweet's full name. And it is a name that is an *aide-memoire* for diagnosis. The onset is usually sudden, though not always. There is usually a prodrome of fever and malaise that alerts you to look for systemic disease. This may range from myelogenous leukemia to colitis. These patients are usually sick. Not only do they have fever but also they have leukocytosis.

A biopsy confirms the clinical diagnosis by revealing dense infiltrates in the dermis. It is these neutrophils that render the skin lesions tender and also responsive to dapsone. But once the diagnosis is made, laboratory study has just begun. It is necessary to search for underlying disease. The blood count, serum protein electrophoresis, and bone marrow examination should rule out hematologic disease. A chest plate may reveal the cause to be a respiratory infection. Check the bowel for colitis. Even a bypass may account for Sweet's syndrome. Order an ANA battery, looking for occult lupus or Sjögren's syndrome. Request appropriate tests to follow any symptoms that might suggest malignant disease. Remember, this is often a **paraneoplastic or preneoplastic syndrome**. Its course may be long, and it may be a recurrent one. Your diagnosis may be a "snap," but finding what's behind the diagnosis may be very difficult.

The easiest **misdiagnosis** for Sweet's syndrome is vasculitis, but this is corrected at once by the biopsy, which shows no vasculitis. An initial cluster of lesions can suggest furunculosis, and indeed the lesions may be pustular. Cellulitis is another diagnostic trap.

Acute febrile neutrophilic dermatosis is usually the face of malignant disease, most commonly myelogenous leukemia. Learn to recognize it by its painful papulonodules, by its "polys" in the blood and skin, and by its paraneoplastic presentation.

Su WPD, Liu H-N H: Diagnostic criteria for **Sweet's syndrome**. Cutis 1986; 37:167–174.

A review of five cases suggests that Sweet's syndrome is a specific reaction pattern triggered by multiple antigens including drugs, insect bites, venipuncture, infection, colon surgery, and leukemia.

Major criteria:

1. Abrupt onset of tender, painful erythematous or violaceous plaques and nodules
2. Skin biopsy showing neutrophilic infiltrates in the dermis, but no leukocytoclastic vasculitis

Minor criteria:

1. Preceding infection or fever
2. Arthralgia, conjunctivitis, fever, or malignant disease
3. Leukocytosis
4. Good response to systemic steroids but not antibiotics

Differential diagnosis:

erythema multiforme	no neutrophilic infiltrate
erythema annulare centrifugum	no neutrophilic infiltrate
erythema nodosum	involves subcutaneous fat
erythema elevatum diutinum	leukocytoclastic vasculitis present, no fever, plaques not tender

granuloma faciale	not tender or painful, no minor criteria
bromoderma	abscesses and pseudoepitheliomatous hyperplasia, serum bromide elevated
bowel bypass syndrome	responds to antibiotics, vesiculopustules, no plaques or nodules

von den Driesch P, Gomez RS, Kiesewetter F, Hornstein OP: **Sweet's syndrome**: Clinical spectrum and associated conditions. Cutis 1989; 44:193–200.

The sudden appearance of **painful raised red plaques** alerts you to the possible presence of Sweet's syndrome. The diagnosis is confirmed by finding fever, leukocytosis, and a dense neutrophil infiltrate on biopsy.

It appears to be a **reactive neutrophil response** to a variety of antigens. Examples are given here of associated preceding disorders:

Crohn's disease
tonsillitis
adenocarcinoma of the colon
urinary tract infection

Although Sweet's syndrome clears rapidly with systemic steroids, each of these patients **deserves elaborate study** to detect underlying chronic inflammatory disease or malignant disease.

Urrutia S, Vazquez F, Requena L, et al: **Fever and painful plaques** on the face, back and extremities. Arch Dermatol 1989; 125:1265–1270.

Tender bluish-red indurated plaques had appeared on the face, neck, upper back, and arms of this 63-year-old man during the past week. The plaques had a sharp border and were studded with vesicles. The man felt sick and was feverish.

X-rays of the chest and abdomen as well as blood and urine cultures were normal. The skin **biopsy** showed an intense inflammatory infiltrate, mainly of neutrophils. There was no vasculitis.

A diagnosis of **acute febrile neutrophilic dermatosis (Sweet's syndrome)** was made. This diagnosis calls for a search for an underlying myeloproliferative disease. Bone marrow aspiration and hematolytic consultation are essential.

In this case, a week of prednisone (60 mg/day) therapy was rapidly followed by complete clearing, suggesting the likelihood that the syndrome in this instance represented a **hypersensitivity reaction** as seen **after respiratory infections**.

Berth-Jones J, Hutchinson PE: **Sweet's syndrome** and malignancy: A case associated with multiple myeloma and review of the literature. Br J Dermatol 1989; 121:123–127.

A **tender rash** on the dorsal aspect of the hands for 4 weeks was the presenting complaint of a 51-year-old man. Examination revealed tender plum-colored erythematous plaques with raised indurated margins. Biopsy showed a dense polymorphonuclear infiltrate and leukocytoclasis in the dermis. Although he had neither fever nor neutrophil leukocytosis, a diagnosis of Sweet's syndrome was made (these features are no longer considered essential).

Since more than 50 patients with Sweet's syndrome have developed **malignant disease**, screening was done. The plasma viscosity was increased, and plasma protein electrophoresis showed a large monoclonal band typed as IgG κ. The serum IgG level was 73 gm/liter (normal 5 to 18 gm/liter). A skeletal survey showed multiple lytic areas in the skull, and bone marrow aspirate showed infiltration with abnormal plasma cells. A diagnosis of **multiple myeloma** was made, this being the third reported case associated with Sweet's syndrome.

All patients with Sweet's syndrome should be **screened** for hematopoietic, plasma cell, and lymphoid neoplasms with a complete blood count, plasma viscosity determination, and plasma protein electrophoresis. If none is found, these patients need regular follow-up for 5 years. Reference is made to 13 cases of malignant disease becoming evident months to years after the dermatosis. Look for clues such as anemia, leukocytosis, and increased erythrocyte sedimentation rate, as well as recurrence or prolonged episodes of Sweet's syndrome.

We must view Sweet's syndrome as another paraneoplastic disorder.

Ilchyshyn A, Smith AG, Phaure TAJ: **Sweet's syndrome** associated with chronic lymphatic leukemia. Clin Exp Dermatol 1987; 12:277–279.

The **crisp definition** of acute febrile neutrophilic dermatosis (Sweet's syndrome) is softening. No longer does it have to be acute or febrile, and the chronic lesions may sport more lymphocytes than neutrophils.

The **hallmark**, however, remains the typical annular erythematous plaques showing central postinflammatory pigmentation.

A 53-year-old man had four attacks of Sweet's syndrome in 12 years, presumably related to IgG paraproteinemia and **chronic lymphatic leukemia** that developed during this time. Previous reports have emphasized an association of Sweet's syndrome with myeloproliferative disease, although the cause of Sweet's syndrome remains unknown.

Alcalay J, Filhaber A, David M, Sandbank M: **Sweet's syndrome** and subacute thyroiditis. Dermatologica 1987; 174:28–29.

In a 63-year-old woman hospitalized with fever and neck pain referred to the lower jaws, subacute thyroiditis was diagnosed. She then developed arthralgias and discrete **erythematous papules and edematous plaques** on the backs of the hands, which later spread to the legs and feet. Skin biopsy revealed a **dense dermal infiltrate of polymorphonuclear leukocytes**, confirming the clinical diagnosis of acute febrile neutrophilic dermatosis (Sweet's syndrome). The ESR was 131 mm/hr, and the WBC count rose to 13,300 with 83% polymorphonuclear neutrophils.

The thyroiditis and skin lesions improved concurrently over a 6-week period with no specific treatment. This suggested that both were of a common origin, possibly an **upper respiratory viral infection**, which commonly precedes subacute **thyroiditis**.

Beutner KR, Packman CH, Markowitch W: **Neutrophilic eccrine hidradenitis** associated with Hodgkin's disease and chemotherapy. A case report. Arch Dermatol 1986; 122:809–811.

Erythematous nonpruritic ill-defined macules and plaques were present for 3 weeks on the face and upper trunk of a 44-year-old man with Hodgkin's disease. They began 2 days after his third course of chemotherapy with doxorubicin, bleomycin, vinblastine, and dacarbazine. **Diagnostic considerations** included drug eruption, erythema multiforme, Sweet's syndrome, and Hodgkin's disease of the skin.

But it was the **pathologist** who made the diagnosis. He saw an infiltrate of neutrophils and histiocytes enveloping the eccrine sweat glands, which showed degenerative changes and mucin.

The cause of **neutrophilic eccrine hidradenitis** remains unknown, but it may represent a reaction pattern to chemotherapy. Think of it when you see puzzling erythematous papules, macules, and plaques in a febrile patient being treated for malignant disease.

Jordaan HF, Cilliers J: **Secondary syphilis** mimicking Sweet's syndrome. Br J Dermatol 1986; 115:495–496.

A 25-year-old woman had three **annular lesions** on the face for 2 weeks, with confluent erythematous papules surrounding central areas of edema and brownish hyperpigmentation. Small ulcers were also noted on the tongue and labia majora. Clinically and histologically the lesions favored a diagnosis of **Sweet's syndrome**. However, serologic tests for syphilis were strongly positive (VDRL 1:256, FTA-ABS positive), leading to a diagnosis of **secondary syphilis**. Weekly injections of benzathine penicillin (2.4 million units IM times 4) led to complete healing and reversal of the VDRL titer.

Dover JS: Case records of the Massachusetts General Hospital: Acute febrile neutrophilic dermatosis (**Sweet's syndrome**). N Engl J Med 1990; 323:254–263.

This is a paradigm of description, differential diagnosis, discussion, and detailed referencing that can be of immense help in preparing for your own local medical grand rounds. Although the author made the correct diagnosis of **Sweet's syndrome** simply by clinical inspection, he marshaled the evidence against the following diagnoses:

    bacterial or viral infection
    erythema multiforme
    Sneddon and Wilkinson dermatosis
    drug eruption
    Behçet's disease
    pyoderma gangrenosum

All in all, a tour de force.

An algorithm takes the art (and joy) out of diagnosis.

Syphilis

A consultant is one who includes syphilis in his differential. He considers syphilis when others see only an upper respiratory infection in an infant with hoarse cry, sniffles, fever, and blisters on the palms. He thinks of syphilis and looks for a chancre on the back of the scrotum when others fail to even take a sexual history. He suspects syphilis when others see only psoriasis in a patient with ham-colored plaques over the trunk.

A consultant is one who never forgets that serpiginous ulcers in old people may be gummas. He is one who looks for the late signs of congenital syphilis as seen in the teeth, the skin, and the clavicle. He is one who thinks of syphilis as an explanation for hair loss, generalized lymphadenopathy, or circinate lesions of the face.

Try being a consultant when you see your next patient and do an STS.

Rudolph AH, Duncan WC, Kettler AH: **Treponemal infections**. J Am Acad Dermatol 1988; 18:1121–1129.

Think of primary syphilis: with any genital lesion appearing 10 to 90 days (average 3 weeks) after sexual contact. The classic chancre is a solitary, nontender, indurated ulcer with painless discrete regional lymphadenopathy. It may occur in mucous membranes, the pharynx, or cervix. The diagnostic window is open for only 1 to 2 months, since spontaneous healing occurs.

Think of secondary syphilis: with any lesion in the at-risk group that is macular, papular, papulosquamous, pustular, acneiform, or follicular, particularly on the palms and soles. Unique annular and arciform lesions with rolled borders and hyperpigmented centers are seen especially on the face in dark-skinned individuals. Also look for:

> mucous patches: painless, dull, erythematous patches or gray-white erosions on any mucous membrane
> alopecia: diffuse or patchy ("moth-eaten")
> condylomata lata: large, pale, flat-topped papules or plaques in intertriginous areas
> generalized lymphadenopathy

Other findings include anemia, leukocytosis, hepatitis, nephropathy, arthritis, bursitis, iritis, and neurologic changes.

Think of late syphilis: with an ulcerative nodule (gumma) that is locally destructive of skin and bones. Cardiovascular involvement is due to aortitis, with aortic regurgitation, aneurysm, or obstruction of the coronary ostium. Neurosyphilis may be asymptomatic prior to causing meningitis, strokes, general paresis, or tabes dorsalis.

Think of congenital syphilis: in an infant who was born healthy, but in the second to sixth week of life developed lesions resembling secondary syphilis: vesiculobullous lesions (especially on the palms and soles), maculopapular eruptions, condylomatous lesions, mucous patches, and "snuffles" due to nasal discharge. Other abnormalities include laryngitis, hepatosplenomegaly, painful bone involvement, renal disease, and central nervous system problems.

Think **late congenital syphilis**: in children over 2 years of age who have Hutchinson's incisors, mulberry or moon molars, and interstitial keratitis.

Laboratory diagnosis:

1. **A darkfield examination** should be performed on a moist cutaneous, nonoral lesion. A negative examination does not exclude the diagnosis of syphilis. Good sources include genital chancres, mucous patches, and condylomata lata.

2. **Nontreponemal serologic tests** used for screening and diagnostic tests:

> VDRL: Venereal Disease Research Laboratory slide test
> USR: unheated serum reagin test
> RPR: rapid plasma reagin card test
> RST: reagin screen test

3. **Treponemal serologic tests** used as confirmation tests:

> FTA-ABS: fluorescent treponemal antibody absorption test
> FTA-ABS DS: fluorescent treponemal antibody absorption test, double-staining test
> MHA-TP: microhemagglutinin assay for *Treponema pallidum* antibodies
> HATTS: hemagglutination treponemal test for syphilis

4. **False-positive reactions**

> Darkfield examination: Oral mucous patches or chancres are not good sources of specimens because of the presence of saprophytic spirochetes in the mouth.
> Nontreponemal tests:
>> acute reactions lasting less than 6 months occur with viral infections, malaria, immunizations, and pregnancy
>> chronic reactions persisting longer than 6 months occur with connective tissue diseases, narcotic addiction, aging, leprosy, malignant disease, and immunoglobulin abnormalities
>
> Treponemal tests: false-positive reactions are rare, but occur with:
> autoimmune or connective tissue diseases
> drug addiction
> Lyme disease
> pregnancy

Luger AFH: **Serological diagnosis of syphilis**: Current methods. *In* Young H, McMillan A (eds): Immunological Diagnosis of Sexually Transmitted Diseases. New York, Marcel Dekker, Inc., 1988, pp 249–274.

A definitive 25-page review.

Tests Using Lipoidal Antigens

In 1941, Mary Pangborn isolated **cardiolipin** from ox hearts. It is a diphospholipid that is inert, but upon the addition of **lecithin and cholesterol** becomes serologically active, reacting with the "**reagins**" or **Wassermann antibodies** in the sera of patients with syphilis. These reagins are autoantibodies against components in mitochondrial membrane.

The one lipoidal antigen test that has supplanted all the rest of the "Wassermann tests" is the **VDRL** (Venereal Disease Research Laboratory) test, developed at the Centers for Disease Control in Atlanta in 1946.

The **antigen** is 0.03% cardiolipin, 0.21% lecithin and 0.9% cholesterol in saline solution. The addition of heated serum containing the antibodies of syphilis induces microscopically visible flocculation. Serially doubling the serum dilution provides a quantitative assay, whereas the highest dilution that can be classified as reactive is reported as the titer. The result is available in 40 minutes. For the rapid plasma reagin test (RPR), charcoal is added to the antigen and the test read on a plastic card in 5 minutes.

The test usually becomes **positive 4 to 5 weeks after infection**. One in a hundred of the patients with secondary syphilis shows a negative test result when undiluted serum is used, but on further dilutions the test becomes positive (**prozone phenomenon**).

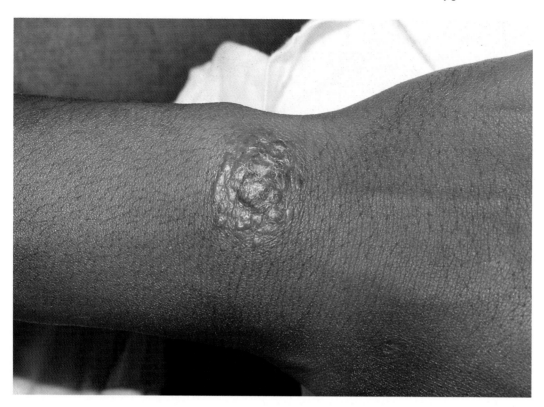

Following adequate treatment of a patient in the first few months of the disease, the VDRL becomes nonreactive in 6 to 12 months. If treatment is given later, the reactivity may be present up to 5 years later. Indeed, one in five may still have reactive tests 30 to 35 years later. **Proper treatment** ordinarily ensures a **fourfold drop in titer at 3 months**, whereas a fourfold increase in titer indicates treatment failure or reinfection.

In the untreated individual, the test will **spontaneously reverse** in 25 to 40% of instances **over a period of years**.

Nonspecific reactivity, i.e., the **biologic false-positive (BFP)**, occurs in less than 1% of all sera examined, but in 5 to 8% of all reactive samples. It is caused mainly by IgM autoantibodies (rheumatoid factor) and is thus seen in autoimmune disease. Nearly half of the patients with systemic lupus erythematosus have a positive VDRL test. It is also found in patients with increased turnover of nucleic acids, as in infectious mononucleosis, viral pneumonia, malignant disease, leprosy, psittacosis, and malaria.

TESTS USING *TREPONEMA PALLIDUM* ANTIGEN

For the greatest sensitivity and specificity, the **pathogen itself** (or fragments) is used **as the antigen**. The test remains positive, since it is so sensitive in detecting the specific diagnostic IgG antibody. The treponemal antigen allows several basic test procedures:

Fluorescent treponema antibody absorption test (FTA-ABS)

In this test, **Treponema pallidum**, harvested from rabbit orchitis and acetone-fixed on slides, is the antigen. The serum to be tested is first diluted in a **sorbent of Reiter treponemes** to remove the antibodies against nonpathogenic treponemes. The serum is then placed on the slide and incubated to allow the antibodies to attach to the pathogenic treponemes. These antibodies are visualized by adding a fluorescein isothiocyanate–labeled antiglobulin, which attaches to them and can be seen by using a **fluorescent microscope**. The intensity of fluorescence is graded from 1 to 4 plus. Quantitation is undertaken by using a serial trebling dilution of sera starting at 1:5, and usually the test is scored only as reactive or nonreactive at a 1:5 dilution.

This test becomes reactive at least 1 to 2 weeks before all other tests. Because of this and its high specificity and sensitivity, it is the **most reliable** test available in doubtful cases.

Treponema pallidum *hemagglutination assay (TPHA) and the microhemagglutination (MHA-TP) test*

In this test, **sheep erythrocytes** treated with formalin and **coated with** an ultrasonicate of orchitis-derived ***T. pallidum*** serves as the antigen. The serum is first incubated in a diluent containing the nonpathogenic (Reiter) treponemes and rabbit testicular tissue, and also extracts of sheep and beef erythrocytes. It is then incubated for 18 hours with the *T. pallidum*–coated red cells, which agglutinate in the presence of the specific antibody to *T. pallidum*. Sera are recovered at 1:80 dilution, with quantitation made by serial doubling dilutions from 1:80 to 1:5120. This test is the most sensitive and most specific method for detecting antibodies to *T. pallidum*. The margin of error is between 0.008% false-nonreactive and 0.07% false-reactive findings. It generally remains positive for life.

A variant of the TPHA test is the microhemagglutination test with *T. pallidum* antigen (MHA-TP), which is much less expensive, as it requires smaller amounts of reagents.

Solid phase hemadsorption test (SPHA)

The same reagents required for the MHA-TP test are used in the solid phase hemadsorption test (SPHA) to detect antitreponemal IgM antibodies (IgM-SPHA). The wells of polystyrene microtiter plates are coated with μ chain-specific serum (anti-IgM). The patient's serum is added and incubated for 30 minutes. After rinsing, the MHA-TP test is performed and serum IgM binds to the walls of the wells, and antitreponemal IgM reacts with the TPHA antigen. The test is reactive if agglutination occurs at a dilution greater than or equal to 1:8.

DETECTION OF IGM ANTIBODIES

Specific tests for IgM antibodies include:

1. 19S–IgM-FTA-ABS
2. IgM-SPHA
3. IgM-ELISA (enzyme-linked immunosorbent assay)

Reactivity indicates either new or active infection and the need for treatment. These **IgM antibodies** are the first demonstrable sign of a humoral response to *T. pallidum* and are detectable at the end of the second week of infection. IgM titers decline rapidly after adequate treatment, and persistence indicates treatment failure. Antitreponemal IgM in the CSF indicates neurosyphilis, providing the blood/CSF barrier function is normal.

DIAGNOSIS OF NEUROSYPHILIS

A lumbar puncture or cisternal puncture is essential in patients with reactive serum tests but no history of infection with *T. pallidum*, particularly if these findings persist unchanged after treatment. The finding of abnormal CSF cytology and an elevated protein level (Dattner-Thomas formula, cell count $> 5 \times 10^6$/liter and total protein above 0.45 gm/liter) indicate inflammation without a specific cause. However, restoration of these findings to normal is the first indication of the effectiveness of treatment. Traditional diagnostic criteria for neurosyphilis are inadequate because of atypical presentations and the finding that CSF VDRL tests are nonreactive in 30 to 47% of patients with active neurosyphilis.

The diagnosis of neurosyphilis can be established by:

1. TPHA index above 100
2. TPA index above 2
3. CSF IgM-SPHA test reactivity
4. CSF IgM-ELISA test reactivity

The diagnosis of neurosyphilis is excluded by:

1. CSF TPHA or CSF MHA-TP tests nonreactive
2. CSF FTA-ABS test nonreactive

DIAGNOSIS OF CONGENITAL SYPHILIS

The detection of IgM antibodies for *T. pallidum* is essential for the diagnosis of congenital syphilis and indicates the need for treatment. IgM reactivity of serum in the newborn is proof of prenatal infection.

Klaus MV, Amarante L, Beam TR Jr: **Routine screening for syphilis** is justified in patients admitted to psychiatric, alcohol, and drug rehabilitation wards of the Veterans Administration Medical Center. Arch Dermatol 1989; 125:1644–1646.

Routine serologic screening of 1515 **drug and alcohol abusers** disclosed 16 had positive test results. Not one of these was suspected to have syphilis on clinical grounds. The value of such screening of a risk group is evident.

Dorfman DH, Glaser JH: **Congenital syphilis** presenting in infants after the newborn period. N Engl J Med 1990; 323:1299–1302.

Although congenital syphilis is ordinarily diagnosed by serologic tests on both mother and infant at the time of delivery, some syphilitic infants are not identified as having syphilis. This is probably because the infection is very recent, and there has been insufficient time for an antibody response to develop. As a result, inclusion of **serologic tests for syphilis** is advisable in the evaluation of **all febrile infants**.

Perine PL, Niemel PLA, St John RK, et al: **Darkfield microscopic technique.** *In* Handbook of Endemic Treponematoses. Geneva, World Health Organization, 1984, pp 39–40.

To view treponemes, an ordinary compound microscope must be equipped with a **darkfield condenser** (which blocks out direct-light rays and allows only peripheral rays to pass through). These rays are then directed onto the specimen at an acute angle and deflected by objects such as red blood cells or treponemes through the barrel of the microscope to the eyepiece. A special eyepiece with a funnel stop is needed to reduce the aperture of the objective lens. The treponemes appear under the microscope as thin, tightly coiled silver threads on a black background.

Chapel TA: The variability of **syphilitic chancres**. Sex Transm Dis 1978; 5:68–70.

A dull red line of hemorrhage and dilated capillaries encircling an ulcer is characteristic of a syphilitic chancre but appears in only 10%. A small percentage (8%) of chancres are nonindurated, and an equal percentage have irregular undermined borders **suggestive of chancroid**.

One in four patients of this series of sixty-four had **three or more chancres**. None had pain, but one of three complained of tenderness. Two patients had noneroded papules as their chancre.

Chancres may show secondary **pyogenic or herpetic infection**. Inguinal adenopathy was found in 81% of these patients.

Echols SK, Shupp DL, Schroeter AL: **Acquired secondary syphilis** in a child. J Am Acad Dermatol 1990; 22:313–314.

A **4-year-old girl** was referred for evaluation of a **rash, hair loss, cough, and sore throat**. On examination, the patient had a low-grade fever, a few enlarged lymph nodes, and scattered white patches of the oral mucosa as well as erythematous denuded areas of the tongue. The scalp hair showed a moth-eaten pattern of alopecia. The palms and soles exhibited hyperpigmented macules with peripheral scales. In the perianal area was a moist verrucous plaque that on scraping gave a positive darkfield examination for spirochetes.

The **VDRL test was positive** at a dilution of 1:64, and the FTA-ABS test was also reactive.

On further questioning, it was found that both parents had been treated for syphilis 3 months earlier. It also revealed that the mother is a prostitute and the father the pimp. The source of the child's **secondary syphilis** was clearly evident, although not the mode of transmission.

Sapra S, Weatherhead L: Extensive **nodular secondary syphilis**. Arch Dermatol 1989; 125:1666–1669.

A 38-year-old man had a widespread symmetrical eruption of the trunk, face, scalp, palms, and soles. The lesions, which had been present for 2 months, were **erythematous papules and scaling nodules**. The glans penis showed the scarring remains of a healed ulcer. Axillary and inguinal lymph nodes were enlarged, firm, and rubbery.

The **differential diagnosis** included nodular secondary syphilis, Kaposi's sarcoma, sarcoidosis, and lymphoma. The diagnosis of secondary syphilis was confirmed not only by a VDRL reactive at 1:256 dilution, but also by visualization of spirochetes in the nodules, using the Steiner silver stain.

Young EJ, Weingarten NW, Baughn RE, Duncan WC: Studies on the pathogenesis of **the Jarisch-Herxheimer reaction**: Development of an animal model and evidence against a role for classical endotoxin. J Infect Dis 1982; 146:606–615.

The diagnosis of syphilis is supported when antitreponemal therapy results in a fever and exacerbation of the skin lesions. This is known as the **Jarisch-Herxheimer reaction** and probably results from **release of antigen** from the dying or dead spirochetes.

Mascola L, Pelosi R, Blount JH, et al: **Congenital syphilis** revisited. Am J Dis Child 1985; 139:575–580.

Major signs:

condylomalata
osteochondritis, periostitis
snuffles, hemorrhagic rhinitis

Minor signs:

fissures of lips
mucous patches
generalized lymphadenopathy
rash

Fiumara NJ, Lessell S: Manifestations of **late congenital syphilis**: An analysis of 271 patients. Arch Dermatol 1970; 102:78–83.

Major stigmata proceeding from common to very rare:

> frontal bossae: rounded, bony prominences due to periostitis of frontal and parietal bones
>
> concave depression of middle of face: rhinitis prevented normal development of maxilla
>
> high palatal arch: due to abnormal development of maxilla
>
> **Hutchinson's triad:**
>
>> upper permanent incisors, seen after the age of 6 years, peg shaped, widely spaced, shorter than lateral incisors; later, development of notch because of defective enamel in middle
>>
>> interstitial keratitis: onset between age 5 and 25 years with signs of iritis (tearing, pain, photophobia) followed by clouding and vascularization of cornea
>>
>> eighth nerve deafness: onset age 5 to 15 years possibly beginning with vertigo; initial loss for high frequencies
>
> saddle nose: another effect of rhinitis on bone and cartilage development
>
> **mulberry molars:** many small cusps on dome-shaped first lower molars; early caries
>
> **Higouménakis' sign:** clavicle on one side enlarged near sternum because of periostitis
>
> bulldog jaw: large appearing mandible because maxilla fails to grow
>
> rhagades: linear scars radiating from mouth, eyes, nose, anus, resulting from linear ulcers appearing in these moist areas at site of syphilitic lesions
>
> **saber shin:** tibia bowed because of thickening following periostitis
>
> scaphoid scapulae: vertebral border of scapulae concave
>
> **Clutton's joint:** doughy swelling of knee at puberty

Browne SG: **Yaws**. Int J Dermatol 1982; 21:220–223.

Yaws can be diagnosed on clinical grounds alone. Although due to a spirochete (***Treponema pertenue***), it is not spread by sexual contact and never affects the nervous system or heart. Nor is it transmitted to the fetus.

Look for it in poor children in tropical areas. The "**mother yaw**" arises at the site of inoculation, in a scratch, bite, or abrasion. Thus the common sites are the legs and buttocks where it appears as a chronic eroded papillomatous mass. This lesion usually heals spontaneously, although it may be secondarily infected.

This is followed by numerous **raspberry-like papules**. The flies that their moist surface attracts serve as a diagnostic feature.

Within months this florid rash involutes, leaving **macules of hyperpigmentation**. Yet periodic recrudescence occurs. Often the new lesions are hyperkeratotic or ulcerative. Indeed, the appearance of this on the soles may make walking impossible. Periostitis occurs with consequent fusiform fingers.

The late stage is more ulceration and **gumma formation**. The central area of the face may be destroyed (**gangosa**). **Ainhum** may occur, as well as juxta-articular nodules. Depigmentation is commonplace.

Perine PL, Hopkins DR, Niemel PLA, et al: Handbook of **endemic treponematoses**: Yaws, endemic syphilis, and pinta. Geneva, World Health Organization, 1984, pp 8–18.

Pinta lesions caused by ***Treponema carateum***:

erythema to squamous plaques
violaceous psoriatic plaques
late pigmented pinta, blue variety
hyperpigmented atrophic skin of late pinta
achromic scars of late pinta
Initial lesion is papule or plaque on uncovered part of body; gradually enlarges with satellite lesions
Three to nine months later **pintids** (disseminated lesions) develop. They become pigmented with age, changing from copper to lead gray to slate blue as a result of photosensitization
Late pinta changes from **dyschromic treponeme-containing lesions** to achromic treponeme-free lesions.

differential diagnosis:
neurodermatitis
psoriasis
tinea versicolor
vitiligo

Yaws caused by *Treponema pertenue*:

differential diagnosis:
impetigo
tinea versicolor
molluscum contagiosum
scabies
lichen planus
tropical ulcer
plantar warts
tungiasis
leishmaniasis
leprosy
psoriasis

In 1987, there were 35,241 cases of primary and secondary syphilis reported in the United States.

Did you miss one in your practice?

Telangiectasia

Many dermatologic problems are poorly named, but not telangiectasia. It is the collective noun for a gathering of the grossly widened and lengthened blood vessels most distant from the heart. Often they fail to reach the diagnostician's awareness level, as in the patient with varicose veins. Or they may be noted as an index of the seriousness of rosacea and its conjunctival component. Their presence may tip our impression of a lesion toward basal cell carcinoma.

Many are brought to us on a silver platter of **cosmetic** demand for help. Other examples have their own prominence as in actinically damaged old skin or as mute evidence of radiation therapy years ago. A few come as an incidental red birth mark. Rarely, other more tufted examples bleed; they were named **Osler** as hereditary hemorrhagic telangiectasia. They are responsible for the nosebleeds that herald bleeding in the gut, kidney, bladder, liver, meninges, or brain.

Other examples of telangiectasia serve as **hallmarks** of poikiloderma vasculare atrophicans, necrobiosis lipoidica, and congenital photosensitivity syndromes. But most dramatic is the widespread telangiectasia that may cover the body in a special form of mastocytosis. **Telangiectasia macularis eruptiva** perstans is a rare telangiectatic subclass of the common form of mastocytosis we see presenting as urticaria pigmentosum. More mysterious is generalized **essential telangiectasia** that usually begins on the lower legs of women and can gradually ascend to involve the entire skin. As its name indicates, its cause is unknown, but extensive telangiectasia may be associated with sinusitis or **dermatomyositis**.

But it is in children, often of consanguineous parentage, that we see the genetic telangiectasia of exposed **photodamaged** skin. Just as there is a poikiloderma of adults with its tracing of dilated vessels on a canvas of atrophy and variable pigmentation, there is poikiloderma congenitale (Rothmund-Thomson syndrome). Usually occurring in young girls, it first becomes apparent at 3 to 6 months of age as pink edematous plaques, which turn into reticulate atrophy and pigmentation traversed by telangiectatic vessels.

A second major form, the **Bloom syndrome**, mimics lupus erythematosus. Again, the LE-like lesions appear early in life. Many other genetic defects become evident, including dwarfism, café au lait spots, and ichthyosis.

A third example of inherited photosensitivity is the center of our understanding of the genetics of sun-damage repair: **xeroderma pigmentosum**. Children with this disease have defects in one or more of seven specific genes that control the repair of the keratinocytes' DNA damaged by ultraviolet light. Unable to properly repair the DNA, the skin quickly devises its own protective freckled, hyperpigmented, thickened epidermis. Such makeshift secondary defenses, however, do not save these children from developing nevi and carcinomas (squamous as well as basal cell). Like the congenital anhidrotic individual who must hide from the heat, these children must hide from the sun.

Finally, there is the child whose early failure to learn to walk normally may lead to the wheelchair by the age of 10 years. This ataxic gait is of cerebellar origin. By the age of 3 years the onset of telangiectasia confirms the diagnosis of **ataxia-telangiectasia** (Louis-Bar syndrome). The dilated vessels come first on the conjunctivae, and then later on the face and ears, on the hard palate, and hands and feet. Death due to bronchiectasis or lymphoma is their later lot.

Along the trail of telangiectasia we see the tracks of developmental defects, atrophy of the collagen support, and the presence of an angiogenic factor. Follow them.

Overview

Shelley WB: **Essential progressive telangiectasia**: Successful treatment with tetracycline. JAMA 1971; 216:1343–1344.

Telangiectasia in the Skin

I. **Component of:**
rosacea
varicose veins
actinic dermatitis
radiodermatitis
xeroderma pigmentosum

II. **Associated with systemic disease:**
lupus erythematosus
dermatomyositis
scleroderma
mastocytosis*
carcinoma telangiectaticum

III. **Hallmark of:**
Basal cell epithelioma
necrobiosis lipoidica diabeticorum
poikiloderma vasculare atrophicans
capillaritis[†]

IV. **Essential primary lesion in vascular nevi**
congenital neuroangiopathies[‡]
hereditary hemorrhagic telangiectasia (Osler)
essential progressive telangiectasia[§]

---

* Telangiectasia macularis eruptiva perstans
[†] Purpura annularis telangiectoides
[‡] e.g., ataxia-telangiectasia
[§] Includes generalized telangiectasia and angioma serpiginosum

Vanderschueren-Lodeweyckx M, Fryns J-P, Van den Berghe H, et al.: **Bloom's syndrome**: Possible pitfalls in clinical diagnosis. Am J Dis Child 1984; 138:812–816.

Low birth weight and **photosensitivity with telangiectatic erythema** in infancy call for a search for immunologic deficiency.

The **three syndromes** to be distinguished include:

Bloom's syndrome
Rothmund-Thomson syndrome
Cockayne's syndrome

Two cases are presented showing the difficulty of diagnosing Bloom's syndrome.

A 15-year-old girl who was small, thin, and delicate had telangiectasia of the conjunctivae (bilateral temporal) and a narrow face with prominent nose and receding chin. The **photosensitivity** of her childhood had faded. Chromosomes showed a high frequency of sister chromatid exchanges (72.1/cell with normal 8 to 12).

An $8\frac{1}{2}$-year-old boy had **photosensitivity** with cracked and crusted lips and eyelids, butterfly erythema since infancy, and erythema without telangiectasia of the forearms, hands, elbows, and knees. His skin was atrophic with bluish mottling and a thin subcutaneous fat layer.

Jones SK, Surbrugg SK, Weston WL: **Bloom's syndrome**. Am J Dis Child 1985; 139:1180.

A baby girl was kept indoors until the age of 14 months because of chronic **candidiasis**, poor health, growth retardation, pneumonia, and low immunoglobulin levels. Following sun exposure she developed red cheeks unresponsive to hydrocortisone, and by age 18 months she had telangiectasia and atrophy of the cheeks and lower eyelids. The diagnosis of **Bloom's syndrome** was confirmed with karyotype analysis for sister chromatid exchanges (SCEs). Cells showed an average of 107 SCEs/metaphase (normal 6 to 9).

Bloom's syndrome should be considered in all children with prenatal and postnatal growth retardation. It is **autosomal recessive** with a 25% recurrence risk and involves a high incidence of malignant disease.

Gretzula JC, Hevia O, Weber PJ: **Bloom's syndrome**. J Am Acad Dermatol 1987; 17:479–488.

1941: David Bloom, M.D., New York University Dermatology Clinic, **sees first case.**

1953: Bloom **sees two additional examples** at a meeting, senses he has an entity, and publishes a paper entitled "**Congenital telangiectatic erythema resembling lupus erythematosus in dwarfs.**"

1966: Chromosomal abnormalities detected (sister chromatid exchanges, quadriradial configurations in lymphocytes). Two patients die of leukemia. From then on, this disease serves as a model for studies relating chromosomal breakage to etiology of neoplasia.

Today the clinical diagnosis remains centered on a **sun-sensitive** telangiectatic facial rash in a patient with **stunted growth**. The rash comes on in the first summer or two of infancy. It not only involves the butterfly distribution of the face but also involves the other sun-exposed areas, i.e., ears, eyelids, forearms, and dorsa of hands.

If the exposure is continued, fissuring, blistering, and hemorrhagic crusting 1193 occur. There is conjunctivitis, even loss of eyelashes. By adulthood the sun sensitivity may lessen, and only **atrophy and depigmentation** remain.

Patients with Bloom's syndrome resemble each other not only in their rash but in their narrow **delicate facies**, prominent nose, small cheek bones, and small mandibles. They may have a variety of congenital malformations ranging from an annular pancreas to a malformed heart. One in four will develop neoplasia, especially **leukemia**.

Any exceedingly small child or infant with telangiectasia is a candidate for the diagnosis of Bloom's syndrome. **Chromosome studies** are needed to confirm it. **Mimics for Bloom's syndrome** are not lacking. Consider

> **ataxia-telangiectasia** (not only a rash but also ataxia)
> poikiloderma congenitale (**Rothmund-Thomson**) (may have telangiectasia also in nonexposed areas)
> **Cockayne's syndrome** (trisomy 10) (photosensitive rash, but with progeria)
> **dyskeratosis congenita:** reticulated telangiectasia, pigmentation, nail dystrophy, leukoplakia

Finally, the rash may not be present, for example in dark sun-protected skin, so that all children with stunted growth deserve chromosomal screening.

Moss C: **Rothmund-Thomson syndrome**: A report of two patients and a review of the literature. Br J Dermatol 1990; 122:821–829.

This 25-year-old man had marked telangiectasia of the face and forearms. Poikiloderma had developed by the age of 1 year. Growth retardation and kyphoscoliosis had been noted at that same time. A diagnosis of **Rothmund-Thomson syndrome** was made.

However, at the age of 3 years, a **laboratory finding** of increased urinary excretion of mucopolysaccharides led to a change in the diagnosis to **Morquio's syndrome**, which was duly reported in the literature. The mucopolysaccharide excretion later proved to be temporary, and since it was uncharacteristic, may have been of urinary bacterial origin. Detailed studies excluded mucolipidosis and sphingolipidosis, as well as the mucopolysaccharidosis. Nor did the urinary amino acid and dipeptide screen show evidence of prolidase deficiency. Endocrine studies as well as collagen typing were normal. The dwarf stature, severe skeletal changes (kyphoscoliosis, genu valgum, and equinus deformity) and lax skin and joints led to a second publication of the problem as seen when he was 18 years old. This time his case and that of his sister, who had similar findings, were **reintroduced** to the world literature as "a **newly recognized syndrome of connective tissue.**"

Now he is 25 years old, and the diagnosis has reverted to the original clinical one of **Rothmund-Thomson**. This is based on the fact that the poikiloderma was not present at birth but arose during infancy. This is the cardinal requirement for a diagnosis of Rothmund-Thomson. Of the 180 cases reported, an unbelievable coterie of associated defects has been described, but always the poikiloderma remains the initial diagnostic determinant. Thus these patients may be photosensitive. They may have dental, nail, and pain perception abnormalities and commonly show a reduction in sweat and sebaceous glands as well as hair. They are **at risk for cataracts** and may develop a saddle nose and widespread cartilaginous and bony abnormalities. Hypogonadism is also a complication in some.

This is an instructive report of how **laboratory data** can blind a diagnostician. In this case, the unaided clinical eye had the best diagnostic vision.

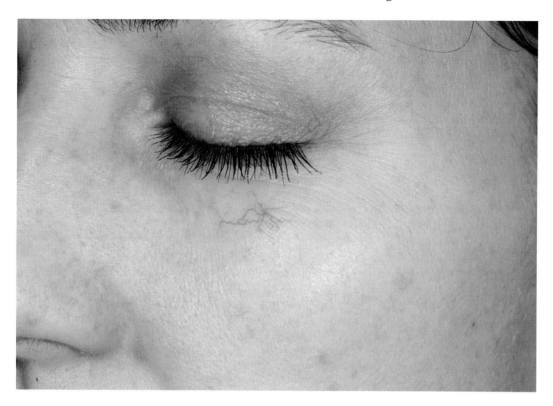

Berg E, Chuang T-Y, Cripps D: **Rothmund-Thomson syndrome**. A case report, photo-testing, and literature review. J Am Acad Dermatol 1987; 17:332–338.

A 25-year-old woman, barely over 4 feet tall, presented for evaluation of a **reticular pattern of mottled hyperpigmentation** and hypopigmentation and telangiectasia of the face, neck, arms, and legs. This had been present since infancy, beginning as a generalized erythema at age 3 months. She had been born with hypoplastic radial and ulnar bones. Indeed, congenitally hypo-plastic thumbs had been amputated when she was 3 years old.

The skin of the extensor surfaces of the joints showed hyperkeratoses. Fi-nally, she gave a history of being sensitive to sunlight.

This patient is a cameo case of the **poikiloderma congenitale** Thomson de-lineated in 1923. It had been originally described by Rothmund over 50 years before that in association with a cataract. The diagnostic poikiloderma develops in the first year of life, whereas the cataracts are not seen until the age of 2 or 3 years.

This patient had escaped the juvenile cataracts, hypogonadism, and mental retardation so often seen in this syndrome. Actually, these dwarf patients can be "dwarfed" in many other developmental ways—nails, teeth, hair, sweat glands, to name a few.

For a **differential** entertain the following: Werner's syndrome, Cockayne's syndrome, Bloom's syndrome, dyskeratosis congenita, and anhidrotic ecto-dermal defect.

Smith LL, Conerly SL: **Ataxia-telangiectasia** or Louis-Bar syndrome. J Am Acad Der-matol 1985; 12:681–696.

A child of a year or so in age who shows a **swaying walk or falls to one side** provides the first sign of this syndrome. The initial gait disturbance may easily be dismissed as an orthopedic abnormality, but it is actually a lack of cerebellar function and hence of control of balance.

The next major sign is the **telangiectasia** of the bulbar conjunctivae, which appears **between the age of 3 and 5 years**. It is not a conjunctivitis, but a symmetrical dilatation of venous vessels extending out from each canthus. It does not extend beyond the limbic region. Once developed it remains for a lifetime. Associated with it are abnormal ocular movements, nystagmus, and frequent blinking.

Next comes the telangiectasia of the sun-exposed areas across the face, in the ears, and around the eyes. It appears by age 10, at which time the child is usually wheelchair bound because of dysarthria. As sun exposure continues, the venous telangiectasia spreads over the neck, dorsa of hands and feet, and antecubital and popliteal fossae. In the sunlight patients easily become freckled and have patchy hypopigmented and hyperpigmented areas. All this photosensitivity reflects a genetic inability in DNA repair.

Atopic dermatitis and seborrheic dermatitis commonly are present. The scalp hair is coarse and brittle and becomes prematurely gray. White patches may be noted. Growth is retarded.

As the child becomes an **adult**, the skin becomes **hidebound**. The fat is lost, and the cutaneous picture is clearly sclerodermoid. Throughout all of this, these patients suffer recurrent respiratory infections and are prey to warts and other viral infections, since their immune system is profoundly depressed. Indeed, a herpes simplex infection is severe and may be fatal. They have but little IgA, an immature thymus, and weak response to antigen challenge.

The neurologic symptoms progress the path of **parkinsonism**. There is a masklike seborrheic facies, constant drooling, and inevitably, choreoathetoid movements, sometimes carelessly dismissed as "cerebral palsy."

These patients with their **progressive cerebellar ataxia** are found to have yet another problem—the risk of cancer. They are 1200 times as likely to develop a malignant disease as the normal person. It is usually leukemia or lymphoma, but the liver, ovary, and other organs may likewise develop malignant change.

The **pathognomic signs of the skin come late**, so the neurologist has a major diagnostic problem in distinguishing this Louis-Bar syndrome from other early ataxias, e.g., Friedreich's ataxia. Once the telangiectasia develops in the skin, the dermatologic **differential** centers on Bloom's syndrome, Rothmund-Thomson syndrome, Cockayne's syndrome, Von Hippel-Lindau disease, and dyskeratosis congenita.

The ataxia-telangiectasia syndrome leaves us in a **diagnostic** "swirl" as its autosomal recessive neurologic and immunologic signs erratically express themselves everywhere. It is a disease for all disciplines and many diagnoses.

Once the syndrome is recognized, alert the parents that the child **must avoid unnecessary sunlight and x-ray exposure**, must wear sunscreen daily, and must avoid contact with children who have colds, cold sores, or warts. Their child's chromosomes make him prone to radiation damage and infection.

Wilkin JK, Smith JG, Cullison DA, et al: Unilateral **dermatomal superficial telangiectasia**: Nine new cases and a review of unilateral dermatomal superficial telangiectasia. J Am Acad Dermatol 1983; 8:468–477.

Since age 12, this 31-year-old woman had noted a rash on the left leg. The redness of the **lesions intensified during** each of two **pregnancies**, returning to a baseline state after each delivery. Examination revealed numerous fine threadlike telangiectasias on the posterior aspect of the left leg in the distribution of S1-2.

A diagnosis of **unilateral dermatomal superficial telangiectasia** was made.

In these patients, **ask:**

> Is it acquired or congenital?
> Is it familial or a somatic mutation?
> Is the patient in a phase of estrogen increase (puberty, pregnancy, adrenarche in males, alcoholism, hepatic disease)?
> Is the redness reduced when the patient takes oral contraceptives that **reduce the estrogen** level?

Although the process is basically dermatomal, recall that lesions may obey only the law of linearity and not involve the entire dermatome.

Cox NH: **Arborizing telangiectasia** with gastrointestinal involvement. Clin Exp Dermatol 1987; 12:273–274.

Rarely does one get to look into the **duodenum** of a patient with telangiectasia. In a 72-year-old woman, however, the endoscopist saw **telangiectases** similar to those on the lower thighs, dorsal area of the hands, and legs, which had been present for 25 years. She had never had gastrointestinal bleeding but did have celiac disease, confirmed by a xylose tolerance test and duodenal biopsy showing villous atrophy. Other medical problems included a past history of anemia, a recently fractured femur, and osteomalacia.

The **arborizing telangiectasia of the skin**, a variant of generalized essential telangiectasia, alerts us to the truism that what's in the skin may be within.

We see what we are ready to see, what we have been taught to see.

J. M. CHARCOT

Acquired

Tatnall FM, Rycroft RJG: **Pityriasis versicolor** with cutaneous atrophy induced by topical steroid application. Clin Exp Dermatol 1985; 10:258–261.

For 4 months a 27-year-old actor had treated a rash on his chest daily with topical fluorinated steroids. He now had numerous **telangiectatic** erythematous scaly lesions on the chest, with cutaneous atrophy limited to each lesion. A scraping showed *Malassezia furfur*. Elimination of the topical steroids and local treatment with clotrimazole 1% cream resulted in clearing of the eruption and reversal of the atrophy within 3 weeks.

Two similar cases are presented in which **pityriasis versicolor** was associated with **selective localization of steroid atrophy**. Possibly the versicolor lesions favor the absorption of steroid or else this may represent an atrophic form of pityriasis versicolor.

Lycka B: **Amyl and butyl nitrites and telangiectasia** in homosexual men. Ann Intern Med 1987; 106:476.

Telangiectasia and erythema on the anterior aspect of the chest of homosexual men, both positive and negative for the human immunodeficiency virus, suggest that the virus is not responsible. Since vasodilating polypeptides such as histamine and serotonin can cause erythema and telangiectases in mastocytosis and carcinoid syndrome, other vasodilating substances should be sought. Patients with such telangiectasia should be questioned about the use of volatile **amyl and butyl nitrites** as aphrodisiacs.

Fried SZ, Lynfield YL: Unilateral facial **telangiectasia macularis eruptiva perstans**. J Am Acad Dermatol 1987; 16:250–252.

A 36-year-old man had over the past 10 years been developing punctate and grouped telangiectatic vessels of the right cheek. There was associated flushing and burning. The patient's concern that this could be the result of exposure to Agent Orange led to a biopsy. This revealed the process to be due to an increase in mast cells around the vessels. This and the clinical feature melded into a diagnosis of **telangiectasia macularis eruptiva perstans**.

In the clinical **differential** one had to consider:

> nevus flammeus, delayed onset
> unilateral nevoid telangiectasia syndrome
> liver disease
> steroid rosacea
> actinic damage
> radiodermatitis
> lupus erythematosus
> poikiloderma vasculare atrophicans
> carcinoid syndrome

Mortensen AC, Kjeldsen H: **Carcinomas following grenz ray treatment** of benign dermatoses. Acta Derm Venereol 1987; 67:523–525.

Over a 5-year period in one hospital in Denmark, 5 patients were seen with **carcinomas** in areas (scalp, lower leg, arms) that had been treated with **grenz rays** 1 to 14 years previously. Ten to thirty thousand rads of grenz radiation given over a period of 8 to 19 years had produced squamous cell carcinomas in four patients and basal cell carcinoma in one.

Grenz rays (Bucky) have been considered relatively safe, causing only minor adverse reactions such as erythema, hyperpigmentation, and telangiectasia.

They are ionizing radiation at 8 to 15 kV with an HVL of 0.018 to 0.036 mm Al and cause radiation effects in a tissue depth of 2 to 3 mm. The first case of a carcinoma from grenz rays occurred as a **squamous cell carcinoma** of the finger in a physician exposed over a 15-year period. The second case was in a dermatologist who eventually lost his thumb.

Caution: If it's radiation, it's carcinogenic.

Forman AB, Garden JM: **Progressive erythematous and atrophic eruption** in a patient with chronic myelogenous leukemia. Arch Dermatol 1989; 125:1265–1270.

A **reticulated erythematous** and violaceous eruption had been present for 3 years on the flanks and lower pelvis of this 71-year-old man. On diascopy there was complete blanching, revealing areas of atrophy and telangiectasia.

A biopsy confirmed the clinical diagnosis of **poikiloderma vasculare atrophicans**. The history revealed the background of chronic myelogenous leukemia, which was in remission.

Poikiloderma is a term from the Greek, meaning "**mottled skin.**" The terms *vasculare* and *atrophicans* refer to the telangiectasia and to the atrophy seen. The diagnosis refers to a reaction pattern. Its presence calls for a search for parapsoriasis, mycosis fungoides, or dermatomyositis.

With no evidence of these, inquiry must be made concerning damage to the skin from radiation, cold, or even heat. Its presence could also be indicative of scleroderma or lupus erythematosus or, as in this case, myeloproliferative disease. One observes it also as a sign of lymphomas, including Hodgkin's disease.

Congenital diseases (**xeroderma pigmentosum, Rothman-Thomson syndrome, Werner's syndrome**) will have poikiloderma vasculare atrophicans in their heraldry. Finally, these skin changes may be a sign of **arsenic** ingestion or of regressing lichen planus.

Poikiloderma vasculare atrophicans always requires a look behind the diagnosis.

Blom WAM, De Wit RFE, Nortier JWR: **Carcinoma telangiectaticum**. Br J Dermatol 1984; 111:495–497.

A 60-year-old woman noticed a **blue-purple discoloration** of the **central forehead**, associated with headache and unexplained 25-kg weight loss. Examination showed a sharply marginated 10 × 7 cm erythematous edematous plaque with prominent telangiectasia and venular dilatation. Skin biopsy revealed dilated vessels with extensive tumor embolism. Telangiectasia was also present on the lateral aspect of the cornea and the epipharynx.

An enlarged supraclavicular node on the right side and a mass in the right breast gave evidence to the source. She proved on **breast biopsy** to have an infiltrating ductal **carcinoma**.

All rosy faces are not rosacea.

Freeman CR, Rozenfeld M, Schopflocher P: **Cutaneous metastases from carcinoma of the cervix**. Arch Dermatol 1982; 118:40–41.

This 69-year-old woman developed a diffuse maculopapular eruption of the lower abdomen that extended down on the right thigh. The right leg was swollen, and inguinal lymphadenopathy was present, being more prominent also on the right.

A biopsy of the skin of the right flank showed **tumor cells filling** not only the **vascular channels**, but also the lymphatics. On pelvic examination a tumor of the cervix was seen that proved to be a **squamous cell carcinoma**. This was thus the source of the metastatic tumor cells seen in the slide.

Remember, not all metastases to the skin present as tumors. Some are sclerodermoid plaques; others are inflammatory telangiectatic lesions suggesting an infectious process. This is the so-called **carcinoma erysipelatoides**. The involved skin in these instances is tender, edematous, and erythematous.

The **location of the metastases** points to the primary site in many instances. In women, skin metastases on the chest are most likely due to a breast tumor, whereas those on the abdomen prompt one to look to the ovary for the primary tumor.

Sartori CR, Baker EJ, Hobbs ER: **Costal fringe**. Arch Dermatol 1991; 127:1201–1202.

Costal fringe (zona corona, Francke's striae) consists of a bandlike pattern of telangiectases across the anterolateral thorax. Usually near the costal margin, it may be bilateral, unilateral, or segmental. Typically it is an acquired finding in elderly men.

These telangiectases represent dilations of the postcapillary venules of superficial cutaneous microvascular plexus. They have no clear relationship to emphysema, congestive heart disease, or internal disease.

Cervical fringe is the term used to denote a similar band of telangiectases occurring in the posterior cervical region.

"Crocks" come from the potter's wheel of chronic, unrecognized disease.

Toxic Epidermal Necrolysis

If you've heard about it, if you've read about it, and if you think about it, you can't miss the diagnosis of toxic epidermal necrolysis. The patient is losing his epidermis like a peach dipped in boiling water. Great **sheets of gray epidermis slide off**, leaving the bare moist surface of the dermis. It is a true acute dermatologic emergency with progression from health to shock and coma in a few hours. It is a bullous disease that often, by the time you see it, is a disease of massive erosions. Without a history, you will think of flash burns.

But what is it? It is the ultimate **drug eruption** in which nearly the entire epidermis, all two square meters, dies within hours. Almost any drug can trigger toxic epidermal necrolysis (TEN), but sulfonamides, anticonvulsants, and nonsteroidal anti-inflammatory drugs head the list of 67 different drugs shown to cause this violent destruction of the patient's epidermis.

And what conditions could ever be mistaken for TEN? The first one, and possibly the only one, is **staphylococcal scalded skin syndrome** (SSSS). This is a disease of childhood in which the skin surface looks scalded. It is due to an enzyme elaborated by *Staphylococcus aureus*. A frozen section will quickly distinguish SSSS from TEN. The separation in the staphylococcic toxin disease is at the granular layer, whereas that in TEN is completely beneath the necrotic epidermis.

We have often said that "bugs and drugs" account for much of your patient's woes. With scalded skin, look for the bugs in the kids and for the drugs in all the others.

Revuz J, Penso D, Roujeau J-C, et al: **Toxic epidermal necrolysis**. Clinical findings and prognosis factors in 87 patients. Arch Dermatol 1987; 123:1160–1165.

Analysis of 87 patients over a 12-year period:

Diffuse deep-red erythema of extensive areas immediately followed by:

> epidermolysis
> crinkled wet cloth appearance of epidermis rubbing off and exposing dermis
> healing within 2 weeks

Erosive mucous membrane lesions:

> oral, ocular, genital (healing of glans penis may take 2 months)

Fever, without documented infection, may last several weeks:

> usually due to drug sensitivity
> mortality 25%:
>> usually due to septicemia: *Staphylococcus aureus, Pseudomonas aeruginosa*
>> prognosis poor: the older the patient, the larger the area involved, the higher the blood urea nitrogen

Long-term sequelae:

> eyes:
>> dry eyes (reduced lacrimal flow)
>> sandy sensation
>> photophobia
>> loss of eyelashes
>> corneal vascularization leading to visual loss (blindness in one case)
> oral: dry mouth (reduced salivary flow), erosions

skin: hypopigmented for many years, rarely hyperpigmented, hyper-hidrosis in some

genital: erosions, phimosis, lichenoid changes occasionally

Differential:

staphylococcal scalded skin syndrome (SSSS)
> no mucous membrane lesions
> no dermis exposed at base of blistering, since only top layer of epidermis peels off
> frozen section of blister roof shows only superficial epidermal blister
> no help from:
>> age: although SSSS usually in child
>> cultures: SSSS may be sterile and TEN colonized

Stevens-Johnson syndrome

target lesions of erythema multiforme

Guillaume J-C, Roujeau J-C, Revuz J, et al: The culprit drugs in 87 cases of **toxic epidermal necrolysis** (Lyell's syndrome). Arch Dermatol 1987; 123:1166–1170.

Mean time from first administration of drug to the onset of toxic epidermal necrolysis, 13.6 ± 8.4 days.

Most **common causes**

sulfonamides
anticonvulsants
nonsteroidal anti-inflammatory drugs

Rare causes

aspirin
allopurinol

Suggestive evidence for specific drug cause

Eruption began 7 to 21 days after first exposure to drug
Eruption began within 48 hours of administration of drug known to have produced previous reaction in that patient
Improvement on withdrawal of drug

Evidence against a specific drug being the cause

Eruption began within 24 hours of first administration of drug
Eruption began more than 21 days after last dose
Improvement despite continuing administration of drug

Roujeau J-C, Guillaume J-C, Fabre J-P, et al: **Toxic epidermal necrolysis** (Lyell syndrome). Incidence and drug etiology in France, 1981–1985. Arch Dermatol 1990; 126:37–42.

Incidence: 1.2 cases/million people/year

Mortality rate: 30% (greater in aged)

Cause: Drugs or chemicals

Most commonly:
nonsteroidal anti-inflammatory drugs
antibacterial agent
anticonvulsants

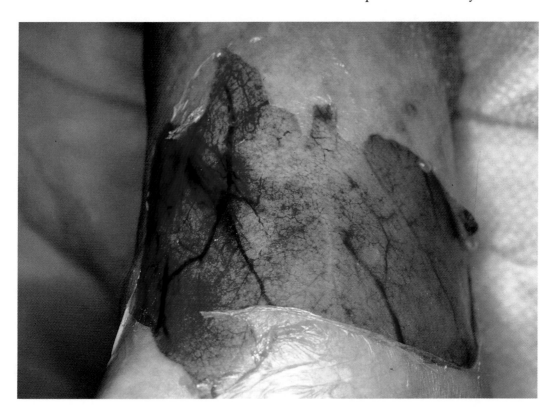

Smith DA, Burgdorf WHC: Universal cutaneous depigmentation following **phenytoin-induced toxic epidermal necrolysis**. J Am Acad Dermatol 1984; 10:106–109.

Three weeks after starting **phenytoin therapy** to control seizures, this 10-year-old black girl developed a generalized erythematous rash that progressed to bullous lesions and desquamation. All of her hair was lost. A diagnosis of phenytoin-induced toxic epidermal necrolysis was made. After 2 months of hospitalization her skin was healed.

Six months later she was referred for study of her **complete lack of skin color** and absence of hair. She had the appearance of an **albino**. No melanocytes could be found on electron microscopy of the biopsy specimens, and later tyrosinase was absent in samples from a sparse regrowth of white hair.

This is the first report of **total loss of all pigmentation** from the skin following **toxic epidermal necrolysis**. Previously, hyperpigmentation, darkening of hair, appearance of new junctional nevi, deformities of eyelashes, a scarred esophagus, loss of hair and nails, and keloids were the litany of sequelae for toxic epidermal necrolysis.

Goldstein SM, Wintroub BW, Elias PM, Wuepper KD: **Toxic epidermal necrolysis**: Unmuddying the waters. Arch Dermatol 1987; 123:1153–1156.

The diagnosis of **toxic epidermal necrolysis** should be limited to patients who meet these four **criteria**:

1. Widespread blisters with morbilliform or confluent erythema and associated skin tenderness
2. Absence of target lesions
3. Sudden onset and generalization within 24 to 48 hours

4. Histologic finding of keratinocyte necrosis that is confluent and extends throughout the full thickness of the epidermis in the virtual absence of dermal infiltrate

Lyell A: Requiem for **toxic epidermal necrolysis**. Br J Dermatol 1990; 122:837–838.

The father of toxic epidermal necrolysis (TEN, Lyell's syndrome) wishes to rename his child *exanthematic necrolysis*. Lyell's son can be distinguished from the other "TEN" siblings, i.e., staphylococcal scalded skin and generalized bullous fixed drug eruption. The exanthematic necrolysis ('EN) boy represents an epidermal necrolysis produced by a **drug acting with a cofactor** such as an upper respiratory infection. Thus the drug is innocuous months later on rechallenge when the infection is no longer present. In contrast, the true bullous drug eruption requires no cofactor, and challenge with the drug at any time will regularly reproduce the blisters.

The concept that a skin disease has a **binomial origin** adds a new dimension of complexity to our thinking. Infection, whether viral, bacterial, or fungal, may be an essential cofactor for certain drug eruptions. In the absence of such infection, the offending drug remains innocuous and a negative rechallenge misleading. Paradoxically, antibiotics are taken by patients with infections, but challenges are made on these patients when free of infection.

Small wonder we see so few successes in fulfilling Koch's postulates. There is greater need to recognize **infection and drug** as partners in crime. There are times when neither alone can rob the skin of its integrity. Learn to recognize this "**dependent drug eruption**" as distinct from the independent drug eruption.

Shearin RS, Boehlke J, Karanth S: **Toxic shock-like syndrome** associated with Bartholin's gland abscess: Case report. Am J Obstet Gynecol 1989; 160:1073–1074.

A 20-year-old white female student presented in a confused, disoriented state. She had shaking chills, was vomiting profusely, and her temperature was 102°. Examination revealed an erythematous, hot, swollen Bartholin cyst on the right labium. The patient was admitted to the hospital with a white blood count of 19,000/mm^3 and a diagnosis of toxic shock syndrome.

Cultures of the Bartholin abscess showed group A β-hemolytic streptococci. Intravenous antibiotics and marsupialization of the abscess led to prompt recovery.

McCarthy VP, Peoples WM: **Toxic shock syndrome** after ear piercing. Pediatr Infect Dis J 1988; 7:741–742.

Five days after having her ears pierced with a spring gun and gold studs, this 6-year-old white girl developed swollen hands and feet as well as a fever and diarrhea. Examination showed injected conjunctivae, cheilitis, strawberry tongue, and a widespread rough erythroderma. The pierced site of the right ear lobe was the source of a purulent discharge from which S. *aureus* was cultured.

A diagnosis of toxic shock syndrome was made. She responded to nafcillin therapy. A similar report of toxic shock syndrome has been made with S. *aureus* infection at the insulin pump infusion sites in a diabetic.

Ulcers

General
Infectious
Drug Induced
Systemic Origin

Ulcers tell the story of what isn't of what was. Diagnosis may range from the obvious **decubitus ulcer** to the occult ulcer of leprosy. We may diagnose the stasis ulcer by a glance from the doorway or the aphthous ulcer by a glance in the mouth. We may recognize the ulcer of basal cell carcinoma by its surroundings. We may know the factitial ulcer by its geometry, the ulcers of excoriation by their pattern, and the ulcer of pyoderma gangrenosum by its history of associated ulcerative colitis.

But we must turn to the **laboratory** for help in making the diagnosis of the ulcers of sickle cell anemia, macroglobulinemia, cryoglobulinemia, and cryofibrinogenemia. We may need to secure a health profile to sense the ulcers of diabetes and gout. We need to secure a proline excretion level to sense the prolidase-deficiency ulcer. We need tuberculin tests and rapid plasma reagin tests for the turberculous and luetic ulcers.

We need to secure **cultures** for identification of a host of ulcers due to infectious disease ranging from sporotrichosis to diphtheritic ulceration. We require the biopsy, sometimes multiple and deep, to sense the deep fungal and the lymphomatous ulcers. We need a **histologic look** for the malignant change at the edge of the chronic ulcer present for decades.

The Oxford English Dictionary records that in 1772 Buchan wrote "Ulcers may be the consequence of wounds, bruises, or imposthumes (abscesses) improperly treated." Today we would write that ulcers are the consequence of a local interruption in the circulation, and whatever their causes may be, we must search for them. We must find the why of what isn't.

General

Krull EA: **Chronic cutaneous ulcerations** and impaired healing in human skin. J Am Acad Dermatol 1985; 12:394–401.

Next time you look into an ulcer, ask: Is it due to:

vascular disease: arteriosclerosis, stasis, vasculitis
hematologic disease: sickle cell anemia, leukemia, cryoglobulinemia
metabolic disease: necrobiosis lipoidica diabeticorum
infection: bacterial, fungal, spirochetal
neoplasm: carcinoma, lymphoma
physical causes: injury, decubitus, factitial
other: pyoderma gangrenosum

Snyderman R: **Behçet's disease**—provocative clues. West J Med 1988; 148:438–439.

The **oral ulcers in Behçet's disease** are present in 99% of cases and are indistinguishable from aphthous stomatitis. They are painful (in contrast to those of Reiter's syndrome) and occur singly or multiply on the mucosa of the tongue, gingiva, lip, or buccal area. The ulcers are rarely confluent and last 7 to 10 days, generally healing without scarring. Ulcers on the palate, pharynx, or tonsils should suggest conditions other than Behçet's disease, such as Stevens-Johnson syndrome or pemphigus. Ulcers on the scrotum, vulva, penis, or perianal area may or may not be painful. In women, such genital lesions are frequently painless.

Pathergy is a phenomenon in which pustules develop on sites of trauma or injections. It indicates hyperactivity of the acute inflammatory response. It is occasionally seen in Behçet's disease, inflammatory bowel disease, and rheumatic diseases.

Inflammatory eye disease occurs in 90% of patients with Behçet's disease, consisting of either anterior or posterior uveitis. Hazy vision due to inflammatory exudation in the anterior chamber is the initial symptom of anterior uveitis, with later formation of hypopyon (pus in the anterior chamber). Posterior uveitis is more ominous, with retinal exudates and bleeding leading to blindness. Usually only one eye is affected during an attack.

It may be difficult to distinguish Behçet's disease from **inflammatory bowel disease**. Gastrointestinal symptoms occur in 50% of patients with Behçet's disease (vomiting, abdominal pain, diarrhea, flatulence, constipation). Discrete inflammatory erosions in the terminal ileum or colon may resemble ulcerative colitis or regional enteritis.

The occurrence of Behçet's disease in discrete **geographic areas** such as the silk route could be due to a neurotropic retrovirus infection. Retroviruses appear to have followed geographic migrations in the past, with HTLV-1 ([human] T-cell lymphotropic virus-1) following the route of Portuguese sailors from Africa to Japan, and HIV (human immunodeficiency virus) going from Africa to other parts of the world. A **neurotropic virus**, as seen with herpes infections, residing primarily in large ganglia such as the trigeminal and pelvic, could account for recurrent ulcerations and inflammatory lesions in the eye, mouth, and genital areas. Viral antigens could then induce circulating immune complexes leading to the other systemic phenomena. Perhaps infection, ingestion of certain foods (such as **English walnuts**), or exposure to various toxic agents (such as **zinc or organophosphate pesticides**) could cause transient immunosuppression and reactivation of an otherwise latent virus.

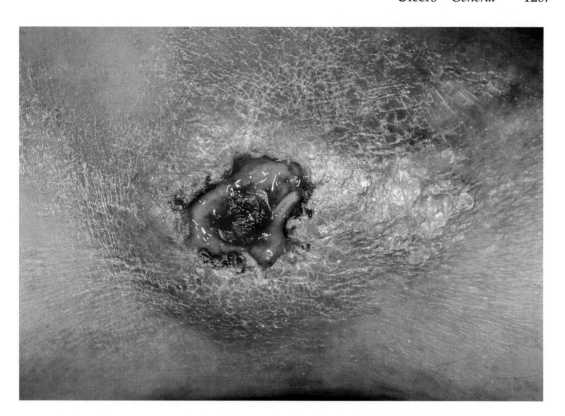

Milligan A, Graham-Brown RAC, Burns DA, Anderson I: **Prolidase deficiency**: A case report and literature review. Br J Dermatol 1989; 121:405–409.

Extensive leg ulcers present for 6 months in an 18-year-old girl were associated with atrophie blanche and multiple telangiectases of the legs. She also had an odd **birdlike facies**, spongy skin texture, and joint hyperextensibility. Chromosome studies were normal, but in searching for a genetic defect, it was found that urinary levels of proline and hydroxyproline were elevated. A collagen disorder such as **Ehlers-Danlos** syndrome was suspected. When the ulcers failed to heal, the limbs were occluded for 3 weeks in the hospital to rule out artifactual interference, which led to an increase in ulcer size. Only prolonged bed rest proved helpful.

Skin biopsies showed nonspecific inflammatory changes with thickened dermal collagen bundles, and collagen studies showed a very low collagen content in skin. Electron microscopy revealed marked cross-banding and shredding of affected skin collagen. **Venograms** showed a paucity of valves, viewed as a contributing factor. As the years went on, her only other medical problem was recurrent sterile erosive cystitis.

After 21 years of observation of the ulcers, the question arose whether she could possibly have the newly described leg ulceration associated with **massive urinary excretion of proline**. She was quickly shown to have just that. Such iminodipeptiduria signals increased collagen breakdown, since proline and hydroxyproline make up 25% of collagen. When present in a massive degree, it is diagnostic for **lack of the enzyme prolidase**, which cleaves dipeptides to release proline for recycling. Absence of prolidase, therefore, depletes the total pool of proline normally used in protein synthesis.

Assays for red cell and fibroblast prolidase were very low. Two brothers had similar low prolidase levels, whereas her sister and mother showed normal values. Clinically, all were normal.

Over a score of patients with prolidase deficiency have been reported. **Screening** is easily done by an assay **for iminodipeptiduria**. Look for it in patients with leg ulcers at an early age, especially if the thighs are also involved. Other **clues** include telangiectasia, prematurely gray hair, hyperextensible joints, lax abdominal wall, low IQ, and characteristic facies (saddle nose, widely spaced eyes).

Strange ulcers call for strange tests.

Weintraub E, Soltani K, Hekmatpanah J, Lorincz AL: **Trigeminal trophic syndrome**. A case and review. J Am Acad Dermatol 1982; 6:52–57.

A 30-year-old Chinese woman developed **right-sided facial paresthesias** and nasal congestion 2 weeks after the third craniotomy for recurrent meningioma and radiation necrosis. She felt as if something were touching her skin and began rubbing and picking at the area. By 6 weeks postoperatively she had a well-circumscribed 2.0- by 2.5-cm ulcer with a crusting bleeding base at the right nasolabial area. There was partial loss of the right ala nasi, and the upper lip was drawn upward by a fibrous band extending from the ulcer to the angle of the mouth. Bacterial culture revealed *Staphylococcus aureus*, and a skin biopsy showed only acute and chronic inflammation. Following treatment with a topical antibiotic ointment, caution against traumatizing the lesion, and use of a protective device to cover the ulcer at night, the ulcer healed in 1 month.

The **trigeminal trophic syndrome (neurotrophic trigeminal ulceration, ulceration *en arc*)** consists of the **triad** of trigeminal **anesthesia**, facial **paresthesias**, and **erosion of the ala nasi** due to scratching or picking at the paresthetic or anesthetic areas. The delusion of nasal congestion may be an important factor. The resulting ulcer of the nasolabial fold may be triangular, crescent, or Y shaped, with a base of crusted dried blood overlying granulation tissue. The ala nasi is often destroyed, and a fibrotic scar may draw the lip up into a sneer. There may also be a fissure in the floor of the nose, usually on the right side. The **differential** diagnosis includes basal cell carcinoma, herpetic ulceration, pyoderma gangrenosum, midline granuloma, and factitial ulcer (dermatitis artefacta).

Specific causes of nerve damage leading to the syndrome include:

nerve resection or alcohol injection for trigeminal neuralgia
postencephalitic parkinsonism
lateral medullary syndrome
acoustic neuroma
syringobulbia
vertebrobasilar insufficiency
amyloid deposits in the trigeminal nerve
meningioma

The name *neurotrophic ulcer* is outmoded, since a nerve has no specific trophic or growth influence. **Sensory loss** anywhere in the skin can **result in ulcers**, such as the trophic ulcers of the feet in diabetes, ulcers of the legs and feet in hereditary sensory radicular neuropathy, and neurotrophic ulcers of the tongue following a lingual nerve block.

Jackson RM, Tucker SB, Abraham JL, Millns JL: **Factitial cutaneous ulcers and nodules**: The use of electron-probe microanalysis in diagnosis. J Am Acad Dermatol 1984; 11:1065–1069.

Year after year, multiple, nonhealing **ulcerations of the hips** and thighs were the presenting complaint of this 36-year-old nurse. They were painful and had required surgical excision, drainage, and numerous hospitalizations. Finally, a biopsy showed foreign body granuloma with polarizable foreign material.

By means of electron-probe microanalysis, talc was identified as being present, and by laser-Raman analysis, cellulose was found. Both are fillers for the drugs (pentazocine, meperidine) she was presumably injecting. A diagnosis of **factitial ulcerations** was made. Such a form is commonly seen in medical personnel who have ready access to drugs.

Think factitial when confronted with that strange lesion in that strange patient.

Guillozet N: **Erosive myiasis**. Arch Dermatol 1981; 117:59–60.

Dozens of **deep punched-out ulcers** covered the trunk of this cachetic 2-year-old African boy. They had been preceded by furunculoid lesions.

The diagnosis of **myiasis** became apparent upon simple expression of the larvae of the tumbu fly from the lesions.

Kofler H, Pichler E, Romani N, et al: **Hemangiosarcoma in chronic leg ulcer**. Arch Dermatol 1988; 124:1080–1082.

An 84-year-old Austrian man had recurrent varicose ulcers at the sites of old gummas. Over a 5-year period a 9- by 15-cm ulcer of the left calf developed, with five solid agminated hemorrhagic necrotic nodules in the center. The surrounding skin was atrophic, edematous, and sclerotic. **Squamous cell carcinoma was suspected**, but repeated punch biopsies revealed only pseudo-epitheliomatous hyperplasia. Only by **deep incisional biopsy** was it possible to diagnose malignancy in the nodular growths. Although malignant fibrous histiocytoma was initially diagnosed, examination of the entire tumor after amputation led to a final diagnosis of **angiosarcoma**.

Angiosarcomas arise in the centers of extensive leg ulcers present for many years. They **resemble hypertrophic granulation tissue** or squamous cell carcinomas, appearing as several dome-shaped agminate nodules.

Other types of angiosarcoma arise on the scalp (elderly people), female breast, liver (after exposure to arsenic oxide or phenyl chloride), and in lymphedema (**Stewart-Treves syndrome**).

Moral: To see the big picture, get the big biopsy.

Shakespearian clues to the diagnosis:
Ay, there's the rub: Intertrigo
More than meets the eye: LE
You'll have to sleep on it and let me know: Decubitus ulcer

Infectious

Greene SL, Su WPD, Muller SA: **Ecthyma gangrenosum**: Report of clinical, histopathologic, and bacteriologic aspects of eight cases. J Am Acad Dermatol 1984; 11:781–787.

Ecthyma gangrenosum is a sign of life-threatening systemic infection with *Pseudomonas aeruginosa.*

Clinical:

> begins as painless, round, erythematous macule
> may develop into vesicle; becomes tender, indurated, then bullous, pustular
> sloughs to form gangrenous ulcer with gray-black eschar and erythematous halo
> often multiple ulcers
> often in gluteal-perineal region

Systemic:

> profound neutropenia or pancytopenia in all
> background drug reaction,, leukemia, systemic lupus erythematosus
> high fever, chills, hypotension

Differential:

> incorrect initial diagnoses:
> > drug eruption
> > pyoderma associated with inflammatory bowel disease
> > perirectal abscess
> > folliculitis
> > herpes simplex
> must consider:
> > cryoglobulinemia
> > periarteritis nodosa
> > necrotizing vasculitis
> > drug eruption
> > ecthyma gangrenosum-like lesions due to *Candida*, aspergillus, and also the gram-negative organisms *Escherichia coli* and *Aeromonas hydrophila*

Diagnostic approach:

> needle aspiration for Gram stain for quick diagnosis
> deep skin biopsy: stain with Gram method, PAS, and acid fast
> second biopsy for culture of bacteria, fungus, yeast, mycobacteria
> blood samples (3): during fever spikes, for bacteria, and sensitivity tests

Early diagnosis and immediate intensive intravenous antibiotic therapy are the only way to save the lives of these patients.

Werman BS, Herskowitz LJ, Olansky S, et al: A clinical variant of **chancroid** resembling granuloma inguinale. Arch Dermatol 1983; 119:890–894.

Basically, **chancroid** is an ulcer, a genital ulcer. It may be shallow, saucer shaped, or deep punched out. Its border is ragged, irregular, and, at times, undermined. The floor of the ulcer is covered with a purulent gray-white exudate. Once you scrape this away, the red granulation tissue becomes evident. Patients complain of pain, and in a large number of patients discrete inguinal nodes develop. In contrast to the chancre of syphilis, the chancroid is a soft lesion.

Typically, **granuloma inguinale** is characterized by one or more soft ulcers of the genitalia. They are painless, have a raised border, and a beefy-red base. Pain and inguinal nodes are not present unless secondary bacterial infection intervenes.

Chancroid may, as in the 16 patients studied, assume the clinical characteristics of granuloma inguinale. Clinical diagnosis has its limitations.

Given a **genital ulcer** that is darkfield negative for *Treponema pallidum*, smear negative for the Donovan bodies of granuloma inguinale, and culture negative for herpes simplex virus, a culture for *Hemophilus ducreyi* should establish or eliminate the diagnosis of chancroid, no matter what the ulcer patterning is.

It is interesting that the **pain and buboes** of chancroid are indicative of the bacterial nature of this infection and that when granuloma inguinale becomes painful and lymphadenopathy appears, one knows that secondary coccal bacterial infection has occurred.

Note: Laboratories can now culture *H. ducreyi* but still cannot culture *Calymmatobacterium (Donovania) granulomatis*.

Held JL, Ross M, Beltrani V Jr, et al: **Noduloulcerative or "malignant" syphilis** occurring in an otherwise healthy woman: Report and review of a dramatic dermatosis. Cutis 1990; 45:119–122.

A **generalized efflorescence** of 100 papules and nodules of only 4 days' duration brought this 53-year-old woman to the emergency room. She was otherwise well, took no medicines, used no intravenous drugs, and never had received a blood transfusion.

On examination the distinctive feature was the **rupioid crusting**, the central necrosis, and ulceration of the lesions. The palms and soles were free of lesions. Biopsy revealed a dense plasma cell and neutrophil infiltrate, but no spirochetes were found on the Warthin-Starry stain. The answer was in the positive serum tests for syphilis. She had a titer of 1:512 and a positive FTA test. A diagnosis of noduloulcerative secondary syphilis was made. It is an entity so rapid in onset, so appalling in appearance, that some have called it **malignant syphilis**. Yet it rapidly clears with penicillin, as did this case.

Lantos G, Fisher BK, Contreras M: **Tuberculous ulcer** of the skin. J Am Acad Dermatol 1988; 19:1067–1072.

For 5 months this 19-year-old Philippine man had had a painful, gradually enlarging **ulcer of the lumbar area**. Systemic steroids and antibiotics given by several physicians had been to no avail.

On examination the ulcer was well demarcated with a violaceous, slighty heaped-up border and deep undermined edges. Granulation tissue at the ulcer base was covered with a scant light-brown, cheesy, purulent discharge. Skin biopsy showed early granuloma formation, but no organism could be seen on acid-fast stains. The picture was suggestive of an **atypical mycobacterial infection**.

However, 6 weeks later the biopsy tissue **culture grew out *Mycobacterium tuberculosis***. Well before this the tuberculin skin test was strongly positive, and by 2 weeks, culture of bronchial washings showed *M. tuberculosis*, thus explaining a dry cough, malaise, and weight loss he had reported.

This patient's lesion best resembled an ulcerated tuberculous **gumma**, resulting from a subcutaneous tuberculous process that leads to a **cold abscess** and later secondary breakdown of the overlying skin.

Fisher MM, McCann W, Michele A: **Foot ulcers** in Hansen's disease. NY State J Med 1964; 64:3021–3025.

Multiple ulcers on the plantar surface of the foot should raise suspicion of **Hansen's disease**.

Kern F, Pedersen JK: **Leishmaniasis** in the United States. A report of ten cases in military personnel. JAMA 1973; 226:872–874.

Ten marines who spent 10 days on military exercises in Panama during one February noted small erythematous papules on the exposed areas of the forearms, wrist, face, or leg. These enlarged despite systemic antibiotics and then developed **central punched-out ulcers** (0.5 to 5.0 cm) covered with thick serosanguineous crusts and indurated thick red-purple rims. Removal of crusts revealed meaty and friable bases. In four patients subcutaneous nodules extended in a linear distribution up the forearm from the primary lesion, resembling sporotrichosis. Two patients had "metastatic type" spread of lesions to various skin areas, long after exposure to the insect vector.

The diagnosis of **leishmaniasis** was suspected by the clinical presentation in individuals exposed in the tropics to sandflies of the genus *Phlebotomus*. The diagnosis was confirmed in six of the ten by seeing Leishman-Donovan bodies in a Giemsa stain of smears taken from the base of the lesions. In an additional case the organisms were seen in the biopsy specimen. The causative organism was *Leishmania brasiliensis*.

Chronic skin ulcerations in patients who have recently been in endemic areas should be highly suspect for leishmaniasis. The diagnosis is easily established by examining **Giemsa-stained smears** taken from the base of the lesions.

Kaiser AB, Rieves D, Price AH, et al: **Tularemia** and rhabdomyolysis. JAMA 1985; 253:241–243.

Two patients with unsuspected tularemia had **ulcers on the hand** along with fever, cough, myalgias, lethargy, and brown urine:

- A 58-year-old man developed a 2-cm ulcer on the right hand with right epitrochlear and axillary lymphadenopathy, beginning 12 days after the illness began. He had **no recognized exposure** for **tularemia**.
- A 63-year-old woman had a 1-cm ulcer on the dorsum of the right hand without associated lymphadenopathy, starting 7 days after becoming ill. She had cooked a **rabbit** 5 days before getting sick. She subsequently died of disseminated intravascular coagulation.

Order:

urine hemoglobin and myoglobin (positive)
creatine kinase ([CPK] elevated)
acute and convalescent tularemia titers (positive for **Francisella tularensis**)

Lambert WC, Pathan AK, Imaeda T, et al: Cultures of *Vibrio extorquens* from severe, **chronic skin ulcers** in a Puerto Rican woman. J Am Acad Dermatol 1983; 9:262–268.

This 48-year-old woman had extensive ulcers on the thighs, buttocks, and right arm. Present for $3\frac{1}{2}$ years, they began as a subcutaneous nodule of the left buttock, which developed a **fistulous drainage**. An enlarging ulcer followed with a similar sequence occurring on the opposite buttock.

Despite surgical excision of both ulcers, as well as systemic antibiotics, the **surgical sites** developed new ulcers. Six months later the nodule-ulcer sequence was repeated on the right arm, and at the time of presentation a new nodule was present on the back.

Biopsies revealed a noncaseating granulomatous process with acid-fast bacilli seen in the cells deep in the tissue. **Cultures** of the ulcers grew out a mucoid colony of aerobic gram-negative rods, identified as *Vibrio extorquens*. On the basis of sensitivity tests, kanamycin (1 gm/day IM) was given. Improvement was noted within a month and cure after $1\frac{1}{2}$ years of this therapy.

The **differential diagnosis** included:

> **mycobacterial infection:** *Mycobacterium tuberculosis, M. leprae, M. ulcerans, M. marinum, M. fortuitum, M. chelonei, M. intracellulare, M. kansasii, M. szulgai, M. scrofulaceum.*
> **mycetoma** (*Actinomyces israelii, Streptomyces madurae*)
> **nocardiosis** (*Nocardia asteroides, Nocardia brasiliensis*)

The absence of undermining of the edges eliminated *M. ulcerans* from serious consideration.

This is the **first report** of *V. extorquens* as a pathogen and stands as a tribute to the microbiology laboratory.

Farge D, Frances C, Vouldoukis I, et al: **Chronic destructive ulcerative lesion** of the midface and nasal cavity due to leishmaniasis contracted in Djibouti. Clin Exp Dermatol 1987; 12:211–213.

A 27-year-old Caucasian man had a 5-year-history of **ulceration** of the right nostril with **septal perforation**. Initially he had a spontaneously resolving erythematous nodule of the right ala nasi, arising 2 years after he completed military service in Djibouti, East Africa. He then had six symptom-free years until another nodule appeared, which over 5 years painlessly destroyed the right ala nasi and nasal septum.

Three biopsies showed epithelial hyperplasia and nonspecific polymorphic infiltrates of lymphocytes, plasma cells, and mast cells. Serodiagnosis for leishmaniasis, using immunofluorescence and counterimmunoelectrophoresis, was negative. **Lethal midline granuloma was suspected**, but no neoplastic, bacterial, or fungal cause could be found.

The answer came with use of a new in vivo technique. Four 50 μl drops of saline serum (0.09%) were left for 5 minutes in contact with the muconasal lesion and then aspirated. Simple air drying of a smear of the aspirate and application of May-Grünwald-Giemsa stain revealed intracellular amastigotes of **Leishmania**. Treatment with antimony was curative.

Marston S: **Wegener's granulomatosis**. J Roy Soc Med 1982; 75:274–276.

A 35-year-old Irish woman developed an **ulcer** on the face, thought to be a **parotid abscess**, which failed to heal despite treatment with antibiotics for 6 weeks. She then developed sterile otitis media, fever, and numerous subcutaneous plaques on the trunk and limbs. Some of the nodules ulcerated and discharged thin brown sterile fluid. At the same time she developed right facial weakness and hoarseness, and the right hemidiaphragm became paralyzed. Laboratory findings included ESR 120 mm/hr, hemoglobin 10 gm/dl, WBC 13,100 with 91% neutrophils, ANA 1:160, and urine with positive protein and 500 WBC/mm^3. Despite prednisolone 60 mg daily for 1 month the skin ulcerations continued, and she developed pulmonary infiltrates suggestive of **Wegener's granulomatosis**. She improved rapidly with cyclophosphamide administration and was finally discharged from the hospital 5 months after admission.

Skin biopsies of subcutaneous nodules were initially interpreted as **Weber-Christian panniculitis**, with a mixed inflammatory infiltrate of the subcutaneous fat and fibrinoid necrosis of vessels. Later review revealed granulomas and leukocytoclastic vasculitis of small and medium vessels in the fat, confirming the diagnosis of Wegener's granulomatosis.

The clinician's laboratory is the clinic.

Drug Induced

Shelley ED, Shelley WB: Inframammary, intertriginous, and decubital **erosions due to etretinate**. Cutis 1990; 45:111–113.

Chronic **erosions** of the buttocks and inframammary area in this 42-year-old woman were viewed as **decubitus ulcers** and erosive intertrigo, respectively. After 3 months of observation, their total resistance to multiple therapies led to the discovery that they **resulted from etretinate**. Discontinuance of this drug led to a rapid cure.

Lawrence CM, Dahl MGC: Two patterns of **skin ulceration induced by methotrexate** in patients with psoriasis. J Am Acad Dermatol 1984; 11:1059–1065.

Methotrexate can be responsible for **ulcerations of the skin.**

Type 1. **Acute erosions** of **psoriatic plaques.** Psoriatic lesions become more reddened and tender, and superficial erosions appear. Rapid healing occurs on stopping methotrexate therapy. These erosions can be confused with an acute episode of **pustular psoriasis**, which could lead to prescribing even more methotrexate.

Type 2. **Ulceration of nonpsoriatic skin.** This ulceration occurs at sites of previous skin damage such as stasis dermatitis, prior leg ulcers, or fistula in ano. These ulcers take several months to heal once the methotrexate is discontinued.

These ulcers can **mimic stasis ulcers**, and the role of methotrexate can then be overlooked. Finally, recall that certain **drugs**, such as aspirin, sulfonamides and their derivatives, and phenytoin, can potentiate the toxic effects of methotrexate simply by displacing it from its albumin-binding sites.

Ramsay B, Bloxham C, Eldred A, et al: **Blistering, erosions, and scarring** in a patient on etretinate. Br J Dermatol 1989; 121:397–400.

Unexplained **ulcers and erosions of the lower back and buttocks** of a 63-year-old woman with psoriasis proved to be due to **etretinate**, which she had been taking for 16 months. Hemorrhagic blisters were seen 11 months after the start of treatment, along with widespread erosions, and many of the erosions developed hypertrophic granulation tissue. Numerous small acral white scars testified to former lesions. The nails had also become brittle. Stopping the drug was followed by improvement in 10 days and complete healing by 36 days. Serum etretinate levels were higher than expected with a dose of 0.5 mg/kg/day.

Sometimes the cure comes not in prescribing a drug, but in *not* prescribing a drug.

Palestine RF, Millns JL, Spigel GT, Schroeter AL: Skin manifestations of **pentazocine abuse.** J Am Acad Dermatol 1980; 2:47–55.

A 51-year-old male physician had **woody sclerosis**, hyperpigmentation, and multiple **ulcerations** with irregular margins and nonpurulent bases on the abdomen, thighs, and buttocks. He had been injecting himself with Talwin (pentazocine) for 9 years to control pain from a gunshot wound of the chest. After 2 years of injections every few hours the skin became sclerotic, rendering injections difficult unless given superficially. In the past year recurrent ulcerations had developed.

Sixteen additional cases of **Talwin abuse** are described; half of them were in persons working in the medical field with easy access to drugs. Symmetrical, deep linear and angulated, sclerotic clean-based ulcers of the thighs and buttocks were typical. They were usually coin sized but sometimes larger and deforming.

In looking at a strange constellation of sclerosis and ulcers in a doctor, nurse, or paramedic, ask yourself if this could be an addictive **factitial dermatitis.**

Mountain JC: **Cutaneous ulceration in Crohn's disease.** Gut 1970; 11:18–26.

Extensive cutaneous **ulceration** was found in 7 of 207 cases of **Crohn's disease** seen in one hospital over an 8-year period. The ulcerations had florid granulation tissue with edematous skin edges and dusky cyanosis of the surrounding skin. The ulceration is usually associated with severe Crohn's disease of the gastrointestinal tract. Biopsy shows a sarcoid granulomatous reaction, which must be distinguished from tuberculosis. Guinea pig inoculation with fresh ulcer tissue may be necessary.

Metastatic ulcerations tend to favor moist intertriginous areas, particularly in obese patients.

Perineal ulceration is the most common site, with wide extension in the perineum, groins, and anterior abdominal wall. Cutaneous ulcerations may erode into surrounding structures, causing a urinary fistula.

Parastomal ulceration is usually associated with recurrent disease of the adjacent bowel.

Gupta AK, Haberman HF, From GLA, Lipa M: Sarcoidosis with extensive **cutaneous ulceration.** Unusual clinical presentation. Dermatologica 1987; 174:135–139.

Ulceration occurred on the lower legs of a 70-year-old white woman with extensive papular and plaque-type **sarcoidosis.** Since she had insulin–resistant diabetes mellitus and the lesions were markedly yellow-orange in the center of the plaques, necrobiosis lipoidica diabeticorum was suspected. However, rapid response to systemic corticosteroid therapy supported the diagnosis of sarcoidal ulcers, as necrobiosis lipoidica is not responsive to systemic steroids.

Other diagnoses considered: actinic granuloma of O'Brien, annular elastolytic giant cell granuloma, Miescher's granuloma.

Lazorik FC, Friedman AK, Leyden JL: Xeroradiographic observation in four patients with chronic renal disease and **cutaneous gangrene.** Arch Dermatol 1981; 117:325–328.

Asymptomatic subcutaneous **nodules** of both knees appeared in this 43-year-old renal transplant patient. Only edema was seen when a 4-mm biopsy punch specimen was obtained and studied. The outcome of the biopsy, however, was a nonhealing enlarging ulcer at the biopsy site.

A second biopsy taken from the edge of the **iatrogenic ulcer** was no more helpful than the first. Cultures isolated not only *Escherichia coli, Enterobacter aerogenes,* and *Bacteroides* sp., but also *Candida albicans.* The key observation remained in the health profile. Here was found an elevated calcium level, a normal phosphorus level, and a parathyroid hormone level elevated to four times normal. Accordingly, a diagnosis of **hyperparathyroidism** was made.

The pathogenesis of the ulcer became further apparent when **roentgenograms** showed **calcification** of medium-sized arteries and when xeroradiograms demonstrated the calcification to extend to small vessels within the skin. Arterioles as small as 0.1 mm could be seen completely calcified in the subcutaneous tissue, not only in the areas of ulceration, but also in clinically normal skin on both knees.

New erythematous mottled **reticulated macules** appeared on the lower right leg, some progressing to deep necrosis and ulceration. A cure was obtained by parathyroidectomy.

The **xeroradiogram** is invaluable in assessing calcification so common in the vessels of the elderly, the diabetic, the patient with chronic renal disease, and in the patient with hyperparathyroidism.

Umbilicus

The umbilicus is the remnant of the once great highway of intrauterine nutritional life. With the opening of the oral route at birth, the umbilical gateway was closed down with only a scarred depression remaining. Yet in the **newborn** or infant, a polyp or **red nodule** in that umbilicus may indicate a yet-patent path to either the intestine or urinary bladder. Mucus, feces, gas, or urine may flow back across it. In others, the polyp may be but sequestered mucosa with no internal connections. No matter, there is still need for radiographic study in search of a fistulous path of an omphalomesenteric duct or of a patent urachus.

Aside from these rare developmental defects that hark back to our intrauterine life, umbilical lesions in the newborn are likely to be **granulation tissue** or a pyogenic granuloma. Before epithelialization has occurred, the umbilicus is a locus minoris resistentiae for impetigo and other bacterial infections as well. The liberal use of talcum powder may also lead to the appearance of a talc granuloma.

As life goes on, a deep umbilicus may be the site of a **foreign body** or of an omphalith of keratin and debris. Warty "growths" may reflect the persistence of scales in an area not well washed.

Almost any disease may develop in this umbilical skin, but seborrheic dermatitis, psoriasis, and candidiasis are commonplace. The scabies mite finds it a protected area in which to tunnel undisturbed. Its unique periumbilical vascular supply may account for the appearance of the lesions of **angiokeratoma** in the umbilical scene.

As the patient ages, watch the umbilicus for **endometriosis** and metastatic tumors, particularly the famed Sister Mary Joseph nodule as a metastatic growth suggesting a primary lesion in the stomach, colon, or ovary.

The umbilicus is also the site of the surgeon's diagnostic aid, **Cullen's sign**. This is a bluish discoloration that may suggest the presence of pancreatitis, a perforated ulcer, or a ruptured ectopic pregnancy.

But most of all, the umbilicus is the quintessential scar that sings the song of the lost cord.

Bean WB: **Omphalosophy:** An inquiry into the inner (and outer) **significance of the belly button**. Arch Intern Med 1974; 134:866–870.

> *"The navel in pathology can make us utter golly, whee!*
> *For it can be the focal place of fistula or wart,*
> *Or calculus or hernia, exposed to sun, sun-burnier,*
> *And polypi may flower up from Solomon's retort.*
>
> *The epitheliomata, ectopic condylomata*
> *And variegated eczemas and nevi find a home*
> *The extrophys and dystrophys, deep esoteric mystrophys*
> *All lesions of exotic type lurk in this catacomb.*
>
> *For those whose itch and urgery leads to omphalic surgery*
> *Cullen's blue belly-button sign's a very handy clue*
> *When scalpels tense are hovering, this sign may aid discovering*
> *The cause of the commotion and exactly what to do."*

de Luna ML, Cicioni V, Herrera A, et al: **Umbilical polyps.** Pediatr Dermatol 1987; 4:341–343.

A 4-day-old boy had a 4-mm **reddish tumor** on the dorsum of the umbilical cord. A small orifice at its vertex could be traced inside the umbilical cord. Radiographic contrast studies demonstrated an **omphalomesenteric fistula** that ended in the small bowel. This was surgically corrected.

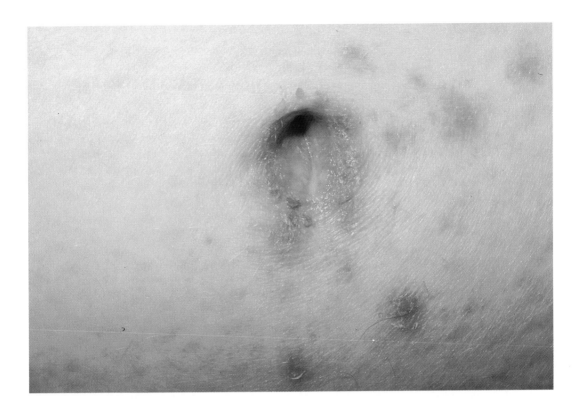

This child's umbilical polyp was more serious than the usual umbilical polyp that shows just sequestered intestinal mucosa, but no connection with the intestine itself.

In newborns or infants, umbilical lesions may reflect a failure to obliterate the once functional route between the midgut and the yolk sac. Later becoming the yolk duct, it normally disappears by the sixth intrauterine week. Failure of resorption results in a **variety of abnormalities** centered on the umbilicus. These include the aforementioned umbilical polyp and enteric fistula, as well as umbilical sinus, vitelline cyst, and Meckel's diverticulum.

The **umbilical polyp** must be **distinguished** from the umbilical granuloma, molluscum contagiosum, angioma, and pyogenic granuloma. In adults, melanomas and metastatic malignant disease must enter the differential.

Shwayder TA: Umbilical nodule and abdominal pain. Arch Dermatol 1987; 123:106–109.

A **brown-blue nodule** with a mamillated surface filled the lower third of the umbilicus of this 42-year-old woman. It resembled seborrheic keratosis, but was tender and had bled once several months before.

The patient's primary problem was unexplained periumbilical, nonradiating pain of a year's duration.

One had to consider in the clinical **differential**:

> nodular melanoma
> pyogenic granuloma
> keloid
> polyp
> carcinoma

metastatic carcinoma (ovary, gastrointestinal tract)
granulomas
embryologic rests (omphaloma, patent urachal duct, persistent vitelline duct)

The **biopsy** showing fragments of **uterine endometrium** within the skin made the diagnosis of **endometriosis**.

It is possible that pluripotential tissue existed in the umbilicus and that under the right stimulus underwent endometrial metaplasia.

Note: The pain that these patients experience need not be at the time of menstruation. Nor does the bleeding from the affected site need be on a regular basis. An "**ectopic uterus**" marches to its own drummer!

Kolbusz RV, Fretzin DF: Bowen's disease of the umbilicus simulating psoriasis vulgaris. Cutis 1988; 42:321–322.

An erythematous **scaly plaque of the umbilicus** failed to respond to topical steroids that controlled lesions of psoriasis elsewhere on the skin of a 56-year-old man. It had slowly enlarged centrifugally for 8 years, and although results of a biopsy several years before had been read as psoriasis, rebiopsy showed **Bowen's disease**.

Beware: All that scales is not psoriasis, even in a patient with psoriasis.

White SW, Meade GG: **A warty condition** of the umbilicus. J Am Acad Dermatol 1983; 8:421–422.

A dirty-looking, irregularly bordered, gray-brown patch in and around the umbilicus of this 17-year-old young man had been present for 4 years.

With the biopsy showing hyperkeratosis, acanthosis, and papillomatosis, the following five **diagnostic categories** were considered:

linear epidermal nevus
acanthosis nigricans
verruca vulgaris
actinic keratosis
seborrheic keratosis

None proved a fit, nor did confluent and reticulated papillomatosis of Gougerot and Carteaud.

Although a **diagnosis was lacking**, the whole area began to peel and flake off, leaving the site essentially clear 2 years later.

(We suspect the process was an example of what we term *keratoderma simplex*, viz., the accumulation of stratum corneum due to failure to wash an area.)

Powell FC, Cooper AJ, Massa MC et al: Sister Mary Joseph's nodule: A clinical and histologic study. J Am Acad Dermatol 1984; 10:610–615.

Sister Mary was the surgical nurse at Mayo Clinic who pointed out that the presence of nodules in the umbilicus of the patients was often a sign of **metastatic disease** and one of ominous prognosis.

The most frequent site of the **primary tumor was within the abdomen**, viz., stomach, bowel, ovary, and pancreas. The secondary umbilical tumors were fissured and ulcerated at times, but once seen, heralded death within a few months. Moreover, in 12 of the 85 cases studied, the Sister Mary Joseph nodule was the very **first sign** of the internal malignant disease.

The best diagnosis over the telephone is an early appointment date.

Of the causes of urticaria, there is no end. But start your search by looking for foods, drugs, and bugs.

Foods are a major cause of acute urticaria. Many examples are solved by the patient who realized the morning after that his hives came on following the shrimp of the night before. For the less dramatic, more prolonged mysterious case of hives, explore foods more in depth. If there was an acute onset, repeatedly quiz the patient for clues as to a new food or food additive. Failing to find one, diagnosis by elimination is next. Have the patient avoid a selected list of known food urticariogens. Center on excluding milk, butter, cheese, eggs, seafood, pork, and tomatoes. Nor can he have coffee, caffeinated drinks, chocolate, and nuts. Yellow-dyed food such as spaghetti and blue-cheese dressing must be removed from the formerly colorful diet. Should the patient complain, the alternative is a 10-day sugar water, rice, and chicken menu.

Drugs must enter as prime suspects from the very first visit. First the obvious troublemakers must be suspected. We have found it difficult to get the patient to indict or suspect aspirin and the swarm of nonsteroidal anti-inflammatory drugs advertised on TV. The reply "I have taken them for years" or a memory-lapse negative reply only deserves further effort on your part to bring these drugs to the level of patient suspicion. Use names—Motrin, Advil, ibuprofen—on direct questioning. Make the patient conscious of each pill, laxative, sedative, or tranquilizer he takes. And make the patient conscious that urticaria can result from eye drops, transdermal patches, suppositories, and douches.

Of all the drugs that may induce urticaria, penicillin and its family probably head the list. Search for occult exposure such as that dental packing 3 weeks ago. In hospital patients, recall the possibility of inadvertent error in medication. At home, medicine cabinet mix-ups are always possible. We have even seen urticaria from the eating of hamburger laced with penicillin to keep the meat fresh looking. And we have seen urticaria in a pharmacist due to airborne penicillin dust.

The sulfa drugs enter the lineup of suspects. Here the patient must be instructed that the diuretic Lasix and the sweetener saccharin are members of this sulfa family and are under suspicion.

We particularly distrust Zyloprim, phenothiazines, and sedatives. Eliminate and wait. There is no rule on how long the body takes to metabolize and degrade a drug to nonantigenicity, but attacks should lessen in severity within days as the inevitable drop in concentration occurs. Be sure the patient eliminates all aspirin and nonsteroidal anti-inflammatory drugs during this period. They not only cause urticaria, but they potentiate the action of urticariogens.

And now to **bugs**. The most common cause of chronic urticaria in women is sensitivity to *Candida albicans*. Ketoconazole can be powerful diagnostic therapy. Dental infection accounts for about 4% of all chronic urticaria. It may be hard to detect. We had one patient whose 9 years of daily hives was terminated only after actual dental probing disclosed an abscessed molar. Repeated x-rays had been normal, and the tooth was painless.

Another **infection** responsible for chronic urticaria is the neglected tinea pedis of onychomycosis. **Look at the feet** before you say you don't know why a patient has hives. Occult infection, whenever you find it, commands attention as a possible cause of hives. Does the patient have sinusitis, cystitis, cholecystitis, or chronic diarrhea?

Intestinal parasites usually signal their presence by eosinophilia but often by hives. Stool examinations are always indicated. Even when they are negative, a course of metronidazole, then chloroquine, and also one of thiabendazole may do wonders in making a diagnosis of urticaria due to giardiasis, amebiasis, or a roundworm infestation.

Note that acute urticaria may be the presenting sign of hepatitis or of viral disease. Systemic disease must receive your attention also. A variety of neoplasms such as lymphoma may surface as urticaria. Look for cryoglobulinemia, gamma globulinemias, collagen vascular disease, lupus, and polycythemia vera. The laboratory will help you sort this out and will provide leads. Measure blood histamine level during an attack to confirm the nature of vessel leakage. Check the IgE for atopy. A chest x-ray may disclose a fractured rib in urticaria due to hyperparathyroidism. Is it hereditary? Biopsy the lesion to detect the presence of vasculitis. Your clinical signal of vasculitic urticaria is the persistence of the lesion for more than 12 hours.

Airborne allergens are next. Inhalants such as dust of both wool and wood, pollens, mold spores, and animal danders account for some urticarias of elusive origins. Even wearing a silk tie may result in urticaria in silk-sensitive patients.

Listen to the patient—he may give you an entry point for diagnosis, such as exercise as the cause, mowing the lawn, working with epoxy resins, going into a florist shop or stable. Is the itch intolerable? Maybe the patient has the occult scabies we miss in the well-washed patient.

Educate your patient to be a fellow sleuth. Point out that urticaria is also acute in nature. Only its persistence is chronic. Alert him to the fact that within minutes, at the most hours, after exposure to an exogenous, external cause, he will develop new hives. It is thus much easier to trap a cause for urticaria than for eczema in which the latent period between exposure and the dermatitis is several days.

Be confident of success. See your patient frequently. Review the history endlessly. Look for new leads. Challenge with foods. Stop all drugs. Treat infections diagnostically. Each patient comes with a hidden cause for his urticaria; you must uncover it.

Finally, avoid the temptation to treat symptomatically with Seldane or Hismanal. They may not make your patient sleepy, but they could put you to sleep diagnostically.

Juhlin L: **Recurrent urticaria**: Clinical investigation of 330 patients. Br J Dermatol 1981; 104:369–381.

A survey of personal observations of 330 patients in Sweden of the most common triggers for their urticaria:

drugs:
    penicillin   aspirin   sulfonamides

foods:
    nuts, fruits, vegetables
    fish, shellfish
    ketchup, spices, vanilla
    egg
    milk products
    cheese

drinks:
    orange or colored drinks   fruit juices   wine

other factors:
    exercise   stress   physical pressure

Several **associated conditions** were seen in many patients:

angioedema	70%
gastritis, diarrhea, abdominal swelling	44%
rhinitis	20%
asthma	11%
depression, psychiatric problems	16%

Many patients were **hospitalized for provocation tests** done with titanium dioxide–whitened gelatin capsules containing either lactose or wheat starch filler. The first dose was given at 8 AM, followed by additional doses at 1-hour intervals. Only one additive was given per day, and the patient was unaware of the compound tested. The test was positive if hives or angioedema developed within 24 hours, although half the patients reacted within 6 hours. About one third of the patients had one or more positive tests, while another one third had totally negative tests. The remaining one third had "uncertain" tests.

The following substances were tested:

SUBSTANCE	DOSE (MG)
Azo dyes:	
Tartrazine	0.1, 1.0, 10*
New coccine	
Sunset yellow	
Benzoates:	
Sodium benzoate	50, 500
4-Hydroxybenzoic acid	50, 200
Carotene	50, 100, 100
Canthaxanthine	10, 200, 200
Annatto	5, 10
BHT-BHA	1, 10, 50, 50
Yeast extract	0.6
Aspirin	0.1, 1, 10, 100, 250, 500[†]
Sorbic acid	50, 200, 200
Sodium nitrate	100
Sodium nitrite	100
Quinoline yellow	1, 5, 10
Sodium glutamate	100, 200

*Only 0.1 mg in patients with asthma.
[†] Only 0.1 mg in patients with asthma; delete 250 and 500 in patients with history of severe aspirin reactions.

Champion RH: **Urticaria**: Then and now. Br J Dermatol 1988; 119:427–436.

An analysis of 1300 cases studied personally by the author indicates that idiopathic urticaria is a disorder of **hidden cause and unpredictable course**.

Investigation centers on the history and exploration of all leads. The duration of wheals, pattern of attacks, provoking factors (including drugs), and associated symptoms should be documented. A **food diary** should be kept in relation to attacks.

The patient and physician must engage in **mutual instruction sessions**. Both must search for the following **flare factors**: aspirin and related compounds, foods and food additives, candidal infection, focal sepsis, systemic illness, psychological.

Shelley ED, Humeniuk HM: **Urticaria**. *In* Newcomer VD, Young EM Jr (eds): Geriatric Dermatology. Clinical Diagnosis and Practical Therapy, New York, Igaku-Shoin, 1989, pp 273–286.

Urticaria in the elderly is not a common problem, possibly because of the decrease in the cutaneous mast cell population with aging.

Most cases of urticaria in the elderly are acute and precipitated by medications. Repeated questioning may be necessary to ferret out both prescription and nonprescription (folk remedies, over the counter) drugs taken for the following common problems:

arthritis	angina
constipation	cold feet
anxiety	calluses
insomnia	incontinence
hemorrhoids	depression
anemia	fatigue
cough	dry skin
leg cramps	glaucoma
digestive disturbances	sore teeth
water retention	vaginal itching
ingrown toenails	

Elderly patients should be specifically quizzed about each of these medications:

antibiotics	mouthwashes
antihistamines	muscle relaxants
cold tablets	rectal medications
cortisone	sedatives
cough medications	sleeping pills
decongestants	thyroid
digitalis	tonic (quinine)
diuretics	tranquilizers
douches	vaginal medications
enemas	vitamins
hormones	water pills
laxatives	weight-control pills
lozenges	

Checklist for urticaria in the elderly:

prescription drugs	candidiasis
injections	tooth abscess
over-the-counter medications	inhalant sprays (perfumes)
health food store products	hidden infection
foods	parasites
alcoholic beverages (wine, beer)	mite bites (scabies)

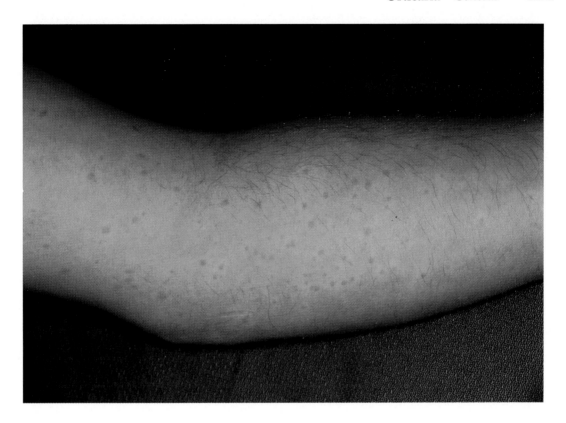

food additives (tartrazine,
   benzoates, sweeteners)
quinine
thyroid disease
x-ray contrast material

implants (teeth, bone,
   intrauterine)
dermographism
malignant disease

Dijkstra JWE, Bergfeld WF, Steck WD, Tuthill RJ: **Eosinophilic cellulitis** associated with urticaria. J Am Acad Dermatol 1986; 14:32–38.

Large deep-red, infiltrated plaques with scattered vesicles on the forearm of this 34-year-old man **appeared to be urticaria**. He had a 10-year history of chronic urticaria. Previous large red swellings of the forearms had lasted 7 to 10 days and were pruritic or painful. Each had coincided with sore throats and upper respiratory infections.

On biopsy a diagnosis of **eosinophilic cellulitis** was made. There was no evidence of vasculitis.

This reemphasizes the need to obtain a biopsy of urticarial lesions that persist more than a day.

Full-screen projection of a 35-mm Kodachrome of your patient's lesion can give new diagnostic insight.

Foods

Monroe EW, Jones HE: **Urticaria**: An updated review. Arch Dermatol 1977; 113:80–90.

Foods are a more important cause of **acute urticaria** than of chronic urticaria. Check on such items in the diet as: nuts, eggs, fish, seafood, and food additives—benzoates, tartrazine.

Keep a food diary to detect relationship to flares or attacks.

Pola J, Subiza J, Armentia A, et al: **Urticaria** caused by caffeine. Ann Allergy 1988; 60:207–208.

A 48-year-old woman carried the diagnosis of chronic **idiopathic urticaria** for over 2 years. The attacks were daily, extremely pruritic, and of an evanescent nature. Once she personally discerned that drinking **coffee** made the hives worse, she was asked to stop all intake of coffee, tea, and chocolate. The following 10 years had been hive free.

Challenge with coffee, tea, or chocolate invariably produced generalized urticaria within 15 minutes. The hives persisted for 12 to 24 hours. A double-blind oral challenge test proved the responsible allergen to be caffeine. The ingestion of 100 mg of caffeine produced generalized hives within 15 minutes, whereas theophylline (300 mg) was without effect. No hives were seen on caffeine challenge, however, if the patient was given 60 mg of terfenadine (Seldane) 3 hours prior to the challenge.

It is noteworthy that **theophylline** and **aminophylline** have been previously reported to cause urticaria.

Years ago, medical students hoped that if they wore neckties that matched those worn by the charismatic clinician, some of his clinical gift for diagnosis might rub off on them.

DUNCAN NEUHAUSER

Chafee FM: **Sensitivity to peanut oil** with the report of a case. Ann Intern Med 1941; 15:1116–1117.

A 32-year-old black woman with hay fever and severe asthma was given **epinephrine in peanut oil** intramuscularly in an emergency room. At the injection site she immediately had a cramplike pain lasting 2 hours, and 4 hours later developed a 2-inch raised red bee-sting–like area that lasted 5 days. Over the next 3 weeks she gave herself at least 10 more similar injections, with similar local reactions as well as flare-ups of all previous injection sites. She stopped the injections after developing **generalized urticaria** that lasted 24 hours. Epinephrine in sesame oil injections were then given and tolerated well. Scratch and intradermal **tests to peanut oil** were strongly positive. She noted that eating peanuts made her wheezy.

Moral: In urticaria, don't forget to ask about injections and then track down the ingredients of each shot.

Note: Dermasmoothe FS/oil contains peanut oil.

Thomas DR, Pursley TV, Jorizzo JL: Chronic urticaria secondary to **aminobenzoic acid**. Arch Dermatol 1984; 120:961–962.

Daily attacks of urticaria for 5 months in this 30-year-old woman proved resistant to avoidance of aspirin, systemic antibiotics, hydroxyzine, cimetidine, a salicylate, and tartrazine-free diet.

Although she had been keeping a food diary and had been repeatedly questioned regarding medication intake, she never disclosed that she had been taking a **vitamin tablet** each night for the past 2 years. Once the vitamin was stopped the hives promptly disappeared.

After being disease free for a month, she was challenged with one tablet of the vitamin. Generalized pruritus immediately occurred, followed by massive urticaria within 24 hours that persisted for 48 hours.

Two months later a challenge with 50 mg of pure **aminobenzoic acid** produced generalized urticaria within 20 minutes. This persisted for 2 days. By avoiding multivitamins, the patient has remained free of hives for over 6 months.

Aminobenzoic acid, although not a vitamin, has been included in certain **multivitamins** in the hope that it would provide a substrate for the consumer's bacteria to synthesize folic acid. It was suspected as the allergen in this patient, since she was sensitive to sulfa drugs, common cross-reactants.

Mayou SC, Kelly SE, McGibbon DH: Local cutaneous **sensitivity to subcutaneous heparin**. Br J Dermatol 1987; 117:664–665.

A 35-year-old woman developed cardiomyopathy at 22 weeks' gestation of her second pregnancy. Anticoagulation with subcutaneous porcine heparin was started, and 5 weeks later she began developing urticated erythematous plaques at the heparin injection site 7 to 36 hours after administration. Bovine heparin caused the same reaction. Since neither heparin contained preservatives, the reaction was felt to represent true local **hypersensitivity to heparin**, and it disappeared after the heparin was discontinued. She delivered a normal baby 2 weeks later.

Orfan N, Patterson R, Dykewicz MS: Severe **angioedema** related to ACE inhibitors in patients with a history of idiopathic angioedema. JAMA 264:1287–1289.

A 36-year-old woman developed **angioedema** of the face, lip, and hands, as   1225 well as generalized urticaria 24 hours after the first dose of the angiotensin–converting enzyme inhibitor, **lisinopril** (10 mg). The lisinopril was discontinued, and the hives abated after a few days of prednisone therapy. Subsequently she had attacks of urticaria about once a month for 4 months. There have been no attacks in the past 5 months.

The past history was instructive. There was a 10-year history of attacks of **angioedema** and generalized urticaria that occurred one or two times a year. They were unrelated to foods, medications, or physical factors. The attacks gradually became less frequent, and for the past 5 years there had been none.

The interpretation of how the **lisinopril** caused hives is fascinating. Lisinopril, as well as its congeners, captopril and enalapril, inhibits the action of the enzyme in the skin (kininase II), which inactivates the powerful inflammatory kinins responsible for urticaria and angioedema. The fortuitous identification of kininase II and ACE (angiotensin-converting enzyme) led to the development of a drug at once capable of controlling hypertension and of inducing angioedema by inhibition of the critical enzyme, ACE, alias kininase II.

Physicists, like patients in a physician's office, only really believe they know what their problem is when it has been given a name.

JOHN A. WHEELER

Tanphaichitr K: **Chronic urticaria** associated with bacterial infection: A case of dental infection. Cutis 1981; 27:653–656.

Two years of chronic urticaria and dermographism led this 35-year-old man to seek medical help. The attacks of swelling appeared once or twice a month with no antecedent factor evident. The urticaria most commonly attacked the lips, palms, and soles.

A food elimination diet gave only modest improvement. The cause of the urticaria remained unknown until 2 years later. At that time he had carious teeth extracted. One hour later he developed generalized urticaria and angioedema. This resolved in 12 hours, and he has had no attacks of hives in the subsequent years.

Thus the cause of the 4 years of hives was shown to be **chronic dental infection**. Other sources of infection causing urticaria include infection of the sinuses, tonsils, adenoids, gallbladder, appendix, pilonidal sinuses, or urinary tract.

The diagnosis of urticaria always calls for the diagnosis of the cause. Here is one avenue to pursue.

James J, Warin RP: An assessment of the role of *Candida albicans* and food yeasts in **chronic urticaria**. Br J Dermatol 1971; 84:227–237.

In this study of 100 patients with chronic urticaria, 26% were found to have significant **Candida albicans sensitivity**. The cross-reactions between this organism and food yeasts supports the finding that anticandida therapy and a low yeast diet help these patients.

Fisher DA: A most memorable case. Cutis 1989; 43:132.

Five physicians over the course of 3 months had failed to free this 52-year-old woman of daily attacks of urticaria. The answer came by following a lead obtained during the taking of an extended **45-minute history**. The patient noted that she had had three or four loose stools daily since vacationing in Mexico. "Yes, the **frequent bowel movements and the hives** came at about the same time, now that I think of it."

A stool culture revealed *Citrobacter fructei*, i.e., an intestinal pathogen. Within 2 days of starting Azulfidine treatment, the urticaria was completely cleared. By the end of 2 weeks of treatment, bowel habits returned to their former chronic state of constipation.

So now, she no longer has either daily hives or daily bowel movements.

Witkowski JA, Parish LC: **Scabies**: A cause of generalized urticaria. Cutis 1984; 33:277–279.

This 22-year-old woman had had **generalized urticaria** and dermographism for 3 months. Initially she had noted only pruritus occurring at night. Now she had daily attacks of hives that were not relieved by a variety of antipruritic lotions and salves as well as systemic antihistamines and steroids.

On examination, scattered punctate and linear crusted lesions attracted attention, since the pruritus of hives rarely produces excoriations. On closer inspection a burrow was found on the side of a finger. A scraping soon demonstrated the mites and ova of *Sarcoptes scabiei* and the diagnosis of urticaria due to scabies was made.

A single 12-hour application of lindane lotion cleared the itch, the dermographism, and hives by the next day.

Making two diagnoses gives one more to treat and more chances of success.

Leighton PM, MacSween HM: *Strongyloides stercoralis*: The cause of an **urticarial-like eruption of 65 years' duration**. Arch Intern Med 1990; 150:1747–1748.

Sixty-five years of intermittent **hives, angioedema, and abdominal pain** had been the plight of this 74-year-old woman. Her emigrant history was of note: Born in Malaysia, she moved to Sri Lanka (Ceylon) at the age of 9 years, then to England at age 16, and then to Canada, where she had lived since she was 17 years old.

Her childhood memories focused on shortness of breath, chest as well as abdominal pain, and hives of all sizes. The hives never abated, continuing throughout her life. They took about 8 hours to peak and lasted up to 3 days. At the age of 59 years she was found to have **eosinophilia**, but no parasites were found in the stool. A diagnosis of **familial angioneurotic edema** was made at that time.

When she was first seen at age 74, eosinophilia was again demonstrated, and another search for stool parasites was unproductive. A negative C1 esterase inhibitor test ruled out angioedema. However, a **duodenal string test** (Entero-test, HDC Corporation, Mountain View, CA) yielded some **larvae of *Strongyloides stercoralis***. Thiabendazole therapy for but 1 day (1250 mg bid) returned the eosinophil level to normal and eliminated the hives. She has now been hive free for 2 years.

The Malay peninsula is an area of high **endemicity** for *S. stercoralis*. Actually, 37% of the laborers on the Burma-Thailand railway in World War II reported having hives or a creeping eruption. In the United States, the junctional area of Kentucky, Virginia, Tennessee, and North Carolina is a strongyloides endemic site. Have a high index of suspicion for this type of parasitic infestation in any patient with hives and eosinophilia who has lived in this area or traveled to Southeast Asia.

Here was a diagnosis that hung by a string, i.e., the duodenal string test.

Hamrick HJ, Moore GW: **Giardiasis** causing urticaria in a child. Am J Dis Child 1983; 137:761–763.

The nature of a 5-year-old girl's urticaria was not evident until a stool specimen was submitted for ova and parasites. It contained numerous cysts of *Giardia lamblia*. Within an hour of the first dose of Flagyl the urticaria worsened, but within 48 hours it had resolved completely.

Humphreys DM, Myers A: **Cytomegalovirus** mononucleosis with urticaria. Postgrad Med J 1975; 51:404–406.

A 25-year-old woman's acute urticaria was associated with colicky abdominal pain and diarrhea. When the condition proved refractory to therapy, numerous studies were done. The bone marrow showed large numbers of atypical mononuclear cells. Complement fixation titers for 13 viruses revealed that she had active infection with cytomegalovirus. Her initial titer on admission was 1:8 and a month later was 1:1024. Steroids were given over a 4-month period with eventual complete resolution of the urticaria.

Stafford CT: **Urticaria** as a sign of systemic disease. Ann Allergy 1990; 64:264–270.

The following are unobvious causes of chronic urticaria:

drugs:
    nonsteroidal anti-inflammatory drugs
    immunoglobulins

infection:

cholecystitis	hepatitis
cystitis	Epstein-Barr virus infections
gingivitis	Coxsackievirus A and B infections
dental abscess	tinea
sinusitis	*Candida* infection

parasitic infestation:

Ascaris	*Schistosoma*
Ancylostoma (hookworm)	*Trichinella*
Strongyloides	*Toxocara*
Filaria	*Fasciola* (liver fluke)
Echinococcus	

diseases:
    serum sickness
    mastocytosis
    hereditary angioedema (deficiency of C1 esterase inhibitor)
    malignant:
        Hodgkin's disease
        tumor of colon, lung, ovary, liver, rectum
    endocrine:

diabetes mellitus	hyperparathyroidism
hypothyroidism	ovarian hormonal effects
hyperthyroidism	

Shornick JK: **Herpes gestationis.** J Am Acad Dermatol 1987; 17:539–556.

Urticarial papules or plaques on the **abdomen** in the second or third trimester of **pregnancy** are the herald signs of this rare affliction of pregnancy. Fifty thousand pregnancies may come and go without its being seen, but once it arrives there is rapid progression to blistering and its terrible itch in days to weeks.

Once the diagnosis is confirmed (complement deposition along basement membrane with subepidermal bulla and eosinophilia) one may **advise** the victim:

It will spare the face.
It may clear before delivery.
It will flare at time of delivery; indeed, this may be its time of onset.
There is a 10% chance the baby will have blisters, but fetal risk is minimal.
It may persist for weeks or months after delivery.
It can reappear during any subsequent pregnancy, usually in a more severe form.
It can flare at the time of menses or if contraceptives are taken.
It responds best to corticosteroids.

Werman BS, Rietschel RL: **Chronic urticaria** from tantalum staples. Arch Dermatol 1981; 117:438–439.

Six months of intractable daily attacks of urticaria in this 39-year-old woman led to hospitalization to find the cause. On examination there were widespread 1- to 3-cm wheals that showed a peculiar tendency to localize on the 1229 legs in the surgical scars of bilateral venous stripping done the year before. There was no dermographism. Single lesions remained for 4 hours before fading, and biopsy showed no vasculitis.

Complete laboratory studies, stool examination, screen for vaginal pathogens, chest and dental x-rays were all negative. A 10-day restricted diet had no effect, nor did challenges with tartrazine, benzoate sodium, or aspirin worsen her urticaria.

Since an x-ray of the legs showed multiple metallic surgical staples, intradermal tests to nickel, copper, chromium, and cobalt were done. Only the **cobalt produced a positive urticarial response**. It was then learned that the staples were pure tantalum. By use of an improvised **tantalum solution**, the patient was found to show a strong urticarial response to the skin test to this metal. A diagnosis was made of **chronic urticaria due to tantalum hypersensitivity**.

Confirmatory evidence came when treatment with a metal chelator (disulfiram [Antabuse]) gave dramatic relief of the hives. Ultimately, conclusive proof of the diagnosis came when surgical removal of the staples from both legs resulted in a cure.

Janier M, Bonvalet D, Blanc M-F, et al: **Chronic urticaria** and macroglobulinemia (**Schnitzler's syndrome**): Report of two cases. J Am Acad Dermatol 1989; 20:206–211.

This 60-year-old man had had **chronic urticaria for 10 years**. He exhibited nonpruritic wheals on the trunk and limbs that in some instances persisted for a few days. He also complained of pain in the lower legs. There was associated intermittent fever, some lymph node enlargement, and hepatomegaly.

Skin biopsy showed leukocytoclastic **vasculitis** with mild fibrinoid necrosis of the vessel wall. Bone x-rays revealed hyperostosis of both tibias. The sedimentation rate was 63 mm/hr, and there was hypergammaglobulinemia as well as hyperfibrinogenemia. On immunoelectrophoresis there was a serum monoclonal $IgM_{-\kappa}$ peak. Both serum and concentrated urine protein electrophoresis disclosed a γ-globulin peak.

The diagnosis of **Schnitzler's syndrome** was made on the basis of the coexistence of urticaria and **macroglobulinemia**. The bone pain is another specific sign of this syndrome. It is refractory to therapy, being indifferent to H_1, H_2 blockers, dapsone, colchicine, chloroquine, cyclophosphamide, chlorambucil, and azathioprine.

This Schnitzler's syndrome is just one of the **cutaneous manifestations** of a **paraproteinemia**. The others are:

1. Plasmacytomas, nodules, plaques
2. Purpura
3. Amyloidosis
4. Papular mucinosis
5. Angioedema
6. Xanthomatosis and necrobiotic xanthogranulomas
7. Cryoglobulinemia
8. Pyoderma gangrenosum
9. Neutrophilic pustulosis and Sneddon-Wilkinson disease
10. Erythema elevation diutinum
11. Vasculitis
12. POEMS syndrome (polyneuropathy, organomegaly, endocrinopathy, M protein, skin changes)
13. Systemic capillary leak syndrome

You can see that serum protein electrophoresis can be worthwhile.

Bisaccia E, Adamo V, Rozan SW: **Urticarial vasculitis** progressing to systemic lupus erythematosus. Arch Dermatol 1988; 124:1088–1090.

Target-shaped urticarial lesions of the legs and large plaques of urticaria on the trunk and arms recurred for over a year in a 30-year-old woman. The urticaria was controlled with diphenhydramine and indomethacin. Lesions lasted 48 to 72 hours and were associated with fever, malaise, arthralgias, photosensitivity, photophobia, and conjunctivitis. Skin biopsy showed leukocytoclastic vasculitis, and repeated blood studies showed only hypocomplementemia. ANA and health profiles remained normal 2 years after the urticaria began, although antimicrosomal and antithyroglobulin antibodies became markedly elevated, indicating **autoimmune thyroiditis**.

Finally, $2\frac{1}{2}$ years after the onset of urticaria, the patient developed nephritis, anemia, and a distinctly positive ANA, permitting a **diagnosis of systemic lupus erythematosus**.

The course of this patient's illness argues forcefully for the need to periodically reevaluate all cases of urticarial vasculitis.

Heskel NS, White CR, Fryberger S, et al: **Aleukemic leukemia cutis**: Juvenile chronic granulocytic leukemia presenting with figurate cutaneous lesions. J Am Acad Dermatol 1983; 9:423–427.

This $3\frac{1}{2}$-year old girl had had persistent, multiple, red annular **urticarial lesions** of the chest, back, and arms for the past 6 months. The biopsy showed a perivascular infiltrate of lymphocytes, large atypical mononuclear cells, and white cell precursors. Although blood counts and a bone marrow study showed no diagnostic abnormality, the **unusual cells in the skin biopsy** suggested the possibility of juvenile chronic granulocytic leukemia.

The skin lesions continued to show an evolution of healing with new erythematous papules becoming annular lesions. However, a year later, hepatosplenomegaly was first noted, and the white count had risen to 24,900/mm³ with 2% blast forms. At this time, a **biopsy of the bone marrow** confirmed the diagnosis of **chronic granulocytic leukemia**, showing as it did 19% blast forms.

This is the first case in which the skin biopsy findings permitted a diagnosis of a preleukemic state long before the bone marrow did.

Wolf C, Pehamberger H, Breyer S, et al: Episodic angioedema with eosinophilia. J Am Acad Dermatol 1989; 20:21–27.

At the age of 30 years, this woman began to have recurrent attacks of pruritic erythema at different body sites. After 6 years, the lesions had become **urticarial** and edematous, affecting the face, arms, legs, and trunk. Several years later, malaise, fevers (temperature up to 39°C), weight gain, and anuria led to hospitalization.

On examination, **greenish-tinted angioedema** and urticarial papules were seen during the attacks. These returned at approximately monthly intervals and lasted 7 to 10 days. The itch led to some lichenification. Notable was the disabling swelling of the arms and legs, leading to temporary inability to walk. Widespread lymph node enlargement was observed, and there was associated fever (with the temperature peaking at 39°C and lasting for 5 days). Finally, a 10% weight gain appeared to be due to a decrease in urine secretion to 100 ml/24 hr. A biopsy of the angiomatous skin showed edema and an eosinophilic infiltrate.

The finding of leukocytosis (up to 31,000 mm³) and eosinophilia (up to 75%) at the times of attack suggested a diagnosis of **eosinophilic leukemia** or possibly hypereosinophilic syndrome. Wells' syndrome (eosinophilic cellulitis) was also considered. Extensive studies, however, ruled these out.

Multiple bone marrow aspirations showed increased numbers of eosinophils but no evidence of malignancy. Serum IgM and IgE levels were elevated, but radioallergosorbent tests and prick skin tests were negative for food, animal, pollen, and mold antigens. Tests for pressure urticaria and dermographism were negative.

Stool samples for ova, parasites, and fungi were negative, as well as serologic tests for leishmaniasis, trichinosis, amebiasis, trypanosomiasis, mononucleosis, *Salmonella, Brucella, Yersinia, Filaria, Toxocara, Echinococcus, Schistosoma, Aspergillus,* and *Borrelia* infection.

Computed tomography, intravenous pyelography, skeletal scans, chest and bone roentgenograms, as well as electrocardiograms and echocardiograms and review by a bevy of consultants revealed no abnormalities.

Serum profiles of sexual hormones were repeatedly normal, and there was no correlation of attacks with the patient's menstrual cycle. Serum levels of renin, aldosterone, and adrenocorticotropic hormone were in the normal range.

Both during attacks and at intervals the following were negative or in the normal range:

> complete blood count
> urinalysis
> Bence Jones protein
> liver and kidney function
> creatinine clearance
> alkaline phosphatase
> serum electrolytes
> creatine kinase
> vitamin B_{12}
> C-reactive protein
> Waaler-Rose test
> latex test
> antibodies:
>> antinuclear
>> antimitochondrial
>> antinative DNA
>> antisingle-stranded DNA
>> antismooth muscle
>> antiskeletal muscle
>> antinuclear (SM, nuclear RNP, Ro, La, scleroderma-70, Jo-1, Laux, Ku)
> circulating immune complexes:
>> complement level (C2, C3, C4, C5, CH_{50})
>> C1 esterase inhibitor
>> cryoglobulins
>> neopterin in both urine and serum

This patient thus had the **very model of a modern major general work-up** and as a **result** her diagnosis became *idiopathic*, **episodic angioedema with eosinophilia.**

Mathias CGT, Frick OL, Caldwell TM, et al: Immediate **hypersensitivity to seminal fluid** and atopic dermatitis. Arch Dermatol 1980; 116:209–212.

Episodic attacks of intense generalized pruritus, **urticaria**, and angioedema of the face occurred in this 26-year-old woman. Severe attacks were anaphylactic, with cyanosis, dyspnea, and collapse requiring emergency room treatment. By history it was discerned that each attack occurred immediately following **intercourse**. Significantly, the attacks did not occur when her husband used a condom.

Intradermal tests with diluted $(10^{-2}-10^{-4})$ **seminal fluid** as well as seminal plasma, not only from her husband but from other males, showed an immediate urticarial reaction.

The patient was successfully desensitized by intradermal injections of seminal plasma but required a maintenance injection of 0.3 ml (1:10 dilution) every 3 weeks.

Here's another example of sex that was never safe without a **condom**.

Parrot J-L, Hébert R, Saindelle A, Ruff F: **Platinum and platinosis**. Allergy and histamine release due to some platinum salts. Arch Environ Health 1969; 19:685–691.

After a lag period of several months, workers in **platinum-refining workshops** may develop asthma and an eczematous or urticarial eruption on the exposed areas of the arms, face, and neck. The culprit is ammonium chloroplatinate, $PtCl_6 (NH_4)_2$, a salt that will cause positive intradermal and patch tests, along with its parent compound, **chloroplatonic acid** $(PtCl_6H_2)$. These chemicals cause immediate histamine release.

Such platonic relationships can be dangerous.

Reichel M, Mauro TM: **Urticaria and hepatitics**. Lancet 1990; 336:822–823.

A 40-year-old black man with sickle cell disease had sudden onset of erythematous **urticarial plaques** that moved on an hourly basis. He had had a blood transfusion 4 weeks earlier. The white count was 24,400/μl and liver enzymes were increased. A diagnosis was made of urticaria due to transfusion-acquired hepatitis.

Hepatitis A IgM antibody was negative, as was the hepatitis B surface antigen. The following week the **hepatitis C** viral (**HCV**) **antibody** became positive. The conclusion was that acute HCV infection may cause acute urticaria. Within 3 weeks of the seroconversion, the hives spontaneously vanished.

Much of the good of diagnosis comes from ruling out that which the patient fears.

Autoimmune

Stephens CJM, Black MM: Autoimmune **progesterone dermatitis**. Br J Dermatol 1989; 121(suppl 34):64.

A review of 26 cases with **autoimmunity to progesterone**:

presentations:
  eczema
  pompholyx
  urticaria
  erythema multiforme
diagnostic tests:
  positive intradermal test in 72%
  exacerbation by oral or intramuscular progesterone challenge
  positive indirect basophil test
  presence of antibodies to corpus luteum
treatment:
  estrogens improved 75%
  danazol
  tamoxifen
  oophorectomy

Mayou SC, Charles-Holmes R, Kenney A, Black MM: A **premenstrual urticarial eruption** treated with bilateral oophorectomy and hysterectomy. Clin Exp Dermatol 1988; 13:114–116.

For 17 years this 42-year-old woman had experienced severe pruritic **urticarial lesions** for the **week before each period**. And during each of three pregnancies she developed an erythematous papular eruption of the abdomen and breasts, which began at the 6th month and disappeared at the 8th month. There was a postpartum flare of but 2 weeks' duration. At no time were there vesicles or bullae, and histologic study showed no evidence of erythema multiforme.

Hormonal studies showed no abnormalities in serum progesterone, estradiol, luteinizing hormone, and follicle-stimulating hormone. Intradermal testing with 0.03 ml of 0.1% aqueous progesterone was negative.

Ethinyl estradiol (30 mg orally) **produced a severe flare** of the eruption, and conversely, danazol (100 mg bid) suppressed ovulation and the rash. The cure came, however, with surgical removal of the ovaries. Significantly, months after the surgery, challenge with **conjugated estrogens** (Premarin 0.625 mg/day) produced a florid reappearance of the hives, whereas a 10-day course of a progesterone (norethisterone 10 mg) produced no effect. She had no further problem until dienoestrol cream was used to treat postoperative atrophic vaginitis. Four days later she experienced urticaria of the groin.

It is important to distinguish this patient's autoimmune **sensitivity to estrogen** from that of **a sensitivity to progesterone**, since levels of each hormone peak just before each menses.

Good diagnosticians have a photographic memory or a good camera.

Shelley WB, Shelley ED: **Adrenergic urticaria**: A new form of stress-induced hives. Lancet 1985; 2:1031–1033.

Five weeks after being in a near-fatal truck accident, this 28-year-old male driver began having hives that have recurred daily for a year. At the time, he developed a **fear of driving**, which was diagnosed by psychological testing as a manifestation of post-traumatic stress disorder.

The hives consisted of multiple 5-mm red macules, as well as 1- to 3-mm red papules with or without a **blanched white halo** 10 to 15 mm in diameter. No lesions showed the erythematous halo characteristic of cholinergic urticaria. In severe attacks he experienced dyspnea and developed very large wheals. Emotional stress, such as that induced by the sight of his truck, triggered attacks. Coffee or chocolate intake also induced the same unique white-halo hives within 10 to 15 minutes.

He claimed also to have developed **vitiligo** following the accident.

Blood studies of vasoactive compounds before and during an attack showed a significant increase in plasma catecholamines and norepinephrine. The diagnostic lesion of this stress type of urticaria could be reproduced by **intradermal injection of** extremely small amounts of **norepinephrine** (<10 ng in 0.02 ml saline). Injections of dilute acetylcholine were without urticarial effect, as was the injection of norepinephrine in normal subjects.

Hirschmann JV, Lawlor F, English JSC, et al: **Cholinergic urticaria**. A clinical and histologic study. Arch Dermatol 1987; 123:462–467.

A review of 61 patients:

> begins with feeling of itching, tingling, burning, warmth, irritation of skin
> occurs at any site: can involve any and all areas, although usually not on palms, soles, face, or axillae
> progresses to punctate erythematous macules, evolving into blotchy macular erythema, then confluent erythema
> development of tiny (1 to 3 mm) **wheals surrounded by erythema**
> duration: 5 minutes to 8 hours
> **elicited by exercise, hot bath, emotional stress, hot or spicy foods**
> not reproducible by intradermal injections of acetylcholine, methacholine, or histamine.

Shelley WB, Shelley ED, Ho AKS: **Cholinergic urticaria**: Acetylcholine-receptor–dependent immediate-type hypersensitivity reaction to copper. Lancet 1983; 1:843–846.

For 6 years this 30-year-old woman had experienced episodic flushing and urticaria. Increasing in intensity and associated with palpitations, headaches, and weakness, these attacks were triggered by exercise, emotional stress, or increased heat.

Examination during an attack showed numerous 1- to 3-mm transitory **papules on an erythematous base**, associated with a large symmetrical plaque of urticaria over the lumbar region. A diagnosis of cholinergic urticaria was made.

Comprehensive studies disclosed a **role for the copper ion** in the pathogenesis of the cholinergic urticaria. The onset was just 2 years after the insertion of a copper intrauterine device (IUD). Repeated patch tests with copper were negative at 48 hours. However, upon exercise or stress these very sites developed small pruritic urticarial papules. The copper ion facilitated or favored the acetylcholine-induced release of mast cell histamine in this patient's cholinergic urticaria.

Contactants

Okano M, Nomura M, Hata S et al: **Anaphylactic symptoms due to chlorhexidine gluconate**. Arch Dermatol 1989; 125:50–52.

A 26-year-old man's penis was disinfected with 1% chlorhexidine gluconate (**Hibiclens**) prior to circumcision. Five minutes later he had wheals and flushing of the face, dyspnea, and numbness. The symptoms resolved following intravenous administration of hydrocortisone.

The diagnosis of a **chlorhexidine urticarial reaction** was confirmed the following day by a positive reaction at 15 minutes to intradermal injection of 0.02 ml of 0.0002% chlorhexidine gluconate.

Not only urticaria and shock may occur in such sensitized patients, but also pruritus and dermatitis. **Patch tests** to a 0.5% solution of the chlorhexidine gluconate are appropriate.

Hibiclens is a cleanser to be avoided in patients with pruritus and excoriated skin. A more common suspect in patients with chronic urticaria is **Peridex**, the chlorhexidine mouthwash prescribed by dentists.

Langeland T, Nyrud M: **Contact urticaria** to wheat bran bath: A case report. Acta Derm Venereol 1982; 62:82–83.

After 4 months of therapeutic wheat bran baths, this 14-month-old atopic boy began to experience wheals and itching within minutes of being placed in such a bath.

Upon challenge, urticaria and severe pruritus developed after a 5-minute exposure to a bran bath. This lasted 1 to 2 hours and involved only the skin in direct contact with the colloidal bran suspension. There was no reaction to a simple water bath. Prick tests as well as the Prausnitz-Küstner test confirmed the diagnosis of immediate-type hypersensitivity to bran.

We can match this with our experience with an erythrodermic patient who came to us having had 11 months of treatment with daily oatmeal baths. Basophil degranulation tests proved him to be exquisitely sensitive to the oatmeal. There was complete remission of the erythroderma on cessation of the baths.

Ask for the specifics of your pruritic patient's bathing habits. And then cross-examine him about soap additives and oils in the bath, as well as what is put on the skin after the bath. Skin disease can have a balneogenesis! One man's pleasure is another man's pathogen.

Grade AC, Martens BPM: **Chronic urticaria** due to dental eugenol. Dermatologica 1989; 178:217–220.

For 2 months this 22-year-old woman had been experiencing generalized urticaria with a **3- to 4-day rhythmic cycle** and an increase toward evenings.

Intradermal tests with inhalant allergens as well as penicillin were negative, but on patch tests there was a 1+ patch test to balsam of Peru and a 2+ reaction to oil of cloves. A 6-week restrictive diet eliminating food additives (azo dyes and benzoates) gave no relief.

In a search for focal infection, **chronic periapical inflammation** was found at the apices of molar 46.

The dentist noted that a root canal preparation had been placed in that tooth as well as a titanium–aluminum metal alloy screw. It had then been crowned with a gold alloy covered with porcelain. An apex resection of the periapical granuloma was done, but to no avail. In the continuing search for a dental cause of the urticaria the crown and screw post were removed. This necessitated further root canal treatment with the same **Grossman's cement** (eugenol in zinc oxide) as used before. Within a few days the urticaria flared markedly.

Eventually the canals were reamed clean and refilled with a different formula (containing sulfonamide, zinc, titanium, and calcium salts). Within a few days the urticaria disappeared. Later, an oral challenge with eugenol oil in tap water reproduced the urticaria about 30 hours after the first dose. Except for this, the patient has remained clear of urticaria despite a new gold and porcelain crown.

Once the **Grossman's cement** was pinpointed as the cause, a search was made for the specific ingredient responsible. This appeared to be eugenol, a liquid used for its antiseptic and anesthetic action. Yet patch tests to this compound, read at both 20 and 48 hours, were entirely negative. It was decided to do an oral provocation test using an incremental series of challenges that started at 0.025 ml emulsified in tap water. The dose was doubled each hour. By the end of the second day the maximum dose of 0.5 ml had been reached, and 7 hours later the urticaria reappeared and persisted for several weeks. Control subjects showed no response to 0.75 ml of eugenol given in 100 ml of tap water. A diagnosis of eugenol urticaria was made with the Grossman's root canal cement the source of exposure.

This returns one to the positive patch test to **balsam of Peru**, a related antigen. It was a diagnostic signpost pointing to the eugenol sensitivity, yet an oral challenge was necessary to pinpoint the sensitivity.

Eugenol is widespread in nature. Sensitized patients should avoid pimento oil (allspice), oil of cloves, oil of bay, and oil of carnation, each of which contains a concentration of up to 80%. Even oil of cinnamon contains it (pointing up the hazard of cinnamon in cookies, candies, and toothpaste). **Perfumes, spices, and dental materials** remain on the to-be-avoided list.

What patients with chronic urticaria need is not strong steroids, but smart sleuthing.

If I were to tell you how uncertain I am of my diagnosis, how little I know about your disease, and how much I know of the adverse effects of the drugs you need, you would run out of my office screaming.

I. M. A. COMPUTER, M.D.

Physical

Dover JS, Kobza Black A, Ward AM, Greaves MW: **Delayed pressure urticaria.** Clinical features, laboratory investigations, and response to therapy of 44 patients. J Am Acad Dermatol 1988; 18:1289–1298.

After a pressure stimulus, the mean onset of whealing was $3\frac{1}{2}$ hours; the mean peak swelling after 10 hours, mean duration 36 hours.

Two thirds had associated generalized flu-like symptoms.

The majority had coexistent chronic idiopathic urticaria as well as delayed dermographism.

One in four had angioedema.

Trigger factors:

standing, walking, sitting on hard surface   dental work
use of screwdriver, hammer   kissing
hand clapping   intercourse
carrying handbag   tampon usage
tight-fitting clothing

Warin RP: Clinical observations on delayed pressure urticaria. Br J Dermatol 1989; 121:225–228.

A study of 48 patients with **delayed pressure urticaria** showed:

All had chronic urticaria and/or angioedema.
Delayed dermographism is the same phenomenon elicited by a slightly different mode of pressure.

Warin RP: A simple outpatient **test for delayed pressure urticaria**. Br J Dermatol 1987; 116:742–743.

The patient places a 1.4-cm marble on the forearm, covers it with a tea towel tied to the handles of a plastic bag suspended below and containing 9 pounds of groceries, a house brick, or three wine bottles full of water. The patient supports this weight for 5 minutes, producing **focal pressure** under the marble. A nice diagram of the arrangement is included.

If the **test** is done 6 hours before the patient is seen by the physician, the delayed pressure urticarial response can be graded at the time of the office visit. A wheal of 3 to 10 cm is considered strongly positive.

Tatnall FM, Gaylarde PM, Sarkany I: Localised **heat urticaria** and its management. Clin Exp Dermatol 1984; 9:367–374.

Contact with heat produced hives for 9 months in a 17-year-old man with a history of atopic eczema and hay fever. He first noted an itchy rash and dizziness after severe exertion, such as cross-country running and playing squash. **Hot drinks** made the lips swell, and a hot bath led to a rash and even fainting. Exercise tests and intradermal carbachol (125 μg) failed to demonstrate cholinergic urticaria. Immersion of the hand in hot water for 1 minute quickly confirmed the diagnosis of **localized heat urticaria**, and in-tradermal atropine (30 μg) failed to inhibit the urticaria induced by heat challenge.

The **critical temperature proved to be 40°C**, as contact for 4 minutes with a beaker filled with water at that temperature elicited a sharply circum-scribed hive. This developed 8 minutes after the beaker was removed and remained for about 20 minutes. Exposure to 39°C was without effect. Plasma histamine was noted to be normal during heat challenge and then to rise with the appearance of the wheal. This suggests that histamine is an impor-

1238

tant mediator, even though the reaction could not be suppressed with oral antihistamines.

It was possible to induce complete **tolerance** by full immersion of the patient in a bath at 40.5°C twice daily. This was gradually reduced to immersion once every 3 days, which kept him symptom free.

Wanderer AA: **Cold urticaria syndromes**: Historical background, diagnostic classification, clinical and laboratory characteristics, pathogenesis, and management. J Allergy Clin Immunol 1990; 85:965–984.

Diagnostic classification of **cold urticaria syndromes**:

I. Acquired Cold Urticaria (ACU) syndromes
    A. Syndromes with a positive cold–contact stimulation test
        1. Primary
        2. Secondary
            Cryoglobulinemia
                Primary
                Secondary
                    Chronic lymphocytic leukemia
                    Lymphosarcoma
                    Leukocytoclastic vasculitis
                    Angioimmunoblastic lymphadenopathy
            Leukocytoclastic vasculitis
            Infectious diseases
                Mononucleosis
                Syphilis
            Cold agglutinins
            Cold hemolysins
            Cold fibrinogens
    B. Atypical Acquired Cold Urticaria syndromes (atypical responses to a cold-contact stimulation test)
        1. Systemic atypical
        2. Cold-dependent dermatographism
        3. Cold-induced cholinergic urticaria
        4. Delayed cold urticaria
        5. Localized cold-reflex urticaria
II. Familial form of cold urticaria
    Delayed cold urticaria (autosomal dominant inheritance)

Neittaanmäki H: **Cold urticaria**: Clinical findings in 220 patients. J Am Acad Dermatol 1985; 13:636–644.

Exposure of skin to cold in these patients results in redness, itching, wheals, and edema. Systemic effects include fatigue, headache, dyspnea, tachycardia, collapse, and anaphylactic shock.

The **diagnostic test** is the application of an ice cube for 20 minutes on the forearm. Ninety per cent of patients with cold urticaria will show a wheal in 10 to 20 minutes. However, in the familial type of cold urticaria or in cold-induced cholinergic urticaria, challenge in a cold room or immersion in cold water is necessary to reproduce the disease. A special form of delayed cold urticaria exists in which the hives do not appear until some time after cold exposure. Blood tests should be done to rule out secondary or acquired cold urticaria. These are tests for: cryoglobulin, cryofibrinogen, cold agglutinin, paroxysmal hemoglobinuria.

In 10 patients the onset of **cold urticaria** was preceded by streptococcal tonsillitis and in 11 others by an upper respiratory infection. Only 1 of the 220 patients showed cryoglobulinemia.

In 30% of the patients with cold urticaria, other forms of physical or chronic urticaria were present. The most common finding was **dermographism**.

Grandel KE, Farr RS, Wanderer AA, et al: Association of platelet-activating factor with primary **acquired cold urticaria**. N Engl J Med 1985; 313:405–409.

Cold urticaria is characterized by **erythema, pruritus, and edema.** Cold challenges were performed in six patients and five controls by submerging one arm below the antecubital fossa in ice water (4 to 8°C) for a minimum of 3 minutes. Blood samples removed via an indwelling catheter in the antecubital vein of the test arm were analyzed for possible mediators, including histamine, neutrophilic chemotactic activity, and platelet-activating factor.

While **controls** developed only erythema, patients with cold urticaria developed either "mild" nonconfluent urticaria with minimal angioedema or "severe" confluent urticaria with severe angioedema and inability to flex the fingers or make a fist.

In four patients with severe edema developing within 10 to 18 minutes after **cold water challenge**, all three mediators were increased. In contrast, they were not increased in the remaining subjects. In three patients, doxepin inhibited release of platelet-activating factor and suppressed the urticaria.

The cause of a cure is as intriguing as the cause of a disease.

Wong RC, Fairley JA, Ellis CN: **Dermographism**: A review. J Am Acad Dermatol 1984; 11:643–652.

Dermographism is a pathologically heightened triple response of Lewis to firm stroking of the skin. In patients with dermographism, the firm stroke produces a wheal 2 to 3 mm in width in about 1 to 3 minutes. The wheal is surrounded by a 5- to 10-mm band of erythema. The wheal reaches its maximum size in 6 to 7 minutes and starts to fade by 10 to 15 minutes, being gone by 30 minutes. There is a refractory period of the area for hours following this.

Pruritus may be severe, especially in the heat or when patients are tired or anxious. This dermographic pruritus may be the presenting complaint, and the patient may not correlate it with such minor shearing forces as rubbing the eyelids, toweling, or even kissing. The ensuing scratching leads to a cycle of more whealing and itching.

Dermographism is seen in nearly all patients with **urticaria pigmentosa** whether it be diffuse or nodular. Here the dermographism is so vivid as to be called Darier's sign. It bespeaks of histamine release from the abnormal aggregates of mast cells responsible for this disease. Thus, papular dermographism may point to the exact sites of these mast cell clusters. In infants the whealing may be so intense that the dermographism is expressed as bullae.

Subclinical drug eruptions may show only dermographism. These include sensitivity reactions to penicillin, aspirin, sulfonamides, and codeine and extend to horse serum and poison ivy sensitization.

Look also for widespread dermographism in **scabies**, *Cheyletiella* **infestations**, or **after wasp and bee stings**. Or one may see dermographism limited to a tattoo site. From the general medical standpoint we may expect to see dermographism and its companion pruritus in the latter half of pregnancy (progesterone sensitivity?) with hepatic cholestasis, hypothyroidism or hyperthyroidism, diabetes mellitus, infectious disease, and phenylketonuria.

In making the diagnosis of dermographism, **reproduce the phenomenon** by using a brisk heavy-pressure stroke employing, for example, the smooth end of a safety pin. The best site is the back. Avoid suntanned areas, since these have reduced capacity to wheal. Rechecking the area at 5 and 30 minutes maximizes the number of positive findings.

In the **differential diagnosis**, remember that angioedema-like reactions can occur with inapparent lip biting or rubbing of the eyelids. Dermographism can mimic all forms of urticaria, and must especially be tested for in presumed cases of contact urticaria or pressure urticaria. Most important, it should be checked for in all patients who have unaccountable itch! They focus on the itch and never talk about the scratch products.

The **dermographic state** persists for days to weeks when associated with a precipitating event such as scabies or acute urticaria. The idiopathic form fades away even more slowly, lasting for years in some patients.

Special forms of dermographism must be recognized.

1. **Follicular dermographism:** Urticarial papules at follicular sites, elicited by wide-band stroking with broad edge of tongue blade.
2. **Delayed dermographism:** Reappearance of wheal 3 to 6 hours later after initial classic stroke-induced wheal. This wheal may last 24 to 48 hours. The delayed wheal is tender and burns. It is to be distinguished from pressure urticaria due to flat pressure rather than the shearing force associated with dermographism. The two may coexist.

3. **Cholinergic dermographism:** Pruritic wheals, 1 to 2 mm, with broad surrounding erythema elicited by stroking. Also known as "beaded" dermographism, it is identical in appearance to cholinergic urticaria and usually coexists with that.

4. **Cold-precipitated dermographism:** Firm stroking of the arm in a patient with cold urticaria was not followed by any whealing, and the site of stroking was inapparent until the arm was immersed in cold water. At that time, well-delineated wheals rose above the background of diffuse cold-induced whealing, revealing the sites of prior strokes. This focal reactivity could be elicited up to 13 hours after the originally negative dermographic stroke test.

5. **Exercise-induced dermographism** with cold-precipitated dermographism: Here the patient had dermographism only following severe exercise and interestingly in sites *after* cold urticaria had been elicited.

6. **Red dermographism:** This is the phenomenon of diffuse whealing in an erythematous band occurring after rubbing in contrast to stroking. The whealing is subtle and best appreciated by stretching the skin. The reaction occurs within a minute or two after rubbing, climaxes at 5 to 6 minutes with the wheals gone in 15 minutes but the erythema persists an hour. Pruritus is of variable degree: scratching produces erythema but no obvious whealing in these patients.

7. **Yellow dermographism:** Occurs in patients with prejaundice state due to extravasated bile pigment.

8. **White dermographism:** It is not truly dermographism, since there is no whealing—only blanching as a result of stroking. It occurs in atopic patients or in association with allergic contact dermatitis. The white line may persist for 20 minutes, coming on within seconds. The phenomenon tends to disappear as the skin heals. It may also be seen in erythrodermas, pityriasis rubra pilaris, seborrheic dermatitis, pityriasis rosea, extenive lichen planus, or even acute graft-versus-host disease.

9. **Black dermographism:** This is a special form of dermographic skin writing in which black or green lines or stains of the stratum corneum occur as a result of contact with metals. Expect it under rings, wristbands, bracelets, or clasps, or in areas where metals rub over medically or cosmetically powdered skin. The color is due to light absorbance by tiny particles of the soft metal abraded off by the rough stratum corneum or powder such as zinc oxide. There is no whealing despite its name.

Scratch your patient and learn something about his itch.

Breathnach SM, Allen R, Ward AM, Greaves MW: **Symptomatic dermographism**: Natural history, clinical features, laboratory investigations and response to therapy. Clin Exp Dermatol 1983; 8:463–476.

Symptomatic dermographism may be differentiated from simple dermographism by the presence of itching and the lower-force threshold required to induce whealing.

A study of 50 patients with symptomatic dermographism showed no association with systemic disease, food allergens, medications, or atopic dermatitis.

The most important finding was a significant reduction in the serum protease inhibitor **alpha$_1$-antitrypsin**. Other protease inhibitors, including C1 esterase inhibitor, were normal.

Shelley WB, Shelley ED: **Follicular dermographism**. Cutis 1983; 32:244–245, 254, 260.

A 43-year-old man complained of widespread pruritus and **transient** "**bumps**" of 4 weeks' duration. On examination, 5- to 10-mm urticarial papules showed precise and consistent localization around the hair follicles.

Stroking, scratching, or rubbing the patient's skin produced similar pruritic papules within a few minutes. **A hair protruded from the center of each.** The lesions never became confluent, but gradually disappeared within a half-hour. Treatment with hydroxyzine prevented their appearance.

A diagnosis of **follicular dermographism** was made. It is to be distinguished from cholinergic urticaria by virtue of the fact that it cannot be elicited by exercise, emotions, or hot baths. Furthermore, its follicular localization is not seen in cholinergic urticaria, nor is follicular dermographism elicited by contact with water as is aquagenic urticaria. Yet both conditions share the follicular localization.

The **best diagnostic test** for follicular dermographism is very firm broadband stroking of the skin in a uniform fashion. This reveals the focal nature of the response.

Mayou SC, Black AK, Eady RAJ, Greaves MW: **Cholinergic dermographism**. Br J Dermatol 1986; 115:371–377.

A 29-year-old woman had a 6-week history of pruritus and cholinergic urticaria. Remarkably, **stroking the skin** elicited both itching and a band of erythema studded with small discrete urticarial wheals.

A pathogenic role of **acetylcholine** in triggering the attacks was proven by showing that topical scopolamine hydrochloride (9% aqueous hyoscine hydrochloride for 5 min) blocked this unique dermographism. A spring-loaded dermographometer was used to produce cholinergic-like wheals in a linear distribution, developing within minutes of stroking or scratching the skin and lasting for approximately 45 minutes. Skin biopsies revealed a moderate perivascular mononuclear cell infiltrate in prechallenge skin and a dense dermal infiltrate of mononuclear cells in a wheal.

McDermott WV, Topol BM: **Systemic mastocytosis** with large cutaneous mastocytomas: Surgical management. J Surg Oncol 1985; 30:221–225.

A 62-year-old white man first developed dermographism in childhood, with wheal and flare responses to skin irritation subsiding slowly over a period of days. At puberty he noted a nonpruritic erythematous macular rash on the trunk that gradually spread over most of the body except for palms, soles, buttocks, and face. By age 42 he had hepatosplenomegaly and had had recurrent peptic ulcer, and at age 47 started to develop nodules on the legs. The nodules, which were **mastocytomas**, grew rapidly and reached 6 to 8 cm in size. They were very vascular and bled frequently after minor trauma. The patient's general health remained good despite extensive infiltration of bone marrow and liver with mast cells. He could not drink alcohol because of an immediate intense uncomfortable flush. Surgical removal of tumor nodules was best accomplished with an ultrasound scalpel.

The diagnosis of pruritus should arouse an itch in you to find the cause.

Urticaria Pigmentosa

Patients with urticaria pigmentosa don't come to you with hives. And most patients with urticaria pigmentosa don't come to you. They are brought, for this is largely a disease of infants. Their problem is **brown bumps**, not urticaria, despite the name of their disease. Actually, the name is an ingenious mnemonic to remind you that you can produce the hive by simply stroking the lesion (Darier's sign). The brown bumps are simply masses of mast cells that, on physical trauma, release their histamine content to induce a local hive. A single lesion merits the name mastocytoma, and multiple lesions in the skin and elsewhere leave dermatologic designation and are called mastocytosis.

As with all diseases, the range of presentation is great. The baby may itch for no apparent reason until a biopsy shows the skin infiltrate of mast cells. The mother may be concerned over a "mole" that swells when rubbed or scratched. There may be yellow plaques that, on biopsy, reveal themselves to be a variant of urticaria pigmentosa called **xanthelasmoidea**. The baby may have blisters or even erythroderma, again explained only on biopsy.

The older patient may come because of **flushing** or because of a rare form of mastocytosis, **telangiectasia macularis eruptiva perstans**. When he is questioned, the patient's complaint of nausea, peptic ulcer, and diarrhea points to mastocytosis of the gastrointestinal tract. The patient may be prodded to recall unusual distress associated with histamine-liberating drugs such as aspirin and codeine. Any organ may be involved. X-rays of the bone may reveal mastocytomas as lytic lesions. The blood count may show basophilia, eosinophilia, or other aberrations. In extensive mastocytosis, the more you look the more you'll find to explain the unexplainable. Remember, your diagnostic entrance point is the pigment spot that urticates.

DiBacco RS, DeLeo VA: **Mastocytoses** and the mast cell. J Am Acad Dermatol 1982; 7:709–722.

I. **Cutaneous Mastocytosis:**

Urticaria pigmentosa:
generalized eruption consisting of multiple red-brown macules and papules distributed usually over the trunk
may consist of lichenoid, plaque-like or nodular lesions
monomorphous lesions that may vary in number from one to several hundred
rare forms presenting as leopard skin
bullae occurring in infants
Telangiectasia macularis eruptiva perstans: numerous, often confluent, telangiectatic hyperpigmented macules that may cover most of the body
Erythroderma: red, thickened, lichenified, skin of doughy consistency; "red leather"
Mastocytoma: red-brown, pink, or yellow nodule, usually solitary lesion present at birth
Xanthelasmoidea: yellow papules resembling xanthoma

II. **Systemic Mastocytosis**

Skeletal: discrete lytic, cystic, or sclerotic lesions, osteoporosis, osteosclerosis
Gastrointestinal: nausea, vomiting, diarrhea, pain, peptic ulcer
Blood: eosinophilia and leukemia, basophilia, anemia, polycythemia vera
Any organ system may be affected.
Diagnostic signs:
cutaneous:

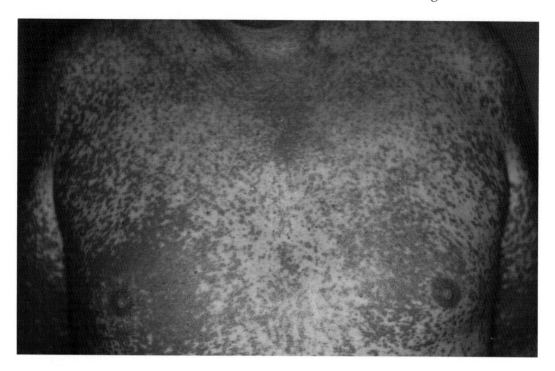

rubbing a lesion will release histamine from mast cell infiltrates, producing wheal and flare response, i.e., **Darier's sign**.

flushing from exercise, hot baths, emotional stress, cold exposure, and intake of aspirin or codeine

dermatographism in clinically uninvolved skin

vesicles and bullae in infants

systemic:

intense **pruritus**, pounding headache, bronchospasm, rhinorrhea, hypotension, tachycardia, dyspnea, and syncope

Differential diagnosis:

isolated mastocytomas: juvenile xanthogranuloma, pigmented nevi, connective tissue nevi

macular form: lentigines, nevi, telangiectasia macularis eruptiva perstans: hereditary hemorrhagic telangiectasia

urticaria pigmentosa: eruptive xanthoma, neurofibroma

systemic mastocytosis: carcinoid syndrome

Laboratory:

mastocytosis: elevated histamine level in blood and urine, occasionally hypocholesterolemia

radiographic study of bone!

In most instances, simply scratching the surface of these patients produced the diagnostic hive.

Rampen F, Westerhof W: The isomorphic (Koebner) phenomenon in cutaneous **mastocytosis**. Acta Derm Venereol 1981; 61:567–569.

Permanent sharply circumscribed reddish-brown discolorations on the right upper arm and right forearm of a 67-year-old man proved to be due to infiltrates of mast cells in two healed **burns** sustained 2 years previously.

The patient had a long history of adult-onset cutaneous mastocytosis, with numerous brownish papules showing the Darier sign. The post-burn mastocytoma was viewed as a **Koebner response** to thermal injury. Similar mastocytosis Koebner responses have been seen following radiation therapy and after the application of Elastoplast tape.

Meneghini CL, Angelini G: Systemic **mastocytosis** with diffuse crocodile-like pachydermic skin, pedunculated pseudofibromas and comedones. Br J Dermatol 1980; 103:329–334.

A 52-year-old woman watched the soft skin of her teens evolve into a brownish, thick, deeply embossed, **crocodile-like pachydermic skin** with numerous pedunculated tumors. The molluscum-like tumors were symmetrical, soft or hard, yellowish or brown lumps, some reminiscent of bunches of small grapes, while others were nodular or flat. Her **leonine facies** stands in startling contrast to her lovely portrait at the age of 19. Numerous large blackheads were present in hair follicles. Pruritus, dermatographism, **elevated blood histamine** levels, **duodenal ulcer**, enlarged liver and spleen, and mastocyte-filled bone marrow completed the extreme picture of **systemic mastocytosis**—all proven by biopsies of skin, liver, marrow, and spleen.

As early as 2 months of age her skin had been brownish with small diffuse raised lesions and episodes of itching. She had also had frequent episodes of diarrhea from a very young age. The slow insidious benign proliferation of mastocytes throughout her life permitted adaptation by her and her fellow office workers to a remarkable degree.

Parks A, Camisa C: Reddish-brown macules with **telangiectasia** and pruritus. Arch Dermatol 1988; 124:429–433.

For 10 years a 75-year-old woman had a pruritic rash of the face, trunk, and proximal area of the extremities as well as periodic nausea, vomiting, abdominal pain, and diarrhea. The skin lesions were **reddish-brown macules** with telangiectasia, which blanched on diascopy and urticated on stroking (**Darier's sign**). Skin biopsy revealed telangiectatic vessels surrounded by collections of mast cells, typical of telangiectasia macularis eruptiva perstans. A bone survey showed osteoporosis and compression fractures of L-1 and L-4, and **bone marrow biopsy** disclosed **increased mast cells**.

In **systemic mastocytosis**, mast cells in the cardiovasculature lead to histamine release with weakness, dizziness, palpitations, and tachycardia. Gastrointestinal involvement can produce anorexia, nausea, vomiting, peptic ulcers, diarrhea, and malabsorption, along with hepatosplenomegaly. In bone, mast cells induce pain, osteoporosis, and osteosclerosis, and mast cell overload in the marrow leads to anemia, leukopenia, and thrombocytopenia.

Truly, urticaria pigmentosa or its variant, telangiectasia macularis eruptiva perstans, is a cutaneous mirror of systemic disease.

Caputo R, Ermacora E, Gelmetti C, et al: Generalized **eruptive histiocytoma** in children. J Am Acad Dermatol 1987; 17:449–454.

In this benign, asymptomatic, self-healing eruption, numerous firm red, bluish-red, brownish papules suddenly appear scattered over the body surface. The biopsy gives the answer: a monotonously monomorphic infiltrate of **histiocytes**. Successive crops appear, but months later spontaneous regression takes place. It is easily **distinguished from**:

> histiocytosis
> juvenile xanthogranuloma
> papular xanthoma
> sinus histiocytosis with massive lymphadenopathy
> urticaria pigmentosa
> benign cephalic histiocytosis (localized to head and neck)

Vasculitis

The clinicians stole the diagnosis of vasculitis from the pathologists. Vasculitis really refers to focal microscopic damage or inflammatory change in the blood vessels. But the clinician has become so adept at recognizing the gross effects of such vasculitis that he uses the term in daily practice.

What are the **lesions** that permit the clinician to anticipate the histopathologic changes of vasculitis? They are the following:

1. Purpura, petechiae, as in Henoch-Schönlein syndrome
2. Palpable purpura
3. Urticarial lesions persisting for more than a day
4. Vesicular, bullous, or pustular lesions with a purpuric base
5. Livedo reticularis
6. Painful retiform macules
7. Necrosis
8. Infarct scars, as in atrophie blanche or Degos' disease (malignant atrophic papulosis)

Vasculitis may involve vessels of any size and any location. As a result, the clinical change may range from the **petechiae of capillaritis** to the **gangrene of arteritis**. Vasculitis may be leukocytoclastic, lymphocytic, granulomatous, or obliterative, the lesions ranging from papules to granulomas and ulcers. With such disparate manifestations, it is small wonder that the clinician grabs the diagnosis of vasculitis as a wide net.

But what may this net catch that looks like vasculitis but isn't? The catch of **nonvasculitis lesions** includes those of the "blue toes" of atheroembolism, as well as the purpuric lesions of scurvy, macroglobulinemia, blood dyscrasias, and factitial dermatitis. Always the biopsy is the arbiter of authenticity.

What do we look for behind the diagnosis of vasculitis? In our experience, **bacterial infection**, focal or otherwise, has been the major cause. The range of organisms is wide, including viruses, rickettsiae, and spirochetes. Reactions to drugs of a wide variety likewise may present as vasculitis. More serious counterparts are **malignant disease** and systemic lupus erythematosus.

We stole the diagnosis of vasculitis from the pathologist, but always we have to go back to him and ask if we stole the real thing.

Overview

Smoller BR, McNutt S, Contreras F: The natural history of **vasculitis**: What the histology tells us about pathogenesis. Arch Dermatol 1990; 126:84–89.

When the **biopsy report** is:

Leukocytoclastic vasculitis:
> look for drug or infection as a cause
> look for coexistent disease:

malignancy	Sjögren's syndrome
systemic lupus erythematosus	rheumatoid arthritis

> anticipate with: urticaria, Henoch-Schönlein purpura

Lymphocytic vasculitis:
> look for:

drug	insect bite, scabies
infection	

> consider:

erythema multiforme	urticarial vasculitis
erythema perstans	pigmented purpuric eruptions

Granulomatous vasculitis:
> think of:

lymphomatoid granulomatosis	temporal arteritis
Wegener's granulomatosis	Takayasu's arteritis
syphilis	

Obliterative vasculitis:
> look for:

syphilis	cholesterol emboli
cryoglobulinemia	thromboembolism
thrombocytopenia	

> think of: Degos' disease, livedo

Chan LS, Cooper KD, Rasmussen JE: Koebnerization as a cutaneous manifestation of **immune complex–mediated vasculitis**. J Am Acad Dermatol 1990; 22:775–781.

To prove that **immune complexes** are the cause of clinical **vasculitic lesions**, it is necessary to show the simultaneous presence of circulating immune complexes (Raji cell assay), tissue-bound vascular immunoreactants (immunofluorescent deposits C3, IgM, etc.), and vascular damage (histologically).

In a 25-year-old woman with a 1-month history of pruritic papules of the ankles, such a demonstration was accomplished. The **papules** that later appeared on the **legs and arms** were either erythematous or yellow-brown with micalike scales and hemorrhagic foci in some. Biopsy showed a pronounced perivascular lymphocytic infiltrate with endothelial cell swelling and proliferation, as well as intravascular fibrin and focal red cell extravasation. C3 and fibrin deposits were seen on immunofluorescence. **Circulating immune complexes** (Raji cell assay positive) were found. A diagnosis of **pityriasis lichenoides et varioliformis** was made, and the vasculitis proved to be immune complex mediated.

Lesions in a scar on the right thigh demonstrated the Koebner phenomenon. Here, the altered vascular anatomy of the scar favored the localization of the immune complex–mediated vasculitis, even as the stasis of dependency favored localization around the ankles.

Diagnostic uncertainty breeds therapeutic uncertainty.

Sanchez NP, Van Hale HM, Su WPD: Clinical and histopathologic spectrum of **necrotizing vasculitis**: Report of findings in 101 cases. Arch Dermatol 1985; 121:220–224.

Clinical:

palpably purpuric	nodular
urticarial	livedoid
infarctive-ulcerative	location: usually lower leg

Pathogenesis: Small postcapillary venules are site of deposition of circulating immune complex that activates complement cascade, leading to migration of polymorphonuclear leukocytes and release of destructive lysosomal enzymes.

drug eruption (13%): penicillin, erythromycin, thiazide, allopurinol, insecticide
Streptococcus (6%) (respiratory tract)
Escherichia coli (3%) (urinary tract)

Jorizzo JL, Daniels JC: Dermatologic conditions reported in patients with **rheumatoid arthritis**. J Am Acad Dermatol 1983; 8:439–457.

When you know the patient has **rheumatoid arthritis**, you know he may have:

Rheumatoid nodules

firm skin-colored, nontender, dome-shaped masses in the subcutaneous tissue
occur at sites of trauma, e.g., elbow, knee, knuckle, scalp, feet
insidious, persistent, may regress
also seen in systemic lupus erythematosus, scleroderma

Rheumatoid vasculitis

digital gangrene
palpable purpura
leukocytoclastic vasculitis, venulitis
nailfold thromboses: paronychial infarcts
erythema elevatum diutinum, erythematous to yellowed plaques on extensor surface of extremities
atrophie blanche, focal purpura progressing to stellate
configurate infarctive lesions representing segmental hyalinizing vasculitis

Pyoderma gangrenosum

acute necrotizing expanding ulcers
undermined edges
commonly on legs or abdomen
"painful pyoderma"
differential diagnosis:
infection: mycobacterial, fungal, amebic, bacterial
haloderma (bromides or iodides)
syphilis
Wegener's granulomatosis
factitial

Leg ulcers
Autoimmune bullous disease
Generalized thinning of skin
Palmar erythema

Much in the skin stems from **deposition of the circulating immune complexes** of rheumatoid arthritis.

1249

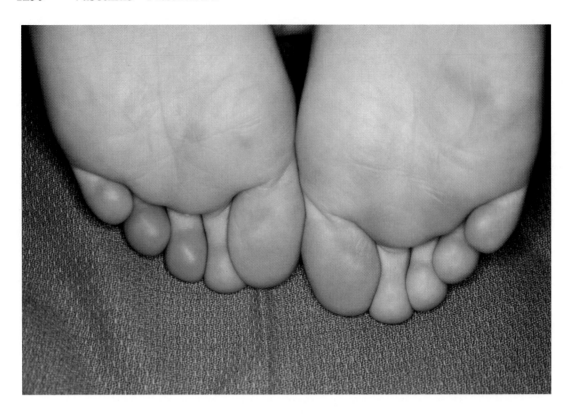

Sánchez JL, Cruz A: **Rheumatoid neutrophilic dermatitis**. J Am Acad Dermatol 1990; 22:922–925.

During recent years this 46-year-old woman had had recurrent **painful erythematous papules** and crusted nodules on the backs of the hands, forearms, and lateral aspect of the thighs. Some of the papules were subcutaneous. The significant finding in the history was the fact that she had had **rheumatoid arthritis** for 13 years.

A **biopsy** revealed a dense infiltrate of neutrophils in the entire dermis. Immunofluorescent studies failed to reveal any immunoglobulins or C3 deposits. A diagnosis of **rheumatoid neutrophilic dermatitis** was made. It has a special predilection for points of trauma on the hands and arms. At times, ulceration occurs, but no vasculitis is found. This distinguishes it from the clinically similar erythema elevatum diutinum characterized by the presence of leukocytoclastic vasculitis. Another clinical diagnostic possibility for the subcutaneous lesions was rheumatoid nodules, but this is readily recognized as a palisading granuloma with abundant fibrin in the center.

Other neutrophil-rich conditions your pathologist can rule out are Sweet's syndrome, pyoderma gangrenosum, and intestinal bypass dermatitis.

Patients with rheumatoid arthritis if not afflicted with neutrophilic dermatosis come to you with **rheumatoid vasculitis**. These are the lesions of purpura, ecchymoses, necrosis, and infarct. These are also the patients with **intractable leg ulcers**.

Walker KD, Badame AJ: **Erythema elevatum diutinum** in a patient with Crohn's disease. J Am Acad Dermatol 1990; 22:948–952.

Dark-brown firm, tender nodules had been present on the **elbows, knees,** and **finger joints** of this 30-year-old woman for the past 5 years. A biopsy revealed leukocytoclastic and angioplastic vasculitis consistent with **erythema elevatum diutinum**.

The pathogenesis was believed to involve the deposition of circulating immune complexes in the skin at the sites of mechanical trauma. Such circulating immune complexes were demonstrated and were felt to arise from the **inflammatory bowel disease (Crohn's)** she had been experiencing for 11 years.

Patients with inflammatory bowel disease may **suffer** not only from erythema elevatum diutinum, but also from erythema nodosum, pyoderma gangrenosum, psoriasis, aphthae, rashes at colostomy site, and malnutritional skin lesions.

Siegel DM, Freeman RG: Fever, **palpable purpura** and a positive Weil-Felix reaction. Arch Dermatol 1986; 122:711–715.

A 17-year-old boy was hospitalized for evaluation of a **painful swollen left foot of 2 days' duration**. The left sole showed multiple exquisitely tender stellate and annular purpuric papules. He also had a small area of subungual purpura and a purpuric papule on the left third finger. In the past 9 days he had had nausea, vomiting, arthralgias, and myalgias, as well as an infected swollen finger with lymphangitis and cellulitis requiring intramuscular penicillin and oral cephalosporin therapy. He denied drug abuse, foreign travel, venereal disease, intravenous medications, or any history of bacterial endocarditis.

In the hospital, new **palpable purpura lesions** appeared, and a biopsy showed leukocytoclastic vasculitis with thrombi of the larger vessels, suggestive of an infectious cause, but no bacteria could be found in the tissue. However, all seven blood cultures taken yielded *Pseudomonas aeruginosa*. An echocardiogram showed aortic valve prolapse without vegetation, confirming *Pseudomonas* **endocarditis**.

Strangely, a Weil-Felix test done on admission was positive with an OX-2 titer of 1:1280 and OX-19 titer of 1:160, but a negative OX-K titer. This suggested Rocky Mountain spotted fever, but was due to cross-reactivity between the *Pseudomonas aeruginosa* surface antigens and the *Proteus* antigens used in the Weil-Felix test.

Finally, the patient in the next bed suspected that there had been tampering with the patient's intravenous unit. A **toxicology serum screen** showed morphine, and the patient then admitted to long-term **intravenous drug abuse**, which explained the presence of small linear and crusted scars on the dorsal aspect of the hands.

This patient had the three classic skin signs of **infective endocarditis**:

> **Osler's nodes:** tender erythematous papules that may necrose
> **Janeway lesions:** nontender hemorrhagic papules
> **splinter hemorrhages:** nontender subungual hemorrhagic streaks

These probably are due not to septic emboli, but rather to immune-mediated vasculitis.

Pseudomonas endocarditis has a predilection for intravenous drug users. Look for it.

Irestedt M, Mansson T, Svensson A: **Vasculitis** simulating eczematous dermatitis due to C2 deficiency. Acta Derm Venereol 1987; 67:265–267.

Pruritic papulovesicular lesions of the elbows, ears, and infragluteal folds in a 26-year-old woman gradually extended to the hands, arms, and lower trunk.

Flares were associated with upper respiratory infections. Three biopsies revealed leukocytoclastic vasculitis, and blood studies showed total absence of the second component of complement. The exacerbations and remissions gave the impression of **eczematous dermatitis** or atopic dermatitis, as well as lupus erythematosus. Plaquenil (400 mg/day) provided prompt improvement.

Demonstration of C2 deficiency was the key to understanding this patient's problem, since the association of **C2 deficiency and leukocytoclastic vasculitis** is well recognized. It also accounts for the correlation between skin symptoms and recurrent upper respiratory infections noted by this and other patients.

The unique feature of this patient was that the **C2 deficiency** did not give dramatic palpable purpura, ulcerations, or systemic vasculitis, but rather only the mildest vasculitic response, a pruritic dermatitis.

Kerdel FA, Fraker DL, Haynes HA: **Necrotizing vasculitis** from radiographic contrast media. J Am Acad Dermatol 1984; 10:25–29.

Within 1 day after cardiac catheterization with the **contrast medium**, Renografin, this 72-year-old man developed a palpable papular purpuric rash of the lower extremities and fever (temperature 39.7°C). A diagnosis of necrotizing vasculitis due to sensitivity to the contrast medium was confirmed by biopsy 2 days later. The eruption spontaneously resolved in the following 2 weeks.

Of special interest was the **complete absence** of the purpuric eruption in a circular **area that had been infiltrated with Xylocaine and 1:100,000 epinephrine** for biopsy of a prior contrast medium eruption 4 hours prior to the Renografin injection. It can be presumed that the epinephrine, which induced vasoconstriction, protected this site by closing off the vessels to the Renografin and its **immune complexes** responsible for the vasculitis.

Some individuals can identify a tree by simply picking up a leaf it has dropped. Others can saw the tree down, have it analyzed chemically, and still not know it is an oak.

Warshauer DM, Hayes ME, Shumer SM: **Scurvy:** A clinical mimic of **vasculitis**. Cutis 1984; 34:539–541.

A 54-year-old woman was referred for evaluation of leukocytoclastic vasculitis. For the past month she had had painful **petechiae and palpable purpura**. These skin lesions had been accompanied by malaise, myalgias, and arthralgias.

The **dietary history** was significant. Because of dyspepsia, she had lived for years on peanut butter sandwiches, and black decaffeinated coffee. She took no vitamins.

On examination, the backs of the hands and feet as well as the soles were **ecchymotic**. The lower legs showed multiple palpable perifollicular petechiae as well as follicular hyperkeratosis. Of special note were corkscrew hairs in these areas.

All laboratory studies, including coagulograms, were normal with the exception of a hemoglobin value of 10 gm/dl. The **serum vitamin C level** was at the low end of normal at 0.2 mg/dl (normal 0.2 to 2 mg/dl). A skin biopsy failed to show any vasculitis.

A **diagnosis of scurvy** was made. This was promptly confirmed by the rapid clearing of all skin lesions as well as dramatic improvement of the myalgias and arthralgias within a week of starting vitamin C therapy (500 mg/day). Indeed, the vitamin C level climbed fivefold after the patient's first hospital meal.

Shelley WB, Wood MG: **Larval papule** as a sign of scabies. JAMA 1976; 236:1144–1145.

A 62-year-old man developed an intensely **pruritic eruption** of the operative area 3 days after insertion of a total hip prosthesis. At first blamed on a known **adhesive tape sensitivity**, the rash spread over the entire body except for the face and neck. After 7 months the lesions were quite variable, being papulovesicles on the hands and feet, papules on the buttocks and thighs, follicular papules on the arms, necrotic papules on the elbows, umbilicated crusted purpuric papules on the legs, and confluent erythematous papules, vesicles, and bullae on the lower two thirds of the body.

Necrotizing vasculitis was diagnosed clinically and histologically, although results of one biopsy also resembled those of **Mucha-Habermann syndrome**. Dermatitis herpetiformis, neurodermatitis, periarteritis, allergic contact dermatitis, and bacterial antigenemia from occult cholecystitis were considered as **diagnostic possibilities**. Patch tests were negative to the prosthesis cement (methyl methacrylate, but strongly positive to epoxy resin and dichromate. Antibiotics were without effect. **Cholecystectomy produced a marked improvement** with clearing of the petechial, purpuric, crusted, necrotic lesions within weeks. However, new pruritic papules continued to appear on the fingers and buttocks. **Biopsy of a new papule** (24 hours old) revealed an **immature scabies** mite. Treatment with Kwell lotion was curative.

Scabies is easily missed when burrows are absent, especially in the **well washed**. It may simulate other diseases, as well as compound them. Topical steroids and immunosuppression also often alter the appearance of scabies.

Brookins-Reddix N, Spivak JL, Watson RM: **Violaceous plaques** on the lower extremities. Arch Dermatol 1988; 124:1853–1856.

A presumptive **clinical diagnosis of vasculitis** failed to explain discrete, nontender, violaceous, blanchable plaques of this 67-year-old woman's feet. Ini- 1253 tially responsive to a course of prednisone, the lesions recurred a year later and were treatment resistant.

The explanation came with the finding of a serum level of IgM of 11.2 gm/liter (normal 1.4 gm/liter) and an infiltrate of small lymphocytes in the bone marrow. The patient had cutaneous **macroglobulinosis**. The macroglobulinemia (**Waldenström's**) was the result of a neoplasm of immature B lymphocytes. In this malignant disease, lymphocytes and plasma cells showed uncontrolled proliferation and synthesis of monoclonal IgM or heavy chain. This leads to the **hyperviscosity syndrome**, in which one may see Raynaud's phenomenon, cryoglobulinemia, hemorrhagic diathesis, and peripheral neuropathy as well as renal failure.

In this patient the lesions were infiltrative plaques of lymphocytes and plasma cells that appeared not only on the extremities, but also on the face and ears.

An alternate form presents as **IgM storage papules**. These are pink, translucent, or flesh-colored papules of the knees, elbows, and buttocks. Central erosion and crusting occur at times. They may also appear on the trunk and face. The biopsy reveals eosinophilic homogeneous deposits of PAS-positive material, which is the IgM. The course of the lesions may be variable, dependent on the activity of the lymphoma.

Longley J, Demar L, Feinstein RP, et al: Clinical and histologic features of **pityriasis lichenoides et varioliformis acuta** in children. Arch Dermatol 1987; 123:1335–1339.

Clinical features of **pityriasis lichenoides et varioliformis acuta (PLEVA)** in five children:

> asynchronous life cycle of individual lesions that can number into the hundreds
> erythematous spots
> erythematous papules: reddish-tan, violaceous puncta in some
> vesiculation, hemorrhage, necrotic crust
> hypopigmented macules or scars

These changes occur in a single lesion within a time window of 2 to 5 weeks. However, the evolution of a given lesion may abort at any time with rapid resolution. The patient thus presents scores of lesions in **varying stages** of **evolution**. They localize on the anterior trunk and proximal rather than distal surface of the extremities. The face, scalp, and mucous membranes were exempt in all five children. This symptomless disease, even as a single lesion, may abort spontaneously or persist for several years.

For diagnosis, a **high index of suspicion** is needed. It must be **considered** in any case of:

> scabies: note absence of itch in PLEVA
> insect bites: exposure history
> varicella: involves scalp, no new lesions after 1 week
> Gianotti-Crosti syndrome: no necrosis occurs, presents acrally, has associated lymphadenopathy
> erythema multiforme: involves mucous membranes

Kisch LS, Bruynzeel DP: Six cases of malignant **atrophic papulosis (Degos' disease)** occurring in one family. Br J Dermatol 1984; 111:469–471.

A 40-year-old healthy man had hundreds of lenticular skin-colored and pink papules spreading over the trunk, arms, and legs for 1 year. Each had a distinctive **central, white, porcelain-like scale** surrounded by a pink ring with telangiectasia. They were completely asymptomatic. **Skin biopsy** showed focal atrophy and an obliterated vessel, leading to a diagnosis of **malignant atrophic papulosis**. Treatment with aspirin (500 mg tid) for 1 year to alter platelet function had no effect on new lesions, which continued to spread on the abdomen, dorsal aspect of the hands, palms, and feet.

Examination of relatives revealed a small number of similar lesions in his mother, two sisters, and two brothers. This suggests that **Degos' disease** may have an autosomal dominant inheritance.

Doutre MS, Beylot C, Bioulac P, et al: Skin lesions resembling malignant **atrophic papulosis** in lupus erythematosus. Dermatologica 1987; 175:45–46.

A 5-mm rounded, **porcelain-white, depressed atrophic lesion** with a red telangiectatic rim was present on the outer surface of the right wrist of a 25-year-old woman with Raynaud's disease for 4 years. It proved not to be **Degos' disease**, but rather a prelude to **systemic lupus erythematosus**. No new skin lesions developed in the following year, but she developed serious proteinuria during pregnancy, leukopenia (WBC 2900/mm^3), ESR 71/94, ANA 1:1000 (homogeneous pattern), decreased complement, and a positive IgG complement Coombs' test.

A diagnosis of **malignant atrophic papulosis** can be made only after systemic lupus erythematosus has been ruled out.

Pursley TV, Jacobson RR, Apisarnthanarax P: **Lucio's phenomenon**. Arch Dermatol 1980; 116:201–204.

Severe **ulcerating skin lesions** of the arms and legs of this 38-year-old woman had been present for 8 years. Clinically, a number of physicians had believed she had leukocytoclastic vasculitis of unknown cause. Some viewed the ulcers as factitial. Others considered collagen vascular disease, erythema multiforme bullosum, or periarteritis to explain the ulcers. Biopsies had also provided a variety of pictures, viz., nonspecific inflammation, periarteritis nodosa, and leukocytoclastic vasculitis. Steroids and antibiotics had been ineffectual.

At the time of this review, it was noted the patient had spent most of her **life in Mexico**. Detailed history taking disclosed the ulcers were always preceded by painful bluish-red macules that lasted a week or so. The ulcers bled quite easily and healed in a few weeks, leaving atrophic scars. The patient had observed that the facial skin was thickening, that the eyebrows were lost, and the bridge of the nose had collapsed with subsequent hemorrhagic nasal discharge. Fever, chills, and fatigue over the 8 years completed the history.

On inspection, one saw a pale, thin woman with a saddle-nose deformity, a perforated septum with hemorrhagic crusting, pendulous earlobes, total loss of eyebrows and eyelashes, and waxy diffusely thickened skin; numerous jagged, angular ulcers were seen on the arms and legs.

Earlobe scrapings as well as biopsies stained with Fite's stain showed numerous acid-fast bacilli and globi, confirming the clinical diagnosis of **lepromatous leprosy**. The unique feature was the ulceration that results from a severe necrotizing reaction. This is termed Lucio's phenomenon. In these patients the absence of the typical lepromatous nodules leads the diagnostician away from leprosy to leukocytoclastic vasculitis. To add to the false leads, the waxy appearance of the skin makes one suspect myxedema.

The **8 years of diagnostic incertitude** with this patient teach us it is not enough to biopsy. One must biopsy the primary painful blue macule, and one must stain for the lepra bacillus.

Warts

Here are some warts that have fooled us:

a solitary wart hiding in thick scalp hair, which, when found, finally accounted for recurrent warts of the fingers

tiny plane warts on the face escaping our attention for lack of good cross-lighting and magnification

mucosal warts resembling punctate leukokeratosis

warts looking like seborrheic keratoses of the genitals

warts hidden under the nail plate, producing onycholysis

warts looking like Bowen's disease

deep warts of palms and soles

hidden perianal warts, insufficient exposure

perianal warts resembling condylomata lata

intraurethral wart, called papilloma

plaque of wart appearing to be keratoderma

wart on sole diagnosed as eccrine poroma

wart simulating malignant melanoma

wart on sole looking like a corn

Cobb MW: **Human papillomavirus infection**. J Am Acad Dermatol 1990; 22:547–566.

SPECIAL POINTS

Only after **application of 5% acetic acid** and the use of magnification can you detect the extent of wart infection in the male genital area. This technique permits you to see small macular and slightly elevated lesions on apparently normal skin. These lesions are verrucae on biopsy, indicating that the area of infected epidermis may be far larger than that suggested by the warts the patient points out.

Warts can present as a **cutaneous horn** or a longer slender filiform process. At times they remain unrecognized, **hidden under the nail plate** or in the scalp.

Pregnancy can stimulate the growth of condylomatous warts to the point of obstructing labor or causing death from sepsis or hemorrhage. Conversely, after birth many warts may regress.

After **inoculation** it takes 1 to 6 months for a clinical wart to become apparent.

At least half of pediatric cases of genital warts are the result of **sexual abuse**.

Mosaic wart is the result of multiple plantar warts coalescing into a plaque. The myrmecia type of plantar wart is the deep endophytic lesion.

Warts may appear as **bowenoid papulosis**, i.e., multiple, small, verrucous or velvety, often pigmented papules of the anogenital region. On typing, HPV (human papillomavirus)-16 is usually found.

Warts may appear as **vulvar papillomatosis**, i.e., a velvety, granular, or cobblestone-like surface of the vulvar vestibule. This condition has been graphically described with terms as diverse as *camel humps*, *cactus bumps*, and *pavement stones*. Remember that "inapparent" warts may account for **vulvodynia**. Acetic acid visualization is necessary.

Warts may appear in the oral mucous membranes. Focal oral hyperplasia has been demonstrated to be due to HPV-13 in American Indian children.

Warts on the larynx can be life threatening by causing **airway obstruction**.

Cervical warts may show endophytic growth patterns and then are known as inverted condylomata. Often cervical warts appear only as white patches seen on colposcopy after acetic acid treatment.

Lifelong, disseminate, flat wartlike lesions and erythematous hyperpigmented or hypopigmented macules are a form of warts known as **epidermodysplasia verruciformis**. It is probably the result of an inborn defect in cell immunity to the papilloma virus. The clinical onset is any time from infancy to adulthood. The papules, when on the knees, are mistaken at times for psoriasis. The pigmentary features may confuse one with tinea versicolor. They can occur on the face, neck, or trunk and have a scale as well as polycyclic borders, but no fungal elements on a KOH examination.

Patients with **epidermodysplasia verruciformis** are at risk for the development of **skin cancer**. The interplay of sunlight and these viral growths results in **Bowen's disease** or invasive squamous cell carcinoma in about a third of these patients. However, metastasis rarely occurs; the lesions are more malignant in histologic appearance than in clinical behavior.

There are now **55 known distinct types of wart viruses**, and 23 of these have been found in epidermodysplasia patients, but HPV-5 is the one type found in warts undergoing malignant change.

The wart **virions** may be seen at times by electron microscopy, most commonly in plantar warts, but rarely in the common wart.

Antisera to the capsid antigens of warts are available, and with immuno-chemical or immunofluorescent techniques, one can show if the infected cells are actively producing viral particles. Common warts react in approximately 90% of the cases.

The **HPV DNA** can be demonstrated in wart tissue, and this allows identification of at least 55 specific types using the hybridization and recombinant techniques of molecular biology.

When it comes to the wart viruses, maybe we still can't grow them, but we sure can number them.

Laffitte F, Chavoin JP, Bonafé JL, Costagliola M: Under heel **foot wart**. Dermatologica 1985; 171:206–208.

With a carbon dioxide laser, it was possible to prove that some plantar warts have **large dermal-epidermal interface extensions** that are completely invisible to the clinician's eye.

A few punctate warts on the surface may be the only evidence of a cigarette paper–thin sheet of wart tissue extending across virtually the entire heel. This "**subepidermal**" **wart** explains the repeated recurrences of certain plantar warts.

Berman A, Domnitz JM, Winkelmann RK: Plantar warts recently turned black: Clinical and histopathologic findings. Arch Dermatol 1982; 118:47–51.

A 12-year-old girl became alarmed when all four of her plantar warts suddenly turned black. Biopsy showed **thrombosed vessels** and necrotic changes in the epidermal cells. Within 2 weeks all of the warts had completely disappeared.

When it comes to warts, black is beautiful.

Stiefler RE, Solomon MP, Shalita AR: **Heck's disease (focal epithelial hyperplasia)**. J Am Acad Dermatol 1979; 1:499–502.

Asymptomatic whitish, clover-shaped 2- to 5-mm **papules on the mucosa** of the lower and upper lips of a 31-year-old Puerto Rican man had been appearing for 6 years. His mother had also developed similar lesions over the past 2 years. Biopsy revealed **focal epithelial hyperplasia** with no viral particles seen on electron microscopy. A diagnosis of **Heck's disease** was made.

This condition has been reported mainly in American Indian children and in Eskimos over 30 years of age. Discrete 1- to 5-mm soft, sessile, papular to nodular elevations occur on the **oral mucosa**. Some have a flat surface, while others are slightly verrucal, keratotic, or finely stippled. They may be whitish, but are usually the color of normal mucosa.

(Oh what the heck, aren't they just mucosal warts?)

Stone MS, Noonan CA, Tschen J, Bruce S: **Bowen's disease** of the feet. Presence of human papillomavirus 16 DNA in tumor tissue. Arch Dermatol 1987; 123:1517–1520.

Hyperkeratotic plaques over several dorsal toes and web spaces of both feet for more than a year in a 36-year-old black man proved to be **intraepidermal squamous cell carcinoma**. DNA hybridization analysis of tumor tissue disclosed HPV-16 DNA, previously reported in other examples of Bowen's disease.

Ross IN, Chesner I, Thompson RA, et al: **Cutaneous viral infection** as a presentation of intestinal lymphangiectasia. Br J Dermatol 1982; 107:357–364.

A 23-year-old woman had **innumerable plane warts** of the face and hands for 6 years, preceded by multiple plantar warts requiring excision. The severity and chronicity of the warts indicated an immunologic deficit, and both humoral and cellular immunity were found to be impaired (low serum IgG, low T-lymphocyte count, reduced peripheral blood lymphocyte transformation on exposure to phytohemagglutinin and other antigens). The source of this defect, however, remained completely hidden until intermittent bouts of colicky gastric pain, nausea, and vomiting were investigated.

A barium enema follow-through examination revealed dilated small-bowel loops with thickened mucosal folds and a polypoid mucosal pattern suggesting lymphoid hyperplasia. On laparotomy the entire small bowel was edematous with prominent surface lymphatics. Although a peroral jejunal biopsy had been normal, wedge resection biopsy of the jejunum during laparotomy showed dilated lymphatic vessels, making the diagnosis **intestinal lymphangiectasia**. Confirming this was the demonstration of increased fecal excretion of both fat and protein ($^{51}CrCl_3$-labeled albumin).

Intestinal lymphangiectasia **impairs immunity** by inducing loss of both immunoglobulins and lymphocytes into the gut. By combating the loss with a low-fat diet and supplementation with medium-chain triglycerides (MCT) (to reduce pressure in the lymphatics by lowering the flow of chyle) this woman's immunologic status improved and the warts cleared over a 2-year period.

A **second case** was in a 46-year-old woman who had presumptive chickenpox for 6 weeks with crops of nonhemorrhagic vesicles and severe scarring. The complete blood count showed only 12% lymphocytes. The patient was found to have a **protein-losing enteropathy** (radiolabeled albumin) and intestinal lymphangiectasia on small-intestine biopsy. A low-fat diet and MCT supplements kept her free of further virus infection for 4 years.

Other **cutaneous signs of intestinal lymphangiectasia** include:

> intermittent asymmetrical edema (due to hypoproteinemia from protein loss in gut)
> stasis dermatitis with skin atrophy and repeated episodes of lymphangitis

The diagnostic studies in these patients provided yet another intriguing way to treat florid recalcitrant warts, i.e., **diet**. The more we know about any patient, the more precise and specific our treatment becomes.

Gardner LW, Acker DW: **Bone destruction** of a distal phalanx caused by periungual warts. Arch Dermatol 1973; 107:275–276.

A biopsy-proven periungual wart on the right index finger of a 39-year-old man resisted seven different local therapeutic measures over a one-year period. Because of the intense pain that developed, a roentgenogram of the finger was taken. It revealed marked tapered loss of bone of the distal phalanx. Once the wart disappeared, after 2,250 rads of x-ray therapy, the bone showed rapid remineralization.

Previously, underlying bone destruction has been associated with subungual epidermoid carcinomas and with keratoacanthomas.

Differential Diagnosis

Himmelstein R, Lynfield YL: **Punctate porokeratosis**. Arch Dermatol 1984; 120:263–264.

The left palm and sole of this 26-year-old man showed numerous discrete 1- to 2-mm **keratotic plugs** arising from hyperkeratotic crypts. Present for 3 years, they could not be related to trauma, but were painful over pressure points. The **differential diagnosis** included warts, arsenical keratoses, and punctate keratoderma palmare et plantare.

A biopsy revealed the diagnostic cornoid lamella of porokeratosis. Such **punctate porokeratosis** is yet another form of a disease that may present as linear, annular, and gyrate plaques as well as verrucous and lichenoid forms.

All punctate keratodermas demand a biopsy for accurate classification.

Nagy-Vezekény K, Makai A, Ambró I, Nagy E: **Histiocytosis X** with unusual skin symptoms. Acta Derm Venereol 1981; 61:447–451.

For 2 years a 4-year-old boy was **thought to have verruca plana** of the lower face and neck, presenting as numerous 2-mm skin-colored to brownish-red or yellowish papules. However, the color play suggested a diagnosis other than plane warts, and a **biopsy showed histiocytosis X** (Letterer-Siwe syndrome). x-Ray of the skull showed radiolucent areas. Vinblastine and prednisone therapy was followed by complete disappearance of the wart-like lesions and the skull lesions.

Ordinarily, histiocytosis X comes in the guise of **seborrheic dermatitis** or **Darier's disease**. But in this little boy, histiocytosis X hid for 2 long years under the mask of warts.

Fujita WH, Barr RJ, Gottschalk HR: **Cutaneous amebiasis**. Arch Dermatol 1981; 117:309–310.

A 3- by 3-cm **odoriferous exudative verrucous plaque** with a necrotic center suddenly appeared in the **gluteal cleft** of a 58-year-old woman. It was bloody and pruritic and had been present for about 1 month. The **diagnoses** considered were: condyloma accuminatum, condyloma latum, pemphigus vegetans, verrucous carcinoma, and amebiasis cutis.

A shave biopsy revealed **amebiasis cutis** with small clusters of trophozoites of *Entamoeba histolytica* seen in the biopsy and subsequently in direct saline mounts of mucus from the ulcer. A cure was accomplished in 10 days with metronidazole (750 mg tid).

Amebic ulcers are oval with irregular necrotic, ragged or verrucous borders that rapidly extend peripherally. In this case the source of amebiasis was probably direct extension from an asymptomatic intestinal infection. Other sources have included direct extension from hepatic abscesses, surgical intervention, venereal transmission, and metastasis during parasitemia (which leads to subcutaneous swellings—"amebomas.")

Look for amebiasis in the tropics, its home territory.

Yesudian P: **Cutaneous rhinosporidiosis** mimicking verruca vulgaris. Int J Dermatol 1988; 27:47–48.

A 30-year-old man from southern India had **six warty lesions** on his face for 1 year. They recurred after local treatment with electrocautery and escharotics and were thought to be warts. Because of the complaint of nasal obstruction and nose bleeding for 3 years, he was sent to the ear, nose, and

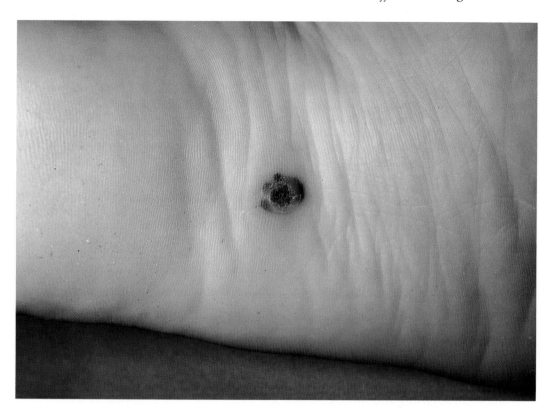

throat clinic, where a diagnosis of **nasal rhinosporidiosis** was made. This prompted a closer look at the "warts" with a hand lens. Under magnification, white spots were seen on the surface of one lesion, typical of rhinosporidiosis. Excisional biopsy of this wart showed the diagnostic sporangia and spores within and below acanthotic epidermis.

Ordinarily, vascular polyps of the nose, soft palate, or nasopharynx clue the physician to the diagnosis of rhinosporidiosis. Often the **polypoid growths** hang down over the upper lip or project into the pharynx. The **key diagnostic sign** is the presence of **white spots on the pink polyps**, representing sporangia filled with the *Rhinosporidium seeberi* **spores**. A sporangium may enlarge up to 3 mm before finally bursting and discharging the spores. The diagnosis may be rapidly confirmed by making a smear of a white spot and staining it with Giemsa. Here, however, no polyps were visible.

The **differential diagnosis** centers on warts, granuloma pyogenicum, and verrucous tuberculosis. In the genital area, confusion may arise with condyloma acuminatum and venereal granuloma.

Thus, look for black dots in verruca vulgaris and white dots in rhinosporidiosis.

When a patient calls on you he is under no obligation to have a simple disease just to please you.

J. M. CHARCOT

Xanthomas

Most diseases have a feature that leads you to a diagnosis. Here it is the color **yellow** (Greek *xanthos*). This is the color of xanthomas. You will see it in the yellowish-tan or orange macules and plaques of plane xanthoma, in the yellow to reddish-brown papules of eruptive xanthoma, and in the bright yellow nodules of tuberous xanthoma. You will see it as yellow streaks in the palms and as yellow papules over the tendons. And you will see it often as the yellowish plaques of the eyelids in xanthelasma. Yellow tonsils are a lead to the diagnosis of Tangier disease. Small yellowish papules may dot the axillae and other folds in xanthoma disseminatum.

All of these lesions are filled with foam cells, loaded with the yellow fats deposited at points of trauma in patients with lipid errors of metabolism. Each calls for cholesterol, triglyceride, and lipoprotein studies. The patient may have primary hyperlipoproteinemia or a secondary form. It may reflect an abnormally large intake of fats, a defect in production, or a defect in the removal of cholesterol or tryglyceride.

In the **secondary hyperlipoproteinemias**, the search is on for biliary cirrhosis with its obstructive effect. Jaundice and hepatomegaly point to this problem. Other causes may be diabetes mellitus, myxedema, renal failure, pancreatitis, and myelomas. Even the drugs isotretinoin and etretinate may elevate triglyceride levels to the point of inducing an eruptive xanthoma.

What about **differential diagnosis** when yellow is the diagnostic flag? In infants, yellow nodules may represent the self-limiting xanthogranulomas that are discerned only on histologic study. A rare and fatal disease, that of Niemann-Pick, comes as a yellowing of the skin, occasionally with plane xanthomas. Here the metabolic defect leads to sphingomyelin and cholesterol deposits in the foam cells. Mastocytosis, at times, has a yellow visage. This variant is called xanthelasmoidea.

The xanthogranulomas may ulcerate and scar and as such are known as **necrobiotic xanthogranulomas**. Yellow is a component of other diseases such as necrobiosis lipoidica diabeticorum. Indeed, diabetics may have the yellow of carotenemia, even as avid drinkers of carrot juice do. Lipoid proteinosis may show yellowish papules on the eyelids, yellow facial plaques, and yellow deposits in the scrotum, axillae, and gluteal folds, as well as the labia. A tied-down wooden tongue and hoarseness cinch this diagnosis.

Last is the **yellow nail** (xanthonychia) syndrome in which the yellowing of the nail often reflects the presence of chronic lymphedema. We suspect this favors leakage of fats and their seepage into the nail plate.

In summary, the clinician can make the diagnosis of xanthoma, but it takes a chemist to define it.

Parker F: **Xanthomas and hyperlipidemias**. J Am Acad Dermatol 1985; 13:1–30.

Xanthomas are the papules, nodules, and plaques that appear as a result of gross accumulation of cholesterol within the histiocytes in the dermis and tendons. Five types can be distinguished clinically.

Planar xanthomas:

xanthelasma: soft yellow macules or plaques on eyelids
xanthoma striatum palmare: yellow to orange linear deposits in creases of the palms
diffuse planar xanthoma: extensive yellow-orange infiltrative lesions that accentuate skin markings, usually on face, neck, and upper trunk

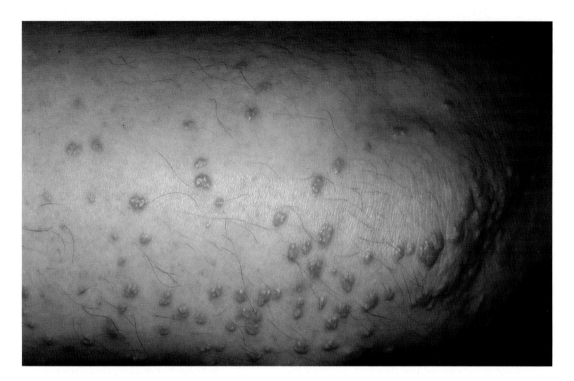

Tuberous xanthomas: yellow-red nodules on elbows, knees, knuckles, buttocks, palms

Eruptive xanthomas: numerous yellow papules with erythematous halo, appearing suddenly on extensor surfaces

Xanthoma disseminatum: yellow-red nodules becoming mahogany color; appears in flexures, eye (cornea, sclera), mucous membranes; may cause dysphagia, dyspnea, and hoarseness. Similar lesions in central nervous system

Tendinous xanthomas: deep smooth nodules within tendon, ligament, or fascia of hands, knees, elbows, and Achilles tendon; skin normal, freely movable over nodules; may be seen with other forms and with coronary arteriosclerosis

All patients with xanthomas must have evaluation of cholesterol, plasma, lipoprotein, and triglyceride levels. All patients with diffuse planar xanthomas must be checked for paraproteinemia.

Cruz PD Jr, East C, Bergstresser PR: Dermal, subcutaneous and tendon xanthomas: Diagnostic markers for specific lipoprotein disorders. J Am Acad Dermatol 1988; 19:95–111.

Here are some pathognomonic skin windows for lipoprotein disorders:

intertriginous xanthomas: familial hypercholesterolemia, homozygous
palmar crease xanthomas: familial dysbetalipoproteinemia type III
eruptive xanthomas: chylomicronemia
tendon xanthomas: familial hypercholesterolemia, heterozygous (elevated LDL); cerebrotendindous xanthomatosis; rarely beta-sitosterolemia; planar xanthomas; cholestasis; diffuse plane xanthomas; paraproteinemias

Know your xanthomas and you will know your patient's chemistry.

Xerosis

Xerosis is simply **dry skin**. Left untended it soon becomes pruritic. It is the itch of old people whose skin has thinned and has been extracted of its protective oils by a thousand baths. It is the itch of the winter months of both the year and the patient. It is the itch that becomes more ferocious with every attack made upon it, whether it be an alcohol rub, a calamine lotion, or a hot bath.

The pruritus of xerosis becomes the picturesque eczema **craquelé** or the staid **asteatotic eczema**. Now redness has developed, and a finely fractured epidermis calls forth the poetic imaging of crackled porcelain. This is most vivid on the shins, but the same process explains the chapped hands of the compulsive hand washer or of those who have to do bare-handed wet work. Such dry-skin eczema is also seen in the one who works with lime or solvents.

Although simple overbathing or tub soaking of an aching back may explain nearly all asteatotic eczema, there are **factors** besides low humidity and drying lotions that favor it. These include hypothyroidism, atopy, and ichthyosis. Certain drugs such as Accutane or Tegison thin the epidermis and lead to xerosis and its sequence of itch and dermatitis. Even Tagamet has been incriminated. Patients who have a low intake of zinc or the essential fatty acids such as linoleic acid are also at risk for xerosis and asteatotic eczema.

Take a careful history and consider zinc and safflower seed oil for diagnosis through therapy. But above all, prove to them that water giveth and water taketh away. Have them raise the room humidity (wet towel, room or central humidifier), but don't let them go near the water except for a short Saturday night bath.

Warin AP: **Eczema craquelé** as a presenting feature of myxoedema. Br J Dermatol 1973; 89:289–291.

A woman, age 80 years, was referred because of a **generalized itchy rash** of 6 months' duration. On examination the arms and legs showed crazy-pavement fissure, discoid eczema, and numerous scratch marks. Laboratory study revealed a total thyroxine of 2.3 μg/dl (normal 5.3 to 12.5 μg/dl).

Within 3 weeks of the start of l-thyroxine therapy, the skin had returned to normal.

Two additional patients with identical findings and therapeutic response are cited to demonstrate that eczema craquelé may be a manifestation of **myxedema**.

The following nine factors are also cited as playing a role in the development of dry itchy skin:

1. Naturally dry skin
2. Decreased sweat and sebaceous gland activity in the aged
3. Decrease in keratin synthesis in the elderly
4. Degreasing by solvents or cleansers, both industrial and domestic
5. Low environmental humidity and dry cold winds
6. Loss of integrity of the water reservoir of horny layer
7. Protein depletion and wasting diseases
8. Strong diuretics
9. Friction

Williams ML, Elias PM: Nature of **skin fragility** in patients receiving retinoids for systemic effect. Arch Dermatol 1981; 117:611–619.

Extensive superficial erosions and dermatitis may occur at the sites of rub-

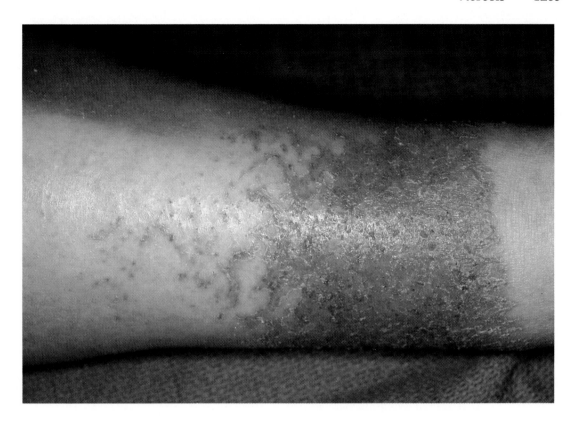

bing or scratching in the skin of patients taking **Accutane** (or other retinoids). It results from a decrease in epidermal cell adhesion.

Greist MC, Epinette WW: Cimetidine-induced **xerosis and asteatotic dermatitis**. Arch Dermatol 1982; 118:253–254.

After 2 weeks of **cimetidine therapy** (300 mg qid) for a gastric ulcer, this 45-year-old man noted his skin was becoming excessively dry. Within another 2 weeks he had multiple erythematous pruritic patches of dermatitis of the upper outer arms. The avoidance of bathing and the use of an oil in water emulsion (Lubriderm) as well as betamethasone valerate cream provided no relief.

A diagnosis of xerosis and asteatotic dermatitis was made, with cimetidine as the likely cause. Cimetidine was discontinued, and the skin returned completely to normal within 3 weeks.

Resumption of the cimetidine 4 months later was followed within a week by recurrence of dry skin.

The pathogenesis of this cimetidine dry skin may reflect the known anti-androgenic activity of this compound. Thus, in the presence of cimetidine, secretion of the natural lubricant, **sebum**, **is** reduced, favoring dry skin.

Weismann K: Generalized **eczema craquelé**: A marker of zinc deficiency? Br J Dermatol 1978; 99:339–340.

Description is given of a widespread **eczema craquelé** occurring in patients with acrodermatitis enteropathica, as well as in chronic alcoholics with malabsorption and gastric resections. This proved to be due to chronic zinc deficiency, as shown by their prompt impressive responses to zinc supplementation.

It is suggested that patients showing widespread recalcitrant eczema craquelé be investigated for possible underlying **zinc deficiency**. A short therapeutic trial with zinc should substantiate or eliminate the role of zinc.

Barker DJ, Cotterill JA: Generalized **eczema craquelé** as a presenting feature of lymphoma. Br J Dermatol 1977; 97:323–326.

A 69-year-old man complained of generalized **itchy dry scaly skin** of a month's duration. The rash had not responded to oil bath treatments and was getting rapidly more extensive. He had noted concurrent anorexia and lassitude. His past history revealed that he had had celiac disease for 12 years. It was successfully being treated with a rigid gluten-free diet.

On examination he had generalized classic **eczema craquelé** of the shins, thighs, shoulders, and back. Enlarged lymph nodes were detected only in the right axilla.

In the hospital, sunflower seed oil applied topically gave no relief. A biopsy of a supraclavicular node gave the diagnosis of **Hodgkin's disease**. Despite chemotherapy the patient later died.

A **second patient**, a 65-year-old man, with identical widespread irregular reticulate dry fissured skin, also proved to have underlying Hodgkin's disease. It was felt that the xerosis and subsequent dermatitis both these patients experienced was due to the **Hodgkin's disease**.

Differential diagnosis included:

the common form of eczema craquelé of the shins due to exercise, bathing, low environmental humidity, and starched sheets
hypothyroidism
peripheral neuropathy
essential fatty acid deficiency

Caplan RM: Superficial **hemorrhagic fissures of the skin**. Arch Dermatol 1970; 101:442–451.

Nine patients are presented with the problem of **parallel and reticulate cracks** on hemorrhagic bases. It appears to be an exaggerated form of **eczema craquelé**. The process may mimic purpura, as the streaks of hemorrhage are due to mechanically ripped capillaries. Histologic evidence of the fissuring of the epidermis is presented.

Often the fissures produce a pattern of irregular polygons. They are analogous to the "**shrinkage cracks**" seen in soil, rocks, concrete, and paint, where drying produces a film inadequate to cover the surface it once did. Inevitably the film is stretched to a breaking point. Similarly, when the dry epidermis is stretched or scratched, fissures will appear.

The secret in diagnosis is to perceive the **linear and polygonal pattern** of the hemorrhage.

Read our book and avoid identity crises in your practice.

This book doesn't cover everything. Rather, it aims to uncover a lot.

If your patient makes you scratch your head for an answer, treat yourself with this book.

Most of what has been written is lost. Use this book as a lost and found department.

If you copy from one author it's plagiarism. If you copy from two, it's research.

We have taken pearls from the journals you never found time to read and put them in a book you must take time to read.

Most of what is written is not read.
Most of what is read is forgotten.
Here's a book to retrieve what you didn't read,
And to recall what you've forgotten.

. . . in short, the most wonderful things can be seen if you have the right sort of eyes for them.

E. T. A. HOFFMAN

And so, adieu, kind reader. May our book bring you:
what you want to know,
what you ought to know,
what you got to know.

Index of Color Plates

1269

1270   Index of Color Plates

How many did you get right?
How many did we get right?

Index

Epilogue

For three full years we breathed this book,
Gaining inspiration from Lisbon to Molokai, Yellowstone to Argentina,
From the majestic mountains of Whistler
To the salty marshes of the Everglades.

It has travelled with us everywhere,
From the libraries of Edinburgh and Cambridge
To the stacks of Uppsala and Irvine,
Our constant consuming companion and jealous mistress.

We have nurtured it with patience,
Fondled and protected it with pride,
Loved it with loyalty and enthusiasm,
And given it nights and weekends to make it grow.

Now it's time to stop, and let it go.
The third and final deadline rushes in.
We must recognize the fringe, and leave our loom,
To pop up elsewhere in another room.

We mourn the missing diagnostic pearls
Lost deep within a sea of library shelves,
Undisturbed by divers in computer suits,
Ever silently waiting to be born again.

Perhaps someday . . .

DERMATOLOGIC VOCABULARY

(What to record when you don't have a camera)

COLOR

Red	Flesh colored	Cyanotic
Brown	Petechial	Plethoric
Golden yellow	Purpuric	Heliotrope
Livid purple	Ecchymotic	Telangiectatic
Gray-black	Icteric	Mottled
Hyperpigmented	Melanotic	Dusky
Hypopigmented	Erythematous	Bright
Leukodermic	Hemorrhagic	Pale
Depigmented		

MORPHOLOGY

Macular	Bullous	Acuminate
Papular	Vesiculobullous	Umbilicated
Nodular	Cystic	Variegated
Multinodular	Dermatitic	Distinctive
Polypoid	Eczematous	Amiantaceous
Pedunculated	Dystrophic	Vascular
Plaquelike	Hypertrophic	Aphthous
Digitate	Alopecic	Indistinct
Urticarial	Agminated	Inapparent
Vesicular	Filiform	Indescribable

SURFACE

Smooth	Pitted	Furrowed
Glossy	Scraped	Depressed
Shiny	Erosive	Scaly
Glazed	Fissured	Desquamating
Wrinkled	Denuded	Furfuraceous
Crinkled	Ulcerative	Powdery
Atrophic	Crusted	Lamellar
Moist	Dimpled	Ostraceous
Macerated	Irregular	Rupioid
Excoriated	Scarred	Ribbed
Abraded		

CONFIGURATION

Punctate	Corymbose	Retiform
Linear	Cocardiform	Guttate
Circinate	Mosaic	Gyrate
Annular	Festooned	Reticulate
Polycyclic	Fusiform	Circumscribed
Multicentric	Angulated	Demarcated
Arcuate	Scalloped	Confluent
Polygonal	Serpiginous	Diffuse
Corymbiform	Racemose	Irregular
Figurate	Stellate	Polymorphic